# Frameworks for Internal Medicine

# Frameworks for Internal Medicine

**André M. Mansoor, MD**
Assistant Professor of Medicine
Division of Hospital Medicine
Director, Procedure Service
Oregon Health & Science University
Portland, Oregon

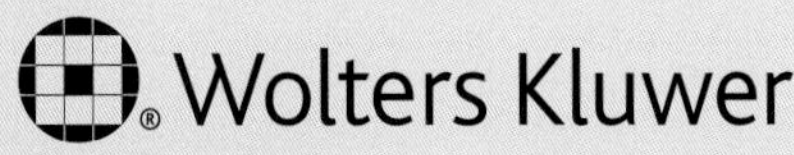


Philadelphia • Baltimore • New York • London
Buenos Aires • Hong Kong • Sydney • Tokyo

*Acquisitions Editor:* Matt Hauber
*Freelance Development Editor:* Tom Conville
*Development Editor:* Andrea Vosburgh
*Editorial Coordinator:* Lindsay Ries
*Marketing Manager:* Mike McMahon
*Production Project Manager:* Kim Cox
*Design Coordinator:* Teresa Mallon
*Manufacturing Coordinator:* Margie Orzech
*Prepress Vendor:* TNQ Technologies



9 8 7 6 5 4

Printed in China

**Library of Congress Cataloging-in-Publication Data**

Names: Mansoor, André M., author.
Title: Frameworks for internal medicine / André M. Mansoor.
Description: Philadelphia : Wolters Kluwer, [2019] | Includes bibliographical references and index.
Identifiers: LCCN 2018041461 | ISBN 9781496359308 (pbk.)
Subjects: | MESH: Internal Medicine | Diagnosis, Differential | Case Reports | Problems and Exercises
Classification: LCC RC71.5 | NLM WB 18.2 | DDC 616.07/5–dc23
LC record available at https://lccn.loc.gov/2018041461



**Cover image:**
Antony Gormley
BUILDING 1-5, 2013
Cast iron
5 elements; dimensions variable
Photograph by Stephen White, London


shop.lww.com

# DEDICATION

*For my mother Salma, and my father Edward. All that I have ever hoped to be, I owe to you.*

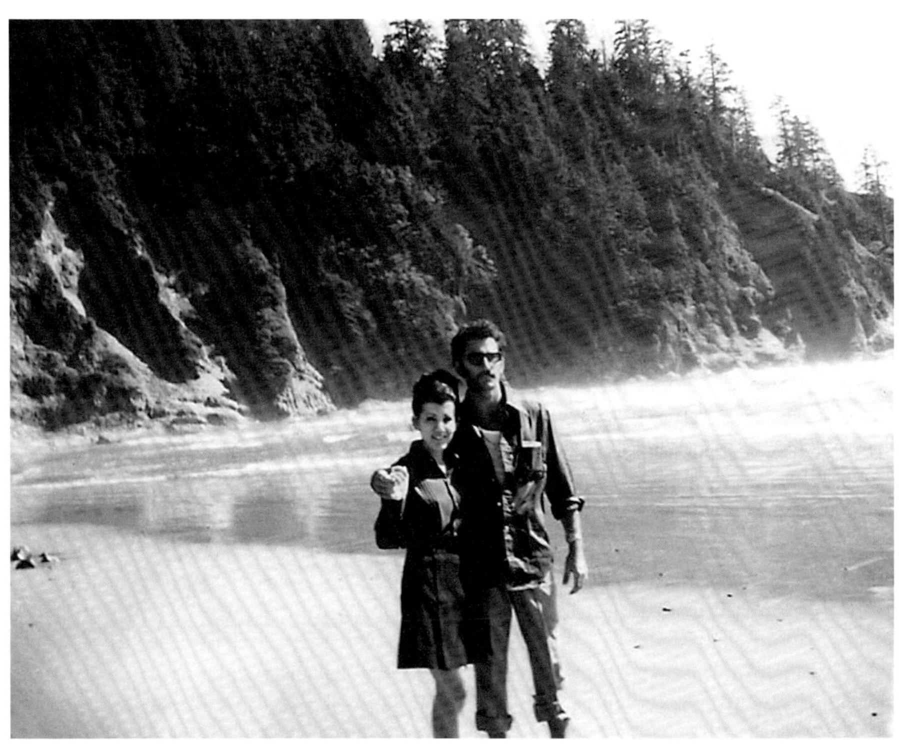

# FOREWORD

In the end, after the "large group learning studios" have fallen silent, the "breakout" rooms are in disarray, and nobody knows that the remotes for the massive TV sets no longer work, medical students will still know 90% of the expected core knowledge. How can this be? It is because these handpicked students are surrounded by handpicked residents, fellows, and junior faculty, all of whom believe it is a fundamental obligation of the profession to teach. They teach all who thirst and most of those who should thirst. It has been this way since the "breakthrough" at Kos. More amazing, the best of these people do not expect any remuneration other than the satisfaction of doing the job well. Education is still the first of the professional expectations at most academic medical centers. These teachers bring the stringent and austere life of physicians-in-training to the task. They can be counted on to teach students what they need to know and, sometimes, what they ought to know.

This task, for which most academic centers pay nothing, is in peril. RVUs, EMRs, "rooming efficiency," and grading scales for "patient satisfaction" all take a toll. These faculty members are expected to recognize "kaizen events" and alert the managers. Some of the managers want to teach the "silver spoon" doctors a lesson or 2 about "hard times." Controversy abides, but the teachers persevere. They are, however, in dire need of help.

Where to start? More than anything else, they need blackboards. Blackboards have disappeared. The boards that fill the old blackboard gaps are white and can be written on only with special order pens. When the pens disappear, "informative flyers" begin to fill the space on the whiteboards. "Quiet please. No one can get well in a noisy place!" Are you sure? Sit and listen to an intensive care unit for an hour. "Wash your hands!" The sinks have all disappeared, too, and the wall "hand wash stations" deliver a foul-smelling liquid that fails to dispatch C-diff spores. It has been labeled toxic for human beings by the FDA. Other messages of importance are an invitation to a potluck lunch. There is an invitation to attend the next art committee meeting. The boards are covered with ephemerata. Doctors need a sacrosanct clean board in every corridor of every ward service in every specialty. What will happen at these boards, should they appear, is an ongoing unscripted discussion of the clinical problems at hand for all to see and hear. Approaches to all of the "slings and arrows that life is heir to" show up on these boards. These challenges to health and happiness are ever-present and countless in number. More appear every day. Doctors learn much of what they know at these vestigial boards. Give them real boards and get out of the way!

This book preserves the art of Socratic teaching, a method that reaches back 2500 years. Not only does the process reveal what is known but, even more clearly, it reveals what is not known. Everybody learns. Students, teachers, and nurses learn. Laboratory personnel and patients learn. All will evolve and grow. It is a powerful thing to witness.

Fifty of the most common clinical problems are illustrated in this book. The cache of questions will evolve as the anatomy of erudition points the way. This book contains frameworks that guide the discussion of the "chosen fifty." The 60-year-old man with hematocrit of 32. The 29-year-old pregnant woman with pitting edema to the axillae. The acutely dyspneic long haul truck driver. The young person with fever of unknown origin. The framework prepares the teacher and the learners. It creates the environment most conducive to high-impact learning efficiency. In the end, it is the *process* rather than the framework. The process becomes generalized. Academia is back on track.

Now that we have the book, the boards will appear, hopefully!

**Lynn Loriaux, MD, PhD**
*Professor of Medicine*
*Oregon Health & Science University*
*Portland, Oregon*

# PREFACE

Twenty: The number of years the average American physician spends as a student before a degree is earned and residency training begins. Experienced physicians would respond to this notion with a grin; medicine is a dynamic field that requires ongoing refinement of those who practice it. For the physician, learning is a *lifelong* endeavor. It does not end after 20 years. However, 20 years does mark an important inflection point in the life of an academic physician: there begins the transition from full-time student to part-time student and part-time educator. For most young doctors, this evolution does not happen naturally. It must be sought.

When I was a third-year medical student on the internal medicine clerkship, I was introduced to the "morning report" case conference, usually led by the chief residents. It was the aspect of the rotation I most enjoyed. I was drawn to the challenge of solving the cases, eventually turning it into a game: I would silently record how long it took for me to guess the correct diagnosis. My record was the time needed for the presenter to finish her opening words, "shortness of breath, facial plethora, and upper extremity swelling" (which I immediately recognized as superior vena cava syndrome). Often I was wrong. However, no one else knew about those mistakes. Then, I became an intern and sat in the same room as before, but my role had changed. As an intern, I was obligated to share my thoughts with the group. Still, it remained simple. I would speak up only when I thought I had a pretty good idea of the correct answer. When I did not, someone else would, and eventually we would get on the right path. On some occasions, however, no one spoke up.

One such occasion involved the case of a middle-aged man with weakness. After time was spent clarifying additional history from the presenter, the chief resident advised that we begin to construct a differential diagnosis. "Stroke," offered a resident in the audience. "Is that all?" asked the chief. The room was quiet. My mind was scrambling to come up with more diagnoses, as it often had when confronted with a problem associated with a broad differential diagnosis. "Does anyone have an approach to weakness?" Meeting more silence, he offered his own method. Breaking it down anatomically, he began to write several headings on the board, including "brain/spinal cord," "anterior horn cell," "peripheral nerve," "neuromuscular junction," and "muscle."

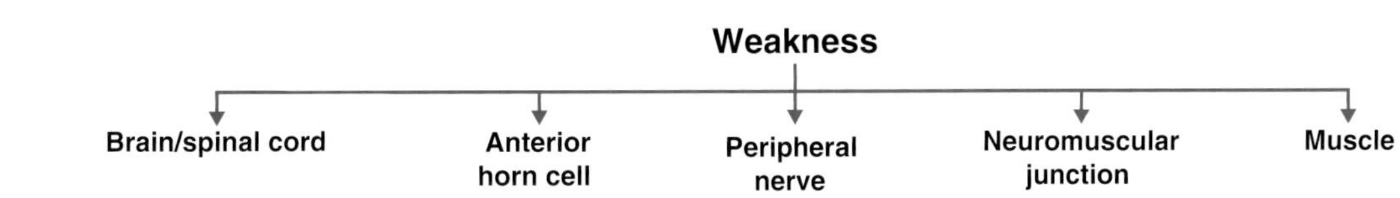


It was as if a light had suddenly turned on in the room. Using this structural format, new possibilities were uncovered. Below the heading "brain/spinal cord," the chief began listing the diagnoses that were now flowing from the audience, including brain tumor, multiple sclerosis, and epidural abscess. Next were lesions of the anterior horn cell. Prompting the group, the chief asked, "Does anyone remember what disease Lou Gehrig had?" Of course, within seconds, ALS appeared on the list. In a similar way, the audience identified diseases of the peripheral nerve, neuromuscular junction, and muscle. With this framework for approaching weakness, we had achieved what seemed impossible moments before.

I left that session with an appreciation of the challenges of leading case conference. When the audience is quiet, the leader must not only determine the direction of the conference but also guide the audience forward. The following year, I was offered one of the future chief resident positions. With joy came some trepidation. One of the concerns on my mind was the idea of leading the case conferences that I always enjoyed as a member of the audience.

I began to strategize. During ensuing conferences, I made note of each case. I soon recognized that certain problems were often at the center of discussion. This list included entities such as dyspnea, acute kidney injury, anemia, hypoxemia, diarrhea, fever of unknown origin, and syncope. Given the frequency with which these entities seemed to appear during case conference, I reasoned that developing an approach to each of them would prove valuable, particularly in moving conference along in front of a reticent audience.

As I began to work toward this goal, I realized that having an approach to a problem in many cases is as simple as constructing a framework that divides the long differential diagnosis into shorter sublists, which are easier for our brains to store and process. Rather than memorize a long list of diagnoses, it is sufficient to remember the headings of a framework, from which many of the diagnoses can then be generated.

I began to build frameworks for all of the common clinical problems in internal medicine. I used various resources, from pages of notes I scribbled at one point or another during residency to textbooks and primary literature. Some frameworks are time-honored and commonly taught, such as those used for acute kidney injury (prerenal, intrarenal, postrenal) and vasculitis (small vessel, medium vessel, large vessel). After a few months, I had accumulated a healthy amount of material. Here is 1 example of the frameworks that I was beginning to assemble:

These frameworks would become the "tip of the spear" when I was faced with silence during case conference. I had accomplished my objective. However, I discovered something much more valuable. I had developed a collection of tools that could be used to teach learners how to approach the clinical problems of internal medicine, beyond the boundaries of case conference.

I spent the rest of my time as a resident using these tools to teach, taking advantage of every opportunity. On the inpatient medical ward, the members of my team were the audience of frequent talks. I discovered that the guidance from the framework alone was enough to result in a meaningful teaching session, but I began to expand the outlines with additional learning points, making each talk healthier and more robust. With each passing month, I sharpened my skills as a resident-teacher. By the end of residency, I had become a nascent teacher. I hope this work can help others reach this point.

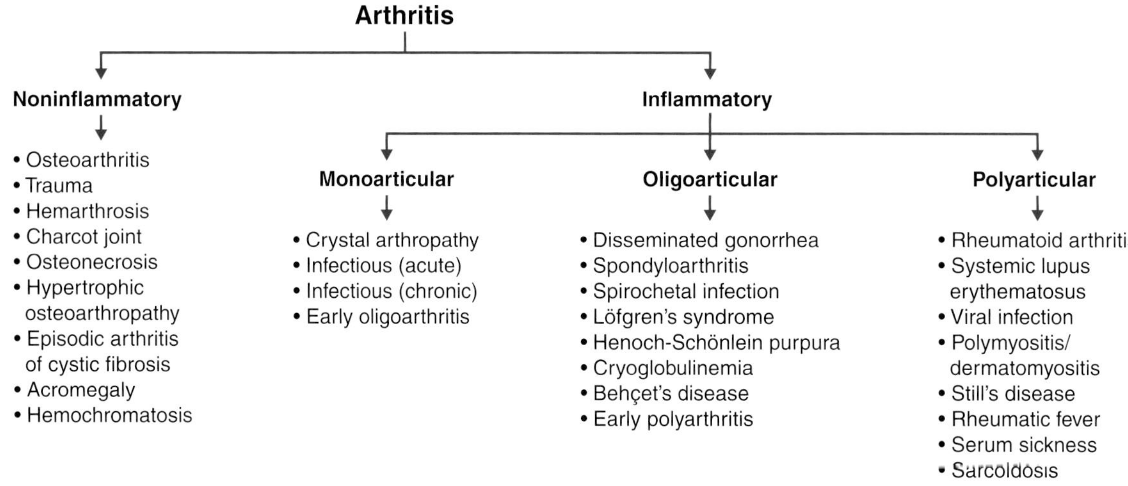

# REVIEWERS

The author would like to thank the following individuals for their time and expertise:

## SECTION 3: Cardiology

**Edward S. Murphy, MD**
Professor of Medicine
Knight Cardiovascular Institute
Oregon Health & Science University
Portland, Oregon

**Khidir Dalouk, MD**
Assistant Professor of Medicine
Clinical Cardiac Electrophysiologist
Knight Cardiovascular Institute
Oregon Health & Science University
Portland, Oregon

## SECTION 4: Endocrinology

**D. Lynn Loriaux, MD, PhD**
Professor of Medicine
Head, Division of Endocrinology, Diabetes, and Clinical Nutrition
Oregon Health & Science University
Portland, Oregon

## SECTION 5: Gastroenterology and Hepatology

**Janice Jou, MD, MHS**
Assistant Professor of Medicine
Division of Gastroenterology and Hepatology
Director, Gastroenterology and Hepatology Fellowship
Oregon Health & Science University
Portland, Oregon

## SECTION 6: General Internal Medicine

**D. Lynn Loriaux, MD, PhD**
Professor of Medicine
Head, Division of Endocrinology, Diabetes, and Clinical Nutrition
Oregon Health & Science University
Portland, Oregon

**David Mansoor, MD**
Associate Professor of Psychiatry
Oregon Health & Science University
Portland, Oregon

## SECTION 7: Hematology

**Thomas DeLoughery, MD, MACP, FAWM**
Professor of Medicine, Pathology, and Pediatrics
Division of Hematology and Oncology
Oregon Health & Science University
Portland, Oregon

## SECTION 8: Infectious Diseases

**Thomas Ward, MD**
Professor Emeritus of Medicine
Division of Infectious Diseases
Oregon Health & Science University
Portland, Oregon

## SECTION 9: Nephrology

**Pavan Chopra, MD, MS**
Assistant Professor of Medicine
Division of Nephrology and Hypertension
Director, Dialysis Services
Oregon Health & Science University
Portland, Oregon

## SECTION 10: Neurology

**Faheem Sheriff, MD**
Fellow of Neurocritical Care
Massachusetts General Hospital
Brigham and Women's Hospital
Boston, Massachusetts

## SECTION 11: Pulmonology

**Alan F. Barker, MD**
Professor of Medicine
Division of Pulmonary and Critical Care
Oregon Health & Science University
Portland, Oregon

## SECTION 12: Rheumatology

**Atul Deodhar, MD, MRCP, FACP, FACR**
Professor of Medicine
Division of Arthritis & Rheumatic Diseases
Director, Rheumatology Clinics
Director, Immunology Infusion Center
Oregon Health & Science University
Portland, Oregon

## Medical Editor

**Margot E. Chase, MPAS, PA-C**
Instructor of Medicine
Division of Hospital Medicine
Oregon Health & Science University
Portland, Oregon

## Additional Faculty Reviewers

**Stephanie A.C. Halvorson, MD, FACP**
Associate Professor of Medicine
Division of Hospital Medicine
Oregon Health & Science University
Portland, Oregon

**Mary Ann Kuzma, MD**
Associate Professor of Medicine
Clerkship Director, Internal Medicine
Drexel University College of Medicine
Philadelphia, Pennsylvania

**Octavian Calin Lucaciu, MD, PhD**
Associate Professor of Anatomy
Canadian Memorial Chiropractic College
Toronto, Ontario, Canada

**Gregory J. Magarian, MD**
Professor of Medicine
Division of Hospital Medicine
Oregon Health & Science University
Portland, Oregon

## Additional Student and Resident Reviewers

Shelby Badani
Cassandra Betts, MD
Karen Bieraugel
Christina B. Cherry
Michael-Hunter Clement
Alexander Connelly
Spencer Degerstedt, MD
Christine Grelpp
Sameer Hirji, MD
Arthur Kehas
Whitney King
Rebecca Levin-Epstein
Aisha Mohammed
Christine Motzkus
Jennifer E. Mustard
Andrew Oehler, MD
Jayoma Perera
Nekeyua N. Richardson
Branden Tarlow
Rachna Unnithan
Cara Varley, MPH

# ACKNOWLEDGEMENTS

I received an incredible amount of support over the 6 years it took me to complete this book. Above all, I am thankful for my mother Salma. I am grateful to my father Edward, siblings Sherri, Steve, Dave, Aimee, and Lori, as well as Sito (grandmother) Margareet Barhoum for encouraging me from the beginning until the end. It is amazing the impact of such a simple question, "How is the book coming along?" My cousins Jamil Mansoor and Joseph Barhoum, and my friend Josh Hughes were always interested in the progress, no matter how fast or how slow.

When I first came to OHSU in 2005, I was introduced to the legend of Lynn Loriaux. So astute a clinician, it was said he needed only a handshake to make a diagnosis. Behind every legend there is a man. Often, they are nothing alike. Sometimes, the man is equal to the legend. Only seldom does he exceed it. When I met the man himself, it was clear just how rare he is. His guidance throughout this process cannot be overstated. And we could not have done it without Julie Walvatne.

I received immeasurable support from Shangar Meman, from the earliest stages of writing until the end (she is a superb agent). The advice of my friend and colleague Christopher "Kwonsult" Kwock was always as effective as it was sarcastic. He was available any time I needed him. This book benefited from exceptional proofreading by Jennifer Mustard and Spencer "274" Degerstedt. Joseph Mabe provided valuable expertise in matters that are beyond me. Christopher Neck always took time to answer questions. Summer Steele contributed countless reference articles. I thank my friends and colleagues Gregory Magarian, Peter Sullivan, Sima Desai, Brian Chan, Elly Karamooz, and Margot Chase for their interest and advice over the years.

I am appreciative of the outstanding team at Wolters Kluwer, in particular Matt Hauber, Tom Conville, Andrea Vosburgh, and Lindsay Ries, first for their patience and second for their innovative ideas that enriched every facet of this book. I would also like to recognize Tari Broderick who first received my proposal and believed in this book from day one.

Finally, and most importantly, I would like to thank all of the patients I have ever had the privilege of caring for, with special attention to those presented in this book. I hope the telling of their stories will serve as a benefit to others.

# CONTENTS


FOREWORD VI

PREFACE VII

REVIEWERS IX

ACKNOWLEDGEMENTS XI

LIST OF COMPLETED FRAMEWORKS XIV

**SECTION 1** How to Use This Book

FOR LEARNERS 1

FOR EDUCATORS 1

- Internal Medicine Residents and Faculty 1
- Internal Medicine Chief Residents 1

**SECTION 2** The Framework System

**SECTION 3** Cardiology

Chapter 1 BRADYCARDIA 5

Chapter 2 CHEST PAIN 15

Chapter 3 HEART BLOCK 29

Chapter 4 HEART FAILURE 37

Chapter 5 PERICARDITIS 55

Chapter 6 TACHYCARDIA 67

**SECTION 4** Endocrinology

Chapter 7 ADRENAL INSUFFICIENCY 78

Chapter 8 CUSHING'S SYNDROME 91

Chapter 9 HYPERCALCEMIA 100

Chapter 10 HYPOCALCEMIA 112

Chapter 11 HYPOTHYROIDISM 125

Chapter 12 THYROTOXICOSIS 137

**SECTION 5** Gastroenterology and Hepatology

Chapter 13 ASCITES 147

Chapter 14 CHOLESTATIC LIVER INJURY 162

Chapter 15 DIARRHEA 176

Chapter 16 GASTROINTESTINAL BLEEDING 198

Chapter 17 HEPATOCELLULAR LIVER INJURY 212

Chapter 18 INTESTINAL ISCHEMIA 223

**SECTION 6** General Internal Medicine

Chapter 19 DELIRIUM 235

Chapter 20 DYSPNEA 248

Chapter 21 FEVER OF UNKNOWN ORIGIN 263

Chapter 22 HYPOTENSION 276

Chapter 23 PERIPHERAL EDEMA 288

Chapter 24 SYNCOPE 300

**SECTION 7** Hematology

Chapter 25 ANEMIA 310

Chapter 26 HEMOLYTIC ANEMIA 326

Chapter 27 PANCYTOPENIA 342

Chapter 28 PLATELET DISORDERS 353

**SECTION 8** Infectious Diseases

Chapter 29 ENDOCARDITIS 365

Chapter 30 MENINGITIS 382

Chapter 31 PNEUMONIA 398

## SECTION 9 Nephrology

Chapter 32 ACID-BASE DISORDERS 414

Chapter 33 ACUTE KIDNEY INJURY 430

Chapter 34 GLOMERULAR DISEASE 445

Chapter 35 HYPERKALEMIA 460

Chapter 36 HYPERNATREMIA 469

Chapter 37 HYPOKALEMIA 479

Chapter 38 HYPONATREMIA 487

Chapter 39 SECONDARY HYPERTENSION 501

## SECTION 10 Neurology

Chapter 40 HEADACHE 510

Chapter 41 POLYNEUROPATHY 525

Chapter 42 SEIZURE 540

Chapter 43 STROKE 557

Chapter 44 WEAKNESS 578

## SECTION 11 Pulmonology

Chapter 45 HEMOPTYSIS 603

Chapter 46 HYPOXEMIA 612

Chapter 47 INTERSTITIAL LUNG DISEASE 631

Chapter 48 PLEURAL EFFUSION 645

## SECTION 12 Rheumatology

Chapter 49 ARTHRITIS 658

Chapter 50 SYSTEMIC VASCULITIS 673

## SECTION 13 Educator's Appendix

A Brief History of Medical Education and Introduction to the Chalk Talk 684

The Seven Tenets of The Chalk Talk 687

Chalk Talks and The Framework System 690

INDEX 693

# LIST OF COMPLETED FRAMEWORKS


**SECTION 3:** Cardiology

BRADYCARDIA 12

CHEST PAIN 25

HEART BLOCK 33

HEART FAILURE 51

PERICARDITIS 64

TACHYCARDIA 75

**SECTION 4:** Endocrinology

ADRENAL INSUFFICIENCY 87

CUSHING'S SYNDROME 97

HYPERCALCEMIA 108

HYPOCALCEMIA 122

HYPOTHYROIDISM 133

THYROTOXICOSIS 143

**SECTION 5:** Gastroenterology and Hepatology

ASCITES 157

CHOLESTATIC LIVER INJURY 172

DIARRHEA 193

GASTROINTESTINAL BLEEDING 208

HEPATOCELLULAR LIVER INJURY 219

INTESTINAL ISCHEMIA 232

**SECTION 6:** General Internal Medicine

DELIRIUM 244

DYSPNEA 259

FEVER OF UNKNOWN ORIGIN 272

HYPOTENSION 285

PERIPHERAL EDEMA 296

SYNCOPE 306

**SECTION 7:** Hematology

ANEMIA 322

HEMOLYTIC ANEMIA 338

PANCYTOPENIA 350

PLATELET DISORDERS 361

**SECTION 8:** Infectious Diseases

ENDOCARDITIS 378

MENINGITIS 394

PNEUMONIA 410

**SECTION 9:** Nephrology

ACID/BASE DISORDERS 427

ACUTE KIDNEY INJURY 442

GLOMERULAR DISEASE 456

HYPERKALEMIA 466

HYPERNATREMIA 476

HYPOKALEMIA 484

HYPONATREMIA 497

SECONDARY HYPERTENSION 507

**SECTION 10:** Neurology

HEADACHE 521

POLYNEUROPATHY 535

SEIZURE 553

STROKE 574

WEAKNESS 598

**SECTION 11:** Pulmonology

HEMOPTYSIS 609

HYPOXEMIA 627

INTERSTITIAL LUNG DISEASE 641

PLEURAL EFFUSION 654

**SECTION 12:** Rheumatology

ARTHRITIS 668

SYSTEMIC VASCULITIS 680

SECTION 1

# How to Use This Book

## FOR LEARNERS

This book is an educational resource and reference tool for those who study internal medicine, including medical students and physician assistant students. Use the frameworks to organize and refine the way you approach clinical problems. The frameworks are easy to understand and will improve your level of comfort with challenging internal medicine topics.

This book offers a general overview of 50 common clinical problems within the discipline of internal medicine, providing teaching pearls along the way. Each chapter may be used as a study guide. Test your knowledge by reviewing the questions in each chapter before revealing the answers, using hints to guide your recall. Understanding the high-yield concepts found within the chapters will help you prepare for standardized tests, such as the internal medicine shelf exam, the United States Medical Licensing Examination (USMLE) Step 2, and the Physician Assistant National Certifying Exam (PANCE). It will also prepare you for daily rounds during the internal medicine clerkship, where there is routine discussion of common clinical problems with an emphasis on differential diagnosis.

Each chapter is associated with a real patient case, demonstrating the relevance and application of the framework system to clinical practice. When evaluating a patient with a clinical problem featured in this book, reference the complete framework to ensure that your approach is sound and that you are not forgetting parts of the differential diagnosis. The frameworks are organized such that entities appear in descending order of prevalence; in some cases, rare conditions are left out entirely. Rather than exhaustive lists of diagnoses, the frameworks provide you with a scaffolding to help you organize your investigation.

Finally, as a student of medicine you will soon become an educator. Use the frameworks found in this book to teach future generations of students how to approach the common clinical problems of internal medicine.

## FOR EDUCATORS

### Internal Medicine Residents and Faculty

This book serves 2 main purposes for educators. First, it is an instructional text. The educator's appendix is designed to improve your level of comfort as an instructor by presenting the teaching method known as the "chalk talk" and offering strategies to maximize its effectiveness. This book is also a resource. Educators can design chalk talks based on the structure and flow of the chapters. Importantly, the hints and questions included in each chapter are not static; depending on audience, time available for teaching, and other factors, you can modify your chalk talk to best serve your needs.

Once you become comfortable with the principles of the chalk talk discussed in the educator's appendix, you can delve into the chapters to design talks for your learners. The inpatient medical ward is an ideal setting to develop as an educator. There, you will lead a team of medical students, interns, and possibly other learners such as physician assistant students and pharmacy students. Talks are most potent when the subject matter is applicable to patients being cared for by the team, although topics can also be generated based on interest from team members. The 50 chapters in this book review the most commonly encountered clinical topics in the field of internal medicine, ensuring you are prepared for what is to come.

Some topics are more challenging than others. Starting with common clinical problems such as anemia or acute kidney injury will allow you to develop your skills in delivering these talks. As your experience grows, challenging topics will become easier to teach. In time, you will be ready to deliver a talk on any internal medicine topic.

### Internal Medicine Chief Residents

At many academic medical centers, chief residents are responsible for leading case conference (or morning report). The traditional format involves the use of a whiteboard to scribe and illustrate key features of the presentation. At some point during the conference, the chief usually leads a discussion of the differential diagnosis. Common clinical problems, such as dyspnea, acute kidney injury, and hypoxemia, are regularly featured in these cases, often at the center of the conversation. It is important to have an approach to these problems to effectively lead the discussion, particularly when the initial differential diagnosis offered by the audience is limited. The framework system described in this book is the ideal tool to ensure that you can lead a discussion that is not only organized, but engages your audience in generating a thoughtful differential diagnosis. When the audience is stuck, you can revive participation by illustrating parts of the framework. For example, in a case of fever of unknown origin, the audience may initially offer only infectious or malignant etiologies. You have an opportunity to resuscitate the discussion by adding a third tier to the differential, "noninfectious inflammatory," from which additional etiologies can be identified. In this way, you gently fuel the discussion, encourage audience participation, and enhance recollection of the differential diagnosis.

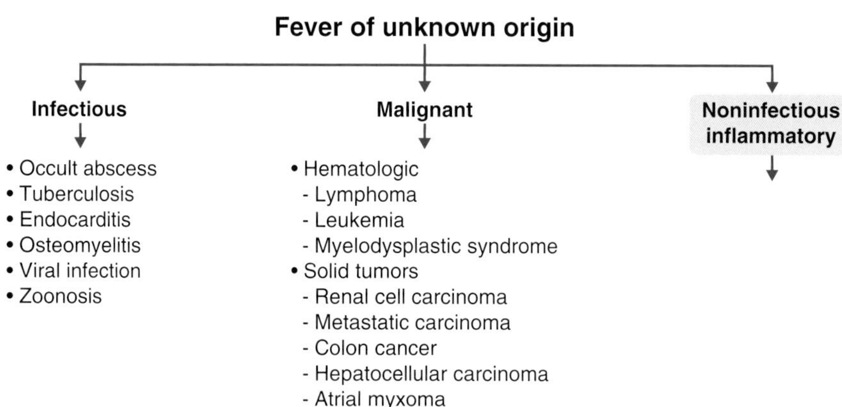

# SECTION 2

# The Framework System

Suppose you were asked to randomly name as many of the states of the United States of America as quickly as you can. How long before the flow of answers would slow to a stutter? What if you approached it methodically, beginning with states that start with the letter A, then B, then C, and so on; or perhaps geographically, grouping states into quadrants such as northwest, northeast, southeast, and southwest? Would you be more successful?

Recall is highly influenced by the way in which memories are organized. It increases significantly when material is structured in a cohesive way. This principle is valuable to anyone who practices medicine. Clinicians are trusted to recall long lists of differential diagnoses for a spectrum of medical problems. This massive undertaking becomes more achievable when problems are organized using the concept of a framework.[1-4]

A framework for a medical topic organizes content in a structured manner that makes it easier for our brains to store and recall. A common example is the organization of a long differential diagnosis into shorter sublists. Consider the topic of systemic vasculitis. Physicians often struggle to recall the list of entities that cause this condition. However, there is a classic framework for this problem that categorizes etiologies by the size of blood vessel involved, namely large, medium, and small. Small vessel vasculitis can be further subdivided by the presence of serologic markers. This organization allows for easier recollection of the differential diagnosis. The framework for systemic vasculitis is illustrated below.

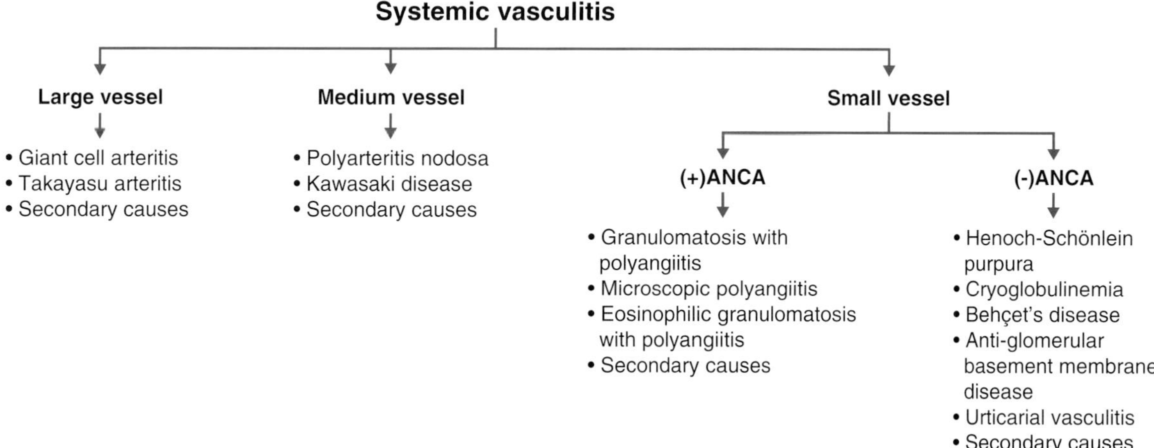


The manner in which a differential diagnosis is organized can vary, depending on the topic. For instance, there is more than 1 suitable way to organize a problem such as abdominal pain. It may be approached anatomically, with subheadings such as liver, gallbladder, stomach, small intestine, pancreas, and so on. Another approach groups diagnoses by region such as right upper quadrant, left lower quadrant, epigastric, and so on. In either model, the long differential has been dramatically reduced to smaller subsets that are easier to memorize and recall.

In addition to this favorable effect on memory, there are other benefits to the framework system. Depending on the organizational approach, it may assist in the diagnostic workup. Referring back to the example of vasculitis, the serologic subdivision of small vessel vasculitis automatically suggests a diagnostic step. A more illustrative model of this benefit is found in the framework for pleural effusion, shown here.

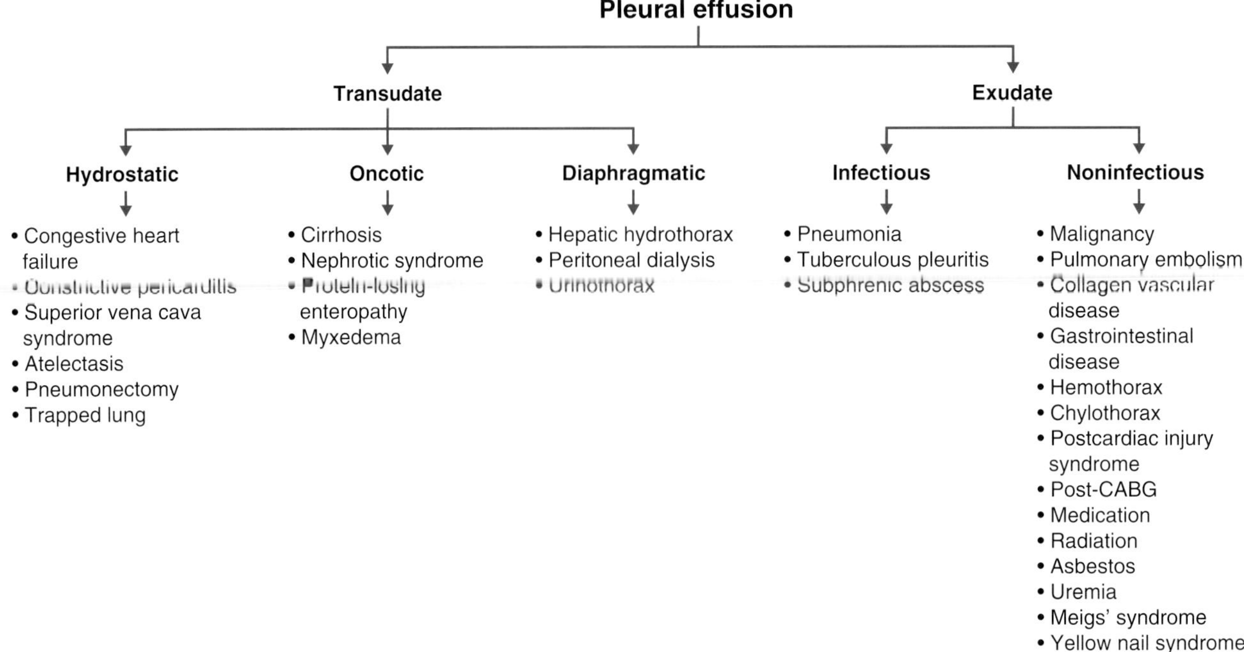


In this framework, the initial division of the differential diagnosis is predicated on diagnostic studies. The calculation of Light's criteria, which is based on laboratory data, is the first step in determining whether pleural fluid is transudative or exudative. Consequently, these studies become seamlessly integrated into the approach to, and investigation of, pleural effusions. With this framework in mind, a clinician is equipped not only with the means to more easily recall the causes of pleural effusion but also the wherewithal to embark on a diagnostic pursuit.

## REFERENCES

1. Bower GH. Memory for scripts with organized vs. randomized presentations. *Br J Psychol.* 1980;71(3):369-377.
2. Bower GHC, Michal C, Lesgold AM, Winzenz D. Hierarchical retrieval schemes in recall of categorized word lists. *J Verbal Learn Verbal Behav.* 1969;8:323-343.
3. Cohen BH. Recall of categorized word lists. *J Exp Psychol.* 1963;66:227-234.
4. Tulving E, Pearlstone Z. Availability versus accessibility of information in memory for words. *J Verbal Learn Verbal Behav.* 1966;5:381-391.

# SECTION 3

# Cardiology

## Chapter 1

## BRADYCARDIA

### Case: An 87-year-old man found down

An 87-year-old man with a history of coronary artery disease, hypertension, and hyperlipidemia is admitted to the hospital after being found down at home. The patient's wife heard a thud in the bathroom where she discovered her husband unresponsive on the floor. The patient regained consciousness and was brought into the hospital for further evaluation. He does not recall any details of the event. He feels light-headed but otherwise has no complaints.

Heart rate is 42 beats per minute, and blood pressure is 85/47 mm Hg. On examination, the pulse is regular and slow. Electrocardiogram (ECG) is shown in Figure 1-1.

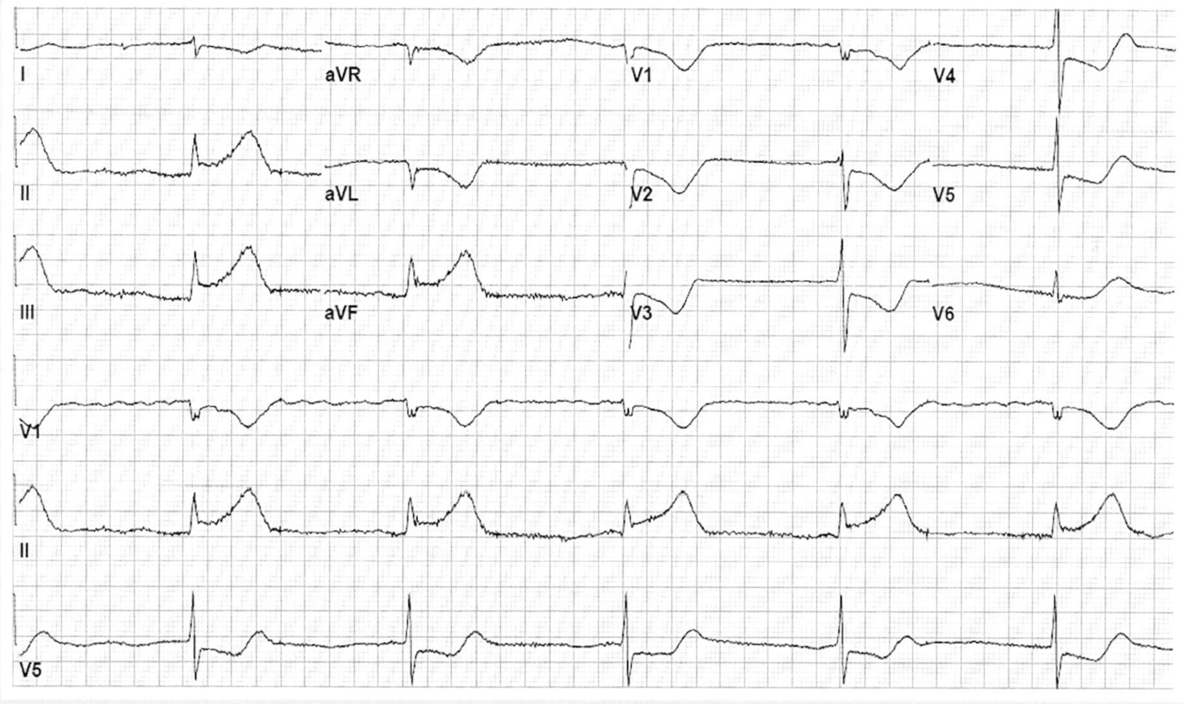


**Figure 1-1.**

***What rhythm disturbance is present in this patient?***

**What is the path of electrical conduction in the normal heart?**

In the normal heart, an impulse spontaneously originates from the sinoatrial (SA) node, which is located in the subepicardial surface at the junction of the right atrium and superior vena cava. The impulse propagates through the myocytes of the right and left atria simultaneously before reaching the atrioventricular (AV) node, which is located in the inferior portion of the right atrium. From there, the impulse is conducted to the bundle of His within the membranous septum, which then separates into the right and left bundle branches supplying the right and left ventricles, respectively (Figure 1-2).

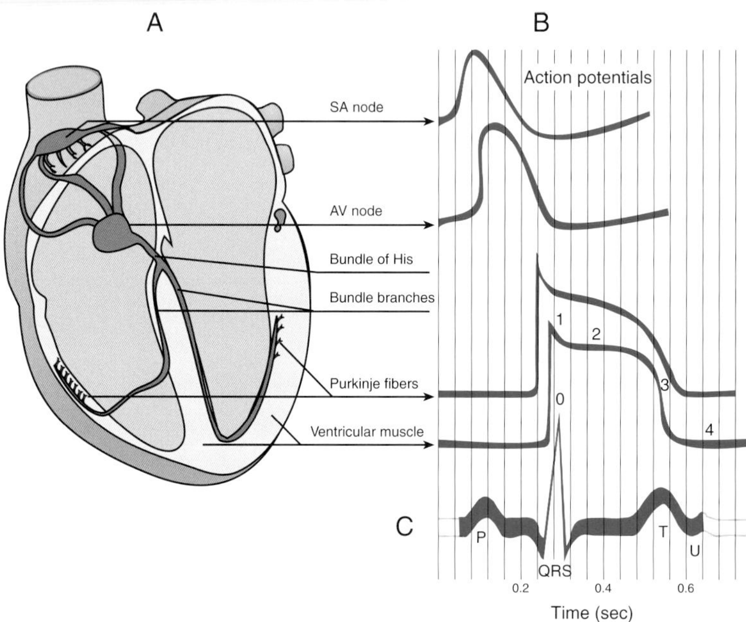


**Figure 1-2.** The cardiac conduction system. A, Cardiac conduction system anatomy. B, Action potentials of specific cardiac cells. C, Relationship of surface electrocardiogram to the action potential.

**Which main coronary artery supplies the SA node in most patients?**

The SA nodal artery originates from the proximal right coronary artery in 65% of patients and the circumflex in 25%; it arises from both in 10% of patients.[1]

**Which main coronary artery supplies the AV node in most patients?**

The AV nodal artery originates from the right coronary artery in 80% of patients and the circumflex in 10%; it arises from both in 10% of patients.[1]

**How is heart rate regulated?**

The sympathetic and parasympathetic nervous systems innervate the conduction system of the heart. Parasympathetic tone decreases SA node automaticity and AV node conduction, whereas sympathetic input increases SA node automaticity and AV node conduction.[1]

**What is the definition of bradycardia in adults?**

The average resting heart rate in adults is 70 beats per minute. Bradycardia is classically defined as a heart rate <60 beats per minute, but there is considerable variation in normal between populations. Age, fitness, and other clinical factors must be taken into consideration.[1,2]

**What is the average drop in heart rate during sleep in young healthy patients and in the elderly?**

During sleep, heart rate in young healthy patients decreases by an average of 24 beats per minute. In the elderly, heart rate decreases by an average of 14 beats per minute.[3,4]

**What is the relationship between cardiac output and heart rate?**

Cardiac output (CO) is equal to the forward stroke volume (SV) of the left ventricle per beat multiplied by heart rate (HR).[1]

$$CO = SV \times HR$$

What are the symptoms of bradycardia?

Patients with bradycardia may be asymptomatic. Symptoms may include fatigue, weakness, light-headedness, and syncope.[1]

What are the physical findings of bradycardia?

The cardinal physical finding of bradycardia is a slow pulse rate, which can be regular or irregular. Additional findings may include hypotension, cool extremities, and cannon A waves (in the setting of AV dissociation).

What are the 2 main electrocardiographic categories of bradycardia?

Bradycardia can be associated with a narrow QRS complex or a wide QRS complex.

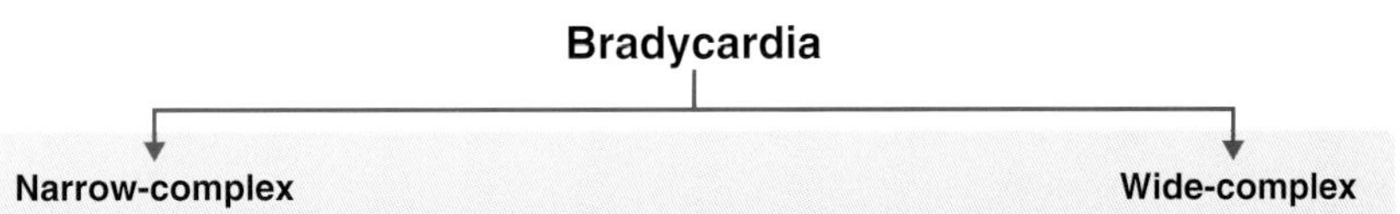


What is the definition of a wide QRS complex?

A wide QRS complex is defined electrocardiographically as QRS duration >120 ms (see Figure 1-2).

The small boxes on the electrocardiogram represent how many milliseconds?

At the standard paper speed of 25 mm/s, each small box (1 mm in width) on the ECG corresponds to 40 ms. Each large box, which is composed of 5 small boxes, represents 200 ms (see Figure 1-2).

## NARROW-COMPLEX BRADYCARDIA

What are the 2 electrocardiographic subcategories of narrow-complex bradycardia?

Narrow-complex bradycardia can be associated with a regular rhythm or an irregular rhythm.

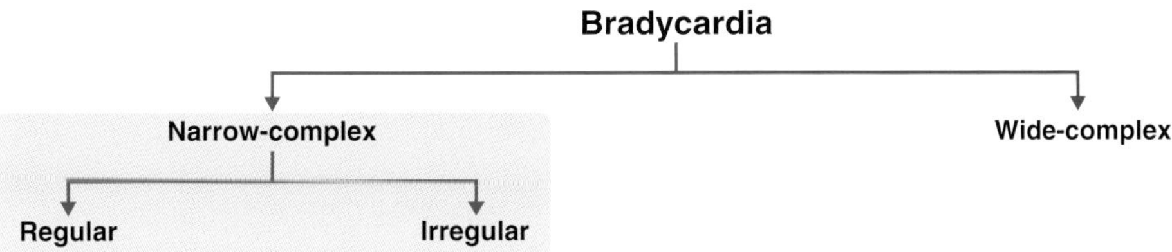


What are the electrocardiographic characteristics of a regular rhythm?

Regular rhythm is defined electrocardiographically by the presence of QRS complexes that are separated by a constant interval (ie, the R-R interval is constant).

## NARROW-COMPLEX BRADYCARDIA WITH REGULAR RHYTHM

### What are the causes of narrow-complex bradycardia with regular rhythm?

A 19-year-old woman with anorexia nervosa and a heart rate of 48 beats per minute.

Sinus bradycardia.

Electrocardiographic sawtooth pattern.

Atrial flutter with AV block and slow ventricular rate (Figure 1-3).

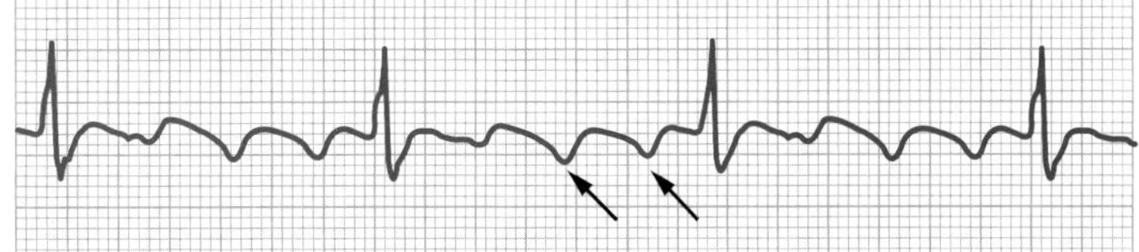

**Figure 1-3.** An example of atrial flutter with 3:1 AV conduction, resulting in bradycardia. Note sawtooth-shaped flutter waves (arrows) with an atrial rate <300 beats per minute. (From De Fer TM. *The Washington Manual of Outpatient Internal Medicine.* Philadelphia, PA: Wolters Kluwer; 2015.)

**This underlying atrial rhythm results in tachycardia when conduction through the AV node is 1:1 and is characterized by the presence of P waves before every QRS complex that are often inverted in leads II, III, and aVF.**

Atrial tachycardia with AV block and slow ventricular rate.

**No visible or discernible P waves before the QRS complexes.**

Junctional escape rhythm.

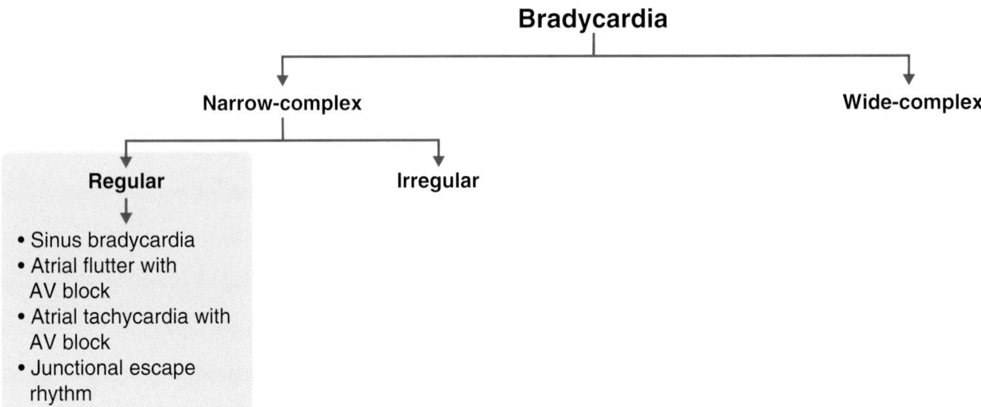


**What are the causes of sinus bradycardia?**

Causes of sinus bradycardia include conditions intrinsic to the SA node, such as idiopathic degeneration (aging), ischemia, infiltrative disorders (eg, amyloidosis), collagen vascular diseases (eg, systemic lupus erythematosus), infectious diseases (eg, Chagas disease), myotonic dystrophy, and surgical trauma (eg, valve replacement), as well as conditions extrinsic to the SA node, including medications (eg, β-blockers), electrolyte disturbances (eg, hypokalemia), neurally-mediated reflexes (eg, carotid sinus hypersensitivity), hypothyroidism, and hypothermia.[1]

**What medications are associated with sinus bradycardia?**

Medications commonly associated with sinus bradycardia include β-blockers, calcium channel blockers, digoxin, clonidine, and antiarrhythmic agents (eg, amiodarone).[1]

**What distinctive pulse-temperature pattern can be observed in some patients with infectious causes of sinus bradycardia?**

Some infections are associated with pulse-temperature dissociation, known as "relative bradycardia." Normally, for each degree Farenheit increase in temperature, there is a corresponding increase in heart rate of 10 beats per minute. Infections associated with relative bradycardia include legionella, psittacosis, Q fever, typhoid fever, typhus, babesiosis, malaria, leptospirosis, yellow fever, dengue fever, viral hemorrhagic fevers, and Rocky Mountain spotted fever.[5]

**What is the mechanism of sinus bradycardia in healthy athletes?**

Well-trained athletes develop sinus bradycardia as a result of increased vagal tone.[1]

**In the setting of atrial flutter with AV block, assuming an atrial rate of 300 beats per minute, what ratio of AV conduction will produce a bradycardic rhythm?**

Assuming an atrial rate of 300 beats per minute, bradycardia is produced when atrial flutter is associated with AV block of at least 5:1 (which corresponds to a ventricular rate of 60 beats per minute). When the atrial rate is <300 beats per minute, ratios of AV block <5:1 may produce bradycardia (see Figure 1-3).

**What is the definition of atrial tachycardia?**

Atrial tachycardia is an atrial rhythm with an atrial rate >100 beats per minute that does not originate in the sinus node (sinus rhythm is associated with P waves that are identical in morphology and upright in leads I and aVF).[6]

**What is the typical rate of a junctional escape rhythm?**

Junctional escape rhythms are associated with a heart rate of 40 to 60 beats per minute; these rhythms are variably responsive to alterations in autonomic tone and pharmacologic agents. *Junctional escape rhythms may originate more distally in the conduction system (eg, in the fascicles or distal Purkinje fibers); these escape rhythms have a wide QRS morphology and slower heart rates.*[1]

## NARROW-COMPLEX BRADYCARDIA WITH IRREGULAR RHYTHM

### What are the causes of narrow-complex bradycardia with irregular rhythm?

**Bradycardia during expiration only.**

Sinus arrhythmia.

**Sinus node intermittently stops firing.**

Sinus arrest (a type of sinus pause due to impulse generation failure in the SA node).

**Sinus node fires normally, but the impulses are intermittently blocked from depolarizing the atria.**

Sinoatrial exit block (a type of sinus pause due to impulse transmission failure).

**No P waves.**

Atrial fibrillation with slow ventricular rate.

**A rhythm that most commonly originates within the right atrium.**

Atrial flutter with variable AV block and slow ventricular rate.

**The following electrocardiographic features are observed in a patient with narrow-complex bradycardia with irregular rhythm: P waves occur regularly at a rate of 120 beats per minute; every QRS complex is preceded by a P wave, but not all P waves are followed by a QRS complex; and P waves are inverted in leads II, III, and aVF.**

Atrial tachycardia with variable AV block and slow ventricular rate.

**Intermittently dropped QRS complexes.**

Mobitz type I (Wenckebach) and Mobitz type II second-degree AV blocks.

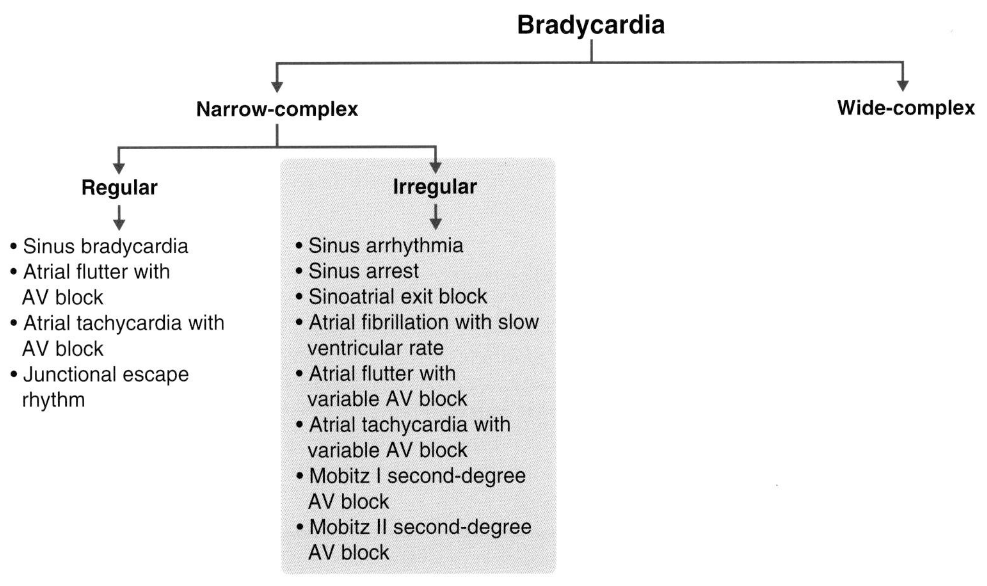


**What is sinus arrhythmia?**

Sinus arrhythmia describes the normal reflex-mediated variability in heart rate during the respiratory cycle in which the heart rate is faster during inspiration and slower during expiration. It may provide certain physiologic advantages, such as enhanced gas exchange by improving ventilation-perfusion matching.[7]

CARDIOLOGY

**What is sinus arrest?**

Sinus arrest is the intermittent failure of the sinus node to generate an impulse (ie, generator failure). The duration of the pause has no relationship to the basic underlying sinus rate, which helps differentiate this entity from second-degree sinoatrial exit block (in which the duration of the pause is a multiple of the basic underlying sinus rate). Sinus arrest longer than 3 seconds in duration requires careful assessment to identify symptomatic correlations and may require intervention (eg, pacemaker placement).[8]

**What is sinoatrial exit block?**

Sinoatrial exit block is the delay or failure of sinus node impulses to propagate through the SA node to neighboring atrial tissue (ie, transmission failure). There are several subtypes. First-degree sinoatrial exit block describes delayed conduction out of the sinus node. It cannot be readily identified electrocardiographically. Second-degree sinoatrial exit block—of which there are 2 subtypes—describes periodic failure of sinus node impulses to exit the sinus node. In second-degree sinoatrial exit block type I, the dropped P wave is preceded by progressively shorter P-P intervals. In second-degree sinoatrial exit block type II, the duration of the pause is a whole number multiple of the immediately preceding P-P interval, a distinctive electrocardiographic finding (Figure 1-4). Third-degree sinoatrial exit block describes complete failure of sinus node impulses to exit the nodal region. Regardless of the subtype, treatment with placement of a permanent pacemaker is usually indicated for symptomatic patients.[8]

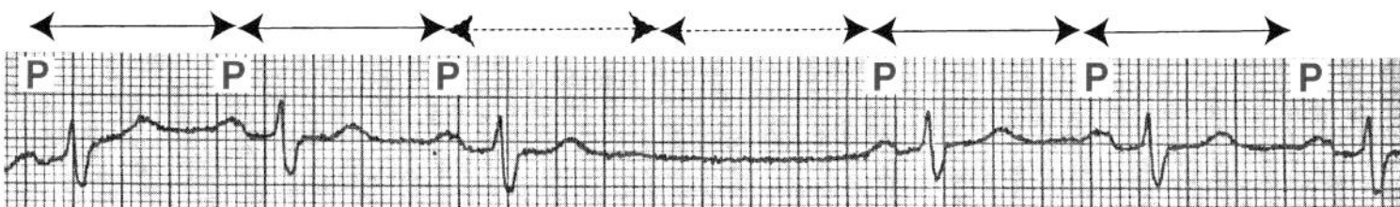


**Figure 1-4.** Second-degree sinoatrial exit block type II (lead II). P waves are regular except after the third QRS complex, where a P wave is dropped. The first P wave after the pause occurs when it would have been expected had there been no interruption in the regular sinus P waves (dashed arrows), a characteristic feature of second-degree sinoatrial exit block type II. (From Katz AM. *Physiology of the Heart*. 5th ed. Philadelphia, PA: Lippincott Williams & Wilkins; 2011.)

**What are the causes of slow ventricular rate in the setting of atrial fibrillation?**

Atrial fibrillation with slow ventricular rate can occur as a result of medication (eg, β-blocker), conduction-system disease (eg, AV block), and increased vagal tone (eg, trained athletes).[9]

**In the setting of atrial flutter with AV block, assuming an atrial rate of 300 beats per minute, what ventricular rates would be expected with the following ratios of AV conduction: 2:1, 3:1, 4:1, and 5:1?**

Atrial flutter with an atrial rate of 300 beats per minute and 2:1, 3:1, 4:1, and 5:1 AV conduction will produce ventricular rates of 150, 100, 75, and 60 beats per minute, respectively.

**What is the prognosis of atrial tachycardia?**

Atrial tachycardia occurs most commonly in patients without heart disease and usually follows a benign course.[10]

**Which type of AV block is characterized electrocardiographically by progressive PR interval lengthening followed by a nonconducted P wave?**

Mobitz I second-degree AV block is characterized by nonconducted (or dropped) beats preceded by progressively lengthening AV conduction intervals (most easily determined on ECG by measuring the PR intervals before and after the nonconducted beat) (see Figure 3-3).

**How often is Mobitz II second-degree AV block associated with a wide QRS complex on ECG?**

Mobitz II second-degree AV block is associated with a wide QRS complex in 80% of cases; the complex is narrow in the remaining 20% (see Figure 3-4).[11]

## WIDE-COMPLEX BRADYCARDIA

**What are the 2 electrocardiographic subcategories of wide-complex bradycardia?**

Wide-complex bradycardia can be associated with a regular rhythm or an irregular rhythm.

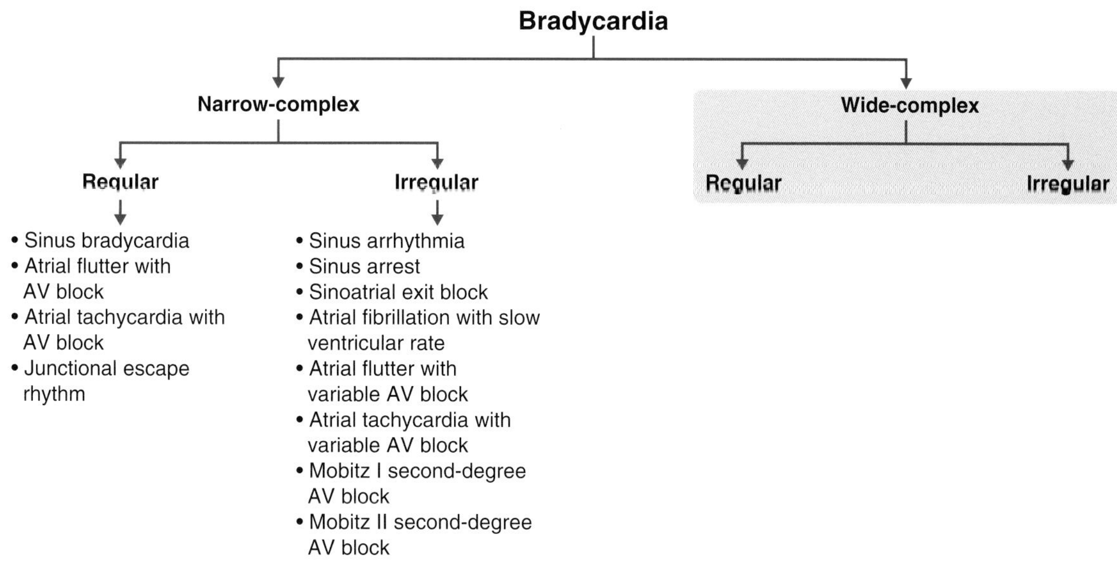


## WIDE-COMPLEX BRADYCARDIA WITH REGULAR RHYTHM

### What are the causes of wide-complex bradycardia with regular rhythm?

**A baseline wide QRS complex.**

Regular supraventricular rhythm (eg, sinus rhythm) with a baseline wide QRS complex (ie, bundle branch block) and slow ventricular rate.

**A 34-year-old man hospitalized with aortic valve endocarditis develops light-headedness and severe bradycardia and is found to have cannon A waves on assessment of the jugular venous waveform.**

Complete heart block with ventricular escape rhythm.

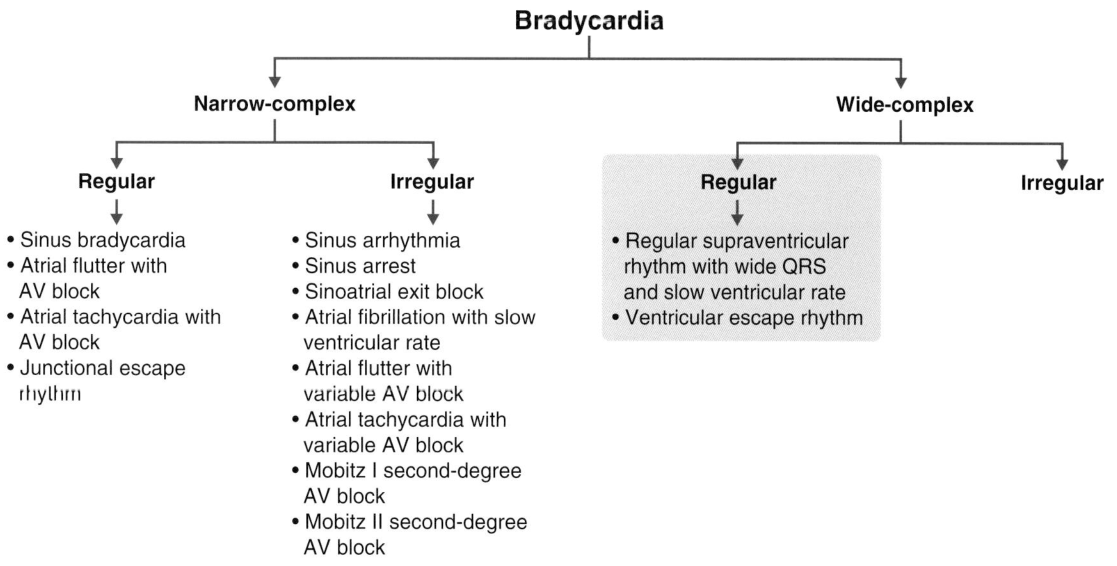


**What electrocardiographic feature can distinguish sinus bradycardia with bundle branch block from a ventricular escape rhythm?**

The presence of AV association (ie, all QRS complexes are preceded by a P wave; all P waves are followed by QRS complexes in regular intervals) would be expected in a patient with sinus bradycardia with a baseline wide QRS complex. Ventricular escape rhythms are characterized by AV dissociation.

**What is the typical rate of a ventricular escape rhythm?**

Ventricular escape rhythms from complete heart block typically occur at a rate between 20 and 40 beats per minute (see Figure 3-6).[12-14]

## WIDE-COMPLEX BRADYCARDIA WITH IRREGULAR RHYTHM

### What are the causes of wide-complex bradycardia with irregular rhythm?

**A baseline wide QRS complex.**

Irregular supraventricular rhythm (eg, atrial fibrillation) with a baseline wide QRS complex (ie, bundle branch block) and slow ventricular rate.

**A 66-year-old woman with symptomatic AV block that worsens with exercise.**

Mobitz II second-degree AV block.

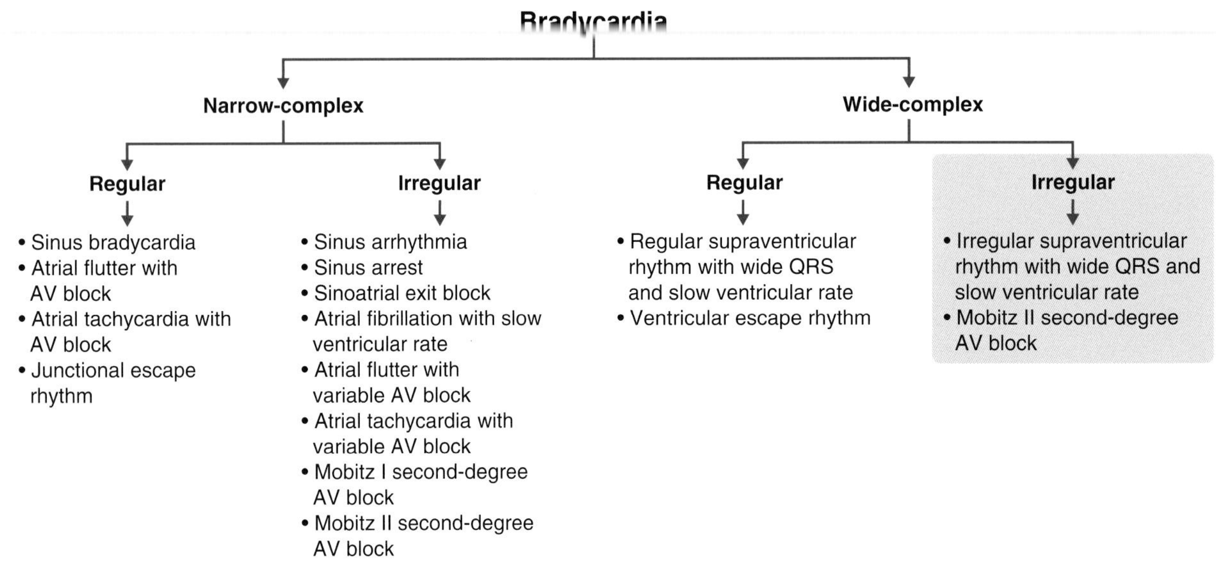


**What is the most likely underlying rhythm if the ECG shows irregular bradycardia with flutter waves and a wide QRS complex?**

Atrial flutter with variable AV block, a baseline wide QRS complex, and slow ventricular rate would present as irregular bradycardia with flutter waves and a wide QRS complex.

**Why is Mobitz II second-degree AV block associated with a wide QRS complex?**

Patients with Mobitz II second-degree AV block usually have preexisting bundle branch blocks (causing a baseline wide QRS complex); the non-conducted beats occur with intermittent failure of the remaining bundle branch.[11,12]

**Can bradycardia occur in pacemaker-dependent patients?**

Pacemakers are programmed to set a "lower rate limit," below which the heart rate should not drop. A drop in heart rate below the lower rate limit can be seen in pacemaker or pacer lead malfunction. Additionally, heart rates that do not meet the definition of bradycardia (ie, rates above 60 beats per minute) in a pacemaker-dependent patient can be considered *relative* bradycardia in clinical scenarios in which the rate is slower than that expected for hemodynamic needs (eg, sepsis).

**What are some clinical scenarios that might result in relative bradycardia in a pacemaker-dependent patient?**

To keep up with the metabolic demand, the heart rate on the pacemaker may need to be increased in patients with sepsis, anemia, hypoxemia, and low cardiac output.

### Case Summary

An 87-year-old man with a history of coronary artery disease, hypertension, and hyperlipidemia presents with syncope and is found to have symptomatic bradycardia.

***What rhythm disturbance is present in this patient?***

Junctional escape rhythm.

### BONUS QUESTIONS

***What electrocardiographic features in this case are suggestive of a junctional rhythm?***

The ECG in this case (see Figure 1-1) demonstrates narrow-complex bradycardia with regular rhythm, which narrows the differential diagnosis to sinus bradycardia, atrial flutter with AV block and slow ventricular rate, atrial tachycardia with AV block and slow ventricular rate, and junctional escape rhythm. The absence of clearly discernible P waves with 1:1 conduction or flutter waves suggests a junctional escape rhythm. If no P waves are discernible, the underlying rhythm is likely sinus arrest with junctional escape. If P waves are discernible but without 1:1 conduction, the underlying rhythm is most likely sinus with complete heart block and junctional escape, or sinus slowing with isorhythmic AV dissociation.

***What other major electrocardiographic finding is present in this case?***

The ECG in this case (see Figure 1-1) demonstrates ST-segment elevation involving the inferior leads, consistent with acute inferior myocardial infarction.

***What is the most likely cause of the junctional escape rhythm in this case?***

The junctional escape rhythm in this case is most likely the result of an inferior myocardial infarction in the distribution of the right coronary artery, which supplies the SA and AV nodes. Possible underlying conduction disturbances include sinus arrest, sinus bradycardia, and heart block. Because appropriately timed P waves are not discernible on the ECG (see Figure 1-1), the underlying conduction disturbance cannot be determined.

***What immediate treatment strategies should be considered in this case?***

Treatment with intravenous fluids, medications, transcutaneous or transvenous temporary pacing, and coronary artery reperfusion strategies (eg, percutaneous coronary intervention or fibrinolytic agents) should be considered in this case.

***What long-term treatment strategy should be offered to the patient in this case if the underlying cause is not reversible and symptomatic bradycardia persists?***

If symptomatic bradycardia persists in the patient in this case, placement of a permanent pacemaker should be considered.[1]

## KEY POINTS

- Bradycardia in the adult is classically defined as heart rate <60 beats per minute, but there is considerable variation in normal between populations.
- Cardiac output is equal to the forward stroke volume of the left ventricle per beat multiplied by heart rate.
- Bradycardia may be asymptomatic or associated with fatigue, weakness, light-headedness, or syncope.
- Physical findings of bradycardia include hypotension, cool extremities, and cannon A waves (in the setting of AV dissociation).
- Bradycardia can be associated with a narrow QRS complex (<120 ms) or a wide QRS complex (>120 ms).
- Narrow-complex bradycardia can be associated with a regular rhythm or an irregular rhythm.
- Wide-complex bradycardia can be associated with a regular rhythm or an irregular rhythm.

### REFERENCES

1. Mangrum JM, DiMarco JP. The evaluation and management of bradycardia. *N Engl J Med*. 2000;342(10):703-709.
2. Berne RML, Levy MN. *Physiology*. 4th ed. St. Louis, MO: Mosby Inc.; 1998.
3. Brodsky M, Wu D, Denes P, Kanakis C, Rosen KM. Arrhythmias documented by 24 hour continuous electrocardiographic monitoring in 50 male medical students without apparent heart disease. *Am J Cardiol*. 1977;39(3):390-395.
4. Kantelip JP, Sage E, Duchene-Marullaz P. Findings on ambulatory electrocardiographic monitoring in subjects older than 80 years. *Am J Cardiol*. 1986;57(6):398-401.
5. Cunha BA. The diagnostic significance of relative bradycardia in infectious disease. *Clin Microbiol Infect*. 2000;6(12):633-634.
6. Page RL, Joglar JA, Caldwell MA, Calkins H, Conti JB, Deal BJ, et al. 2015 ACC/AHA/HRS guideline for the management of adult patients with supraventricular tachycardia: a report of the American College of Cardiology/American Heart Association Task Force on Clinical Practice Guidelines and the Heart Rhythm Society. *Circulation*. 2016;133(14):e506-e574.

7. Yasuma F, Hayano J. Respiratory sinus arrhythmia: why does the heartbeat synchronize with respiratory rhythm? *Chest*. 2004;125(2): 683-690.
8. Benditt DG, Gornick CC, Dunbar D, Almquist A, Pool-Schneider S. Indications for electrophysiologic testing in the diagnosis and assessment of sinus node dysfunction. *Circulation*. 1987;75(4 Pt 2):III93-III102.
9. Falk RH. Atrial fibrillation. *N Engl J Med*. 2001;344(14):1067-1078.
10. Levine HD, Smith C Jr. Repetitive paroxysmal tachycardia in adults. *Cardiology*. 1970;55(1):2-21.
11. Dreifus LS, Likoff W, eds. *Cardiac Arrhythmias*. New York: Grune and Stratton; 1973.
12. Merideth J, Pruitt RD. Cardiac arrhythmias. 5. Disturbances in cardiac conduction and their management. *Circulation*. 1973;47(5): 1098-1107.
13. Riera AR, Barros RB, de Sousa FD, Baranchuk A. Accelerated idioventricular rhythm: history and chronology of the main discoveries. *Indian Pacing Electrophysiol J*. 2010;10(1):40-48.
14. Vogler J, Breithardt G, Eckardt L. Bradyarrhythmias and conduction blocks. *Rev Esp Cardiol (Engl Ed)*. 2012;65(7):656-667.

Chapter 2

# CHEST PAIN

## Case: A 76-year-old woman with an extra heart sound

A 76-year-old woman with a history of hypertension and hyperlipidemia presents to the clinic with increasingly frequent episodes of chest pain over the course of a few months. The episodes occur several times per day, lasting for up to 15 minutes. The pain is "squeezing" in quality. The episodes occur most frequently when she walks around the grocery store. Rest alleviates the discomfort. She reports recent episodes of light-headedness on standing and has lost consciousness on 2 occasions. She underwent coronary angiography 2 years ago that showed no evidence of coronary artery disease (CAD).

Blood pressure is 102/85 mm Hg. An extra heart sound is heard just before S1 with the bell of the stethoscope over the apex; S2 is obliterated by a grade III/VI late-peaking crescendo-decrescendo systolic murmur best heard over the right upper sternal border, with radiation to the carotids. The peripheral pulse is difficult to find and its contour is prolonged (slow rise and fall).

Electrocardiogram (ECG) is shown in Figure 2-1.

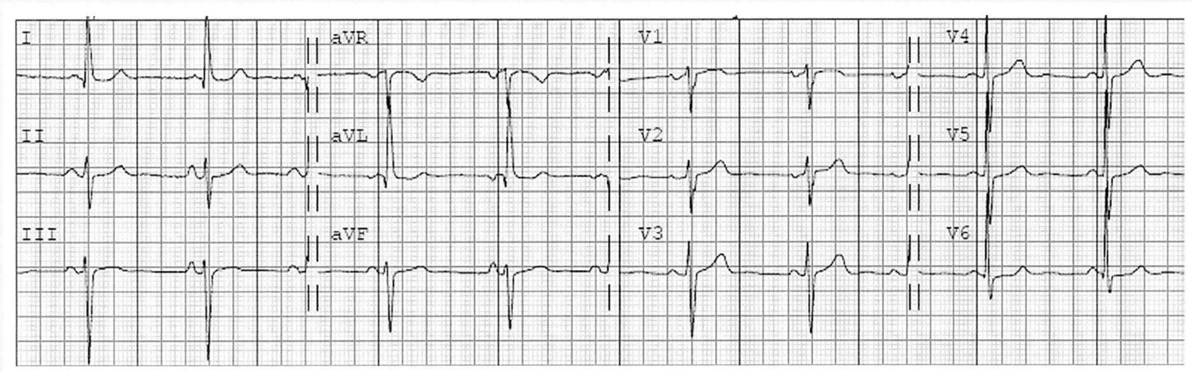


**Figure 2-1.**

***What is the most likely cause of chest pain in this patient?***

What are the 2 general sources of chest pain? Sources of chest pain can be cardiac or noncardiac.

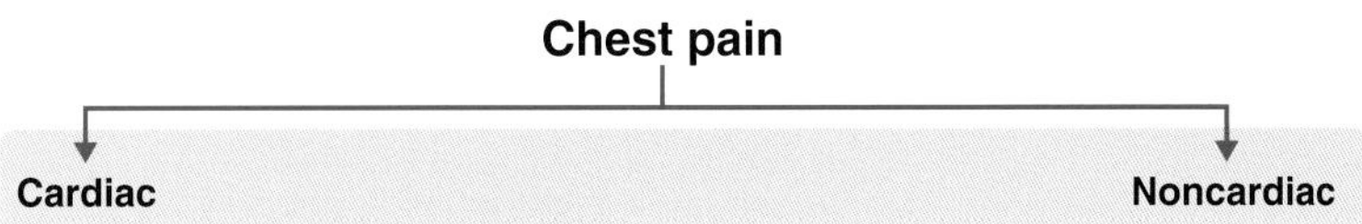


Is chest pain more often cardiac or noncardiac in nature? Most cases of chest pain are noncardiac in nature.[1]

## CARDIAC CAUSES OF CHEST PAIN

What are the 2 general subcategories of cardiac chest pain? Cardiac chest pain can be related to acute coronary syndrome (ACS) or unrelated to ACS.

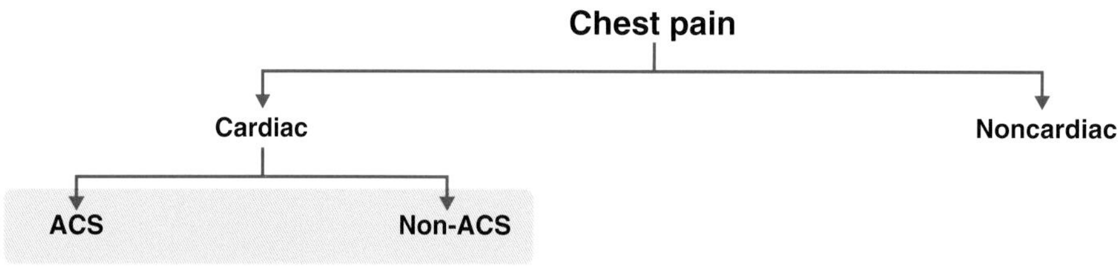


## ACUTE CORONARY SYNDROME

**What is acute coronary syndrome?**

ACS describes a range of clinical syndromes that result in myocardial ischemia with or without infarction. The diagnosis relies on the identification of characteristic clinical features, including a compatible history, electrocardiographic findings, and biochemical markers.[2]

**What are the characteristic symptoms of acute coronary syndrome?**

Patients with ACS often experience chest, upper extremity, mandibular, or epigastric discomfort that occurs with exertion or at rest, and typically lasts >20 minutes. These symptoms may be associated with diaphoresis, nausea, or syncope. Some patients experience "angina equivalent" symptoms such as dyspnea or fatigue. *Symptoms of myocardial ischemia may be atypical in certain populations, particularly women, diabetics, and postoperative patients.*[3]

**What differentiates acute myocardial infarction from myocardial ischemia?**

Acute myocardial infarction is defined as myocardial necrosis that occurs as a result of myocardial ischemia, and can be identified by the rise and fall of cardiac biomarkers in the blood (eg, cardiac-specific troponin) along with other supportive evidence (eg, characteristic electrocardiographic changes).[4]

**What are the 3 subtypes of acute coronary syndrome?**

The subtypes of ACS are ST-elevation myocardial infarction (STEMI), unstable angina (UA), and non–ST-elevation myocardial infarction (NSTEMI).

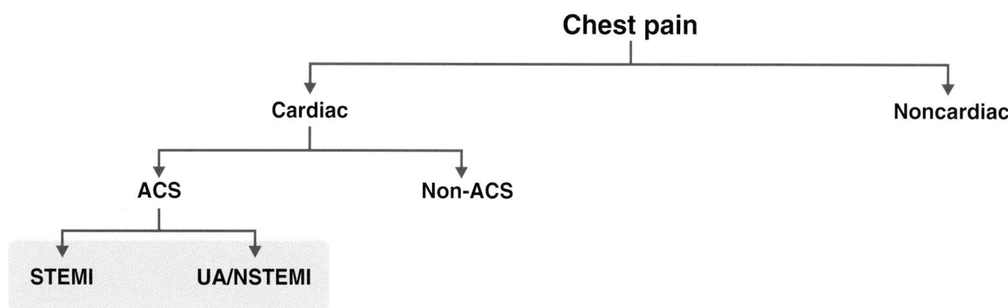


**Why is it important to differentiate STEMI from UA/NSTEMI?**

STEMI and UA/NSTEMI are differentiated based on the presence of characteristic electrocardiographic findings. The distinction is important because acute treatment strategies differ between them. Immediate reperfusion therapy (eg, percutaneous coronary intervention or fibrinolytics) has been shown to be beneficial in patients with STEMI.[2,3]

**What are the earliest electrocardiographic manifestations of STEMI?**

An ECG should be obtained promptly for any patient suspected of having acute myocardial infarction. An early electrocardiographic manifestation of STEMI can be the presence of hyperacute (ie, broad-based, tall, symmetrical) T-waves in at least 2 contiguous leads (Figure 2-2). Transient Q waves may also be observed in acute myocardial ischemia.[3]

**What electrocardiographic findings are diagnostic of STEMI?**

In the appropriate clinical context, the presence of new ST-segment elevation at the J point in 2 contiguous leads of ≥0.1 mV (except in leads $V_2$-$V_3$ where it must be ≥0.2 mV in men ≥40 years of age, ≥0.25 mV in men <40 years of age, or ≥0.15 mV in women) is diagnostic of STEMI (see Figure 2-2). *It is important to recognize that ST-segment elevation can occur as a result of conditions other than myocardial infarction (eg, acute pericarditis).*[3]

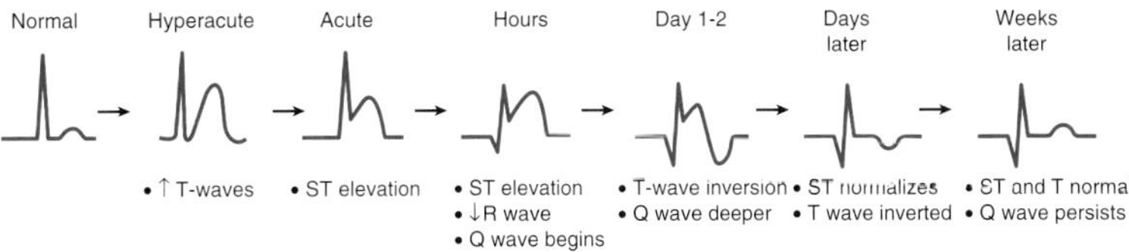


**Figure 2-2.** The evolution of ECG changes associated with STEMI. (From Lilly LS. *Pathophysiology of Heart Disease: A Collaborative Project of Medical Students and Faculty*. 6th ed. Philadelphia, PA: Wolters Kluwer Health; 2016.)

**What are the characteristic electrocardiographic findings of UA/NSTEMI?**

Electrocardiographic findings characteristic of UA/NSTEMI include new horizontal or downsloping ST-segment depression ≥0.05 mV in 2 contiguous leads and/or T-wave inversion ≥0.1 mV in 2 contiguous leads with prominent R wave or R/S ratio >1 (Figure 2-3).[3]

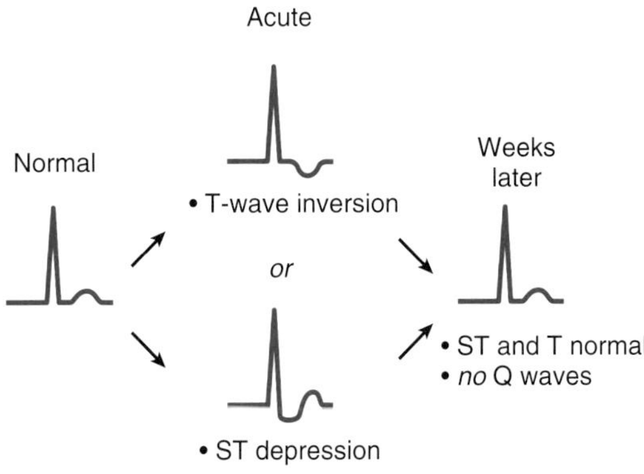


**Figure 2-3.** ECG abnormalities associated with UA/NSTEMI. (From Lilly LS. *Pathophysiology of Heart Disease: A Collaborative Project of Medical Students and Faculty*. 6th ed. Philadelphia, PA: Wolters Kluwer Health; 2016.)

**Which groups of ECG leads are considered contiguous?**

Contiguous ECG leads include the anterior leads ($V_1$-$V_6$), inferior leads (II, III, aVF), and the lateral/apical leads (I, aVL). Additional leads such as $V_3R$ and $V_4R$ reflect the free wall of the right ventricle, and $V_7$-$V_9$ the infero-basal wall. ST-segment elevation or diagnostic Q waves in contiguous leads are more specific than ST-segment depression in localizing the region of myocardial ischemia or infarction.[3]

**What baseline conditions make electrocardiographic interpretation of ischemia unreliable?**

False-positive electrocardiographic features of ischemia may occur in the setting of early repolarization, left ventricular hypertrophy, left bundle branch block, ventricular paced rhythm, preexcitation, J-point elevation syndromes (eg, Brugada syndrome), acute pericarditis, myocarditis, subarachnoid hemorrhage, metabolic disturbances (eg, hyperkalemia), stress cardiomyopathy, and cholecystitis. False-negative findings may occur in the setting of prior myocardial infarction with Q waves and/or persistent ST-segment elevation, ventricular paced rhythm, and left bundle branch block.[3]

**How are UA and NSTEMI distinguished?**

UA and NSTEMI are subtypes of ACS, but can be differentiated based on the degree of myocardial injury, reflected by the presence of serum biomarkers (eg, troponin). Unlike UA, NSTEMI is associated with elevated serum troponin. The diagnosis of UA relies mostly upon the clinical history; electrocardiographic features of ischemia may or may not be present.[3]

## What are the causes of acute coronary syndrome?

**The prototypical and most common mechanism of ACS.**

Rupture of an atherosclerotic plaque (Figure 2-4).[3]

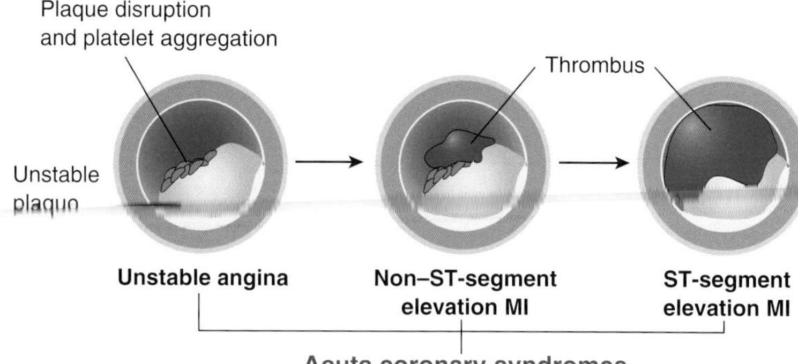


**Figure 2-4.** Unstable atherosclerotic plaque with plaque disruption and platelet aggregation in the acute coronary syndromes. (From Porth CM. *Essentials of Pathophysiology: Concepts of Altered Health States*. 4th ed. Philadelphia, PA: Wolters Kluwer; 2015.)

**Consider this etiology in patients who recently underwent primary coronary intervention.**

Stent thrombosis.

**A traveling clot.**

Coronary artery embolism.

**A 32-year-old man presents with crushing substernal chest pain, ST-segment elevation on ECG, positive serum biomarkers, and positive urine drug screen.**

Coronary artery vasospasm, including Prinzmetal's (ie, variant) angina.

**Consider this etiology in pregnant women who present with ACS.**

Coronary artery dissection.

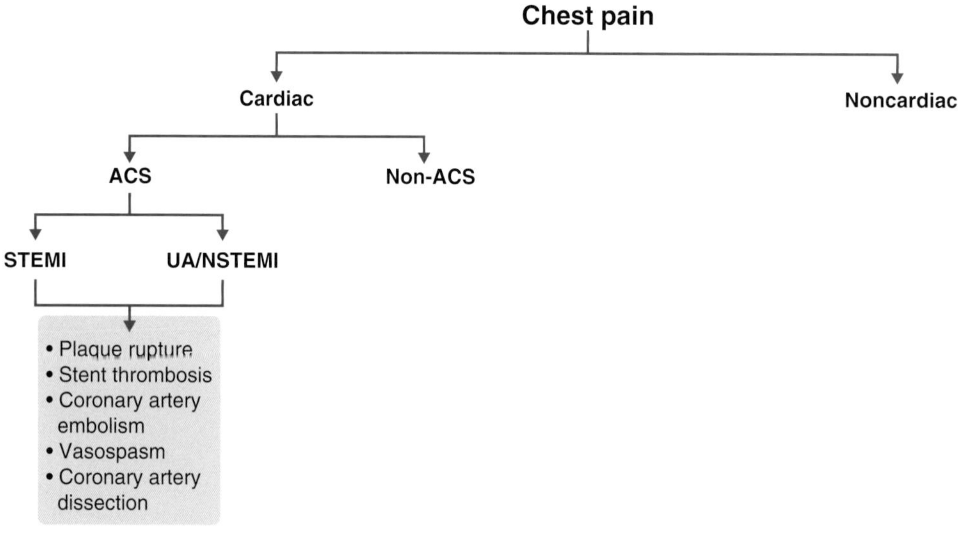


**What are the risk factors for coronary artery disease?**

Risk factors for CAD include older age, male sex, smoking, hyperlipidemia, diabetes, physical inactivity, family history of premature CAD, and chronic inflammatory conditions.[5]

What criteria are used to establish a positive family history of premature coronary artery disease?

A family history of premature CAD is established when there is definite myocardial infarction or sudden death before 55 years of age in a first-degree male relative, or before 65 years of age in a first-degree female relative.[5]

How does the timing of stent thrombosis differ between bare metal stents and drug-eluting stents?

Stent thrombosis is largely an early complication of bare metal stents (within 30 days); it tends to be a late complication of drug-eluting stents (after several years).[6]

What is the most common risk factor for coronary artery embolism?

Atrial fibrillation is the most common risk factor for coronary artery embolism.[7]

In patients with coronary artery vasospasm, what risk factor is associated with myocardial infarction (as opposed to myocardial ischemia)?

Coronary artery vasospasm is more likely to result in myocardial infarction in patients with underlying CAD.[8]

What proportion of cases of coronary artery dissection occur in the peripartum period?

The majority of coronary artery dissections occur in women. Among them, one-third of cases occur in the peripartum period.[9]

## CARDIAC CAUSES OF CHEST PAIN UNRELATED TO ACUTE CORONARY SYNDROME

### What are the cardiac causes of chest pain unrelated to acute coronary syndrome?

A 62-year-old man complains of episodes of substernal chest pressure that reliably occur 10 minutes after he begins to mow the lawn, and resolve with rest.

Stable angina pectoris.

Pulsus parvus et tardus.

Aortic stenosis.

Pleuritic chest pain that is relieved by leaning forward.

Acute pericarditis.

"Ripping" chest pain associated with pulse discrepancies between extremities and dense mediastinum on chest radiography.

Aortic dissection.

Recurrent episodes of substernal chest pain at rest in the early morning hours in a patient with a negative cardiac stress test.

Coronary artery vasospasm, including Prinzmetal's angina.

Commonly caused by viral infections and may be associated with diffuse ST-segment elevation on ECG; some patients go on to develop dilated cardiomyopathy and chronic systolic heart failure.

Myocarditis.

A 22-year-old man presents with several episodes of syncope and chest pain during exercise and is found to have a systolic ejection murmur on examination that intensifies with Valsalva.

Hypertrophic obstructive cardiomyopathy (HOCM).

A 26-year-old woman with an asthenic body type presents with recurrent episodes of anxiety, heart palpitations, and chest pain, and is found to have a midsystolic click followed by a murmur best heard over the apex of the heart.

Mitral valve prolapse (MVP).

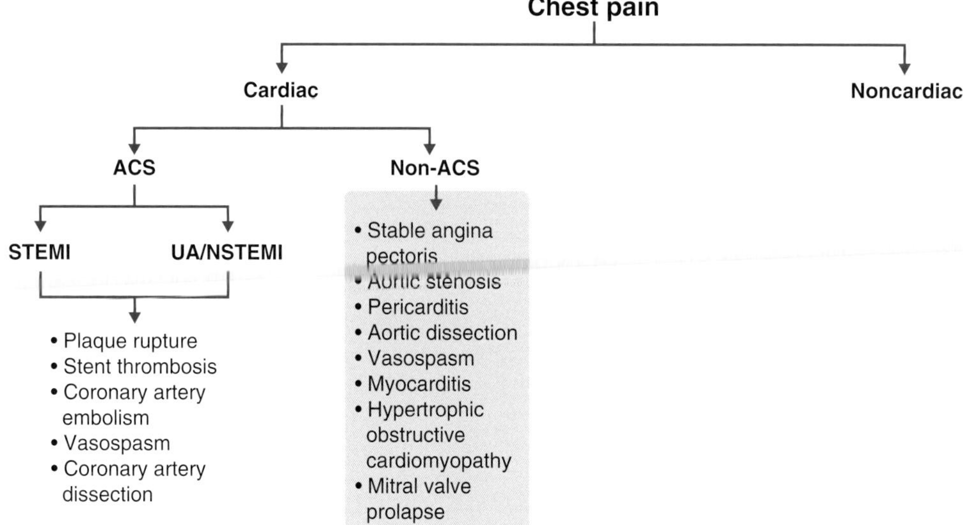


**What is the mechanism of stable angina?**

Stable angina occurs when there is an obstructive but stable atherosclerotic plaque within a coronary artery that leads to relative myocardial hypoperfusion and ischemia in the territory it supplies when myocardial oxygen demand increases. In ambulatory patients, this can occur with light physical activity such as mowing the lawn. Hospitalized patients with stable angina may experience "supply/demand mismatch" when myocardial oxygen demand increases as a result of conditions such as tachycardia, hypotension, hypertension, congestive heart failure, anemia, hypoxemia, and sepsis (Figure 2-5).

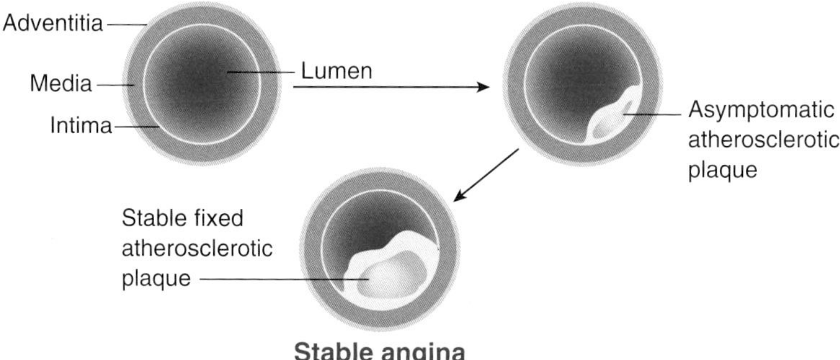


**Figure 2-5.** Stable fixed atherosclerotic plaque in stable angina. (From Porth CM. *Essentials of Pathophysiology: Concepts of Altered Health States*. 4th ed. Philadelphia, PA: Wolters Kluwer; 2015.)

**Without treatment, what is the mean survival in patients with severe aortic stenosis associated with angina?**

Without treatment, mean survival in patients with severe aortic stenosis associated with angina is 5 years.[10]

**What are the electrocardiographic findings of acute pericarditis?**

The typical electrocardiographic findings of acute pericarditis include diffuse ST-segment elevation, diffuse PR-segment depression, and PR-segment elevation in lead aVR.[11]

**What risk factors are associated with acute aortic dissection?**

Risk factors for acute aortic dissection include male sex, age in the 60s and 70s, hypertension, prior cardiac surgery (particularly aortic valve repair), bicuspid aortic valve, connective tissue diseases (eg, Marfan syndrome), and aortitis (eg, giant cell arteritis, syphilis).[12,13]

What substances are associated with coronary artery vasospasm?

Coronary artery vasospasm can be provoked by a number of substances, including cocaine, amphetamines, marijuana, 5-fluorouracil, and sumatriptan. The cause of spontaneous coronary artery vasospasm (ie, Prinzmetal's angina) has not been completely elucidated, but genetic and environmental factors may play a role. Active smokers constitute the majority of patients who suffer from spontaneous coronary artery vasospasm.[14]

How often do patients with myocarditis present with chest pain?

Dyspnea is the most frequent symptom of acute or chronic myocarditis, reported by most patients on presentation. Around one-third of patients report chest pain on presentation.[15]

What is the expected change in quality of the murmur caused by hypertrophic obstructive cardiomyopathy when patients move from a standing to squatting position?

Moving from a standing to squatting position increases preload, which results in a decrease in the intensity of the murmur associated with HOCM.

Why do patients with symptomatic mitral valve prolapse often have persistent episodes of chest pain and palpitations after undergoing mitral valve replacement?

Symptoms experienced by patients with MVP, including chest pain and palpitations, are often related to associated autonomic dysfunction that persists after the valvular lesion is addressed.[16]

## NONCARDIAC CAUSES OF CHEST PAIN

The causes of noncardiac chest pain can be separated into which system-based subcategories?

The causes of noncardiac chest pain can be separated into the following subcategories: pulmonary, gastrointestinal, musculoskeletal, and other.

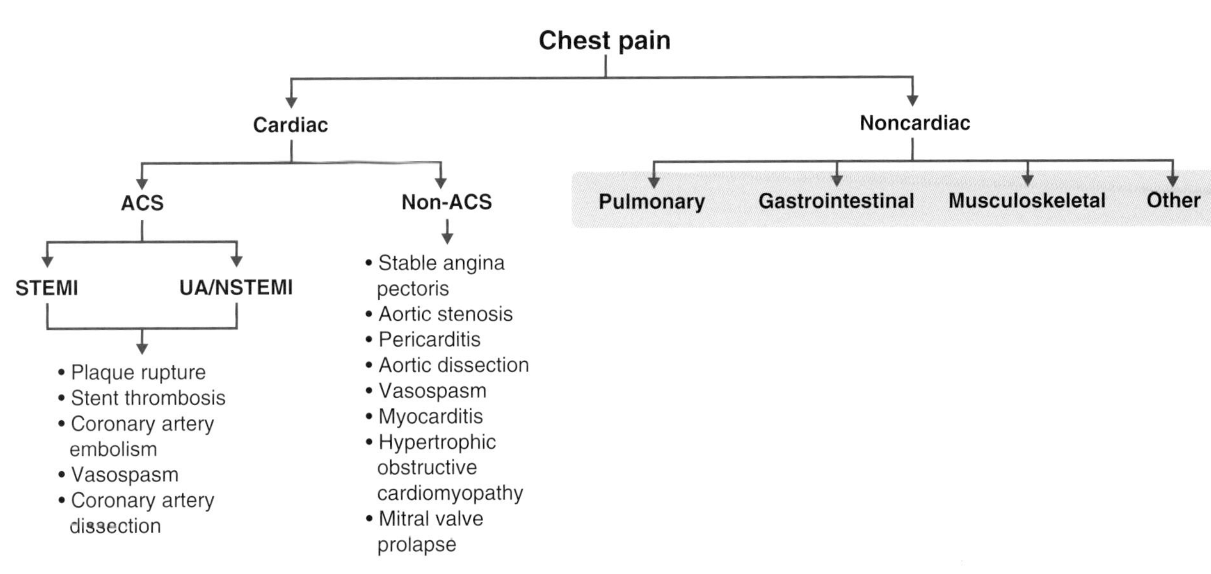


## PULMONARY CAUSES OF CHEST PAIN

### What are the pulmonary causes of chest pain?

This condition is associated with an auscultatory sound akin to walking on fresh snow.

Pleurisy.

Fever, purulent cough, and pleuritic chest pain.

Pneumonia.

A 46-year-old woman from California with a history of ovarian cancer presents with sudden onset pleuritic chest pain after returning home from a trip to Thailand.

Pulmonary embolism (PE).

Hyperresonance to percussion of the chest over the affected area.

Pneumothorax.

A previously healthy 36-year-old woman presents with dyspnea on exertion and is found to have elevated jugular venous pressure (JVP), a right ventricular heave, and a loud pulmonic component of the second heart sound (P2).

Pulmonary hypertension.

A 24-year-old man from Saudi Arabia with a known blood disorder (he cannot recall the name) presents with diffuse arthralgias and sudden-onset chest pain.

Acute chest syndrome (related to sickle cell disease).

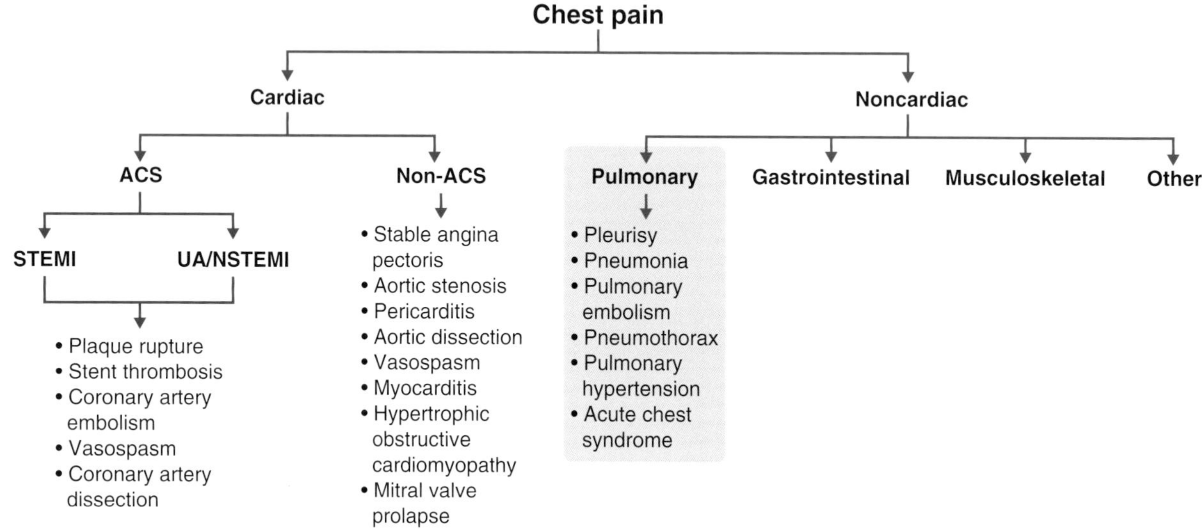


What is pleurisy?

Pleurisy describes inflammation of the pleura and is associated with numerous conditions (eg, infection, medication, rheumatologic disease). The chest pain is typically pleuritic in nature, exacerbated by deep breathing, coughing, or sneezing. In addition to addressing the underlying cause, first-line pharmacologic treatment for the symptoms of pleurisy is nonsteroidal anti-inflammatory drugs.[17]

Does tactile fremitus increase or decrease over an area of pneumonia?

Tactile fremitus increases over an area of consolidation related to pneumonia. Other physical findings of consolidation include dullness to percussion, egophony (when the patient says the word "bee," the "e" sounds more like an "a"), and whispered pectoriloquy ("chest-speaking"), which refers to an increase in volume and clarity of whispered sounds while listening to the chest with the stethoscope.[18]

What are the electrocardiographic findings of acute pulmonary embolism?

Electrocardiographic manifestations of acute PE include sinus tachycardia, new atrial fibrillation, and evidence of right ventricular strain such as T-wave inversion in the anteroseptal leads, right axis deviation, new right bundle branch block, and S1Q3T3 pattern (S wave in lead I, Q wave in lead III, and inverted T wave in lead III). The ECG may be normal in up to one-quarter of patients.[19]

What is the immediate treatment for tension pneumothorax?

Tension pneumothorax (see Figure 24-3) should immediately be treated by placing a large-bore needle/catheter through the second anterior intercostal space. The catheter should remain in place until a thoracostomy tube can be inserted.

What is the definitive diagnostic study to evaluate for pulmonary hypertension?

History, physical examination, electrocardiography, and echocardiography can provide information suggestive of pulmonary hypertension. The gold standard diagnostic study to evaluate for pulmonary hypertension is right heart catheterization with direct measurement of pulmonary pressures.

In a patient with acute chest syndrome, what finding is often present on chest imaging?

Consolidation is a common finding on chest imaging in patients with acute chest syndrome.

## GASTROINTESTINAL CAUSES OF CHEST PAIN

### What are the gastrointestinal causes of chest pain?

**A 48-year-old man with obesity presents to his primary care physician with complaints of chest pain and an acidic taste in his mouth after large meals.**

Gastroesophageal reflux disease (GERD).

**A 42-year-old woman who has been taking increasing doses of nonsteroidal anti-inflammatory drugs for chronic low back pain complains of episodes of epigastric and retrosternal chest discomfort after meals.**

Peptic ulcer disease (PUD).

**Pain associated with this entity is typically located in the right upper quadrant of the abdomen but may radiate to the chest and right scapular region.**

Biliary colic.

**Painful contractions of the esophagus.**

Esophageal spasm.

**A 39-year-old man with a history of severe hypertriglyceridemia presents with epigastric and retrosternal chest pain that radiates to the back.**

Acute pancreatitis.

**A 36-year-old man with a history of heavy alcohol use is admitted for chest pain following an episode of violent retching and is found to have subcutaneous emphysema of the chest and a left-sided pleural effusion.**

Esophageal rupture (Boerhaave syndrome).

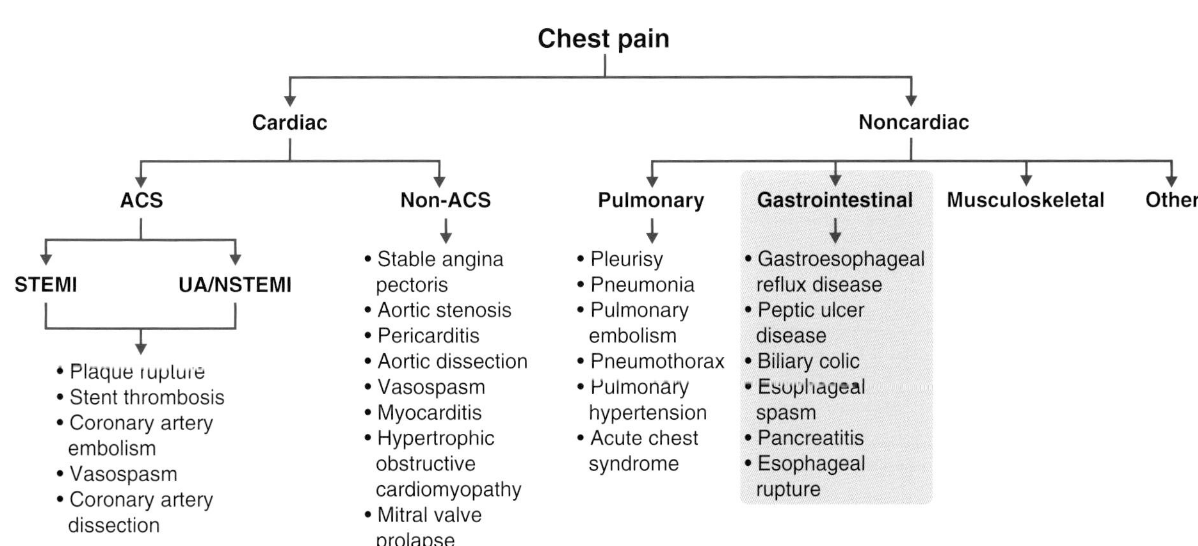


**What lifestyle modifications are helpful in treating gastroesophageal reflux disease?**

Lifestyle modifications that may help treat GERD include avoidance of foods that are acidic or irritating (eg, citrus fruits, tomatoes, onions, spicy foods), avoidance of foods that cause gastric reflux (eg, fatty or fried foods, coffee, tea, caffeinated beverages, chocolate, mint), reduction of alcohol consumption, smoking cessation, and weight loss. Patients with post-prandial symptoms may benefit from smaller and more frequent meals, and refraining from lying down after meals. For patients with nocturnal symptoms, food should not be consumed within 3 hours of bedtime, and the head of the bed should be elevated.[20]

**Which type of peptic ulcer disease often presents with pain that worsens with meals?**

Pain that worsens with meals is suggestive of gastric PUD. Pain that improves with meals is suggestive of duodenal PUD.

**How common is cholelithiasis?**

In the industrialized world, 10% to 15% of adults develop gallstones. Asymptomatic patients develop symptoms at a rate of 1% to 4% per year. Risk factors for developing cholelithiasis include older age, female sex, obesity, family history, pregnancy, rapid weight loss, and parenteral nutrition.[21]

**How is the diagnosis of esophageal spasm made?**

The diagnosis of esophageal spasm can be made with the combination of barium swallow and esophageal manometry testing. Pharmacologic treatment strategies include proton pump inhibitors, calcium channel blockers, nitrates, and phosphodiesterase inhibitors.[22]

**How is the diagnosis of acute pancreatitis made?**

The diagnosis of acute pancreatitis requires at least 2 of the following 3 features: (1) characteristic abdominal pain (eg, postprandial, epigastric, radiating to the back); (2) serum lipase or amylase levels at least 3 times the upper limit of normal; or (3) evidence of acute pancreatitis on cross-sectional imaging.[23]

**What is the most common cause of esophageal rupture?**

The most common cause of esophageal rupture is medical instrumentation (eg, esophageal dilators for achalasia). Other causes are related to a variety of conditions that increase intraabdominal pressure, including intense vomiting or retching, weight lifting, parturition, and status epilepticus.[24]

## MUSCULOSKELETAL CAUSES OF CHEST PAIN

### What are the musculoskeletal causes of chest pain?

**These 3 related disorders typically respond well to nonsteroidal anti-inflammatory drugs.**

Costochondritis, chest wall trauma, and rib fracture.

**Often associated with neck pain.**

Radiculopathy (ie, cervical angina).

**A 33-year-old man with a history of groin sarcoma presents with chest wall pain, and cross-sectional imaging of the chest reveals multiple nodules and masses throughout the mediastinum, pleurae, and osseous structures.**

Chest wall tumor.

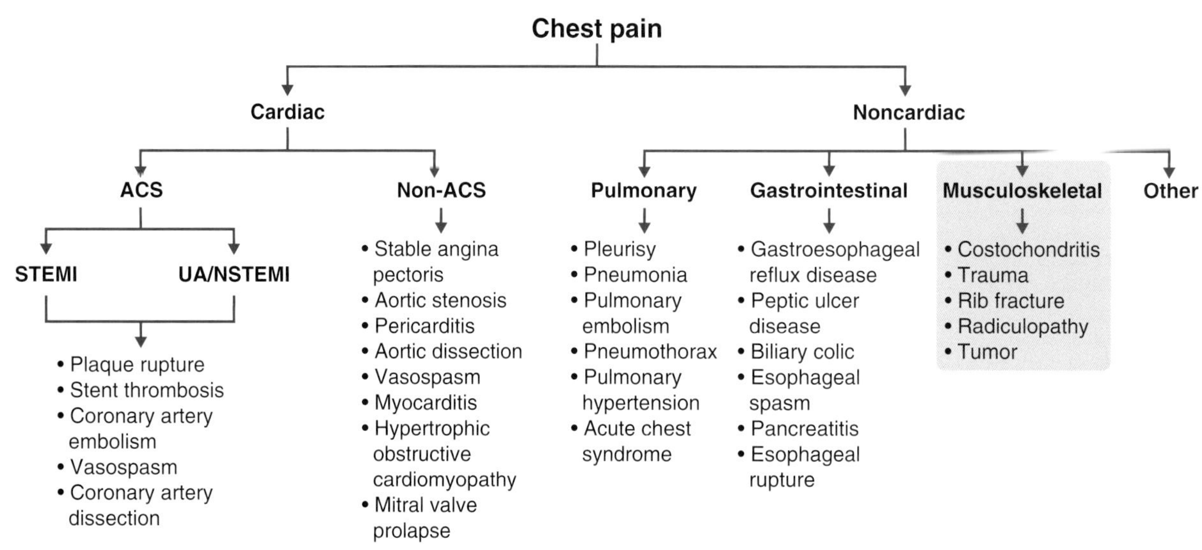

**What physical finding is often present in patients with costochondritis, chest wall trauma, or rib fracture that can help differentiate these conditions from angina?**

Pain is often reproducible with palpation of the chest in patients with costochondritis, chest wall trauma, and rib fracture.

**What causes cervical angina?**

The majority of cases of cervical angina are caused by cervical nerve root compression (C4-C8) associated with conditions such as degenerative disc disease.[25]

**What is the most common primary malignant tumor of the chest wall?**

Soft tissue sarcoma is the most common primary malignant tumor of the chest wall. Other types of tumors include chondrosarcoma, osteosarcoma, small round cell tumor, plasmacytoma, and giant cell tumor.[26]

## OTHER CAUSES OF CHEST PAIN

### What are the other causes of chest pain?

**Patients with this condition may also suffer from agoraphobia, major depression, and substance abuse.**

Anxiety (panic disorder).[1]

**During finals week of his first year in college, a previously healthy 18-year-old man presents to the clinic with pain over the right side of the chest associated with vesicular skin lesions on an erythematous base.**

Herpes zoster.

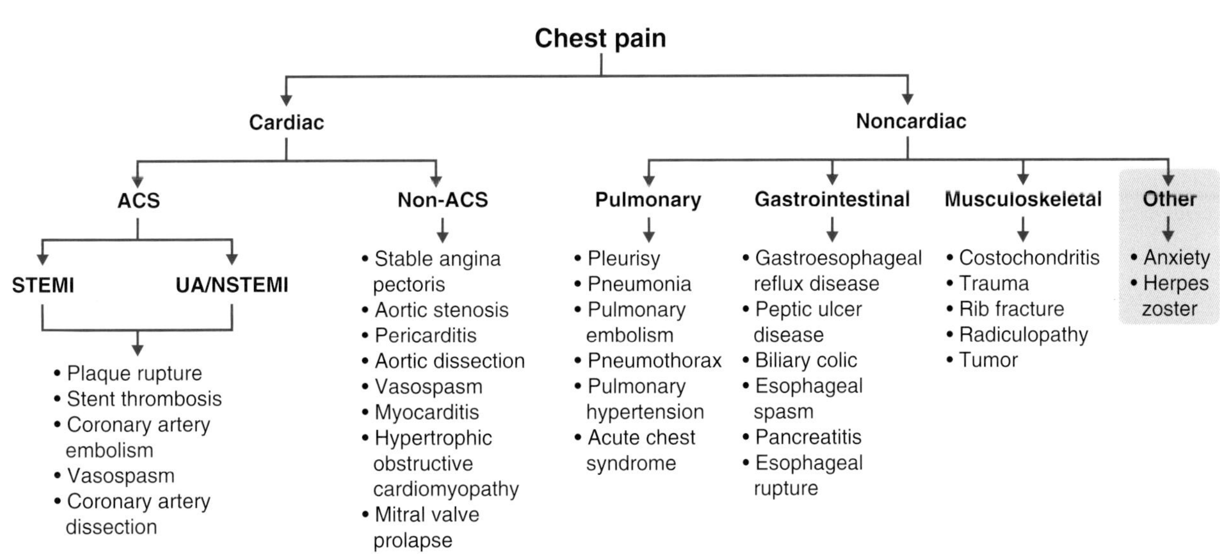


**What is the treatment for panic disorder?**

The majority of patients with panic disorder (with or without agoraphobia) can be effectively treated with either nonpharmacologic modalities such as cognitive and behavioral techniques, or pharmacologic modalities such as selective serotonin reuptake inhibitors.[1]

**What is the typical distribution of herpes zoster?**

The rash of herpes zoster tends to be asymmetric, following a unilateral dermatomal distribution.

CARDIOLOGY

## Case Summary

A 76-year-old woman with hypertension and hyperlipidemia presents with escalating episodes of exertional chest pain and is found to have narrow pulse pressure, a late-peaking systolic ejection murmur, a weak and delayed peripheral pulse, and an abnormal ECG.

***What is the most likely cause of chest pain in this patient?***

Severe aortic stenosis.

### BONUS QUESTIONS

***How common is aortic stenosis?***

In the industrialized world, aortic stenosis occurs in 1% to 3% of the general population over 70 years of age. It is the most common cause of valvular heart disease in this population.[27]

***What is the most likely source of the extra heart sound in this case?***

Extra heart sounds that occur near S1 include split S1, S4 gallop, and ejection clicks. The extra sound in this case is most likely an S4 gallop, based on location, pitch, and clinical history (see Figure 4-4). An S4 often occurs in the setting of concentric ventricular hypertrophy, an expected sequela of severe aortic stenosis. An ejection click might also be expected in the setting of aortic stenosis, but this sound is appreciated over the base of the heart.[28]

***What relevant electrocardiographic findings are present in this case?***

The ECG in this case (see Figure 2-1) demonstrates left ventricular hypertrophy and left axis deviation, findings that are compatible with the underlying diagnosis of aortic stenosis. There are several different criteria used to diagnose left ventricular hypertrophy on ECG. In this case, the ECG meets the "R in aVL" score (R in aVL ≥11 mm), for example.[27,29]

***What physical findings correlate with the severity of aortic stenosis?***

Physical findings that predict greater severity of aortic stenosis include a narrow pulse pressure, pulsus parvus et tardus (small, slowly rising and falling pulse), brachioradial pulse delay, diminished or inaudible aortic component of the second heart sound (A2), and a late-peaking systolic murmur. As the degree of stenosis worsens, the murmur peaks progressively later in systole. The intensity of the murmur does not correlate with severity.[28]

***What is the most likely cause of aortic stenosis in this case?***

In the industrialized world, age-related calcific degeneration of aortic leaflets—an inflammatory process similar to atherosclerosis—is the most common underlying cause of aortic stenosis in patients >70 years of age. Other causes include congenital disease (eg, bicuspid aortic valve) and rheumatic heart disease, but these conditions tend to present in younger patients.[28]

***If the patient in this case were age 46 instead of age 76, what would be the most likely cause of aortic stenosis?***

Congenital bicuspid aortic valve is the most common cause of aortic stenosis in younger patients. This is a condition in which the valve is composed of 2 leaflets instead of 3. It affects 1% to 2% of the general population in the industrialized world. Because of abnormal hemodynamics across the bicuspid valve, these patients develop degenerative changes at an earlier age.[27]

***What are the typical clinical manifestations of aortic stenosis?***

The 3 classic manifestations of aortic stenosis are angina, presyncope/syncope, and dyspnea related to heart failure; symptoms typically develop in that order as the disease progresses. When untreated, mean survival is 5 years in patients with severe aortic stenosis associated with angina, 3 years in patients with syncope, and 2 years in patients with heart failure.[10,27]

***What is the mechanism of chest pain in patients with aortic stenosis?***

Severe aortic stenosis results in compensatory ventricular hypertrophy as a means to maintain cardiac output. This leads to decreased compliance and diastolic dysfunction. Eventually, the hypertrophied myocardium is unable to keep up with increasing oxygen demands, resulting in myocardial ischemia.[27]

***How should patients with asymptomatic aortic stenosis be monitored?***

Patients with asymptomatic aortic stenosis and preserved cardiac function should be monitored with serial echocardiography (every 5 years for mild disease, every 3 years for moderate disease, and annually for severe disease).[27]

***What is the treatment for symptomatic severe aortic stenosis?***

The definitive treatment for symptomatic severe aortic stenosis is aortic valve replacement. Options include conventional aortic valve replacement (with either a mechanical or bioprosthetic valve) or transcatheter aortic valve replacement.[27]

## KEY POINTS

- Sources of chest pain can be cardiac or noncardiac.
- The majority of cases of chest pain are noncardiac in nature.
- Cardiac chest pain can be related to ACS or unrelated to ACS.
- The symptoms of ACS include chest, upper extremity, mandibular, or epigastric discomfort that occurs with exertion or at rest, and typically lasts >20 minutes; associated symptoms may include diaphoresis, nausea, or syncope.
- ACS includes the following distinct clinical entities: STEMI, UA, and NSTEMI.
- The electrocardiographic features of STEMI include hyperacute T waves and ST-segment elevation in at least 2 contiguous leads.
- The electrocardiographic features of UA/NSTEMI include ST-segment depression and T-wave inversion in at least 2 contiguous leads.
- STEMI and NSTEMI are associated with elevated serum biomarkers.
- Acute plaque rupture is the prototypical and most common mechanism of ACS.
- The causes of noncardiac chest pain can be separated into the following system-based subcategories: pulmonary, gastrointestinal, musculoskeletal, and other.

## REFERENCES

1. Fleet RP, Beitman BD. Unexplained chest pain: when is it panic disorder? *Clin Cardiol.* 1997;20(3):187-194.
2. Smith JN, Negrelli JM, Manek MB, Hawes EM, Viera AJ. Diagnosis and management of acute coronary syndrome: an evidence-based update. *J Am Board Fam Med.* 2015;28(2):283-293.
3. Thygesen K, Alpert JS, Jaffe AS, et al. Third universal definition of myocardial infarction. *Circulation.* 2012;126(16):2020-2035.
4. Alpert JS, Thygesen K, Antman E, Bassand JP. Myocardial infarction redefined—a consensus document of The Joint European Society of Cardiology/American College of Cardiology Committee for the redefinition of myocardial infarction. *J Am Coll Cardiol.* 2000;36(3):959-969.
5. National Cholesterol Education Program Expert Panel on Detection, Evaluation, and Treatment of High Blood Cholesterol in Adults. Third report of the National Cholesterol Education Program (NCEP) Expert Panel on Detection, Evaluation, and Treatment of High Blood Cholesterol in Adults (Adult Treatment Panel III) final report. *Circulation.* 2002;106(25):3143-3421.
6. Kirtane AJ, Stone GW. How to minimize stent thrombosis. *Circulation.* 2011;124(11):1283-1287.
7. Shibata T, Kawakami S, Noguchi T, et al. Prevalence, clinical features, and prognosis of acute myocardial infarction attributable to coronary artery embolism. *Circulation.* 2015;132(4):241-250.
8. Walling A, Waters DD, Miller DD, Roy D, Pelletier GB, Theroux P. Long-term prognosis of patients with variant angina. *Circulation.* 1987;76(5):990-997.
9. DeMaio SJ Jr, Kinsella SH, Silverman ME. Clinical course and long-term prognosis of spontaneous coronary artery dissection. *Am J Cardiol.* 1989;64(8):471-474.
10. Ross J Jr, Braunwald E. Aortic stenosis. *Circulation.* 1968;38(1 suppl):61-67.
11. Spodick DH. *The Pericardium: A Comprehensive Textbook.* New York, NY: Marcel Dekker, Inc.; 1997.
12. Criado FJ. Aortic dissection: a 250-year perspective. *Tex Heart Inst J.* 2011;38(6):694-700.
13. Nienaber CA, Clough RE. Management of acute aortic dissection. *Lancet.* 2015;385(9970):800-811.
14. Lanza GA, Careri G, Crea F. Mechanisms of coronary artery spasm. *Circulation.* 2011;124(16):1774-1782.
15. Hufnagel G, Pankuweit S, Richter A, Schonian U, Maisch B. The European Study of Epidemiology and Treatment of Cardiac Inflammatory Diseases (ESETCID). First epidemiological results. *Herz.* 2000;25(3):279-285.
16. Gaffney FA, Karlsson ES, Campbell W, et al. Autonomic dysfunction in women with mitral valve prolapse syndrome. *Circulation.* 1979;59(5):894-901.
17. Kass SM, Williams PM, Reamy BV. Pleurisy. *Am Fam Physician.* 2007;75(9):1357-1364.
18. Sapira JD. *The Art & Science of Bedside Diagnosis.* Baltimore, MD: Urban & Schwarzenberg Inc.; 1990.
19. Sreeram N, Cheriex EC, Smeets JL, Gorgels AP, Wellens HJ. Value of the 12-lead electrocardiogram at hospital admission in the diagnosis of pulmonary embolism. *Am J Cardiol.* 1994;73(4):298-303.
20. Kahrilas PJ. Clinical practice. Gastroesophageal reflux disease. *N Engl J Med.* 2008;359(16):1700-1707.
21. Sanders G, Kingsnorth AN. Gallstones. *BMJ.* 2007;335(7614):295-299.
22. Tutuian R, Castell DO. Review article: oesophageal spasm—diagnosis and management. *Aliment Pharmacol Ther.* 2006;23(10):1393-1402.
23. Forsmark CE, Vege SS, Wilcox CM. Acute pancreatitis. *N Engl J Med.* 2016;375(20):1972-1981.
24. Soreide JA, Viste A. Esophageal perforation: diagnostic work-up and clinical decision-making in the first 24 hours. *Scand J Trauma Resusc Emerg Med.* 2011;19:66.

25. Sussman WI, Makovitch SA, Merchant SH, Phadke J. Cervical angina: an overlooked source of noncardiac chest pain. *Neurohospitalist*. 2015;5(1):22-27.
26. Bagheri R, Haghi SZ, Kalantari MR, et al. Primary malignant chest wall tumors: analysis of 40 patients. *J Cardiothorac Surg*. 2014;9:106.
27. Zakkar M, Bryan AJ, Angelini GD. Aortic stenosis: diagnosis and management. *BMJ*. 2016;355:i5425.
28. Marriott HJL. *Bedside Cardiac Diagnosis*. Philadelphia, PA: Lippincott Company; 1993.
29. Casiglia E, Schiavon L, Tikhonoff V, et al. Electrocardiographic criteria of left ventricular hypertrophy in general population. *Eur J Epidemiol*. 2008;23(4):261-271.

Chapter 3

# HEART BLOCK

## Case: An 82-year-old man with an abnormal jugular venous waveform

An 82-year-old man with a history of coronary artery disease, hypertension, and hyperlipidemia is admitted to the hospital with episodes of light-headedness over the past few days. Symptoms occur at rest and with activity and are associated with palpitations.

Heart rate is 48 beats per minute, and blood pressure is 140/40 mm Hg. Jugular venous pressure is estimated to be 8 cm $H_2O$. Qualitative analysis of the jugular venous waveform reveals a large outward pulsation that occurs intermittently.

Laboratory studies are unremarkable. The rhythm strip of the electrocardiogram (ECG) is shown in Figure 3-1.

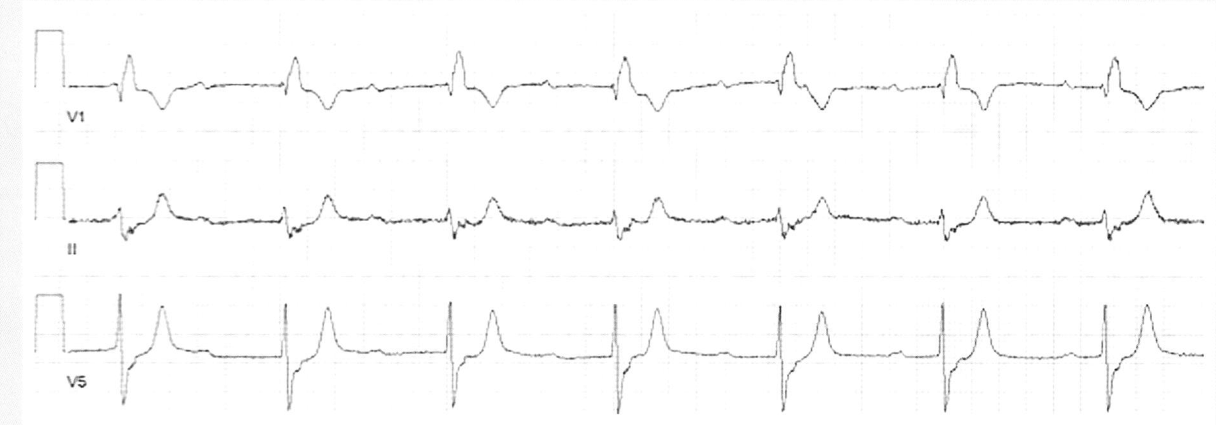


**Figure 3-1.**

***What is the most likely cause of light-headedness in this patient?***

**What is heart block?**

Heart block refers to disruption of electrical conduction that normally occurs sequentially from the atria to the ventricles.

**What is the path of electrical conduction in the normal heart?**

In the normal heart, an impulse spontaneously originates from the sinoatrial (SA) node, which is located in the subepicardial surface at the junction of the right atrium and superior vena cava. The impulse propagates through the myocytes of the right and left atria simultaneously before reaching the atrioventricular (AV) node, which is located in the inferior portion of the right atrium. From there, the impulse is conducted to the bundle of His within the membranous septum, which then separates into the right and left bundle branches supplying the right and left ventricles, respectively (see Figure 1-2).

**How is heart rate regulated?**

The sympathetic and parasympathetic nervous systems innervate the conduction system of the heart. Parasympathetic tone decreases SA node automaticity and AV node conduction, whereas sympathetic input increases SA node automaticity and AV node conduction.[1]

**What is the relationship between cardiac output and heart rate?**

Cardiac output (CO) is equal to the forward stroke volume (SV) of the left ventricle per beat multiplied by heart rate (HR).[1]

$$CO = SV \times HR$$

**What are the symptoms of heart block?**

Many patients with heart block are asymptomatic. Symptoms depend on the type of heart block; however in general, may include fatigue, dyspnea, weakness, light-headedness, and syncope.[2]

**What are the physical findings of heart block?**

Physical findings of heart block may include hypotension, cool extremities, and qualitative changes in the jugular venous waveform (eg, cannon A waves if there is AV dissociation).

**What are the 3 general types of heart block?**

The 3 general types of heart block are first-degree AV block, second-degree AV block, and third-degree AV block (ie, complete heart block).

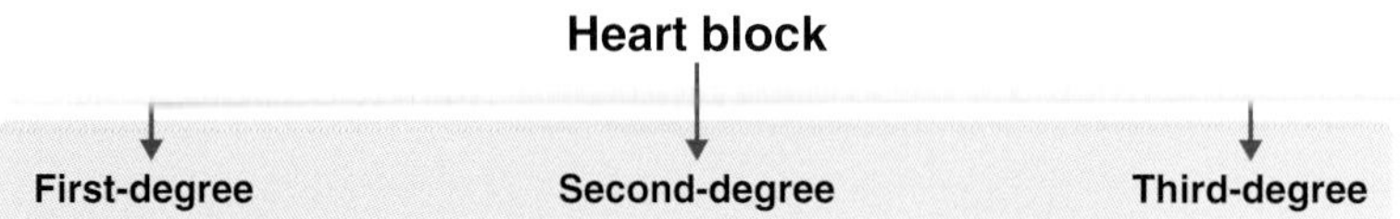


## FIRST-DEGREE ATRIOVENTRICULAR BLOCK

**What electrocardiographic finding is diagnostic of first-degree AV block?**

First-degree AV block is defined by a PR interval >200 ms on ECG (Figure 3-2).[3]

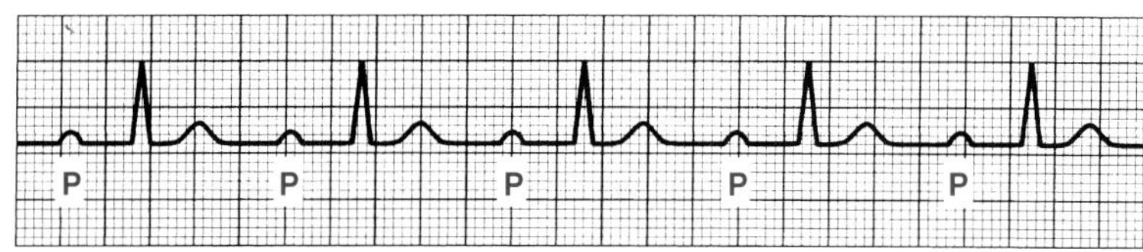


**Figure 3-2.** First-degree AV block. The PR interval is >200 ms in duration. (From Lilly LS. *Pathophysiology of Heart Disease: A Collaborative Project of Medical Students and Faculty*. 6th ed. Philadelphia, PA: Wolters Kluwer Health; 2016.)

**What does the PR interval measure?**

The PR interval measures the time between the onset of atrial depolarization and the onset of ventricular depolarization (see Figure 1-2).

**What structure regulates conduction between the atria and the ventricles?**

The AV node regulates conduction between the atria and the ventricles (see Figure 1-2).

**Which main coronary artery supplies the AV node in most patients?**

The AV nodal artery originates from the right coronary artery in 80% of patients and the circumflex in 10%; it arises from both in 10% of patients.[1]

**Is first-degree AV block associated with nonconducted (or dropped) beats?**

First-degree AV block is not associated with nonconducted beats. The term is somewhat of a misnomer because there is only delayed AV conduction without actual block.[4]

**How common is first-degree AV block?**

In the industrialized world, the prevalence of first-degree AV block in the general population is approximately 1% in individuals <60 years of age, and 6% in individuals >60 years of age. Nonmodifiable risk factors include male sex, increasing age, and genetic factors.[5,6]

**What are the symptoms of first-degree AV block?**

First-degree AV block is generally asymptomatic. However, more severe cases (ie, PR interval >300 ms) can be associated with symptoms of dyspnea and light-headedness that usually worsen with exercise as a result of the loss of AV synchrony.[2,4]

**What are the acquired causes of first-degree AV block?**

Acquired causes of first-degree AV block include idiopathic progressive degeneration of the cardiac conduction system (ie, Lenègre's disease and Lev's disease), medications (eg, β-blockers), procedures (eg, postcatheter ablation), enhanced vagal tone (eg, athletes), electrolyte disturbances (eg, hypokalemia), myocardial ischemia (most commonly inferior territory), endocarditis, myocarditis, infections (eg, Lyme disease), certain muscular dystrophies (eg, myotonic muscular dystrophy), and infiltrative diseases (eg, amyloidosis). Any reversible secondary causes that are identified should be addressed.[2,3,6]

**What is the prognosis of first-degree AV block?**

Generally, first-degree AV block is a benign condition with an excellent prognosis. However, there is some evidence that these patients are at slightly increased risk of developing more serious conduction abnormalities (eg, atrial fibrillation) and all-cause mortality.[4,7]

**What is the treatment for first-degree AV block that is unrelated to a reversible cause?**

Most patients with first-degree AV block are asymptomatic and prognosis is excellent without treatment. However, in patients with symptoms related to severe PR prolongation (>300 ms), implantation of a pacemaker may be considered (although there is no evidence that pacemakers improve survival in this setting).[2,4]

## SECOND-DEGREE ATRIOVENTRICULAR BLOCK

**What are the 2 general types of second-degree AV block?**

The 2 general types of second-degree AV block are Mobitz type I (Wenckebach) and Mobitz type II.

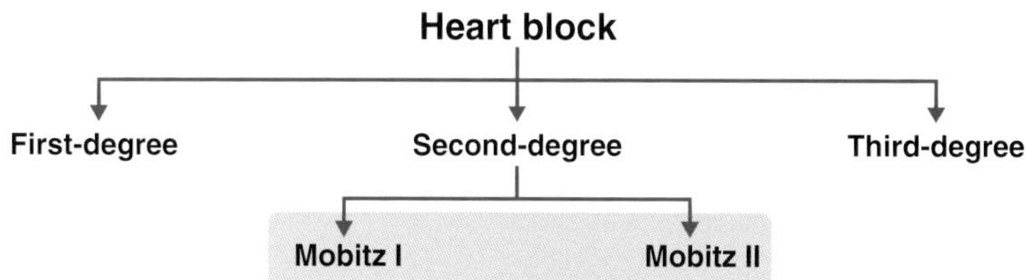


## MOBITZ I SECOND-DEGREE ATRIOVENTRICULAR BLOCK

**What electrocardiographic findings are diagnostic of Mobitz I second-degree AV block?**

Second-degree AV block is characterized by the presence of both conducted beats (ie, P wave followed by an associated QRS complex) and nonconducted (or dropped) beats (ie, P wave not followed by an associated QRS complex). Mobitz I is defined by the presence of nonconducted beats that are preceded by conducted beats associated with progressively longer PR intervals on ECG. This is most easily appreciated by measuring the PR intervals before and after the nonconducted beat. The PR interval immediately after the nonconducted P wave returns to its baseline value and is shorter than the PR interval before the nonconducted beat (Figure 3-3). *Mobitz I was originally described by Wenckebach using tracings of the jugular venous waveform. He observed A-C prolongation leading up to dropped beats.*[3]

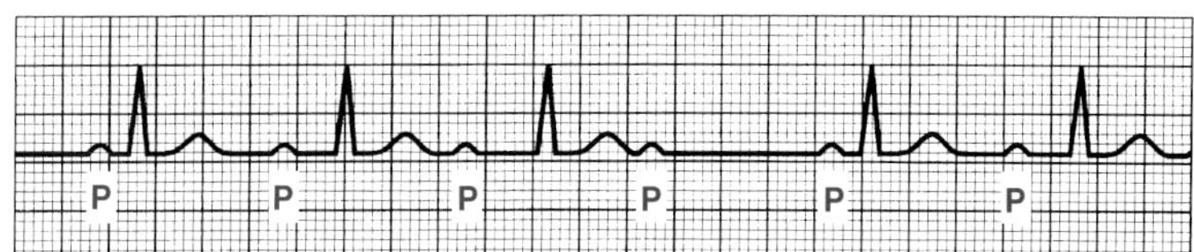


**Figure 3-3.** Mobitz I second-degree AV block. The P-wave rate is constant, but the PR interval progressively lengthens until a QRS is completely blocked (after the fourth P wave). (From Lilly LS. *Pathophysiology of Heart Disease: A Collaborative Project of Medical Students and Faculty*. 6th ed. Philadelphia, PA: Wolters Kluwer Health; 2016.)

**What is the typical location of block within the conduction system in Mobitz I second-degree AV block?**

The typical location of block in Mobitz I is the AV node.[8]

**Mobitz I second-degree AV block is most commonly associated with myocardial infarction involving which vascular territory?**

Mobitz I is most commonly associated with myocardial infarction involving the distribution of the right coronary artery, which supplies the AV node in most patients. Look for corresponding ST-segment elevation in the inferior leads (II, III, aVF) accompanying the rhythm disturbance.[9]

**What are the symptoms of Mobitz I second-degree AV block?**

Mobitz I is generally asymptomatic. Symptoms such as dyspnea, palpitations, and light-headedness are rare.[3,8]

**What are the acquired causes of Mobitz I second-degree AV block?**

The acquired causes of Mobitz I are similar to those of first-degree AV block. Any reversible secondary causes that are identified should be addressed.[2,3,6]

**What is the prognosis of Mobitz I second-degree AV block?**

Mobitz I is generally associated with a good prognosis; progression to higher degrees of AV block is uncommon. However, factors such an infranodal location of block may be associated with higher risk.[2,3]

**What is the treatment for Mobitz I second-degree AV block that is unrelated to a reversible cause?**

Treatment for Mobitz I is usually unnecessary in asymptomatic patients. In rare cases when patients are symptomatic and hemodynamically unstable, urgent pharmacologic treatment (eg, atropine) or temporary cardiac pacing should be pursued. Placement of a permanent pacemaker may be necessary in cases of symptomatic Mobitz I.[2,3]

## MOBITZ II SECOND-DEGREE ATRIOVENTRICULAR BLOCK

**What electrocardiographic findings are diagnostic of Mobitz II second-degree AV block?**

Mobitz II is characterized by the presence of conducted beats (with a constant PR interval) followed by sudden failure of P wave conduction (ie, a nonconducted beat) (Figure 3-4).[3]

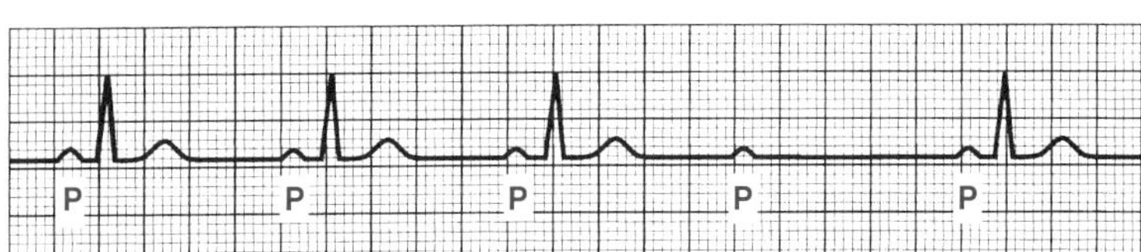


**Figure 3-4.** Mobitz II second-degree AV block. A QRS complex is blocked (after the fourth P wave) without gradual lengthening of the preceding PR intervals. Although the QRS width in this example is narrow, it is often widened in patients with Mobitz II. (From Lilly LS. *Pathophysiology of Heart Disease: A Collaborative Project of Medical Students and Faculty*. 6th ed. Philadelphia, PA: Wolters Kluwer Health; 2016.)

**What is the typical location of block within the conduction system in Mobitz II second-degree AV block?**

The typical location of block in Mobitz II is below the AV node, within the His-Purkinje system or bundle branches.[3,8]

**Mobitz II second-degree AV block is most commonly associated with myocardial infarction involving which vascular territory?**

Mobitz II is most commonly associated with myocardial infarction involving the distribution of the left anterior descending artery, which supplies the His-Purkinje system and bundle branches in most patients. Look for corresponding ST-segment elevation in the anterior leads ($V_1$-$V_4$) accompanying the rhythm disturbance.[9]

**What are the symptoms of Mobitz II second-degree AV block?**

Patients with Mobitz II are frequently symptomatic and may complain of dyspnea, palpitations, light-headedness, and syncope.[3,8]

**What are the acquired causes of Mobitz II second-degree AV block?**

The acquired causes of Mobitz II are similar to those of first-degree AV block and Mobitz I second-degree AV block. Any reversible secondary causes that are identified should be addressed.[2]

**What is the prognosis of Mobitz II second-degree AV block?**

Mobitz II is associated with a high rate of progression to third-degree AV block, and increased mortality.[2,3]

**What is the treatment for Mobitz II second-degree AV block that is unrelated to a reversible cause?**

Treatment for Mobitz II is virtually always necessary. In cases when patients are symptomatic and hemodynamically unstable, urgent pharmacologic treatment (eg, dopamine) or temporary cardiac pacing should be pursued. Given its unstable nature, placement of a permanent pacemaker is typically necessary in patients with Mobitz II.[2,3]

**What ratio of AV conduction makes the electrocardiographic distinction between Mobitz I and Mobitz II second-degree AV blocks challenging?**

It is difficult to distinguish between Mobitz I and Mobitz II electrocardiographically in the presence of second-degree 2:1 AV block.

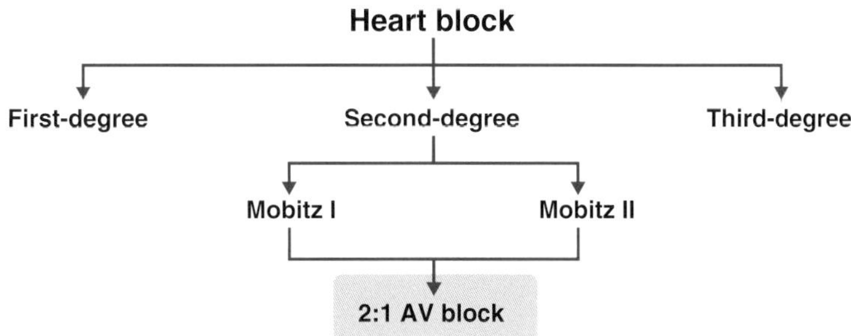


## SECOND-DEGREE 2:1 ATRIOVENTRICULAR BLOCK

**What are the electrocardiographic findings of second-degree 2:1 AV block?**

Second-degree 2:1 AV block is defined by a pattern of alternating conducted and nonconducted beats (Figure 3-5). This pattern makes it impossible to define the underlying rhythm as Mobitz I or Mobitz II electrocardiographically because an assessment of sequential PR intervals cannot be made. However, it is important to determine the level of block (ie, nodal or infranodal) because of prognostic and therapeutic implications. Infranodal block carries a poorer prognosis, and placement of a permanent pacemaker is indicated.[1,2]

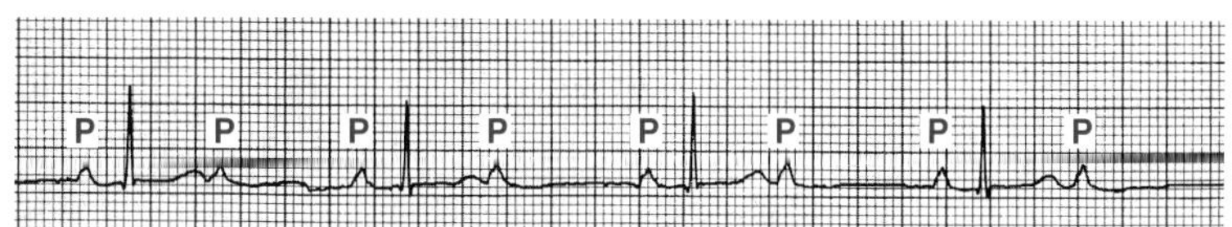


**Figure 3-5.** Second-degree AV block with 2:1 AV conduction. There are twice as many P waves (P) as QRS complexes, indicating that every other atrial impulse is blocked. (From Katz AM. *Physiology of the Heart*. 5th ed. Philadelphia, PA: Lippincott Williams & Wilkins; 2011.)

**When there is 2:1 AV block, what electrocardiographic features can help determine the level of AV block?**

In the setting of 2:1 AV block, several electrocardiographic features can help distinguish the level of block: (1) When 2:1 AV block is associated with a narrow QRS complex, it is likely that the level of block is in the AV node, whereas a wide QRS suggests that the level of block is infranodal. (2) Fixed 2:1 AV block with a PR interval longer than 280 ms suggests block at the level of the AV node, whereas a PR interval shorter than 160 ms suggests infranodal block. (3) Presence of Mobitz I AV block before or after episodes of 2:1 AV block is highly suggestive of block at the level of the AV node.[2,3,10]

**When there is 2:1 AV block, what maneuvers can be performed to help determine the level of AV block?**

In the setting of 2:1 AV block, maneuvers that increase heart rate and AV conduction (eg, exercise) typically improve conduction when the level of block is nodal (eg, the ratio of AV conduction may improve from 2:1 to 1:1), but worsen conduction when the level of block is infranodal (eg, the ratio of AV conduction may worsen from 2:1 to 3:1). Maneuvers that decrease heart rate and AV conduction (eg, carotid massage) typically worsen conduction when the level of block is nodal, but improve conduction when the level of block is infranodal.[2,3]

## THIRD-DEGREE ATRIOVENTRICULAR BLOCK

**What electrocardiographic findings are diagnostic of third-degree AV block?**

Third-degree AV block is defined by a total lack of AV conduction. This is characterized electrocardiographically by the presence of regular P-P and R-R intervals but with complete dissociation of P waves and QRS complexes (usually atrial rate > ventricular rate) (Figure 3-6).

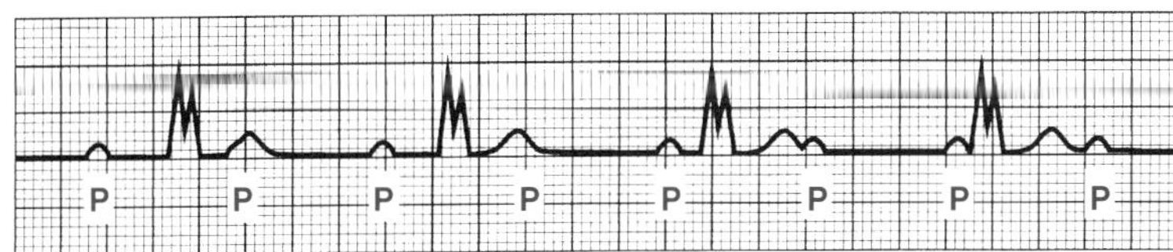


**Figure 3-6.** Third-degree AV block. The P wave and QRS rhythms are independent of one another. The QRS complexes are widened because they originate within the distal ventricular conduction system, not at the bundle of His. The second and fourth P waves are superimposed on normal T waves. (From Lilly LS. *Pathophysiology of Heart Disease: A Collaborative Project of Medical Students and Faculty*. 6th ed. Philadelphia, PA: Wolters Kluwer Health; 2016.)

**Is the QRS complex narrow or wide in the setting of third-degree AV block?**

Third-degree AV block can produce either a narrow or wide QRS complex, depending on the location of the escape rhythm. If the escape rhythm originates above the level of the bundle of His, the QRS complex will usually be narrow (with a rate between 40-60 beats per minute); if it is generated below the level of the bundle of His, the QRS complex will be wide (with a rate between 20-40 beats per minute).[2,3]

**What are the symptoms of third-degree AV block?**

Patients with third-degree AV block are usually symptomatic, and may complain of dyspnea, palpitations, light-headedness, and syncope.[3,8]

**What are the acquired causes of third-degree AV block?**

The acquired causes of third-degree AV block are similar to those of first-degree and second-degree AV block. Any reversible secondary causes that are identified should be addressed.[2,3]

**What is the prognosis of third-degree AV block?**

The prognosis of third-degree AV block is generally poor, particularly when patients are symptomatic. In patients with syncope related to third-degree AV block, the 1-year mortality rate can be as high as 50%.[2,3]

**What is the treatment for third-degree AV block that is unrelated to a reversible cause?**

Treatment for third-degree AV block is virtually always necessary. In cases when patients are symptomatic and hemodynamically unstable, urgent pharmacologic treatment (eg, dopamine) or temporary cardiac pacing should be pursued. Given its unstable nature, placement of a permanent pacemaker is typically necessary in patients with third-degree AV block.[2,3]

### Case Summary

An 82-year-old man presents with episodes of light-headedness and is found to have bradycardia, wide pulse pressure, and large intermittent venous pulsations in the neck.

***What is the most likely cause of light-headedness in this patient?***

Third-degree AV block.

#### BONUS QUESTIONS

***What are the relevant electrocardiographic findings in this case?***

The ECG in this case (see Figure 3-1) demonstrates wide-complex bradycardia with regular P-P and R-R intervals. The P waves are dissociated from the QRS complexes, consistent with third-degree AV block.

| | |
|---|---|
| ***What is the significance of the blood pressure in this case?*** | Wide pulse pressure can be a manifestation of third-degree AV block. Other hemodynamic consequences of third-degree AV block include elevated right-sided cardiac pressures, increased systemic and pulmonary vascular resistance, and reduced cardiac output despite increased stroke volume.[11] |
| ***What abnormality of the jugular venous waveform is described in this case?*** | The large intermittent venous pulsations described in this case are most likely cannon A waves. |
| ***Why is third-degree AV block associated with cannon A waves?*** | The A wave of the jugular venous waveform occurs as a result of right atrial contraction. In the setting of third-degree AV block, when there is atrioventricular dyssynchrony, the right atrium intermittently contracts against a closed tricuspid valve, producing a spike in pressure within the right atrium, which is then transmitted to the jugular vein as a large positive wave. *For a video of cannon A waves, see the associated reference.*[12] |
| ***Is the escape rhythm in this case more likely arising from above or below the bundle of His?*** | The ECG in this case (see Figure 3-1) demonstrates a wide QRS complex, indicative of a focus below the bundle of His. Notably, the heart rate is slightly higher than expected for a ventricular escape rhythm. |
| ***What is the most likely cause of third-degree AV block in this case?*** | The most common cause of third-degree AV block is idiopathic progressive degeneration of the cardiac conduction system (ie, Lenègre's disease and Lev's disease), which is indeed the most likely cause in this case. A thorough investigation into other potentially reversible secondary causes should be pursued.[2,3] |
| ***What long-term treatment strategy should be offered to the patient in this case if no reversible cause of third-degree AV block is identified?*** | If no reversible cause of third-degree AV block is identified, the patient in this case would benefit from placement of a permanent pacemaker.[2,3] |

## KEY POINTS

- Heart block can be asymptomatic or associated with fatigue, weakness, dyspnea, light-headedness, or syncope.
- Physical findings of heart block include hypotension, cool extremities, and cannon A waves (in the setting of AV dissociation).
- The 3 general types of heart block are first-degree AV block, second-degree AV block, and third-degree AV block.
- Second-degree AV block can be subdivided into Mobitz I and Mobitz II.
- Electrocardiography is the simplest method to distinguish between the various types of AV block.
- First-degree heart block is defined by a PR interval >200 ms.
- Mobitz I second-degree AV block is defined electrocardiographically by nonconducted beats preceded by conducted beats with progressively longer PR intervals.
- Mobitz II second-degree AV block is defined electrocardiographically by the presence of conducted beats with a constant PR interval, followed by sudden failure of P wave conduction (ie, nonconducted beats).
- Second-degree 2:1 AV block is defined electrocardiographically by a pattern of alternating conducted and nonconducted beats. It is imperative to determine the level of block (ie, nodal or infranodal) because of therapeutic implications.
- Third-degree AV block is defined electrocardiographically by regular P-P and R-R intervals, but with complete dissociation of P waves and QRS complexes.
- There are a variety of reversible causes of each type of AV block.
- Hemodynamically unstable AV block requires acute treatment with medications (eg, atropine) and/or temporary pacing.
- AV block, particularly when it is of higher grade, often requires treatment with placement of a permanent pacemaker.



## REFERENCES

1. Mangrum JM, DiMarco JP. The evaluation and management of bradycardia. *N Engl J Med*. 2000;342(10):703-709.
2. Vogler J, Breithardt G, Eckardt L. Bradyarrhythmias and conduction blocks. *Rev Esp Cardiol*. 2012;65(7):656-667.

3. Merideth J, Pruitt RD. Cardiac arrhythmias. 5. Disturbances in cardiac conduction and their management. *Circulation*. 1973;47(5):1098-1107.
4. Holmqvist F, Daubert JP. First-degree AV block-an entirely benign finding or a potentially curable cause of cardiac disease? *Ann Noninvasive Electrocardiol*. 2013;18(3):215-224.
5. Kwok CS, Rashid M, Beynon R, et al. Prolonged PR interval, first-degree heart block and adverse cardiovascular outcomes: a systematic review and meta-analysis. *Heart*. 2016;102(9):672-680.
6. Nikolaidou T, Ghosh JM, Clark AL. Outcomes related to first-degree atrioventricular block and therapeutic implications in patients with heart failure. *JACC Clin Electrophysiol*. 2016;2(2):181-192.
7. Cheng S, Keyes MJ, Larson MG, et al. Long-term outcomes in individuals with prolonged PR interval or first-degree atrioventricular block. *JAMA*. 2009;301(24):2571-2577.
8. Dhingra RC, Denes P, Wu D, Chuquimia R, Rosen KM. The significance of second degree atrioventricular block and bundle branch block. Observations regarding site and type of block. *Circulation*. 1974;49(4):638-646.
9. Langendorf R, Pick A. Atrioventricular block, type II (Mobitz)–its nature and clinical significance. *Circulation*. 1968;38(5):819-821.
10. Josephson ME. *Clinical Cardiac Electrophysiology: Techniques and Interpretations*. 4th ed. Philadelphia, PA: Lippincott Williams & Wilkins; 2008.
11. Stack MF, Rader B, Sobol BJ, Farber SJ, Eichna LW. Cardiovascular hemodynamic functions in complete heart block and the effect of isopropylnorepinephrine. *Circulation*. 1958;17(4, Part 1):526-536.
12. Tung MK, Healy S. Images in clinical medicine. Cannon A waves. *N Engl J Med*. 2016;374(4):e4.

Chapter 4

# HEART FAILURE

## Case: A 66-year-old woman with orthostatic hypotension

A 66-year-old woman with a history of hypertension, carpal tunnel syndrome, and heart failure of unknown etiology is referred to cardiology for evaluation. Her symptoms first began 6 months ago with progressive dyspnea on exertion, orthopnea, and paroxysmal nocturnal dyspnea. At that time, echocardiography revealed biventricular concentric hypertrophy with normal systolic function. She was diagnosed with congestive heart failure thought to be related to hypertension, and has since been treated symptomatically with diuretics. Blood pressure has been well controlled with antihypertensive medications. Progressive symptoms and recent episodes of syncope prompted referral to cardiology for evaluation.

In the recumbent position, heart rate is 90 beats per minute and blood pressure is 118/84 mm Hg. On standing, heart rate is 89 beats per minute and blood pressure is 92/60 mm Hg. Jugular venous pressure (JVP) is 16 cm $H_2O$. An extra heart sound is heard just before S1 with the bell of the stethoscope over the apex.

Electrocardiogram (ECG) is shown in Figure 4-1.

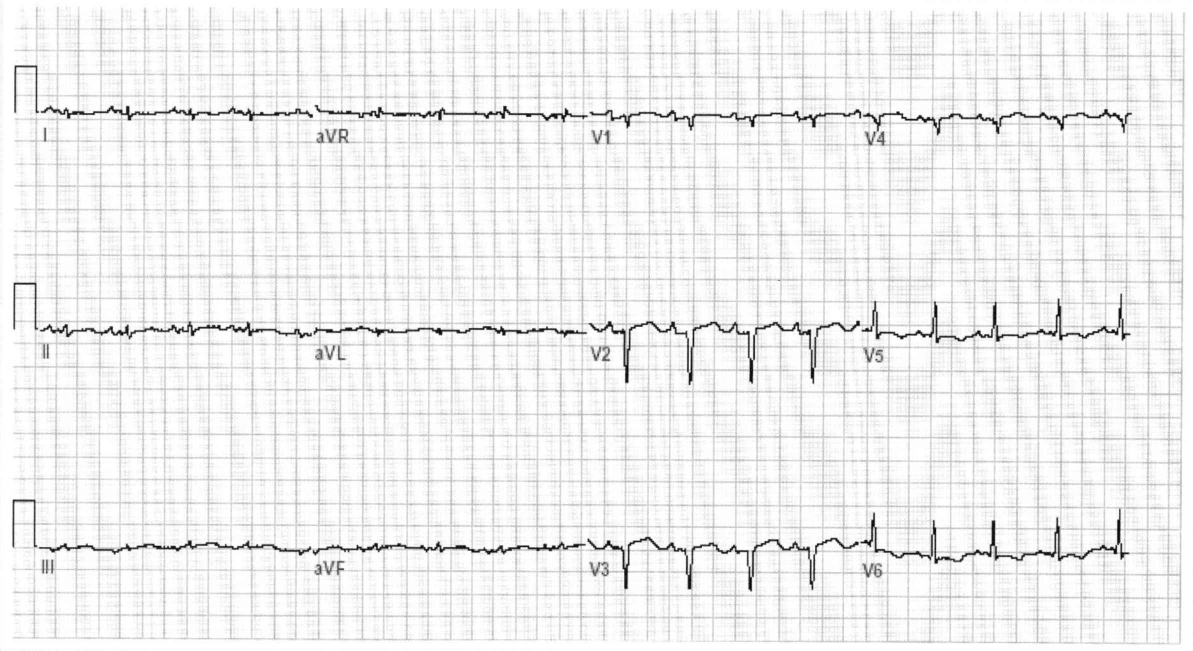


**Figure 4-1.** (From Moscucci M. *Grossman & Baim's Cardiac Catheterization, Angiography, and Intervention*. 8th ed. Philadelphia, PA: Lippincott Williams & Wilkins; 2014.)

Repeat echocardiography shows progressive biventricular concentric hypertrophy with preserved systolic function. Cardiac magnetic resonance imaging (MRI) demonstrates restriction of diastolic filling, normal systolic function, and diffuse biventricular wall thickening with heterogeneous enhancement on delayed contrast exposure. Endomyocardial biopsy with Congo red staining demonstrates extracellular amorphous hyaline deposits that turn an apple-green color under polarized light.

***What is the most likely cause of heart failure in this patient?***

**What is heart failure?**

Heart failure is a clinical syndrome that develops as a result of structural or functional impairment of ventricular filling or the ejection of blood.[1]

**What modifiable risk factors are associated with heart failure?**

Heart failure occurs more frequently in patients with hypertension, diabetes mellitus, metabolic syndrome, and atherosclerotic disease.[1]

**How common is heart failure?**

In the industrialized world, heart failure is estimated to affect 2% of individuals 65 to 69 years of age, and 8% of individuals ≥80 years of age. Black patients are disproportionately affected.[1]

**What are the symptoms of heart failure?**

Symptoms of heart failure may include dyspnea, cough, orthopnea, paroxysmal nocturnal dyspnea, fatigue or lethargy, weight gain, light-headedness, nausea, early satiety, and abdominal discomfort.[1]

**What are the physical findings of right-sided heart failure?**

Physical findings of right-sided heart failure may include tachycardia, hypotension, elevated JVP, right ventricular heave, right-sided gallop (heard best at the left lower sternal border), ascites, and lower extremity edema.[1]

**What are the physical findings of left-sided heart failure?**

Physical findings of left-sided heart failure may include tachycardia, hypotension, narrow pulse pressure, end-inspiratory crepitant rales on auscultation of the lungs, diffuse expiratory wheeze (ie, cardiac asthma), left-sided gallop (heard best at the apex), laterally displaced apical impulse, pulsus alternans (in end-stage disease), and cool extremities (in cardiogenic shock).[1]

**Are inspiratory rales always present in patients with left-sided heart failure?**

In patients with chronic left-sided heart failure, the lungs may be clear as a result of adaptive dilation of the pulmonary lymphatic vessels, which prevents the development of pulmonary edema despite the presence of an elevated wedge pressure and pulmonary congestion.[1]

**What is the prognosis of heart failure?**

The prognosis of heart failure depends on patient-specific factors and the underlying cause of heart failure but, overall, half of patients die within 5 years of diagnosis.[1]

**What are the 2 general categories of heart failure based on left ventricular function?**

Heart failure can be associated with reduced left ventricular systolic function (ie, systolic dysfunction) or preserved left ventricular systolic function (ie, diastolic dysfunction).

*Other common categorizations of heart failure include right-sided or left-sided heart failure, dilated or restrictive cardiomyopathy, and ischemic or nonischemic cardiomyopathy.*

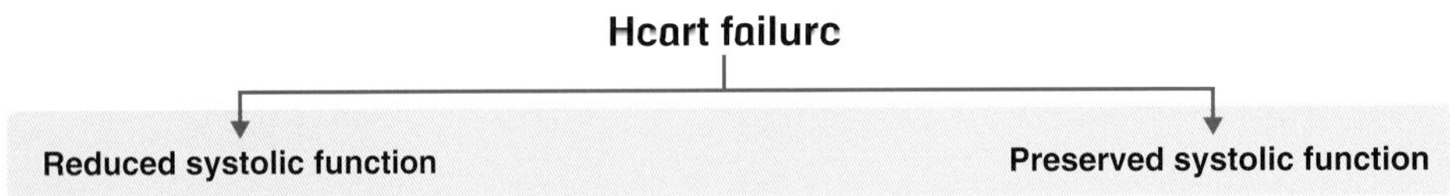


**What is the definition of heart failure with preserved systolic function?**

Heart failure with preserved systolic function is defined as the presence of the clinical syndrome of heart failure with normal or near-normal left ventricular ejection fraction (>50%).[2]

**Is heart failure more often associated with reduced systolic function or preserved systolic function?**

Patients with heart failure are equally divided between those with reduced systolic function and those with preserved systolic function.[2]

*It is important to note that there is considerable overlap between these categories of heart failure. In patients with reduced systolic function, there is often concomitant diastolic dysfunction. Furthermore, many diseases that are classified under heart failure with preserved systolic function can and often do eventually lead to heart failure with reduced systolic function.*

## HEART FAILURE WITH REDUCED LEFT VENTRICULAR SYSTOLIC FUNCTION

**What type of myocardial hypertrophy is typically associated with heart failure with reduced systolic function?**

Heart failure with reduced systolic function is associated with eccentric hypertrophy. The chambers of the heart dilate and the myocardial walls thin (Figure 4-2).

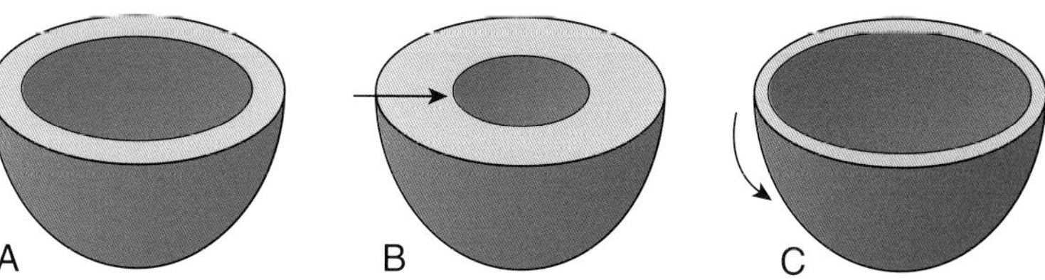


**Figure 4-2.** Different types of myocardial hypertrophy. A, Normal symmetric hypertrophy with proportionate increases in myocardial wall thickness and length. B, Concentric hypertrophy with a disproportionate increase in wall thickness, resulting in a decrease in chamber size (arrow). C, Eccentric hypertrophy with ventricular dilation and a decrease in wall thickness (curved arrow), resulting in an increase in chamber size. (From Porth CM. *Essentials of Pathophysiology Concepts of Altered Health States*. 2nd ed. Philadelphia: Lippincott Williams & Wilkins; 2007.)

**What is the manifestation of eccentric hypertrophy on chest radiography?**

Eccentric hypertrophy manifests as an enlarged cardiac silhouette on chest radiography. In adults, an enlarged cardiac silhouette is generally defined by a cardiothoracic ratio ≥0.5. The cardiothoracic ratio is measured by dividing the transverse diameter of the heart by the maximum internal diameter of the thoracic cavity. *Be careful not to diagnose "cardiomegaly" on the chest radiograph, as there are other conditions that can cause an enlarged cardiac silhouette (eg, pericardial effusion).*[3]

**Is heart failure with reduced systolic function typically associated with dilated or restrictive cardiomyopathy?**

Heart failure with reduced systolic function is typically associated with dilated cardiomyopathy. Eccentric hypertrophy results in thinned ventricular myocardium with reduced contractility (ie, the heart becomes "big and floppy").

**What extra heart sound is commonly associated with heart failure with reduced systolic function?**

An S3 gallop is a common finding in patients with heart failure with reduced systolic function and is highly specific in the appropriate clinical context. The S3 is a low-frequency early diastolic sound that is best appreciated over the apex of the heart with the bell of the stethoscope (Figure 4-3).[4,5]

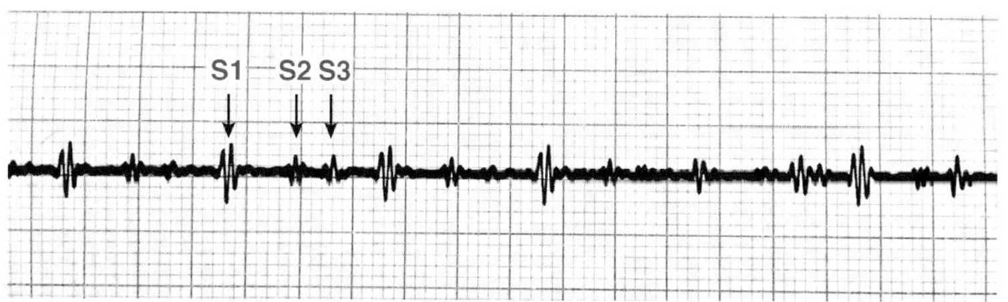


**Figure 4-3.** Phonocardiographic tracing of an S3 gallop recorded over the apex (heart rate 100 beats per minute).

**What pharmacologic agents improve symptoms in patients with heart failure with reduced systolic function, regardless of underlying etiology?**

Patients with heart failure with reduced systolic function from any cause experience improved symptoms with the use of diuretics (when indicated), β-blockers, angiotensin-converting enzyme (ACE) inhibitors or angiotensin II receptor blockers (ARBs) or angiotensin receptor-neprilysin inhibitors (ARNi), the combination of hydralazine and a nitrate, digoxin, and aldosterone antagonists. Decisions regarding choice of agents depend on patient-specific factors (eg, renal function) and disease-specific factors (eg, stage and class of heart failure).[1,6]

**What pharmacologic agents improve survival in patients with heart failure with reduced systolic function, regardless of underlying etiology?**

Survival is improved in patients with heart failure with reduced systolic function from any cause with the use of certain β-blockers (eg, metoprolol succinate), an ACE inhibitor or ARB or ARNi, the combination of hydralazine and a nitrate (particularly in black patients), and an aldosterone antagonist. Decisions regarding choice of agents depend on patient-specific factors (eg, renal function) and disease-specific factors (eg, stage and class of heart failure).[1,6]

**The causes of heart failure with reduced left ventricular systolic function can be separated into which general subcategories?**

The causes of heart failure with reduced left ventricular systolic function can be separated into the following subcategories: cardiovascular, toxic, infectious, and other.

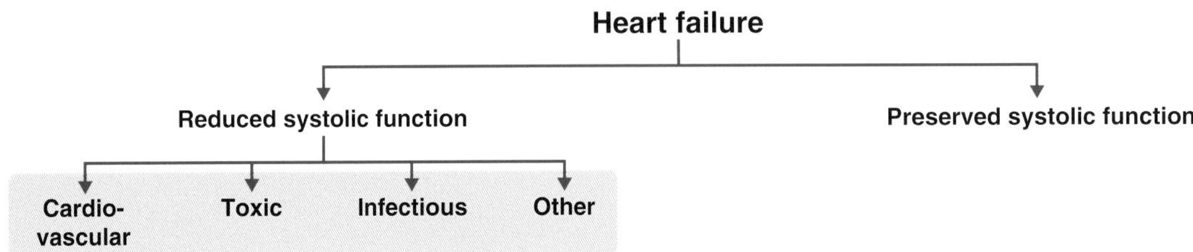


## CARDIOVASCULAR CAUSES OF HEART FAILURE WITH REDUCED SYSTOLIC FUNCTION

### What are the cardiovascular causes of heart failure with reduced systolic function?

**The presence of electrocardiographic Q waves are a clue to this underlying condition.**

Ischemic cardiomyopathy.

**The "go-fasts."**

Tachyarrhythmia-induced cardiomyopathy.

**A valvular condition associated with wide pulse pressure.**

Aortic regurgitation.

**Associated with a holosystolic murmur over the apex that radiates to the axilla and increases in intensity with handgrip.**

Mitral regurgitation.

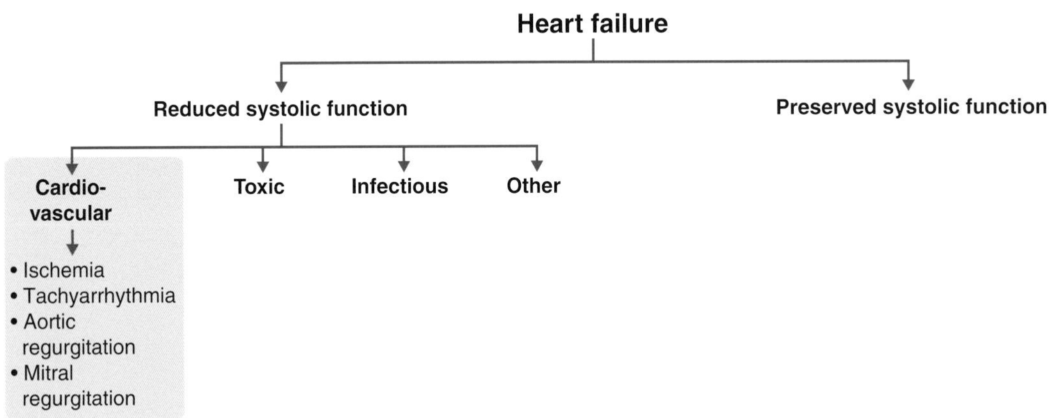


**How is ischemic cardiomyopathy defined?**

Ischemic cardiomyopathy is defined as left ventricular systolic dysfunction with at least one of the following: (1) a history of prior myocardial revascularization or myocardial infarction; (2) >75% stenosis of the left main or left anterior descending coronary arteries; or (3) 2 vessels or more with >75% stenosis.[7]

**What is tachyarrhythmia-induced cardiomyopathy?**

Tachyarrhythmia-induced cardiomyopathy describes the development of left ventricular dysfunction related to chronic tachyarrhythmia that improves or resolves after the tachyarrhythmia is controlled (usually within 4 weeks). Atrial fibrillation with rapid ventricular response is the most common cause of tachyarrhythmia-induced cardiomyopathy. Other causative tachyarrhythmias include atrial flutter, atrial tachycardia, reentrant supraventricular tachycardia, frequent premature ventricular contractions, and ventricular tachycardia.[8,9]

**What are the characteristics of the murmur of aortic regurgitation?**

The murmur of aortic regurgitation typically begins early in diastole, is decrescendo in shape, and is best heard over the third intercostal space along the left sternal border (Erb's point). Maneuvers that increase blood flow to the heart (eg, moving from standing to squatting) can intensify the murmur. There is often an associated systolic ejection murmur that occurs as the regurgitant bolus of blood generates turbulence on its way back through the aortic valve (technically a flow murmur). Aortic regurgitation may be associated with a low-pitched, "blubbering," mid-to-late diastolic murmur heard over the apex, known as the Austin Flint murmur. Severe aortic regurgitation is associated with numerous peripheral findings (eg, Corrigan's pulse [a bounding carotid pulse]). *Acute regurgitant lesions can be associated with preserved left ventricular systolic function.*[10]

**What is the most common cause of primary mitral regurgitation in the industrialized world?**

The most common cause of primary mitral regurgitation in the industrialized world is mitral valve prolapse secondary to myxomatous degeneration (ie, degenerative changes of the tissues of the mitral valve and chordae tendineae, usually idiopathic in nature).[11]

## TOXIC CAUSES OF HEART FAILURE WITH REDUCED SYSTOLIC FUNCTION

### What are the toxic causes of heart failure with reduced systolic function?

**A middle-aged man with a long history of "morning shakes" develops dyspnea with exertion, orthopnea, and elevated JVP.**

Alcohol.

**Often snorted.**

Cocaine.

**Known on the street as "speed."**

Amphetamines.

**These agents are used for the treatment of malignancies such as breast cancer, leukemia, and lymphoma.**

Anthracycline chemotherapeutic agents (eg, doxorubicin).

**An endocrinopathy.**

Thyrotoxicosis.

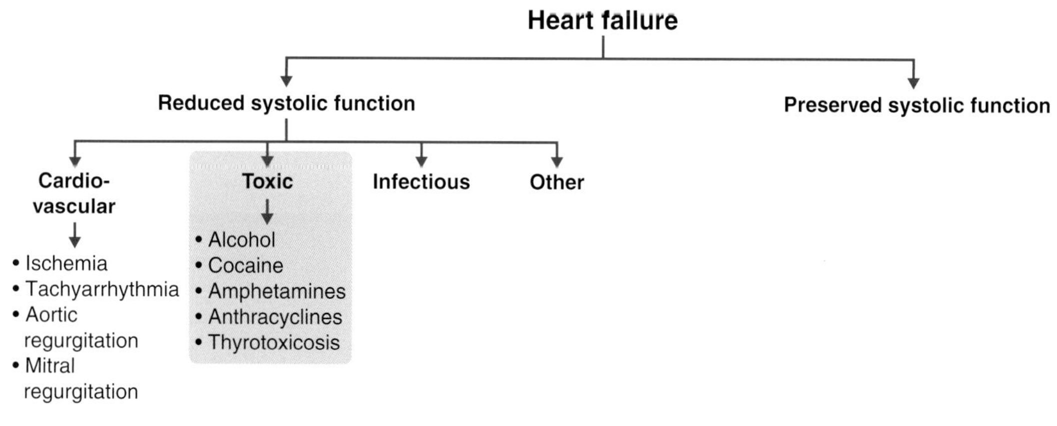

**What threshold of alcohol consumption is associated with the development of cardiomyopathy?**

Mild to moderate alcohol consumption is thought to be protective against the development of heart failure (the low point of a J-shaped curve). The risk of alcoholic cardiomyopathy is increased in those who consume >90 g of alcohol (7-8 drinks) per day for >5 years. It is most common in men 30 to 55 years of age who have consumed heavy amounts of alcohol for >10 years. Only 15% of patients with alcoholic cardiomyopathy are women. Biventricular failure is typical.[1]

**How does the acute management of myocardial infarction change when it is related to acute cocaine toxicity?**

In patients with myocardial ischemia or infarction related to cocaine use, β-blocker medications must be avoided, as unopposed α-receptor stimulation can worsen vasospasm. Cocaine can contribute to the development of heart failure in a number of ways, including infarction related to vasospasm, premature coronary artery disease, vasculitis, and dilated cardiomyopathy. Up to one-fifth of asymptomatic cocaine abusers may have left ventricular dysfunction.[1]

**Is methamphetamine-associated cardiomyopathy reversible?**

Methamphetamine-associated cardiomyopathy is reversible if it is recognized early and there is no delay in treatment. The mechanism of heart failure in these patients is thought to be multifactorial with contributions from vasospasm, direct myocyte toxicity, and catecholamine excess. Cor pulmonale related to pulmonary hypertension can also develop in methamphetamine users.[12]

**How common is anthracycline-associated cardiomyopathy?**

Overall, an estimated 10% of patients treated with anthracyclines will develop cardiomyopathy within 5 years of completing treatment, with most cases developing within 1 year. All patients undergoing treatment with anthracycline agents should be monitored for the development of cardiotoxicity. There is potential for reversibility if the diagnosis is made early, and treatment is promptly initiated.[13]

**What cardiovascular conditions are associated with thyrotoxicosis?**

Heart failure typically occurs in hyperthyroid patients with coexistent atrial fibrillation. Other cardiovascular manifestations of hyperthyroidism include pulmonary hypertension and valvular heart disease (usually functional mitral and tricuspid regurgitation). The cardiovascular conditions associated with hyperthyroidism generally reverse with adequate treatment.[14]

## INFECTIOUS CAUSES OF HEART FAILURE WITH REDUCED SYSTOLIC FUNCTION

### What are the infectious causes of heart failure with reduced systolic function?

**This condition is most often caused by viral infection and typically presents with chest pain, troponin elevation, and diffuse ST-segment elevation.**

Myocarditis.

**This infectious disease is endemic in South and Central America and is transmitted through the bite of a triatomine bug, also known as the "kissing bug."**

Chagas disease (caused by *Trypanosoma cruzi*).[15]

**This viral infection is highly prevalent in sub-Saharan Africa and is associated with an elevated serum protein gap.**

Human immunodeficiency virus (HIV).[16]

**Treatment for this systemic condition often involves intravenous fluids, broad-spectrum antibiotics, and vasopressor medications.**

Sepsis.

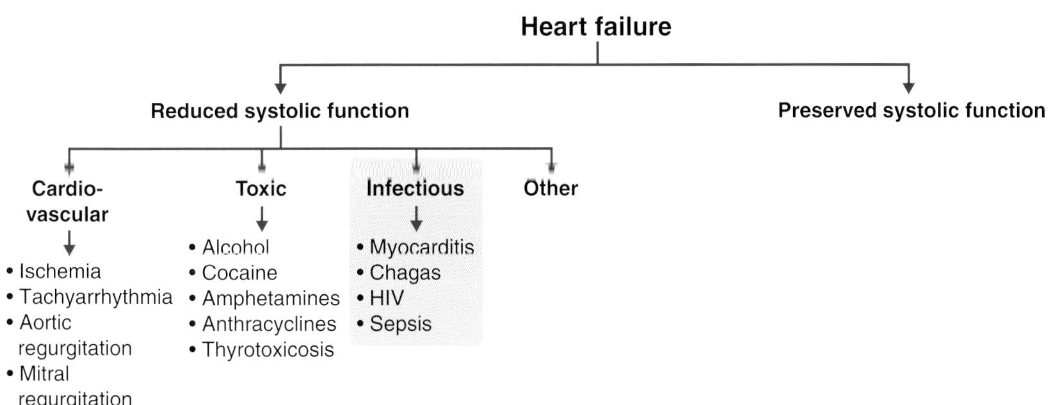


**What proportion of patients with acute myocarditis will go on to develop chronic heart failure?**

Approximately one-third of patients with acute myocarditis develop chronic dilated cardiomyopathy, which is associated with a poor prognosis. In addition to viruses, myocarditis can also be caused by other infectious organisms (eg, *Staphylococcus aureus*), systemic diseases (eg, systemic lupus erythematosus), and toxins (eg, amphetamines). The clinical presentation can vary considerably and endomyocardial biopsy is the diagnostic gold standard.[17]

**What proportion of patients with acute Chagas disease will progress to chronic Chagas disease with associated cardiomyopathy?**

Approximately one-third of patients with acute Chagas disease will progress to the chronic form with associated cardiomyopathy. It is the leading cause of nonischemic cardiomyopathy in Latin America.[15]

**How has antiretroviral therapy (ART) changed the characteristics of HIV-associated cardiomyopathy?**

In the pre-ART era, HIV-associated cardiomyopathy was characterized by severe systolic dysfunction and grim prognosis. In the developing world, where ART is not widely available, this type of presentation remains common. In populations where ART is widely used, HIV-associated cardiomyopathy has become less prevalent. When it does occur, it more commonly manifests with diastolic dysfunction. Notably, ART is associated with a higher incidence of coronary artery disease.[16]

**What is the prognosis of sepsis-associated cardiomyopathy?**

Sepsis-associated cardiomyopathy typically resolves within 7 to 10 days. Although sepsis can be a cause of Takotsubo cardiomyopathy, sepsis-associated cardiomyopathy is a distinct entity. Initial management is the same as in sepsis without cardiomyopathy, with careful attention to volume status.[18]

## OTHER CAUSES OF HEART FAILURE WITH REDUCED SYSTOLIC FUNCTION

### What are the other causes of heart failure with reduced systolic function?

**Always take a family history in a patient presenting with heart failure.**

Familial dilated cardiomyopathy.

**This cause of cardiomyopathy only occurs in women.**

Peripartum cardiomyopathy.

**"Wet beriberi."**

Thiamine deficiency.

**"Broken-heart" syndrome.**

Takotsubo cardiomyopathy.

**A primary disorder of the muscle.**

Muscular dystrophy.

**A middle-aged man develops heart failure with reduced systolic function of unknown etiology, and endomyocardial biopsy reveals the presence of multinucleated giant cells.**

Giant cell myocarditis.

**An underlying cause cannot be identified despite a complete workup.**

Idiopathic dilated cardiomyopathy.

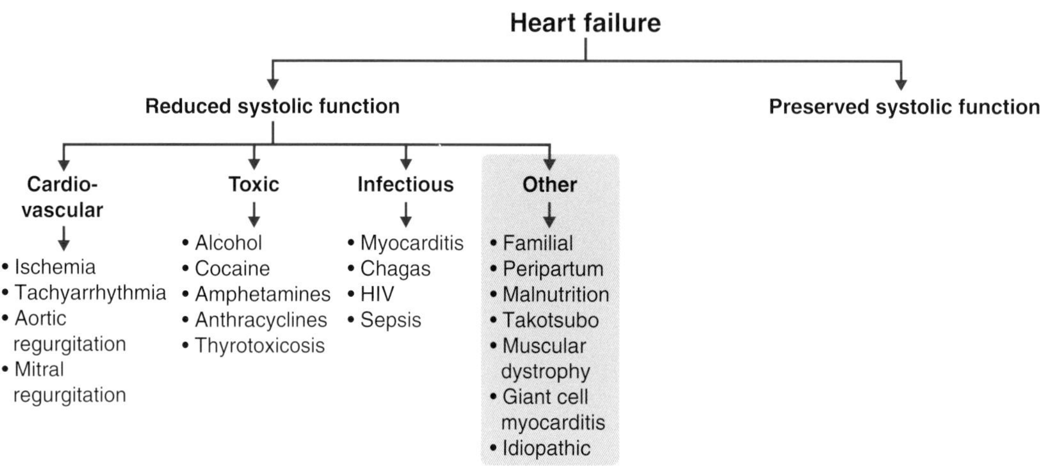


**What criteria are used to diagnose familial dilated cardiomyopathy?**

Familial dilated cardiomyopathy can be diagnosed in an individual with known idiopathic dilated cardiomyopathy and at least one of the following: (1) at least 1 relative also diagnosed with idiopathic dilated cardiomyopathy, or (2) at least 1 first-degree relative with an unexplained sudden death under 35 years of age.[19]

**When does peripartum cardiomyopathy usually present?**

The majority of patients with peripartum cardiomyopathy (approximately 80%) present within 3 months of delivery; 10% present during the last month of pregnancy, and 10% present 4 to 5 months postpartum.[20]

**What nutritional deficiencies are associated with heart failure with reduced systolic function?**

Deficiencies of thiamine, carnitine, selenium, zinc, or copper can result in heart failure with reduced systolic function.[21]

**What echocardiographic finding is characteristic of Takotsubo cardiomyopathy?**

Echocardiographic apical ballooning in association with basilar hyperkinesis is characteristic of Takotsubo cardiomyopathy.

**What types of muscular dystrophy are associated with heart failure with reduced systolic function?**

Heart failure with reduced systolic function can be associated with Duchenne muscular dystrophy, Becker muscular dystrophy, Emery-Dreifuss muscular dystrophy, limb-girdle muscular dystrophy, and myotonic dystrophy.[22]

**What is the treatment for and prognosis of giant cell myocarditis?**

Giant cell myocarditis is treated with combinations of immunosuppressive medications including glucocorticoids, azathioprine, and cyclosporine. Transplant-free survival is estimated to be 70% at 1 year, and 50% at 5 years from symptom onset. A significant proportion of survivors go on to experience sustained ventricular tachyarrhythmias.[23]

**How common is idiopathic dilated cardiomyopathy?**

Approximately one-half of all cases of dilated cardiomyopathy remain idiopathic.[24]

## HEART FAILURE WITH PRESERVED LEFT VENTRICULAR SYSTOLIC FUNCTION

**What type of myocardial hypertrophy is associated with heart failure with preserved systolic function?**

Heart failure with preserved systolic function is associated with concentric hypertrophy. The chambers of the heart remain similar or decrease in size, but the myocardial walls thicken (see Figure 4-2).

**Is heart failure with preserved systolic function associated with an enlarged cardiac silhouette on chest radiography?**

Concentric hypertrophy is generally not associated with an enlarged cardiac silhouette on chest radiography.

**Is heart failure with preserved systolic function typically associated with dilated or restrictive cardiomyopathy?**

Heart failure with preserved systolic function is typically associated with restrictive cardiomyopathy. Concentric hypertrophy results in thickened ventricular myocardium with preserved contractility but impaired diastolic filling (ie, compliance is decreased).

**What extra heart sound is commonly associated with heart failure with preserved systolic function?**

An S4 gallop is a common finding in patients with heart failure with preserved systolic function. The S4 is a low-frequency late diastolic sound that is best appreciated over the apex of the heart with the bell of the stethoscope (Figure 4-4).[5,10]

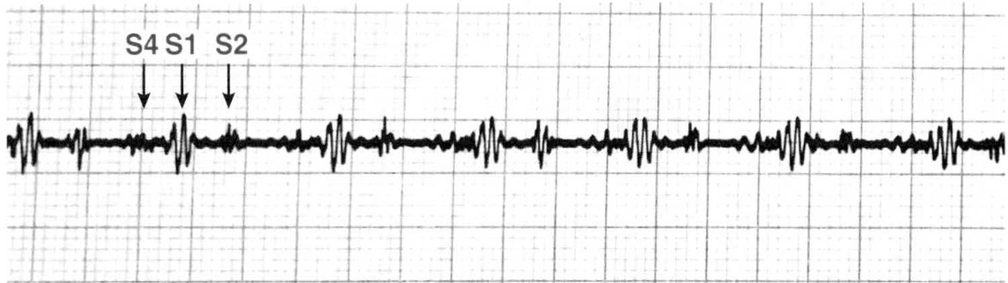


**Figure 4-4.** Phonocardiographic tracing of an S4 gallop recorded over the apex (heart rate 100 beats per minute).

**What is the treatment for heart failure with preserved systolic function?**

Unlike the myriad pharmacologic agents that improve mortality in patients with heart failure with reduced systolic function, no such agents have been proven effective in patients with heart failure with preserved systolic function. Treatment focuses on underlying or associated conditions (eg, hypertension) and symptom management (eg, diuretics).[1]

**The causes of heart failure with preserved left ventricular systolic function can be separated into which general subcategories?**

The causes of heart failure with preserved left ventricular systolic function can be separated into the following subcategories: increased afterload, valvular disease, infiltrative disorders, genetic conditions, and other.

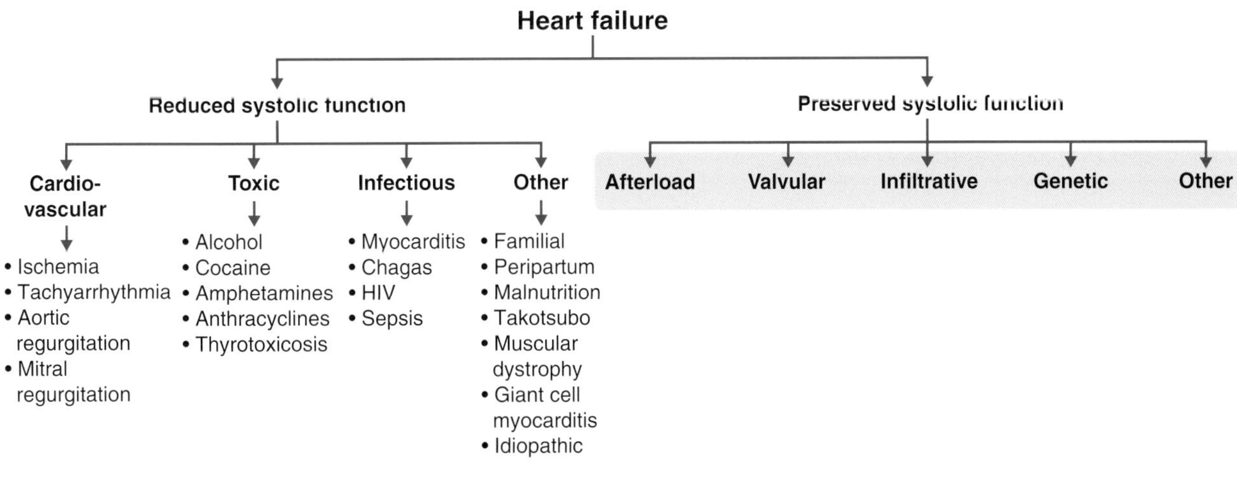


CARDIOLOGY

## CAUSES OF HEART FAILURE WITH PRESERVED SYSTOLIC FUNCTION RELATED TO INCREASED AFTERLOAD

**What is afterload in cardiac physiology?**

For cardiac muscle, afterload is the force against which the myocardial fibers contract during systole. This force is a product of left ventricular systolic pressure and the internal dimension of the left ventricular cavity.[25]

### What are the causes of heart failure with preserved systolic function related to increased afterload?

**Colloquially referred to as the "silent killer."**

Hypertension.

**Right-sided heart failure related to the lungs or pulmonary vessels.**

Cor pulmonale.

**Associated with hypertrophic cardiomyopathy.**

Hypertrophic obstructive cardiomyopathy (HOCM).

**Brachial-femoral pulse delay and rib notching on chest radiography.**

Coarctation of the aorta.

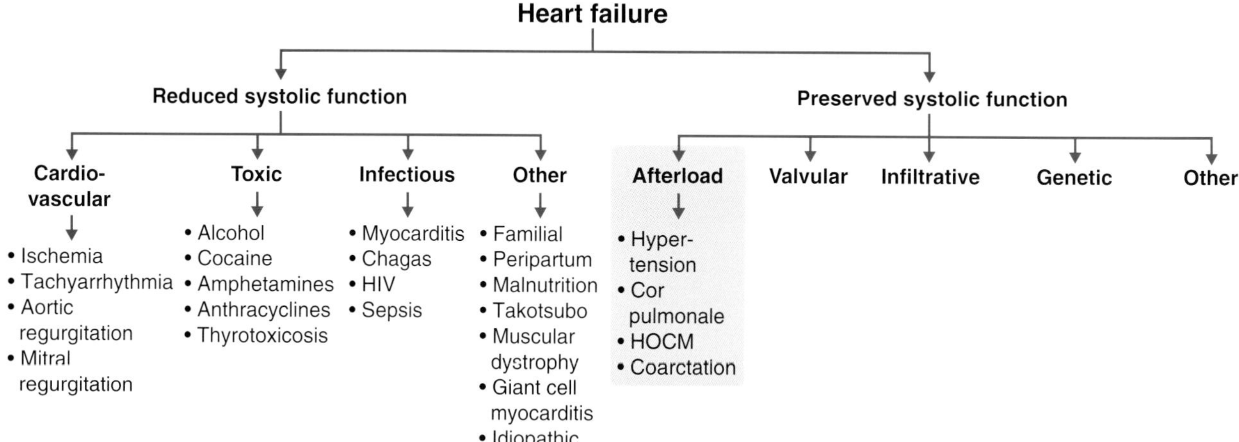


**How common is hypertension in patients with heart failure with preserved systolic function?**

Hypertension is present in the vast majority of patients with heart failure with preserved systolic function. The use of β-blockers, ACE inhibitors, and ARBs to control blood pressure in patients with heart failure with preserved systolic function is reasonable. However, no particular class of antihypertensive medications has been shown to improve outcomes in these patients.[1,2]

**What is the final common pathway of all processes that lead to cor pulmonale?**

Pulmonary hypertension, which increases afterload of the right ventricle, is the final common pathway of all processes that lead to cor pulmonale.

**How does the quality of the murmur associated with hypertrophic obstructive cardiomyopathy change with Valsalva maneuver?**

The left ventricular outflow tract obstruction of HOCM is dynamic, varying according to several factors, including cardiac preload. When preload is increased, the degree of obstruction is decreased; when preload is decreased, the degree of obstruction is increased. Preload is decreased during the straining phase of the Valsalva maneuver, which leads to an increase in the degree of outflow obstruction with an associated increase in the intensity of the murmur.[10]

**What are the management strategies for patients with coarctation of the aorta?**

In patients with coarctation of the aorta, hypertension should be controlled with β-blockers, ACE inhibitors, or ARBs as first-line medications. Intervention (eg, percutaneous catheter intervention or surgical repair) should be considered in patients with a peak-to-peak coarctation gradient ≥20 mm Hg or in those with a gradient <20 mm Hg who have evidence of significant collateral blood flow (which can decrease the gradient and mask severe obstruction).[26]

## VALVULAR CAUSES OF HEART FAILURE WITH PRESERVED SYSTOLIC FUNCTION

**What general type of valvular lesion is associated with concentric hypertrophy and heart failure with preserved systolic function?**

In general, concentric hypertrophy and heart failure with preserved systolic function are associated with stenotic valvular lesions. In contrast, eccentric hypertrophy and heart failure with reduced systolic function are associated with regurgitant valvular lesions. *Right-sided valvular lesions, both regurgitant and stenotic, are generally associated with preserved left ventricular function.*

### What are the valvular causes of heart failure with preserved systolic function?

**A late-peaking crescendo-decrescendo systolic murmur best heard over the right upper sternal border with radiation to the carotids and the apex where the murmur takes on a musical quality (ie, Gallavardin phenomenon).**

Aortic stenosis.

**A low-pitched rumbling diastolic murmur with presystolic accentuation.**

Mitral stenosis.

**A 26-year-old woman with a history of intravenous drug use presents with fever and heart failure and is found to have a holosystolic murmur best heard over the left lower sternal border that augments with inspiration (ie, Carvallo's sign).**

Tricuspid regurgitation.

**Similar in quality to aortic stenosis, but Carvallo's sign is present.**

Pulmonic stenosis.

**A short, late diastolic murmur with positive Carvallo's sign.**

Tricuspid stenosis.

**A decrescendo diastolic murmur with positive Carvallo's sign.**

Pulmonic regurgitation.

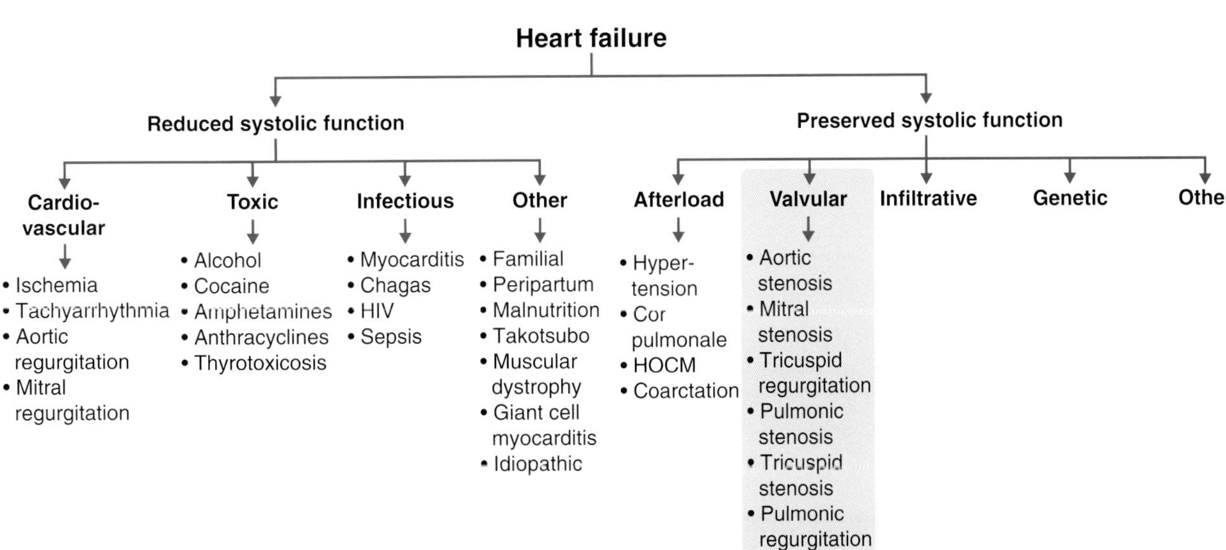


**What are the echocardiographic criteria for severe aortic stenosis?**

Severe aortic stenosis is defined by an aortic jet velocity >4.0 m/s or mean gradient >40 mm Hg. Aortic valve area is typically <1 $cm^2$ but this finding is not required for diagnosis.[27]

**Why is mitral stenosis often associated with embolic events such as stroke and renal infarction?**

Mitral stenosis is associated with atrial fibrillation in almost half of all cases, and the risk of embolic events in the setting of valvular atrial fibrillation is higher than in patients with atrial fibrillation alone.[28]

**What characteristic finding of the jugular venous waveform is associated with severe tricuspid regurgitation?**

Severe tricuspid regurgitation causes a CV fusion wave in the jugular venous waveform, known as Lancisi's sign. *For a video of Lancisi's sign, see the associated reference.*[29]

**What causes pulmonic stenosis?**

Pulmonic stenosis is almost always congenital in nature and is more common in males. When mild (ie, transpulmonary gradient <25 mm Hg), the clinical course is typically benign. However, more severe degrees of pulmonic stenosis (ie, gradient >50 mm Hg) may necessitate valvuloplasty or valvotomy. Prognosis in patients who undergo such a procedure is excellent.[30]

**What finding of the jugular venous waveform is associated with tricuspid stenosis?**

Tricuspid stenosis causes a giant A wave in the jugular venous waveform. In the normal waveform, the A wave is caused by an increase in pressure associated with right atrial contraction. When the atrium contracts against a stenotic valve, a large positive pressure wave is generated, producing the giant A wave. *For a video of giant A waves, see the associated reference.*[31]

**What is a Graham Steell murmur?**

A Graham Steell murmur describes the murmur of pulmonic regurgitation when it occurs as a result of pulmonary hypertension.[10]

*Aortic stenosis and pulmonic stenosis, which are listed under the valvular category, cause heart failure with preserved systolic function as a result of increased afterload.*

## INFILTRATIVE CAUSES OF HEART FAILURE WITH PRESERVED SYSTOLIC FUNCTION

### What are the infiltrative causes of heart failure with preserved systolic function?

**A middle-aged man with macroglossia and large shoulders.**

Amyloidosis.

**A granulomatous disease.**

Sarcoidosis.

**Infiltration of a metallic element.**

Iron overload.

**Generalized lymphadenopathy and elevated serum lactate dehydrogenase.**

Lymphoma.

**Infiltration of "acid-loving" cells.**

Eosinophilia.

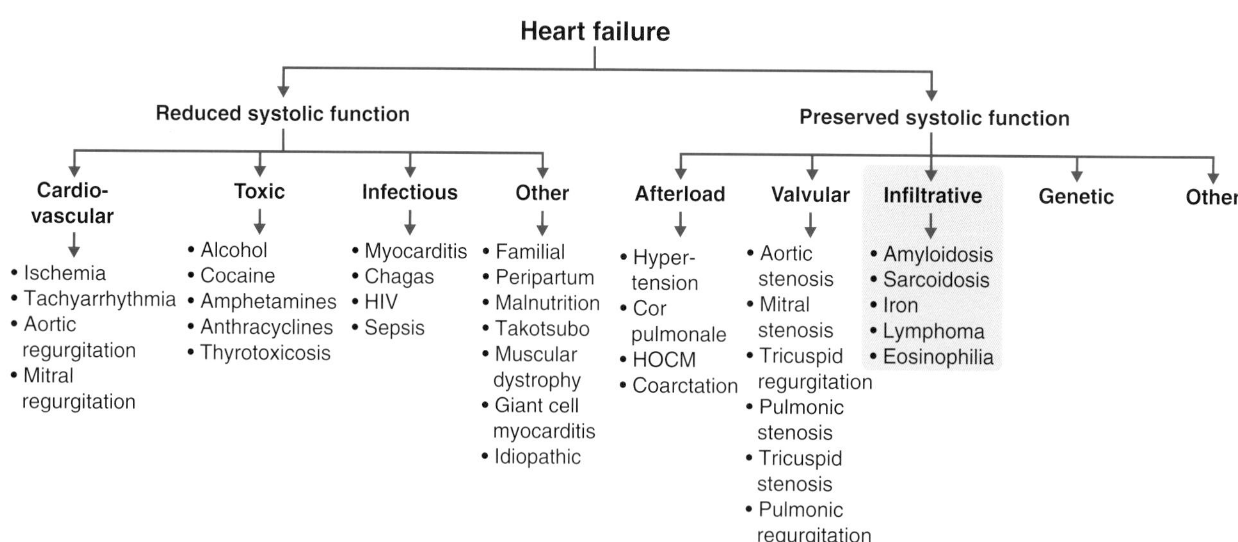


**How common is cardiac disease in patients with amyloidosis?**

Cardiac involvement can occur in all forms of amyloidosis but is most common in patients with immunoglobulin light chain (AL) amyloidosis and transthyretin amyloidosis (wild-type and hereditary). Approximately one half of patients with AL amyloidosis develop cardiac disease, including heart failure in around one-quarter.[32,33]

**How common is cardiac sarcoidosis?**

Cardiac sarcoidosis affects up to one-quarter of patients with systemic sarcoidosis. Manifestations most commonly include conduction disease (eg, atrioventricular block) and heart failure. Treatment with high-dose glucocorticoids may halt progression or reverse heart disease.[1]

**What are the causes of secondary iron overload?**

Causes of secondary iron overload include excess dietary intake of iron, severe and chronic hemolysis of any cause, and multiple blood transfusions.

**In addition to myocardial infiltration, how can lymphoma cause the clinical syndrome of heart failure?**

Lymphoma can cause the clinical syndrome of heart failure as a result of pericardial infiltration and pericardial effusion.

**What is Löffler endocarditis?**

Löffler endocarditis (ie, eosinophilic myocarditis) describes the development of endocardial fibrosis in association with hypereosinophilic syndrome (HES), which is defined as persistent hypereosinophilia with an eosinophil count >1500/μL for ≥6 months with evidence of organ damage by eosinophils. HES can be primary (ie, neoplastic), secondary (eg, parasitic infection), or idiopathic (most common). Idiopathic HES is significantly more common in men than women, generally affecting men between the ages of 20 and 50 years. Conditions closely related to Löffler endocarditis include endomyocardial fibrosis and eosinophilic granulomatosis with polyangiitis (EGPA, or Churg-Strauss syndrome). Endomyocardial fibrosis is a disease of the tropics that affects men and women equally; its pathophysiology is unknown.[34,35]

## GENETIC CAUSES OF HEART FAILURE WITH PRESERVED SYSTOLIC FUNCTION

### What are the genetic causes of heart failure with preserved systolic function?

**Cyanosis in the newborn.**

Congenital heart disease.

**The leading cause of sudden cardiac death in young athletes; this condition follows an autosomal dominant inheritance pattern.**

Hypertrophic cardiomyopathy.[36]

**"Bronze diabetes."**

Hemochromatosis.

**Inborn error of metabolism.**

Glycogen storage disease.

**An X-linked lysosomal storage disorder related to deficiency of the enzyme α-galactosidase A.**

Fabry disease.[37]

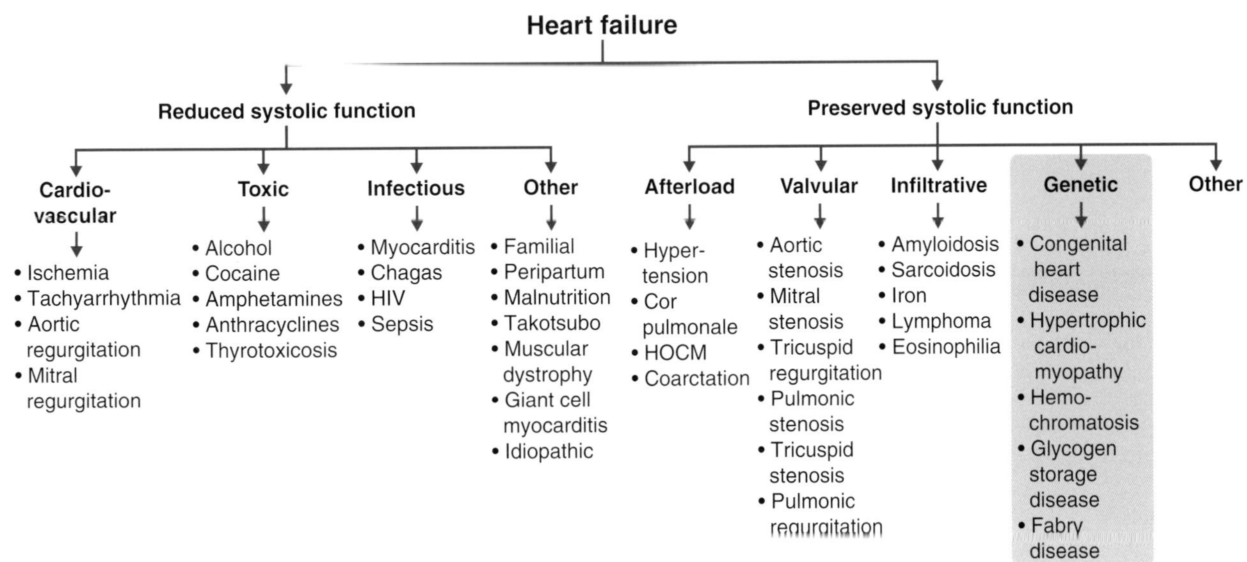

**Which common congenital heart defect is associated with a fixed split second heart sound (S2) and may lead to right heart failure?**

Atrial septal defect (ASD) is associated with a fixed split S2. Over time, as a result of left-to-right shunt, an uncorrected large ASD can lead to right-sided volume overload, flow-related pulmonary hypertension, and eventual right heart failure. Other cardiac manifestations include atrial dysrhythmias such as atrial flutter, atrial fibrillation, and sick sinus syndrome. Small atrial septal defects can remain asymptomatic into the fourth and fifth decades of life.[26]

**How common is heart failure in patients with hypertrophic cardiomyopathy without associated outflow obstruction?**

Approximately one-third of patients with hypertrophic cardiomyopathy without obstruction develop heart failure with preserved systolic function. Most patients experience a relatively stable course without significant symptoms of heart failure. A small minority of patients develops "burned-out" disease characterized by the conversion to heart failure with reduced systolic function.[36]

**What is the treatment of choice in patients with cardiac hemochromatosis?**

Phlebotomy is first-line treatment for cardiac hemochromatosis in patients without coexistent anemia. Initially, it is typically scheduled every 4 to 14 days as tolerated. Therapeutic targets include ferritin level <50 ng/mL and transferrin saturation <30%. Once the target is reached, maintenance phlebotomy is titrated to keep the ferritin level between 50 and 100 ng/mL and transferrin saturation <50%. Phlebotomy has been shown to improve cardiac parameters in patients with cardiac hemochromatosis, including left ventricular mass and ejection fraction.[38]

**In patients with glycogen storage disease who present with loss of consciousness, what noncardiac cause should immediately be considered?**

Hypoglycemia is a common manifestation of glycogen storage diseases given the inability to store glycogen, and patients may present with loss of consciousness.

**How common is cardiac involvement in Fabry disease?**

More than half of patients with Fabry disease develop cardiac involvement, most frequently concentric left ventricular hypertrophy. Improvement in cardiac disease can be expected when enzyme replacement therapy is started early.[37]

## OTHER CAUSES OF HEART FAILURE WITH PRESERVED SYSTOLIC FUNCTION

### What are the other causes of heart failure with preserved systolic function?

**External cardiac restraint.**

Pericardial disease.

**A 42-year-old woman of the Oklahoma Choctaw Native American tribe presents with episodes of discoloration of the fingers on cold exposure and progressive skin tightening.**

Scleroderma (ie, systemic sclerosis).[39]

**A patient with a history of mediastinal lymphoma presents with dyspnea and is found to have elevated JVP, Kussmaul's sign, and marker tattoos on the anterior chest.**

Mediastinal radiation therapy.

**Anemia, thyrotoxicosis, arteriovenous shunt, cirrhosis, Paget disease, acromegaly, and beriberi.**

High-output heart failure.

**An underlying cause cannot be identified despite a complete workup.**

Idiopathic restrictive cardiomyopathy.

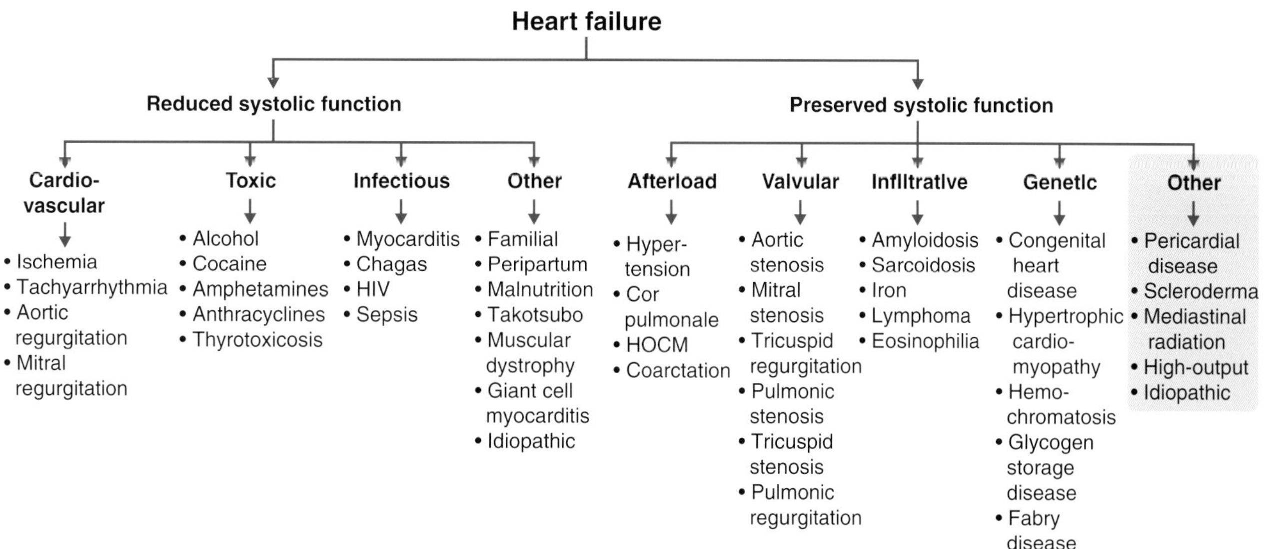


**What 2 eponymous findings of the jugular venous waveform can be seen in constrictive pericarditis?**

Constrictive pericarditis is associated with Kussmaul's sign (a paradoxical increase in JVP with inspiration) and Friedreich's sign (a sharp and deep Y descent). *For a video of Kussmaul's sign, see the associated reference.*[40]

**How does scleroderma affect the heart?**

Cardiac involvement in scleroderma can occur in a variety of ways, including cor pulmonale from lung disease or isolated pulmonary hypertension, acute pericarditis, constrictive pericarditis, pericardial effusion, premature coronary artery disease, myocarditis, nonbacterial thrombotic (marantic) endocarditis, and conduction system abnormalities.[41]

**In addition to the myocardium, what other cardiac structures can be affected by radiation therapy?**

The spectrum of radiation-induced cardiac disease includes premature coronary artery disease, pericardial disease (eg, pericardial effusion), myocardial disease (eg, myocarditis), valvular disease (eg, aortic stenosis), and conduction system abnormalities (eg, atrioventricular block).[42]

**What are the physical findings of high-output states?**

Physical findings of high-output states may include elevated JVP, warm extremities, widened pulse pressure (with associated findings such as Quincke's pulse or bounding pulses), hyperdynamic precordium, and a systolic flow murmur. Other findings of heart failure may also be present.

**What is the prognosis of idiopathic restrictive cardiomyopathy?**

Idiopathic restrictive cardiomyopathy is associated with poor prognosis: overall 5-year survival in patients of all ages is 65%; 10-year survival is 35%. Men older than 70 years of age with idiopathic restrictive cardiomyopathy have a particularly high rate of mortality.[44]

## Case Summary

A 66-year-old woman with a history of hypertension and carpal tunnel syndrome is referred to cardiology for evaluation of chronic heart failure of unknown etiology and is found to have an extra heart sound on examination, an abnormal ECG, evidence of concentric hypertrophy with preserved systolic function on echocardiography, diffuse biventricular wall thickening with heterogeneous enhancement on contrast-enhanced cardiac MRI, and positive Congo red staining with apple-green birefringence under polarized light on endomyocardial biopsy.

***What is the most likely cause of heart failure in this patient?***

Amyloidosis.

### BONUS QUESTIONS

***Which parts of the history and physical examination in this case offer clues to the diagnosis of amyloidosis?***

Amyloidosis is often associated with carpal tunnel syndrome as a result of soft tissue infiltration. The orthostatic hypotension (with stable heart rate) in this case is suggestive of autonomic peripheral neuropathy, which is also associated with amyloidosis.[32]

CARDIOLOGY

| | |
|---|---|
| ***What is the most likely source of the extra heart sound in this case?*** | Extra heart sounds that occur near S1 include split S1, S4 gallop, and ejection clicks. The extra sound in this case is most likely an S4 gallop, based on location, pitch, and clinical history (see Figure 4-4). An S4 often occurs in the setting of restrictive cardiomyopathy, which is associated with cardiac amyloidosis.[10] |
| ***Which electrocardiographic feature in this case argues against hypertension as the underlying cause of heart failure?*** | The low-voltage QRS complexes on the ECG in this case (see Figure 4-1) would be highly atypical of hypertensive heart disease, which is usually associated with concentric left ventricular hypertrophy and increased voltage. Infiltrative disorders, such as amyloidosis, on the other hand, are associated with decreased QRS voltage on ECG.[32] |
| ***What are all of the relevant electrocardiographic findings in this case?*** | The ECG in this case (see Figure 4-1) demonstrates reduced limb lead QRS voltage (all limb leads ≤0.5 mV) with preserved precordial voltage, P-wave prominence, and poor R-wave progression in the precordial leads (ie, pseudoinfarction pattern). These findings are characteristic of cardiac amyloidosis.[21,32] |
| ***What biochemical tests are helpful when cardiac amyloidosis is suspected?*** | In the appropriate clinical setting, the presence of elevated brain natriuretic peptide (BNP) or its N-terminal fragment (NT-pro-BNP) and cardiac troponins is suggestive of cardiac amyloidosis and is associated with a significantly increased rate of mortality in these patients.[32] |
| ***How can cardiac MRI distinguish the hypertrophy related to amyloidosis from that of long-standing hypertension?*** | On cardiac MRI, late contrast enhancement of the thickened myocardium is highly characteristic of cardiac amyloidosis but is absent in patients with myocardial hypertrophy related to hypertension.[32] |
| ***What is the significance of the endomyocardial biopsy in this case?*** | The histologic demonstration of extracellular deposits with Congo red staining that turn apple-green in color under polarized light is pathognomonic for amyloidosis and is the diagnostic gold standard.[32] |
| ***What is the prognosis of cardiac amyloidosis?*** | In general, cardiac amyloidosis is associated with a poor prognosis. The median survival of patients with AL amyloidosis without cardiac involvement is 4 years. Median survival declines to 8 months in patients with advanced cardiac involvement.[32] |

## KEY POINTS

- Heart failure is a clinical syndrome that develops as a result of structural or functional impairment of ventricular filling, or the ejection of blood.
- Symptoms of heart failure include dyspnea, cough, orthopnea, paroxysmal nocturnal dyspnea, fatigue or lethargy, weight gain, nausea, early satiety, and abdominal discomfort.
- Physical findings of right-sided heart failure include elevated JVP, right ventricular heave, right-sided gallop, ascites, and lower extremity edema.
- Physical findings of left-sided heart failure include end-inspiratory crepitant rales on auscultation of the lungs, left-sided gallop, laterally displaced apical impulse, pulsus alternans, and cool extremities.
- The lungs may be clear in the context of chronic left-sided heart failure.
- Heart failure can be associated with reduced left ventricular systolic function or preserved left ventricular systolic function (ejection fraction >50%).
- Heart failure with reduced systolic function is associated with eccentric hypertrophy, whereas heart failure with preserved systolic function is associated with concentric hypertrophy.
- The causes of heart failure with reduced systolic function can be separated into the following subcategories: cardiovascular, toxic, infectious, and other.
- The causes of heart failure with preserved systolic function can be separated into the following subcategories: increased afterload, valvular disease, infiltrative disorders, genetic conditions, and other.
- Specific pharmacologic agents have been shown to improve survival in patients with heart failure with reduced systolic function; outcomes have been largely neutral in patients with preserved systolic function.

## REFERENCES


1. Yancy CW, Jessup M, Bozkurt B, et al. 2013 ACCF/AHA guideline for the management of heart failure: executive summary: a report of the American College of Cardiology Foundation/American Heart Association Task Force on practice guidelines. *Circulation*. 2013;128(16):1810-1852.
2. Volpe M, McKelvie R, Drexler H. Hypertension as an underlying factor in heart failure with preserved ejection fraction. *J Clin Hypertens*. 2010;12(4):277-283.
3. Mensah YB, Mensah K, Asiamah S, et al. Establishing the cardiothoracic ratio using chest radiographs in an indigenous Ghanaian population: a simple tool for cardiomegaly screening. *Ghana Med J*. 2015;49(3):159-164.
4. Inamdar AA, Inamdar AC. Heart failure: diagnosis, management and utilization. *J Clin Med*. 2016;5(7).
5. Tavel ME. *Clinical Phonocardiography and External Pulse Recording*. 2nd ed. Chicago, IL: Year Book Medical Publishers, Inc.; 1967.
6. Yancy CW, Jessup M, Bozkurt B, et al. 2017 ACC/AHA/HFSA focused update of the 2013 ACCF/AHA guideline for the management of heart failure: a report of the American College of Cardiology/American Heart Association Task Force on clinical practice guidelines and the Heart Failure Society of America. *Circulation*. 2017.
7. Briceno N, Schuster A, Lumley M, Perera D. Ischaemic cardiomyopathy: pathophysiology, assessment and the role of revascularisation. *Heart*. 2016;102(5):397-406.
8. Anter E, Jessup M, Callans DJ. Atrial fibrillation and heart failure: treatment considerations for a dual epidemic. *Circulation*. 2009;119(18):2516-2525.
9. Ellis ER, Josephson ME. What about tachycardia-induced cardiomyopathy? *Arrhythm Electrophysiol Rev*. 2013;2(2):82-90.
10. Marriott HJL. *Bedside Cardiac Diagnosis*. Philadelphia, PA: Lippincott Company; 1993.
11. Enriquez-Sarano M, Akins CW, Vahanian A. Mitral regurgitation. *Lancet*. 2009;373(9672):1382-1394.
12. Won S, Hong RA, Shohet RV, Seto TB, Parikh NI. Methamphetamine-associated cardiomyopathy. *Clin Cardiol*. 2013;36(12):737-742.
13. Groarke JD, Nohria A. Anthracycline cardiotoxicity: a new paradigm for an old classic. *Circulation*. 2015;131(22):1946-1949.
14. Merce J, Ferras S, Oltra C, et al. Cardiovascular abnormalities in hyperthyroidism: a prospective Doppler echocardiographic study. *Am J Med*. 2005;118(2):126-131.
15. Benziger CP, do Carmo GA, Ribeiro AL. Chagas cardiomyopathy: clinical presentation and management in the Americas. *Cardiol Clin*. 2017;35(1):31-47.
16. Remick J, Georgiopoulou V, Marti C, et al. Heart failure in patients with human immunodeficiency virus infection: epidemiology, pathophysiology, treatment, and future research. *Circulation*. 2014;129(17):1781-1789.
17. Caforio AL, Pankuweit S, Arbustini E, et al. Current state of knowledge on aetiology, diagnosis, management, and therapy of myocarditis: a position statement of the European Society of Cardiology Working Group on Myocardial and Pericardial Diseases. *Eur Heart J*. 2013;34(33):2636-2648, 2648a-2648d.
18. Sato R, Nasu M. A review of sepsis-induced cardiomyopathy. *J Intensive Care*. 2015;3:48.
19. Mestroni L, Maisch B, McKenna WJ, et al. Guidelines for the study of familial dilated cardiomyopathies. Collaborative Research Group of the European Human and Capital Mobility Project on Familial Dilated Cardiomyopathy. *Eur Heart J*. 1999;20(2):93-102.
20. Givertz MM. Cardiology patient page: peripartum cardiomyopathy. *Circulation*. 2013;127(20):e622-e626.
21. Marinescu V, McCullough PA. Nutritional and micronutrient determinants of idiopathic dilated cardiomyopathy: diagnostic and therapeutic implications. *Expert Rev Cardiovasc Ther*. 2011;9(9):1161-1170.
22. Verhaert D, Richards K, Rafael-Fortney JA, Raman SV. Cardiac involvement in patients with muscular dystrophies: magnetic resonance imaging phenotype and genotypic considerations. *Circ Cardiovasc Imaging*. 2011;4(1):67-76.
23. Kandolin R, Lehtonen J, Salmenkivi K, Raisanen-Sokolowski A, Lommi J, Kupari M. Diagnosis, treatment, and outcome of giant-cell myocarditis in the era of combined immunosuppression. *Circ Heart Fail*. 2013;6(1):15-22.
24. Felker GM, Thompson RE, Hare JM, et al. Underlying causes and long-term survival in patients with initially unexplained cardiomyopathy. *N Engl J Med*. 2000;342(15):1077-1084.
25. Tarazi RC, Levy MN. Cardiac responses to increased afterload. State-of-the-art review. *Hypertension*. 1982;4(3 Pt 2):8-18.
26. Warnes CA, Williams RG, Bashore TM, et al. ACC/AHA 2008 guidelines for the management of adults with congenital heart disease: executive summary: a report of the American College of Cardiology/American Heart Association Task Force on practice guidelines (writing committee to develop guidelines for the management of adults with congenital heart disease). *Circulation*. 2008;118(23):2395-2451.
27. Nishimura RA, Otto CM, Bonow RO, et al. 2014 AHA/ACC guideline for the management of patients with valvular heart disease: a report of the American College of Cardiology/American Heart Association Task Force on practice guidelines. *J Am Coll Cardiol*. 2014;63(22):e57-185.
28. Carabello BA. Modern management of mitral stenosis. *Circulation*. 2005;112(3):432-437.
29. Mansoor AM, Mansoor SE. Images in clinical medicine. Lancisi's Sign. *N Engl J Med*. 2016;374(2):e2.
30. Almeda FQ, Kavinsky CJ, Pophal SG, Klein LW. Pulmonic valvular stenosis in adults: diagnosis and treatment. *Catheter Cardiovasc Interv*. 2003;60(4):546-557.
31. Burgess TE, Mansoor AM. Giant a waves. *BMJ Case Rep*. 2017;2017.
32. Banypersad SM, Moon JC, Whelan C, Hawkins PN, Wechalekar AD. Updates in cardiac amyloidosis: a review. *J Am Heart Assoc*. 2012;1(2):e000364.
33. Hassan W, Al-Sergani H, Mourad W, Tabbaa R. Amyloid heart disease. New frontiers and insights in pathophysiology, diagnosis, and management. *Tex Heart Inst J*. 2005;32(2):178-184.
34. Ginsberg F, Parrillo JE. Eosinophilic myocarditis. *Heart Fail Clin*. 2005;1(3):419-429.
35. Valent P, Klion AD, Horny HP, et al. Contemporary consensus proposal on criteria and classification of eosinophilic disorders and related syndromes. *J Allergy Clin Immunol*. 2012;130(3):607-612.e9.
36. Maron BJ, Ommen SR, Semsarian C, Spirito P, Olivotto I, Maron MS. Hypertrophic cardiomyopathy: present and future, with translation into contemporary cardiovascular medicine. *J Am Coll Cardiol*. 2014;64(1):83-99.
37. Seydelmann N, Wanner C, Stork S, Ertl G, Weidemann F. Fabry disease and the heart. *Best Pract Res Clin Endocrinol Metab*. 2015;29(2):195-204.

38. Gulati V, Harikrishnan P, Palaniswamy C, Aronow WS, Jain D, Frishman WH. Cardiac involvement in hemochromatosis. *Cardiol Rev*. 2014;22(2):56-68.
39. Arnett FC, Howard RF, Tan F, et al. Increased prevalence of systemic sclerosis in a Native American tribe in Oklahoma. Association with an Amerindian HLA haplotype. *Arthritis Rheum*. 1996;39(8):1362-1370.
40. Mansoor AM, Karlapudi SP. Images in clinical medicine. Kussmaul's sign. *N Engl J Med*. 2015;372(2):e3.
41. Champion HC. The heart in scleroderma. *Rheum Dis Clin North Am*. 2008;34(1):181-190; viii.
42. Yusuf SW, Sami S, Daher IN. Radiation-induced heart disease: a clinical update. *Cardiol Res Pract*. 2011;2011:317659.
43. Stern AB, Klemmer PJ. High-output heart failure secondary to arteriovenous fistula. *Hemodial Int*. 2011;15(1):104-107.
44. Ammash NM, Seward JB, Bailey KR, Edwards WD, Tajik AJ. Clinical profile and outcome of idiopathic restrictive cardiomyopathy. *Circulation*. 2000;101(21):2490-2496.

Chapter 5

# PERICARDITIS

## Case: A 32-year-old man with positional chest pain

A 32-year-old man presents to the emergency department with increasing episodes of chest discomfort over the course of several days. The pain is located in the center of the chest and radiates to the shoulders. It is sharp in quality, worsens when the patient lies flat, and improves when he leans forward. He reports a history of recurrent painful oral and genital ulcers and inflamed joints over the course of a year.

Cardiac auscultation is notable for the presence of 3 distinct scratchy sounds occurring in concert with the cardiac cycle. Ulcers are present on the oral mucosa, and there are several tender erythematous nodules over the anterior shins.

Electrocardiogram (ECG) is shown in Figure 5-1.

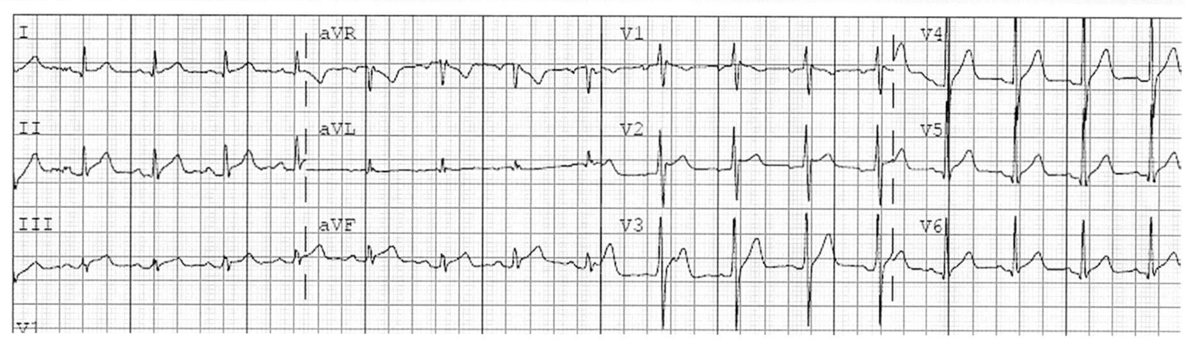


**Figure 5-1.**

***What is the most likely cause of chest pain in this patient?***

**What is pericarditis?**

Pericarditis describes inflammation of the pericardium, the fibrous sac that surrounds the heart. Pericarditis is most often an acute process, but acute pericarditis from virtually any cause can become chronic and evolve into constrictive pericarditis. Pericarditis may or may not be associated with a pericardial effusion.[1]

**What are the symptoms of acute pericarditis?**

Symptoms of acute pericarditis may include pleuritic chest pain, nonproductive cough, hiccups, and odynophagia.[1]

**What are the characteristics of pleuritic chest pain?**

Pleuritic chest pain is sharp or stabbing in quality, positional, and exacerbated by breathing or coughing.

**What are the characteristic features of the chest pain associated with acute pericarditis?**

The pleuritic chest pain of acute pericarditis often radiates to the trapezius ridges, is exacerbated by recumbence, and is improved by leaning forward.[1]

**What are the physical findings of acute pericarditis?**

Physical findings of acute pericarditis may include fever and a pericardial friction rub (a high-pitched scratchy sound that may have 1, 2, or 3 components). The friction rub occurs as a result of friction between inflamed pericardial surfaces and is the cardinal sign of pericarditis.[1]

**What are the electrocardiographic manifestations of acute pericarditis?**

Electrocardiographic changes associated with acute pericarditis occur as a result of superficial myocarditis. Manifestations include diffuse ST-segment elevation, diffuse PR-segment depression, and PR-segment elevation in lead aVR. In patients with cardiac tamponade, there may be reduced voltage or the presence of electrical alternans (ie, alternating amplitude of the QRS complex).[1]

**Is acute pericarditis more common in men or women?**

Acute pericarditis occurs more commonly in men at a ratio of 4:1.[1]

**What other pericardial process can occur in association with acute pericarditis?**

Acute pericarditis may be either "dry" or associated with pericardial effusion, the size of which can range from trivial without hemodynamic significance, to large and associated with cardiac tamponade.[1]

**What is cardiac tamponade?**

Cardiac tamponade describes external cardiac compression by abnormal pericardial content (usually fluid) that results in hemodynamic changes, the most significant of which is hypotension (Figure 5-2). Virtually any cause of acute pericarditis can be associated with cardiac tamponade.[1]

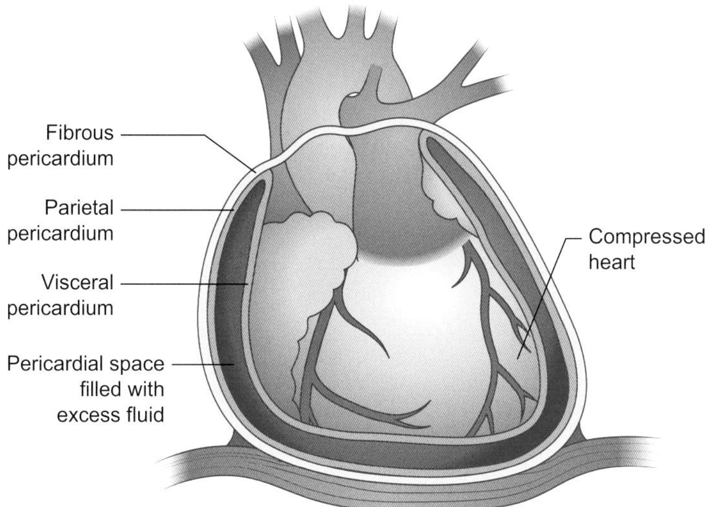


**Figure 5-2.** In cardiac tamponade, blood or fluid fills the pericardial space, compressing the heart chambers, increasing intracardiac pressure, and obstructing venous return. As blood flow into the ventricles falls, so does cardiac output. (Adapted from *Cardiovascular Care Made Incredibly Visual!* Philadelphia, PA: Lippincott Williams & Wilkins; 2011.)

**Which diagnostic and therapeutic procedure can be performed to sample and drain pericardial fluid?**

Pericardial fluid may be sampled by performing a pericardiocentesis. The fluid can generally be described as transudative or exudative in nature, depending on fluid characteristics such as protein and lactate dehydrogenase (LDH) content. However, unlike fluid from pleural effusions, there is considerable biochemical overlap between pericardial transudates and exudates. Nevertheless, fluid characteristics such as appearance, cholesterol content, LDH content, total protein content, cell count, glucose content, Gram stain, culture, and other studies (eg, polymerase chain reaction, cytology) can be helpful in establishing the underlying diagnosis.[1]

**What is the utility of chest radiography in patients with pericardial disease?**

An enlarged cardiac silhouette on chest radiography, particularly if it is acute, can be a diagnostic clue to the presence of a pericardial effusion. For the cardiac silhouette to be changed, effusions must be large, typically >250 mL. Significantly smaller effusions can be detected by echocardiography.[1]

**What is constrictive pericarditis?**

Constrictive pericarditis describes external cardiac compression by diseased or scarred pericardium (see Figure 5-2). Virtually any cause of acute pericarditis can result in constrictive pericarditis, usually after months to years.[1]

**In patients with constrictive pericarditis, what respiratory change in jugular venous pressure may be observed?**

Normally, jugular venous pressure decreases with inspiration. In patients with constrictive pericarditis it often increases with inspiration. This finding is known as Kussmaul's sign and occurs as a result of decreased right ventricular compliance. *For a video of Kussmaul's sign, see the associated reference.*[2]

**The causes of pericarditis can be separated into which general categories?**

The causes of pericarditis can be separated into the following categories: infectious, malignant, connective tissue disease (CTD), cardiac, metabolic, and other.

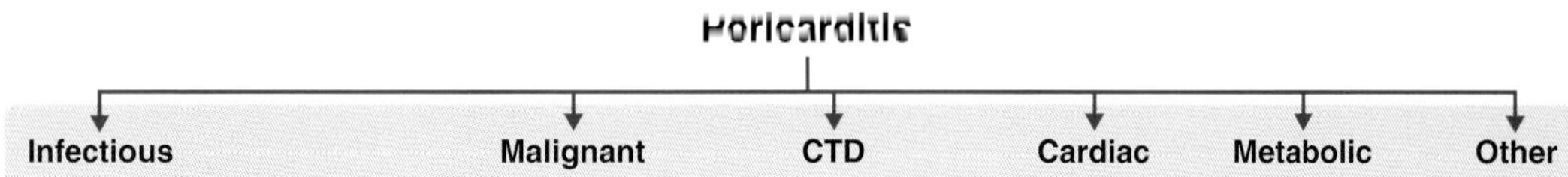


## INFECTIOUS CAUSES OF PERICARDITIS

**What are the 3 main groups of organisms that cause infectious pericarditis?**

Infectious pericarditis can be caused by viral, bacterial, or fungal organisms.

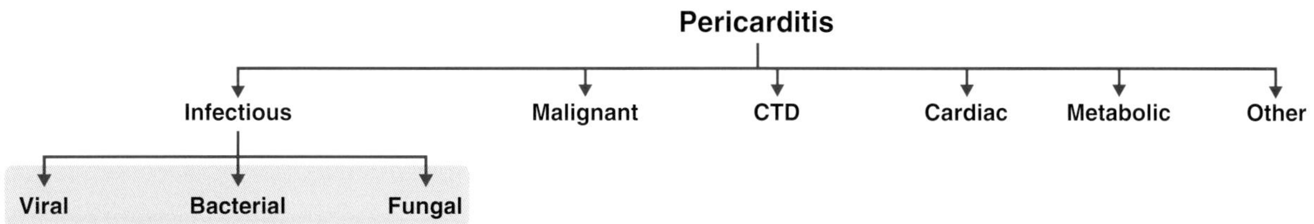


**What are the differences in clinical presentation between viral, bacterial, and fungal pericarditis?**

Viral pericarditis is more likely to present with the full spectrum of symptoms and physical findings of acute pericarditis, whereas bacterial (particularly tuberculosis) and fungal causes of acute pericarditis are often insidious and overshadowed by other systemic manifestations of the infection.[1]

## VIRAL CAUSES OF PERICARDITIS

**When does pericarditis usually occur during the course of a viral illness?**

Acute pericarditis may develop during the initial viral infection but more often appears 1 to 3 weeks later (usually following an upper respiratory or gastrointestinal illness).[1]

**What is the natural progression of acute viral pericarditis?**

Viral pericarditis is self-limited, typically resolving within 2 weeks.[1]

**What are the most common causes of viral pericarditis?**

Many viruses are capable of causing pericarditis, but the most common offenders include coxsackieviruses, echoviruses, adenoviruses, Epstein-Barr virus (EBV), cytomegalovirus (CMV), human immunodeficiency virus (HIV), influenza A and B viruses, herpes simplex virus, respiratory syncytial virus, and hepatitis A and B viruses.[1]

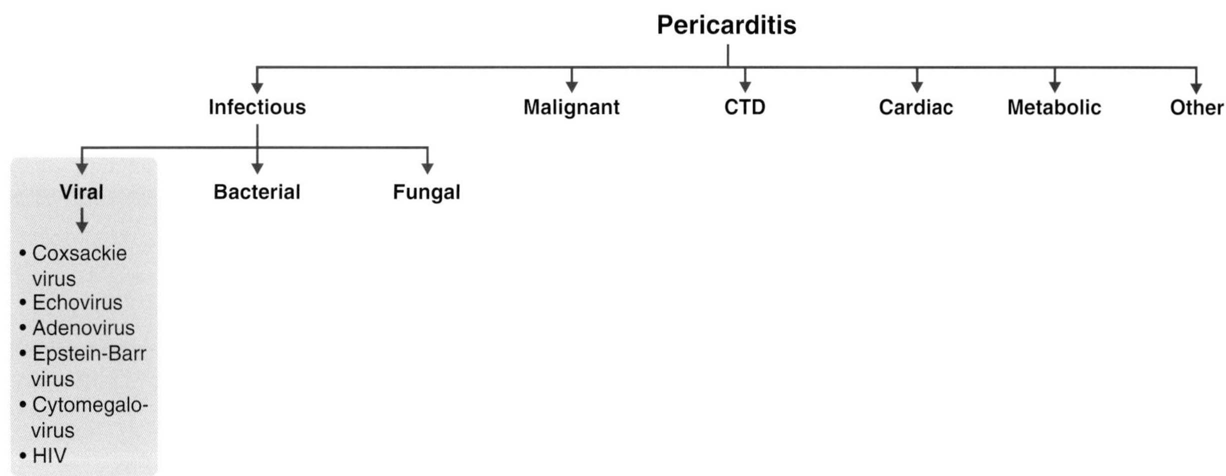


CARDIOLOGY

**Which viruses are most likely to cause pericarditis during the spring and fall seasons?**

Peak incidence of pericarditis during the spring and fall seasons is characteristic of enteroviruses, particularly group A and B coxsackieviruses, adenoviruses, rhinoviruses, echoviruses, and influenza viruses.[1]

**What characteristics make patients particularly susceptible to pericarditis related to EBV and CMV?**

Pericarditis related to EBV and CMV tends to occur in patients with compromised immune systems.[1]

**What are the characteristics of pericarditis and/or pericardial effusion associated with acquired immunodeficiency syndrome (AIDS)?**

Pericardial involvement in patients with HIV/AIDS tends to be a late manifestation. Effusions are small in the vast majority of patients, but tamponade can occur. Survival is significantly better in those without pericardial involvement; only around one-third of patients with pericardial involvement related to HIV are alive at 6 months.[3]

*Viral infections probably account for the majority of cases of "idiopathic" pericarditis.[1]*

## BACTERIAL CAUSES OF PERICARDITIS

**How does bacterial infection cause pericarditis?**

The mechanisms of pericarditis related to bacterial infection include direct invasion of the pericardium from contiguous foci (eg, infective endocarditis) and hematogenous spread (ie, preexisting noninfectious pericardial effusions can become secondarily infected via hematogenous spread).[1]

**What are the characteristics of pericardial fluid in the setting of acute bacterial pericarditis?**

Pericardial fluid related to acute bacterial pericarditis is often turbid in appearance and contains a predominance of polymorphonuclear leukocytes, elevated lactate dehydrogenase, and decreased glucose.[1]

**How should bacterial pericarditis be managed?**

Effective management of bacterial pericarditis typically requires the combination of pericardial drainage and systemic antimicrobial agents. Pericardiectomy may be necessary when adhesions and loculations occur.[1]

### What are the bacterial causes of pericarditis?

**A common cause of bacterial pericarditis worldwide, particularly in endemic regions.**

*Mycobacterium tuberculosis* (TB).

**Before the antibiotic era, this organism was a common cause of pericarditis, usually associated with pneumonia.**

*Streptococcus pneumoniae*.

**Gram-positive cocci in clusters.**

*Staphylococcus aureus*.

**Inquiring about travel history and exposure to animals is helpful in identifying the possibility of infection caused by this general group of organisms.**

Zoonoses.

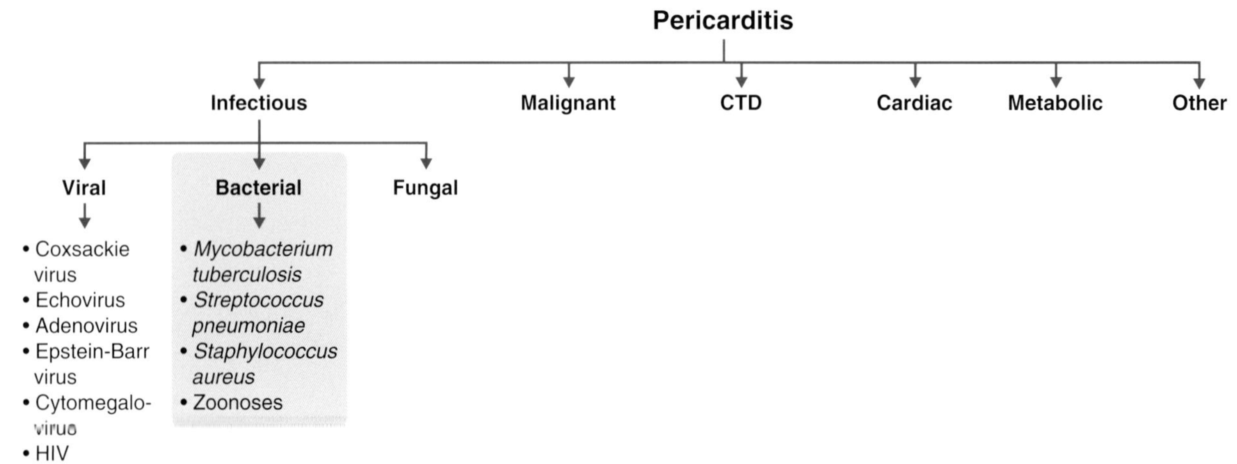

**What are the characteristics of tuberculous pericardial effusions?**

Tuberculous effusions are typically exudative with elevated protein content and leukocyte count (typically with a lymphocytic predominance >50%). Identification of *Mycobacterium* by smear, culture, or polymerase chain reaction is sufficient for the diagnosis, but a negative result does not rule out tuberculous pericarditis. High levels of adenosine deaminase activity (ie, >40 U/L) can be suggestive of tuberculous pericarditis.[1]

**What are the mechanisms of pericarditis caused by streptococcal and staphylococcal species?**

A common mechanism of pericarditis related to streptococcal and staphylococcal species is contiguous spread from infective endocarditis, especially with *Streptococcus viridans* and *Staphylococcus aureus* infections. Spread from other intrathoracic foci also occurs, including pneumonia (particularly cases caused by *Streptococcus pneumoniae*), mediastinitis, wound infection, myocardial abscess (including infected myocardial infarction), and subdiaphragmatic abscess. Hematogenous spread to the pericardium also occurs with bacteremia from streptococcal and staphylococcal species.[1]

**What are some of the zoonotic organisms associated with pericarditis?**

Zoonoses associated with pericarditis include *Rickettsia rickettsii* (Rocky Mountain spotted fever), *Borrelia burgdorferi* (Lyme disease), and *Coxiella burnetii* (Q fever).[1]

## FUNGAL CAUSES OF PERICARDITIS

**What are the 2 epidemiologic categories of fungi?**

It is helpful to categorize fungi as either endemic or ubiquitous. Endemic fungi frequently affect both immunocompromised and immunocompetent hosts, whereas ubiquitous fungi predominantly affect immunocompromised hosts.

### What are the fungal causes of pericarditis?

**This fungus is endemic near the Ohio River Valley and the lower Mississippi River.**

*Histoplasma capsulatum.*

**This fungus is endemic near the San Joaquin River Valley.**

*Coccidioides immitis.*

**These 2 ubiquitous fungi are opportunistic and associated with pericarditis in immunocompromised hosts.**

*Candida* and *Aspergillus* species.

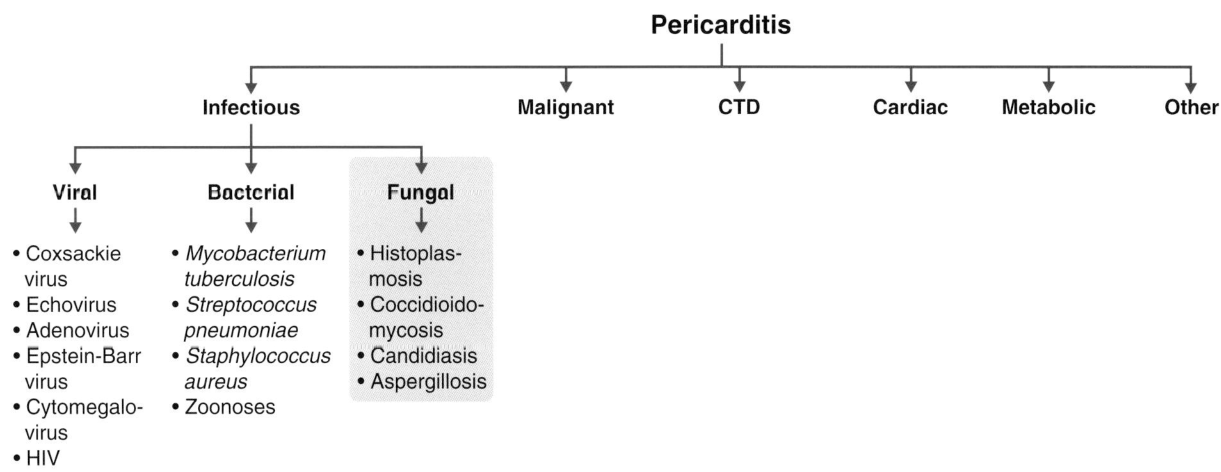


**What is the prognosis of pericarditis caused by histoplasmosis?**

In general, pericarditis caused by histoplasmosis is self-limited; however, it may run a protracted course in some cases. Most patients recover, although recurrences are common.[4]

**What concurrent site of infection is common in patients with pericardial coccidioidomycosis?**

Pericardial coccidioidomycosis often occurs with pneumonia.[1]

CARDIOLOGY

**What are the predisposing factors for the development of pericardial *Candida* and *Aspergillus* infections?**

Risk factors for developing pericardial candidiasis and aspergillosis include recent antibiotic treatment for bacterial infection, immunocompromised status, and the presence of indwelling catheters.[1]

## MALIGNANT CAUSES OF PERICARDITIS

**In addition to routine fluid analysis, what additional pericardial studies can be helpful in evaluating for malignancy?**

Cytology and flow cytometry of the pericardial fluid and biopsy of the pericardial tissue can be helpful in establishing the diagnosis of malignant pericarditis.[1]

**In patients presenting with acute pericardial disease, what clinical characteristics tend to favor underlying malignancy?**

Malignant pericarditis becomes more likely when there is a history of malignancy, cardiac tamponade at presentation, a lack of response to non-steroidal anti-inflammatory drugs, and recurrent pericarditis.[5]

**What are the 3 ways in which malignancy can cause pericarditis?**

Malignant pericarditis can occur as a result of metastatic disease (most common), reaction to distant malignancy (ie, non-neoplastic pericardial effusion associated with malignancy elsewhere in the body), and primary pericardial tumor (rare).[1]

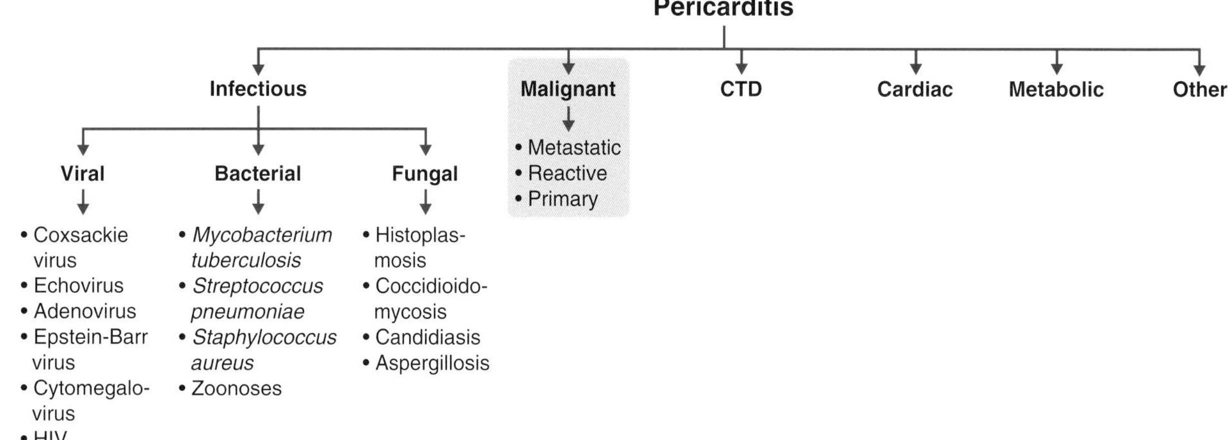


**Which malignancies most commonly metastasize to the pericardium?**

Malignancies that most commonly metastasize to the pericardium include melanoma, lymphoma, leukemia, and lung, breast, and esophageal cancer.[6]

**What are the 2 most common types of primary pericardial malignancy?**

Mesotheliomas and sarcomas are the most common primary pericardial malignancies. These tumors tend to be aggressive, often spreading through the pericardium to invade the myocardium.[1]

## PERICARDITIS RELATED TO CONNECTIVE TISSUE DISEASE

**Which gender is disproportionally affected by pericardial involvement of connective tissue disease?**

Although connective tissue diseases tend to be more prevalent in women, pericardial involvement related to these conditions occurs more frequently in men.[1]

### What are the connective tissue diseases that cause pericarditis?

**A 48-year-old woman with symmetric inflammatory polyarticular arthritis is found to have serum anti-cyclic citrullinated peptide (anti-CCP) antibodies.**

Rheumatoid arthritis.

**A 31-year-old woman with recurrent episodes of acute pericarditis associated with serum anti–double-stranded DNA antibodies and low complement levels.**

Systemic lupus erythematosus (SLE).

**This disease can be either diffuse or limited, both types of which can be associated with pericardial disease.**

Scleroderma (ie, systemic sclerosis).

**An overlap syndrome with features of SLE, scleroderma, and dermatomyositis/ polymyositis.**

Mixed connective tissue disease (MCTD).

**Oligoarticular inflammatory arthritis, often involving the axial skeleton, with negative serum rheumatoid factor.**

Seronegative spondyloarthritides.

**May be associated with palpable purpura.**

Vasculitis.

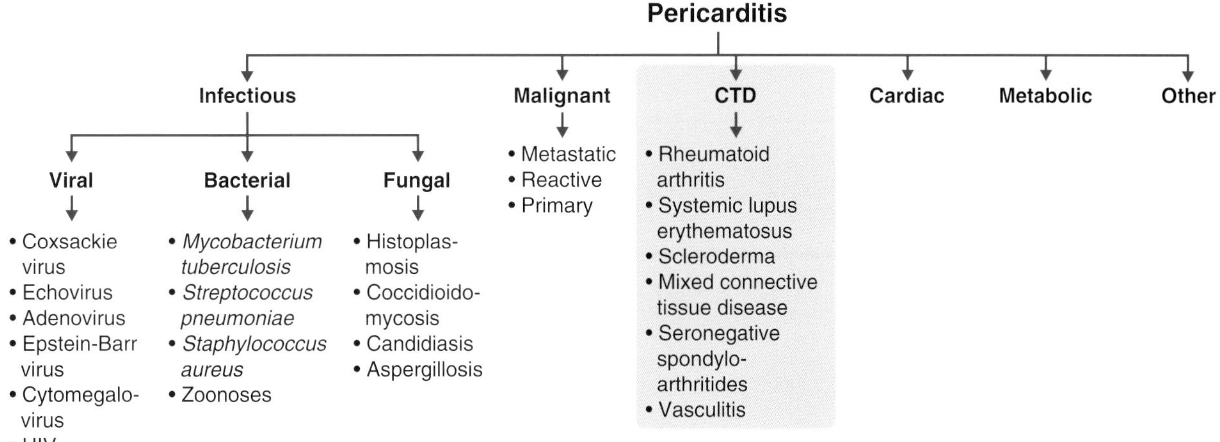


**What are the clinical features of the pericardial involvement that occurs with rheumatoid arthritis?**

Around half of patients with RA have increased pericardial fluid on echocardiography, and nearly half have significant pericardial adhesions at autopsy. Patients most commonly present with either an asymptomatic pericardial friction rub or an asymptomatic effusion on echocardiography. Most effusions are serous with low glucose, increased protein, increased cholesterol, and decreased complement.[1]

**What are the clinical features of the pericardial involvement that occurs with systemic lupus erythematosus?**

Some form of pericarditis develops in the majority of patients with SLE, particularly men. SLE can cause a spectrum of pericardial abnormalities, from large pericardial effusions to constrictive pericarditis. Pericardial involvement is often the first manifestation of SLE and should trigger an investigation to evaluate for the disease in select patients (eg, young women).[1]

**What are the clinical features of the pericardial involvement that occurs with scleroderma?**

Pericardial involvement is frequent in patients with scleroderma and can take many forms, including acute pericarditis, large pericardial effusion, and constrictive pericarditis. Pericardial effusion is present on echocardiography in close to one-half of patients, and pericardial disease is present in most patients at autopsy. Despite these high rates, most patients do not experience significant clinical manifestations.[1]

**What are the clinical features of the pericardial involvement that occurs with mixed connective tissue disease?**

Pericarditis is the most frequent cardiac manifestation of MCTD and can be a presenting feature. The electrocardiographic manifestations of pericarditis (eg, diffuse ST-segment elevation) are more frequent in patients with MCTD than other connective tissue diseases. Prognosis is generally good with most cases being responsive to short courses of glucocorticoid therapy.[1]

**Of the seronegative spondyloarthritides, which is most frequently associated with pericarditis?**

Pericardial involvement occurs frequently in reactive arthritis, particularly acute pericarditis with or without pericardial effusion.[1]

**Which vasculitides are associated with pericarditis?**

Among the vasculitides, pericardial involvement is most common in patients with granulomatosis with polyangiitis (GPA, or Wegener's granulomatosis), but it also occurs with giant cell arteritis, eosinophilic granulomatosis with polyangiitis (EGPA, or Churg-Strauss syndrome), polyarteritis nodosa, and Behçet's disease.[1]

## CARDIAC CAUSES OF PERICARDITIS

### What are the cardiac causes of pericarditis?

**An umbrella term describing the development of pericarditis following various types of cardiac injury.**

Postcardiac injury syndrome (PCIS).

**A 54-year-old man with arachnodactyly (Figure 5-3) and a high-arched palate presents with tearing substernal chest pain that radiates to the back, and is found to have a blood pressure of 183/98 mm Hg in the right upper extremity and 104/65 mm Hg in the left upper extremity.**

Aortic dissection.

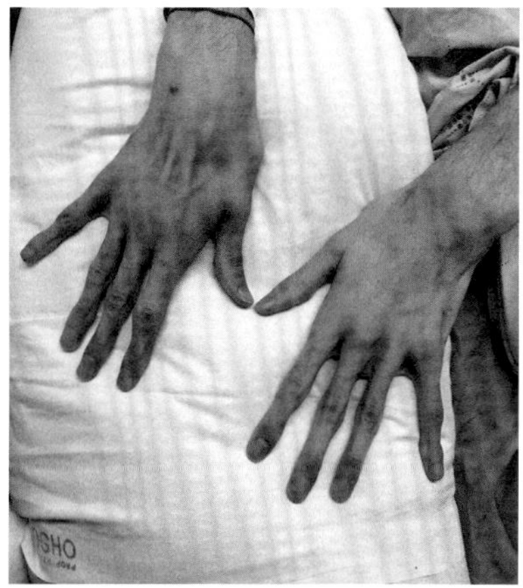

**Figure 5-3.** Long and slender fingers (arachnodactyly) in a patient with Marfan syndrome.

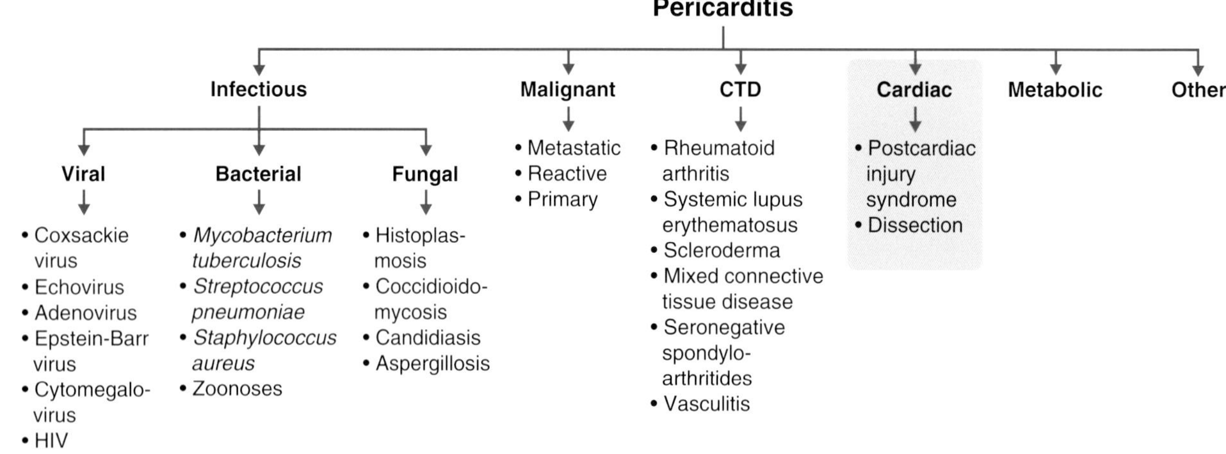

**What are the various causes of postcardiac injury syndrome?**

PCIS can be caused by myocardial infarction (ie, infarct pericarditis), Dressler's syndrome (ie, postmyocardial infarction syndrome), trauma, and postpericardiotomy syndrome.[1]

**What are the clinical features of infarct pericarditis?**

Infarct pericarditis (ie, pericarditis epistenocardica) occurs when there is transmural or near transmural infarction. It is limited to the pericardium adjacent to the zone of infarction and occurs early in the course of myocardial infarction (unlike Dressler's syndrome, which is delayed). Pericardial friction rubs are usually present and tend to be monophasic, with a peak incidence between the first and third days.[1]

**What are the clinical features of Dressler's syndrome?**

Dressler's syndrome is characterized by severe pleuritic chest pain, fever, pericardial friction rub, and elevated erythrocyte sedimentation rate. It can develop even without transmural infarction. Onset is typically 1 week to several months after infarction. Pericardial effusion occurs in around half of patients, and concurrent pleural involvement is common.[1]

**What is the mechanism of pericardial disease associated with aortic dissection?**

Dissecting aortic aneurysms can rupture into the pericardium, which may lead to sudden death via cardiac tamponade. Pericardial effusion may also develop slowly over a longer period of time (weeks to months), allowing massive amounts of blood (as much as 1500 mL) to encase the heart. Surgical drainage is required.[1]

## METABOLIC CAUSES OF PERICARDITIS

### What are the metabolic causes of pericarditis?

**Asterixis and a pericardial friction rub.**

Uremia.

**Associated with treatment for uremia.**

Dialysis-related pericarditis.

**The development of pericarditis and associated pericardial effusion in this condition is often slow, mirroring its effect on metabolism.**

Hypothyroidism.[1]

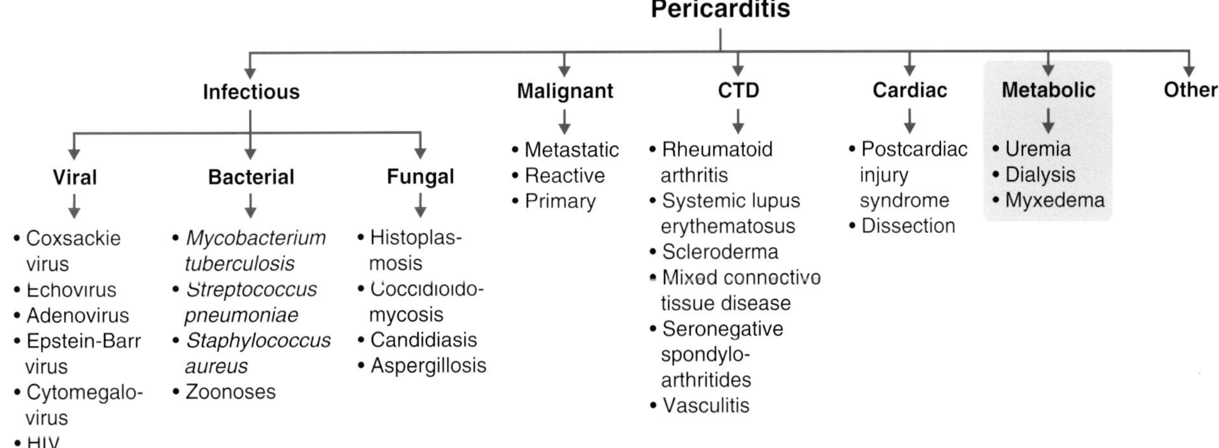


**What are the clinical features of uremic pericarditis?**

Uremic pericarditis generally does not occur unless blood urea nitrogen levels are >60 mg/dL (although this relationship is not strict). It does not discriminate between the underlying causes of renal failure. The typical electrocardiographic features of pericarditis are often absent. There is an increased risk of bleeding into the pericardium with associated cardiac tamponade in patients with uremic pericarditis.[1]

**What is dialysis-related pericarditis?**

Dialysis-related pericarditis describes the development of pericarditis in dialysis patients despite good biochemical control of renal failure. Its pathogenesis is not known, but it is significantly less common in patients who receive peritoneal dialysis compared with those who receive hemodialysis. Precipitants include inadequate dialysis, volume overload, and systemic infection.[1]

**What are the clinical features of the pericardial involvement that occurs with hypothyroidism?**

Pericardial involvement occurs in severe cases of hypothyroidism (ie, myxedema). It typically manifests as a pericardial effusion; signs of pericardial inflammation are almost always absent. Pericardial involvement is virtually always completely reversed with adequate thyroid hormone replacement therapy.[1]

## OTHER CAUSES OF PERICARDITIS

### What are the other causes of pericarditis?

**Iatrogenic complications.**

Medication and radiation therapy.

**No underlying cause is identified despite a thorough workup.**

Idiopathic.

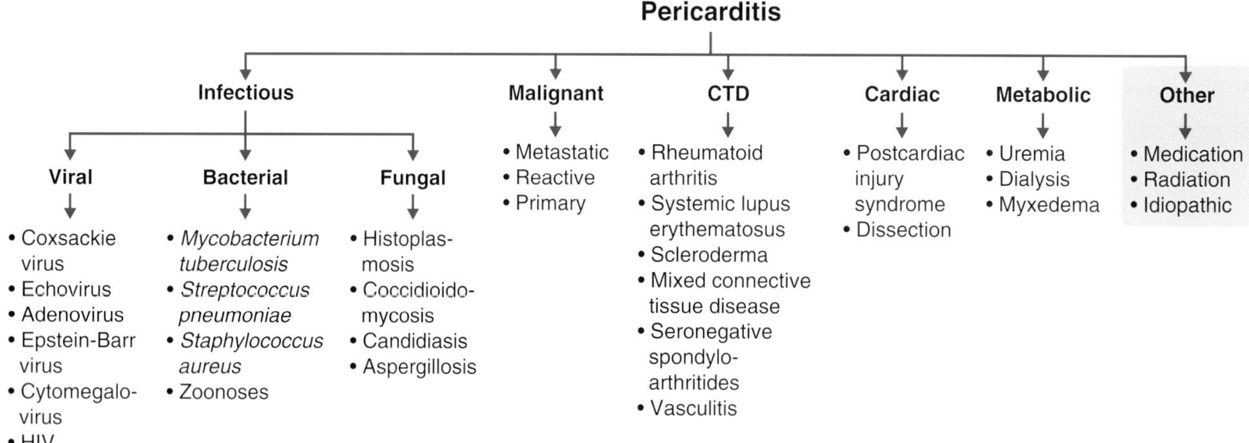


**What medications are associated with pericarditis?**

Numerous medications can be associated with pericardial disease, typically manifesting as acute pericarditis or inflammatory pericardial effusion. Some of the more widely used agents include penicillins (eg, ampicillin), sulfa drugs, thiazides, amiodarone, procainamide, cyclosporine, sirolimus, minoxidil, hydralazine, and doxorubicin. Anticoagulants and thrombolytics can precipitate bleeding into the pericardial space when there is preexisting pericarditis.[1]

**What are the clinical features of pericardial disease related to radiation therapy?**

Radiation therapy for diseases arising in the vicinity of the pericardium, such as mediastinal lymphoma, breast cancer, and lung cancer, frequently leads to pericardial disease. Severity depends on radiation dose, duration of treatment, and extent of the radiation field. While acute pericarditis can develop at the time of therapy, pericardial disease related to radiation is most commonly delayed, sometimes for many years, and most often presents as a chronic effusion or constrictive pericarditis.[1]

**What proportion of cases of acute pericarditis is idiopathic?**

A definitive underlying diagnosis is elusive in around 80% of cases of acute pericarditis. The majority of these cases are likely viral in nature.[7,8]

## Case Summary

A 32-year-old man with a history of recurrent painful oral and genital ulcers and arthritis presents with acute-onset pleuritic chest pain and is found to have oral ulcers and tender erythematous nodules over the anterior shins.

| | |
|---|---|
| ***What is the most likely cause of chest pain in this patient?*** | Acute pericarditis. |

BONUS QUESTIONS

| | |
|---|---|
| ***What is the nature of the extra heart sounds described in this case?*** | The patient in this case has a pericardial friction rub, the cardinal sign of pericarditis. The "scratchy" sounds occur as a result of friction between inflamed pericardial surfaces and are generally best appreciated with the diaphragm of the stethoscope along the left mid- to lower-sternal border. Rubs may be transient and often change with position or respiration. *Except when palpable in uremic pericarditis, friction rubs can only be appreciated by auscultation, one of many reasons the stethoscope is an irreplaceable tool in the arsenal of the skilled clinician.*[1] |
| ***What cardiac events generate the 3 components of the pericardial friction rub?*** | The complete 3-component friction rub is the result of 2 diastolic events (passive ventricular filling and atrial contraction) and 1 systolic event (ventricular contraction).[1] |
| ***What electrocardiographic findings are present in this case?*** | The ECG in this case (see Figure 5-1) demonstrates diffuse ST-segment elevation, diffuse PR-segment depression, and PR-segment elevation in aVR. These findings are consistent with acute pericarditis. |
| ***What is the most likely underlying cause of acute pericarditis in this case?*** | The patient in this case most likely has Behçet's disease, given the recurrent oral and genital ulcers, arthralgias/arthritis, and erythema nodosum (see Figure 15-3). |
| ***What are clinical features of the pericardial involvement that occurs with Behçet's disease?*** | The pericardium is the most common site of cardiac involvement in Behçet's disease. Manifestations include acute pericarditis, pericardial effusions ranging from small and asymptomatic to large with associated tamponade, and constrictive pericarditis. Of note, Behçet's disease can provoke thromboses of the major veins, mimicking pericardial constriction.[1] |
| ***How should this patient be treated?*** | Pericarditis related to Behçet's disease is generally self-limited and responsive to anti-inflammatory medications used to treat the disease itself.[1] |

## KEY POINTS

- Pericarditis describes inflammation of the pericardium, the fibrous sac that surrounds the heart.
- Pericarditis is most often an acute process but can become chronic and evolve into constrictive pericarditis.
- Acute pericarditis may be "dry" or associated with pericardial effusion, the size of which can range from trivial without hemodynamic significance to large and associated with cardiac tamponade.
- Symptoms of acute pericarditis include pleuritic chest pain, nonproductive cough, hiccups, and odynophagia.
- Physical findings of acute pericarditis include fever and pericardial friction rub, a high-pitched scratchy sound that may have 1, 2, or 3 components.
- The electrocardiographic findings of acute pericarditis include diffuse ST-segment elevation, diffuse PR-segment depression, and PR-segment elevation in lead aVR.
- The causes of pericarditis can be separated into the following categories: infectious, malignant, connective tissue disease, cardiac, metabolic, and other.
- Infectious pericarditis is most often viral in nature, but bacterial and fungal cases do occur.
- Cytology and flow cytometry of the pericardial fluid and biopsy of the pericardial tissue can be helpful in establishing the diagnosis of malignant pericarditis.
- Men are more likely than women to develop pericardial involvement from connective tissue disease.
- Postcardiac injury syndrome is an umbrella term that describes the development of pericarditis following cardiac injury.
- Uremia is the most common metabolic cause of pericarditis.
- The majority of cases of acute pericarditis are idiopathic, which are most likely undiagnosed viral infections.

## REFERENCES


1. Spodick DH. *The Pericardium: A Comprehensive Textbook*. New York, NY: Marcel Dekker, Inc.; 1997.
2. Mansoor AM, Karlapudi SP. Images in clinical medicine. Kussmaul's sign. *N Engl J Med*. 2015;372(2):e3.
3. Heidenreich PA, Eisenberg MJ, Kee LL, et al. Pericardial effusion in AIDS. Incidence and survival. *Circulation*. 1995;92(11):3229-3234.
4. Picardi JL, Kauffman CA, Schwarz J, Holmes JC, Phair JP, Fowler NO. Pericarditis caused by Histoplasma capsulatum. *Am J Cardiol*. 1976;37(1):82-88.
5. Imazio M, Demichelis B, Parrini I, et al. Relation of acute pericardial disease to malignancy. *Am J Cardiol*. 2005;95(11):1393-1394.
6. Klatt EC, Heitz DR. Cardiac metastases. *Cancer*. 1990;65(6):1456-1459.
7. Permanyer-Miralda G, Sagrista-Sauleda J, Soler-Soler J. Primary acute pericardial disease: a prospective series of 231 consecutive patients. *Am J Cardiol*. 1985;56(10):623-630.
8. Zayas R, Anguita M, Torres F, et al. Incidence of specific etiology and role of methods for specific etiologic diagnosis of primary acute pericarditis. *Am J Cardiol*. 1995;75(5):378-382.

# Chapter 6

# TACHYCARDIA

## Case: A 65-year-old woman with palpitations

A 65-year-old woman with a history of coronary artery disease presents to the emergency department with chest palpitations. She had an ST-elevation myocardial infarction at 62 years of age, and underwent percutaneous coronary intervention with deployment of a drug-eluting stent to the circumflex artery. There was no evidence of left ventricular systolic dysfunction at the time of discharge or at any time during her follow-up with cardiology. She has been adherent to medications including aspirin, atorvastatin, metoprolol succinate, and lisinopril. She began feeling chest palpitations on the day of presentation. She has not experienced chest pain or light-headedness.

Heart rate is regular and 144 beats per minute, and blood pressure is 118/69 mm Hg. Jugular venous pressure is estimated to be 7 cm $H_2O$ with intermittent large outward pulsations. No murmurs are appreciated. The lungs are clear.

Electrocardiogram (ECG) is shown in Figure 6-1.

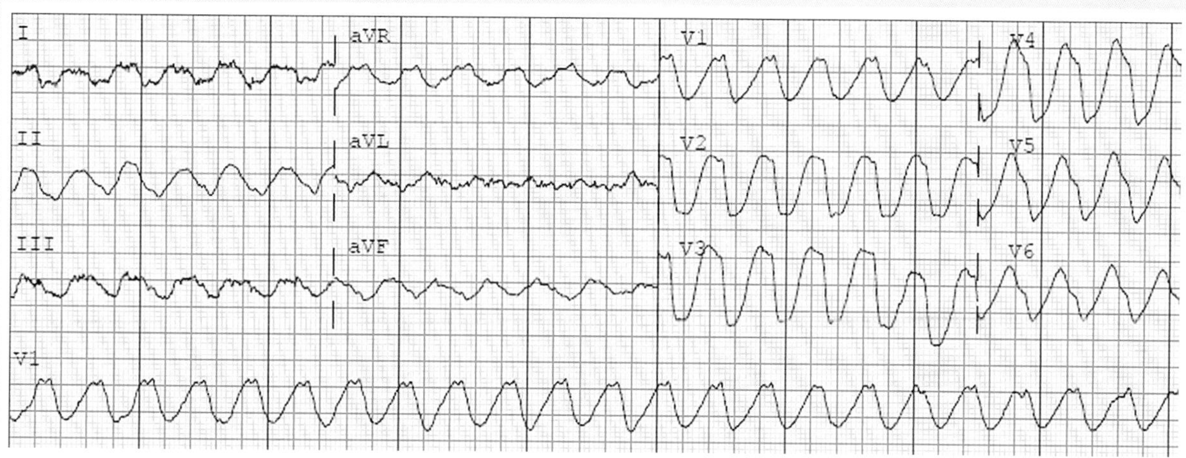


**Figure 6-1.**

Serum biomarkers are negative, and repeat transthoracic echocardiography shows an area of lateral wall akinesis but preserved left ventricular systolic function. Coronary angiography demonstrates a patent stent in the circumflex and patent native vessels.

***What rhythm disturbance is present in this patient?***

**What is the path of electrical conduction in the normal heart?**

In the normal heart, an impulse spontaneously originates from the sinoatrial (SA) node, which is located in the subepicardial surface at the junction of the right atrium and superior vena cava. The impulse propagates through the myocytes of the right and left atria simultaneously before reaching the atrioventricular (AV) node, which is located in the inferior portion of the right atrium. From there, the impulse is conducted to the bundle of His within the membranous septum, which then separates into the right and left bundle branches supplying the right and left ventricles, respectively (see Figure 1-2).

**How is heart rate regulated?**

The sympathetic and parasympathetic nervous systems innervate the conduction system of the heart. Parasympathetic tone decreases SA node automaticity and AV node conduction, whereas sympathetic input increases SA node automaticity and AV node conduction.[1]

**What is the definition of tachycardia in adults?**

The average resting heart rate in adults is 70 beats per minute. Tachycardia is classically defined by a heart rate greater than 100 beats per minute.[2,3]

**What are the 3 basic mechanisms of tachycardia?**

Tachycardia can occur as a result of increased pacemaker automaticity (eg, sinus tachycardia), triggered activity outside of the normal conduction system (eg, ectopic impulses), or reentry (eg, AV nodal reentrant tachycardia [AVNRT]).[3]

**What is the relationship between cardiac output and heart rate?**

Cardiac output (CO) is equal to the forward stroke volume (SV) of the left ventricle per beat multiplied by heart rate (HR).[1]

$$CO = SV \times HR$$

**What are the symptoms of tachycardia?**

Patients with tachycardia may be asymptomatic. Symptoms may include palpitations, light-headedness, syncope, chest pain, and dyspnea.

**What are the physical findings of tachycardia?**

The cardinal physical finding of tachycardia is a fast pulse rate, which can be regular or irregular. Additional findings may include hypotension and cool extremities.

**What are the 2 electrocardiographic categories of tachycardia?**

Tachycardia can be associated with a narrow QRS complex or a wide QRS complex.

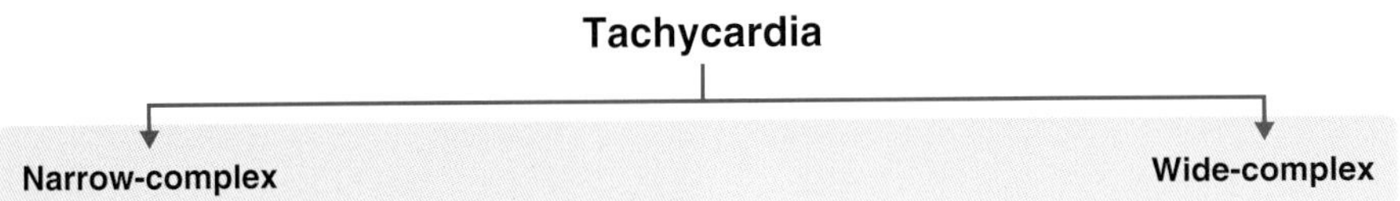


**What is the definition of a wide QRS complex?**

A wide QRS complex is defined electrocardiographically as QRS duration >120 ms (see Figure 1-2).

**The small boxes on the electrocardiogram represent how many milliseconds?**

At the standard paper speed of 25 mm/s, each small box (1 mm in width) on the ECG corresponds to 40 ms. Each large box, which is composed of 5 small boxes, represents 200 ms (see Figure 1-2).

## NARROW-COMPLEX TACHYCARDIA

**What are the 2 subcategories of narrow-complex tachycardia?**

Narrow-complex tachycardia can be associated with a regular rhythm or an irregular rhythm.

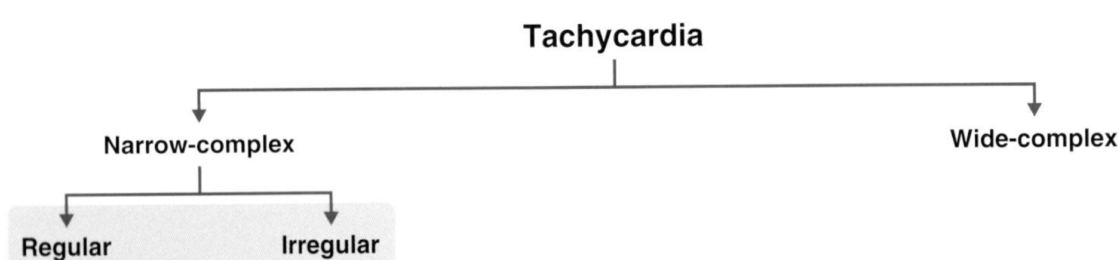


**What are the electrocardiographic characteristics of a regular rhythm?**

Regular rhythm is defined electrocardiographically by the presence of QRS complexes that are separated by a constant interval (ie, the R-R interval is constant).

## NARROW-COMPLEX TACHYCARDIA WITH REGULAR RHYTHM

### What are the causes of narrow-complex tachycardia with regular rhythm?

**A 34-year-old man presents with purulent cough, fever, leukocytosis, and a heart rate of 125 beats per minute.**

Sinus tachycardia related to infection.

**This rhythm most commonly originates in the right atrium.**

Atrial flutter.

**Dual AV nodal pathways physiology is required for this type of tachycardic rhythm.**

Atrioventricular nodal reentrant tachycardia (AVNRT).

**Wolff-Parkinson-White syndrome.**

Atrioventricular reentrant tachycardia (AVRT).

**This rhythm originates from a focus within the atria rather than the SA node.**

Atrial tachycardia.

**No visible or discernible P waves associated with the QRS complexes.**

Junctional tachycardia.

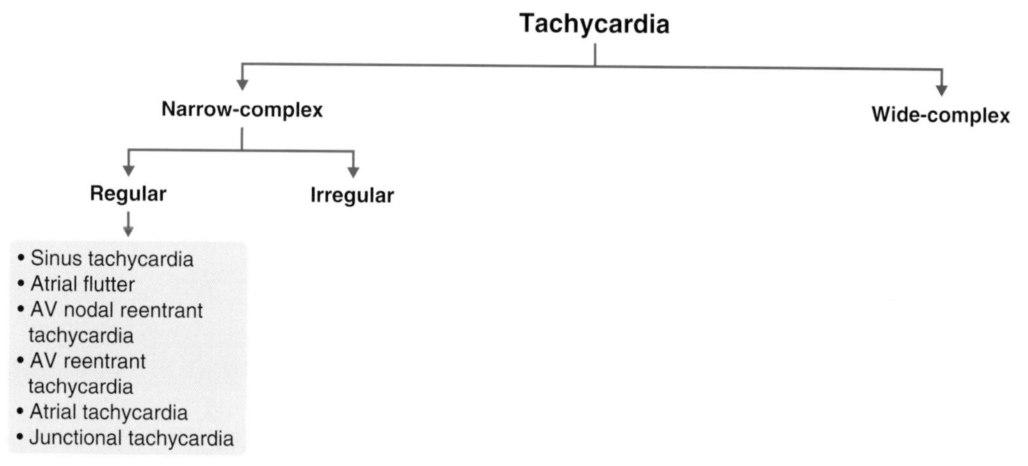


**What are the characteristics of sinus tachycardia?**

Sinus tachycardia is characterized by gradual onset with heart rates generally between 100 and 140 beats per minute (maximum HR is approximately 220 beats per minute minus the patient's age). Rhythms that are generated from the SA node are electrocardiographically characterized by P waves that are morphologically identical and upright (ie, positive) in leads I and aVF.

**What are the characteristics of atrial flutter?**

Atrial flutter is a type of a reentrant circuit that involves an area near the tricuspid valve in the right atrium, called the cavotricuspid isthmus, as an essential part of its circuit. The atrial rate is typically 240 to 350 beats per minute. Commonly, the atrial rate is 300 beats per minute, and there is 2:1 conduction within the AV node, resulting in a ventricular rate of 150 beats per minute, which can be a clue to the diagnosis.[4]

**What are the characteristics of atrioventricular nodal reentrant tachycardia?**

AVNRT typically occurs in patients without evidence of structural heart disease. Onset is abrupt with ventricular rates generally between 150 and 250 beats per minute. AVNRT requires dual AV nodal physiology (2 pathways with different electrophysiologic properties), 1 slow (with a shorter refractory period) and 1 fast (with a longer refractory period). Dual pathways are present in up to one-third of the general population. Normal sinus rhythm usually conducts through the fast pathway, whereas competing anterograde/retrograde conduction nullifies transmission through the slow pathway. Typical AVNRT (common) is triggered by atrial premature depolarization with anterograde conduction through the slow pathway (while the fast pathway remains refractory). Atypical AVNRT (uncommon) is triggered by ventricular premature depolarization with retrograde conduction through the slow pathway (Figure 6-2).[3,5]

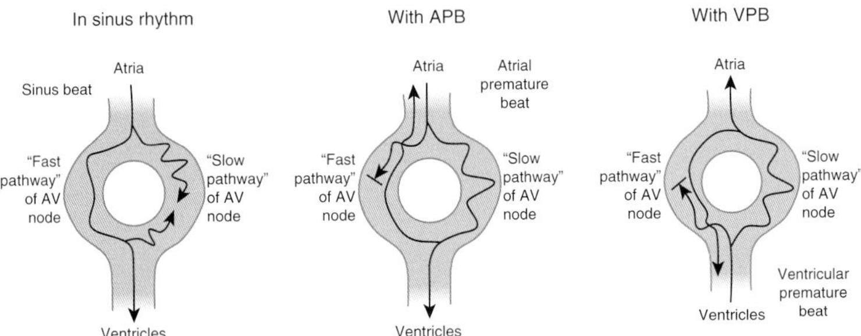


**Figure 6-2.** Model of dual AV nodal pathways physiology in sinus rhythm (left), with an atrial premature beat (APB), which initiates typical "slow-fast" AVNRT (middle), and with a ventricular premature beat (VPB), which initiates atypical "fast-slow" AVNRT (right). (Adapted from Mani BC, Pavri BB. Dual atrioventricular nodal pathways physiology: a review of relevant anatomy, electrophysiology, and electrocardiographic manifestations. *Indian Pacing Electrophysiol J.* 2014;14(1):12-25.)

**What are the characteristics of atrioventricular reentrant tachycardia?**

AVRT is a type of reentrant tachycardia that requires the presence of a bypass tract (ie, accessory pathway) between the atria and ventricles that is capable of conducting in the anterograde direction, in the retrograde direction, or in both directions. When the reentrant loop is characterized by anterograde conduction down the AV node and retrograde conduction through the bypass tract (orthodromic), the QRS complex is narrow. When it is characterized by anterograde conduction through the bypass tract and retrograde conduction through the AV node (antidromic), the QRS complex is wide. Onset is abrupt with ventricular rates generally between 150 and 250 beats per minute. In sinus rhythm, when there is anterograde conduction down the accessory pathway, an initial slurring of the QRS complex can be seen and is known as a delta wave (Figure 6-3).[4]

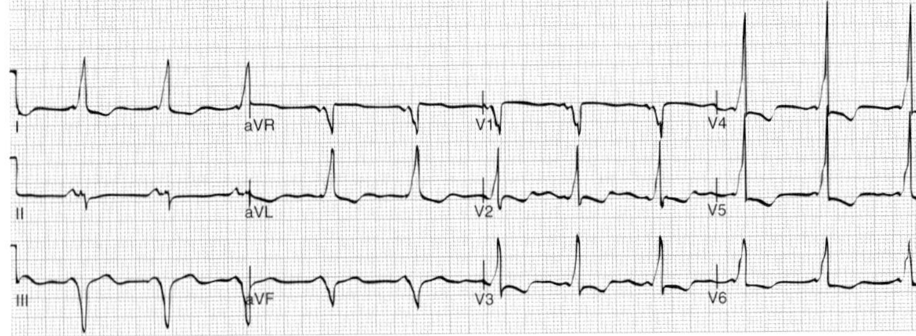


**Figure 6-3.** Sinus rhythm with short PR interval and delta wave (ie, pre-excitation pattern) consistent with the presence of an accessory pathway. The delta wave is positive in all leads except aVR and $V_1$ where it is negative. (From Woods SL, Froelicher ES, Motzer SA, Bridges EJ. *Cardiac Nursing*. 6th ed. Philadelphia, PA: Wolters Kluwer Health; 2010.)

**What are the characteristics of atrial tachycardia?**

Atrial tachycardia is defined as an atrial rhythm with a rate greater than 100 beats per minute originating outside the SA node. Mechanisms can be reentry (micro- or macroreentrant circuits) or focal activity (automatic or triggered) within the atria. Onset is abrupt with ventricular rates generally between 150 and 250 beats per minute. Atrial tachycardia tends to occur in repetitive short bursts, usually preceded by a "warm up" period in which the atrial rate increases over a period of 5 to 10 seconds before stabilizing.[4]

**Junctional tachycardia can occur as a result of what commonly prescribed cardiac medication?**

Junctional tachycardia is associated with digitalis toxicity.[6]

## NARROW-COMPLEX TACHYCARDIA WITH IRREGULAR RHYTHM

### What are the causes of narrow-complex tachycardia with irregular rhythm?

**No P waves on ECG.**

Atrial fibrillation.

**This rhythm is strongly associated with lung disease, particularly chronic obstructive pulmonary disease.**

Multifocal atrial tachycardia (MAT).[7]

**You are confused because you identify the presence of flutter waves on ECG, but the rhythm is irregular.**

Atrial flutter with variable AV conduction.

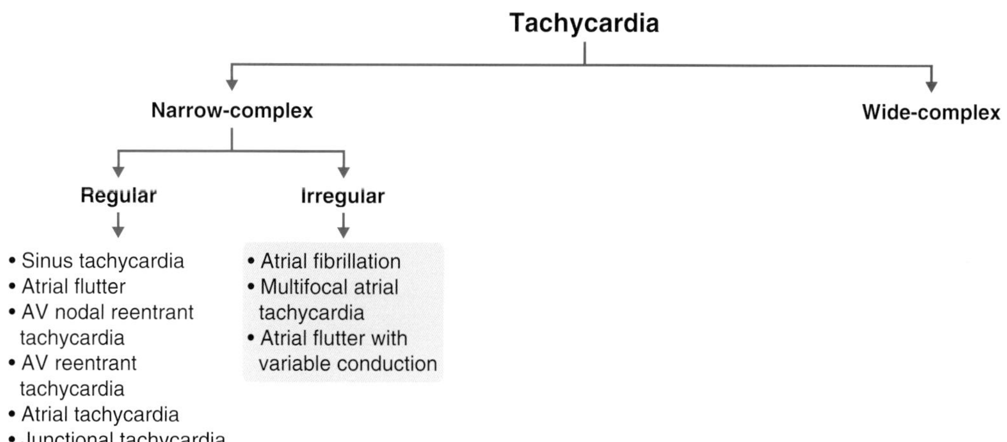


**What are the characteristics of atrial fibrillation?**

Atrial fibrillation is the most common dysrhythmia. It is the result of multiple electrical wavelets in the atria occurring simultaneously so that there is no coordinated atrial contraction. Risk factors include older age, male sex, hypertension, and underlying cardiac disease. The onset of rapid heart rates can be sudden, particularly in patients with acute atrial fibrillation, or gradual, which usually occurs in patients with chronic atrial fibrillation, with ventricular rates generally between 100 and 220 beats per minute. In older patients with chronic atrial fibrillation, rate control and rhythm control strategies are associated with equivalent outcomes.[4,8]

**What are the characteristics of multifocal atrial tachycardia?**

MAT is the result of increased atrial automaticity, most commonly related to hypoxia, increased atrial pressure, or theophylline treatment. Onset is gradual with ventricular rates generally between 100 and 150 beats per minute. MAT is defined electrocardiographically by the following features: atrial rate greater than 100 beats per minute, at least 3 morphologically distinct P waves associated with variable P-P intervals, and an isoelectric baseline between P waves.[4,9]

CARDIOLOGY

**Does flutter wave morphology change in patients with atrial flutter with variable AV conduction?**

In atrial flutter with variable AV conduction, flutter wave morphology remains the same, but the rate at which the waves conduct through the AV node changes. Flutter waves can be identified between the QRS complexes to determine the flutter rate (the interval between 2 flutter waves). The ratio of AV conduction can then be calculated by dividing the flutter rate by the ventricular rate.

## WIDE-COMPLEX TACHYCARDIA

**What are the 2 types of QRS morphologies associated with wide-complex tachycardia?**

Wide-complex tachycardia can be associated with uniform QRS morphology (monomorphic) or variable QRS morphology (polymorphic).

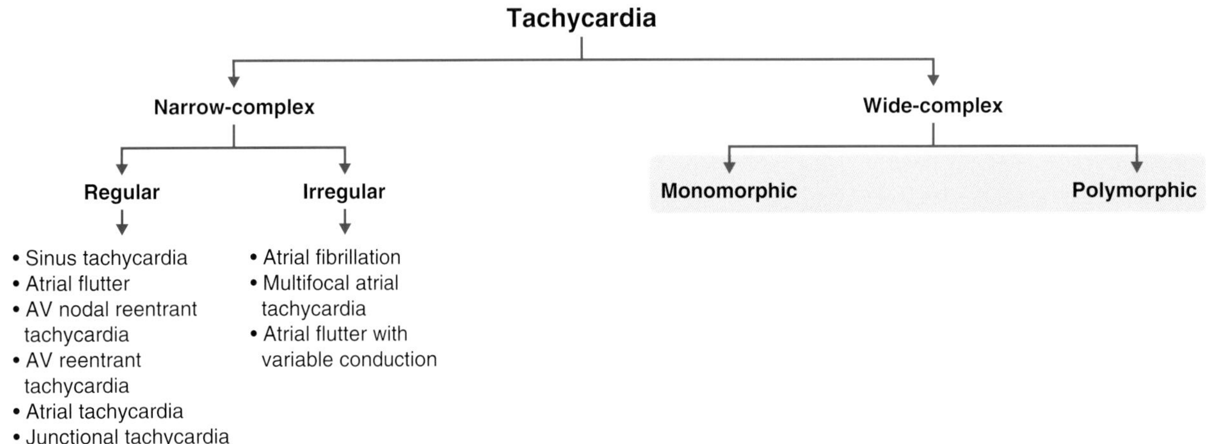


## MONOMORPHIC WIDE-COMPLEX TACHYCARDIA

**What are the 2 subcategories of monomorphic wide-complex tachycardia?**

Monomorphic wide-complex tachycardia can be associated with a regular rhythm or an irregular rhythm.

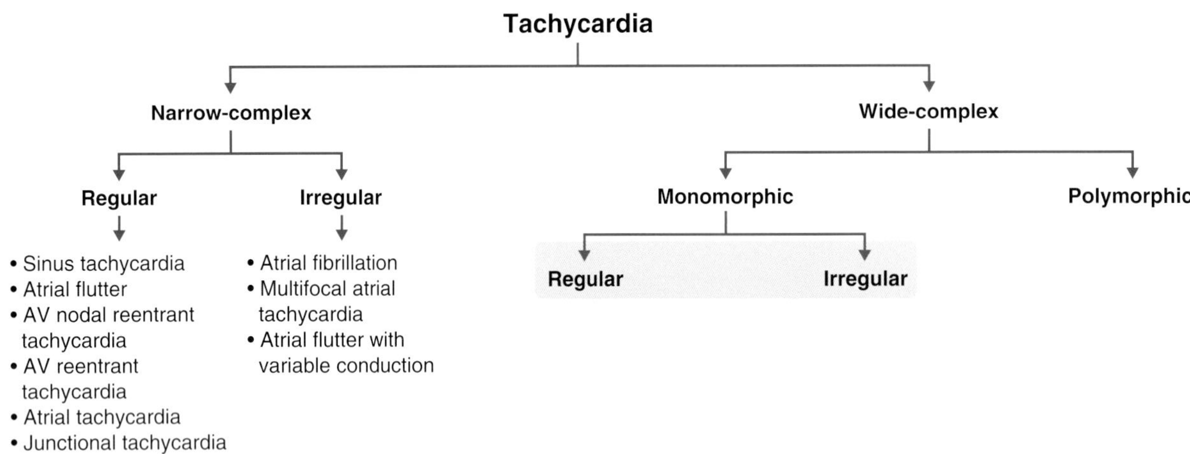


## MONOMORPHIC WIDE-COMPLEX TACHYCARDIA WITH REGULAR RHYTHM

### What are the causes of monomorphic wide-complex tachycardia with regular rhythm?

**Often associated with a myocardial scar.**

Monomorphic ventricular tachycardia (VT).

**These rhythms originate above the ventricles.**

Regular supraventricular tachycardia (SVT) with a baseline wide QRS complex (ie, bundle branch block) and regular SVT with aberrant conduction (eg, rate related).

**This rhythm is generated from a device.**

Pacemaker-facilitated tachycardia.

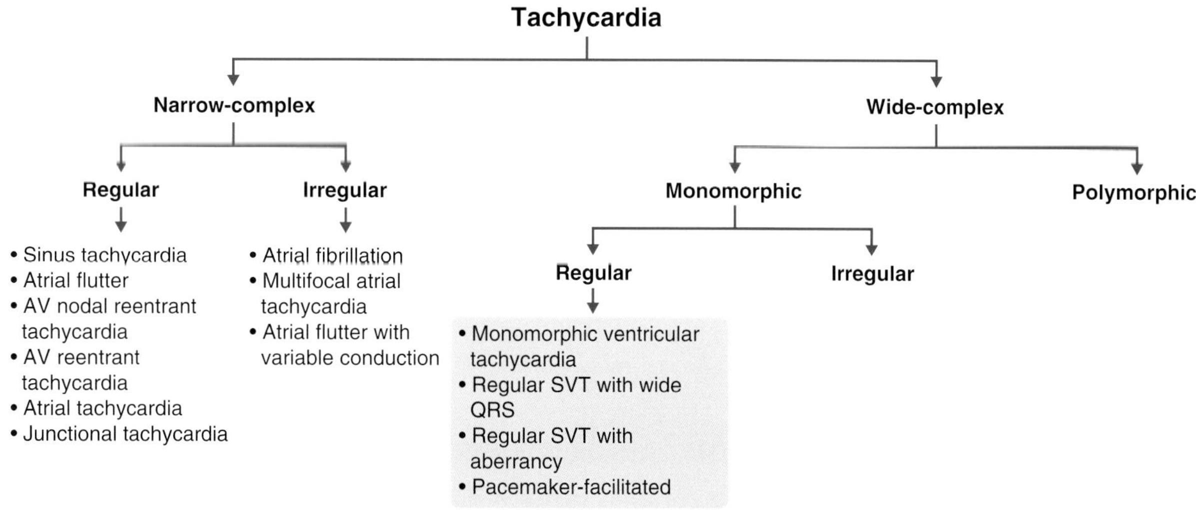


**What are the characteristics of monomorphic VT?**

Monomorphic VT most commonly occurs in association with myocardial scarring (from prior myocardial infarction), but also occurs in the setting of dilated cardiomyopathy, prior cardiac surgery, infiltrative disorders, and hypertrophic cardiomyopathy. It may also occur in the structurally normal heart. It is sustained when it lasts at least 30 seconds or is associated with hemodynamic instability. Patients with hemodynamic instability should immediately be treated with synchronized direct current cardioversion.[3,10,11]

**What is the difference between SVT with a baseline wide QRS complex and SVT with aberrancy?**

SVT with a baseline wide QRS complex refers to a baseline block in one of the bundle branches (right bundle branch or left bundle branch). SVT with aberrancy, on the other hand, refers to a "functional" block that occurs in one of the bundle branches only in certain circumstances (eg, tachycardia-related aberrancy).[12]

**What validated electrocardiographic algorithm can distinguish VT from either regular SVT with a baseline wide QRS complex or regular SVT with aberrancy?**

The Brugada criteria is the most commonly used ECG algorithm to distinguish VT from either regular SVT with a baseline wide QRS complex or regular SVT with aberrancy (Figure 6-4). The majority of wide-complex tachycardias are VTs.[13]

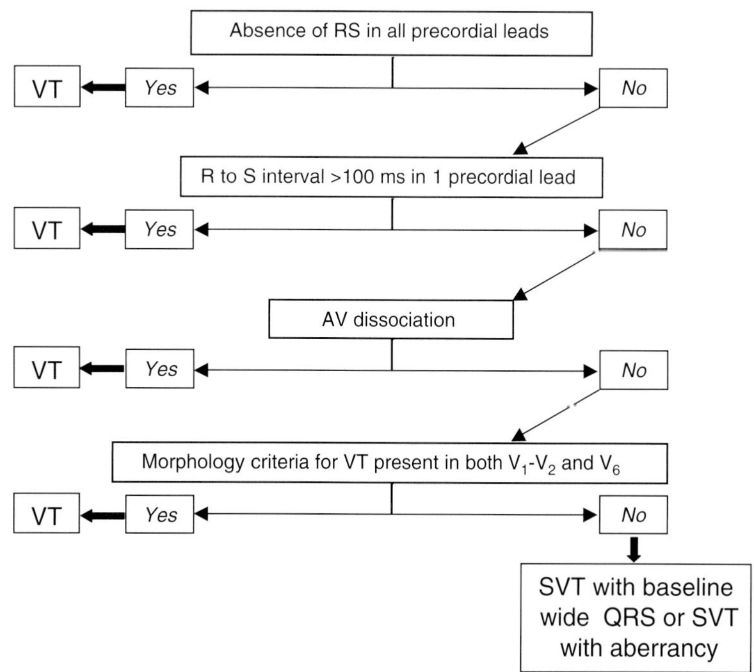


**Figure 6-4.** Brugada criteria for distinguishing ventricular tachycardia (VT) from either supraventricular tachycardia (SVT) with a baseline wide QRS complex or SVT with aberrancy. (Adapted from Brugada P, Brugada J, Mont L, Smeets J, Andries EW. A new approach to the differential diagnosis of a regular tachycardia with a wide QRS complex. *Circulation*. 1991;83(5):1649-1659. Copyright © 1991, American Heart Association.)

CARDIOLOGY

**What are the mechanisms of pacemaker-facilitated tachycardia?**

Pacemaker-facilitated tachycardia occurs either as a result of pacemaker-mediated tachycardia (PMT), or as a result of tracking of an atrial rhythm. Between the two, PMT is more common. It occurs in patients with dual-chamber pacemakers and intact retrograde conduction when a ventricular contraction (either spontaneous or paced) is conducted retrograde through the AV node, where it depolarizes the atria. The retrograde P wave is then sensed by the atrial lead. The pacemaker waits for the programmed AV interval and then triggers ventricular pacing. However, retrograde conduction through the AV node occurs again, followed by paced ventricular activation in an endless loop. Pacemaker-facilitated tachycardia due to tracking of an atrial rhythm occurs when a supraventricular tachyarrhythmia (eg, atrial tachycardia) is sensed by the atrial lead, which attempts to maintain atrioventricular synchrony by triggering ventricular pacing at the same atrial rate.[14]

## MONOMORPHIC WIDE-COMPLEX TACHYCARDIA WITH IRREGULAR RHYTHM

### What are the causes of monomorphic wide-complex tachycardia with irregular rhythm?

**These rhythms originate above the ventricles.**

Irregular SVT with a baseline wide QRS complex and irregular SVT with aberrant conduction.

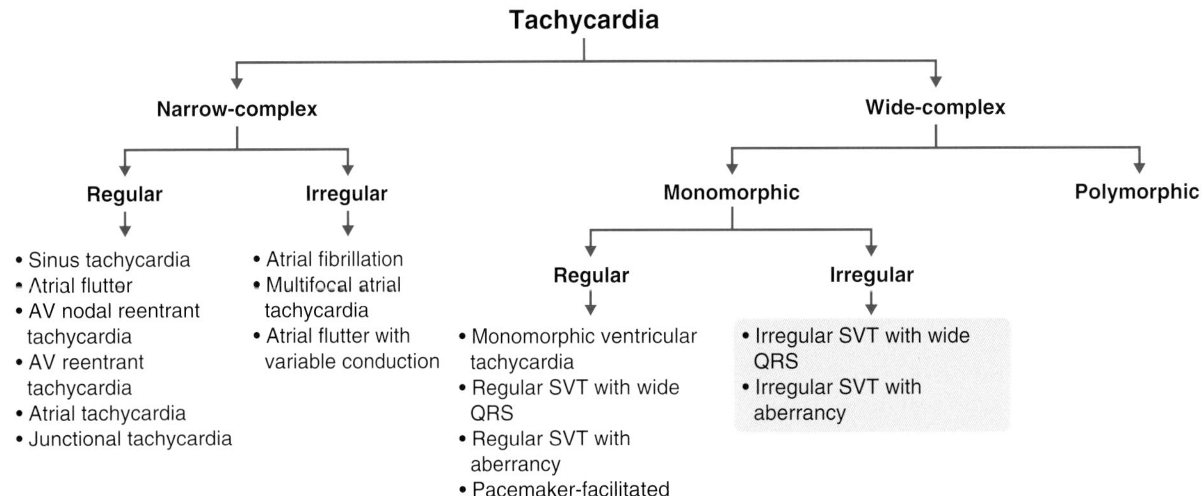


**What are some examples of irregular SVT with a wide QRS complex?**

Examples of irregular SVT with a wide QRS complex include the following: atrial fibrillation with an accessory pathway (known as preexcited atrial fibrillation); atrial flutter with variable conduction and a baseline bundle branch block; and multifocal atrial tachycardia with a baseline bundle branch block.

**Does aberrant conduction occur more commonly in the pattern of a right or left bundle branch block?**

Aberrant conduction most commonly occurs in a right bundle branch block pattern because the refractory period of the right bundle is longer than that of the left.[15]

## POLYMORPHIC WIDE-COMPLEX TACHYCARDIA

### What are the causes of polymorphic wide-complex tachycardia?

**A ventricular rhythm with variable QRS morphology most commonly associated with ischemia.**

Polymorphic VT.

**A type of polymorphic VT described by the phrase, "twisting around the points."**

Torsades de pointes (Figure 6-5).[3]

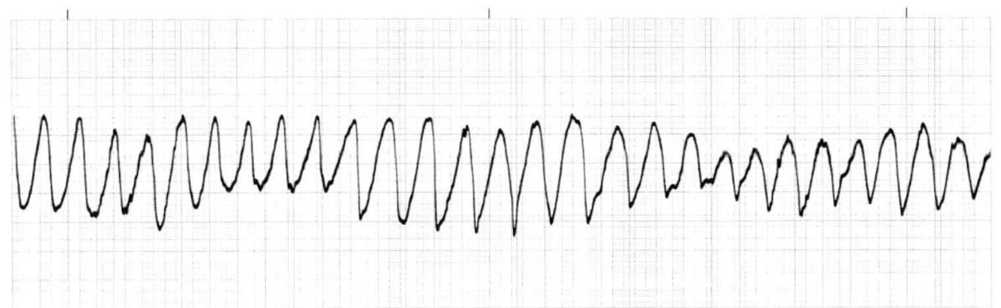

**Figure 6-5.** Torsades de pointes. The QRS changes from negative to positive polarity and appears to twist around the isoelectric line. (From Huff J. *ECG Workout Exercises in Arrythmia Interpretation*. 7th ed. Philadelphia, PA: Wolters Kluwer; 2017.)

**Disorganized ventricular electrical activity that is invariably fatal without prompt treatment.**

Ventricular fibrillation (VF). *VF does not produce true QRS complexes per se because there is no coordinated ventricular contraction.*

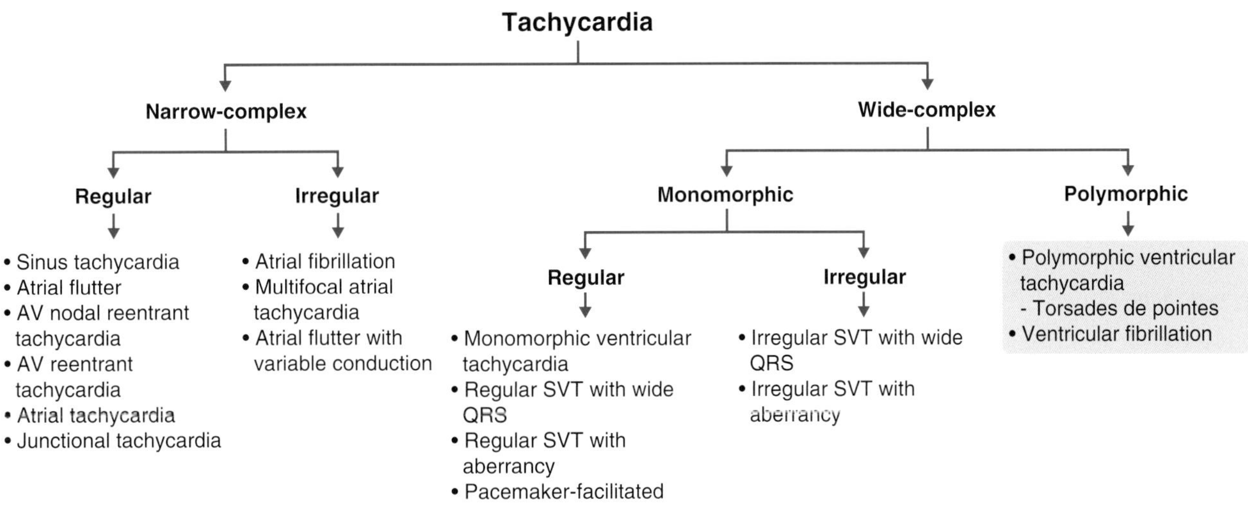


**What are the characteristics of polymorphic VT?**

Polymorphic VT most commonly occurs in the context of acute ischemia, but also occurs in patients with electrolyte disturbances, long QT syndrome, Brugada syndrome, and structurally normal hearts. Evaluation for underlying coronary artery disease is important in patients with polymorphic VT. Patients with hemodynamic instability should immediately be treated with defibrillation.[10,11]

**What are the characteristics of torsades de pointes?**

Torsades de pointes is a type of polymorphic VT that occurs in the setting of a prolonged QT interval, such as in genetic syndromes or exposure to QT-prolonging medications. It can be short and self-terminating, causing palpitations and syncope, or if sustained it can deteriorate into VF and cardiac arrest. Intravenous magnesium can be used to terminate torsades de pointes. Patients with hemodynamic instability should immediately be treated with defibrillation.[10,16]

**What are the characteristics of ventricular fibrillation?**

VF is an unstable and pulseless condition characterized by rapid and disorganized ventricular electrical activity resulting in the absence of coordinated ventricular contraction. The electrocardiographic features of VF include irregular QRS complexes of variable morphology and amplitude. Patients should immediately be treated with defibrillation.[10]

## Case Summary

A 65-year-old woman with a history of ST-elevation myocardial infarction was admitted with palpitations and hemodynamically stable tachycardia.

***What rhythm disturbance is present in this patient?***

Monomorphic ventricular tachycardia.

### BONUS QUESTIONS

***What are the electrocardiographic characteristics of the tachycardia in this case?***

The ECG in this case (see Figure 6-1) demonstrates a wide-complex tachycardia with uniform QRS morphology (monomorphic) and regular rhythm.

***What are the possible causes of monomorphic wide-complex tachycardia with regular rhythm?***

The differential diagnosis for monomorphic wide-complex tachycardia with regular rhythm includes monomorphic VT, regular SVT with a baseline wide QRS complex, regular SVT with aberrancy, and PMT. This patient does not have a pacemaker, so the differential diagnosis can be narrowed to monomorphic VT or SVT with a wide QRS complex. The Brugada criteria can be used to differentiate these conditions (see Figure 6-4).

***After which step in the Brugada criteria is the diagnosis of VT made in this case?***

The diagnosis of VT is made after the first step in the Brugada algorithm (see Figure 6-4). There is no RS complex in any of the precordial leads.

***What is the most likely cause of monomorphic VT in this patient?***

The most common substrate for monomorphic VT is myocardial scarring related to infarction. Indeed, it the most likely explanation in this case given the history of myocardial infarction.[11]

***What effective strategy can be used to prevent sudden death related to VT in patients with heart disease?***

Implantable cardioverter-defibrillators reduce mortality as a method of primary prevention in select patients with reduced systolic function.[11]

***When is it appropriate to treat acute sustained monomorphic VT with pharmacologic cardioversion instead of electrical cardioversion?***

When there is hemodynamic stability, monomorphic VT can be treated with pharmacologic cardioversion, using agents such as lidocaine, procainamide, and amiodarone. If pharmacologic conversion of VT is unsuccessful, synchronized electrical cardioversion can be attempted.[11]

***What long-term treatment options are available for patients with a history of sustained monomorphic VT?***

There are a variety of modalities available to treat patients who survive an episode of sustained monomorphic VT. If the episode was unrelated to a clear reversible cause (eg, electrolyte disturbance), then patients should receive an implantable cardioverter-defibrillator for secondary prevention. Patients with recurrent episodes of sustained monomorphic VT can be treated with pharmacologic agents (eg, β-blocker, amiodarone) and radiofrequency catheter ablation.[11]

## KEY POINTS

- Tachycardia in adults is defined as a heart rate >100 beats per minute.
- The mechanisms of tachycardia include increased pacemaker automaticity (eg, sinus tachycardia), triggered activity outside of the normal conduction system (eg, ectopic impulses), and reentry.
- Tachycardia can be asymptomatic or associated with palpitations, light-headedness, syncope, or dyspnea.
- The treatment and prognosis of tachycardia vary widely depending on the underlying condition.
- Tachycardia can be associated with a narrow QRS complex (<120 ms) or a wide QRS complex (>120 ms).
- Narrow-complex tachycardia can be associated with a regular rhythm or an irregular rhythm.
- Wide-complex tachycardia can associated with uniform QRS morphology (monomorphic) or variable QRS morphology (polymorphic).
- Monomorphic wide-complex tachycardia can be associated with a regular rhythm or an irregular rhythm.
- Idioventricular tachycardia always presents with a wide QRS complex, whereas SVT can present with a narrow or wide QRS complex.

## REFERENCES


1. Mangrum JM, DiMarco JP. The evaluation and management of bradycardia. *N Engl J Med.* 2000;342(10):703-709.
2. Berne RML, Levy MN. *Physiology*. 4th ed. St. Louis, MO: Mosby, Inc.; 1998.
3. Marino PL. *The ICU Book*. 3rd ed. Philadelphia, PA: Lippincott Williams & Wilkins—a Wolters Kluwer business; 2007.
4. Link MS. Clinical practice. Evaluation and initial treatment of supraventricular tachycardia. *N Engl J Med.* 2012;367(15):1438-1448.
5. Mani BC, Pavri BB. Dual atrioventricular nodal pathways physiology: a review of relevant anatomy, electrophysiology, and electrocardiographic manifestations. *Indian Pacing Electrophysiol J.* 2014;14(1):12-25.
6. Barold SS, Hayes DL. Non-paroxysmal junctional tachycardia with type I exit block. *Heart.* 2002;88(3):288.
7. McCord J, Borzak S. Multifocal atrial tachycardia. *Chest.* 1998;113(1):203-209.
8. Wyse DG, Waldo AL, DiMarco JP, et al. A comparison of rate control and rhythm control in patients with atrial fibrillation. *N Engl J Med.* 2002;347(23):1825-1833.
9. Shine KI, Kastor JA, Yurchak PM. Multifocal atrial tachycardia. Clinical and electrocardiographic features in 32 patients. *N Engl J Med.* 1968;279(7):344-349.
10. Link MS, Berkow LC, Kudenchuk PJ, et al. Part 7: Adult advanced cardiovascular life support: 2015 American Heart Association guidelines update for cardiopulmonary resuscitation and emergency cardiovascular care. *Circulation.* 2015;132(18 suppl 2):S444-S464.
11. Roberts-Thomson KC, Lau DH, Sanders P. The diagnosis and management of ventricular arrhythmias. *Nat Rev Cardiol.* 2011;8(6):311-321.
12. Eckardt L, Breithardt G, Kirchhof P. Approach to wide complex tachycardias in patients without structural heart disease. *Heart.* 2006;92(5):704-711.
13. Brugada P, Brugada J, Mont L, Smeets J, Andries EW. A new approach to the differential diagnosis of a regular tachycardia with a wide QRS complex. *Circulation.* 1991;83(5):1649-1659.
14. Ip JE, Markowitz SM, Liu CF, Cheung JW, Thomas G, Lerman BB. Differentiating pacemaker-mediated tachycardia from tachycardia due to atrial tracking: utility of V-A-A-V versus V-A-V response after postventricular atrial refractory period extension. *Heart Rhythm.* 2011;8(8):1185-1191.
15. Myerburg RJ, Stewart JW, Hoffman BF. Electrophysiological properties of the canine peripheral A-V conducting system. *Circ Res.* 1970;26(3):361-378.
16. Pellegrini CN, Scheinman MM. Clinical management of ventricular tachycardia. *Curr Probl Cardiol.* 2010;35(9):453-504.

SECTION 4

# Endocrinology

Chapter 7

## ADRENAL INSUFFICIENCY

### Case: A 44-year-old man with acute abdominal pain

A 44-year-old man is admitted to the hospital for evaluation of acute, cramping abdominal pain associated with nausea, vomiting, and watery diarrhea.

Heart rate is 130 beats per minute and blood pressure is 90/52 mm Hg. Generalized hyperpigmentation is present (Figure 7-1A). For comparison, the patient provided an old photograph (Figure 7-1B). Scattered patches of hypopigmentation are also present on the trunk. The abdomen is diffusely tender to palpation.

The patient first noted skin changes 8 years ago. He also describes weight loss, fatigue, and episodes of light-headedness over the past few years. Several physicians evaluated him over this time, but no diagnosis was made.

Peripheral white blood cell count is 13 K/μL, serum sodium is 126 mEq/L, and serum glucose is 68 mg/dL. Cross-sectional imaging of the abdomen shows diffuse thickening of the terminal ileum and ascending, transverse, and descending colon, consistent with infectious or inflammatory ileocolitis. Serum cortisol level is 4.4 μg/dL 60 minutes after a 250 μg injection of synthetic adrenocorticotropic hormone (ACTH). Plasma ACTH level drawn prior to the stimulation test is 872 pg/mL (reference range 10-60 pg/mL). Closer review of the abdominal imaging reveals diminutive adrenal glands.

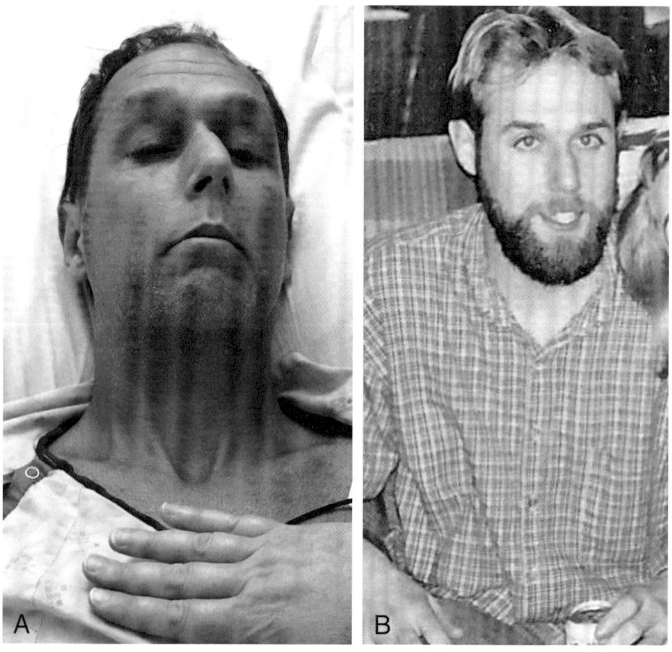


**Figure 7-1.**

***What is the most likely underlying diagnosis in this patient?***

**What is adrenal insufficiency?**

Adrenal insufficiency is a clinical condition that results from deficient production or action of glucocorticoids, with or without mineralocorticoid or androgen deficiency.[1]

**What is the normal hormonal cycle of the hypothalamic pituitary adrenal axis?**

The hypothalamus produces corticotropin-releasing hormone (CRH), which stimulates the pituitary to secrete ACTH, which stimulates the adrenal glands to secrete cortisol, which then provides negative feedback to both the hypothalamus and pituitary (Figure 7-2). Cortisol is essential for life owing to its many functions, including maintenance of glucose production from protein, facilitation of fat metabolism, augmentation of vascular tone, modulation of central nervous system function, and modulation of the immune system.[2]

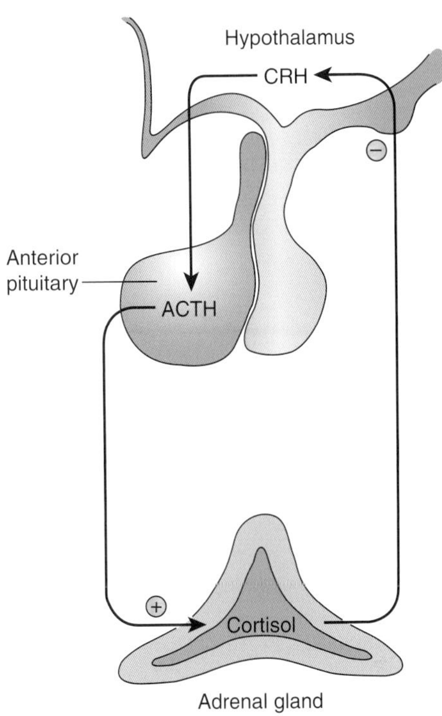


**Figure 7-2.** Schematic of the hypothalamic-pituitary-adrenal axis. Regulatory feedback relationships are designated with arrows. (From Mulholland MW, Lillemoe KD, Doherty GM, Maier RV, Simeone DM, Upchurch GR, eds. *Greenfield's Surgery: Scientific Principles & Practice*. 5th ed. Philadelphia, PA: Lippincott Williams & Wilkins; 2011.)

**Are serum cortisol levels constant throughout the day?**

In healthy adults, secretion of cortisol is pulsatile and highest in the early morning.[1]

**What conditions normally stimulate the hypothalamus to secrete corticotropin-releasing hormone?**

Stimulants of CRH secretion include stress (eg, trauma, surgery, infection), psychiatric disturbance (eg, depression, anxiety), sleep-wake transition, and low serum cortisol.[2]

**What hormones are secreted by the adrenal gland?**

The adrenal cortex secretes glucocorticoids, mineralocorticoids, and androgens, while the adrenal medulla secretes catecholamines.[2]

**How common is adrenal insufficiency?**

In the industrialized world, the incidence of adrenal insufficiency is rising; it is currently associated with a prevalence of up to 40 per 100,000 persons in the general population.[1]

**What are the clinical manifestations of chronic adrenal insufficiency?**

Clinical manifestations of chronic adrenal insufficiency reflect the consequences of deficient adrenocortical hormones (cortisol, aldosterone, and androgens) and may include fatigue, weakness, malaise, weight loss, nausea, vomiting, hypoglycemia, loss of libido (in women), orthostatic hypotension, loss of axillary or pubic hair (in women), and generalized hyperpigmentation of the skin and mucous membranes (only in chronic primary adrenal insufficiency).[1]

**What are the clinical manifestations of acute adrenal insufficiency?**

Acute adrenal insufficiency (ie, adrenal crisis) is usually triggered by acute illness. Manifestations include abdominal pain, nausea, vomiting, fever, confusion, hypotension (usually shock), and hypoglycemia. Many of the symptoms and signs can be mistakenly attributed to the acute illness that triggers the adrenal crisis.[1]

**If adrenal insufficiency is suspected based on the clinical evaluation, what is the next diagnostic step?**

In patients with a clinical condition compatible with adrenal insufficiency, an ACTH stimulation test should be performed to confirm the diagnosis of adrenal insufficiency. *Before the ACTH stimulation test is performed, a baseline plasma ACTH level should be drawn, which may later prove useful.*[1]

**What are the steps of the ACTH stimulation test?**

To perform an ACTH stimulation test, a standard dose of synthetic ACTH (250 μg IV or IM) is given to the patient, and a total serum cortisol level is drawn 60 minutes later. A baseline cortisol level is not necessary because neither the absolute value nor the percentage change between basal and postinjection cortisol has any impact on the interpretation of the ACTH stimulation test.[1,3-5]

**Does the ACTH stimulation test need to be performed at a particular time of day?**

The ACTH stimulation test can be done at any time of day.[3]

**How should the results of the ACTH stimulation test be interpreted?**

Normal adrenal function is established when serum cortisol level is ≥18 μg/dL after ACTH is administered.[6]

**In what scenario might the ACTH stimulation test yield a false-negative result?**

The ACTH stimulation test may yield a false-negative result (ie, serum cortisol concentration rises to ≥18 μg/dL after ACTH is administered in a patient with adrenal insufficiency) in the setting of central adrenal insufficiency of recent onset, as there may be incomplete atrophy of the adrenal glands. In such patients, the ACTH stimulation test should be repeated a few weeks later. A false-negative result may also occur in patients treated with exogenous glucocorticoids, particularly hydrocortisone (prednisone and dexamethasone typically do not interfere with modern cortisol assays). The morning dose of hydrocortisone should be held before performing the ACTH stimulation test. It can be given as soon as the blood samples are drawn.[1]

**Does a positive ACTH stimulation test distinguish between primary and central adrenal insufficiency?**

A positive ACTH stimulation test (ie, serum cortisol concentration remains <18 μg/dL after ACTH administration) is the expected result in any patient with chronic adrenal insufficiency; it does not distinguish between primary and central adrenal insufficiency.[1]

**If the ACTH stimulation test is positive, what is the next step to determine whether adrenal insufficiency is primary or central?**

Plasma ACTH level (which should have been drawn before the ACTH stimulation test) determines whether adrenal insufficiency is ACTH-independent (ACTH level is elevated) or ACTH-dependent (ACTH level is low or normal).

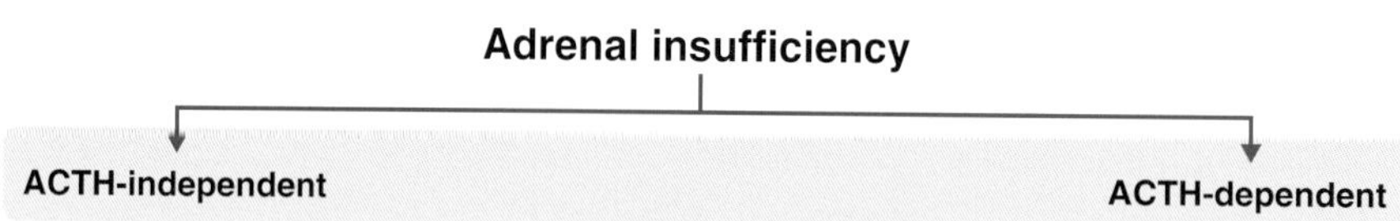


**In the setting of adrenal insufficiency, why does a normal plasma ACTH value implicate an ACTH-dependent process?**

When there is cortisol deficiency, pituitary ACTH secretion should increase in an attempt to return serum cortisol levels to normal. Therefore, an ACTH level within the normal range is "inappropriately normal."

Why is it helpful to separate the causes of adrenal insufficiency into ACTH-independent and ACTH-dependent categories?

ACTH-independent adrenal insufficiency indicates intrinsic dysfunction of the adrenal glands (primary), whereas ACTH-dependent adrenal insufficiency indicates a dysfunctional hypothalamic-pituitary axis (central).

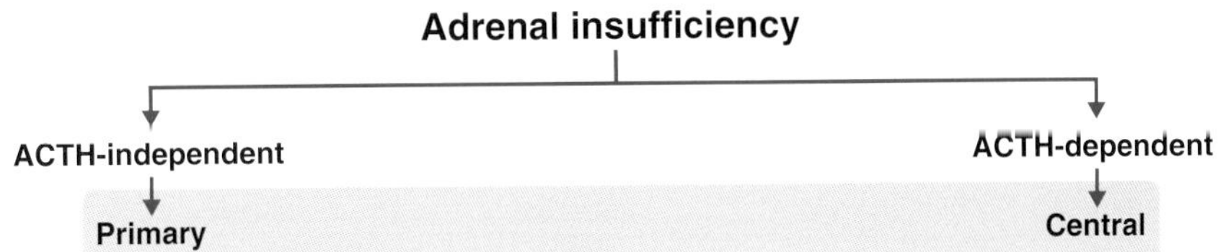


## PRIMARY ADRENAL INSUFFICIENCY

What is the fundamental mechanism of primary adrenal insufficiency?

Primary adrenal insufficiency occurs when the adrenal glands fail to produce adequate hormones despite increased ACTH stimulation.

How much adrenal cortical tissue must be destroyed to result in clinically apparent adrenal insufficiency?

Clinically evident adrenal insufficiency occurs when ≥90% of adrenal cortical tissue has been destroyed.[7]

In addition to cortisol, patients with primary adrenal insufficiency should be evaluated for what other hormonal deficiency?

Mineralocorticoid deficiency may be present in cases of primary adrenal insufficiency, and should be investigated by measuring simultaneous plasma renin activity and serum aldosterone concentration. Mineralocorticoid deficiency due to primary adrenal insufficiency should result in low serum aldosterone levels with elevated plasma renin activity. In such patients, mineralocorticoid replacement therapy will prevent sodium loss, intravascular volume depletion, and hyperkalemia; it is given in the form of fludrocortisone (9-α-fluorohydrocortisone), and the dose is titrated according to blood pressure, serum sodium and potassium concentrations, and plasma renin activity.[1,2]

The causes of primary adrenal insufficiency can be separated into which general subcategories?

The causes of primary adrenal insufficiency can be separated into the following subcategories: autoimmune, infectious, hemorrhagic, infiltrative, and other.

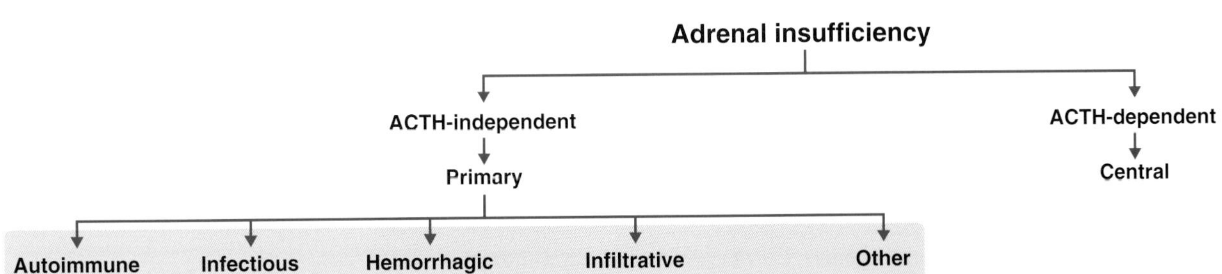


## AUTOIMMUNE CAUSES OF PRIMARY ADRENAL INSUFFICIENCY

### What are the autoimmune causes of primary adrenal insufficiency?

This condition is the most common cause of primary adrenal insufficiency in the industrialized world.

Isolated autoimmune adrenalitis.[1]

**Autoimmune conditions often coexist within individuals and families.**

Polyglandular autoimmune syndrome type 1 (PAS-1) and polyglandular autoimmune syndrome type 2 (PAS-2).

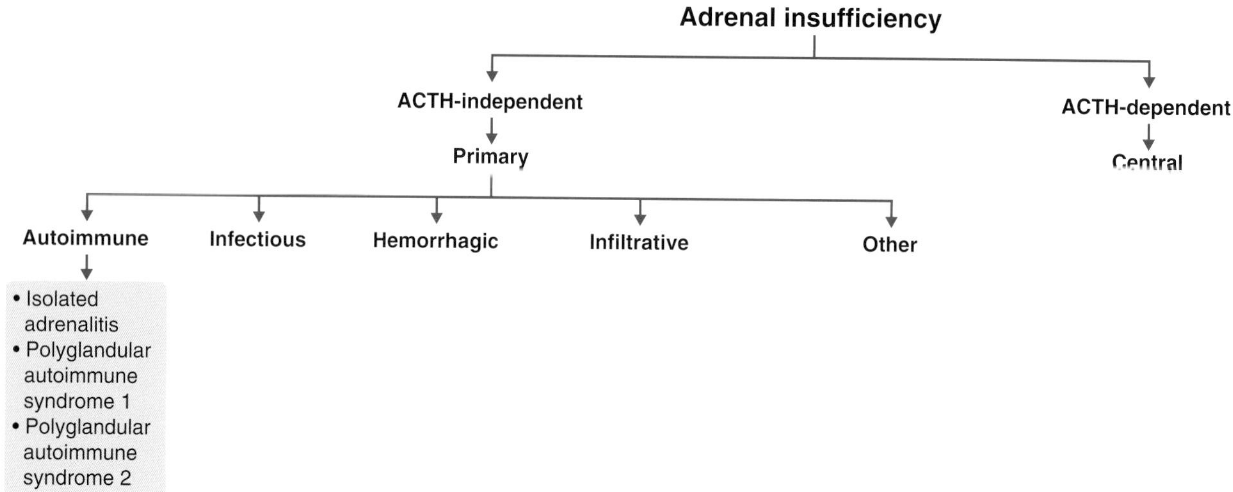


**How common is autoimmune adrenalitis?**

Autoimmune adrenalitis accounts for up to 90% of cases of primary adrenal insufficiency in the industrialized world. Serum autoantibodies to the adrenal cortex or 21-hydroxylase are present in the vast majority of cases. The finding of small adrenal glands on imaging can be a clue to the diagnosis.[1,8,9]

**What are the characteristics of polyglandular autoimmune syndrome type 1?**

PAS-1 is a rare autosomal recessive disorder that disproportionately affects certain populations, such as patients from Sardinia and Finland. Main features include chronic mucocutaneous candidiasis, autoimmune hypoparathyroidism, and autoimmune adrenalitis. Confirmatory testing includes measurement of serum antibodies and gene mutation analysis.[1]

**What are the characteristics of polyglandular autoimmune syndrome type 2?**

PAS-2 is more common than PAS-1. It occurs more frequently in women than men and often presents in the fourth decade of life. Main features include autoimmune adrenalitis, autoimmune thyroid disease, and type 1 diabetes mellitus.[1]

## INFECTIOUS CAUSES OF PRIMARY ADRENAL INSUFFICIENCY

### What are the infectious causes of primary adrenal insufficiency?

**A 58-year-old man from Mexico presents with chronic abdominal pain, weight loss, and night sweats, and is found to have calcified and atrophic adrenal glands on cross-sectional imaging.**

Tuberculosis.

**Consider these infections in immunocompromised hosts or anyone with exposure to endemic regions.**

Disseminated fungal infection.

**Associated with a low CD4 cell count.**

Human immunodeficiency virus and acquired immunodeficiency syndrome (HIV/AIDS).

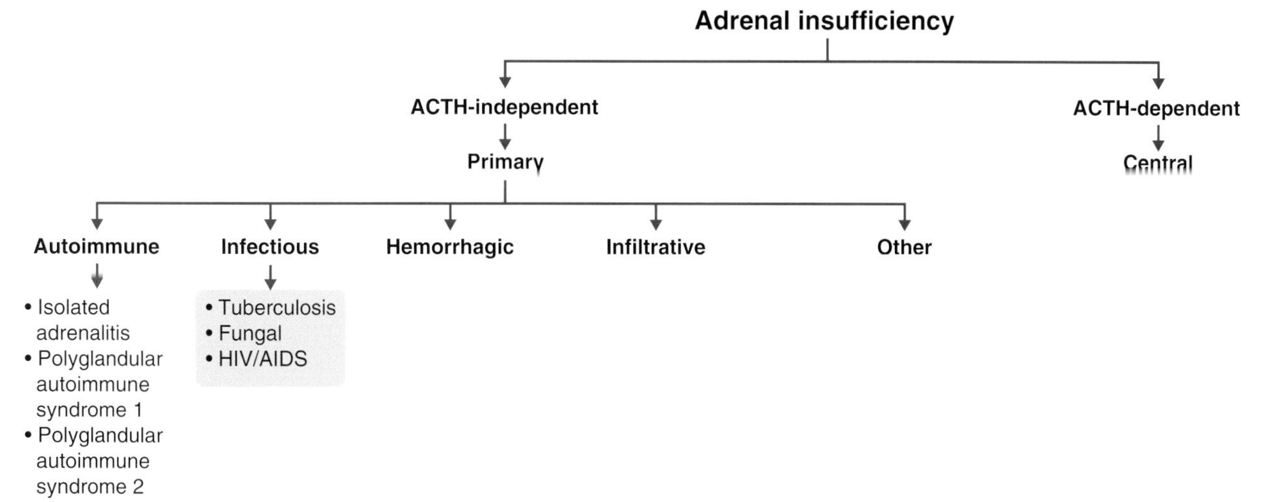

**What percentage of cases of primary adrenal insufficiency are related to tuberculosis?**

When Thomas Addison first described adrenal insufficiency, most cases were related to tuberculosis. It remains a common cause of adrenal insufficiency in the developing world, accounting for up to one-third of cases. In the industrialized world, it accounts for up to 15% of cases. Infection with *Mycobacterium tuberculosis* involves the adrenal gland via hematogenous spread. Imaging findings consistent with recently acquired disease (<2 years) include bilateral adrenal enlargement, whereas the dominant findings in patients with infection of longer duration are calcification and atrophy.[1,10]

**Which disseminated fungal infections are associated with the development of adrenal insufficiency?**

Virtually any disseminated fungal infection can involve the adrenal gland and lead to primary adrenal insufficiency, but the most common include histoplasmosis, paracoccidioidomycosis (South American blastomycosis), cryptococcosis, blastomycosis, and coccidioidomycosis. In patients with adrenal involvement of disseminated fungal infection, imaging often reveals adrenal gland enlargement; image-guided biopsy can be performed to confirm the diagnosis.[10]

**What are the major mechanisms of adrenal insufficiency related to HIV/AIDS?**

Adrenal insufficiency occurs in up to one-fifth of patients admitted to the hospital with AIDS, and is related to a variety of mechanisms including infiltration of the glands with opportunistic infection (eg, cytomegalovirus) or HIV-associated malignancy (eg, Kaposi sarcoma, lymphoma), and as a side effect of medications used to treat HIV/AIDS (eg, ketoconazole, fluconazole, rifampin).[10]

## HEMORRHAGIC CAUSES OF PRIMARY ADRENAL INSUFFICIENCY

**Why is the adrenal gland vulnerable to hemorrhage?**

The adrenal gland is intrinsically susceptible to hemorrhage because of its unique vascular anatomy. Three suprarenal arteries supply the gland with a high volume of blood flow, but only 1 vein provides drainage, creating a "vascular dam." During periods of hemodynamic stress, such as increased perfusion pressure, rupture of the capillaries can result in hemorrhage into the gland.[7]

**What clinical clues suggest the diagnosis of bilateral adrenal hemorrhage?**

The combination of hypotension, acute decline in hematocrit, and signs of adrenal insufficiency (eg, hyperkalemia, hyponatremia, hypovolemia) should prompt consideration of bilateral adrenal hemorrhage. Major risk factors include thromboembolic disease, coagulopathy, and the postoperative state.[11]

**How is the diagnosis of bilateral adrenal gland hemorrhage confirmed?**

Because the clinical manifestations of bilateral adrenal hemorrhage can overlap with concurrent critical illness, diagnosis is often missed or delayed. Diagnosis is confirmed with biochemical evidence of adrenal insufficiency and imaging evidence of adrenal hemorrhage (via computed tomography imaging, ultrasonography, or magnetic resonance imaging).[7]

**What is the prognosis of bilateral adrenal gland hemorrhage?**

Bilateral adrenal gland hemorrhage is associated with a high mortality rate, largely because of missed or delayed diagnosis. In those who survive after treatment with glucocorticoid replacement, the development of chronic primary adrenal insufficiency is virtually universal.[7]

## What are the causes of bilateral adrenal gland hemorrhage?

**A 32-year-old man is admitted with epistaxis and petechial skin rash following an upper respiratory tract infection and subsequently develops hypotension, hyperkalemia, and hyponatremia.**

Immune thrombocytopenic purpura.

**A vascular complication that can occur in patients with underlying thrombophilia (eg, antiphospholipid antibody syndrome).**

Adrenal vein thrombosis.

**Adrenal hemorrhage in the intensive care unit.**

Critical illness, including the postoperative state, myocardial infarction, congestive heart failure, and sepsis.

**An 18-year-old woman with headache, photophobia, and neck stiffness.**

Waterhouse-Friderichsen syndrome related to meningococcemia.

**A 32-year-old woman is brought to the emergency department after a motor vehicle accident, and cross-sectional imaging of the abdomen reveals bilateral adrenal hemorrhage.**

Trauma.

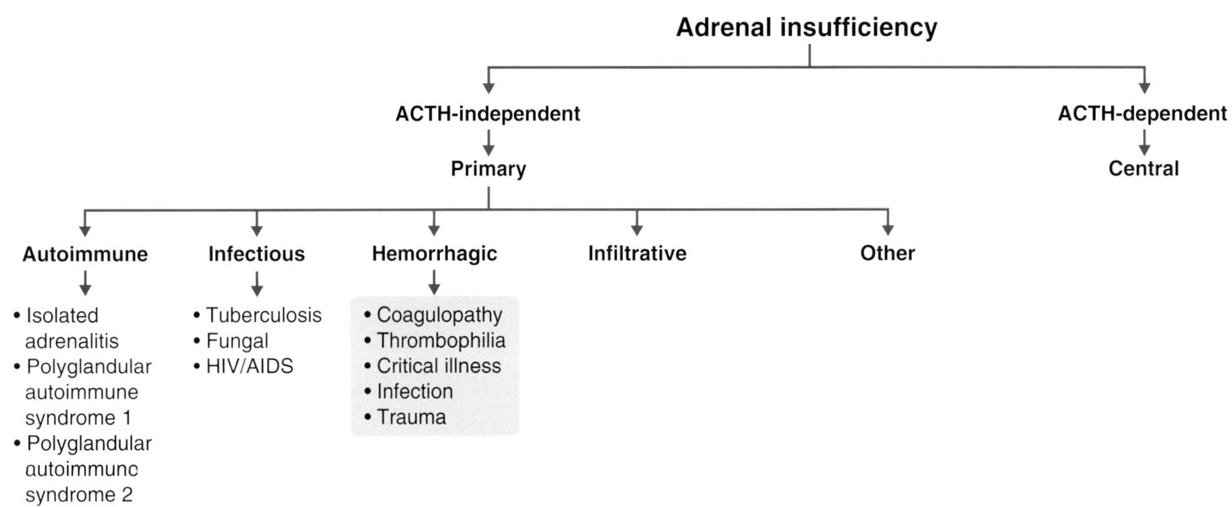


**Which causes of coagulopathy are most often associated with bilateral adrenal hemorrhage?**

Thrombocytopenia and the use of anticoagulant medications are the coagulopathies most frequently associated with bilateral adrenal hemorrhage.[7,11]

**What is the mechanism of adrenal hemorrhage in the setting of adrenal vein thrombosis?**

The combination of rich arterial blood flow to the adrenal gland and decreased venous drainage related to adrenal vein thrombosis results in increased pressure and subsequent capillary rupture with intraglandular hemorrhage.[12]

**What is the mechanism of bilateral adrenal hemorrhage in the setting of critical illness?**

It is theorized that surges in ACTH levels during acute illness increase blood flow to the adrenal glands, which overwhelms the drainage capability of the adrenal vein, resulting in capillary rupture and intraglandular hemorrhage.[7]

**What infections are associated with Waterhouse-Friderichsen syndrome?**

Waterhouse-Friderichsen syndrome most commonly occurs in association with sepsis from *Neisseria meningitidis*. However, infection with other bacteria can also lead to adrenal hemorrhage, including *Rickettsia rickettsii*, *Streptococcus pneumoniae*, group A streptococcus, and *Staphylococcus aureus*.[13]

**What types of traumatic injuries are most commonly associated with adrenal hemorrhage?**

Motor vehicle accidents, falls, and sports injuries are the most common traumatic causes of adrenal hemorrhage. Most cases involve the right adrenal gland, in part because of its anatomic location between the liver and spine (Figure 7-3). Bilateral adrenal hemorrhage should be suspected in trauma patients who present with symptoms and signs of adrenal insufficiency. Imaging of the adrenal glands can confirm the diagnosis.[14]

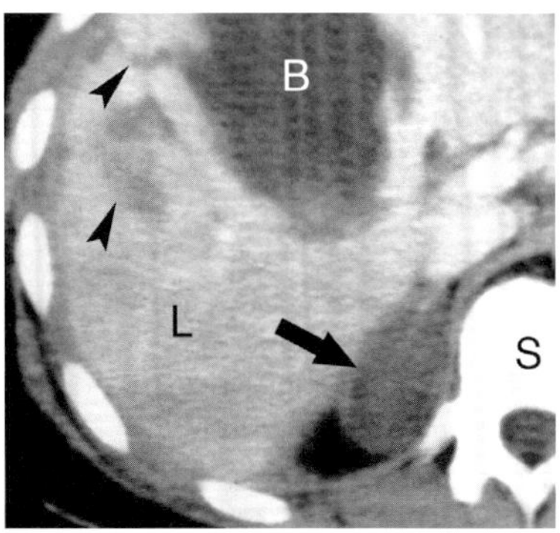


**Figure 7-3.** Postcontrast CT shows posttraumatic hemorrhage (arrow) into the right adrenal gland. Blunt trauma to the abdomen can compress the right adrenal gland between the liver (L) and the spine (S), resulting in adrenal hemorrhage. This patient also has areas of fracture and hemorrhage (arrowheads) within the liver, as well as a biloma (B). (From Brant W, Helms CA. *Fundamentals of Diagnostic Radiology*. 3rd ed. Philadelphia, PA: Lippincott Williams & Wilkins; 2007.)

## INFILTRATIVE CAUSES OF PRIMARY ADRENAL INSUFFICIENCY

### What are the infiltrative causes of primary adrenal insufficiency?

**Diffuse lymphadenopathy and elevated serum lactate dehydrogenase.**

Lymphoma.

**A common histologic feature of sarcoidosis and tuberculosis.**

Granulomatous disease.

**Think of this entity in patients with multiple myeloma or chronic inflammatory conditions.**

Amyloidosis.

**Another reason to have bronzed skin.**

Hemochromatosis.

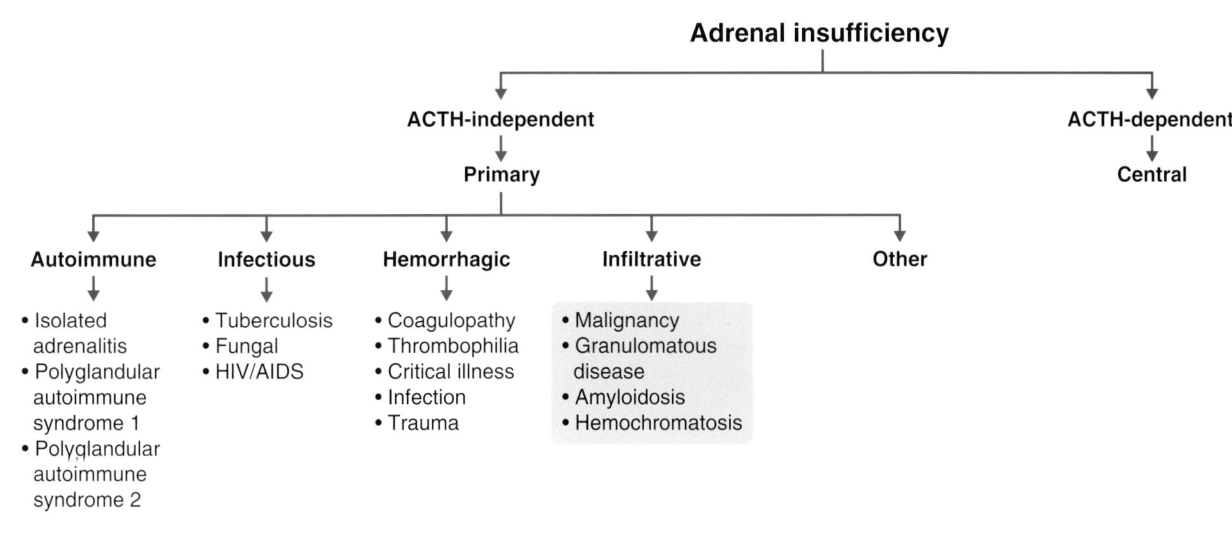

**What are the characteristics of adrenal infiltration related to malignancy?**

Metastatic infiltration is the primary mechanism by which malignancy involves the adrenal gland. Adrenal metastasis occurs most frequently in patients with lung, breast, gastric, and colorectal cancer, melanoma, and lymphoma. Up to one-third of patients with bilateral adrenal metastases develop adrenal insufficiency. Patients with malignancy can also develop adrenal insufficiency as a result of hemorrhagic necrosis, impaired adrenal synthesis due to antineoplastic agents, and central adrenal insufficiency from malignant infiltration of the hypothalamus or pituitary or discontinuation of glucocorticoids used in the antineoplastic treatment protocol.[15,16]

**What are the characteristics of adrenal insufficiency related to sarcoidosis?**

In patients with sarcoidosis, the adrenal gland can become infiltrated with granulomatous lesions and eventually replaced by dense fibrosis. However, the occurrence of primary adrenal insufficiency is rare in sarcoidosis. Patients generally respond well to glucocorticoid replacement (and mineralocorticoid replacement, if necessary). In addition to its effects on the adrenal glands via granulomatous infiltration, there is an association between sarcoidosis and autoimmune adrenalitis.[17]

**How common is adrenal insufficiency in patients with systemic amyloidosis with renal involvement?**

Primary or central adrenal insufficiency occurs in almost one-half of patients with renal amyloidosis. It occurs in both immunoglobulin light chain (AL) amyloidosis and inflammatory (AA) amyloidosis. Symptoms and signs of adrenal insufficiency in these patients may be confused for those of uremia, a common comorbidity in this population.[18,19]

**What are the characteristics of adrenal insufficiency related to hemochromatosis?**

Iron deposition within the adrenal gland occurs more frequently with secondary hemochromatosis; primary hemochromatosis tends to cause central adrenal insufficiency. In patients with primary adrenal insufficiency related to hemochromatosis, computed tomography imaging shows characteristic hyperdense adrenal glands with normal or reduced size and preserved contours.[20,21]

## OTHER CAUSES OF PRIMARY ADRENAL INSUFFICIENCY

### What are the other causes of primary adrenal insufficiency?

**Iatrogenesis (at least 3 answers are correct).**

Bilateral adrenalectomy, radiotherapy, and medication.

**An X-linked disease that can be diagnosed by measuring the serum concentration of very long-chain fatty acids.**

Adrenoleukodystrophy (ALD).

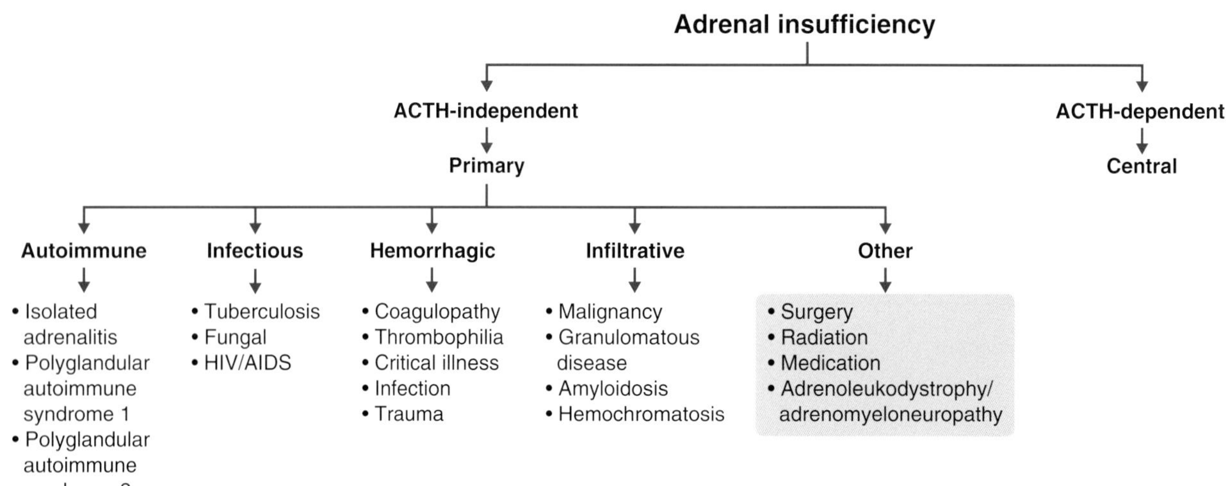

**What type of hormone replacement is necessary in patients who have undergone bilateral adrenalectomy?**

Lifelong replacement of both glucocorticoids and mineralocorticoids is necessary in all patients who have undergone bilateral adrenalectomy.[22]

**Is external beam radiation therapy most often associated with primary or central adrenal insufficiency?**

Primary adrenal insufficiency related to external beam radiation is relatively rare. In contrast, central adrenal insufficiency occurs in up to one-half of patients treated with radiation to the hypothalamic-pituitary region. Median time to occurrence is 5 years.[23]

**What are the 2 main mechanisms through which medications result in primary adrenal insufficiency?**

Medication-induced primary adrenal insufficiency can occur as a result of (1) inhibition of cortisol biosynthesis (eg, ketoconazole), and (2) acceleration of the metabolism of cortisol (eg, phenytoin).[24,25]

**What is adrenoleukodystrophy?**

ALD is an X-linked genetic condition characterized by impaired peroxisomal β-oxidation of very long-chain fatty acids, resulting in accumulation within the tissues, including the adrenal cortex. ALD presents with a spectrum of phenotypes, including adrenomyeloneuropathy (AMN), which generally develops in adults in the third and fourth decades of life. The majority of patients with AMN develop adrenal insufficiency.[26]

## CENTRAL ADRENAL INSUFFICIENCY

**What is the fundamental mechanism of central adrenal insufficiency?**

Central adrenal insufficiency occurs as a result of inadequate ACTH stimulation of the adrenal glands.

**What are the clues to the presence of a central process in patients with adrenal insufficiency?**

In patients with adrenal insufficiency, a central process is suggested by preexisting hypothalamic or pituitary disease, history of head trauma, headaches, visual field defects, and focal neurologic findings.[27]

**Which glands are involved in central adrenal insufficiency?**

Central adrenal insufficiency can occur as a result of pituitary gland dysfunction (ie, secondary adrenal insufficiency) or hypothalamic dysfunction (ie, tertiary adrenal insufficiency).

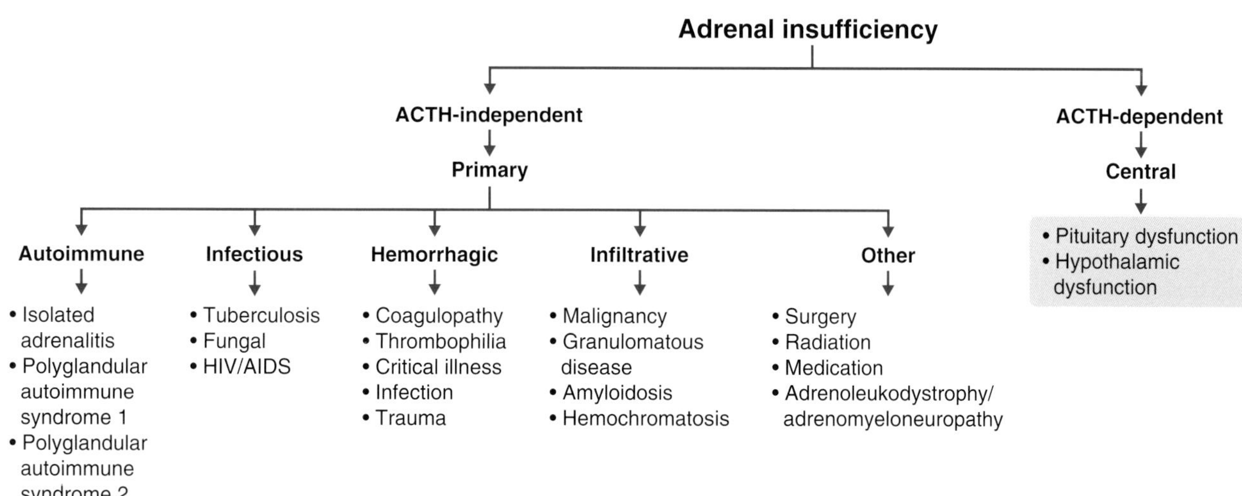


**Is mineralocorticoid deficiency associated with central adrenal insufficiency?**

In general, the adrenal glands remain responsive to renin activity in patients with central adrenal insufficiency. However, mineralocorticoid deficiency can develop in cases of longstanding ACTH deficiency.[1]

**What general processes can cause pituitary and/or hypothalamic dysfunction?**

Pituitary and/or hypothalamic dysfunction can be caused by medication (eg, glucocorticoids), mass lesion (eg, brain metastasis), traumatic brain injury, subarachnoid hemorrhage, infection/abscess, stroke, external beam radiation, pituitary apoplexy, Sheehan's syndrome, autoimmune disease (eg, lymphocytic hypophysitis), and infiltrative disease (eg, hemochromatosis).[27]

**What is the most common cause of central adrenal insufficiency?**

Chronic exposure to excessive glucocorticoids, either from an exogenous source (eg, glucocorticoid medication) or from an endogenous source (eg, Cushing's disease), results in persistent suppression of hypothalamic secretion of CRH. An abrupt decrease in exposure to glucocorticoids, such as when medication is stopped or Cushing's syndrome is treated, can result in central adrenal insufficiency.[1]

**How long can it take for hypothalamic function to recover once exposure to supraphysiologic doses of glucocorticoids has ceased?**

Recovery of the hypothalamus can take up to 9 months following cessation of exposure to excess glucocorticoids.[28]

## Case Summary

A 44-year-old man with chronic generalized hyperpigmentation, weight loss, and fatigue is admitted to the hospital with an acute gastrointestinal illness and is found to have tachycardia, hypotension, hypoglycemia, and hyponatremia.

***What is the most likely underlying diagnosis in this patient?***

Primary adrenal insufficiency.

### BONUS QUESTIONS

***Which features of this case make primary adrenal insufficiency more likely than central adrenal insufficiency?***

The presence of generalized hyperpigmentation (see Figure 7-1A) is the first clue to the diagnosis of chronic primary adrenal insufficiency in this case. Elevated plasma ACTH in the setting of a compatible clinical syndrome and biochemical evidence of adrenal insufficiency clinches the diagnosis of primary adrenal insufficiency.

***What is the mechanism of hyperpigmentation from chronic primary adrenal insufficiency?***

High levels of ACTH found in patients with primary adrenal insufficiency stimulate the melanocortin-1 receptor in the skin, resulting in hyperpigmentation. It tends to first occur in areas of the skin under pressure, including elbows, knuckles, palmar creases, lips, and buccal mucosa.[1]

***What is the best explanation for the patchy areas of skin hypopigmentation described in this case?***

The patchy areas of hypopigmentation described in this case are most likely manifestations of vitiligo, an autoimmune condition that tends to accompany other autoimmune conditions such as autoimmune adrenalitis.

***What is the most likely cause of primary adrenal insufficiency in this case?***

Isolated autoimmune adrenalitis is the most likely cause of primary adrenal insufficiency in this case. In general, it is the most common cause of primary adrenal insufficiency, and there are other clues to the diagnosis (eg, vitiligo). There is no evidence of a polyglandular syndrome based on the information provided.

***Is the patient in this case in adrenal crisis?***

The patient in this case is in adrenal crisis, likely triggered by the underlying inflammatory gastrointestinal condition. Adrenal crisis is a life-threatening condition characterized by abdominal pain, vomiting, myalgias, arthralgias, severe hypotension, and hypovolemic shock.[1]

***Which urgent treatment should be provided to the patient in this case?***

Patients with adrenal crisis should be treated with stress-dose glucocorticoid replacement (typically given as hydrocortisone 50-100 mg intravenously or intramuscularly every 6 hours, depending on age and body surface area), until clinical stability is achieved. At that point, a maintenance dose of glucocorticoid should be started.[1]

***What is the physiologic replacement dose of glucocorticoids?***

The physiologic replacement dose (ie, maintenance dose) of glucocorticoids is 10 to 12 mg/m$^2$ per day of hydrocortisone or equivalent.[29]

***Does the patient in this case require mineralocorticoid replacement?***

The patient in this case might require mineralocorticoid replacement, as mineralocorticoid deficiency occurs in some cases of primary adrenal insufficiency. Testing should be done with simultaneous plasma renin activity and serum aldosterone concentration.[1]

## KEY POINTS

- Adrenal insufficiency is a clinical condition that results from deficient production or action of glucocorticoids, with or without mineralocorticoid or androgen deficiency.
- Clinical manifestations of chronic adrenal insufficiency include fatigue, weakness, malaise, weight loss, nausea, vomiting, hypoglycemia, loss of libido (in women), orthostatic hypotension, loss of axillary or pubic hair (in women), and generalized hyperpigmentation of the skin and mucous membranes (only in chronic primary adrenal insufficiency).
- When adrenal insufficiency is suspected clinically, an ACTH stimulation test should be performed to confirm the diagnosis.
- The plasma ACTH level determines whether adrenal insufficiency is ACTH-independent (primary) or ACTH-dependent (central).
- The causes of primary adrenal insufficiency can be separated into the following subcategories: autoimmune, infectious, hemorrhagic, infiltrative, and other.
- Central adrenal insufficiency occurs as a result of pituitary dysfunction (secondary) or hypothalamic dysfunction (tertiary).
- The most common causes of adrenal insufficiency include abrupt withdrawal of glucocorticoid therapy, autoimmune adrenalitis, and tuberculosis.
- Acute adrenal insufficiency (ie, adrenal crisis) must be treated with high-dose glucocorticoids.
- Treatment for chronic adrenal insufficiency includes maintenance-dose glucocorticoid replacement and may include mineralocorticoid replacement in some patients.

## REFERENCES

1. Charmandari E, Nicolaides NC, Chrousos GP. Adrenal insufficiency. *Lancet*. 2014;383(9935):2152-2167.
2. Berne RML, Levy MN. *Physiology*. 4th ed. St. Louis, MO: Mosby, Inc.; 1998.
3. Dorin RI, Qualls CR, Crapo LM. Diagnosis of adrenal insufficiency. *Ann Intern Med*. 2003;139(3):194-204.
4. Oelkers W. Adrenal insufficiency. *N Engl J Med*. 1996;335(16):1206-1212.
5. Zueger T, Jordi M, Laimer M, Stettler C. Utility of 30 and 60 minute cortisol samples after high-dose synthetic ACTH-1-24 injection in the diagnosis of adrenal insufficiency. *Swiss Med Wkly*. 2014;144:w13987.
6. Longo DL, Fauci AS, Kasper DL, Hauser SL, Jameson JL, Loscalzo J, eds. *Harrison's Principles of Internal Medicine*. 18th ed. New York, NY: McGraw-Hill; 2012.
7. Kovacs KA, Lam YM, Pater JL. Bilateral massive adrenal hemorrhage. Assessment of putative risk factors by the case-control method. *Medicine*. 2001;80(1):45-53.
8. Kasperlik-Zaluska AA, Migdalska B, Czarnocka B, Drac-Kaniewska J, Niegowska E, Czech W. Association of Addison's disease with autoimmune disorders—a long-term observation of 180 patients. *Postgrad Med J*. 1991;67(793):984-987.
9. Zelissen PM, Bast EJ, Croughs RJ. Associated autoimmunity in Addison's disease. *J Autoimmun*. 1995;8(1):121-130.
10. Upadhyay J, Sudhindra P, Abraham G, Trivedi N. Tuberculosis of the adrenal gland: a case report and review of the literature of infections of the adrenal gland. *Int J Endocrinol*. 2014;2014:876037.
11. Rao RH, Vagnucci AH, Amico JA. Bilateral massive adrenal hemorrhage: early recognition and treatment. *Ann Intern Med*. 1989;110(3):227-235.
12. Presotto F, Fornasini F, Betterle C, Federspil G, Rossato M. Acute adrenal failure as the heralding symptom of primary antiphospholipid syndrome: report of a case and review of the literature. *Eur J Endocrinol*. 2005;153(4):507-514.
13. Guarner J, Paddock CD, Bartlett J, Zaki SR. Adrenal gland hemorrhage in patients with fatal bacterial infections. *Mod Pathol*. 2008;21(9):1113-1120.
14. Sinelnikov AO, Abujudeh HH, Chan D, Novelline RA. CT manifestations of adrenal trauma: experience with 73 cases. *Emerg Radiol*. 2007;13(6):313-318.
15. Carvalho F, Louro F, Zakout R. Adrenal insufficiency in metastatic lung cancer. *World J Oncol*. 2015;6(3):375-377.
16. Yeung SCJ, Escalante CP, Gagel RF, eds. *Medical Care of Cancer Patients*. Shelton, CT: People's Medical Publishing House; 2009.
17. Porter N, Beynon HL, Randeva HS. Endocrine and reproductive manifestations of sarcoidosis. *QJM*. 2003;96(8):553-561.
18. Arik N, Tasdemir I, Karaaslan Y, Yasavul U, Turgan C, Caglar S. Subclinical adrenocortical insufficiency in renal amyloidosis. *Nephron*. 1990;56(3):246-248.
19. Danby P, Harris KP, Williams B, Feehally J, Walls J. Adrenal dysfunction in patients with renal amyloid. *Q J Med*. 1990;76(281):915-922.
20. Doppman JL, Gill Jr JR, Nienhuis AW, Earll JM, Long Jr JA. CT findings in Addison's disease. *J Comput Assist Tomogr*. 1982;6(4):757-761.
21. Kannan CR. *The Adrenal Gland*. New York, NY: Plenum Publishing Corporation; 1988.
22. Loriaux L. The diagnosis and differential diagnosis of Cushing's syndrome. *N Engl J Med*. 2017:376;1451-1459.
23. Kufe DW, Pollock RE, Weichselbaum RR, et al, eds. *Cancer Medicine*. 6th ed. Hamilton (ON): BC Decker; 2003.
24. Elias AN, Gwinup G. Effects of some clinically encountered drugs on steroid synthesis and degradation. *Metabolism*. 1980;29(6):582-595.
25. Sonino N. The use of ketoconazole as an inhibitor of steroid production. *N Engl J Med*. 1987;317(13):812-818.

26. Engelen M, Kemp S, de Visser M, et al. X-linked adrenoleukodystrophy (X-ALD): clinical presentation and guidelines for diagnosis, follow-up and management. *Orphanet J Rare Dis*. 2012;7:51.
27. Persani L. Clinical review: central hypothyroidism: pathogenic, diagnostic, and therapeutic challenges. *J Clin Endocrinol Metab*. 2012;97(9):3068-3078.
28. Byyny RL. Withdrawal from glucocorticoid therapy. *N Engl J Med*. 1976;295(1):30-32.
29. Gupta P, Bhatia V. Corticosteroid physiology and principles of therapy. *Indian J Pediatr*. 2008;75(10):1039-1044.

Chapter 8

# CUSHING'S SYNDROME

## Case: A 43-year-old man with delusions

A previously healthy 43-year-old man is brought to the emergency department for evaluation of confusion. The patient has complained to his wife of weight gain and frequent urination for the past several months. Over the same period, he has had progressive weakness in his shoulders and legs, recently requiring help to rise from a seated position. The patient's wife became more concerned when he told her he is a secret agent of the Federal Bureau of Investigation. The patient has never smoked and does not drink alcohol or use illicit substances.

Heart rate is 110 beats per minute and blood pressure is 188/104 mm Hg. There are scattered ecchymoses, abdominal striae (Figure 8-1), and hyperpigmentation of the knuckles, palmar creases, and elbows. Proximal muscle weakness and atrophy are present.

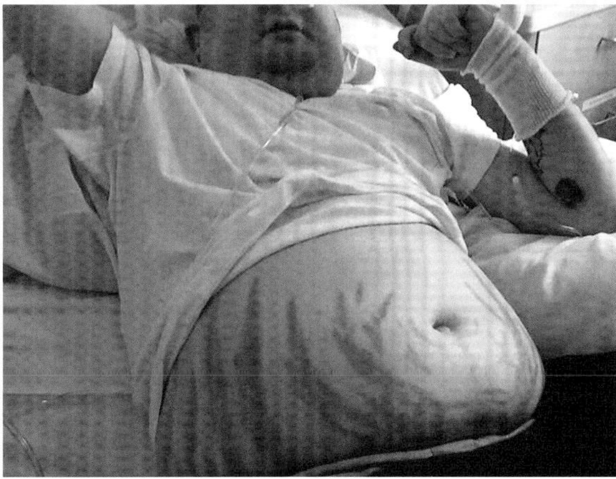

**Figure 8-1.**

Serum glucose is 525 mg/dL and serum potassium is 2.1 mg/dL. Urine free cortisol is measured at 645 μg/day (reference range <50 μg/day). Plasma adrenocorticotropic hormone (ACTH) is 1000 pg/mL (reference range 10-60 pg/mL). Simultaneous sampling of the inferior petrosal sinus and peripheral blood is performed and reveals a central-to-peripheral ACTH concentration ratio of 0.6. Cross-sectional imaging of the chest reveals an endobronchial nodule within the left main bronchus (arrow, Figure 8-2).

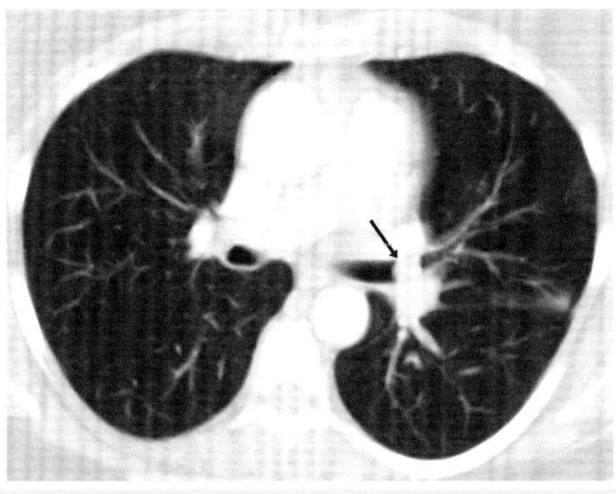

**Figure 8-2.** (Courtesy of Cristina Fuss, MD.)

***What is the most likely diagnosis in this patient?***

**What is Cushing's syndrome?**

Cushing's syndrome is a clinical condition that results from cortisol excess.

**What is the normal hormonal cycle of the hypothalamic-pituitary-adrenal axis?**

The hypothalamus produces corticotropin-releasing hormone (CRH), which stimulates the pituitary to secrete ACTH, which stimulates the adrenal glands to secrete cortisol, which then provides negative feedback to both the hypothalamus and pituitary (see Figure 7-2).[1]

**Are serum cortisol levels constant throughout the day?**

In healthy adults, secretion of cortisol is pulsatile and highest in the early morning.[2]

**What conditions normally stimulate the hypothalamus to secrete corticotropin-releasing hormone?**

Stimulants of CRH secretion include stress (eg, trauma, surgery, infection), psychiatric disturbance (eg, depression, anxiety), sleep-wake transition, and low serum cortisol.[1]

**How common is Cushing's syndrome?**

Cushing's syndrome is present in up to 8 per 100,000 persons in the general population. It is estimated that an equal number of cases are undiagnosed. The median age of diagnosis is 40 years with a 3:1 female-to-male predominance.

**What are the clinical manifestations of Cushing's syndrome?**

Clinical manifestations of Cushing's syndrome (Figure 8-3) may include central obesity, "moon facies" (rounded face due to fat deposition), "buffalo hump" (increased fat deposition between the shoulders), thin skin, bruising, abdominal striae, hyperpigmentation (ACTH-dependent causes only), hirsutism, oligomenorrhea, psychosis, proximal myopathy, arterial hypertension, polycythemia, hyperglycemia (with associated polyuria), hypokalemia, and osteopenia. The manifestations of hypercortisolism can generally be divided into anabolic (eg, polycythemia) and antianabolic effects (eg, thin skin).[3]

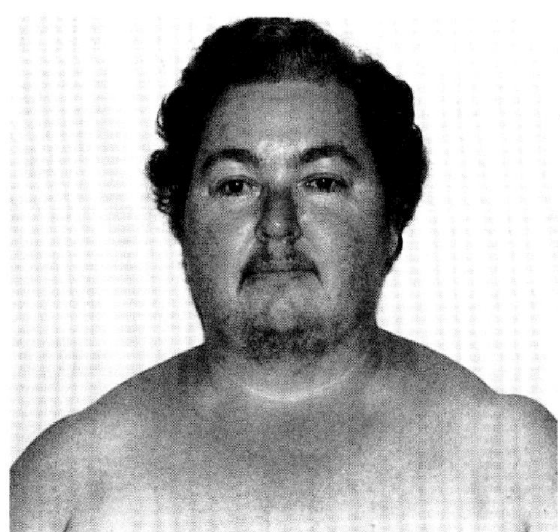

**Figure 8-3.** A woman with Cushing's syndrome. Note the moon facies (rounded face due to fat deposition), reddened cheeks, hirsutism, and buffalo hump (increased fat deposition between the shoulders). (From Rubin E. *Essential Pathology*. 3rd ed. Philadelphia: Lippincott Williams & Wilkins; 2000.)

**What condition, which is on the rise in the industrialized world, is often confused for Cushing's syndrome?**

The metabolic syndrome of obesity is associated with the same anabolic signs as the syndrome of glucocorticoid excess. A focus on the antianabolic effects of cortisol excess is useful for differentiating Cushing's syndrome from simple obesity. The probability of Cushing's syndrome exceeds 90% in the obese population when the triad of thin skin (established when a skin fold over the proximal phalanx of the middle finger of the nondominant hand is <2 mm thick), osteoporosis, and ecchymoses is present.[3]

**If Cushing's syndrome is suspected based on the clinical evaluation, what is the next diagnostic step?**

In patients with a clinical condition compatible with Cushing's syndrome, a confirmatory laboratory test should be obtained. When carefully performed, the urine free cortisol (UFC) test, which measures the quantity of free cortisol secreted in the urine in a 24-hour period, is the most reliable confirmatory test. The upper limit of the normal reference range for this test should be increased slightly in patients with depression. When renal function is abnormal, UFC is less reliable. In such patients, confirmatory tests of salivary cortisol may be helpful.[3,4]

Cushing's syndrome

Confirmatory test

Negative Positive

**What are the possible explanations for patients who have a clinical condition compatible with Cushing's syndrome but a negative confirmatory test?**

If Cushing's syndrome is present clinically, then a negative confirmatory test (ie, UFC is not elevated) indicates either exposure to exogenous glucocorticoids or a false-negative confirmatory study.[3]

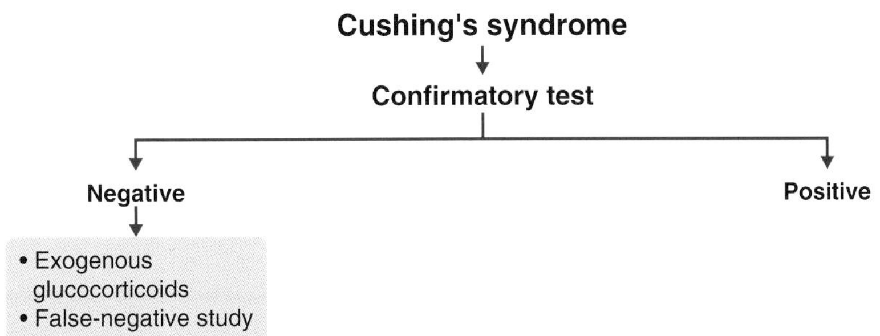


**In patients with Cushing's syndrome related to exogenous glucocorticoids, what are the dangers of abrupt glucocorticoid cessation?**

In patients with Cushing's syndrome related to exogenous glucocorticoids, the danger of abrupt glucocorticoid cessation is twofold. First, recrudescence of the underlying condition being treated (eg, rheumatoid arthritis) may occur. Second, chronic exposure to supraphysiologic levels of glucocorticoids can lead to the development of central adrenal insufficiency, which will become unmasked if glucocorticoids are stopped abruptly. For these reasons, it is preferred that exogenous glucocorticoids are tapered over a period of time.

**How can exogenous glucocorticoids be discontinued safely?**

Exogenous glucocorticoids can be safely and efficiently discontinued using the following strategy: (1) reduce the glucocorticoid to physiologic dose (10-12 mg/m$^2$ per day of hydrocortisone or equivalent); (2) obtain an ACTH stimulation test (before the morning dose of glucocorticoid) every 3 months; (3) stop all glucocorticoids when there is an adequate response to the ACTH stimulation test (ie, cortisol levels rise to ≥18 µg/dL). The hypothalamic-pituitary-adrenal axis eventually recovers in the vast majority of patients.[5]

**What strategies can minimize the risk of a false-negative urine free cortisol test?**

To minimize the chance of a false-negative result, UFC samples must be complete (ie, all urine must be collected over a full 24-hour period) and measured with high-performance liquid chromatography and mass spectrometry in patients with normal renal function. The most reliable way to confirm that a complete 24-hour urine collection has been obtained is to measure urinary creatinine. Urinary creatinine <1.5 g per day for men and <1.0 g per day for women indicates incomplete collection, and the test should be repeated.[3]

**If the confirmatory test is positive, what is the next diagnostic step in the evaluation of Cushing's syndrome?**

In a patient with a clinical condition compatible with Cushing's syndrome, a positive confirmatory test (ie, UFC is elevated) should prompt measurement of plasma ACTH levels. The plasma ACTH level determines whether Cushing's syndrome is ACTH-dependent (ACTH level is elevated or normal) or ACTH-independent (ACTH level is low).

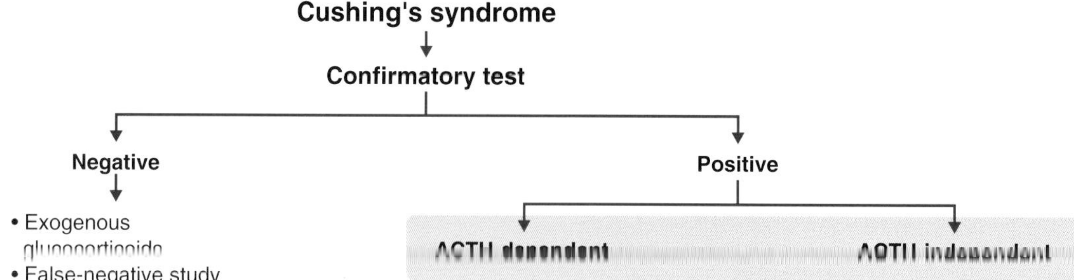


**In the setting of cortisol excess, why does a normal plasma ACTH value imply an ACTH-dependent process?**

When there is cortisol excess, negative feedback to the hypothalamus and pituitary should decrease ACTH secretion in an attempt to return serum cortisol levels to normal. Therefore, an ACTH level within the normal range is "inappropriately normal."

**What is the relative prevalence of ACTH-dependent and ACTH-independent causes of Cushing's syndrome?**

ACTH-dependent causes of Cushing's syndrome represent 80% of cases, whereas ACTH-independent causes make up the remaining 20%.[6]

## ACTH-DEPENDENT CUSHING'S SYNDROME

**What is the fundamental mechanism of hypercortisolism in patients with ACTH-dependent Cushing's syndrome?**

ACTH-dependent Cushing's syndrome occurs as a result of excess ACTH stimulation of the adrenal glands that then respond by producing excess cortisol.

**In patients with ACTH-dependent Cushing's syndrome, what is the next diagnostic step in evaluation?**

Patients with ACTH-dependent Cushing's syndrome should undergo inferior petrosal sinus sampling to determine if the excess ACTH is eutopic (from the pituitary gland) or ectopic (from elsewhere). Following direct stimulation of the pituitary gland with CRH, ACTH plasma levels from the inferior petrosal sinus and periphery (eg, antecubital vein) are simultaneously measured. Eutopic ACTH secretion is associated with a central-to-peripheral ACTH ratio ≥3. Ectopic ACTH secretion is associated with a central-to-peripheral ACTH ratio <3.[3]

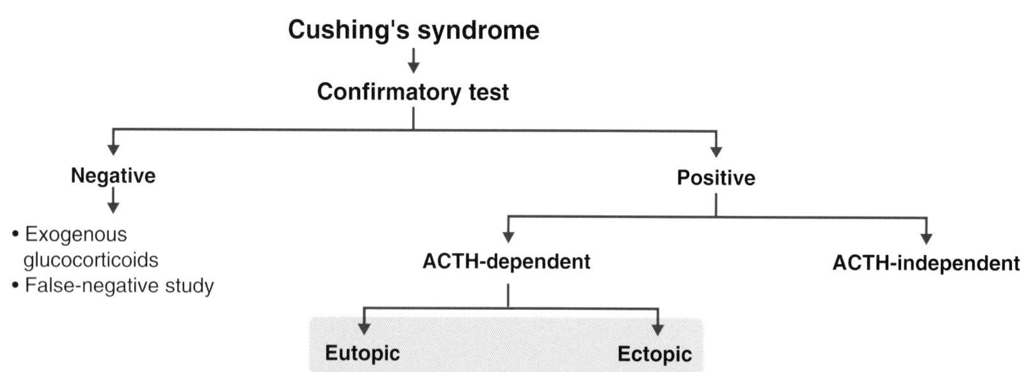


## CUSHING'S SYNDROME CAUSED BY EUTOPIC ACTH PRODUCTION

### What are the causes of eutopic ACTH production?

**When caused by this underlying condition, Cushing's syndrome is known as "Cushing's disease."**

Pituitary adenoma.

**The pituitary is overstimulated.**

Excess CRH.

Cushing's syndrome
↓
Confirmatory test

- Negative
  - Exogenous glucocorticoids
  - False-negative study
- Positive
  - ACTH-dependent
    - Eutopic
      - Pituitary adenoma
      - Excess corticotropin-releasing hormone
    - Ectopic
  - ACTH-independent

**What are the characteristics of ACTH-secreting pituitary adenomas?**

Pituitary adenoma is the most common cause of ACTH-dependent Cushing's syndrome, about 7 times more common than ectopic sources of ACTH. It is more common in women by a ratio of 4:1, with a peak incidence in the third and fourth decades of life. About half of ACTH-secreting pituitary adenomas are visible on magnetic resonance imaging (MRI) of the brain (Figure 8-4). Transsphenoidal adenectomy is the initial treatment of choice for Cushing's disease. If successful, the plasma cortisol level on the morning after transsphenoidal adenectomy will be zero. Glucocorticoid replacement is necessary until the hypothalamic-pituitary-adrenal axis regains function, which typically takes a year or longer. Up to one-third of patients will eventually experience a recurrence.[3,6]

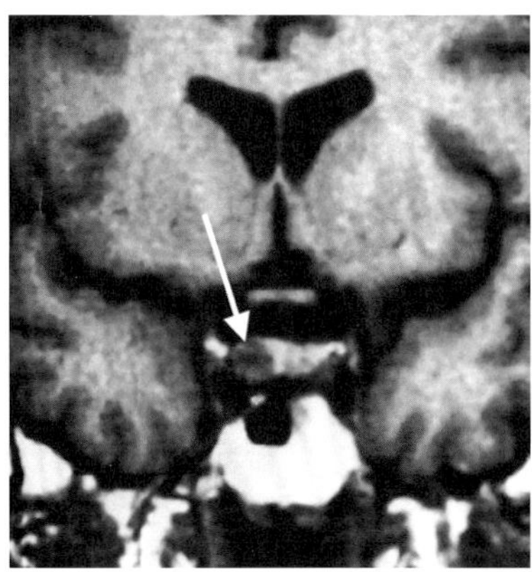

**Figure 8-4.** Pituitary adenoma. T1-weighted coronal MRI after gadolinium enhancement demonstrates a discrete focus of hypointensity (arrow) involving the right side of the pituitary gland, most consistent with pituitary adenoma. (Courtesy of Dr S. Chan.)

**What are the sources of excess corticotropin-releasing hormone?**

Excess CRH can be caused by pseudo-Cushing's syndrome or ectopic CRH production from a tumor (rare).

**What is the most common cause of pseudo-Cushing's syndrome?**

Chronic alcohol use is the most common cause of pseudo-Cushing's syndrome. Investigation into the possibility of alcohol-induced pseudo-Cushing's syndrome begins with a period of abstinence from alcohol, followed by clinical monitoring.[3]

## CUSHING'S SYNDROME CAUSED BY ECTOPIC ACTH PRODUCTION

**What electrolyte disturbance is associated with Cushing's syndrome caused by ectopic ACTH production?**

Hypokalemia is present in the majority of patients with Cushing's syndrome related to ectopic ACTH production but is only rarely seen in patients with Cushing's disease. This observation has several explanations. First, compared with those with Cushing's disease, patients with ectopic ACTH production generally have higher circulating levels of cortisol, which has activity at the mineralocorticoid receptor (which, when activated, promotes renal potassium excretion). Second, the activity of 11β-hydroxysteroid dehydrogenase type 2, which is essential in preventing the mineralocorticoid activity of cortisol, is decreased in patients with ectopic ACTH production.[7]

## What are the causes of ectopic ACTH production?

**Smoking is the most important risk factor for the development of this malignancy.**

Small cell lung cancer.

**This neuroendocrine tumor, when located in the gastrointestinal tract, can be associated with flushing and diarrhea.**

Carcinoid tumor.

**A pancreatic mass is identified on cross-sectional imaging in a patient with Cushing's syndrome.**

Pancreatic islet cell tumor (ie, pancreatic neuroendocrine tumor).

**A type of thyroid cancer that originates from the parafollicular cells (C cells).**

Medullary thyroid carcinoma.

**A 32-year-old man presents with episodes of headache, chest pressure, tachycardia, and hypertension.**

Pheochromocytoma.

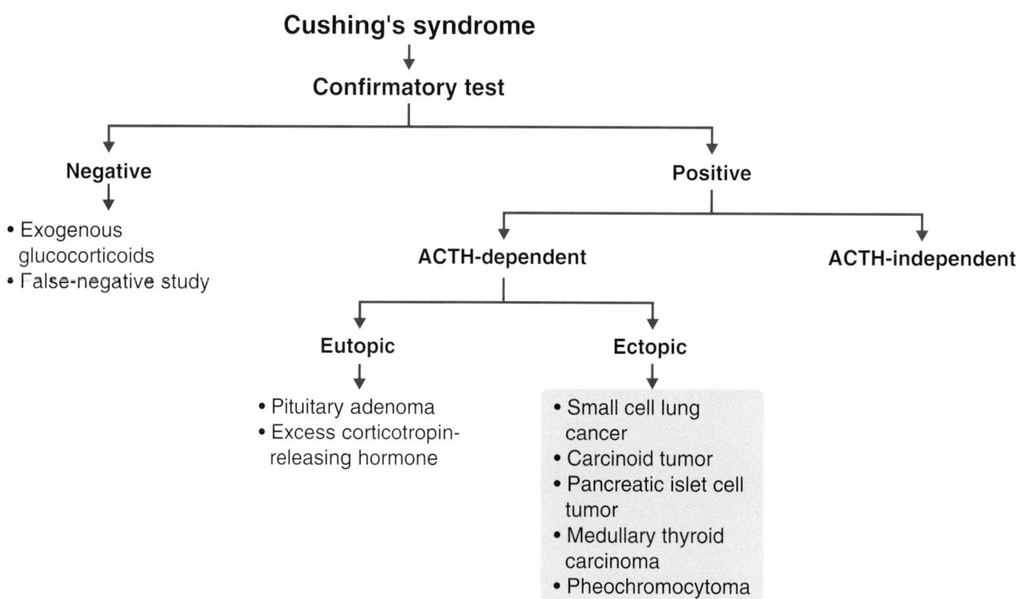


**What are the characteristics of Cushing's syndrome related to small cell lung cancer?**

Patients with ectopic ACTH production from small cell lung cancer are more likely to present with weight loss, hypokalemia, abnormal glucose tolerance, and edema rather than the more classic manifestations of Cushing's syndrome. In addition to ectopic ACTH production, small cell lung cancer can cause other paraneoplastic endocrine syndromes, including the syndrome of inappropriate antidiuretic hormone (SIADH), and hypercalcemia via parathyroid hormone–related peptide (PTHrP). Treatment of Cushing's syndrome related to small cell lung cancer includes radical excision of the tumor, chemotherapy, and pharmacologic cortisol inhibition (eg, ketoconazole). Prognosis is poor.[8]

**What are the most common locations of carcinoid tumors associated with ectopic production of ACTH?**

Carcinoid tumors of the lung, thymus, and pancreas are most often associated with ectopic ACTH production. Thymic carcinoid tumors in particular are associated with poor prognosis.[7]

**What are the characteristics of pancreatic islet cell tumors that secrete ACTH?**

Pancreatic islet cell tumors account for up to 3% of pancreatic tumors. These tumors are capable of secreting various hormones, including insulin, gastrin, glucagon, and ACTH. When the tumor is limited to the pancreas, secreted ACTH enters the enterohepatic circulation and is rapidly metabolized by the liver, preventing the clinical syndrome from developing. By the time Cushing's syndrome has become apparent, most ACTH-secreting pancreatic islet cell tumors are advanced, with hepatic metastases, and are associated with poor prognosis.[9]

**Which genetic syndrome is associated with the development of both medullary thyroid carcinoma and pheochromocytoma?**

Medullary thyroid carcinoma and pheochromocytoma can occur together in multiple endocrine neoplasia types 2a and 2b but are most often sporadic. These entities are relatively rare sources of ectopic ACTH production.[6]

**In patients with Cushing's syndrome caused by ectopic ACTH production, what is the next diagnostic step?**

Patients with ectopic sources of ACTH production should undergo an imaging study guided by the clinical presentation (eg, a patient with a history and examination compatible with pheochromocytoma should undergo imaging of the adrenal glands). When there are no clinical clues to a possible tumor site, patients should first undergo computed tomography imaging or MRI of the chest; a tumor will be found in the majority of patients. If a tumor is not identified in the chest, then MRI of the abdomen and pelvis should be performed next.[3]

**If the source of ectopic ACTH production cannot be identified after imaging the chest, abdomen, and pelvis, what treatment options are available?**

If a tumor cannot be identified in patients with ectopic ACTH production, there are 2 options for management: pharmacologic blockade of cortisol synthesis or bilateral adrenalectomy.[3]

## ACTH-INDEPENDENT CUSHING'S SYNDROME

**What is the fundamental mechanism of hypercortisolism in patients with ACTH-independent Cushing's syndrome?**

ACTH-independent Cushing's syndrome occurs as a result of excess cortisol production by the adrenal glands, independent of ACTH stimulation.

### What are the ACTH-independent causes of Cushing's syndrome?

**Cross-sectional imaging of the adrenal glands can be helpful in distinguishing these 2 causes of ACTH-independent Cushing's syndrome.**

Adrenal tumor and adrenal hyperplasia.

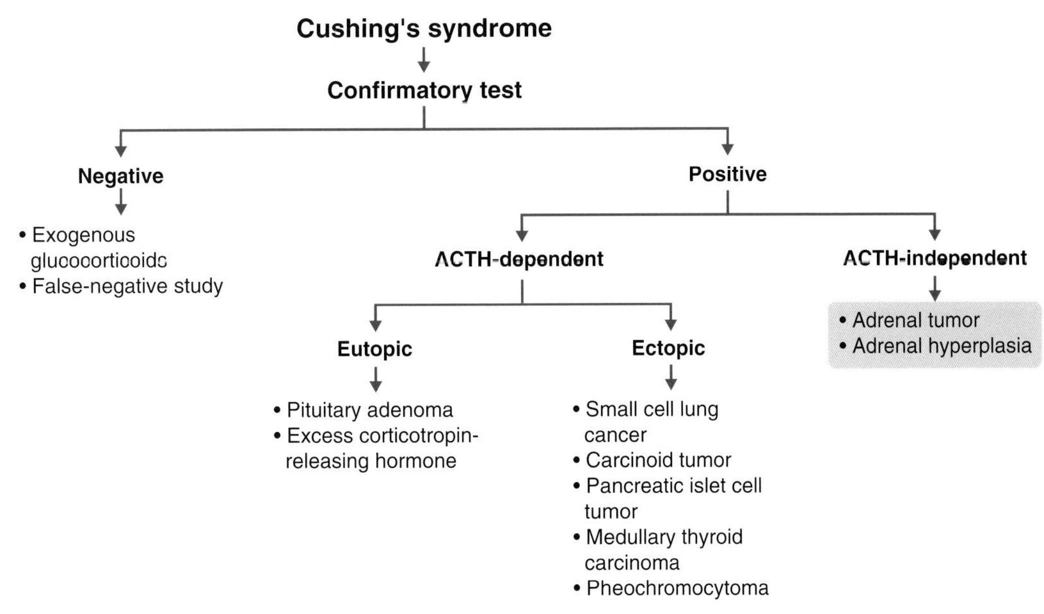

**What are the characteristics of adrenal tumors that cause Cushing's syndrome?**

Adrenal tumors capable of causing Cushing's syndrome via secretion of excess cortisol include both adenomas (benign) and carcinomas (malignant). Benign tumors tend to be smaller in size (<5 cm) and secrete only 1 hormone (eg, cortisol). These tumors are treated with laparoscopic adrenalectomy with a high rate of success. Malignant tumors tend to be larger in size (>5 cm) and secrete more than 1 hormone (eg, cortisol and androgen). Surgical removal of all detectable tissue, including metastases, should be pursued.[3]

**What are the 2 general types of ACTH-independent adrenal hyperplasia?**

Cushing's syndrome can occur as a result of micronodular adrenal hyperplasia or bilateral macronodular adrenal hyperplasia. These entities typically affect both adrenal glands. Bilateral adrenalectomy is curative. All patients who undergo bilateral adrenalectomy must be treated with lifelong glucocorticoid and mineralocorticoid replacement.[3]

## Case Summary

A 43-year-old man presents with weight gain, polyuria, and confusion, and is found to have ecchymoses, abdominal striae, and hyperpigmentation on examination and an endobronchial nodule within the left main bronchus on cross-sectional imaging of the chest.

***What is the most likely diagnosis in this patient?***

Cushing's syndrome related to ectopic ACTH production.

### BONUS QUESTIONS

***Which clinical features in this case suggest the diagnosis of Cushing's syndrome?***

Features of Cushing's syndrome in this case include central obesity, psychosis, ecchymoses, abdominal striae (see Figure 8-1), polyuria (from hyperglycemia), arterial hypertension, proximal myopathy, hyperpigmentation, and hypokalemia.

***What is the significance of the hyperpigmentation in this case?***

Hyperpigmentation is associated only with ACTH-dependent Cushing's syndrome. High levels of ACTH stimulate the melanocortin-1 receptor in the skin, resulting in hyperpigmentation. It tends to first occur in areas of the skin under pressure, including elbows, knuckles, palmar creases, lips, and buccal mucosa.[2]

***What is the most likely cause of Cushing's syndrome in this case?***

The patient in this case has ACTH-dependent Cushing's syndrome based on the elevated plasma ACTH level. Inferior petrosal sinus sampling demonstrates a central-to-peripheral ACTH ratio <3, implying an ectopic source of ACTH production. In such patients, cross-sectional imaging of the chest often reveals the source. In this case, the endobronchial nodule within the left main bronchus (see Figure 8-2, arrow) is most likely a bronchial carcinoid tumor. Bronchoscopy with biopsy would confirm the diagnosis.

***What other type of lung cancer is associated with ectopic ACTH production?***

Cushing's syndrome can also occur in patients with small cell lung cancer. However, these patients are less likely to present with the classic manifestations of Cushing's syndrome. Bronchial carcinoid tumors tend to follow a more chronic and indolent course, which allows for full development of Cushing's syndrome.[8]

***What is the treatment of choice for Cushing's syndrome related to ectopic ACTH production?***

Cushing's syndrome related to ectopic ACTH production should be treated with surgical removal of the tumor if it can be located. If surgery is not possible or the tumor cannot be located, other treatment options include pharmacologic cortisol synthesis blockade (eg, ketoconazole), and bilateral adrenalectomy.[3]

## KEY POINTS

- Cushing's syndrome is a clinical condition that results from cortisol excess.
- Clinical manifestations of Cushing's syndrome include central obesity, moon facies, buffalo hump, thin skin, bruising, abdominal striae, hyperpigmentation, hirsutism, oligomenorrhea, psychosis, proximal myopathy, arterial hypertension, hyperglycemia, hypokalemia, and osteopenia.
- When Cushing's syndrome is suspected clinically, it should be confirmed with the UFC test.
- If the UFC test is negative, it may be a false-negative result or the patient may be receiving exogenous glucocorticoids.
- Plasma ACTH level determines whether Cushing's syndrome is ACTH-dependent (80% of cases) or ACTH-independent (20% of cases).
- ACTH-dependent Cushing's syndrome occurs as a result of eutopic (pituitary) or ectopic ACTH excess. Inferior petrosal sinus sampling is used to distinguish eutopic and ectopic sources of ACTH production.
- ACTH-independent Cushing's syndrome occurs as a result of cortisol excess from the adrenal gland(s).
- Treatment for Cushing's syndrome may involve surgical and pharmacologic modalities, depending on the underlying cause.

## REFERENCES


1. Berne RML, Levy MN. *Physiology*. 4th ed. St. Louis, MO: Mosby, Inc.; 1998.
2. Charmandari E, Nicolaides NC, Chrousos GP. Adrenal insufficiency. *Lancet*. 2014;383(9935):2152-2167.
3. Loriaux DL. Diagnosis and differential diagnosis of Cushing's syndrome. *N Engl J Med*. 2017;376(15):1451-1459.
4. Loriaux DL. Diagnosis and differential diagnosis of Cushing's syndrome. *N Engl J Med*. 2017;377(2):e3.
5. Nieman LK, Biller BM, Findling JW, et al. Treatment of Cushing's syndrome: an Endocrine Society Clinical Practice Guideline. *J Clin Endocrinol Metab*. 2015;100(8):2807-2831.
6. Lacroix A, Feelders RA, Stratakis CA, Nieman LK. Cushing's syndrome. *Lancet*. 2015;386(9996):913-927.
7. Salgado LR, Fragoso MC, Knoepfelmacher M, et al. Ectopic ACTH syndrome: our experience with 25 cases. *Eur J Endocrinol*. 2006;155(5):725-733.
8. Gandhi L, Johnson BE. Paraneoplastic syndromes associated with small cell lung cancer. *J Natl Compr Canc Netw*. 2006;4(6):631-638.
9. Byun J, Kim SH, Jeong HS, Rhee Y, Lee WJ, Kang CM. ACTH-producing neuroendocrine tumor of the pancreas: a case report and literature review. *Ann Hepatobiliary Pancreat Surg*. 2017;21(1):61-65.

Chapter 9

# HYPERCALCEMIA

## Case: A 71-year-old man with confusion

A 71-year-old black man with a history of coronary artery disease and hypertension is brought to the emergency department for evaluation of confusion. Symptoms of malaise and fatigue began several weeks ago. More recently, he developed abdominal pain and frequent urination. Medications include aspirin, simvastatin, hydrochlorothiazide, and metoprolol.

Heart rate is 110 beats per minute. The patient appears ill. Jugular venous pressure is 4 cm $H_2O$. Mucous membranes and axillae are dry.

Hematocrit is 28%, serum sodium 134 mEq/L, serum chloride 110 mEq/L, serum bicarbonate 22 mEq/L, serum creatinine 2.3 mg/dL, total serum calcium 14.6 mg/dL (reference range 8.6-10.4 mg/dL), serum albumin 2.5 g/dL, and total serum protein 8.4 g/dL. Serum parathyroid hormone (PTH) is undetectable. Chest radiograph demonstrates a peripheral density with smooth borders (arrow, Figure 9-1).

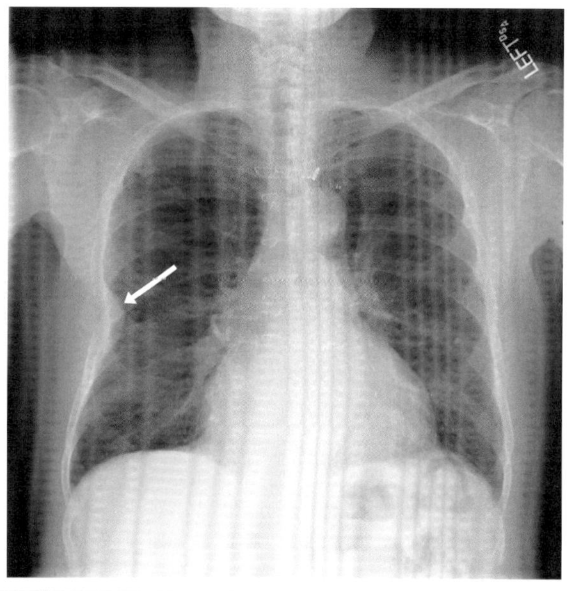


**Figure 9-1.**

***What is the most likely cause of hypercalcemia in this patient?***

What is the normal range for total serum calcium concentration?

Normal total serum calcium in adults is 8.6 to 10.4 mg/dL. Severity of hypercalcemia is variably defined, but the following thresholds provide a rule of thumb: total serum calcium 10.5 to 11.9 mg/dL is mild, total calcium 12.0 to 13.9 mg/dL is moderate, and total serum calcium >14.0 mg/dL is severe.[1,2]

How is calcium distributed in the body?

The vast majority of calcium (99%) is stored within bone, while approximately 1% is found within intracellular fluid, and about 0.1% in extracellular fluid. Total body calcium is determined by gastrointestinal absorption and renal excretion.[3]

How is calcium distributed within blood?

Under normal conditions, total serum calcium is divided between 3 forms: roughly 45% of total serum calcium is bound to plasma proteins (mostly albumin), 10% is bound to anions (eg, phosphate and citrate), and 45% is ionized (unbound). Only ionized calcium is biologically active.[1]

**What conditions may result in a change in ionized calcium but not total serum calcium concentration?**

Conditions that may change ionized calcium without changing total calcium concentration include alkalemia (decreases ionized fraction), acidemia (increases ionized fraction), and the presence of calcium chelators (decreases ionized fraction). *When these conditions are suspected, ionized calcium should be measured directly.*[1,2]

**What conditions may result in a change in total serum calcium but not ionized calcium concentration?**

Conditions that may change total calcium without changing ionized calcium concentration include hypoalbuminemia (decreases total calcium), hyperalbuminemia (increases total calcium), and multiple myeloma (increases total calcium).[1,2]

**How should the measurement of total serum calcium concentration be adjusted in the setting of hypoalbuminemia?**

Corrected total serum calcium (g/dL) = measured total serum calcium (g/dL) + (0.8 × [4 – serum album concentration (g/dL)]). *When significant changes in serum protein levels are suspected, ionized calcium should be measured directly.*[1,2]

**What processes are responsible for regulating serum calcium concentration?**

Serum ionized calcium concentration is tightly regulated by the actions of PTH and activated vitamin D (ie, $1,25(OH)_2D$, or 1,25-dihydroxyvitamin D). Hypocalcemia stimulates the secretion of PTH from the parathyroid glands and the production of activated vitamin D within the proximal tubule cells of the kidney. PTH acts directly at 2 sites in the body to increase serum calcium: the bone (by stimulating osteoclasts) and the kidney (by increasing calcium reabsorption). By stimulating production of $1,25(OH)_2D$, PTH acts indirectly in the GI tract to increase calcium absorption. Through a negative-feedback mechanism, PTH secretion from the parathyroid glands is turned off when calcium levels are normal or elevated (Figure 9-2).[3]

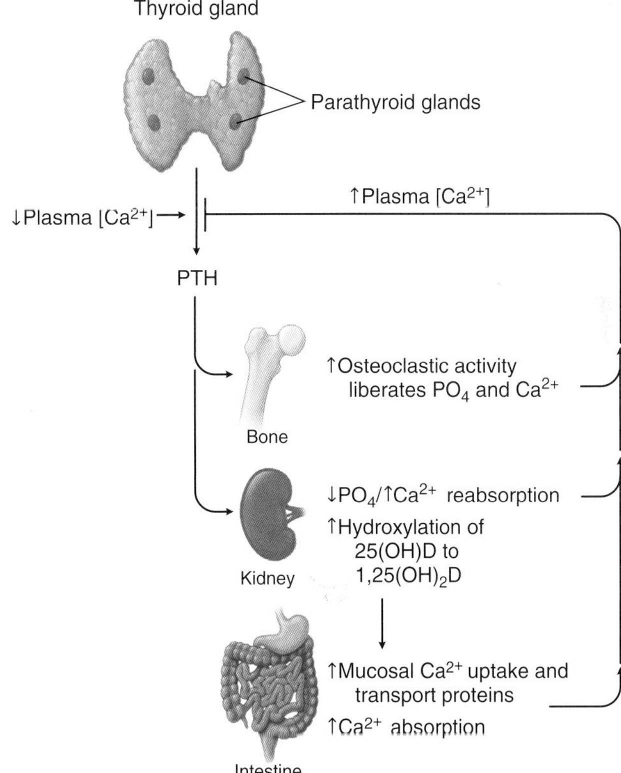


**Figure 9-2.** Summary of the actions of PTH on bones, kidneys, and intestines. Decreased serum calcium concentration is the primary stimulus for PTH secretion by the parathyroid glands. PTH raises serum calcium levels through its effects on bones, kidneys, and intestines. (From Golan DE, Armstrong EJ, Armstrong AW. *Principles of Pharmacology: The Pathophysiologic Basis of Drug Therapy*. 4th ed. Philadelphia, PA: Wolters Kluwer Health; 2017.)

**Why is it important to maintain normal serum calcium concentration?**

Hypocalcemia increases the excitability of nerve and muscle cells, which can lead to tetany; hypercalcemia decreases neuromuscular excitability, which can lead to cardiac dysrhythmias, lethargy, disorientation, and death. Clinical manifestations associated with hypercalcemia increase in severity based on not only the degree of elevation in serum calcium, but also the rate at which it develops. Moreover, older patients with preexisting cognitive dysfunction may experience neurologic complications with milder degrees of hypercalcemia compared with younger, previously healthy patients.[1-3]

**What are the symptoms of hypercalcemia?**

Mild and moderate hypercalcemia are commonly asymptomatic, depending on the rate of development and other patient-specific factors. Hypercalcemia typically affects the neuropsychiatric, gastrointestinal, and renal systems. Neuropsychiatric symptoms may include anxiety, mood changes, and decreased cognitive function. Gastrointestinal symptoms may include anorexia, constipation, abdominal pain, nausea, and vomiting. Renal symptoms may include polyuria, polydipsia, and symptoms of nephrolithiasis.[1,2,4]

**What are the electrocardiographic manifestations of hypercalcemia?**

Hypercalcemia typically causes shortening of the QT interval. Severe cases can mimic the changes associated with ST-elevation myocardial infarction. Cardiac dysrhythmias can occur, including highly unstable rhythms such as ventricular fibrillation.[4]

**What is the first step in determining the etiology of hypercalcemia?**

Serum PTH level determines whether hypercalcemia is PTH-dependent (PTH level is elevated or normal) or PTH-independent (PTH level is low).

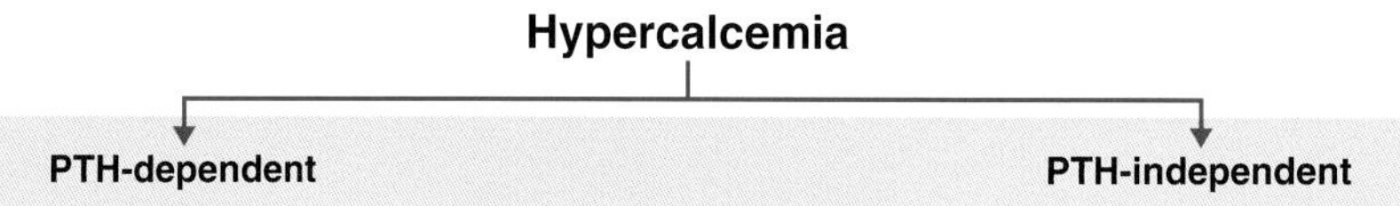


**In the setting of hypercalcemia, why does a normal serum PTH value implicate a PTH-dependent process?**

When serum calcium is elevated, negative feedback to the parathyroid glands should turn off PTH secretion in an attempt to return serum calcium levels to normal. Therefore, a PTH level within the normal range is "inappropriately normal."

## PTH-DEPENDENT HYPERCALCEMIA

**What is the fundamental mechanism of PTH-dependent hypercalcemia?**

PTH-dependent hypercalcemia occurs as a result of excess PTH secretion from the parathyroid glands despite elevated serum calcium levels.

### What are the causes of PTH-dependent hypercalcemia?

**The single most common cause of hypercalcemia.**

Primary hyperparathyroidism.[5]

**Associated with end-stage renal disease.**

Tertiary hyperparathyroidism.

**This genetic syndrome is associated with low urine calcium concentration.**

Familial hypocalciuric hypercalcemia (FHH).

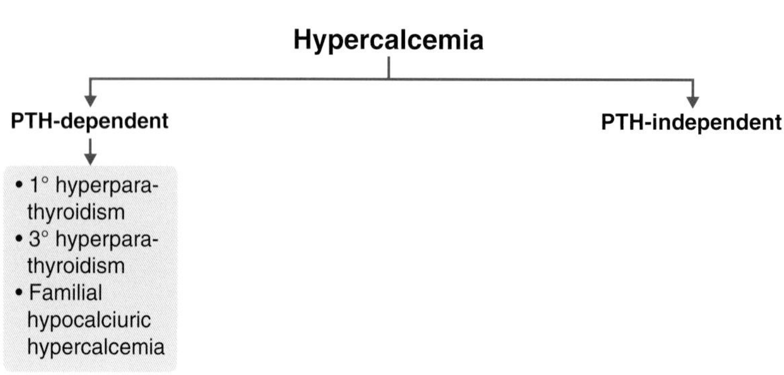

**What are the characteristics of primary hyperparathyroidism?**

Primary hyperparathyroidism can occur as a result of parathyroid adenoma, hyperplasia, or carcinoma (rare). It can be sporadic or part of the multiple endocrine neoplasia (MEN) types 1 and 2a syndromes. The majority of cases occur in women, and incidence peaks in the seventh decade of life (incidence is similar between men and women before 45 years of age). In the industrialized world, most patients are asymptomatic and the disease is discovered with routine laboratory evaluation, although worldwide, a significant proportion of patients are symptomatic. Treatment is surgical. Asymptomatic patients can be monitored over time.[5]

**What clinical features raise suspicion that primary hyperparathyroidism may be part of an underlying multiple endocrine neoplasia syndrome?**

The possibility that primary hyperparathyroidism is part of an underlying MEN syndrome increases with the presence of skin lesions associated with MEN (eg, angiofibroma) and when patients are young (<30 years), have a family history of hypercalcemia, and have a personal or family history of neuroendocrine tumors.[5]

**What clinical features raise suspicion that primary hyperparathyroidism is caused by parathyroid carcinoma?**

The possibility that primary hyperparathyroidism is caused by parathyroid carcinoma increases when there is a palpable neck mass, severe hypercalcemia (>14 mg/dL), and markedly elevated PTH levels (greater than 3-10 times the upper limit of normal). Parathyroid carcinoma is a rare cause of hypercalcemia (<1% of cases).[5]

**Is secondary hyperparathyroidism associated with hypercalcemia?**

Secondary hyperparathyroidism is not associated with hypercalcemia. In fact, it is usually associated with normal or low serum calcium levels. Secondary hyperparathyroidism occurs in patients with compromised renal function. In these patients, PTH secretion is stimulated in response to phosphate retention and decreased activated vitamin D levels. Serum calcium levels may be preserved initially, but as renal dysfunction progresses, the compensatory response begins to fail.[6]

**What is tertiary hyperparathyroidism?**

Tertiary hyperparathyroidism can occur after chronic secondary hyperparathyroidism is corrected. Long-standing secondary hyperparathyroidism (usually from renal failure) results in hypertrophy of the parathyroid glands, which can continue to secrete PTH in excess for prolonged periods after the underlying cause of secondary hyperparathyroidism has been corrected (eg, hemodialysis is started).

**What is the underlying mechanism of hypercalcemia in familial hypocalciuric hypercalcemia?**

In FHH, a mutation in the calcium-sensing receptor expressed in parathyroid tissue causes decreased sensitivity to serum calcium levels. This results in an increase in the "set point" of serum calcium, leading to inappropriate secretion of PTH despite elevated serum calcium.[5]

## PTH-INDEPENDENT HYPERCALCEMIA

**What is the fundamental mechanism of PTH-independent hypercalcemia?**

PTH-independent hypercalcemia occurs despite normal parathyroid gland function and decreased (often undetectable) serum PTH levels.

**The causes of PTH-independent hypercalcemia can be separated into which general subcategories?**

The causes of PTH-independent hypercalcemia can be separated into the following subcategories: medication, malignancy, granulomatous disease, endocrinopathy, and other.

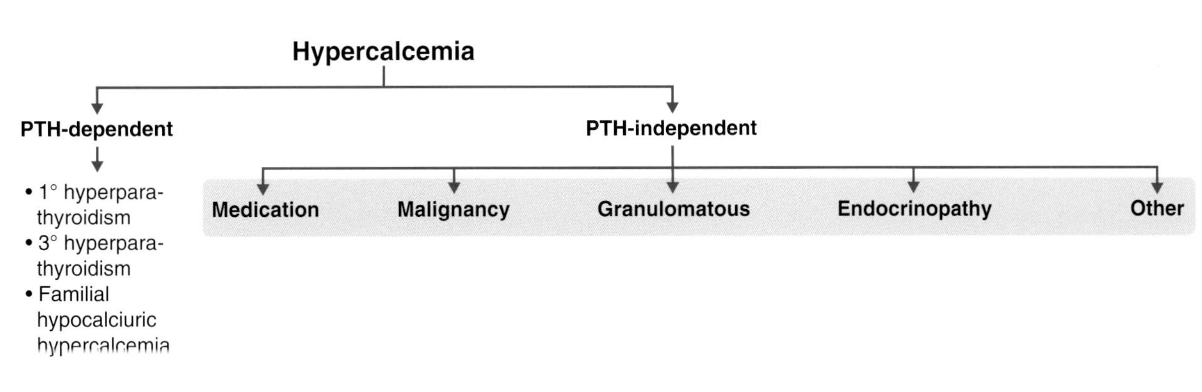


ENDOCRINOLOGY

## PTH-INDEPENDENT HYPERCALCEMIA RELATED TO MEDICATION

### Which medications cause PTH-independent hypercalcemia?

**A 40-year-old woman uses over-the-counter medication to treat severe acid reflux disease.**

Milk-alkali syndrome.

**Vitamins.**

Vitamins D and A.

**A 52-year-old man develops hypercalcemia after starting treatment for hypertension.**

Thiazide diuretics.

**Hypercalcemia in a patient with bipolar disorder.**

Lithium.

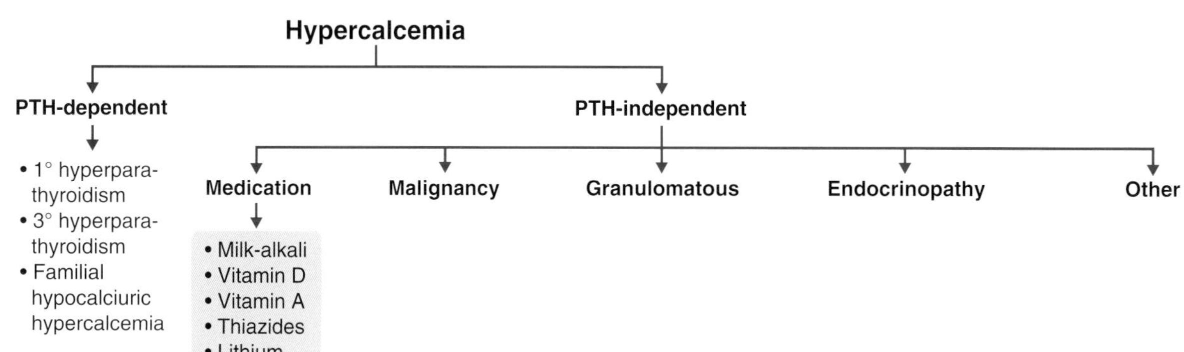


**What is the milk-alkali syndrome?**

Milk-alkali syndrome is characterized by the development of hypercalcemia with hypercalciuria and renal dysfunction in patients who consume large quantities of calcium (at least 2 g of elemental calcium per day) and absorbable alkali (eg, calcium carbonate). The history may be readily informative, but sometimes the nature of the dietary source may be harder to recognize (eg, the combination of betel nuts with oyster shell powder). In some cases, the patient may intentionally or unintentionally conceal the ingestion.[7,8]

**What is the safe limit for daily vitamin D intake?**

The dose at which vitamin D becomes toxic is not clearly known, but the recommended upper limit of daily intake is 100 μg (4000 IU).[9]

**What are the dietary sources of preformed vitamin A?**

The most common dietary sources of preformed vitamin A include multivitamins, fish liver oil, animal liver, and fortified foods including milk, butter, margarine, and breakfast cereals. Chronic toxicity develops when patients consume large amounts of preformed vitamin A over months to years.[10]

**What is the mechanism of hypercalcemia related to thiazide diuretic use?**

Thiazide diuretics can increase the reabsorption of calcium in the kidney. Hypercalcemia occurs in up to 8% of patients taking thiazides.[1]

**What is the problem with relying on symptoms to diagnose hypercalcemia related to lithium use in bipolar patients?**

The symptoms of hypercalcemia can mimic those of the underlying mental health disorder being treated with lithium. Hypercalcemia occurs in approximately 15% of patients taking lithium. The mechanisms of lithium-induced hypercalcemia are direct stimulation of PTH secretion and increased renal calcium reabsorption. It is reversible with careful discontinuation of the drug.[1,11]

## PTH-INDEPENDENT HYPERCALCEMIA RELATED TO MALIGNANCY

### What are the 3 main mechanisms of PTH-independent hypercalcemia related to malignancy?

**The most common mechanism of hypercalcemia associated with malignancy, responsible for 80% of cases.**

Secretion of parathyroid hormone–related peptide (PTHrP).[4]

**Sometimes visible on imaging; this condition is responsible for 20% of cases of hypercalcemia related to malignancy.**

Osteolytic metastases.[4]

**This is also the mechanism of hypercalcemia related to sarcoidosis.**

Ectopic 1,25$(OH)_2$D secretion.

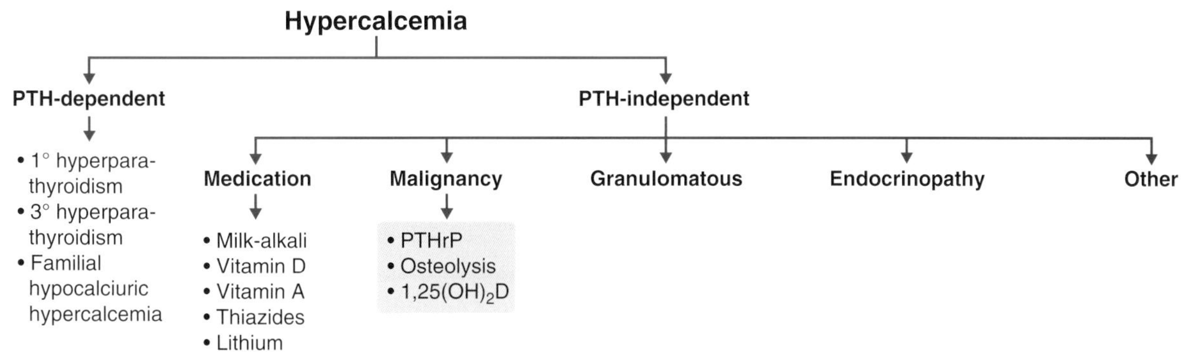


**Which malignancies are most commonly associated with hypercalcemia?**

Malignancies most frequently associated with hypercalcemia include breast cancer, lung cancer, and multiple myeloma.[12]

**What is the mechanism of PTHrP-induced hypercalcemia?**

PTHrP is close in structure to PTH and acts on the same receptors, with overlapping effects. Most cases of hypercalcemia related to PTHrP are associated with breast cancer, squamous cell cancer, renal cell carcinoma, bladder cancer, ovarian cancer, non-Hodgkin's lymphoma, and endometrial cancer.[2,4]

**Which malignancies are capable of causing hypercalcemia through local osteolysis?**

Most cases of hypercalcemia related to local osteolysis are associated with breast cancer and multiple myeloma (Figure 9-3). Lymphoma is also capable of causing hypercalcemia through this mechanism.[2,4]

**Which malignancies are capable of causing hypercalcemia through the production of 1,25$(OH)_2$D?**

Most cases of hypercalcemia from ectopic production of 1,25$(OH)_2$D are related to lymphoma and some ovarian germ cell tumors.[2,4]

**Figure 9-3.** Lateral radiograph of the distal femur of a 65-year-old woman with multiple myeloma showing multiple lytic lesions, which produce a characteristic "moth-eaten" appearance. (From Greenspan A. *Orthopedic Imaging: A Practical Approach*. 5th ed. Philadelphia, PA: Lippincott Williams & Wilkins; 2011.)

## PTH-INDEPENDENT HYPERCALCEMIA RELATED TO GRANULOMATOUS DISEASE

**What is the mechanism of hypercalcemia related to granulomatous disease?**

Granulomatous diseases can cause hypercalcemia as a result of ectopic secretion of 1,25$(OH)_2$D. The hypercalcemia of granulomatous disease can be aggravated by a diet rich in vitamin D and excessive sun exposure. Serum levels of 1,25$(OH)_2$D can be measured to support the diagnosis.[13]

**What medication can be helpful in treating the hypercalcemia associated with granulomatous disease?**

Glucocorticoids can treat the hypercalcemia associated with granulomatous disease by decreasing the production of 1,25$(OH)_2$D through the inhibition of 1-α-hydroxylase and stimulating its metabolism through the activation of 24-hydroxylase.[1,14]

### What are the granulomatous causes of PTH-independent hypercalcemia?

**A 52-year-old woman presents with chronic fatigue and dyspnea and is found to have hypercalcemia and bilateral hilar lymphadenopathy (see Figure 21-4).**

Sarcoidosis.

**A 39-year-old expatriate of Mexico presents with weight loss, night sweats, and hemoptysis.**

Tuberculosis (TB).

**Saddle nose deformity (see Figure 50-4).**

Granulomatosis with polyangiitis (GPA, or Wegener's granulomatosis).

**A 34-year-old spelunker presents with fever and cough.**

Histoplasmosis.

**Abdominal pain and diarrhea.**

Crohn's disease.

**Between lithium and boron.**

Berylliosis.

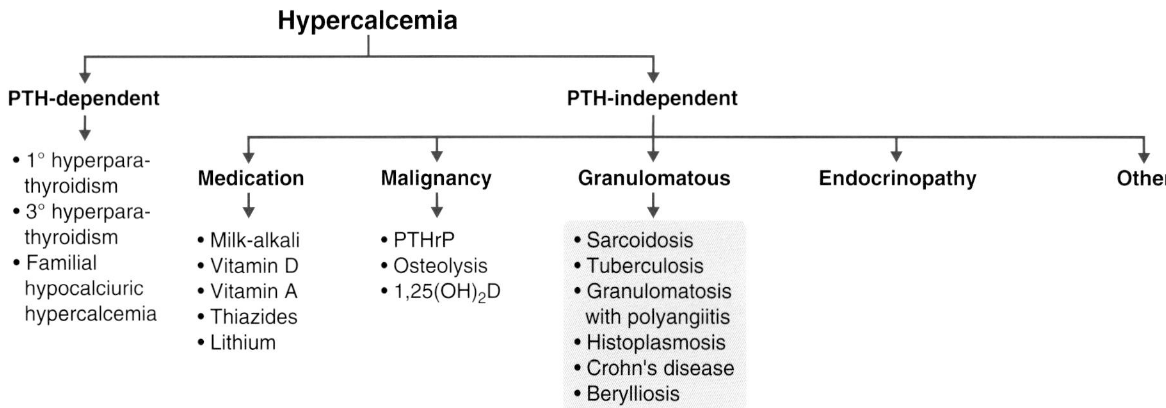


**What are the characteristics of hypercalcemia related to sarcoidosis?**

Hypercalcemia occurs in around one-fifth of patients with sarcoidosis. It can develop in any patient with sarcoidosis regardless of race, age, or sex. It occurs more frequently in patients with systemic sarcoidosis compared with those with limited disease. Most patients have mild hypercalcemia, but severe life-threatening hypercalcemia can occur.[15]

**What medication can be added to the antimicrobial treatment for tuberculosis to lower calcium levels?**

In patients with hypercalcemia related to TB, glucocorticoids can be added to the antituberculosis regimen to control calcium levels.[13]

**What is the prognosis of hypercalcemia related to granulomatosis with polyangiitis?**

The hypercalcemia of GPA is responsive to treatment for the underlying condition with glucocorticoids and cyclophosphamide.[13]

**Where is *Histoplasma capsulatum* endemic?**

*Histoplasma capsulatum* is endemic to the Midwestern and South Central regions of the United States, and most cases originate there. Histoplasmosis has also been reported in Southeast Asia (eg, Indonesia, Thailand, Vietnam).[16]

**Is Crohn's disease more commonly associated with hypercalcemia or hypocalcemia?**

Although Crohn's disease can be associated with hypercalcemia, hypocalcemia is more common because of poor calcium intake and vitamin D deficiency related to malabsorption.[17]

**Beryllium exposure most frequently occurs in what industries?**

Beryllium is used in automotive electronics, telecommunications, computers, aerospace, and defense equipment. Many workers are unaware of the exposure.[18]

**What other granulomatous conditions can cause hypercalcemia?**

Other granulomatous conditions associated with hypercalcemia include fungal infections (eg, coccidioidomycosis), leprosy, and foreign-body granulomatous reactions (eg, silicosis).[13]

## PTH-INDEPENDENT HYPERCALCEMIA RELATED TO ENDOCRINOPATHY

### What are the endocrinologic causes of PTH-independent hypercalcemia?

**Associated with a fine tremor.**

Thyrotoxicosis.

**Hypoglycemia, hyponatremia, and hypercalcemia.**

Adrenal insufficiency.

**A disease that does not respond well to β-blocker monotherapy.**

Pheochromocytoma.

**A 43-year-old woman goes up in shoe size for the first time in 30 years.**

Acromegaly.

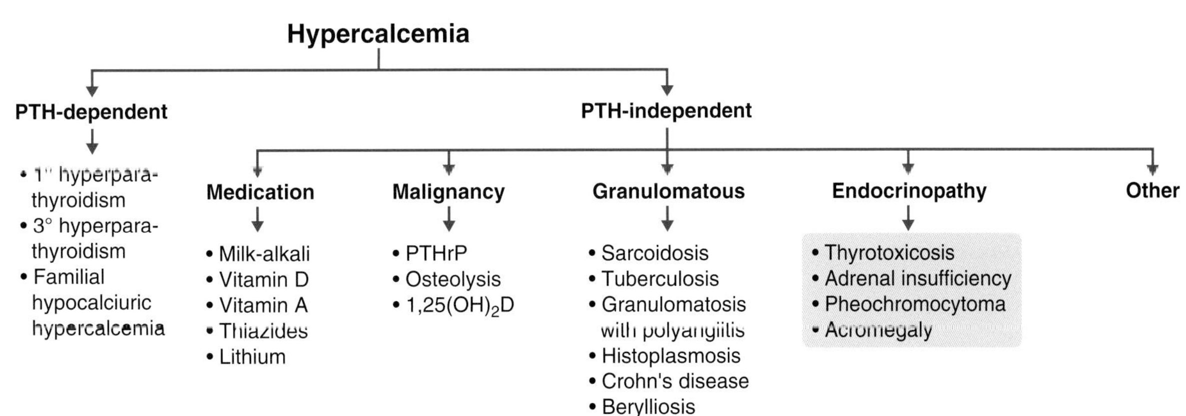


ENDOCRINOLOGY

**What are the characteristics of hypercalcemia related to thyrotoxicosis?**

Hypercalcemia occurs in around one-fifth of patients with thyrotoxicosis and is typically mild to moderate in severity. The mechanism of hypercalcemia related to thyrotoxicosis is thought to be increased bone turnover. It is reversible with treatment of thyrotoxicosis.[19]

**What are the characteristics of hypercalcemia related to adrenal insufficiency?**

Hypercalcemia is not uncommon in patients with adrenal insufficiency, particularly during acute episodes (ie, adrenal crisis). Volume contraction results in hemoconcentration and increased renal calcium reabsorption. It is reversible with treatment of adrenal insufficiency.[20]

**What are the mechanisms of hypercalcemia related to pheochromocytoma?**

Hypercalcemia can develop in patients with pheochromocytoma as a result of ectopic secretion of PTHrP, catecholamine-induced osteoclastic bone resorption, and catecholamine-induced PTH secretion. It is reversible with removal of the tumor.[21]

**What is the most common cause of hypercalcemia in patients with acromegaly?**

Hypercalcemia related to acromegaly is most commonly the result of coexisting primary hyperparathyroidism. However, when it occurs independently, the mechanism is thought to be overproduction of 1,25(OH)$_2$D. It is typically mild in severity and, in most cases, resolves with treatment of acromegaly.[22]

*Some endocrinopathies occur in association with multiple endocrine neoplasia syndromes, and hypercalcemia may be driven by primary hyperparathyroidism in those cases.*

## OTHER CAUSES OF PTH-INDEPENDENT HYPERCALCEMIA

### What are the other causes of PTH-independent hypercalcemia?

**A 25-year-old man develops hypercalcemia 2 months after a car accident that has left him bedbound.**

Immobility.

**A patient with a crush injury initially presents with hypocalcemia but subsequently develops hypercalcemia.**

Rhabdomyolysis.

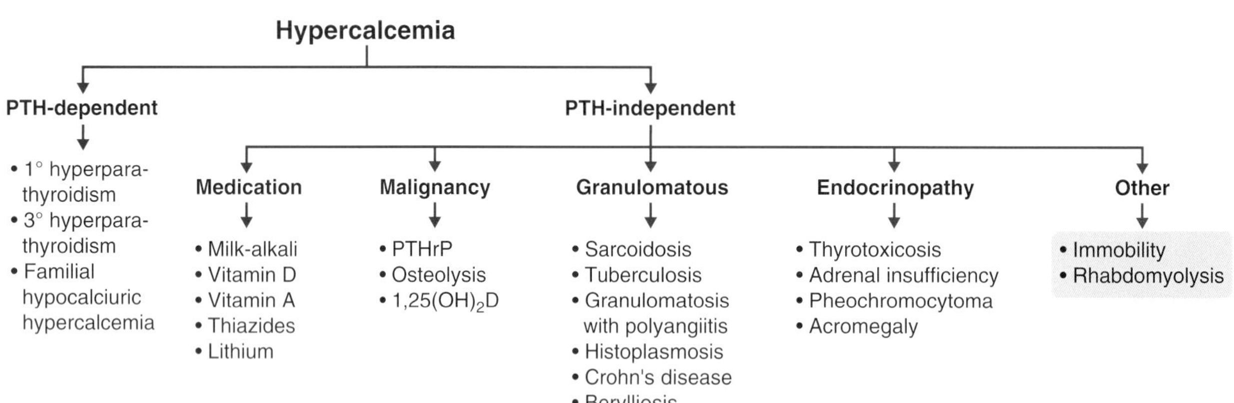


**What are the characteristics of hypercalcemia related to immobilization?**

Hypercalcemia from immobilization typically affects children or young adults during the first 4 to 6 weeks after an inciting event; however, it can happen months later. It is caused by increased bone resorption. Bisphosphonates are useful in treating this condition. Physical therapy should also be used to improve the underlying condition.[23]

**What are the characteristics of hypercalcemia related to rhabdomyolysis?**

Calcium dysregulation occurs in patients with rhabdomyolysis complicated by acute kidney injury. Hypocalcemia is the dominant finding in early rhabdomyolysis, during the oliguric phase of kidney injury; it is likely related to calcium deposition in injured tissues. Around one-third of these patients develop hypercalcemia during the diuretic phase of acute kidney injury related to the remobilization of calcium from the soft tissues. Increased $1,25(OH)_2D$ levels may also play a role.[24]

## Case Summary

A 71-year-old black man with a history of hypertension treated with a thiazide diuretic presents with confusion and is found to have anemia, kidney injury, hypercalcemia, elevated protein gap, and an abnormal chest radiograph.

***What is the most likely cause of hypercalcemia in this patient?***

Multiple myeloma.

BONUS QUESTIONS

***What is multiple myeloma?***

Multiple myeloma is a clonal plasma cell malignant neoplasm with characteristic clinical manifestations. Multiple myeloma occurs more frequently in men and blacks, and is almost always preceded by monoclonal gammopathy of unknown significance. The median age at onset is 66 years. The most common clinical manifestations are fatigue, bone pain, anemia, kidney injury, hypercalcemia, and osteolytic skeletal lesions (see Figure 9-3).[25]

***What is the significance of the anion gap in this case?***

Because of the presence of cationic paraproteins, the anion gap is frequently low or negative in patients with multiple myeloma. In this case, the low anion gap of 2 mEq/L is a clue to the diagnosis.[26]

***Which laboratory tests should be ordered to investigate the elevated total protein in this case?***

The diagnosis of multiple myeloma is based on the presence of a monoclonal protein in serum or urine and the presence of ≥10% monoclonal bone marrow plasma cells. Serum protein electrophoresis can be used to identify a monoclonal (M) protein, which is characterized as a narrow spike in the $\gamma$ zone of the gel. Serum immunofixation can then confirm that the gammopathy is monoclonal rather than polyclonal in nature. A monoclonal protein is identified on serum protein electrophoresis in 80% of patients with multiple myeloma. Adding serum immunofixation and the serum free light chain assay (or 24-hour urinary protein electrophoresis with immunofixation) will identify a monoclonal protein in nearly all cases. About 2% to 3% of cases are not associated with a detectable monoclonal protein and are referred to as "nonsecretory multiple myeloma." In such cases, the diagnosis is based on the presence of ≥30% monoclonal bone marrow plasma cells, or a biopsy-proven plasmacytoma.[25,27]

***What is the significance of the radiographic abnormality in this case?***

The peripheral density in the chest radiograph in this case (see Figure 9-1, arrow) has a "ball-under-the-rug" appearance, which indicates that the lesion arises from outside the parietal pleura of the lung (eg, rib metastasis, nerve sheath tumor, lipoma). In this case, the most likely explanation is a plasmacytoma arising from the chest wall or rib.[20]

***What is the significance of the use of hydrochlorothiazide by the patient in this case?***

Although it is not the principal cause of hypercalcemia in this case, thiazide diuretics can contribute to hypercalcemia and should be stopped in patients with hypercalcemia from other causes.

***What is the corrected serum total calcium concentration in this case?***

Corrected total serum calcium (g/dL) = 14.6 g/dL + (0.8 × [4 − 2.5 g/dL]) = 15.8 g/dL.

| | |
|---|---|
| ***What treatment(s) can be used to acutely lower serum calcium levels?*** | Patients with hypercalcemia are often dehydrated as a result of hypercalcemia-mediated nephrogenic diabetes insipidus, and decreased oral intake related to gastrointestinal symptoms. Intravenous crystalloid solutions can be used to expand intravascular volume and decrease reabsorption of calcium in the proximal tubule. Calcitonin can also be used to acutely decrease serum calcium by inhibiting bone resorption and decreasing renal tubular calcium reabsorption.[1] |
| ***Which class of medications can be used for long-term management of hypercalcemia in this case (not including treatment for the underlying disease)?*** | Bisphosphonates are the long term treatment of choice for hypercalcemia and act by decreasing bone resorption through the inhibition of osteoclast activity. The calcium-lowering effect of bisphosphonates typically requires several days.[1] |

## KEY POINTS

- Serum calcium levels are tightly regulated by the actions of PTH and the active form of vitamin D.
- Hypercalcemia decreases neuromuscular excitability with manifestations that include anxiety, mood changes, decreased cognitive function, anorexia, constipation, abdominal pain, nausea, vomiting, polyuria, polydipsia, QT shortening, and cardiac dysrhythmia.
- Clinical manifestations associated with hypercalcemia increase in severity based on not only the degree of elevation in serum calcium, but also the rate at which it develops.
- Serum PTH level determines whether hypercalcemia is PTH-dependent or PTH-independent.
- The most common cause of PTH-dependent hypercalcemia (and of hypercalcemia overall) is primary hyperparathyroidism.
- The causes of PTH-independent hypercalcemia can be separated into the following subcategories: medication, malignancy, granulomatous disease, endocrinopathy, and other.
- Intravenous fluids and calcitonin can be used to acutely decrease serum calcium levels.
- Hypercalcemia can be managed long-term with bisphosphonates and by treating the underlying condition.

## REFERENCES


1. Minisola S, Pepe J, Piemonte S, Cipriani C. The diagnosis and management of hypercalcaemia. *BMJ.* 2015;350:h2723.
2. Stewart AF. Clinical practice. Hypercalcemia associated with cancer. *N Engl J Med.* 2005;352(4):373-379.
3. Berne RML, Levy MN. *Physiology.* 4th ed. St. Louis, MO: Mosby, Inc.; 1998.
4. Mirrakhimov AE. Hypercalcemia of malignancy: an update on pathogenesis and management. *N Am J Med Sci.* 2015;7(11):483-493.
5. Marcocci C, Cetani F. Clinical practice. Primary hyperparathyroidism. *N Engl J Med.* 2011;365(25):2389-2397.
6. de Francisco AL. Secondary hyperparathyroidism: review of the disease and its treatment. *Clin Ther.* 2004;26(12):1976-1993.
7. Jacobs TP, Bilezikian JP. Clinical review: rare causes of hypercalcemia. *J Clin Endocrinol Metab.* 2005;90(11):6316-6322.
8. Orwoll ES. The milk-alkali syndrome: current concepts. *Ann Intern Med.* 1982;97(2):242-248.
9. Ross AC, Manson JE, Abrams SA, et al. The 2011 report on dietary reference intakes for calcium and vitamin D from the Institute of Medicine: what clinicians need to know. *J Clin Endocrinol Metab.* 2011;96(1):53-58.
10. Penniston KL, Tanumihardjo SA. The acute and chronic toxic effects of vitamin A. *Am J Clin Nutr.* 2006;83(2):191-201.
11. Twigt BA, Houweling BM, Vriens MR, et al. Hypercalcemia in patients with bipolar disorder treated with lithium: a cross-sectional study. *Int J Bipolar Disord.* 2013;1:18.
12. Seccareccia D. Cancer-related hypercalcemia. *Can Fam Physician.* 2010;56(3):244-246, e90–e92.
13. Sharma OP. Hypercalcemia in granulomatous disorders: a clinical review. *Curr Opin Pulm Med.* 2000;6(5):442-447.
14. Kallas M, Green F, Hewison M, White C, Kline G. Rare causes of calcitriol-mediated hypercalcemia: a case report and literature review. *J Clin Endocrinol Metab.* 2010;95(7):3111-3117.
15. Winnacker JL, Becker KL, Katz S. Endocrine aspects of sarcoidosis. *N Engl J Med.* 1968;278(8):427-434.
16. Liu JW, Huang TC, Lu YC, et al. Acute disseminated histoplasmosis complicated with hypercalcaemia. *J Infect.* 1999;39(1):88-90.
17. Tuohy KA, Steinman TI. Hypercalcemia due to excess 1,25-dihydroxyvitamin D in Crohn's disease. *Am J Kidney Dis.* 2005;45(1):e3-e6.
18. Balmes JR, Abraham JL, Dweik RA, et al. An official American Thoracic Society statement: diagnosis and management of beryllium sensitivity and chronic beryllium disease. *Am J Respir Crit Care Med.* 2014;190(10):e34-e59.
19. Chen K, Xie Y, Zhao L, Mo Z. Hyperthyroidism-associated hypercalcemic crisis: a case report and review of the literature. *Medicine.* 2017;96(4):e6017.
20. Muls E, Bouillon R, Boelaert J, et al. Etiology of hypercalcemia in a patient with Addison's disease. *Calcif Tissue Int.* 1982;34(6):523-526.
21. Kannan CR. *The Adrenal Gland.* New York, NY: Plenum Publishing Corporation; 1988.

22. Shah R, Licata A, Oyesiku NM, Ioachimescu AG. Acromegaly as a cause of 1,25-dihydroxyvitamin D-dependent hypercalcemia: case reports and review of the literature. *Pituitary*. 2012;15 suppl 1:S17-S22.
23. Cano-Torres EA, Gonzalez-Cantu A, Hinojosa-Garza G, Castilleja-Leal F. Immobilization induced hypercalcemia. *Clin Cases Miner Bone Metab*. 2016;13(1):46-47.
24. Akmal M, Bishop JE, Telfer N, Norman AW, Massry SG. Hypocalcemia and hypercalcemia in patients with rhabdomyolysis with and without acute renal failure. *J Clin Endocrinol Metab*. 1986;63(1):137-142.
25. Rajkumar SV, Kumar S. Multiple myeloma: diagnosis and treatment. *Mayo Clin Proc*. 2016;91(1):101-119.
26. Murray T, Long W, Narins RG. Multiple myeloma and the anion gap. *N Engl J Med*. 1975;292(11):574-575.
27. Palumbo A, Anderson K. Multiple myeloma. *N Engl J Med*. 2011;364(11):1046-1060.
28. Hsu CC, Henry TS, Chung JH, Little BP. The incomplete border sign. *J Thorac Imaging*. 2014;29(4):W48.

ENDOCRINOLOGY

Chapter 10

# HYPOCALCEMIA

## Case: An 18-year-old man with chest pain

A previously healthy 18-year-old man presents to the emergency department for evaluation of chest pain and other symptoms. Just before arrival, he was playing basketball with his cousins when he complained of chest discomfort and difficulty breathing. He then developed numbness around his mouth and had difficulty freely move his hands and feet. The patient does not drink alcohol or use illicit substances. He is starting college soon and has been dealing with the recent death of his father.

Heart rate is 120 beats per minute and regular, respiratory rate is 38 breaths per minute, and blood pressure is 155/89 mm Hg. Hemoglobin oxygen saturation by pulse oximetry is normal on room air. The patient is in extremis, with increased work of breathing. The lungs are clear to auscultation. There are spasms of the hands and feet. Tapping the facial nerve elicits upward movement of the lips on the ipsilateral side.

Serum albumin is 4.2 g/dL, total serum calcium is 9.6 mg/dL (reference range 8.6-10.4 mg/dL), and ionized calcium is 3.1 mg/dL (reference range 4.6-5.08 mg/dL). Arterial blood gas measurement shows pH 7.71, partial pressure of carbon dioxide 18 mm Hg, and bicarbonate 22 mg/dL. Serum parathyroid hormone (PTH) is elevated.

***What is the most likely cause of hypocalcemia in this patient?***

**What is the normal range for total serum calcium concentration?**

Normal total serum calcium in adults is 8.6 to 10.4 mg/dL.[1]

**How is calcium distributed in the body?**

The vast majority of calcium (99%) is stored within bone, while 1% is found within intracellular fluid, and about 0.1% in extracellular fluid. Total body calcium is determined by gastrointestinal absorption and renal excretion.[2]

**How is calcium distributed in blood?**

Under normal conditions, total serum calcium is divided between 3 forms: roughly 45% of total calcium is bound to plasma proteins (mostly albumin), 10% is bound to anions (eg, phosphate and citrate), and 45% is ionized (unbound). Only ionized calcium is biologically active.[1]

**What conditions may result in a change in ionized calcium but not total serum calcium concentration?**

Conditions that may change ionized calcium without changing total calcium concentration include alkalemia (decreases ionized fraction), acidemia (increases ionized fraction), and the presence of calcium chelators (decreases ionized fraction). *When these conditions are suspected, ionized calcium should be measured directly.*[1,3]

**What conditions may result in a change in total serum calcium but not ionized calcium concentration?**

Conditions that may change total calcium without changing ionized calcium concentration include hypoalbuminemia (decreases total calcium), hyperalbuminemia (increases total calcium), and multiple myeloma (increases total calcium).[1-3]

**How should the measurement of total serum calcium concentration be adjusted in the setting of hypoalbuminemia?**

Corrected total serum calcium (g/dL) = measured total serum calcium (g/dL) + (0.8 × [4 − serum album concentration (g/dL)]). *When significant changes in serum protein levels are suspected, ionized calcium should be measured directly.*[1,3]

**What processes are responsible for regulating serum calcium concentration?**

Serum ionized calcium concentration is tightly regulated by the actions of PTH and activated vitamin D (ie, $1,25(OH)_2D$, or 1,25-dihydroxyvitamin D). Hypocalcemia stimulates the secretion of PTH from the parathyroid glands and the production of activated vitamin D within the proximal tubule cells of the kidney. PTH acts directly at 2 sites in the body to increase serum calcium: the bone (by stimulating osteoclasts) and the kidney (by increasing calcium reabsorption). By stimulating production of $1,25(OH)_2D$, PTH acts indirectly in the GI tract to increase calcium absorption. Through a negative feedback mechanism, PTH secretion from the parathyroid glands is turned off when calcium levels are normal or elevated (see Figure 9-2).[2]

**Why is it important to maintain normal serum calcium concentration?**

Hypocalcemia increases the excitability of nerve and muscle cells, which can lead to tetany; hypercalcemia decreases neuromuscular excitability, which can lead to cardiac dysrhythmias, lethargy, disorientation, and death. Clinical manifestations associated with hypocalcemia increase in severity based on not only the degree of elevation in serum calcium, but also the rate at which it develops.[1,4]

**What are the clinical manifestations of hypocalcemia?**

Mild and moderate hypocalcemia are commonly asymptomatic, depending on the rate of development and other patient-specific factors. Hypocalcemia can lead to neuromuscular excitability with manifestations that may include muscle twitching and spasm (eg, carpopedal spasm), tingling, numbness, hyperreflexia, tetany, seizure, QT prolongation, and cardiac dysrhythmia. Physical findings include Chvostek's sign and Trousseau's sign.[4]

**What is Chvostek's sign?**

Chvostek's sign describes facial muscle contraction on tapping the parotid gland over the facial nerve.[4]

**What is Trousseau's sign?**

Trousseau's sign describes the development of carpal spasms after inflating a sphygmomanometer cuff over the brachial artery above systolic blood pressure. It is more specific for hypocalcemia than Chvostek's sign.[4]

**What is the first step in determining the etiology of hypocalcemia?**

Serum PTH level determines whether hypocalcemia is PTH-dependent (PTH level is low or normal) or PTH-independent (PTH level is elevated).

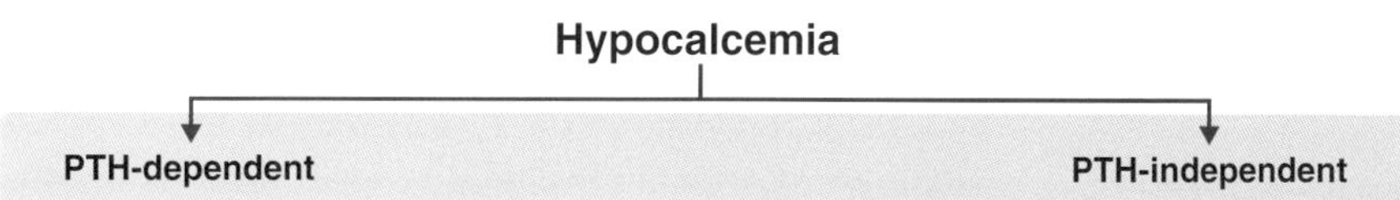


**In the setting of hypocalcemia, why does a normal serum PTH value implicate a PTH-dependent process?**

When serum calcium is low, PTH secretion from the parathyroid glands should increase in an attempt to return serum calcium levels to normal. Therefore, a PTH level within the normal range is "inappropriately normal."

## PTH-DEPENDENT HYPOCALCEMIA

**What is the fundamental mechanism of PTH-dependent hypocalcemia?**

PTH-dependent hypocalcemia occurs as a result of impaired secretion of PTH from the parathyroid glands (ie, hypoparathyroidism) despite low serum calcium levels.

**What general laboratory pattern is associated with hypoparathyroidism?**

Hypoparathyroidism is generally associated with low serum calcium level, low or normal serum PTH level, and elevated serum phosphorus level.

**The causes of hypoparathyroidism can be separated into which general subcategories?**

The causes of hypoparathyroidism can be separated into the following subcategories: iatrogenic, autoimmune, infiltrative, and other.

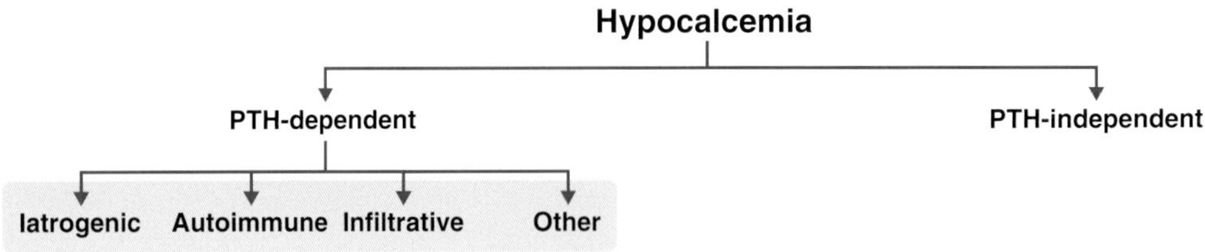


## IATROGENIC CAUSES OF HYPOPARATHYROIDISM

### What are the iatrogenic causes of hypoparathyroidism?

| | |
|---|---|
| **You will find a transverse incision scar over the anterior neck.** | Surgical removal. |
| **Nonsurgical therapy for head and neck cancers.** | Ionizing radiation therapy. |
| **Used in the treatment for renally-induced secondary hyperparathyroidism.** | Calcimimetics. |

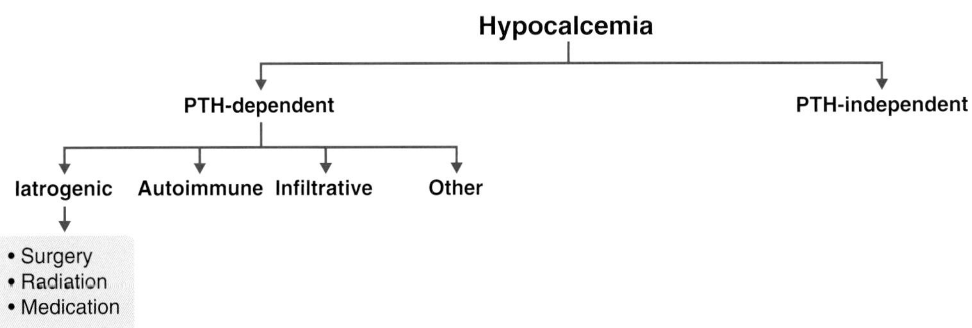


| | |
|---|---|
| **What types of surgeries can lead to hypoparathyroidism?** | Postsurgical hypoparathyroidism is the most common cause of hypoparathyroidism in adults. It typically results from the inadvertent or unavoidable removal of or damage to the parathyroid glands or the blood supply of the glands during surgeries such as thyroidectomy, parathyroidectomy, and radical neck dissection for head and neck cancer. Most cases are temporary, attributed to "stunning" of the glands, with patients regaining function within weeks to months after surgery. Chronic postsurgical hypoparathyroidism, defined as persistent hypoparathyroidism 6 months after surgery, is relatively rare.[5] |
| **What are the 2 scenarios in which the parathyroid glands may become damaged as a result of ionizing radiation therapy?** | Iatrogenic hypoparathyroidism can occur following external beam radiation therapy for head and neck cancers, and radioactive iodine therapy for hyperthyroidism (rare).[6] |
| **What is the mechanism of PTH-dependent hypocalcemia related to cinacalcet?** | Cinacalcet, used in the treatment for renally-induced secondary hyperparathyroidism, decreases PTH secretion by activating the calcium-sensing receptors within the parathyroid gland. Patients with hypocalcemia should not receive cinacalcet.[7] |

## AUTOIMMUNE CAUSES OF HYPOPARATHYROIDISM

| | |
|---|---|
| **What are the 2 general mechanisms of autoimmune-related hypoparathyroidism?** | Hypoparathyroidism can occur via immune-mediated destruction of parathyroid tissue, or activation of the calcium-sensing receptor (CaSR) within the parathyroid glands. |

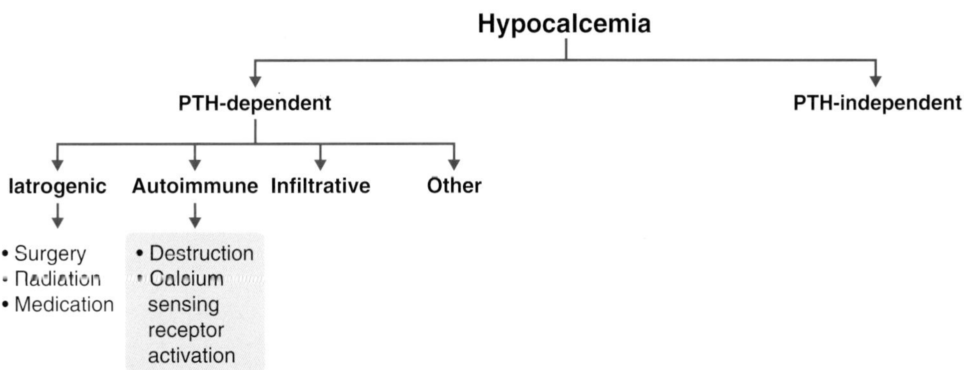


**What are the characteristics of immune-mediated parathyroid gland destruction?**

Immune-mediated parathyroid destruction is the second most common cause of hypoparathyroidism in adults. It can occur in isolation or as part of a polyglandular syndrome. The vast majority of patients with polyglandular autoimmune syndrome type 1 have hypoparathyroidism; other main features include chronic mucocutaneous candidiasis and adrenal insufficiency.[5]

**Why does activation of the calcium-sensing receptor result in decreased PTH secretion?**

The CaSR is part of a negative feedback loop and is normally activated by elevated serum ionized calcium levels, which, in turn, decreases PTH release from the parathyroid glands, returning serum calcium levels to normal. Antibody-mediated activation of these receptors provides persistent negative feedback, resulting in inappropriately low PTH levels and hypocalcemia.[5]

## INFILTRATIVE CAUSES OF HYPOPARATHYROIDISM

### What are the infiltrative causes of hypoparathyroidism?

**A 21-year-old man with a history of thalassemia, requiring multiple blood transfusions over his lifetime, is found to have hypocalcemia on routine laboratory evaluation.**

Iron deposition.

**Characteristic apple-green color when tissue is stained with Congo red and viewed with polarized light.**

Amyloidosis.

**A common histopathologic finding of various infectious and autoimmune diseases.**

Granulomatous disease.

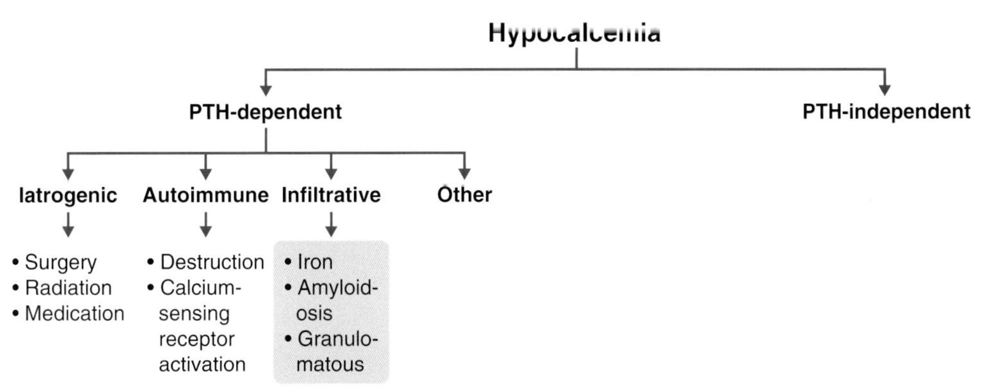


ENDOCRINOLOGY

**What are the characteristics of hypoparathyroidism related to iron infiltration?**

Hypoparathyroidism occurs most commonly as a result of secondary iron overload (eg, after multiple blood transfusions in a patient with thalassemia) and only rarely as a result of primary hemochromatosis. It occurs more frequently in male patients with peak prevalence around 20 years of age. It does not regress with iron chelation therapy. Hypoparathyroidism related to other heavy metals (eg, copper deposition in patients with Wilson's disease) is exceedingly rare.[6]

**What are the characteristics of hypoparathyroidism associated with amyloidosis?**

Infiltration of the parathyroid gland with amyloid occurs in primary (AL) amyloidosis as well as secondary (AA) amyloidosis, but it rarely causes a reduction in PTH production. More often, amyloidosis is associated with hypercalcemia as a result of its link to multiple myeloma.[6]

**Which granulomatous diseases can cause hypoparathyroidism?**

Sarcoidosis, tuberculosis, and syphilis are rare causes of hypoparathyroidism via gland infiltration. More commonly, granulomatous diseases cause hypercalcemia via ectopic production of $1,25(OH)_2D$.[6]

*Infiltration of the parathyroid gland with malignancy (eg, metastatic disease or lymphoma) is a rare cause of hypoparathyroidism.*

## OTHER CAUSES OF HYPOPARATHYROIDISM

### What are the other causes of hypoparathyroidism?

**Another electrolyte is to blame.**

Magnesium derangement.

**A persistently stimulated negative feedback loop.**

Activating mutation of the calcium-sensing receptor.

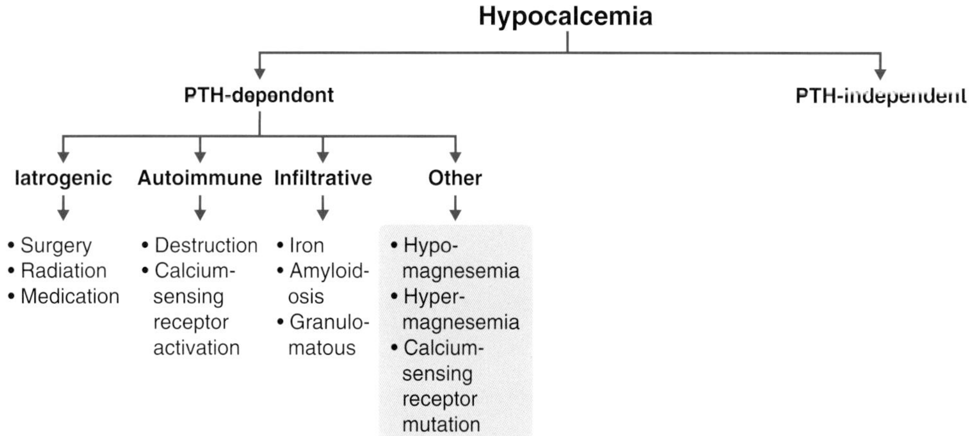


**What is the mechanism of hypoparathyroidism related to hypomagnesemia?**

The synthesis, release, and peripheral action of PTH are dependent on magnesium. Hypocalcemia related to magnesium deficiency is not responsive to exogenous administration of PTH, calcium, or vitamin D. The cornerstone of treatment is magnesium repletion.[6]

**What is the mechanism of hypoparathyroidism related to hypermagnesemia?**

Hypermagnesemia inhibits PTH secretion. The hypoparathyroidism caused by hypermagnesemia is mild, typically asymptomatic, and reversible with normalization of magnesium levels.[6]

**What are the clinical manifestations of activating mutations of the calcium-sensing receptor?**

A variety of gain-of-function genetic mutations of the CaSR have been described. The degree of hypocalcemia and resultant clinical manifestations are variable, even between individuals with the same mutation. Most patients are asymptomatic until adulthood, but some present with severe manifestations of hypocalcemia, including seizures. Patients are at risk for nephrocalcinosis related to hypercalciuria, which occurs because the combination of low serum PTH and activation of the CaSR in the renal tubule decreases tubular reabsorption of calcium. This risk escalates when serum calcium levels increase from treatment, and such patients should be monitored closely.[8]

## PTH-INDEPENDENT HYPOCALCEMIA

**What is the fundamental mechanism of PTH-independent hypocalcemia?**

PTH-independent hypocalcemia occurs despite normal parathyroid gland function and increased serum PTH levels.

**What general laboratory pattern is associated with PTH-independent hypocalcemia?**

PTH-independent hypocalcemia is generally associated with low serum calcium level, elevated serum PTH level, and low serum phosphorus level.

**The causes of PTH-independent hypocalcemia can be separated into which general subcategories?**

The causes of PTH-independent hypocalcemia can be separated into the following subcategories: vitamin D deficiency, consumption, and other.

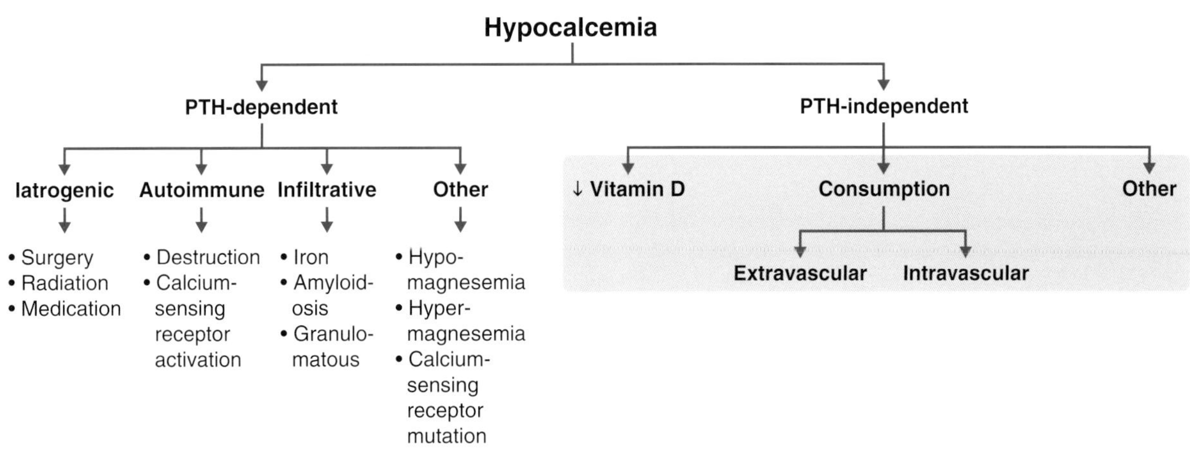


## PTH-INDEPENDENT HYPOCALCEMIA RELATED TO VITAMIN D DEFICIENCY

**What are the 2 main forms of biologically inactive vitamin D?**

Vitamin $D_2$ (ie, ergocalciferol) and vitamin $D_3$ (ie, cholecalciferol) are the main forms of inactive vitamin D (both forms are referred to as vitamin D). Sources of vitamin D include diet, dietary supplements, and sunlight exposure.[2,9]

**What is the biologically active form of vitamin D?**

$1,25(OH)_2D$ is biologically active. It primarily acts to increase gastrointestinal calcium absorption and calcium resorption from bone.[2,9]

**How can vitamin D deficiency be confirmed?**

The measurement of low serum 25-hydroxyvitamin D (ie, 25(OH)D) concentration confirms the diagnosis of vitamin D deficiency.[1]

**What effect can chronic vitamin D deficiency have on bones?**

Chronic vitamin D deficiency can result in deficient bone growth and mineralization. Rickets, which occurs in children, refers to deficient mineralization at the growth plates and is characterized by various bone deformities (Figure 10-1). Osteomalacia, which occurs in both children and adults, refers to impaired mineralization of the bone matrix and is characterized by pain, vertebral collapse, and fractures along stress lines.[2,10]

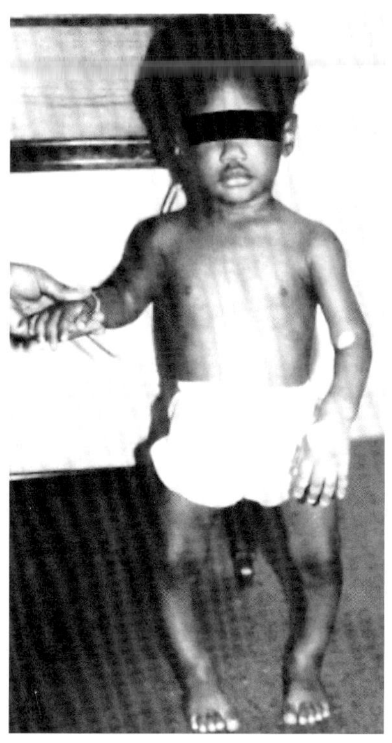

**Figure 10-1.** A young child with rickets. Note the bowed legs and thickening of the wrist and ankles. (From Becker KL, Bilezikian JP, Brenner WJ, et al. *Principles and Practice of Endocrinology and Metabolism*. 3rd ed. Philadelphia, PA: Lippincott Williams & Wilkins; 2001.)

## What are the causes of vitamin D deficiency?

**This occurs during the many rainy months of Portland, Oregon.**

Sunlight deprivation.

**Jaundice, spider angiomas, and palmar erythema.**

Liver disease.

**Chronic anemia and shrunken kidneys on ultrasound.**

Chronic kidney disease.

**A 24-year-old man with Crohn's disease presents with perioral numbness and is found to have hypocalcemia.**

Gastrointestinal malabsorption.

**A 42-year-old woman with a history of epilepsy develops hypocalcemia.**

Antiepileptic medication.

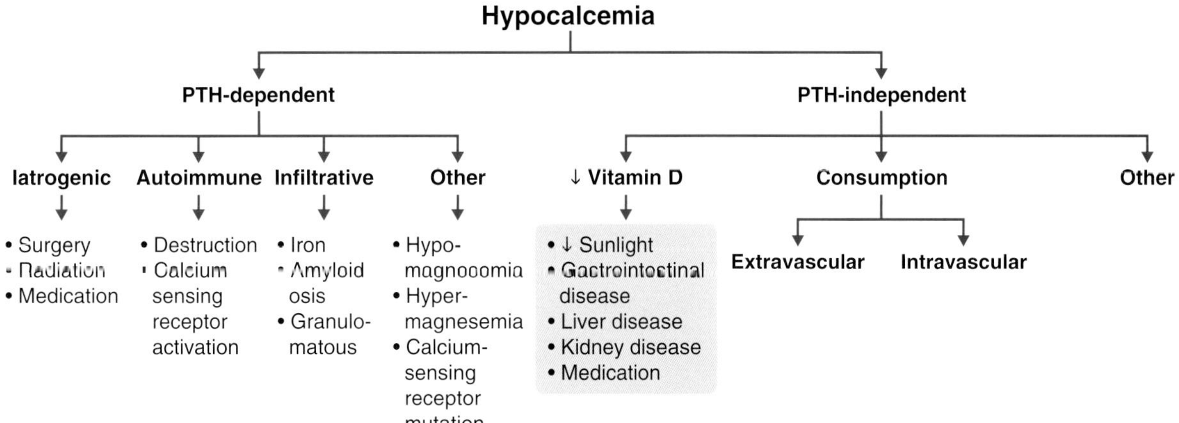


**What is the role of sunlight in vitamin D metabolism?**

Ultraviolet B radiation induces the production of vitamin $D_3$ from 7-dehydrocholesterol in the epidermis (Figure 10-2). At moderate to high latitudes, decreased solar intensity and cold temperatures (particularly during the winter season) lead to reduced skin exposure to ultraviolet B radiation. In addition to sunlight deprivation, increased skin pigmentation and skin thinning with age can contribute to vitamin D deficiency. In these populations, dietary sources of vitamin D become increasingly important.[1,2,11]

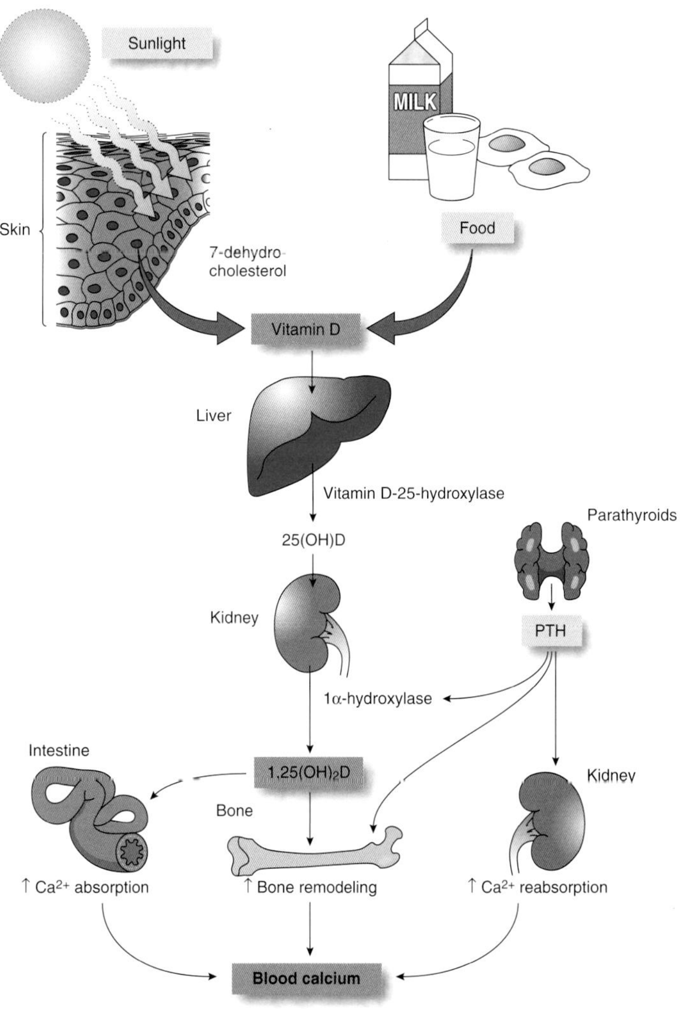


**Figure 10-2.** Metabolism of vitamin D and the regulation of serum calcium. (From Rubin R, Strayer DS. *Rubin's Pathology: Clinicopathologic Foundations of Medicine.* 5th ed. Philadelphia, PA: Lippincott Williams & Wilkins; 2008.)

**How is vitamin D absorbed in the gastrointestinal tract?**

The jejunum and ileum absorb vitamin D from dietary sources. Because it is fat soluble, absorption of vitamin D is facilitated by bile salts. Excess vitamin D is stored in adipose tissue and the liver, and can last for several months.[2]

**How does the liver affect vitamin D metabolism?**

Vitamin $D_2$ and $D_3$ are converted to 25(OH)D in the liver (see Figure 10-2). The liver is also a storage site of excess vitamin D.[2]

**How does the kidney affect vitamin D metabolism?**

The kidney converts 25(OH)D to the metabolically active $1,25(OH)_2D$, which then primarily acts in the gastrointestinal tract and bone to increase serum calcium concentration (see Figure 10-2). Serum PTH, calcium, and phosphorus levels regulate renal production of $1,25(OH)_2D$.[2,9]

**What is the mechanism of vitamin D deficiency caused by medication?**

Various drugs accelerate the metabolism of vitamin D via activation of the xenobiotic receptor. Activation of the xenobiotic receptor results in increased synthesis of enzymes that degrade 25(OH)D and $1,25(OH)_2D$. Common medications that act through this mechanism include phenytoin, carbamazepine, cyclophosphamide, dexamethasone, nifedipine, and spironolactone.[9,12]

## PTH-INDEPENDENT HYPOCALCEMIA RELATED TO EXTRAVASCULAR CONSUMPTION

### What are the causes of PTH-independent hypocalcemia related to extravascular consumption?

**Alcohol and gallstones are common causes of this condition.**

Acute pancreatitis.

**Consumed by another electrolyte.**

Hyperphosphatemia.

**A patient with dialysis-dependent renal failure, complicated by secondary hyperparathyroidism with associated osteitis fibrosa cystica, undergoes parathyroidectomy and subsequently suffers from severe hypocalcemia for weeks despite elevated levels of serum PTH.**

Hungry bone syndrome.

**A certain type of metastatic bone lesion.**

Osteoblastic bone metastases.

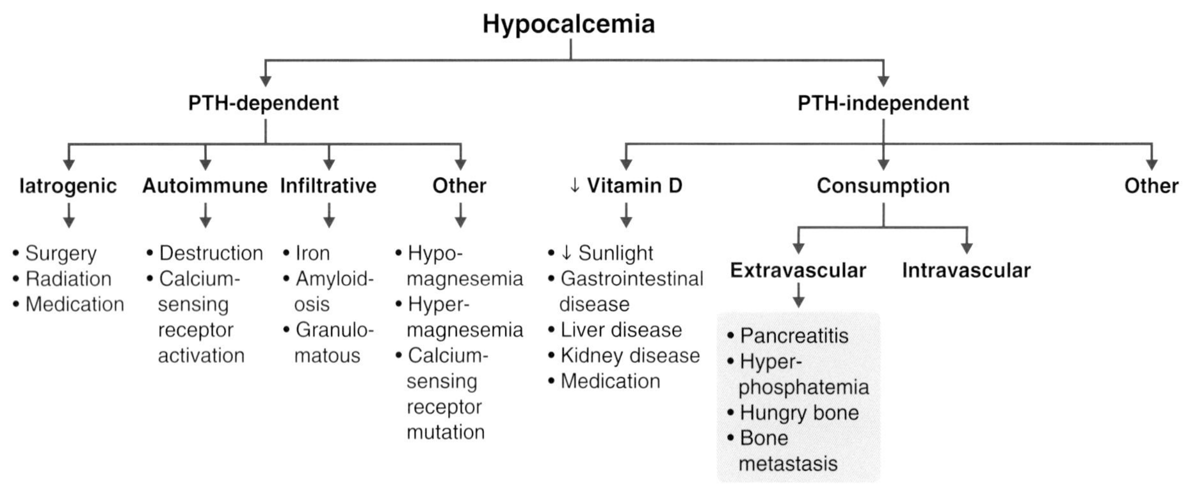

**What are the characteristics of hypocalcemia related to acute pancreatitis?**

The mechanism of hypocalcemia in acute pancreatitis is thought to be related to autodigestion of mesenteric fat with release of free fatty acids, which consume calcium during the formation of calcium salts. Hypocalcemia is more likely to develop in severe cases of acute pancreatitis, and is a poor prognostic marker. Correction of hypocalcemia in patients with acute pancreatitis must be done cautiously as calcium plays a role in acinar cell injury and death.[13]

**What is the mechanism of hypocalcemia related to hyperphosphatemia?**

Hyperphosphatemia may lead to the precipitation of calcium phosphate in soft tissues, resulting in hypocalcemia. Acute hyperphosphatemia most commonly occurs as a result of cell breakdown (eg, tumor lysis syndrome, rhabdomyolysis) or increased intake of phosphate (eg, increased dietary intake, phosphate-containing enemas). Caution should be exercised in correcting hypocalcemia in the setting of hyperphosphatemia given the possibility of hastening widespread soft tissue calcium phosphate precipitation.[14]

**What is hungry bone syndrome?**

Hungry bone syndrome describes rapid onset of severe and prolonged hypocalcemia following parathyroidectomy for severe hyperparathyroidism associated with high bone turnover. It usually lasts for 4 days or more, and is also characterized by hypophosphatemia and hypomagnesemia. The pathophysiology is thought to be increased skeletal uptake of calcium following removal of high circulating levels of PTH. Hungry bone syndrome may last for months, requiring ongoing electrolyte monitoring and replacement.[15]

**What are the characteristics of hypocalcemia related to osteoblastic bone lesions?**

Hypocalcemia occurs in patients with osteoblastic bone lesions as a result of calcium consumption during formation of new bone around the metastatic lesions. Malignancies most commonly associated with osteoblastic metastases include prostate and breast cancer. *Hypercalcemia is the most common calcium disturbance in patients with malignancy.*[16]

## PTH-INDEPENDENT HYPOCALCEMIA RELATED TO INTRAVASCULAR CONSUMPTION

### What are the causes of PTH-independent hypocalcemia related to intravascular consumption?

**Hypocalcemia develops after intense vomiting in a patient with viral gastroenteritis.**

Alkalemia.

**Hypocalcemia develops in a trauma patient after receiving massive amounts of blood products.**

Citrate.

**Used in the treatment for lead poisoning.**

Ethylenediaminetetraacetic acid (EDTA).

**A product of tissue ischemia.**

Lactate.

**An antiviral medication.**

Foscarnet.

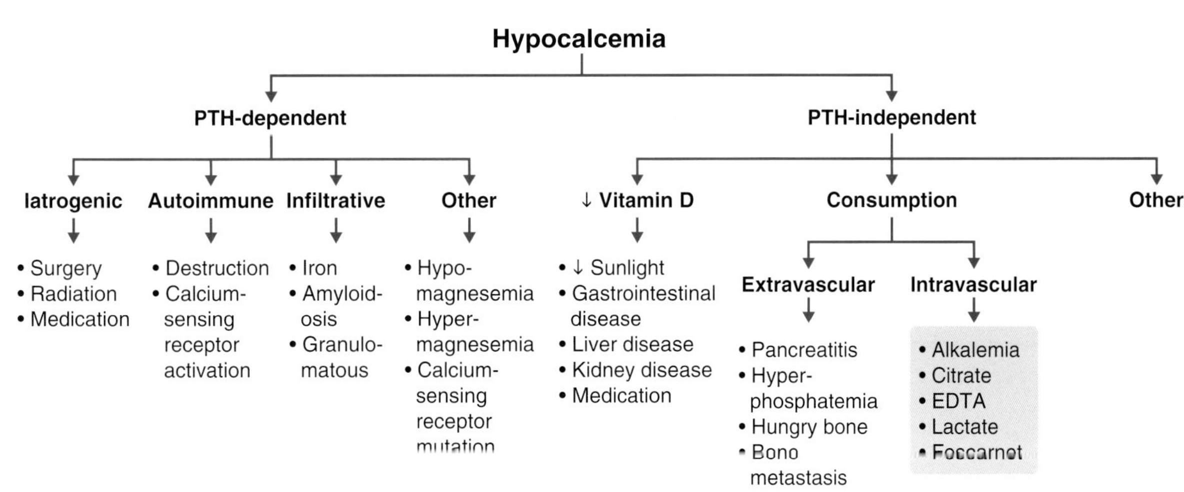

**What is the mechanism of hypocalcemia in the setting of alkalemia?**

Alkalemia enhances binding between albumin and calcium, thereby decreasing the ionized calcium levels (total calcium level remains unchanged).[1,3]

**What is the mechanism of hypocalcemia in the presence of citrate, EDTA, lactate, and foscarnet?**

Citrate, EDTA, lactate, and foscarnet chelate calcium, thereby decreasing the ionized calcium level (total calcium level remains unchanged).[17-19]

## OTHER CAUSES OF PTH-INDEPENDENT HYPOCALCEMIA

### What are the other causes of PTH-independent hypocalcemia?

**Chronic alcohol consumption and gastrointestinal malabsorption are common causes of this electrolyte disorder.**

Hypomagnesemia.

**Iatrogenesis.**

Medication.

**Genetic renal and bone insensitivity to PTH.**

Pseudohypoparathyroidism.

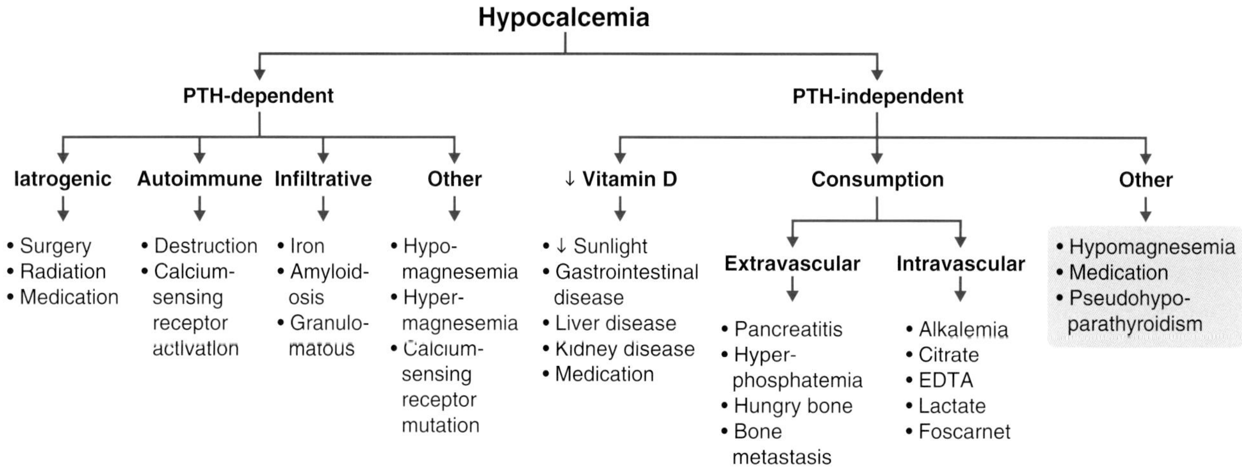


**What is the mechanism of PTH-independent hypocalcemia related to hypomagnesemia?**

Hypomagnesemia causes peripheral PTH resistance. The cornerstone of treatment for hypocalcemia related to magnesium deficiency is magnesium repletion.[6]

**Which class of medication commonly used to treat hypercalcemia is associated with PTH-independent hypocalcemia?**

Bisphosphonates cause hypocalcemia as a result of potent inhibition of osteoclastic bone resorption. This effect is potentiated in patients with compromised renal function and in those with vitamin D deficiency.[20]

**What general laboratory pattern is associated with pseudohypoparathyroidism?**

Pseudohypoparathyroidism describes various disorders defined by end-organ resistance to PTH. It is associated with low serum calcium and elevated serum PTH levels; unlike most causes of PTH-independent hypocalcemia, it is associated with hyperphosphatemia.[5]

## Case Summary

An 18-year-old man with recent life stressors presents with acute-onset chest pain, perioral numbness, and carpopedal spasms and is found to have decreased serum ionized calcium with normal total serum calcium concentration.

***What is the most likely cause of hypocalcemia in this patient?***

Alkalemia.

### BONUS QUESTIONS

***Which specific acid-base disturbance is present in this case?***

The patient in this case has primary acute respiratory alkalosis. The history suggests acute-onset respiratory distress. Primary respiratory alkalosis is confirmed by the combination of alkalemia (arterial blood pH >7.45) and low partial pressure of carbon dioxide in arterial blood. Serum bicarbonate is only mildly low, reflecting the expected degree of renal compensation for acute respiratory alkalosis.

***What is the most likely underlying condition in this case?***

The patient in this case most likely experienced a panic attack related to life stressors that resulted in hyperventilation syndrome and respiratory alkalosis.

***What is hyperventilation syndrome?***

Hyperventilation syndrome describes a constellation of clinical manifestations that occurs when minute ventilation exceeds metabolic needs. Episodes are often triggered by stress. Symptoms of the syndrome may include dyspnea, light-headedness, numbness, paresthesias, and chest pain. These symptoms are the result of physiologic responses to hypocapnea and alkalemia, including cerebral vasoconstriction, the Bohr effect, hypocalcemia, and hypophosphatemia.[21]

***What is the importance of measuring serum ionized calcium concentration in this case?***

Normal total serum calcium levels may mask true hypocalcemia in certain circumstances, such as alkalemia or the presence of calcium chelators. Alkalemia promotes the binding of ionized calcium and albumin, thereby reducing serum ionized calcium without altering total serum calcium concentration.[1,3]

***What is the treatment of choice for acute hyperventilation syndrome?***

Reassurance and counseling on behavioral modification is the cornerstone of management of hyperventilation syndrome. Patients may be more receptive to the diagnosis after provocation of symptoms with a "hyperventilation trial." After breathing deeply at a rate of 30 to 40 breaths per minute, most patients will experience recurrent symptoms within seconds to minutes.[21]

***What are the principles of the management of hypocalcemia?***

Hypocalcemia is best managed by treating the underlying cause (eg, hyperventilation syndrome). Patients with hypocalcemia complicated by neuromuscular irritability require hospitalization and treatment with intravenous calcium. Asymptomatic patients with corrected total serum calcium <7.6 mg/dL may develop serious complications and hospitalization should be considered. Intravenous calcium gluconate is preferred over calcium chloride because it is less likely to cause local irritation at the infusion site.[4]

## KEY POINTS

- Serum calcium levels are tightly regulated by the actions of PTH and the active form of vitamin D.
- Hypocalcemia can lead to neuromuscular excitability with manifestations that include muscle twitching and spasm, tingling, numbness, hyperreflexia, tetany, seizure, QT prolongation, and cardiac dysrhythmia.
- Clinical manifestations associated with hypocalcemia increase in severity based on not only the degree of elevation of serum calcium, but also the rate at which it develops.
- Physical findings of hypocalcemia include Chvostek's sign and Trousseau's sign.
- Serum PTH level determines whether hypocalcemia is PTH-dependent or PTH-independent.
- The causes of PTH-dependent hypocalcemia (ie, hypoparathyroidism) can be separated into the following subcategories: iatrogenic, autoimmune, infiltrative, and other.
- The causes of PTH-independent hypocalcemia can be separated into the following subcategories: vitamin D deficiency, consumption, and other.
- Patients with symptomatic hypocalcemia should be hospitalized and treated with intravenous calcium.
- The long-term management of hypocalcemia depends on the underlying cause.

## REFERENCES


1. Minisola S, Pepe J, Piemonte S, Cipriani C. The diagnosis and management of hypercalcaemia. *BMJ*. 2015;350:h2723.
2. Berne RML, Levy MN. *Physiology*. 4th ed. St. Louis, MO: Mosby, Inc.; 1998.
3. Stewart AF. Clinical practice. Hypercalcemia associated with cancer. *N Engl J Med*. 2005;352(4):373-379.
4. Cooper MS, Gittoes NJ. Diagnosis and management of hypocalcaemia. *BMJ*. 2008;336(7656):1298-1302.
5. Bilezikian JP, Khan A, Potts JT Jr, et al. Hypoparathyroidism in the adult: epidemiology, diagnosis, pathophysiology, target-organ involvement, treatment, and challenges for future research. *J Bone Miner Res*. 2011;26(10):2317-2337.
6. Brandi ML, Brown EM, eds. *Hypoparathyroidism*. Milan, Italy: Springer-Verlag Italia; 2015.
7. Poon G. Cinacalcet hydrochloride (Sensipar). *Bayl Univ Med Cent Proc*. 2005;18(2):181-184.
8. Lienhardt A, Bai M, Lagarde JP, et al. Activating mutations of the calcium-sensing receptor: management of hypocalcemia. *J Clin Endocrinol Metab*. 2001;86(11):5313-5323.
9. Holick MF. Vitamin D deficiency. *N Engl J Med*. 2007;357(3):266-281.
10. Sahay M, Sahay R. Rickets-vitamin D deficiency and dependency. *Indian J Endocrinol Metab*. 2012;16(2):164-176.
11. Engelsen O. The relationship between ultraviolet radiation exposure and vitamin D status. *Nutrients*. 2010;2(5):482-495.
12. Grober U, Kisters K. Influence of drugs on vitamin D and calcium metabolism. *Dermatoendocrinol*. 2012;4(2):158-166.
13. Ahmed A, Azim A, Gurjar M, Baronia AK. Hypocalcemia in acute pancreatitis revisited. *Indian J Crit Care Med*. 2016;20(3):173-177.
14. Sutters M, Gaboury CL, Bennett WM. Severe hyperphosphatemia and hypocalcemia: a dilemma in patient management. *J Am Soc Nephrol*. 1996;7(10):2056-2061.
15. Witteveen JE, van Thiel S, Romijn JA, Hamdy NA. Hungry bone syndrome: still a challenge in the post-operative management of primary hyperparathyroidism: a systematic review of the literature. *Eur J Endocrinol*. 2013;168(3):R45-R53.
16. Kassi E, Kapsali I, Kokkinos M, Gogas H. Treatment of severe hypocalcaemia due to osteoblastic metastases in a patient with post-thyroidectomy hypoparathyroidism with 153Sm-EDTMP. *BMJ Case Rep*. 2017;2017.
17. Cairns CB, Niemann JT, Pelikan PC, Sharma J. Ionized hypocalcemia during prolonged cardiac arrest and closed-chest CPR in a canine model. *Ann Emerg Med*. 1991;20(11):1178-1182.
18. Giancarelli A, Birrer KL, Alban RF, Hobbs BP, Liu-DeRyke X. Hypocalcemia in trauma patients receiving massive transfusion. *J Surg Res*. 2016;202(1):182-187.
19. Jacobson MA, Gambertoglio JG, Aweeka FT, Causey DM, Portale AA. Foscarnet-induced hypocalcemia and effects of foscarnet on calcium metabolism. *J Clin Endocrinol Metab*. 1991;72(5):1130-1135.
20. Do WS, Park JK, Park MI, Kim HS, Kim SH, Lee DH. Bisphosphonate-induced severe hypocalcemia—a case report. *J Bone Metab*. 2012;19(2):139-145.
21. Magarian GJ. Hyperventilation syndromes: infrequently recognized common expressions of anxiety and stress. *Medicine*. 1982;61(4):219-236.

# Chapter 11

# HYPOTHYROIDISM

## Case: A 38-year-old woman with bradycardia

A previously healthy 38-year-old woman is brought to the hospital for confusion. Her husband provides most of the history. She has complained of fatigue, weight gain, and constipation for several months. Over the past few weeks, the patient's husband has noticed episodes of drowsiness, forgetfulness, and inability to concentrate that have been occurring with increasing frequency. She was much drowsier on the day of presentation, prompting her husband to bring her in for evaluation.

Temperature is 35.3°C, and heart rate is 46 beats per minute. The patient is somnolent but arouses when prompted. She is easily distracted and oriented to self but not place or time. A photo of the patient is shown in Figure 11-1. There is non-pitting edema of the lower extremities. There are 5 vitiliginous patches on the trunk. Reflexes are symmetric with a delayed relaxation phase.

Laboratory evaluation is notable for serum sodium of 118 mEq/L, thyroid stimulating hormone of 192 mIU/L (reference range 0.4-4.2 mIU/L), and free thyroxine of 0.12 ng/dL (reference range 0.6-1.2 ng/dL).

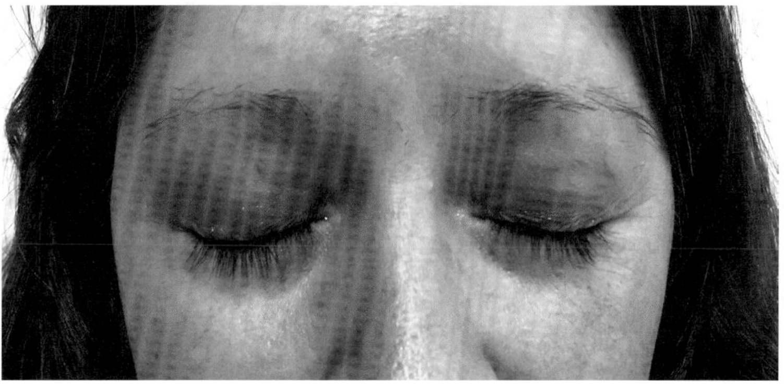

**Figure 11-1.**

***What is the most likely diagnosis in this patient?***

**What is hypothyroidism?**

Hypothyroidism is a clinical condition that results from thyroid hormone deficiency.

**What is the normal hormonal cycle of the hypothalamic-pituitary-thyroid axis?**

The hypothalamus produces thyroid-releasing hormone (TRH), which stimulates the pituitary to secrete thyroid-stimulating hormone (TSH). The thyroid gland responds to TSH stimulation by secreting thyroxine ($T_4$) and triiodothyronine ($T_3$), which then provide negative feedback to both the hypothalamus and pituitary (Figure 11-2).

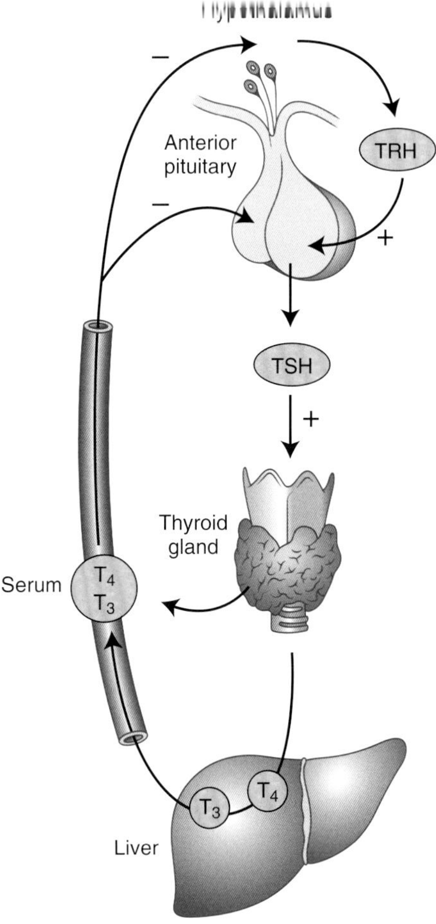


**Figure 11-2.** Schematic of the hypothalamic-pituitary-thyroid axis. Regulatory feedback relationships are designated with arrows.

**What is the relationship between $T_3$ and $T_4$?**

$T_3$ and $T_4$ are both produced in the thyroid gland by the follicular cells, although the vast majority of thyroid output is in the form of $T_4$. Peripheral conversion of $T_4$ to $T_3$ occurs in the liver and kidney (see Figure 11-2). The relative potency of $T_3$ is several times greater than that of $T_4$, and it is more biologically active.[1]

**How common is hypothyroidism?**

The prevalence of hypothyroidism in the general population varies by sex and age. It is more common in women with an overall prevalence of up to 5% in the industrialized world. Incidence in women rises with age, particularly after 45 years.[2,3]

**What are the symptoms of hypothyroidism?**

Symptoms of hypothyroidism depend on the age and sex of the patient but in general may include weight gain, fatigue, poor concentration, depression, constipation, cold intolerance, dry skin, proximal muscle weakness, hair thinning or loss, and menorrhagia.[4]

**What are the physical findings of hypothyroidism?**

Physical findings of hypothyroidism depend on the age and sex of the patient but in general may include hypothermia, bradycardia, diastolic hypertension, cognitive impairment, coarse facies, lateral eyebrow thinning (ie, Queen Anne's sign), periorbital edema, goiter (see Figure 12-2), dry or coarse skin, hoarse voice, delayed relaxation phase of deep tendon reflexes, nonpitting peripheral edema, and macroglossia.[4]

**What life-threatening complication can occur in patients with untreated hypothyroidism?**

Myxedema coma is a severe and life-threatening complication of hypothyroidism, usually associated with a precipitating factor such as infection. It is more common in older patients, particularly women. Patients present with mental status changes and other severe manifestations of hypothyroidism, such as lethargy, cognitive dysfunction and psychosis, hypothermia, bradycardia, hyponatremia, and hypoventilation. Myxedema coma requires prompt recognition and treatment.[5]

**If hypothyroidism is suspected clinically, what is the next diagnostic step?**

In patients with a clinical condition compatible with hypothyroidism, low serum free $T_4$ will confirm the diagnosis. Concurrent measurement of serum TSH level can distinguish whether the process is TSH-independent (TSH is elevated) or TSH-dependent (TSH is low or normal).

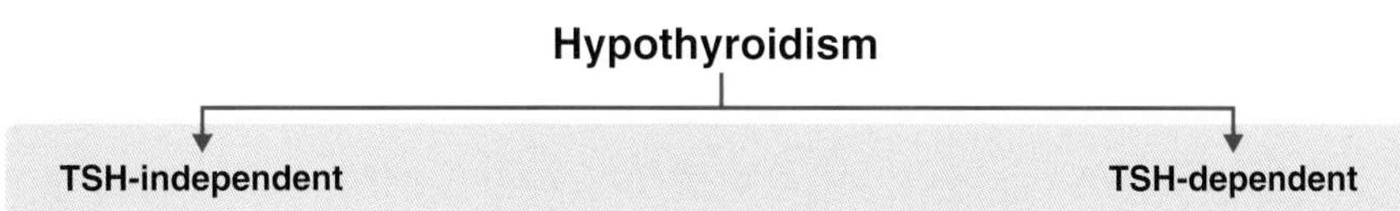


**In the setting of hypothyroidism, why does a normal serum TSH value implicate a TSH-dependent process?**

When there is thyroid hormone deficiency, pituitary TSH secretion should increase in an attempt to return serum thyroid hormone levels to normal. Therefore, a TSH level within the normal range is "inappropriately normal."

**Which coexisting conditions can make the interpretation of thyroid function studies difficult?**

Pregnancy, nonthyroid acute illness, medications (eg, glucocorticoids), and recovery from thyrotoxicosis can make the interpretation of thyroid function studies challenging.[6]

**What clinical entity is characterized by the combination of normal serum free $T_4$ and elevated serum TSH?**

Subclinical hypothyroidism is defined by the presence of normal serum free $T_4$ with elevated serum TSH. This diagnosis is valid only when such results have been demonstrated over the course of at least several weeks, the hypothalamic-pituitary-thyroid axis is normal, and there is no recent or ongoing nonthyroidal illness.[7]

**How common is subclinical hypothyroidism?**

Subclinical hypothyroidism is present in up to 8% of the general population in the industrialized world.[7]

**In patients with subclinical hypothyroidism, what is the risk of developing overt hypothyroidism over time?**

In women with subclinical hypothyroidism, the risk of developing overt hypothyroidism is 2% to 3% per year, and this rises to 4% per year when serum antithyroid peroxidase antibodies are present. The relative risk of progression is even higher in men, but the overall prevalence of overt hypothyroidism in men remains significantly lower than in women.[7]

**Should patients with subclinical hypothyroidism be treated with thyroid hormone?**

It remains unclear whether there are benefits to treating patients with subclinical hypothyroidism with thyroid hormone. Treatment should be considered for symptomatic patients and in those who are pregnant or attempting to conceive.[4,7]

**Why is it helpful to separate the causes of hypothyroidism into TSH-independent and TSH-dependent processes?**

TSH-independent hypothyroidism indicates intrinsic dysfunction of the thyroid gland (ie, primary hypothyroidism), whereas TSH-dependent hypothyroidism suggests dysfunction in the hypothalamic or pituitary components of the regulatory axis (ie, central hypothyroidism).

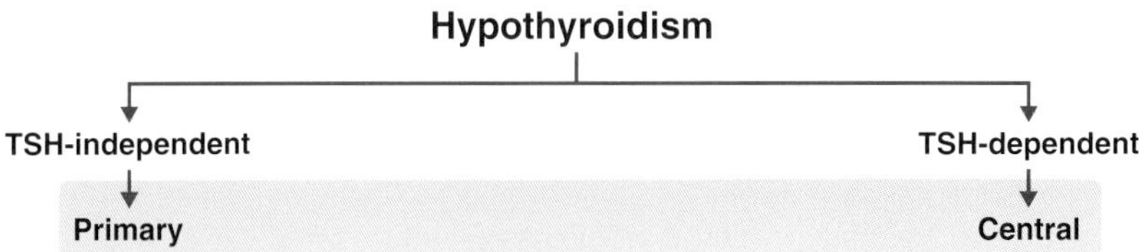


**What is the relative prevalence of primary and central hypothyroidism?**

Central hypothyroidism is rare, accounting for <1% of all cases, and estimated to be 1000 times less common than primary hypothyroidism.

## PRIMARY HYPOTHYROIDISM

**What is the fundamental mechanism of primary hypothyroidism?**

Primary hypothyroidism occurs as a result of failure of the thyroid gland to produce adequate thyroid hormones despite stimulation from increased TSH.

**The causes of primary hypothyroidism can be separated into which general subcategories?**

The causes of primary hypothyroidism can be separated into the following subcategories: thyroiditis, iodine-related, iatrogenic, and infiltrative.

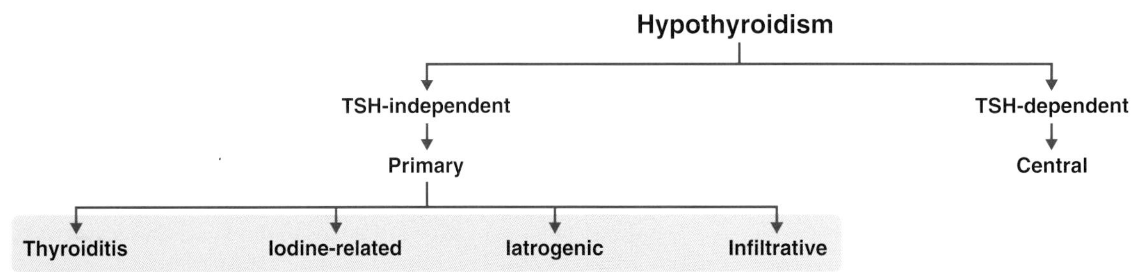


## PRIMARY HYPOTHYROIDISM RELATED TO THYROIDITIS

**What is thyroiditis?**

Thyroiditis refers to a group of disorders that produce inflammation of the thyroid gland, which may lead to the destruction of follicular cells (thyrocytes) and unregulated release of preformed thyroid hormones into the circulation. There is typically a phase of excess circulating thyroid hormone (ie, thyrotoxicosis) followed by either normal thyroid function or hypothyroidism, which may be temporary or permanent.[9,10]

**During the phase of thyrotoxicosis in patients with thyroiditis, what is the typical result of a radioactive iodine uptake test?**

Thyroiditis is generally associated with decreased radioiodine uptake (see Figure 12-3). *The thyrotoxic phase of Hashimoto's thyroiditis (ie, Hashitoxicosis) can be associated with normal or even increased radioactive iodine uptake.*[9,11]

### What causes of thyroiditis can lead to hypothyroidism?

**Responsible for the vast majority of cases of primary hypothyroidism in iodine-sufficient parts of the world; this condition is associated with other autoimmune diseases, such as vitiligo, pernicious anemia, celiac disease, autoimmune adrenalitis, and type 1 diabetes mellitus.**

Hashimoto's thyroiditis.[2]

**Two months after giving birth, a 29-year-old woman experiences a period of restlessness, tremor, and weight loss, followed by weight gain, constipation, and dry skin.**

Postpartum thyroiditis.

A 50-year-old woman presents during the summer with anterior neck pain after a recent upper respiratory tract infection and is found to have a painful goiter on examination.

Subacute thyroiditis (ie, de Quervain's thyroiditis).

Iatrogenic causes of thyroiditis.

Drug-induced thyroiditis and radiation-induced thyroiditis.

Mild symptoms of hyperthyroidism followed by transient hypothyroidism in a patient with a nontender thyroid gland.

Painless thyroiditis (ie, silent thyroiditis).

A 62-year-old woman with rheumatoid arthritis treated with immunosuppressive medications presents with left anterior neck pain and is found to have an exquisitely tender thyroid gland with overlying erythema, fever, and positive blood cultures.

Infectious thyroiditis.

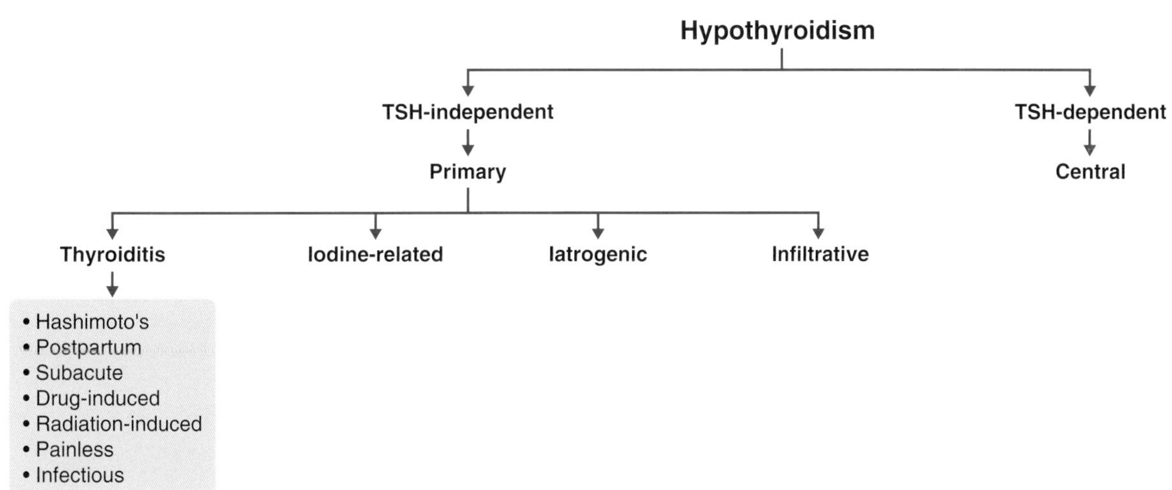


What serologic studies are supportive of the diagnosis of Hashimoto's thyroiditis?

Thyroid autoantibodies (eg, antithyroid peroxidase antibodies and antithyroglobulin antibodies) are present in the majority of patients with Hashimoto's thyroiditis. *Unlike most other causes of thyroiditis, Hashimoto's thyroiditis virtually always causes permanent hypothyroidism.*[2]

What are the characteristics of postpartum thyroiditis?

Postpartum thyroiditis occurs during the first postpartum year with a mean prevalence of 10%. It is a manifestation of an underlying but previously clinically silent autoimmune thyroiditis, which becomes unmasked by "immunologic rebound" after pregnancy. The most common presentation is isolated hypothyroidism, but it can also present with transient hyperthyroidism with or without subsequent hypothyroidism. The majority of patients are euthyroid within 1 year postpartum; however, permanent hypothyroidism develops in some.[12]

What are the characteristics of subacute thyroiditis?

Subacute thyroiditis is most likely caused by viral infection and commonly presents with a tender thyroid gland and associated systemic manifestations. Symptoms typically last for weeks to months but can be improved with nonsteroidal anti-inflammatory drugs along with glucocorticoids in severe cases. The majority of patients fully recover, but some develop permanent hypothyroidism.[13]

**What medications can cause thyroiditis?**

Medications associated with thyroiditis include amiodarone, interferon-α, interleukin-2, lithium, and tyrosine kinase inhibitors. Medication-induced thyroiditis is usually painless.[14]

**What are the 2 main types of radiation-induced thyroiditis?**

Patients treated with radioactive iodine therapy for hyperthyroidism rarely develop radiation-induced thyroiditis. When it does occur, symptoms usually present 5 to 10 days after exposure. Thyroiditis may also be caused by external beam radiation therapy for head and neck cancers. Risk factors include high-dose therapy, young age, female sex, and preexisting hypothyroidism.[14]

**What are the characteristics of painless thyroiditis?**

Painless thyroiditis is an autoimmune condition similar to postpartum thyroiditis, although the affected populations include men and women who are not within the peripartum period. It typically presents with transient hyperthyroidism, which can be followed by thyroid recovery or hypothyroidism. The majority of patients who experience hypothyroidism recover completely after 3 months, but up to one-fifth will develop permanent hypothyroidism.[15]

**What are the risk factors for developing infectious thyroiditis?**

Infectious thyroiditis is a rare condition but occurs more frequently in patients with certain congenital abnormalities (eg, persistent thyroglossal duct), those who are older in age, and those who are immunocompromised. Pathogens include bacteria (eg, *Streptococcus pyogenes*, *Staphylococcus aureus*, *Streptococcus pneumoniae*), fungi, and parasites.[14]

## PRIMARY HYPOTHYROIDISM RELATED TO IODINE

**What is the role of iodine in thyroid physiology?**

Iodine is an essential element of the $T_4$ and $T_3$ hormones, and most of the body's iodine stores are contained within the thyroid gland. Iodide, the reduced form of iodine, modulates thyroid function and is capable of decreasing thyroid hormone production and release. Both iodine deficiency and excess can lead to thyroid dysfunction.[16]

### What are the iodine-related causes of hypothyroidism?

**Dietary fortification has decreased the burden of this condition, but it remains prevalent in some parts of the world, including Africa and Asia.**

Iodine deficiency.[2]

**A 34-year-old woman with subclinical hypothyroidism develops symptoms and signs of hypothyroidism after undergoing an imaging study with iodinated intravenous contrast.**

Iodine excess (Wolff-Chaikoff effect).

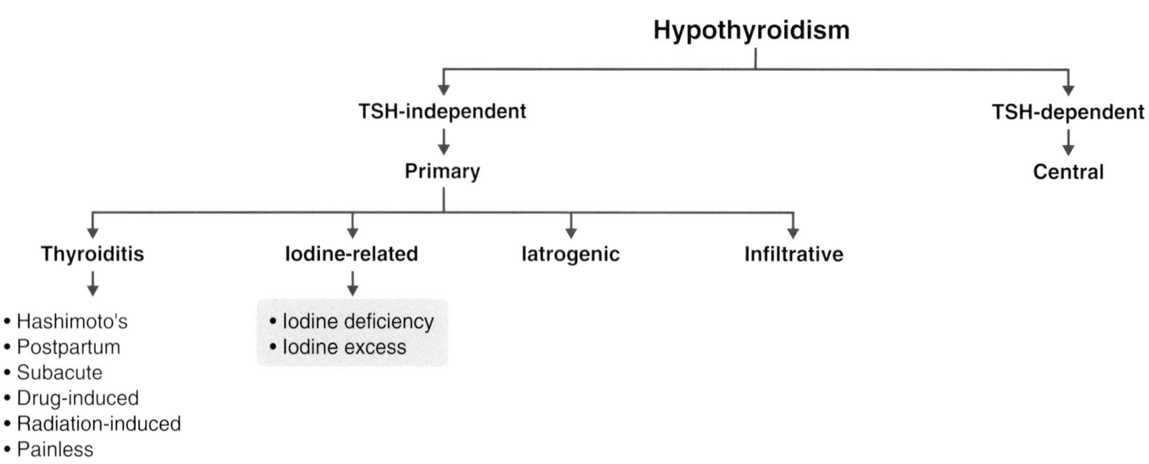

**How common is hypothyroidism caused by iodine deficiency?**

Iodine deficiency is the most common cause of hypothyroidism in the developing world. Patients commonly develop a large goiter as a result of TSH-mediated adaptation to iodine deficiency.[7]

**What are the characteristics of iodine-induced hypothyroidism?**

Sources of excess iodine include diet, medications (eg, amiodarone), and iatrogenic administration of a radiocontrast agent. Iodine excess can activate an autoregulatory phenomenon known as the Wolff-Chaikoff effect that inhibits iodination of thyroglobulin to prevent thyrotoxicosis. Usually, this effect only lasts for a few days, but in some individuals, the hypothyroid state persists. Patients at highest risk include the elderly, those with underlying thyroid disease (eg, subclinical hypothyroidism), and those with chronic nonthyroidal illness (eg, cystic fibrosis). Thyroid function usually returns to baseline within 2 to 8 weeks of iodine withdrawal (although cases of amiodarone-induced hypothyroidism may be prolonged because of the long half-life of the drug).[17]

## PRIMARY HYPOTHYROIDISM RELATED TO IATROGENESIS

### What are the iatrogenic causes of hypothyroidism?

**Definitive treatment for hyperthyroidism.**

Thyroidectomy or radioactive iodine ablation.

**A 46-year-old man with bipolar disorder develops weight gain, cold intolerance, and hair loss a few months after starting a mood-stabilizing medication.**

Lithium.

**Look for tattoo marks over the anterior neck.**

External beam radiation therapy.

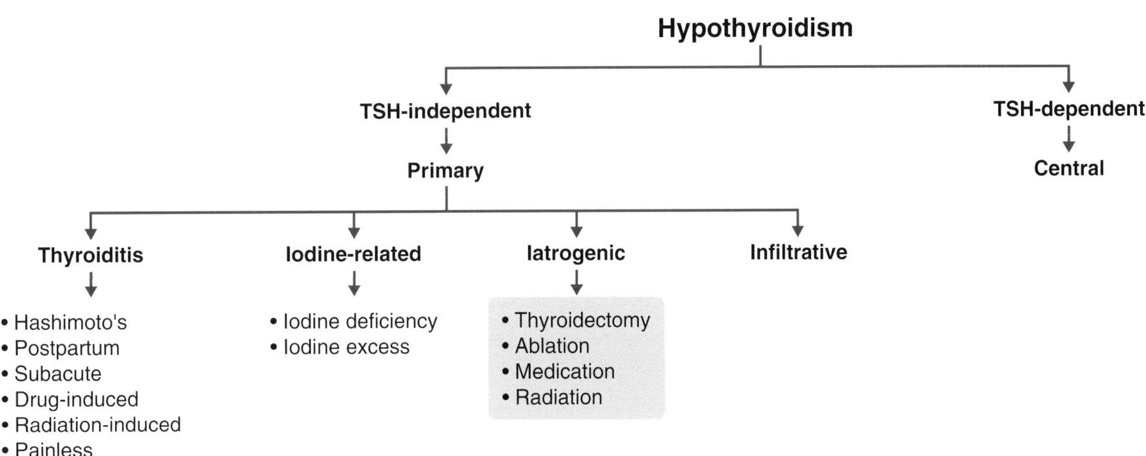


**How common is permanent hypothyroidism after thyroidectomy?**

Hypothyroidism is inevitable after total thyroidectomy but also occurs in up to one-third of patients who undergo hemithyroidectomy. Risk factors include preexisting thyroid disease such as subclinical hypothyroidism or Hashimoto's thyroiditis. Hypothyroidism begins 2 to 4 weeks after total thyroidectomy; in cases of hemithyroidectomy, it can develop months or years following the procedure.[18]

**How common is permanent hypothyroidism after radioactive iodine therapy for Graves' disease?**

The development of hypothyroidism after radioactive iodine ablation is dose-dependent, but the majority of patients develop hypothyroidism within the first year. After the first year, the incidence is 2% to 3% per year.[19]

**How common is hypothyroidism caused by lithium?**

Lithium interferes with thyroid hormone secretion, causing an increase in TSH and hypertrophy of thyroid tissue. Long-term lithium therapy results in a goiter in up to one-half of patients, subclinical hypothyroidism in up to one-third, and overt hypothyroidism in up to 15%. *Other medications that can cause hypothyroidism include tyrosine kinase inhibitors, interferon-α, thalidomides, and antiepileptic drugs (eg, valproate).*[2,20]

**What are the characteristics of hypothyroidism related to external beam radiation of the neck?**

Hypothyroidism is the most common late clinical sequela of external beam radiation to the neck. It is dose-dependent and occurs more commonly in women and in patients who undergo combined neck surgery and radiation. Patients can develop subclinical or overt hypothyroidism; patients who develop subclinical hypothyroidism progress to overt hypothyroidism at a high rate over time.[21]

## PRIMARY HYPOTHYROIDISM RELATED TO INFILTRATIVE DISORDERS

### What are the infiltrative causes of hypothyroidism?

**Patients who have received numerous blood transfusions, such as those with thalassemia, are at risk for developing this condition.**

Hemochromatosis.

**Characterized by the accumulation of amorphous, proteinaceous material.**

Amyloidosis.

**Noncaseating granulomas on histologic evaluation.**

Sarcoidosis.

**A fibrotic condition originally described with the German term "eisenharte," which means iron-hard, to denote the fixed hard enlargement of the thyroid gland.**

Riedel's thyroiditis.[22]

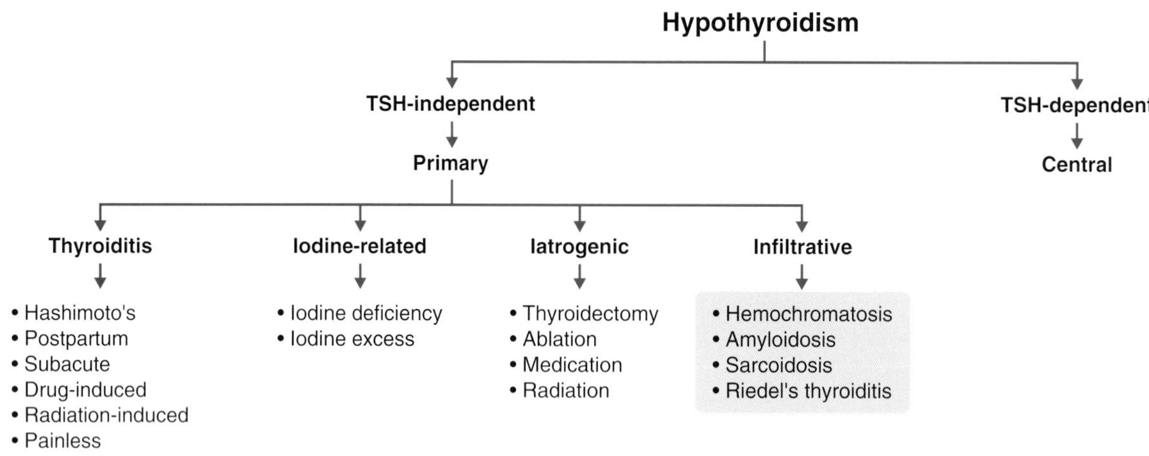


**How common is hypothyroidism in patients with hemochromatosis?**

Endocrine disorders are common in patients with hemochromatosis; the most frequent disorders are diabetes mellitus and hypogonadism. Hypothyroidism occurs in 10% of men with hemochromatosis. Iron loss through menstruation is protective against iron accumulation in women with hemochromatosis, which delays the onset of clinical sequelae.[23]

**How common is hypothyroidism in patients with amyloidosis?**

Clinically significant thyroid involvement (ie, amyloid goiter) is uncommon in patients with systemic amyloidosis. However, patients who do develop amyloid goiter are frequently hypothyroid. Treatment is aimed at the underlying condition.[24]

**How common is hypothyroidism in patients with sarcoidosis?**

Thyroid infiltration from sarcoidosis is rare. Although there is evidence of thyroid involvement on autopsy in 4% of patients with sarcoidosis, it is clinically significant in <1% of cases.[25]

**What imaging finding can be helpful in distinguishing Riedel's thyroiditis from other infiltrative disorders?**

The extension of fibrotic changes on imaging beyond the thyroid capsule to adjacent structures, such as encasement of the carotid artery, can be a clue to Riedel's thyroiditis.[22]

**What other infiltrative disorders can involve the thyroid gland and result in hypothyroidism?**

Hypothyroidism from infiltration of the thyroid gland can occur in patients with scleroderma, lymphoma, leukemia, and cystinosis.[26]

## CENTRAL HYPOTHYROIDISM

**What is the fundamental mechanism of central hypothyroidism?**

Central hypothyroidism occurs as a result of understimulation of the thyroid gland due to inadequate production of TSH.

**What are some clues to the presence of central hypothyroidism?**

In patients presenting with the typical manifestations of hypothyroidism, a central process is more likely in those with preexisting hypothalamic or pituitary disease, history of head trauma, headaches, visual field defects, and focal neurologic findings.[8]

**Which glands are involved in central hypothyroidism?**

Central hypothyroidism can occur as a result of pituitary gland dysfunction (ie, secondary hypothyroidism) or hypothalamic dysfunction (ie, tertiary hypothyroidism).

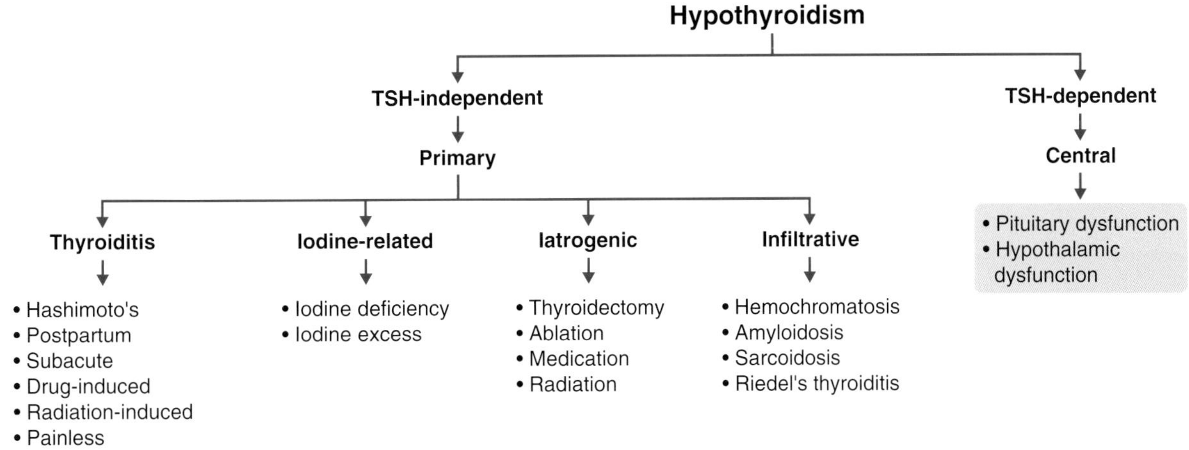


**What general processes can cause pituitary and/or hypothalamic dysfunction?**

Pituitary and/or hypothalamic dysfunction can be caused by medication (eg, glucocorticoids), mass lesion (eg, brain metastasis), traumatic brain injury, subarachnoid hemorrhage, infection/abscess, stroke, external beam radiation, pituitary apoplexy, Sheehan's syndrome, autoimmune disease (eg, lymphocytic hypophysitis), and infiltrative disease (eg, hemochromatosis).[2,8]

**What is the most common cause of central hypothyroidism?**

Pituitary macroadenomas (eg, prolactinoma) are responsible for more than half of cases of central hypothyroidism.[8]

## Case Summary

A 38-year-old woman with recent weight gain and constipation presents with confusion and is found to have hypothermia, bradycardia, nonpitting peripheral edema, abnormal neurologic reflexes, hyponatremia, low serum free $T_4$, and elevated serum TSH.

***What is the most likely diagnosis in this patient?***

Primary hypothyroidism.

### BONUS QUESTIONS

***What physical finding of hypothyroidism is seen in the photograph of the patient in this case?***

The photograph of the patient in this case (see Figure 11-1) shows thinning of the eyebrows, particularly the lateral third (known as the Sign of Hertoghe or Queen Anne's sign).

***What is the significance of the thyroid biochemical profile in this case?***

The patient in this case has TSH-independent (primary) hypothyroidism, which is characterized by the combination of elevated serum TSH and depressed serum free $T_4$. In TSH-dependent (central) hypothyroidism, serum TSH would be low or normal in the setting of low serum free $T_4$.

***What type of primary hypothyroidism is most likely in this case?***

Hashimoto's thyroiditis causes the vast majority of cases of primary hypothyroidism in the industrialized world and is statistically most likely in this case. The presence of serum thyroid autoantibodies would support the diagnosis.[2]

***How should the patient in this case be managed?***

The patient in this case has myxedema coma based on the presence of somnolence and delirium. The cornerstone of therapy is immediate thyroid hormone replacement. Synthetic $T_4$ may be given alone or in combination with $T_3$. Intravenous administration is recommended initially because the presence of bowel edema may limit absorption. In cases of secondary hypothyroidism or polyglandular autoimmune syndrome, baseline cortisol should always be obtained to evaluate for coexistent adrenal insufficiency. If present, glucocorticoids should be given before thyroid replacement.[5]

***What is the initial management of permanent hypothyroidism when myxedema coma is not present?***

Patients with permanent hypothyroidism should be started on oral synthetic thyroxine (ie, levothyroxine) according to body mass. A daily dose of 1.6 μg/kg body mass (equivalent to 100 μg daily for the average-sized woman) is sufficient for most adults. Older patients (>60 years of age) or those with ischemic heart disease should be started on a lower dose of levothyroxine (eg, 25-50 μg daily) and titrated up gradually. For optimal and consistent absorption, levothyroxine should be taken on an empty stomach, usually 60 minutes before breakfast or at bedtime (at least 3 hours after dinner).[27,28]

***After starting replacement hormone, how should patients with primary hypothyroidism be monitored?***

After starting therapy for primary hypothyroidism, serum TSH and free $T_4$ levels should be measured after 4 to 6 weeks, with adjustments made to the dose accordingly. Serum TSH should be rechecked in 4 to 6 week intervals after any dose adjustment. The "goal" serum TSH level is within the lower half of the reference range. Once a dose is found that achieves a serum TSH level within the goal, it can be measured annually. Dose adjustments may need to be considered sooner for weight changes or pregnancy.[27]

***How soon do patients with hypothyroidism notice an improvement after thyroid hormone replacement has been started?***

The half-life of levothyroxine is 7 days, so it takes at least a week for the symptoms of hypothyroidism to begin to improve. Muscle weakness and cognitive deficits may take up to 6 months to fully recover.[28]

## KEY POINTS

- Hypothyroidism is a clinical condition that results from thyroid hormone deficiency.
- Hypothyroidism is more common in women than men.
- Symptoms of hypothyroidism include weight gain, fatigue, poor concentration, depression, constipation, cold intolerance, dry skin, proximal muscle weakness, hair thinning or loss, and menorrhagia.
- Physical findings of hypothyroidism include hypothermia, bradycardia, diastolic hypertension, cognitive impairment, coarse facies, lateral eyebrow thinning, goiter, dry or coarse skin, hoarse voice, delayed relaxation phase of deep tendon reflexes, nonpitting peripheral edema, and macroglossia.
- Myxedema coma is a severe and life-threatening complication of hypothyroidism, usually associated with a precipitating factor such as infection.
- When hypothyroidism is suspected clinically, it is confirmed with a low serum free $T_4$.
- Serum TSH level determines whether hypothyroidism is TSH-independent (primary) or TSH-dependent (central).
- The causes of primary hypothyroidism can be separated into the following subcategories: thyroiditis, iodine-related, iatrogenic, and infiltrative.
- The most common causes of primary hypothyroidism are Hashimoto's thyroiditis (in the industrialized world) and iodine deficiency (in the developing world).
- Central hypothyroidism is rare and caused by pituitary and/or hypothalamic dysfunction.
- Synthetic thyroxine is the treatment of choice for primary hypothyroidism; most adults require a daily dose of 1.6 μg/kg body mass.

## REFERENCES

1. Berne RML, Levy MN. *Physiology*. 4th ed. St. Louis, MO: Mosby, Inc.; 1998.
2. Chaker L, Bianco AC, Jonklaas J, Peeters RP. Hypothyroidism. *Lancet*. 2017;390(10101):1550-62.
3. Tunbridge WM, Evered DC, Hall R, et al. The spectrum of thyroid disease in a community: the Whickham survey. *Clin Endocrinol*. 1977;7(6):481-493.
4. Gaitonde DY, Rowley KD, Sweeney LB. Hypothyroidism: an update. *Am Fam Physician*. 2012;86(3):244-251.
5. Mathew V, Misgar RA, Ghosh S, et al. Myxedema coma: a new look into an old crisis. *J Thyroid Res*. 2011;2011:493462.
6. Koulouri O, Moran C, Halsall D, Chatterjee K, Gurnell M. Pitfalls in the measurement and interpretation of thyroid function tests. *Best Pract Res Clin Endocrinol Metab*. 2013;27(6):745-762.
7. Garber JR, Cobin RH, Gharib H, et al. Clinical practice guidelines for hypothyroidism in adults: cosponsored by the American Association of Clinical Endocrinologists and the American Thyroid Association. *Endocr Pract*. 2012;18(6):988-1028.
8. Persani L. Clinical review: central hypothyroidism: pathogenic, diagnostic, and therapeutic challenges. *J Clin Endocrinol Metab*. 2012;97(9):3068-3078.
9. De Leo S, Lee SY, Braverman LE. Hyperthyroidism. *Lancet*. 2016;388(10047):906-918.
10. Pearce EN, Farwell AP, Braverman LE. Thyroiditis. *N Engl J Med*. 2003;348(26):2646-2655.
11. Intenzo CM, Capuzzi DM, Jabbour S, Kim SM, dePapp AE. Scintigraphic features of autoimmune thyroiditis. *Radiographics*. 2001;21(4):957-964.
12. Stagnaro-Green A. Clinical review 152: postpartum thyroiditis. *J Clin Endocrinol Metab*. 2002;87(9):4042-4047.
13. Fatourechi V, Aniszewski JP, Fatourechi GZ, Atkinson EJ, Jacobsen SJ. Clinical features and outcome of subacute thyroiditis in an incidence cohort: olmsted County, Minnesota, study. *J Clin Endocrinol Metab*. 2003;88(5):2100-2105.
14. Bindra A, Braunstein GD. Thyroiditis. *Am Fam Physician*. 2006;73(10):1769-1776.
15. Mittra ES, McDougall IR. Recurrent silent thyroiditis: a report of four patients and review of the literature. *Thyroid*. 2007;17(7):671-675.
16. Chung HR. Iodine and thyroid function. *Ann Pediatr Endocrinol Metab*. 2014;19(1):8-12.
17. Markou K, Georgopoulos N, Kyriazopoulou V, Vagenakis AG. Iodine-Induced hypothyroidism. *Thyroid*. 2001;11(5):501-510.
18. Stoll SJ, Pitt SC, Liu J, Schaefer S, Sippel RS, Chen H. Thyroid hormone replacement after thyroid lobectomy. *Surgery*. 2009;146(4):554-558, discussion 8-60.
19. Mumtaz M, Lin LS, Hui KC, Mohd Khir AS. Radioiodine I-131 for the therapy of graves' disease. *Malays J Med Sci*. 2009;16(1):25-33.
20. George J, Joshi SR. Drugs and thyroid. *J Assoc Physicians India*. 2007;55:215-223.
21. Vogelius IR, Bentzen SM, Maraldo MV, Petersen PM, Specht L. Risk factors for radiation-induced hypothyroidism: a literature-based meta-analysis. *Cancer*. 2011;117(23):5250-5260.
22. Hennessey JV. Clinical review: Riedel's thyroiditis: a clinical review. *J Clin Endocrinol Metab*. 2011;96(10):3031-3041.
23. Edwards CQ, Kelly TM, Ellwein G, Kushner JP. Thyroid disease in hemochromatosis. Increased incidence in homozygous men. *Arch Intern Med*. 1983;143(10):1890-1893.
24. Kimura H, Yamashita S, Ashizawa K, Yokoyama N, Nagataki S. Thyroid dysfunction in patients with amyloid goitre. *Clin Endocrinol*. 1997;46(6):769-774.

25. Kmiec P, Lewandowska M, Dubaniewicz A, et al. Two cases of thyroid sarcoidosis presentation as painful, recurrent goiter in patients with Graves' disease. *Arq Bras Endocrinol Metabol.* 2012;56(3):209-214.
26. Braverman LE, Cooper DS, eds. *Werner and Ingbar's the Thyroid: A Fundamental and Clinical Text.* 10th ed. Philadelphia: Lippincott Williams & Wilkins; 2013.
27. Jonklaas J, Bianco AC, Bauer AJ, et al. Guidelines for the treatment of hypothyroidism: prepared by the american thyroid association task force on thyroid hormone replacement. *Thyroid.* 2014;24(12):1670-1751.
28. Vaidya B, Pearce SH. Management of hypothyroidism in adults. *BMJ.* 2008;337:a801.

Chapter 12

# THYROTOXICOSIS

## Case: A 64-year-old woman with palpitations

A previously healthy 64-year-old woman presents to the clinic with several weeks of intermittent palpitations. The episodes seem to occur randomly, including when she is at rest. When symptomatic, she does not have chest pain but does feel short of breath. She has had an unintentional weight loss of 10 pounds over this time. Her husband reports she has seemed more irritable lately.

Heart rate is 120 beats per minute and irregular, and blood pressure is 150/70 mm Hg. There is a fine tremor of the hands. The eyes appear to bulge anteriorly. The tissue over the anterior neck is generous in appearance, and a continuous bruit is heard when the diaphragm of the stethoscope is placed over it.

Serum thyroid-stimulating hormone is measured at 0.01 mIU/L (reference range 0.4-4.2 mIU/L). Free thyroxine is 6.8 ng/dL (reference range 0.6-1.2 ng/dL). A radioactive iodine uptake test with thyroid scan shows diffusely increased uptake (Figure 12-1).

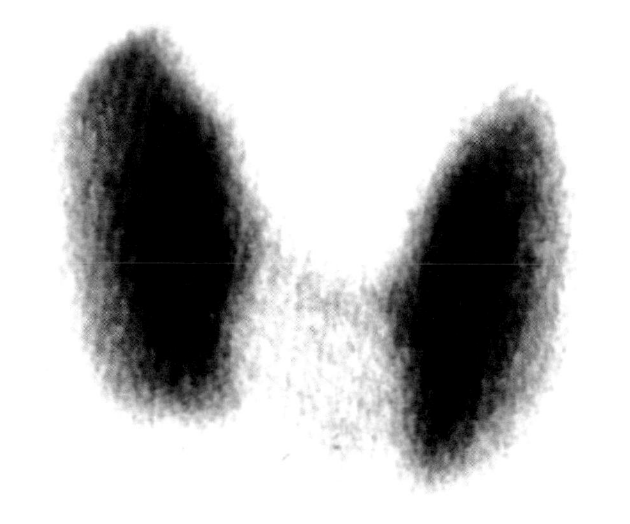

**Figure 12-1.** (Courtesy of Mary H. Samuels, MD.)

***What is the most likely diagnosis in this patient?***

**What is thyrotoxicosis?**

Thyrotoxicosis is a clinical condition that results from excess circulating thyroid hormones from any source. Hyperthyroidism specifically refers to increased thyroid hormone synthesis from the thyroid gland.[1]

**What is the normal cycle of the hypothalamic-pituitary-thyroid axis?**

The hypothalamus produces thyroid-releasing hormone (TRH), which stimulates the pituitary to secrete thyroid-stimulating hormone (TSH). The thyroid gland responds to TSH stimulation by secreting thyroxine ($T_4$) and triiodothyronine ($T_3$), which then provide negative feedback to both the hypothalamus and pituitary (see Figure 11-2).[2]

**What is the relationship between $T_3$ and $T_4$?**

$T_3$ and $T_4$ are both produced in the thyroid gland by the follicular cells, although the vast majority of thyroid output is in the form of $T_4$. Peripheral conversion of $T_4$ to $T_3$ occurs in the liver and kidney (see Figure 11-2). The relative potency of $T_3$ is several times greater than that of $T_4$, and it is more biologically active.[2]

**How common is thyrotoxicosis?**

In the industrialized world, thyrotoxicosis affects 1 in 2000 persons per year.[3]

**What are the symptoms of thyrotoxicosis?**

Symptoms of thyrotoxicosis depend on underlying cause, duration of disease, and patient-specific factors such as age and sex but in general may include heat intolerance, sweating, nervousness, irritability, anxiety, fatigue, poor concentration, palpitations, dyspnea, hyperdefecation, nausea, vomiting, menstrual irregularities, diplopia, and eye discomfort.[1]

**What are the physical findings of thyrotoxicosis?**

Physical findings of thyrotoxicosis depend on the underlying cause, duration of disease, and patient-specific factors such as age and sex but in general may include weight loss, tremor of the extremities, hyperreflexia, tachycardia, systolic hypertension, tachypnea, goiter (with or without bruit), abdominal tenderness, pelvic and shoulder muscle weakness, warm and moist skin, exophthalmos (ie, proptosis) (Figure 12-2), eyelid retraction and lag, periorbital edema, and ophthalmoplegia.[1]

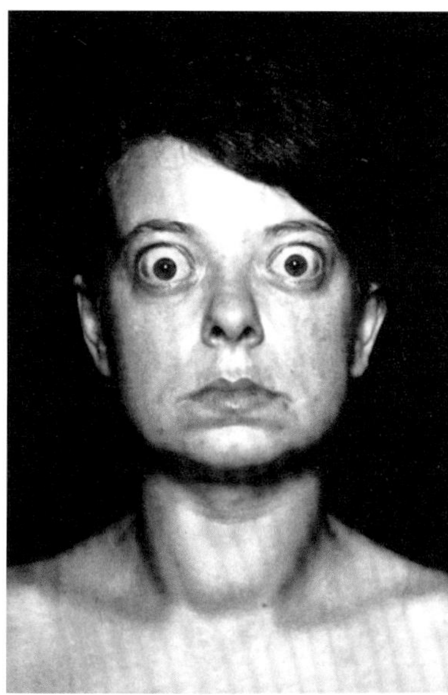

**Figure 12-2.** A young woman with hyperthyroidism. Note the anterior neck mass (goiter) and bulging of the eyes (exophthalmos). (Reprinted with permission from Rubin E, Farber JL. *Pathology*. 3rd ed. Philadelphia, PA: Lippincott Williams & Wilkins; 1999.)

**How does the presentation of thyrotoxicosis vary with age?**

Younger patients with thyrotoxicosis are more likely to have hyperadrenergic manifestations (eg, anxiety, restlessness, tremor); older patients tend to be less symptomatic but are more likely to develop cardiovascular complications (eg, dysrhythmia).[1]

**What life-threatening complication can occur in patients with untreated thyrotoxicosis?**

Thyroid storm describes a severe and life-threatening form of thyrotoxicosis with extreme signs and symptoms of hypermetabolism, including tachycardia, fever, perspiration, diarrhea, anxiety, seizure, delirium, and coma. There is often a precipitating factor, such as discontinuation of antithyroid drugs, infection, trauma, stress, or pregnancy. The distinction is clinical, as thyroid hormone levels are comparable to those in patients with compensated thyrotoxicosis. The condition is life-threatening; up to one-quarter of patients die.[1]

**If thyrotoxicosis is suspected based on the clinical evaluation, what is the next diagnostic step?**

In patients with a clinical condition compatible with thyrotoxicosis, elevated serum free $T_4$ will confirm the diagnosis. Concurrent measurement of serum TSH can distinguish whether the process is TSH-independent (TSH level is low) or TSH-dependent (TSH level is elevated or normal).

Thyrotoxicosis

TSH-independent | TSH-dependent

**In the setting of thyrotoxicosis, why does a normal serum TSH value implicate a TSH-dependent process?**

When there is thyroid hormone excess, negative feedback to the hypothalamus and pituitary should turn off TSH secretion in an attempt to return serum thyroid hormone levels to normal. Therefore, a TSH level within the normal range is "inappropriately normal."

**Which coexisting conditions can make the interpretation of thyroid function studies difficult?**

Pregnancy, nonthyroid acute illness, medications (eg, glucocorticoids), and recovery from thyrotoxicosis can make the interpretation of thyroid function studies challenging.[4]

**What condition is characterized by the combination of normal serum thyroid hormone levels and suppressed TSH?**

Subclinical hyperthyroidism is defined by the presence of low serum TSH with normal serum levels of thyroid hormone. Over time, patients with subclinical hyperthyroidism may remain stable, progress to overt thyrotoxicosis, or revert to euthyroid state. Risk of progression is increased when serum TSH levels are <0.1 mIU/L. There is an increased risk of atrial fibrillation in patients with subclinical hyperthyroidism. The decision to treat is controversial and depends on the patient's age and degree of TSH suppression.[5]

**What condition is characterized by the combination of normal serum free $T_4$, suppressed TSH, and elevated total $T_3$ or free $T_3$?**

$T_3$ toxicosis describes the combination of normal serum free $T_4$, suppressed TSH, and elevated total $T_3$ or free $T_3$. This pattern can be seen early in the course of hyperthyroidism. It also occurs with a higher frequency in patients with the combination of hyperthyroidism (eg, Graves' disease) and concurrent iodine deficiency.[6,7]

## TSH-INDEPENDENT THYROTOXICOSIS

**What is the fundamental mechanism of TSH-independent thyrotoxicosis?**

TSH-independent thyrotoxicosis occurs as a result of the presence of excess thyroid hormones independent of TSH stimulation of the thyroid gland.

**Once TSH-independent thyrotoxicosis is established, what is the next diagnostic step?**

Patients with TSH-independent thyrotoxicosis should undergo a radioactive iodine uptake test. Patients are given radioactive iodine and then a $\gamma$ probe is used to detect how much of it is taken up by the thyroid gland. Uptake can be normal, increased, or decreased. *True hyperthyroidism (ie, increased thyroid hormone synthesis from the thyroid gland) results in increased radioactive iodine uptake, whereas thyrotoxicosis without hyperthyroidism results in decreased uptake.*

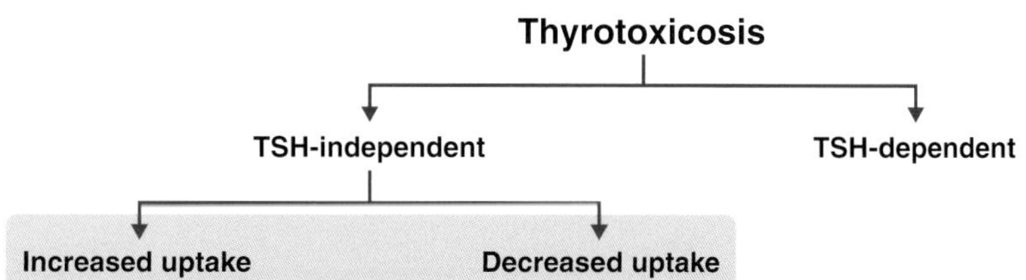

## TSH-INDEPENDENT THYROTOXICOSIS WITH INCREASED RADIOACTIVE IODINE UPTAKE

What are the 2 general patterns of increased radioactive iodine uptake?

When radioactive iodine uptake is increased, a diffuse or focal pattern of uptake can be identified by thyroid scintigraphy (ie, thyroid scan) (Figure 12-3). *Thyroid scintigraphy is different than, but adjunctive to, the radioactive iodine uptake test.*

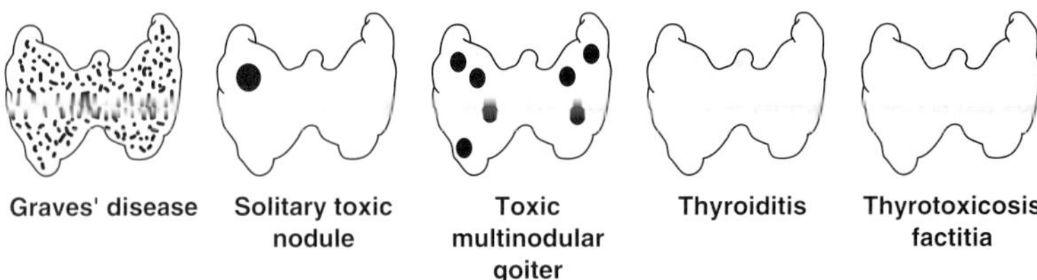


**Figure 12-3.** An illustration depicting the patterns of radioactive iodine uptake by thyroid scan in patients with various forms of thyrotoxicosis. One important exception is the thyrotoxic phase of Hashimoto's thyroiditis (ie, Hashitoxicosis), which can be associated with normal or even increased radioactive iodine uptake. (From Chowdhury SH, Cozma AI, Chowdhury JH. *Essentials for the Canadian Medical Licensing Exam*. 2nd ed. Philadelphia, PA: Wolters Kluwer Health; 2017.)

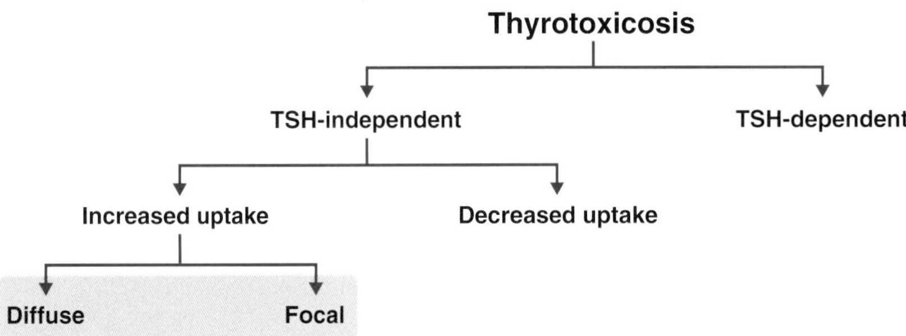


## TSH-INDEPENDENT THYROTOXICOSIS WITH DIFFUSELY INCREASED RADIOACTIVE IODINE UPTAKE

### What are the causes of TSH-independent thyrotoxicosis with diffusely increased radioactive iodine uptake?

Associated with TSH-receptor antibodies, this condition is the most common cause of thyrotoxicosis in iodine-sufficient parts of the world.

Graves' disease.

A hormone produced during pregnancy with a subunit that is identical to that of TSH.

Human chorionic gonadotropin (hCG).

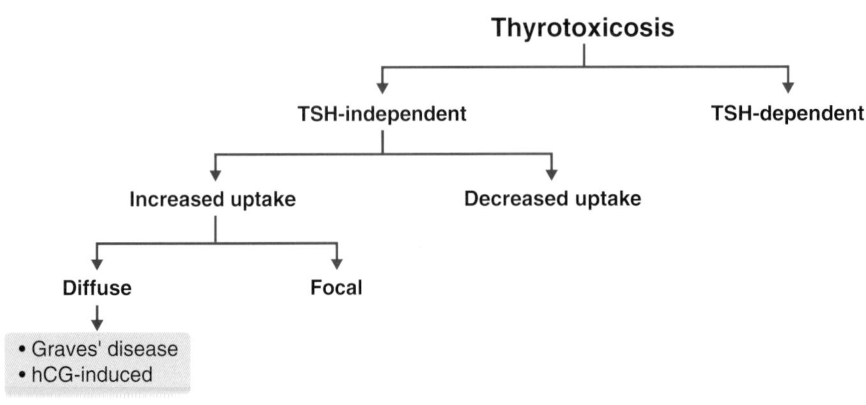

**What are the characteristics of Graves' disease?**

Graves' disease accounts for the majority of cases of thyrotoxicosis in iodine-sufficient parts of the world. Its cause is multifactorial but involves the development of autoantibodies that activate the TSH receptor and stimulate thyroid follicular cells. There is a higher prevalence of Graves' disease in women. Clinical manifestations specific to Graves' disease include Graves' ophthalmopathy, including exophthalmos (see Figure 12-2), pretibial myxedema (ie, thyroid dermopathy) (see Figure 23-6), and a systolic or continuous bruit over the thyroid gland.[1,8]

**What are the sources of hCG-induced hyperthyroidism?**

Because of its structural similarity to TSH, hCG can stimulate thyroid TSH receptors, causing hyperthyroidism. The most common causes of hCG-induced hyperthyroidism include pregnancy (typically multiple gestation) and gestational trophoblastic tumors.[1]

## TSH-INDEPENDENT THYROTOXICOSIS WITH FOCALLY INCREASED RADIOACTIVE IODINE UPTAKE

### What are the causes of TSH-independent thyrotoxicosis with focally increased radioactive iodine uptake?

**Multiple focal areas of uptake.**

Toxic multinodular goiter (TMNG).

**A "hot nodule."**

Toxic adenoma.

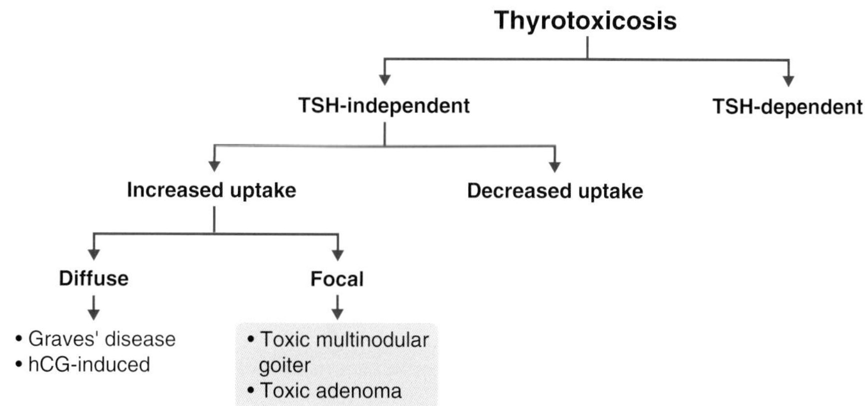


**What are the characteristics of toxic multinodular goiter?**

TMNG is the most common cause of thyrotoxicosis in iodine-deficient parts of the world and is more frequent in women and the elderly. In the setting of iodine deficiency, chronic TSH stimulation results in the growth of thyroid tissue that can produce thyroid hormone autonomously, independent from stimulation by TSH. This usually results in suppression of the surrounding normal thyroid tissue. Patients typically develop TMNG after a long history of euthyroid multinodular goiter. Thyrotoxicosis occurs when the autonomous nodules "tip the balance" toward excess thyroid hormone. TMNG is best treated with radioactive iodine ablation or surgery, as antithyroid drugs alone are unlikely to achieve remission.[1,9]

**Do all thyroid adenomas result in thyrotoxicosis?**

Thyroid adenomas are present in around one-half of the general population at autopsy, although the majority are never diagnosed. Adenomas typically present as palpable nodules discovered by the patient or physician but are also discovered incidentally during imaging studies. The vast majority of adenomas are clinically silent or "cold." Only 5% of thyroid nodules are functional or "hot" and capable of causing thyrotoxicosis (see Figure 12-3). The majority of all thyroid nodules are benign. However, malignancy is more likely in patients with a thyroid nodule when serum TSH is not suppressed. Such cold nodules should be evaluated with biopsy. Although far less likely, malignancy can occur in patients with functional adenomas. Thyrotoxicosis related to thyroid adenoma is best treated with radioactive iodine ablation or surgery, as antithyroid drugs alone are unlikely to achieve remission.[1,9,10]

## TSH-INDEPENDENT THYROTOXICOSIS WITH DECREASED RADIOACTIVE IODINE UPTAKE

### What are the causes of TSH-independent thyrotoxicosis with decreased radioactive iodine uptake?

**A 25-year-old woman with a history of anorexia nervosa presents with symptoms and signs of thyrotoxicosis.**

Exposure to exogenous thyroid hormone.

**Typically characterized by a phase of thyrotoxicosis followed by either normal thyroid function or hypothyroidism, which may be temporary or permanent.**

Thyroiditis.

**Jod-Basedow phenomenon.**

Iodine exposure.

**The thyroid gland is an innocent bystander.**

Extraglandular production of thyroid hormone.

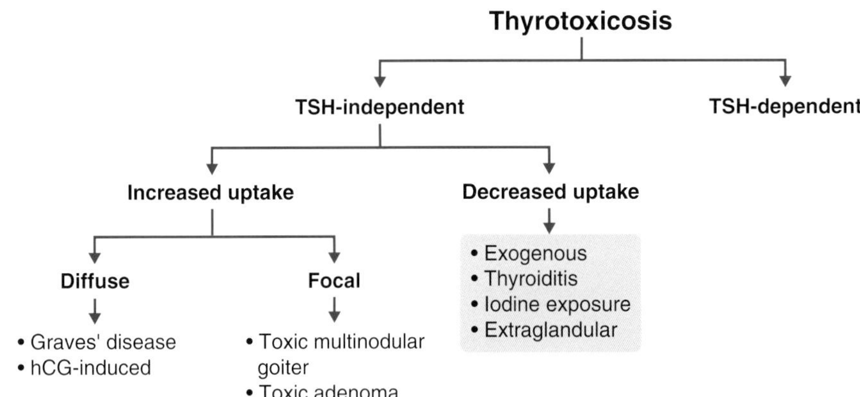


**For what reason might a young woman take thyroid medication surreptitiously?**

Surreptitious thyroid hormone ingestion, known as thyrotoxicosis factitia, is often used to augment weight loss. The finding of undetectable serum thyroglobulin levels can distinguish thyrotoxicosis factitia from other causes of TSH-independent thyrotoxicosis. However, the presence of thyroglobulin antibodies can interfere with the assay, producing misleading results. In such cases, increased fecal thyroxine levels suggest the diagnosis.[11,12]

**What is thyroiditis?**

Thyroiditis refers to a group of disorders that produce inflammation of the thyroid gland, which may lead to destruction of thyrocytes and the unregulated release of preformed thyroid hormones into the circulation. There are several distinct clinical entities that cause painful thyroiditis, such as subacute thyroiditis (ie, de Quervain's thyroiditis), infectious thyroiditis (ie, suppurative thyroiditis), radiation-induced thyroiditis, and trauma-induced thyroiditis. Those that are not painful include Hashimoto's thyroiditis, painless thyroiditis (ie, silent thyroiditis), postpartum thyroiditis, drug-induced thyroiditis, and fibrous thyroiditis (ie, Riedel's thyroiditis). *The thyrotoxic phase of Hashimoto's thyroiditis (ie, Hashitoxicosis) can be associated with normal or even increased radioactive iodine uptake.*[1,13,14]

**What is the Jod-Basedow phenomenon?**

The Jod-Basedow phenomenon refers to iodine-induced hyperthyroidism. It typically occurs in patients with preexisting autonomous thyroid tissue related to iodine deficiency (eg, multinodular goiter). When the iodine supply is increased, the autonomous regions begin to increase thyroid hormone synthesis independent of autoregulatory mechanisms, resulting in thyrotoxicosis within weeks to months. Sources of iodine include radiographic contrast media and medications (eg, amiodarone). It is typically self-limited once the source of excess iodine has been removed (cases of amiodarone-induced hyperthyroidism may be particularly prolonged because of the long half-life of the drug).[15]

**What source of extraglandular thyroid hormone production occurs only in women?**

Extraglandular thyroid hormone production is very rare. Struma ovarii describes an ovarian tumor that contains functioning thyroid tissue[1]

## TSH-DEPENDENT THYROTOXICOSIS

**What is the fundamental mechanism of TSH-dependent thyrotoxicosis?**

TSH-dependent thyrotoxicosis occurs as a result of excess TSH stimulation of the thyroid gland that responds by producing excess thyroid hormones.

**What general term is used to describe thyrotoxicosis related to excess TSH?**

Thyrotoxicosis related to excess TSH is referred to as TSH-induced hyperthyroidism.

### What are the causes of TSH-induced hyperthyroidism?

**A 55-year-old man presents with weight loss, headache, and tremor and is found to have a visual field defect on examination.**

Pituitary adenoma.

**The hypothalamus and pituitary do not respond to negative feedback.**

Impaired sensitivity to thyroid hormone.

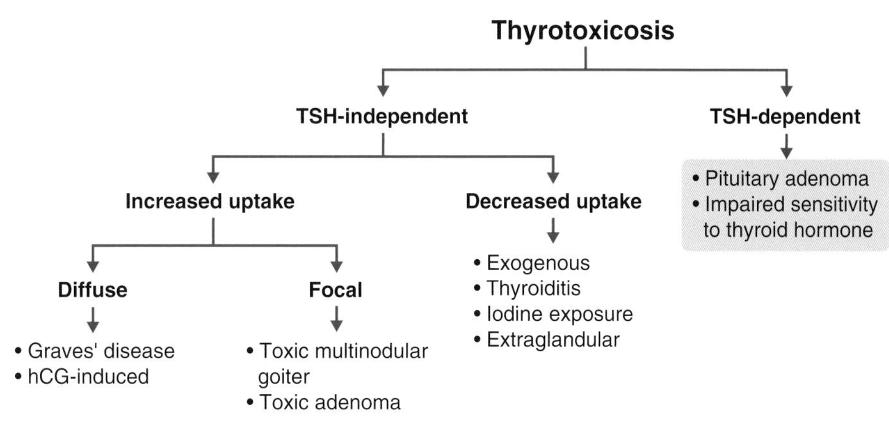

What are the characteristics of TSH-induced hyperthyroidism caused by pituitary adenoma?

TSH-secreting pituitary adenomas are rare, representing 0.5% to 3% of all pituitary adenomas. Both genders are equally affected, and most patients are diagnosed in the fifth to sixth decades of life. The clinical manifestations tend to be mild compared with other forms of thyrotoxicosis. Some tumors secrete both TSH and growth hormone, giving rise to a mixed clinical picture of thyrotoxicosis and acromegaly. The majority of TSH-secreting pituitary adenomas are large and invasive, with associated headache, visual field defects, and loss of vision. Magnetic resonance imaging of the brain should be performed in patients suspected of having a TSH-secreting pituitary adenoma.[16]

What is impaired sensitivity to thyroid hormone?

Impaired sensitivity to thyroid hormone describes any condition that reduces the effectiveness of thyroid hormone. Resistance to thyroid hormone is the most common subtype and usually occurs as a result of an inherited mutation in the thyroid hormone receptor. The degrees of thyroid hormone resistance and TSH-mediated compensation vary between patients, but there are also considerable differences within each individual's own peripheral tissues, giving rise to a unique mixture of clinical features of hyperthyroidism and hypothyroidism. The most common manifestations of thyrotoxicosis in these patients include goiter, sinus tachycardia, and hyperactivity.[17,18]

## Case Summary

A 64-year-old woman presents with palpitations, weight loss, and dyspnea and is found to have irregularly irregular tachycardia, wide pulse pressure, elevated serum free $T_4$, suppressed serum TSH, and diffusely increased radioiodine uptake as measured by a radioactive iodine uptake test and thyroid scan.

***What is the most likely diagnosis in this patient?***

Graves' disease.

### BONUS QUESTIONS

***What heart rhythm is most likely present in this case?***

The irregularly irregular tachycardia described in this case is most likely atrial fibrillation, which occurs at a higher rate in patients with thyrotoxicosis.[1]

***Which features in this case are specifically suggestive of Graves' disease?***

Weight loss, irritability, palpitations, and tremor may be features of thyrotoxicosis from any cause. However, the exophthalmos (bulging of the eyes anteriorly) and bruit over the thyroid gland (systolic or continuous in nature) described in this case are specific for Graves' disease. Another finding specific to Graves' disease (not present in this case) is pretibial myxedema (ie, thyroid dermopathy), characterized by pigmented and thickened skin, most evident over the shins (see Figure 23-6).[1,8]

***What causes Graves' ophthalmopathy?***

In some patients with Graves' disease, autoimmune-mediated lymphocytic infiltration of the orbital tissues (including adipose tissue and the extraocular muscles) leads to deposition of glycosaminoglycans, resulting in edema and increased orbital volume. Over time, this process leads to fibrosis and scarring within the orbital tissues. The most common manifestations include exophthalmos, periorbital edema, and diplopia.[1,19]

***What measurable autoantibody is present in patients with Graves' disease?***

Antibodies against the TSH receptor are present in the serum of patients with Graves' disease and can be measured to confirm the diagnosis when radioactive iodine uptake testing is unavailable or contraindicated.[1]

***What class of medication can be used to treat the hyperadrenergic manifestations of thyrotoxicosis?***

Thyrotoxicosis leads to an increase in β-adrenergic receptors in peripheral tissues, resulting in manifestations such as anxiety, tachycardia, and palpitations. β-Blockers can be used to ameliorate these manifestations.[20,21]

***What options are available for long-term treatment of hyperthyroidism caused by Graves' disease?***

Options for long-term treatment of Graves' disease generally include antithyroid drugs (eg, thionamides), radioactive iodine ablation, and surgery. Treatment approach depends on regional practice, patient-specific factors (eg, age, severity of symptoms), and patient preference. Several modalities may ultimately be necessary to achieve remission.[1]

| | |
|---|---|
| ***How effective are the antithyroid drugs?*** | The thionamide agents (eg, methimazole) treat hyperthyroidism by inhibiting the synthesis of thyroid hormones. These drugs are effective in achieving remission in patients with Graves' disease, but relapse rates are high when discontinued, particularly within the first year. The risk for recurrence is greater in those with severe hyperthyroidism, large goiter, high $T_4$:$T_3$ ratios, persistently suppressed TSH, and high baseline titers of TSH-receptor antibodies. In patients with toxic adenomas and TMNG, remission is rarely achieved with antithyroid drugs alone; however, these agents can be useful in combination with definitive therapy (eg, radioactive iodine ablation or surgery). The most common major side effect of the thionamides is agranulocytosis, which can be life-threatening.[1] |
| ***When can radioactive iodine therapy be used to treat hyperthyroidism?*** | Radioactive iodine therapy can be used as first-line treatment in patients with Graves' disease, toxic adenoma, and TMNG. Absolute contraindications include pregnancy, breastfeeding, and planned pregnancy. Radioactive iodine therapy can make Graves' ophthalmopathy worse and should be avoided in most patients with this condition. The choice between radioactive iodine therapy and thyroidectomy depends on regional practice, patient-specific factors, and patient preference.[1] |
| ***When can thyroidectomy be used to treat hyperthyroidism?*** | Thyroidectomy can be used to treat Graves' disease, toxic adenoma, and TMNG. Thyroidectomy is generally recommended in patients with large goiters, low uptake of radioactive iodine, suspected or documented thyroid cancer, and moderate to severe ophthalmopathy. Major adverse effects include hypothyroidism, hypoparathyroidism, and recurrent laryngeal nerve injury.[1] |

## KEY POINTS

- Thyrotoxicosis is a clinical condition that results from thyroid hormone excess.
- Symptoms of thyrotoxicosis include heat intolerance, sweating, nervousness, irritability, anxiety, fatigue, poor concentration, palpitations, dyspnea, hyperdefecation, nausea, vomiting, menstrual irregularities, diplopia, and eye discomfort.
- Physical findings of thyrotoxicosis include weight loss, tremor of the extremities, hyperreflexia, tachycardia, systolic hypertension, tachypnea, goiter with or without bruit, abdominal tenderness, pelvic and shoulder muscle weakness, warm and moist skin, exophthalmos, eyelid retraction and lag, periorbital edema, and ophthalmoplegia.
- Younger patients with thyrotoxicosis are more likely to have hyperadrenergic manifestations (eg, anxiety, restlessness, tremor); older patients tend to be less symptomatic but are more likely to develop cardiovascular complications (eg, dysrhythmia).
- Thyroid storm describes a severe and life-threatening form of thyrotoxicosis with extreme signs and symptoms of hypermetabolism.
- When thyrotoxicosis is suspected clinically, it is confirmed with an elevated serum free $T_4$.
- Serum TSH level determines whether thyrotoxicosis is TSH-independent or TSH-dependent.
- TSH-independent thyrotoxicosis can be associated with increased or decreased radioactive iodide uptake.
- Increased radioactive iodine uptake can occur in a diffuse or focal pattern, which informs the differential diagnosis.
- β-Blockers can be used to ameliorate the hyperadrenergic manifestations of thyrotoxicosis (eg, anxiety, tachycardia).
- Options for the long-term treatment for hyperthyroidism related to Graves' disease, toxic adenoma, and toxic multinodular goiter generally include antithyroid drugs (eg, thionamides), radioactive iodine ablation, and/or surgery. Choice of modality depends on underlying cause, regional practice, patient-specific factors, and patient preference.

ENDOCRINOLOGY

## REFERENCES

1. De Leo S, Lee SY, Braverman LE. Hyperthyroidism. *Lancet*. 2016;388(10047):906-918.
2. Berne RML, Levy MN. *Physiology*. 4th ed. St. Louis, Missouri: Mosby, Inc.; 1998.
3. Vaidya B, Pearce SH. Diagnosis and management of thyrotoxicosis. *BMJ*. 2014;349:g5128.
4. Koulouri O, Moran C, Halsall D, Chatterjee K, Gurnell M. Pitfalls in the measurement and interpretation of thyroid function tests. *Best Pract Res Clin Endocrinol Metab*. 2013;27(6):745-762.

5. Biondi B, Bartalena L, Cooper DS, Hegedus L, Laurberg P, Kahaly GJ. The 2015 European Thyroid Association Guidelines on diagnosis and treatment of endogenous subclinical hyperthyroidism. *Eur Thyroid J*. 2015;4(3):149-163.
6. Figge J, Leinung M, Goodman AD, et al. The clinical evaluation of patients with subclinical hyperthyroidism and free triiodothyronine (free T3) toxicosis. *Am J Med*. 1994;96(3):229-234.
7. Hollander CS, Mitsuma T, Shenkman L, Stevenson C, Pineda G, Silva E. T3 toxicosis in an iodine-deficient. *Lancet*. 1972;2(7790):1276-1278.
8. Williams E, Chillag S, Rizvi A. Thyroid bruit and the underlying 'inferno'. *Am J Med*. 2014;127(6):489-490.
9. Krohn K, Fuhrer D, Bayer Y, et al. Molecular pathogenesis of euthyroid and toxic multinodular goiter. *Endocr Rev*. 2005;26(4):504-524.
10. Mirfakhraee S, Mathews D, Peng L, Woodruff S, Zigman JM. A solitary hyperfunctioning thyroid nodule harboring thyroid carcinoma: review of the literature. *Thyroid Res*. 2013;6(1):7.
11. Bouillon R, Verresen L, Staels F, Bex M, De Vos P, De Roo M. The measurement of fecal thyroxine in the diagnosis of thyrotoxicosis factitia. *Thyroid*. 1993;3(2):101-103.
12. Mariotti S, Martino E, Cupini C, et al. Low serum thyroglobulin as a clue to the diagnosis of thyrotoxicosis factitia. *N Engl J Med*. 1982;307(7):410-412.
13. Pearce EN, Farwell AP, Braverman LE. Thyroiditis. *N Engl J Med*. 2003;348(26):2646-2655.
14. Intenzo CM, Capuzzi DM, Jabbour S, Kim SM, dePapp AE. Scintigraphic features of autoimmune thyroiditis. *Radiographics*. 2001;21(4):957-964.
15. El-Shirbiny AM, Stavrou SS, Dnistrian A, Sonenberg M, Larson SM, Divgi CR. Jod-Basedow syndrome following oral iodine and radioiodinated-antibody administration. *J Nucl Med*. 1997;38(11):1816-1817.
16. Beck-Peccoz P, Lania A, Beckers A, Chatterjee K, Wemeau JL. 2013 European thyroid association guidelines for the diagnosis and treatment of thyrotropin-secreting pituitary tumors. *Eur Thyroid J*. 2013;2(2):76-82.
17. De Groot LJ, Chrousos G, Dungan K, et al, eds. *Endotext*. South Dartmouth, MA: MDText.com, Inc.; 2000.
18. Refetoff S, DeWind LT, DeGroot LJ. Familial syndrome combining deaf-mutism, stuppled epiphyses, goiter and abnormally high PBI: possible target organ refractoriness to thyroid hormone. *J Clin Endocrinol Metab*. 1967;27(2):279-294.
19. Maheshwari R, Weis E. Thyroid associated orbitopathy. *Indian J Ophthalmol*. 2012;60(2):87-93.
20. Bilezikian JP, Loeb JN. The influence of hyperthyroidism and hypothyroidism on alpha- and beta-adrenergic receptor systems and adrenergic responsiveness. *Endocr Rev*. 1983;4(4):378-388.
21. Geffner DL, Hershman JM. Beta-adrenergic blockade for the treatment of hyperthyroidism. *Am J Med*. 1992;93(1):61-68.

SECTION 5

# Gastroenterology and Hepatology

## Chapter 13

## ASCITES

### Case: A 54-year-old woman with shortness of breath

A 54-year-old woman with a remote history of Hodgkin's lymphoma treated with mantle-field radiation is admitted to the hospital with progressive shortness of breath over the past few months. She also describes an enlarging abdomen and bilateral lower extremity swelling. She has gained 20 pounds since these symptoms began. The patient is an avid bicyclist but has been forced to give it up in recent weeks because she can no longer keep up. The lymphoma has been in remission since treatment without evidence of recurrence. Social history is notable for the consumption of 1 to 2 glasses of wine with dinner on a nightly basis.

There is symmetric distention of the abdomen with bulging flanks and the presence of shifting dullness to percussion. There are tattoo marks on the anterior chest, consistent with prior radiation therapy. Neither palmar erythema nor spider angiomas are present. Jugular venous pressure (JVP) is estimated at 16 cm $H_2O$ and is noted to increase with inspiration. An extra heart sound after S2 is heard best with the diaphragm of the stethoscope over the apex and is recorded with a phonocardiograph machine (Figure 13-1). Lungs are clear to auscultation bilaterally.

Hematocrit is 32% and platelet count is 210 K/µL. Aspartate aminotransferase (AST) is 67 U/L, alanine aminotransferase (ALT) is 78 U/L, total bilirubin is 2.3 mg/dL, and international normalized ratio (INR) is 1.1. A diagnostic paracentesis is performed, and the ascitic albumin concentration is 2.5 g/dL with a total protein of 4.3 g/dL. Serum albumin is 3.8 g/dL.

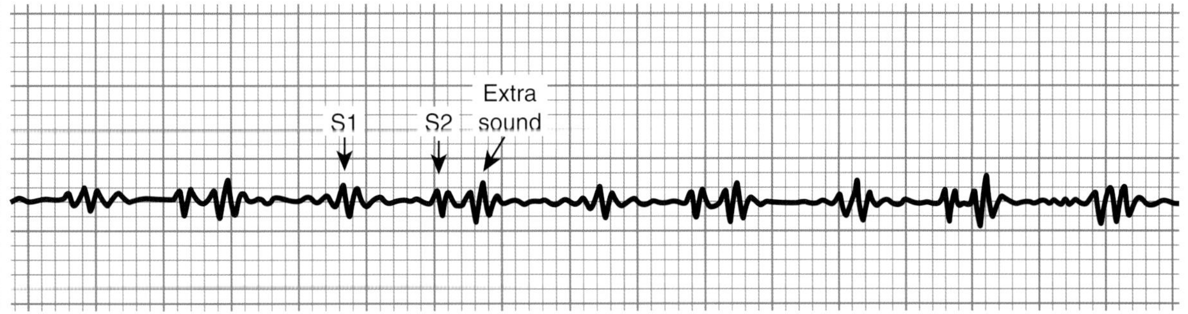


**Figure 13-1.**

***What is the most likely cause of ascites in this patient?***

**What is ascites?**

Ascites is the abnormal accumulation of fluid within the peritoneal cavity. Normally, the peritoneal cavity contains 25 to 50 mL of serous fluid, which allows the bowels to move around with less friction. Normal intraperitoneal pressure is 5 to 10 mm Hg.[1]

**What mechanisms maintain peritoneal fluid volume?**

The balance between fluid entering the peritoneal cavity from the mesenteric capillaries and fluid absorbed by the lymphatic system normally maintains a constant volume of peritoneal fluid. The maximum absorption capacity of the lymphatic system is 850 mL/d.[1]

**What are the symptoms of ascites?**

Symptoms of ascites depend on volume, rate of accumulation, and other factors but may include increased abdominal girth, abdominal fullness, abdominal discomfort, dyspnea, early satiety, and a sense of decreased mobility.[1]

**What physical findings are associated with ascites?**

Physical findings of ascites may include abdominal distention (usually symmetric), bulging flanks, shifting dullness to percussion, and the presence of a fluid wave.[1]

**What is the role of ultrasonography in the evaluation of ascites?**

Ultrasonography is a bedside imaging modality that is sensitive for detecting the presence of ascites ≥100 mL in volume. Simple ascites is anechoic and appears between the abdominal wall and loops of bowel (Figure 13-2).[1]

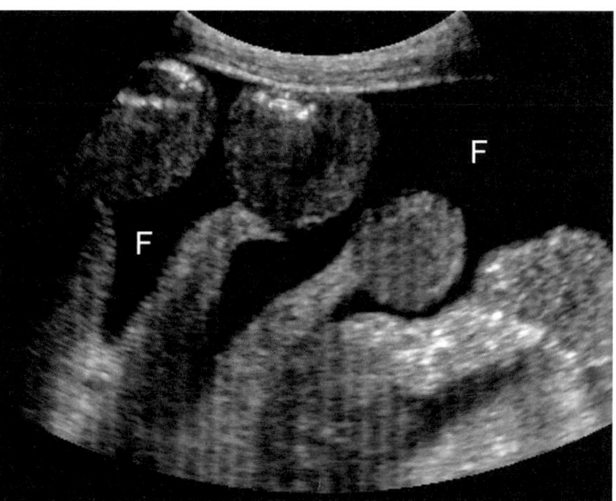


**Figure 13-2.** Abdominal ultrasound (sagittal view) demonstrating loops of bowel and mesentery floating freely within anechoic peritoneal fluid (F). (Courtesy of Philips Medical Systems, Bothell, WA.)

**How is the severity of ascites defined?**

Grade I ascites is ≥100 mL in volume; grade II ascites is ≥1000 mL; and grade III ascites describes a grossly distended abdomen, which indicates the presence of liters of fluid.[1]

**What are the 2 general categories of ascites?**

Ascites can be related to portal hypertension or unrelated to portal hypertension.

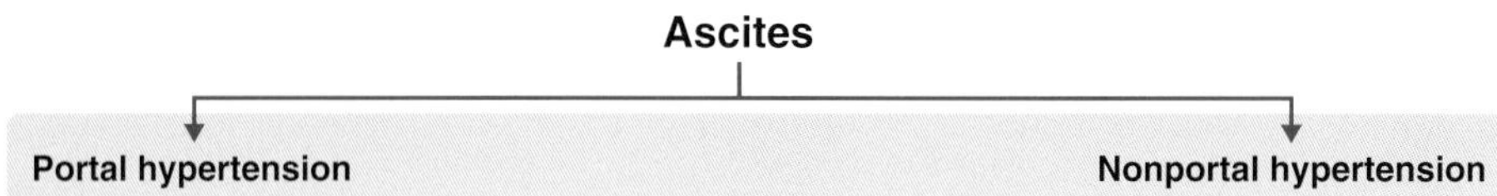


**Which laboratory result indicates whether ascites is caused by portal hypertension?**

A diagnostic paracentesis with calculation of the serum-ascites albumin gradient (SAAG) determines whether or not ascites is the result of portal hypertension. The SAAG is calculated by subtracting the concentration of albumin in ascitic fluid from the concentration of albumin in serum (each in g/dL). SAAG ≥1.1 (high gradient) indicates that the fluid is related to portal hypertension, whereas SAAG <1.1 (low gradient) indicates that the fluid is unrelated to portal hypertension.[2,3]

**What basic fluid characteristics can be helpful in the evaluation of ascites?**

Routine ascitic fluid evaluation includes gross appearance (eg, color, turbidity, viscosity), total and differential cell counts, total protein concentration, albumin concentration, Gram stain, and culture. Other tests are available and should be used in the appropriate settings (eg, cytology if there is a concern for malignancy).[4]

**What is the significance of the gross appearance of ascitic fluid?**

The gross appearance of ascitic fluid can help narrow the differential diagnosis. Uncomplicated ascites is typically clear and a pale straw-colored yellow. Hazy, cloudy, or bloody fluid is suggestive of infection. Frank blood indicates hemorrhagic ascites. Milky fluid suggests chylous ascites. Brown fluid can occur in patients with significantly elevated serum bilirubin. However, if the bilirubin concentration of ascitic fluid is greater than that of serum, a ruptured gallbladder or perforated duodenal ulcer should be suspected.[4-7]

**What is the significance of the differential cell count in evaluating ascitic fluid?**

The predominant cell type in ascitic fluid can help narrow the differential diagnosis. For example, a predominance of mononuclear leukocytes (ie, lymphocytes and monocytes) is suggestive of tuberculous ascites. Measurement of the cell count and differential is also necessary to make the diagnosis of spontaneous bacterial peritonitis (SBP), which is defined by the presence of an ascitic polymorphonucleocyte (PMN) count ≥250/µL with or without a positive culture.[4]

**What is the significance of the total protein concentration in ascitic fluid?**

In ascitic fluid, total protein concentration <1.0 g/dL is associated with a higher risk of developing SBP. Total protein concentration is also helpful for differentiating cirrhotic ascites (total protein <2.5 g/dL) from cardiac ascites and other causes of posthepatic portal hypertension (total protein ≥2.5 g/dL).[8,9]

**What is the significance of ascitic fluid glucose and lactate dehydrogenase (LDH) concentrations?**

Ascitic fluid glucose concentration tends to be similar to that of serum except in the setting of peritoneal infection or malignancy, where it is lower as a result of consumption. The LDH concentration of ascitic fluid tends to be higher in patients with infection or malignancy (ascites-to-serum LDH ratio of around 1.0) compared with that in cirrhotics (ascites-to-serum LDH radio of around 0.4).[4,10]

**What ascitic fluid findings are helpful in distinguishing spontaneous bacterial peritonitis from secondary bacterial peritonitis related to bowel perforation into preexisting ascites?**

Patients with ascites who develop bowel perforation often do not manifest the typical symptoms and signs of a surgical abdomen (eg, rigidity) because the ascitic fluid separates the surfaces of the visceral and parietal peritoneum. In patients with an ascitic fluid PMN count ≥250/µL, secondary bacterial peritonitis from bowel perforation into preexisting ascites is more likely than SBP when any 2 of the following 3 criteria are met: (1) ascitic fluid total protein >1 g/dL, (2) ascitic fluid glucose <50 mg/dL, and (3) ascitic fluid LDH >upper limit of normal for serum.[11,12]

**What is the significance of Gram stain and culture of ascitic fluid?**

Gram stain and culture of ascitic fluid should be included in any infectious workup. There is an increased diagnostic yield when culture bottles are inoculated at the bedside without delay. Special smears and cultures may be indicated based on other clinical data (eg, acid-fast smear if tuberculosis is suspected).[13]

**What is the significance of cytologic examination of ascitic fluid?**

Cytologic examination of ascitic fluid can establish a diagnosis of malignancy. Yield is variable and dependent on the type of cancer and the mechanism of ascites formation. Sensitivity approaches 100% for peritoneal carcinomatosis but is lower for other causes of malignancy-related ascites, such as liver metastases.[14,15]

## ASCITES RELATED TO PORTAL HYPERTENSION

**What is the fundamental mechanism of ascites related to portal hypertension?**

Portal hypertension leads to increased hydrostatic pressure within the portal capillaries, which favors the movement of fluid out of the capillaries and into the peritoneum.

**What is the gold standard for diagnosing portal hypertension?**

SAAG ≥1.1 is highly suggestive of portal hypertension. The diagnosis can be confirmed by measuring the hepatic venous pressure gradient (HVPG), which is the difference between wedged hepatic venous pressure (an approximation of portal venous pressure) and free hepatic venous pressure (an approximation of inferior vena cava pressure). A normal HVPG is 3 to 5 mm Hg. Portal hypertension is defined by an HVPG ≥6 mm Hg. Clinically significant portal hypertension occurs when the HVPG is ≥10 to 12 mm Hg. *In cases of posthepatic portal hypertension (eg, heart failure), there is a comparable increase in free hepatic venous pressure and wedged hepatic venous pressure such that the HVPG is not elevated.*[16-18]

**What are the clinical sequelae of portal hypertension?**

Portal hypertension can cause splenomegaly with hypersplenism (leading to anemia and thrombocytopenia), portosystemic collaterals, esophageal and gastric varices, ascites, and hepatocellular carcinoma.[17,18]

**What are the anatomic subcategories of portal hypertension?**

Portal hypertension can be prehepatic, hepatic, or posthepatic.

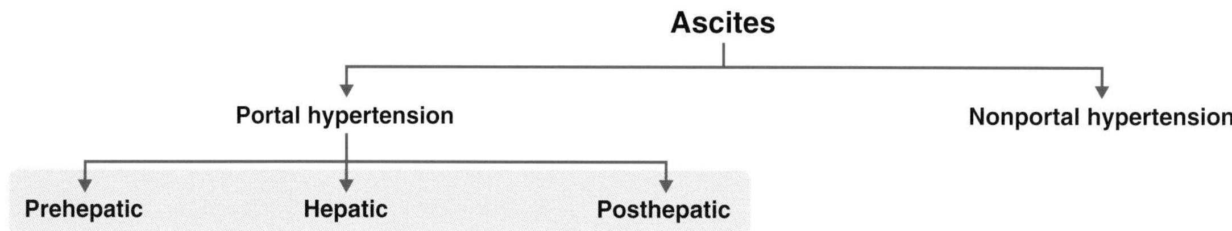


*In this framework, the term prehepatic refers to circulation of the portal side of the liver, while posthepatic refers to circulation of the systemic side.*

## PREHEPATIC PORTAL HYPERTENSION

### What are the prehepatic causes of portal hypertension?

**Intraluminal vascular obstruction.**

Portal vein thrombosis (PVT) and splenic vein thrombosis.

**Obstruction of the portal system originating outside the vessel walls.**

Extrinsic compression of the portal system.

**Listen for a bruit.**

Splanchnic arteriovenous fistula.

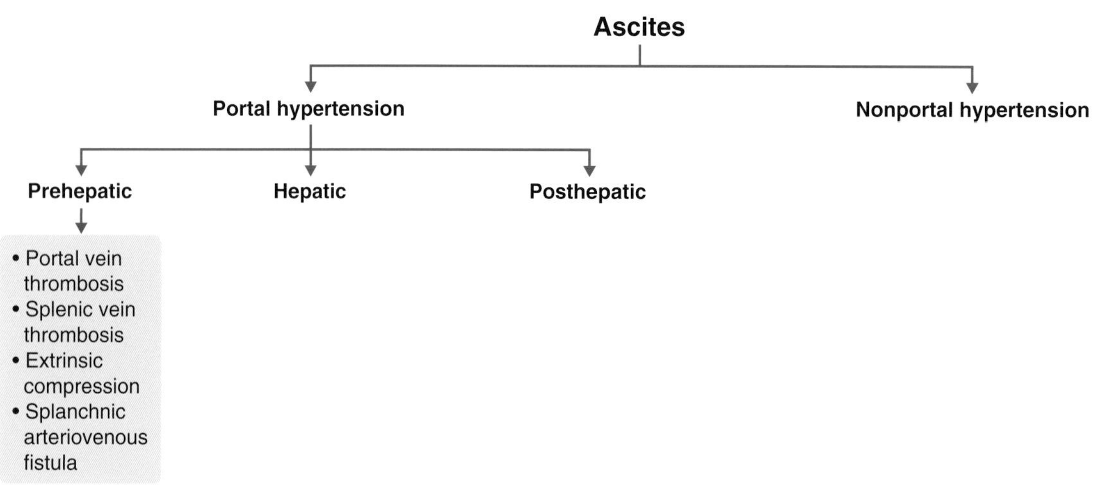

**What are the characteristics of portal vein thrombosis?**

Cirrhosis is a significant predisposing factor for PVT; risk increases with disease severity and in those with concomitant hepatocellular carcinoma. PVT also occurs in noncirrhotic patients; often in association with one or more of Virchow's triad: underlying thrombophilia (eg, primary myeloproliferative disorder), endothelial injury (eg, abdominal trauma), and reduced portal blood flow (eg, external compression by a mass). PVT may be acute or chronic, the latter of which can lead to portosystemic collateral circulation that is visible on imaging. The most common manifestations of acute PVT include abdominal pain, fever, ascites, and variceal bleeding (in patients with coexistent cirrhosis). Chronic PVT is frequently asymptomatic, and the diagnosis is often made incidentally on abdominal imaging. When symptomatic, the most common clinical manifestations of chronic PVT are related to portal hypertension and include variceal bleeding, splenomegaly, anemia, and thrombocytopenia. Intestinal ischemia can be a major complication of both acute and chronic PVT. The initial diagnostic study of choice for acute or chronic PVT is Doppler ultrasonography. Anticoagulation is the cornerstone of medical therapy for patients with acute PVT, and some patients with chronic PVT.[19]

**What condition is most frequently associated with splenic vein thrombosis?**

Chronic pancreatitis is the most common cause of splenic vein thrombosis, accounting for more than one-half of all cases. Splenic vein thrombosis is associated with gastric and esophageal varices. Patients may be asymptomatic. Gastrointestinal bleeding and splenomegaly are the most common clinical manifestations. Splenectomy is indicated in symptomatic patients.[20]

**What are potential causes of external compression of the portal vein?**

Portal hypertension can develop as a result of external compression (or invasion) of the portal vein related to tumor (benign or malignant), bulky lymphadenopathy, or hematoma. There may be a role for portal stent placement in some cases.[21]

**What are the causes of splanchnic arteriovenous fistula?**

Splanchnic arteriovenous fistulae are rare. They are most often acquired as a result of abdominal trauma or spontaneous rupture of splenic artery aneurysms, the latter of which occurs with higher frequency in pregnant women. The increase in portal blood flow related to the shunt leads to a sudden increase in portal pressures.[22,23]

## HEPATIC PORTAL HYPERTENSION

### What are the hepatic causes of portal hypertension?

**The most common cause of portal hypertension worldwide.**

Cirrhosis.[17]

**A parasitic infection.**

Schistosomiasis.

**A patient with chronic hepatitis B infection is found to have several hepatic masses that enhance during the late arterial phase and washout in the delayed phases of a contrast-enhanced computed tomography imaging study.**

Hepatocellular carcinoma.

**A 38-year-old woman with a history of depression complicated by previous suicide attempts presents with marked aminotransferase elevation, elevated INR, delirium, and ascites.**

Acute (fulminant) liver failure likely from overdose with acetaminophen (or other toxin).

**A 40-year-old woman presents with pruritis and is found to have mild cholestatic liver injury and positive serum antimitochondrial antibodies.**

Primary biliary cholangitis (PBC).

**Associated with ulcerative colitis.**

Primary sclerosing cholangitis (PSC).

**Despite a complete workup, the cause of portal hypertension cannot be identified.**

Idiopathic noncirrhotic portal hypertension (ie, nodular regenerative hyperplasia).

**A 58-year-old woman develops hepatomegaly, jaundice, and ascites 12 days after undergoing allogeneic hematopoietic stem cell transplantation for acute myeloid leukemia.**

Sinusoidal obstruction syndrome (SOS).

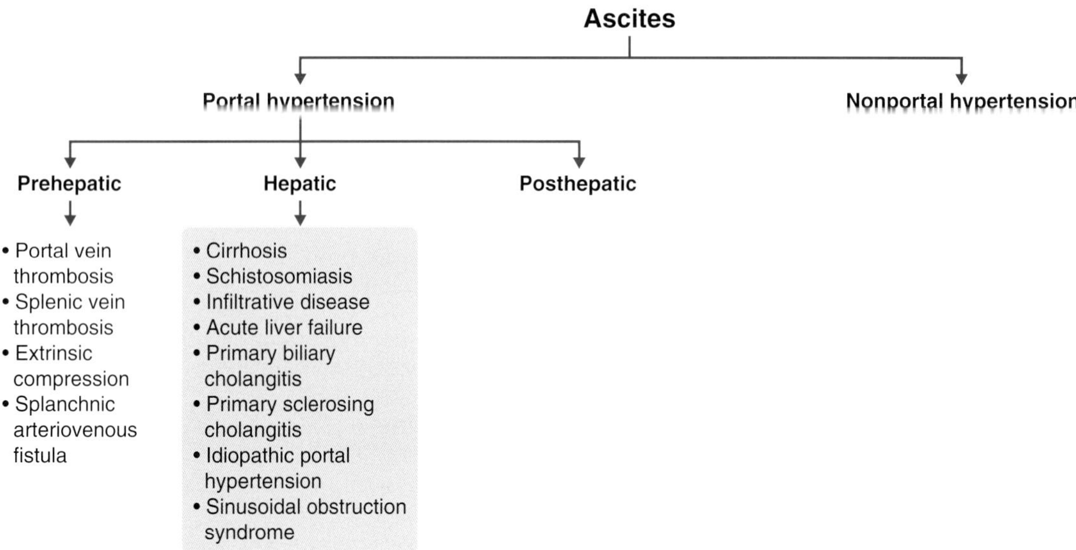


**How common is ascites in patients with cirrhosis?**

Ascites is a frequent complication of cirrhosis, developing in up to one-half of patients within 10 years of diagnosis. Ascites develops predominantly as a result of portal hypertension, but there are other contributing factors, such as decreased capillary oncotic pressure and sodium and fluid retention (Figure 13-3). SBP is a common complication of cirrhotic ascites and should be considered in patients with compatible clinical features such as abdominal pain, fever, delirium, and peripheral leukocytosis.[4]

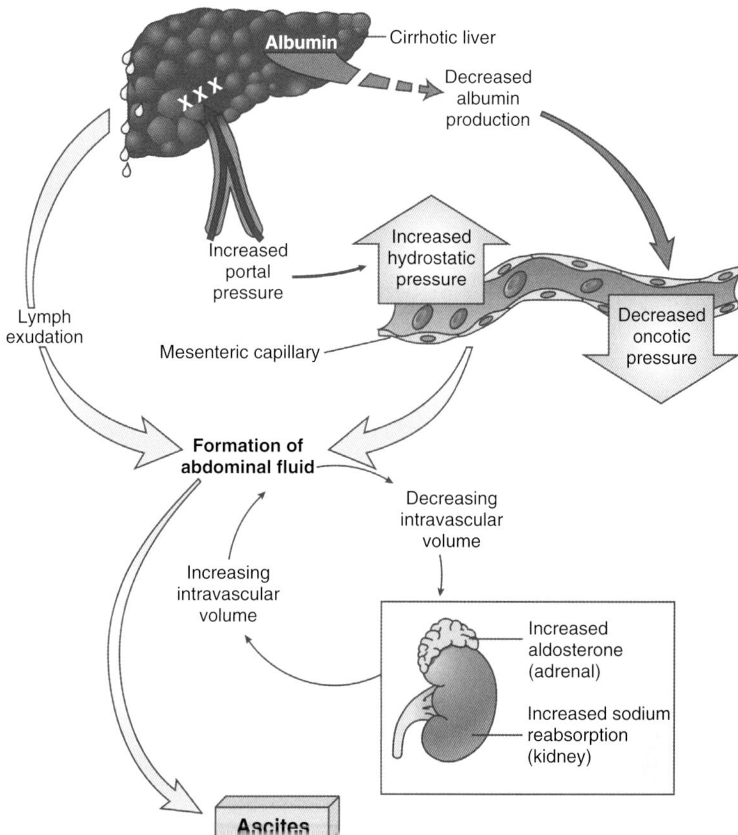


**Figure 13-3.** Mechanisms of ascites formation in cirrhosis. (From Rubin E, Farber JL. *Pathology*. 3rd ed. Philadelphia, PA: Lippincott Williams & Wilkins; 1999.)

**What are the characteristics of portal hypertension caused by schistosomiasis?**

Schistosomiasis is endemic to Asia, Africa, and South America. It is the second most common cause of portal hypertension worldwide. The preservation of hepatic function helps to distinguish schistosomiasis from cirrhosis. Schistosomal ova become lodged in the periportal space, triggering an immune-mediated response that leads to hepatic fibrosis, portal hypertension, and splenomegaly, which are the dominant features of the disease. The diagnosis can be made with identification of schistosomal ova in stool. Praziquantel is the treatment of choice for chronic schistosomiasis. Liver damage is at least partially reversible with treatment in the early stages of the disease.[17,21]

**In addition to hepatocellular carcinoma, what other infiltrative conditions can cause portal hypertension?**

Liver metastases, lymphoma, sarcoidosis, amyloidosis, myelofibrosis, mastocytosis, and Gaucher disease are some of the infiltrative causes of portal hypertension. These conditions can lead to cirrhosis but are also capable of causing portal hypertension independently.[17]

**How common is ascites in patients with acute liver failure?**

Acute liver failure is characterized by signs of advanced liver disease (eg, synthetic dysfunction) and encephalopathy over a course of days to months, most often occurring in patients without preexisting liver disease. Portal hypertension is present in the vast majority of patients, and ascites develops in over one-half. Kidney injury is common in these patients, most often related to acute tubular necrosis or hemodynamic changes similar to the hepatorenal syndrome.[25]

**What is primary billiary cholangitis?**

PBC is an autoimmune disease characterized by progressive destruction of intrahepatic bile ducts, which can lead to cholestasis, portal inflammation, and fibrosis. It most frequently occurs in women in the fourth and fifth decades of life. If untreated, PBC may progress to cirrhosis. However, patients may develop portal hypertension with ascites and esophageal varices before progressing to cirrhosis. The mainstay of treatment for PBC is ursodeoxycholic acid.[26]

**What is primary sclerosing cholangitis?**

PSC is an idiopathic chronic disease that results in fibrosis and strictures of the intrahepatic and/or extrahepatic biliary tract, with associated cholestatic liver injury. PSC is frequently associated with inflammatory bowel disease (ulcerative colitis in particular) and, in this population, most often affects men in the fourth and fifth decades of life. The diagnostic test of choice is magnetic resonance cholangiopancreatography (MRCP). PSC is generally a progressive disease that leads to cirrhosis. A minority of patients will develop portal hypertension without cirrhosis.[27]

**What is idiopathic noncirrhotic portal hypertension?**

Idiopathic noncirrhotic portal hypertension has been referred to by a variety of names, including nodular regenerative hyperplasia, idiopathic portal hypertension, and hepatoportal sclerosis. The etiology is unknown, but it is associated with various conditions including infections, medications or toxins, and thrombophilia. Diagnosis is based on the identification of portal hypertension in patients without cirrhosis or other causes of noncirrhotic portal hypertension (eg, portal vein thrombosis). The appearance of the liver is indistinguishable from cirrhosis on imaging; histology is often necessary to make the distinction. Compared with cirrhotics, prognosis is more favorable because there is preservation of hepatic function. However, these patients can still develop severe sequelae of portal hypertension, including variceal bleeding.[28]

**What is sinusoidal obstruction syndrome?**

SOS is a disease that occurs after hematopoietic stem cell transplantation, usually within 30 days. SOS develops when the conditioning regimen results in sinusoidal endothelial cell damage. Severity and clinical course are variable, with some cases being self-limited and others resulting in multiorgan failure and death.[29]

## POSTHEPATIC PORTAL HYPERTENSION

### What are the posthepatic causes of portal hypertension?

**An S3 gallop heard over the left lower sternal border.**

Right-sided heart failure.

**A 42-year-old woman with a history of systemic lupus erythematosus complicated by recurrent bouts of acute pericarditis presents with dyspnea and is found to have elevated JVP, Kussmaul's sign (inspiratory increase in JVP), and ascites.**

Constrictive pericarditis.

**Vascular structures.**

Thrombosis of the hepatic vein (Budd-Chiari syndrome) and obstruction of the inferior vena cava (IVC).

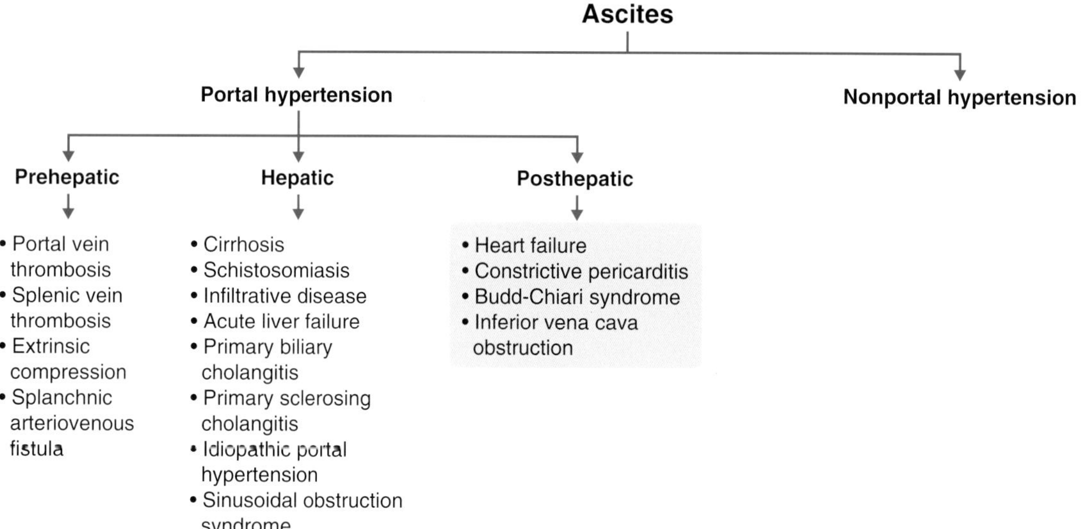


**Which cause of right-sided heart failure often presents with a pulsatile liver?**

Congestive hepatopathy and portal hypertension can develop in patients with right-sided heart failure from various causes, including cor pulmonale, valvular disease, ischemic disease, and cardiomyopathy. Severe tricuspid regurgitation results in retrograde blood flow from the right ventricle to the right atrium, which is transmitted to the venous system, producing characteristic physical findings. Lancisi's sign (CV fusion wave) can be visualized in the jugular venous waveform in the neck, and a pulsatile liver can be palpated in the abdomen. *For a video of Lancisi's sign, see the associated reference.*[30]

**How common is ascites in patients with constrictive pericarditis?**

Ascites occurs in almost one-half of patients with constrictive pericarditis. The most common physical finding in these patients is elevated JVP, which serves as an important clue that ascites may be primarily driven by cardiac disease rather than liver disease.[31]

**What classic triad of clinical manifestations is associated with Budd-Chiari syndrome?**

Acute Budd-Chiari syndrome classically presents with abdominal pain, ascites, and hepatomegaly. Chronic Budd-Chiari syndrome is often asymptomatic but can be associated with the sequelae of portal hypertension. Most cases are associated with underlying thrombophilia, usually a primary myeloproliferative disorder (eg, polycythemia vera). Doppler ultrasonography of the liver is the initial diagnostic test of choice. Without treatment, Budd-Chiari syndrome is associated with poor prognosis. Anticoagulation is the cornerstone of treatment and significantly improves survival rates.[32]

**What are the causes of inferior vena cava obstruction?**

IVC obstruction can occur as a result of thrombosis related to underlying thrombophilia, extrinsic compression by tumor, infective phlebitis, and regional inflammation from trauma or surgery. It may be acute or chronic. Abdominal pain, ascites, and lower extremity edema are typical clinical manifestations. Chronic cases are more insidious due to the development of collateral circulation. Doppler ultrasonography is the initial diagnostic test of choice. Treatment depends on the underlying cause but includes anticoagulation, procedures such as balloon dilation and stenting, and surgery.[33]

## ASCITES UNRELATED TO PORTAL HYPERTENSION

**When portal hypertension is absent, what are the 2 main types of ascitic fluid produced?**

Ascitic fluid unrelated to portal hypertension can be protein-poor (total protein generally <2.5 g/dL) or protein-rich (total protein generally ≥2.5 g/dL). *Ascitic fluid should not be categorized as protein-poor or protein-rich before first determining that it is unrelated to portal hypertension based on the SAAG.*[34]

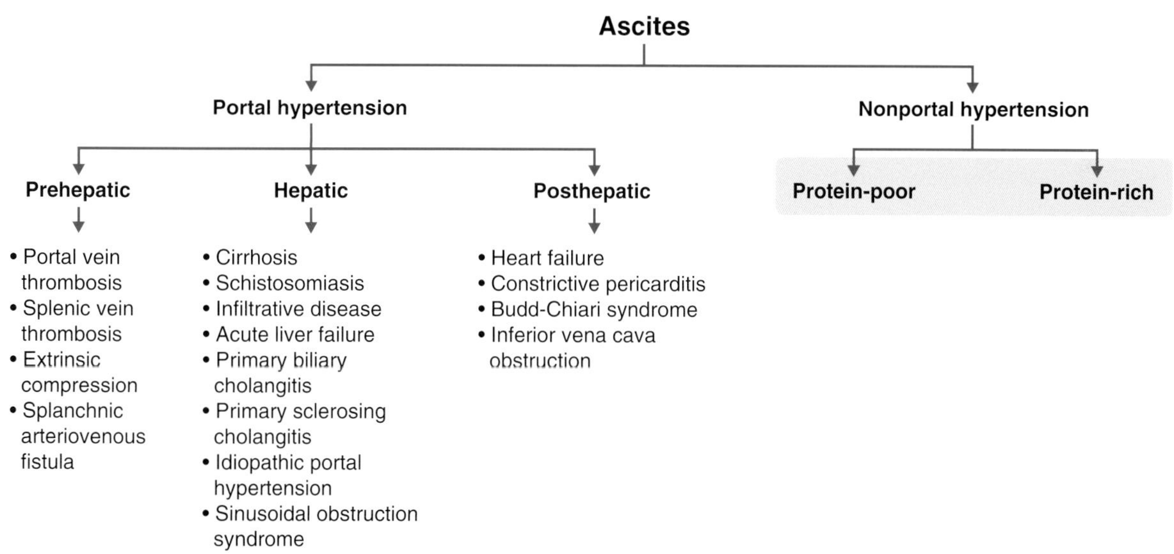


## PROTEIN-POOR ASCITES UNRELATED TO PORTAL HYPERTENSION

**What fundamental mechanism underlies the development of protein-poor ascites unrelated to portal hypertension?**

Decreased oncotic pressure within the portal capillaries favors the movement of protein-poor fluid out of the capillaries and into the peritoneum.

**What is the principal contributor to capillary oncotic pressure?**

Large nonfiltered proteins, primarily albumin, contribute the bulk of capillary oncotic pressure.[35]

### What are the causes of ascites related to low capillary oncotic pressure?

**Foamy urine.**

Nephrotic syndrome.

**An impoverished child with a protuberant abdomen.**

Protein-calorie malnutrition.

**Increased fecal α-1 antitrypsin clearance.**

Protein-losing enteropathy.

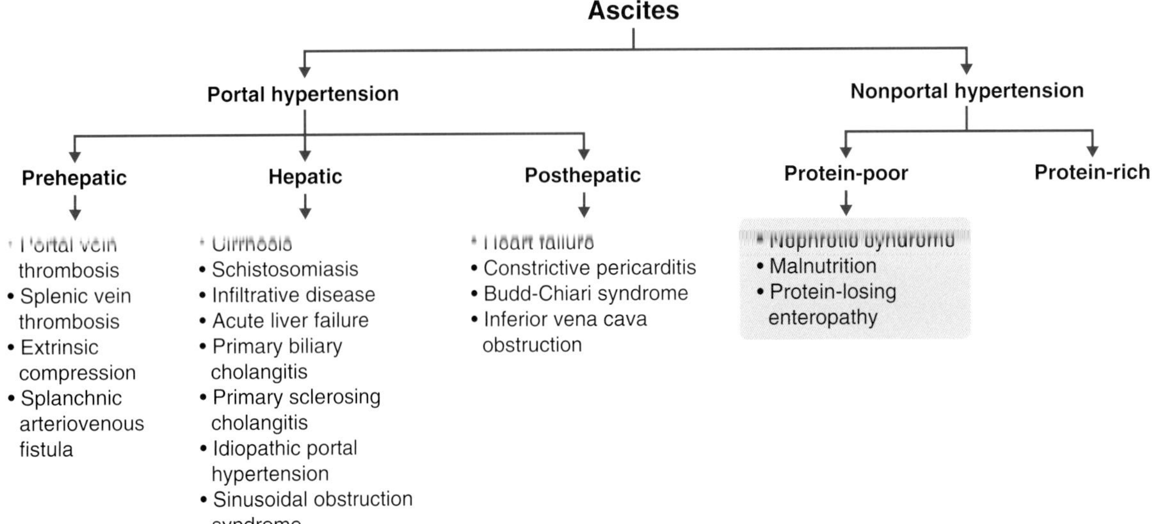


**What are the general treatment strategies for ascites related to nephrotic syndrome?**

In addition to addressing the underlying disease, patients with ascites caused by nephrotic syndrome tend to respond to salt restriction and diuretics. This is in contrast to most other causes of ascites unrelated to portal hypertension, in which salt restriction and diuretics have unpredictable results.[36]

**What pediatric condition is associated with severe protein-calorie malnutrition and protuberant abdomen?**

Severe protein-calorie malnutrition can result in kwashiorkor, a condition with clinical manifestations such as lethargy, dermatitis, thinning hair, protuberant abdomen, and lower extremity edema (Figure 13-4). Abdominal distention in these patients is primarily related to hepatomegaly from fatty infiltration, with or without ascites. Severe protein-calorie malnutrition is common in patients with cirrhosis, where it contributes to morbidity and mortality, including the development of refractory ascites.[37,38]

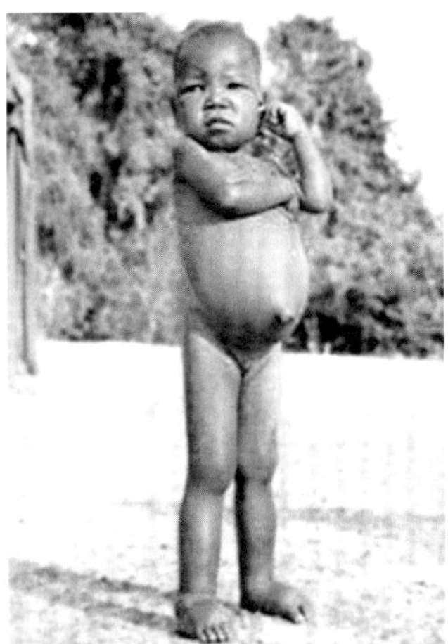

**Figure 13-4.** A child with kwashiorkor. Notice the thinning hair, protuberant abdomen, and lower extremity edema. (From Ferrier DR. *Lippincott's Illustrated Reviews: Biochemistry*. 6th ed. Philadelphia, PA: Lippincott Williams & Wilkins; 2014.)

**What is protein-losing enteropathy?**

Protein-losing enteropathy is a rare condition that develops when protein is lost in the gastrointestinal tract, resulting in hypoalbuminemia, which leads to peripheral edema, ascites, and pleural and pericardial effusions. It can be caused by a variety of conditions, most commonly cardiac (eg, after the Fontan procedure for congenital single ventricle) or gastrointestinal (eg, inflammatory bowel disease) in nature. The initial diagnostic test of choice is measurement of fecal clearance of α-1 antitrypsin, which is elevated in patients with protein-losing enteropathy. Treatment for this condition is aimed at the underlying cause, but a high protein diet is generally recommended.[39]

*Cirrhosis can contribute to low capillary oncotic pressure (see Figure 13-3). However, despite the mixed nature of the fluid, it is typically associated with elevated SAAG and is therefore classified as a cause of ascites related to portal hypertension.*[34]

## PROTEIN-RICH ASCITES UNRELATED TO PORTAL HYPERTENSION

**What mechanisms underlie the development of protein-rich ascites unrelated to portal hypertension?**

When portal hypertension is absent, protein-rich ascites develops via one or more of the following mechanisms: increased capillary permeability, increased fluid production, and impaired fluid reabsorption from lymphatic obstruction.

### What are the causes of protein-rich ascites unrelated to portal hypertension?

**May be discovered on cytologic analysis of peritoneal fluid.**

Intraperitoneal malignancy.

**Alcohol and gallstones account for most cases.**

Pancreatitis.

**An infection that most often involves the upper lobes of the lungs (see Figure 31-3).**

Tuberculosis.

**A 49-year-old man with cirrhosis develops hypotension and an acute drop in hematocrit after a paracentesis procedure.**

Hemoperitoneum.

**Milky ascites.**

Chylous ascites.

**A 44-year-old woman presents with weight gain, constipation, and cold intolerance.**

Myxedema.

**Peritoneal signs are present on abdominal examination.**

Perforated viscus.

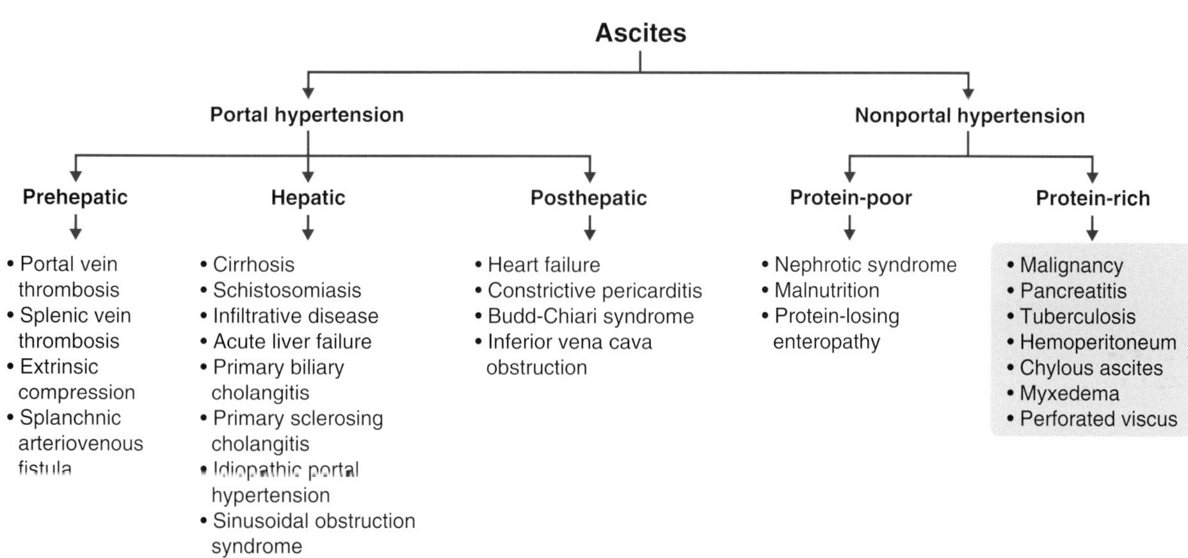


**What are the characteristics of malignant ascites?**

Malignant ascites is indicative of peritoneal carcinomatosis: the presence of malignant cells in the peritoneal cavity. It accounts for about 10% of all cases of ascites and is most commonly associated with lymphoma, peritoneal mesothelioma, and ovarian, uterine, colorectal, pancreatic, lung, and breast cancers. Several mechanisms are responsible for malignant ascites related to peritoneal carcinomatosis, including altered capillary permeability and lymphatic obstruction, both of which contribute to the accumulation of peritoneal exudate. Prognosis is poor, with most patients surviving only weeks to months after the diagnosis is made. Malignancy, particularly lymphoma, is a common cause of chylous ascites, resulting from lymphatic infiltration and obstruction. *When malignancy-related ascites occurs as a result of massive liver metastases, it is often protein-poor and associated with a high gradient (SAAG ≥1.1).*[4,15,40]

**What is pancreatic ascites?**

Pancreatic ascites is an uncommon complication of pancreatic disease that refers to the accumulation of pancreatic fluid within the peritoneal cavity as a result of pancreatic ductal disruption or pseudocyst leakage. It most commonly occurs in men with alcohol-related chronic pancreatitis who are between 20 and 50 years of age, but can also occur as a result of abdominal trauma or ampullary stenosis. Ascitic fluid is protein-rich (typically >3 g/dL) with elevated amylase (typically >1000 U/L). Conservative management includes bowel rest, somatostatin analogues, and large-volume paracentesis, repeated as necessary. In some patients, more invasive options may be necessary, including pancreatic duct stent placement and surgery.[41]

**What diagnostic studies are available for peritoneal tuberculosis?**

Peritoneal tuberculosis is typically associated with a primary site of tuberculosis elsewhere in the body, most commonly the lungs. However, only one-third of patients with peritoneal tuberculosis have clinical or radiographic evidence of pulmonary disease. Ascitic fluid is protein-rich (typically >3 g/dL) with an elevated total cell count with a lymphocytic predominance (>70%). Acid-fast bacilli smear is positive in <3% of cases; culture yield is higher, but results can take weeks to return. Ascitic fluid adenosine deaminase levels are useful; however, false negatives occur in patients with concurrent HIV infection or cirrhosis, and false positives occur in malignant ascites. Ascitic fluid polymerase chain reaction for *Mycobacterium tuberculosis* has been shown to be highly sensitive and specific. Laparoscopy may reveal characteristic macroscopic findings (eg, thickened peritoneum with tubercles), and peritoneal biopsy yields a histologic diagnosis in most cases.[42-44]

**What is chylous ascites?**

Chylous ascites describes the presence of thoracic or intestinal lymphatic fluid within the peritoneal cavity that occurs as a result of disruption to the lymphatic system, usually from trauma or obstruction. Chylous ascites has a creamy or milky appearance and is rich in triglycerides (>200 mg/dL). A wide range of conditions can result in chylous ascites, including cirrhosis, malignancy (particularly lymphoma), infection, and trauma. In the industrialized world, cirrhosis and malignancy account for the majority of cases; in the rest of the world, tuberculosis and filariasis are more common.[45]

**What are the causes of hemoperitoneum?**

In the general population, hemoperitoneum most commonly occurs as a result of abdominal trauma or nonmalignant gynecologic conditions. In patients with preexisting ascites, hemorrhagic ascites is defined by an RBC count >50,000/μL (hematocrit 0.5%). It most often develops spontaneously or secondary to iatrogenic abdominal trauma from diagnostic or therapeutic procedures. Spontaneous hemorrhagic ascites in cirrhotics usually develops insidiously without hemodynamic instability or clinical evidence of bleeding. However, acute and massive hemoperitoneum (with hematocrit values that approach 40%) can occur with rupture of hepatocellular carcinoma or an intra-abdominal varix, requiring prompt surgical management. Abdominal trauma (eg, injury to the inferior epigastric artery during paracentesis) can also result in acute and massive hemoperitoneum.[5]

**How common is myxedema ascites?**

Ascites is a rare complication of hypothyroidism; however, hypothyroidism is a common condition. Myxedema ascites is thought to develop as a result of increased capillary permeability. The fluid is virtually always protein-rich (typically ≥2.5 g/dL). However, the SAAG is sometimes unexpectedly increased (≥1.1) despite the absence of portal hypertension. Myxedema ascites resolves with thyroid replacement therapy.[46,47]

What are the characteristics of ascites caused by viscus perforation?

In addition to causing secondary peritonitis in patients with preexisting ascites, viscus perforation can cause de novo ascites. Fluid is usually blood-tinged with an elevated white blood cell count. The combination of a PMN count ≥250/μL and a polymicrobial Gram stain or culture is suggestive of bowel perforation (SBP is polymicrobial in only 10% of cases). The combination of a PMN count <250/μL and a polymicrobial Gram stain or culture (ie, polymicrobial bacterascites) is suggestive of a traumatic paracentesis during which the needle entered the bowel.[48,49]

## Case Summary

A 54-year-old woman with a remote history of Hodgkin's lymphoma treated with mediastinal radiation presents with dyspnea and is found to have ascites, elevated JVP, and the presence of an extra heart sound.

***What is the most likely cause of ascites in this patient?***

Constrictive pericarditis.

### BONUS QUESTIONS

***Which clinical features in this case make cirrhosis less likely than constrictive pericarditis?***

Cirrhosis is the most common cause of ascites, and the patient in this case does consume significant amounts of alcohol. However, the elevated JVP is suggestive of right-sided heart failure or constrictive pericarditis. Hepatic fibrosis may develop during the later stages of congestive hepatopathy (known as "cardiac cirrhosis"). However, the preservation of hepatic synthetic function and the absence of characteristic physical findings (eg, spider angiomas) suggest that advanced liver disease is not present.[50]

***What are the significant characteristics of the ascitic fluid in this case?***

The ascitic fluid in this case is associated with a high gradient (SAAG ≥1.1), indicating that it is related to portal hypertension. In this setting, elevated ascitic fluid total protein ≥2.5 g/dL is suggestive of cardiac ascites, which can be related to right-sided heart failure or constrictive pericarditis, or other post-hepatic causes of portal hypertension (eg, Budd-Chiari syndrome).[9]

***What is the most likely cause of constrictive pericarditis in this case?***

As part of the treatment for Hodgkin's lymphoma, the patient in this case received external beam radiation therapy to the mediastinum, which can result in constrictive pericarditis, often many years after treatment. When the history is unavailable or unreliable, the presence of tattoo markers on the skin can be a helpful clue to previous external beam radiation therapy.

***What is the most likely source of the extra heart sound in this case?***

Extra heart sounds that occur near S2 include split S2, S3 gallop, opening snap, and pericardial knock. The extra sound in this case (see Figure 13-1) is most likely a pericardial knock, based on location, pitch, and clinical history. The pericardial knock is thought to arise from the abrupt cessation of early diastolic ventricular filling because of noncompliant pericardium. It tends to occur earlier than the S3 gallop and is higher in pitch.[51]

***What is the significance of the change in jugular venous pressure with inspiration in this case?***

Paradoxical rise in JVP with inspiration, known as Kussmaul's sign, is suggestive of impaired filling of the right ventricle. It is a common finding in patients with constrictive pericarditis. *For a video of Kussmaul's sign, see the associated reference.*[52]

***What additional diagnostic studies can help confirm the diagnosis in this case?***

In patients with constrictive pericarditis, cardiac computed tomography or magnetic resonance imaging may reveal pericardial thickening and calcification. Hemodynamic assessment with right and left cardiac catheterization may demonstrate characteristic findings of constriction, including abrupt and rapid early diastolic filling, elevated and equal end-diastolic pressures in all 4 chambers, and discordance between the peak inspiratory pressures of the right ventricle compared with the left.[50]

***What options are available to treat ascites related to constrictive pericarditis?***

Conservative management of ascites related to constrictive pericarditis includes dietary restriction, diuretic medication, and large-volume paracentesis, which can be repeated as necessary. Surgical pericardiectomy is the only definitive treatment for constrictive pericarditis.[50]

## KEY POINTS

- Ascites is the abnormal accumulation of fluid within the peritoneal cavity.
- Symptoms of ascites include increased abdominal girth, abdominal fullness, abdominal discomfort, dyspnea, early satiety, and a sense of decreased mobility.
- Physical findings of ascites include abdominal distention, bulging flanks, shifting dullness to percussion, and the presence of a fluid wave.
- Ascites can be related to portal hypertension (SAAG ≥1.1) or unrelated to portal hypertension (SAAG <1.1).
- Portal hypertension can be prehepatic, hepatic, or posthepatic.
- Ascites unrelated to portal hypertension can be protein-poor or protein-rich.
- Ascitic fluid analysis, including gross appearance, cell count and differential, total protein, Gram stain and culture, cytology, and other ancillary tests, can be helpful in determining the etiology of ascites.
- In addition to addressing the underlying cause, management of ascites includes salt restriction, diuretics, and large-volume paracentesis.

## REFERENCES


1. Moore CM, Van Thiel DH. Cirrhotic ascites review: pathophysiology, diagnosis and management. *World J Hepatol*. 2013;5(5):251-263.
2. Pare P, Talbot J, Hoefs JC. Serum-ascites albumin concentration gradient: a physiologic approach to the differential diagnosis of ascites. *Gastroenterology*. 1983;85(2):240-244.
3. Runyon BA, Montano AA, Akriviadis EA, Antillon MR, Irving MA, McHutchison JG. The serum-ascites albumin gradient is superior to the exudate-transudate concept in the differential diagnosis of ascites. *Ann Intern Med*. 1992;117(3):215-220.
4. Huang LL, Xia HH, Zhu SL. Ascitic fluid analysis in the differential diagnosis of ascites: focus on cirrhotic ascites. *J Clin Transl Hepatol*. 2014;2(1):58-64.
5. Akriviadis EA. Hemoperitoneum in patients with ascites. *Am J Gastroenterol*. 1997;92(4):567-575.
6. Chinnock B, Hendey GW. Can clear ascitic fluid appearance rule out spontaneous bacterial peritonitis? *Am J Emerg Med*. 2007;25(8):934-937.
7. Runyon BA. Ascitic fluid bilirubin concentration as a key to choleperitoneum. *J Clin Gastroenterol*. 1987;9(5):543-545.
8. Runyon BA. Low-protein-concentration ascitic fluid is predisposed to spontaneous bacterial peritonitis. *Gastroenterology*. 1986;91(6):1343-1346.
9. Runyon BA. Cardiac ascites: a characterization. *J Clin Gastroenterol*. 1988;10(4):410-412.
10. Runyon BA, Hoefs JC. Ascitic fluid chemical analysis before, during and after spontaneous bacterial peritonitis. *Hepatology*. 1985;5(2):257-259.
11. Akriviadis EA, Runyon BA. Utility of an algorithm in differentiating spontaneous from secondary bacterial peritonitis. *Gastroenterology*. 1990;98(1):127-133.
12. Runyon BA, Hoefs JC. Ascitic fluid analysis in the differentiation of spontaneous bacterial peritonitis from gastrointestinal tract perforation into ascitic fluid. *Hepatology*. 1984;4(3):447-450.
13. Runyon BA, Antillon MR, Akriviadis EA, McHutchison JG. Bedside inoculation of blood culture bottles with ascitic fluid is superior to delayed inoculation in the detection of spontaneous bacterial peritonitis. *J Clin Microbiol*. 1990;28(12):2811-2812.
14. DiBonito L, Falconieri G, Colautti I, Bonifacio D, Dudine S. The positive peritoneal effusion. A retrospective study of cytopathologic diagnoses with autopsy confirmation. *Acta Cytol*. 1993;37(4):483-488.
15. Runyon BA, Hoefs JC, Morgan TR. Ascitic fluid analysis in malignancy-related ascites. *Hepatology*. 1988;8(5):1104-1109.
16. Pinzani M, Rosselli M, Zuckermann M. Liver cirrhosis. *Best Pract Res Clin Gastroenterol*. 2011;25(2):281-290.
17. Berzigotti A, Seijo S, Reverter E, Bosch J. Assessing portal hypertension in liver diseases. *Expert Rev Gastroenterol Hepatol*. 2013;7(2):141-155.
18. Bari K, Garcia-Tsao G. Treatment of portal hypertension. *World J Gastroenterol*. 2012;18(11):1166-1175.
19. Chawla YK, Bodh V. Portal vein thrombosis. *J Clin Exp Hepatol*. 2015;5(1):22-40.
20. Sakorafas GH, Sarr MG, Farley DR, Farnell MB. The significance of sinistral portal hypertension complicating chronic pancreatitis. *Am J Surg*. 2000;179(2):129-133.
21. Sakurai K, Amano R, Yamamoto A, et al. Portal vein stenting to treat portal vein stenosis in a patient with malignant tumor and gastrointestinal bleeding. *Int Surg*. 2014;99(1):91-95.
22. Johnston GW, Gibson JB. Portal hypertension resulting from splenic arteriovenous fistulae. *Gut*. 1965;6(5):500-502.
23. Siablis D, Papathanassiou ZG, Karnabatidis D, Christeas N, Katsanos K, Vagianos C. Splenic arteriovenous fistula and sudden onset of portal hypertension as complications of a ruptured splenic artery aneurysm: successful treatment with transcatheter arterial embolization. A case study and review of the literature. *World J Gastroenterol*. 2006;12(26):4264-4266.
24. Elbaz T, Esmat G. Hepatic and intestinal schistosomiasis: review. *J Adv Res*. 2013;4(5):445-452.
25. Navasa M, Garcia-Pagan JC, Bosch J, et al. Portal hypertension in acute liver failure. *Gut*. 1992;33(7):965-968.
26. Selmi C, Bowlus CL, Gershwin ME, Coppel RL. Primary biliary cirrhosis. *Lancet*. 2011;377(9777):1600-1609.
27. Lindor KD, Kowdley KV, Harrison ME, American College of Gastroenterology. ACG Clinical Guideline: primary sclerosing cholangitis. *Am J Gastroenterol*. 2015;110(5):646-659; quiz 60.

28. Schouten JN, Garcia-Pagan JC, Valla DC, Janssen HL. Idiopathic noncirrhotic portal hypertension. *Hepatology*. 2011;54(3):1071-1081.
29. Mohty M, Malard F, Abecassis M, et al. Sinusoidal obstruction syndrome/veno-occlusive disease: current situation and perspectives-a position statement from the European Society for Blood and Marrow Transplantation (EBMT). *Bone Marrow Transplant*. 2015;50(6):781-789.
30. Mansoor AM, Mansoor SE. Images in clinical medicine. Lancisi's sign. *N Engl J Med*. 2016;374(2):e2.
31. Howard JP, Jones D, Mills P, Marley R, Wragg A. Recurrent ascites due to constrictive pericarditis. *Frontline Gastroenterol*. 2012;3(4):233-237.
32. Darwish Murad S, Plessier A, Hernandez-Guerra M, et al. Etiology, management, and outcome of the Budd-Chiari syndrome. *Ann Intern Med*. 2009;151(3):167-175.
33. Srinivas BC, Dattatreya PV, Srinivasa KH, Prabhavathi, Manjunath CN. Inferior vena cava obstruction: long-term results of endovascular management. *Indian Heart J*. 2012;64(2):162-169.
34. Rector Jr WG, Reynolds TB. Superiority of the serum-ascites albumin difference over the ascites total protein concentration in separation of "transudative" and "exudative" ascites. *Am J Med*. 1984;77(1):83-85.
35. Weisberg HF. Osmotic pressure of the serum proteins. *Ann Clin Lab Sci*. 1978;8(2):155-164.
36. Runyon BA. Management of adult patients with ascites caused by cirrhosis. *Hepatology*. 1998;27(1):264-272.
37. Eghtesad S, Poustchi H, Malekzadeh R. Malnutrition in liver cirrhosis:the influence of protein and sodium. *Middle East J Dig Dis*. 2013;5(2):65-75.
38. Tierney EP, Sage RJ, Shwayder T. Kwashiorkor from a severe dietary restriction in an 8-month infant in suburban Detroit, Michigan: case report and review of the literature. *Int J Dermatol*. 2010;49(5):500-506.
39. Umar SB, DiBaise JK. Protein-losing enteropathy: case illustrations and clinical review. *Am J Gastroenterol*. 2010;105(1):43-49; quiz 50.
40. Sangisetty SL, Miner TJ. Malignant ascites: a review of prognostic factors, pathophysiology and therapeutic measures. *World J Gastrointest Surg*. 2012;4(4):87-95.
41. Kanneganti K, Srikakarlapudi S, Acharya B, Sindhaghatta V, Chilimuri S. Successful management of pancreatic ascites with both conservative management and pancreatic duct stenting. *Gastroenterol Res*. 2009;2(4):245-247.
42. Hillebrand DJ, Runyon BA, Yasmineh WG, Rynders GP. Ascitic fluid adenosine deaminase insensitivity in detecting tuberculous peritonitis in the United States. *Hepatology*. 1996;24(6):1408-1412.
43. Mimidis K. Peritoneal tuberculosis. *Ann Gastroenterol*. 2005;18(3):325-3295.
44. Uzunkoy A, Harma M, Harma M. Diagnosis of abdominal tuberculosis: experience from 11 cases and review of the literature. *World J Gastroenterol*. 2004;10(24):3647-3649.
45. Cardenas A, Chopra S. Chylous ascites. *Am J Gastroenterol*. 2002;97(8):1896-1900.
46. de Castro F, Bonacini M, Walden JM, Schubert TT. Myxedema ascites. Report of two cases and review of the literature. *J Clin Gastroenterol*. 1991;13(4):411-414.
47. Ji JS, Chae HS, Cho YS, et al. Myxedema ascites: case report and literature review. *J Korean Med Sci*. 2006;21(4):761-764.
48. Cappell MS. Intestinal (mesenteric) vasculopathy. I. Acute superior mesenteric arteriopathy and venopathy. *Gastroenterol Clin North Am*. 1998;27(4):783-825, vi.
49. Runyon BA, Hoefs JC, Canawati HN. Polymicrobial bacterascites. A unique entity in the spectrum of infected ascitic fluid. *Arch Intern Med*. 1986;146(11):2173-2175.
50. Kwan DM, Dhaliwal G, Baudendistel TE. Thinking inside the box. *J Hosp Med*. 2008;3(1):71-76.
51. Marriott HJL. *Bedside Cardiac Diagnosis*. Philadelphia, PA: Lippincott Company; 1993.
52. Mansoor AM, Karlapudi SP. Images in clinical medicine. Kussmaul's sign. *N Engl J Med*. 2015;372(2):e3.

Chapter 14

# CHOLESTATIC LIVER INJURY

## Case: A 48-year-old woman with pruritis

A previously healthy 48-year-old woman presents to the clinic with 8 months of progressive fatigue and generalized itching. The fatigue has prevented her from activities she previously enjoyed, such as gardening and going on walks. The itching, which involves the whole body, has gotten worse over the past few months. The patient has never smoked cigarettes, and does not consume alcohol regularly or use illicit drugs. Urine and stool have been normal in quality.

Vital signs are unremarkable. The abdomen is nontender, and the liver is normal in size. Murphy's sign is negative. There are yellow-orange papules and nodules over the extensor surfaces of both elbows, and around the eyelids (Figure 14-1).

Aspartate aminotransferase (AST) is 52 U/L; alanine aminotransferase (ALT), 71 U/L; total bilirubin, 1.8 mg/dL (direct bilirubin, 1.4 mg/dL); alkaline phosphatase (ALP), 340 U/L (reference range 30-120 U/L); $\gamma$-glutamyl transferase (GGT), 290 U/L (reference range 2-30 U/L); albumin, 3.6 mg/dL; and international normalized ratio (INR), 0.9. Transcutaneous abdominal ultrasound shows normal liver size and contour and no biliary dilation.

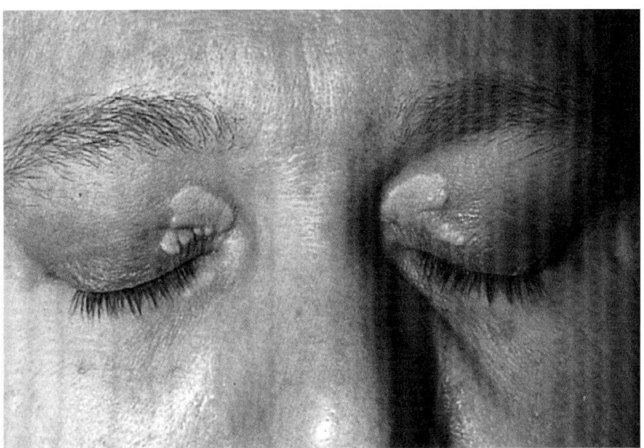

**Figure 14-1.** (From Elder DE, Elenitsas R, Rubin AI, et al. *Atlas and Synopsis of Lever's Histopathology of the Skin*. 3rd Edition. Philadelphia, PA: Lippincott Williams & Wilkins; 2012.)

***What is the most likely cause of cholestatic liver injury in this patient?***

**What biochemical laboratory pattern describes cholestatic liver injury?**

Diseases of the liver produce characteristic biochemical patterns of injury. Distinguishing cholestatic liver injury from hepatocellular liver injury can be helpful in narrowing the differential diagnosis. Cholestatic liver injury refers to the predominance of serum ALP elevation compared with serum aminotransferases. Serum bilirubin levels are usually also elevated.[1,2]

**What demographic groups tend to have higher serum alkaline phosphatase levels at baseline?**

Blacks tend to have slightly higher serum ALP values than whites; smokers have slightly higher values than nonsmokers; and pregnant women have higher values than nonpregnant women.[2]

**What are the sources of alkaline phosphatase in the body?**

In addition to the hepatobiliary system, ALP is present in bone, intestine, kidney, placenta, and white blood cells. Diseases of the hepatobiliary system and bone are the most common causes of elevated serum ALP.[2]

**When serum alkaline phosphatase levels are elevated, what other laboratory result is suggestive of a hepatic source?**

When serum ALP is elevated, concomitant elevation of either serum GGT or serum 5′-nucleotidase (5′-NT) is suggestive of hepatobiliary disease. The combination of elevated serum ALP and normal serum GGT or 5′-NT should shift attention from the liver to the bone or elsewhere. Fractionating serum ALP isoenzymes can aid in identifying the source but is usually not necessary.[2]

**What is the role of alkaline phosphatase in hepatic metabolism?**

ALP is an enzyme found on the surface of cells that transports metabolites across the membrane. In the liver, it is found on the surface of bile duct epithelia. Cholestasis and accumulating bile salts augment the synthesis and release of ALP, resulting in increased serum levels.[1,3,4]

**Compared with the aminotransferases, why are serum alkaline phosphatase levels typically late to rise in the setting of acute liver injury and slow to fall after it has resolved?**

Unlike the aminotransferases, which are immediately leaked into the circulation upon hepatocyte necrosis, ALP is synthesized in response to cholestasis and accumulating bile salts, which requires additional time. This makes ALP late to rise when there is acute liver injury; its long serum half-life (around 1 week) makes it slower to peak and fall after liver injury resolves.[1]

**How does bilirubin end up in bile?**

Water-insoluble unconjugated (indirect) bilirubin is a product of hemoglobin breakdown within the reticuloendothelial system. It travels to the liver where it is converted to water-soluble conjugated (direct) bilirubin, which is then excreted into bile.[1]

**Is cholestasis associated with elevated serum levels of unconjugated or conjugated bilirubin?**

Cholestasis predominantly results in elevated conjugated bilirubin, which typically occurs when the liver has lost at least half of its excretory capacity.[1]

**What are the clinical manifestations of cholestasis?**

Clinical manifestations of cholestasis depend on the underlying cause but may include pruritis, fatigue, dark-colored urine, acholic (pale or light-colored) stools, jaundice, and palpable dilation of the gallbladder (Courvoisier sign).[2]

**What are the 2 general categories of cholestatic liver injury?**

Cholestatic liver injury can occur as a result of extrahepatic or intrahepatic cholestasis.

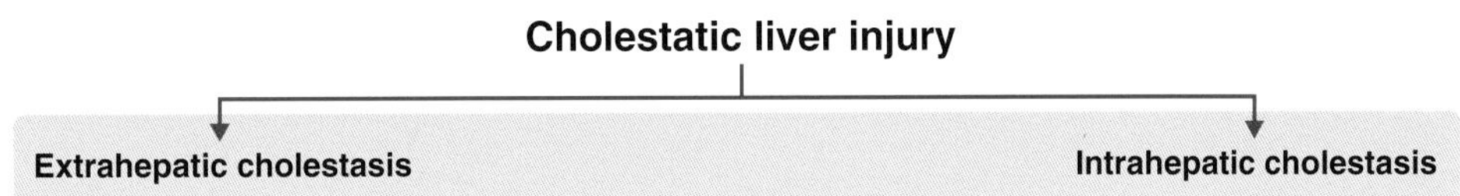


**What is the anatomic distinction between intrahepatic and extrahepatic cholestasis?**

Intrahepatic causes of cholestasis occur at the hepatocellular level and generally result in impaired bilirubin transport from hepatocytes to the bile canaliculi and intrahepatic ducts. Extrahepatic causes of cholestasis involve the larger bile ducts.

**What is the fundamental mechanism of extrahepatic cholestasis?**

Extrahepatic cholestasis occurs when large bile ducts become obstructed, either intrinsically or by external compression, resulting in impaired excretion of bile into the small intestine.

**What first-line imaging modality is used to distinguish extrahepatic from intrahepatic cholestasis?**

Transcutaneous abdominal ultrasonography (TUS) can be helpful in differentiating extrahepatic and intrahepatic cholestasis. Biliary duct dilation is suggestive of an extrahepatic process (ie, biliary obstruction) but typically does not identify the cause. The overall sensitivity of TUS is limited, particularly in obese patients. Furthermore, biliary duct dilation may be entirely absent in some cases of obstruction (eg, partial obstruction). *Insignificant biliary duct dilation unrelated to obstruction can be seen in patients with a history of cholecystectomy.*[2,5]

**What additional information can be obtained with computed tomography (CT) imaging in a patient with cholestatic liver injury?**

CT imaging has similar sensitivity compared with TUS for identifying biliary duct dilatation, but it can provide additional information about the liver parenchyma and may be more helpful in identifying mass lesions (eg, pancreatic tumor).[2]

**If transcutaneous abdominal ultrasonography and CT imaging are negative for biliary duct dilation, what additional imaging modalities can be used to detect the presence of extrahepatic cholestasis?**

Given the limited sensitivities of TUS and CT imaging, negative studies in patients strongly suspected of extrahepatic cholestasis should be followed by further imaging, including magnetic resonance cholangiopancreatography (MRCP) or endoscopic ultrasound (EUS), which are significantly more sensitive.[2]

**What is the gold standard for evaluation of the biliary tract?**

ERCP is the gold standard for evaluating the biliary tract and can identify the cause and level of obstruction. It offers additional diagnostic information via brushings and biopsies as well as therapeutic interventions such as stone extraction, sphincterotomy, dilation of strictures, and stent placement.[2]

## EXTRAHEPATIC CHOLESTASIS

**What life-threatening condition can develop in patients with extrahepatic cholestasis?**

Extrahepatic cholestasis can lead to ascending cholangitis, a life-threatening infection of the biliary tract. Charcot's triad of fever, right upper quadrant abdominal pain, and jaundice is present in most patients.[2]

**What are the 2 anatomic subcategories of extrahepatic cholestasis?**

Obstruction of the large bile ducts can occur as a result of processes associated with the biliary system or the adjacent pancreas.

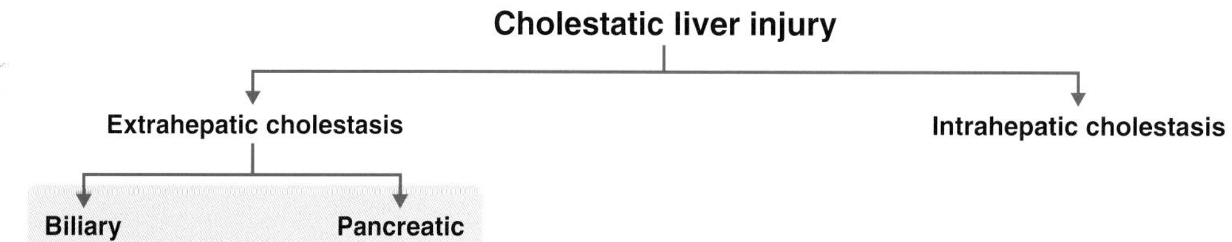


**What is the anatomic relationship between the extrahepatic biliary tree and the pancreas?**

In most patients, the common bile duct passes posterior to the head of the pancreas on its way to the duodenum, becoming at least partially covered by pancreatic tissue. This is referred to as the intrapancreatic portion of the common bile duct (Figure 14-2).[6]

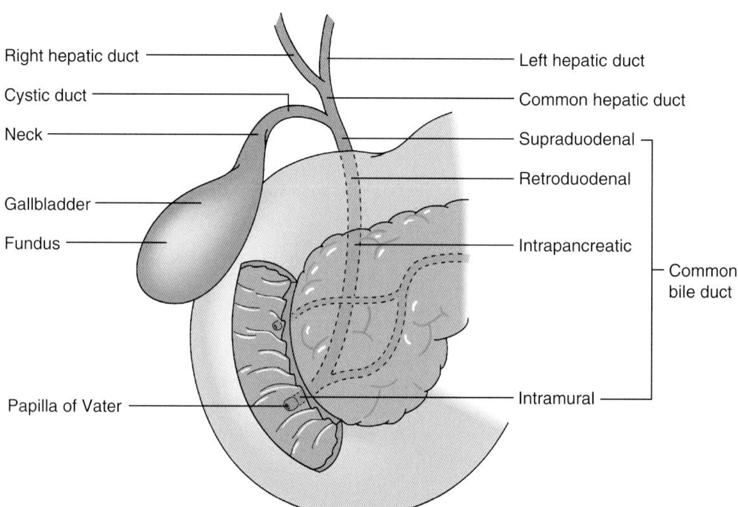


**Figure 14-2.** Anatomy of the extrahepatic biliary tree and its relationship to the pancreatic head. (From Mulholland MW, et al. *Greenfield's Surgery: Scientific Principles and Practice*. 6th ed. Philadelphia, PA: Wolters Kluwer Health; 2017.)

## EXTRAHEPATIC CHOLESTASIS RELATED TO THE BILIARY SYSTEM

### What are the biliary causes of extrahepatic cholestasis?

**A 42-year-old obese woman presents with right upper quadrant abdominal pain and jaundice.**

Choledocholithiasis.

**Narrowing of bile duct lumen that can occur as a result of a variety of conditions.**

Biliary stricture.

**ERCP brushings of a biliary stricture identifies the presence of atypical cells.**

Malignancy.

**Parasites.**

Liver flukes and *Ascaris lumbricoides*.

**A 19-year-old Asian woman presents with abdominal pain and jaundice and is found to have several saccular outpouchings of the biliary tree on cross-sectional imaging.**

Choledochal cyst.

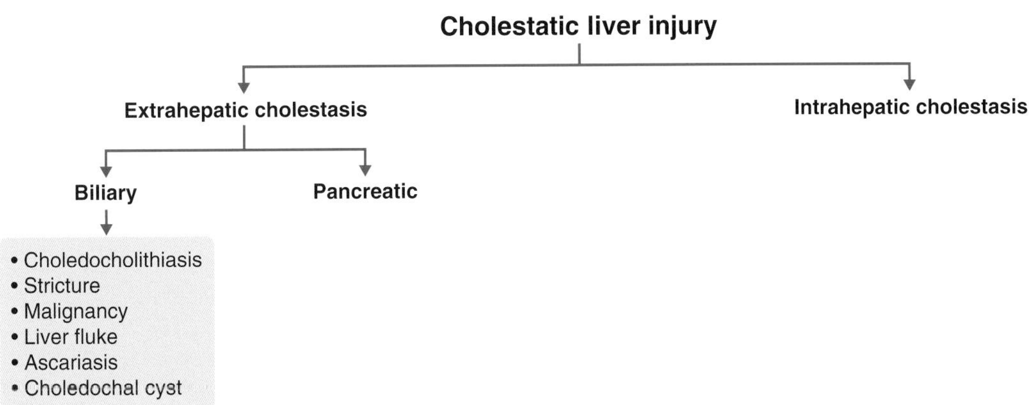


**What is choledocholithiasis?**

Choledocholithiasis describes the presence of gallstones within the common bile duct, which occurs in up to one-fifth of patients with cholelithiasis (Figure 14-3). Most patients are symptomatic with right upper quadrant abdominal pain, nausea, and vomiting. TUS is the initial diagnostic imaging study of choice, which can visualize the stone or show common bile duct dilation. The main advantage of ERCP over MRCP in patients with choledocholithiasis is the ability to perform therapeutic interventions (eg, stone retrieval). Complications of choledocholithiasis include acute pancreatitis and ascending cholangitis.[2]

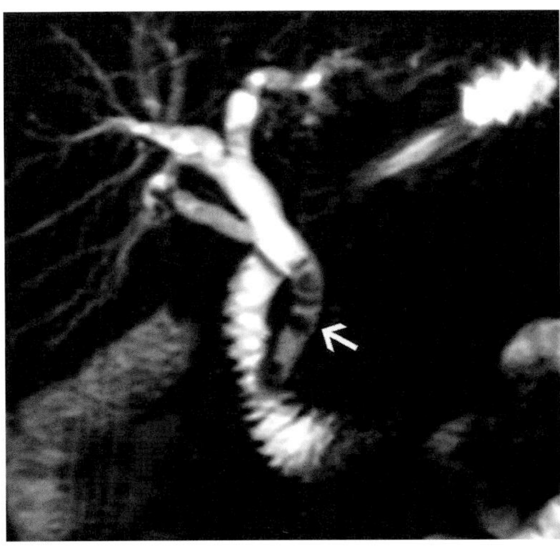

**Figure 14-3.** Coronal MRCP image shows multiple filling defects (arrow) within the distal common bile duct causing intrahepatic and extrahepatic biliary duct dilation. (From Zyromski NJ. *Handbook of Hepato-Pancreato-Biliary Surgery*. Philadelphia, PA: Wolters Kluwer Health; 2015.)

**What are the causes of biliary stricture?**

Biliary strictures can be benign or malignant. Causes include bile duct injury related to surgery (eg, cholecystectomy), recurrent choledocholithiasis, primary sclerosing cholangitis (PSC), acquired immunodeficiency syndrome (AIDS) cholangiopathy, radiation therapy, cholangiocarcinoma, chronic pancreatitis, pancreatic cancer, and a history of blunt trauma to the abdomen.[2]

**What are the mechanisms of cholestasis caused by malignancy of the biliary tract?**

Cancer of the gallbladder, cholangiocarcinoma, and cancer of the ampulla of Vater cause cholestasis because of obstruction by tumor or secondary stricture. Cytologic evaluation of brushings obtained during ERCP can be helpful in making the diagnosis. Techniques such as digital image analysis and fluorescence in situ hybridization have markedly increased the diagnostic yield of ERCP brushings for cholangiocarcinoma.[2]

**What are liver flukes?**

Liver flukes are endemic trematodes that infect the bile ducts. Species that most commonly cause human infection include *Clonorchis sinensis* (Chinese liver fluke), *Opisthorchis viverrini* (Southeast Asian liver fluke), *Opisthorchis felineus* (Siberian liver fluke), and *Fasciola hepatica* (common liver fluke). Humans acquire the infection after ingesting raw fluke-infested freshwater fish. The flukes travel to the bile ducts where they remain for decades. Most patients are asymptomatic, but those with a large fluke burden can experience mechanical obstruction of the bile ducts and nonspecific gastrointestinal discomfort. Chronic inflammation of the bile ducts can result in stone formation, suppurative cholangitis, and the development of cholangiocarcinoma. Peripheral eosinophilia may provide a clue, although diagnosis is based on identification of eggs from samples of stool, duodenal aspirate, or bile. Praziquantel is the treatment of choice.[7,8]

**What are the clinical features of ascariasis?**

Ascariasis is the gastrointestinal infection with the nematode *Ascaris lumbricoides*, which can include intestinal, hepatobiliary, and pancreatic manifestations. Pulmonary manifestations are also possible early in the course of the infection. It is found most commonly in tropical countries and is estimated to affect up to one-third of the world's population. Risk factors for hepatobiliary involvement include female sex, prior biliary surgery (eg, endoscopic sphincterotomy), and pregnancy. Most patients are asymptomatic, but those with heavy worm loads can experience mechanical obstruction of the bile ducts and nonspecific gastrointestinal discomfort. Complications include biliary colic, acute cholangitis, acute cholecystitis, and hepatic abscess. Peripheral eosinophilia is common. Diagnosis requires visualization of the parasite in the biliary tree. TUS is the initial study of choice. ERCP can be diagnostic and therapeutic. Oral antihelminthic medications can also be used to treat ascariasis.[9]

**What are choledochal cysts?**

Choledochal cysts are the defining feature of a rare condition characterized by the presence of one or more cystic dilations of the intrahepatic and/or extrahepatic ducts. Asians and women are disproportionately affected. Clinical manifestations may include abdominal pain, jaundice, and a palpable right upper quadrant abdominal mass. Most cases are diagnosed in childhood. Certain types of cysts are associated with a significant risk of developing cholangiocarcinoma; surgical resection is recommended in these cases to lower the risk.[2]

*Cholelithiasis and acute cholecystitis are not usually associated with cholestatic liver injury because biliary obstruction is limited to the gallbladder. However, a minority of patients may experience a complication known as Mirizzi syndrome in which a gallstone in the neck of the gallbladder or cystic duct causes external compression of the adjacent common hepatic duct. This leads to biliary obstruction proximal to the common hepatic duct along with a cholestatic pattern of liver injury.*[10]

## EXTRAHEPATIC CHOLESTASIS RELATED TO THE PANCREAS

### What are the pancreatic causes of extrahepatic cholestasis?

**A 38-year-old man with active alcohol abuse presents with nausea, vomiting, and epigastric abdominal pain that radiates to the back.**

Acute pancreatitis.

**A 46-year-old man with a history of recurrent acute pancreatitis has chronic abdominal pain, weight loss, and pancreatic parenchymal calcifications on cross-sectional imaging.**

Chronic pancreatitis.

**A late complication of acute pancreatitis, typically developing over the course of a few weeks.**

Pancreatic pseudocyst.

**A 60-year-old man with a heavy smoking history presents with painless jaundice and a palpable gallbladder.**

Pancreatic cancer.

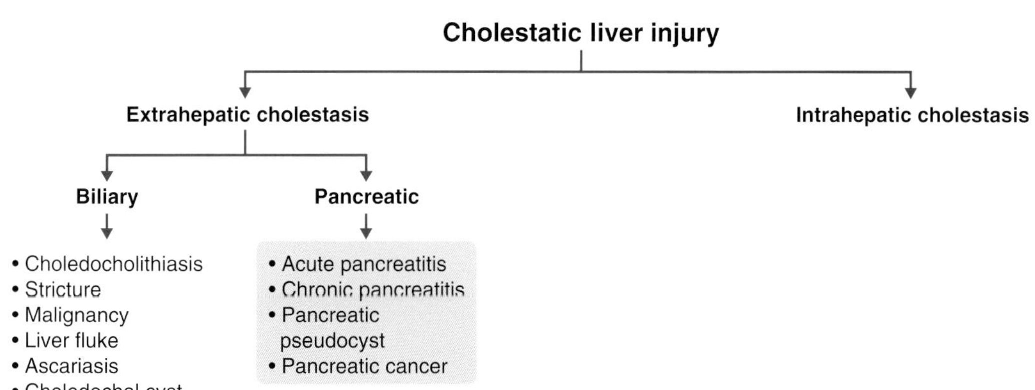


**What are the mechanisms of cholestasis caused by acute and chronic pancreatitis?**

In the setting of acute pancreatitis, tissue edema or abscess can compress the intrapancreatic portion of the common bile duct; in chronic pancreatitis, compression of the duct occurs as a result of encroaching pancreatic fibrosis. Patients with chronic pancreatitis often experience recurrent cholestasis during episodes of acute pancreatitis when a partially compressed duct becomes further compromised by tissue edema. This can eventually lead to common bile duct stricture. Surgical intervention should be considered for patients with persistent cholestasis related to chronic pancreatitis.[6]

**What are pancreatic pseudocysts?**

Pancreatic pseudocysts arise when there is disruption of the pancreatic duct, resulting in leakage of pancreatic fluid into the surrounding tissues that develops an encapsulating fibrous wall over time. Pseudocysts occur in up to one-fifth of patients with acute pancreatitis but also occur in patients with chronic pancreatitis. Most pseudocysts resolve spontaneously, although rupture can occur, resulting in pancreatic ascites, and the potential for the formation of fistulae to other viscera. Pseudocysts can also cause extrahepatic biliary obstruction from extrinsic common bile duct obstruction (Figure 14-4). Patients with biliary obstruction should be considered for cyst drainage.[6,11]

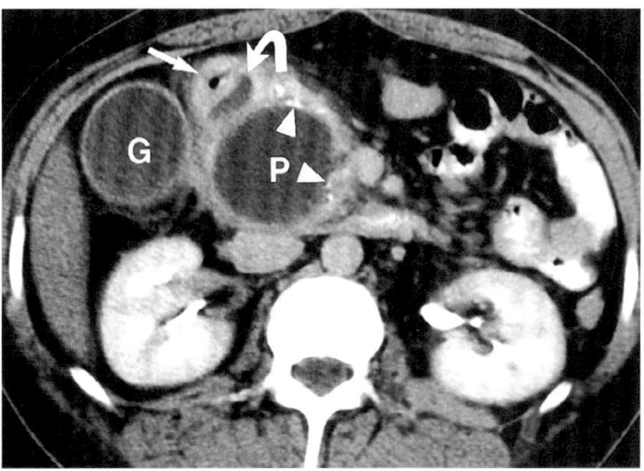


**Figure 14-4.** Enhanced CT image through the pancreatic head shows a mature pancreatic pseudocyst (P). Note the distended gallbladder (G), compressed duodenum (straight arrow), and distended common bile duct (curved arrow). Several small pancreatic calcifications (arrowheads) are seen adjacent to the pseudocyst, indicative of chronic pancreatitis. (From Pope TL, Harris JH. *Harris & Harris' The Radiology of Emergency Medicine*. 5th ed. Philadelphia, PA: Lippincott Williams & Wilkins; 2012.)

**What are the risk factors for pancreatic cancer?**

The strongest risk factors for pancreatic cancer are family history (lifetime risk for a patient with ≥3 affected first-degree relatives is about 40%), advanced age, cigarette smoking, and a history of chronic pancreatitis. Cancers that arise near the head of the pancreas present with obstructive jaundice in most cases; other manifestations include weight loss, abdominal pain, and new-onset diabetes. Prognosis is poor, with 5-year survival rates <10%.[12]

## INTRAHEPATIC CHOLESTASIS

**What are the main clinical features of chronic intrahepatic cholestasis?**

Most patients with chronic intrahepatic cholestasis experience fatigue and pruritis. Hypercholesterolemia is common, often producing xanthomas (cholesterol deposits in tendon sheaths and bony prominences) and xanthelasma (cholesterol deposits around the eyelids).[2]

**What diagnostic studies are helpful in the workup of intrahepatic cholestasis?**

Once extrahepatic cholestasis has been ruled out with imaging, investigation into intrahepatic causes of cholestasis should begin. Occasionally, the cause of intrahepatic cholestasis is identified during the initial workup (eg, hepatocellular carcinoma detected on initial imaging). Otherwise, history and physical examination should direct a serologic workup. Liver biopsy may ultimately be necessary in some cases.[2]

**What are the general mechanisms of intrahepatic cholestasis?**

Intrahepatic cholestasis can be obstructive, toxic, or infectious.

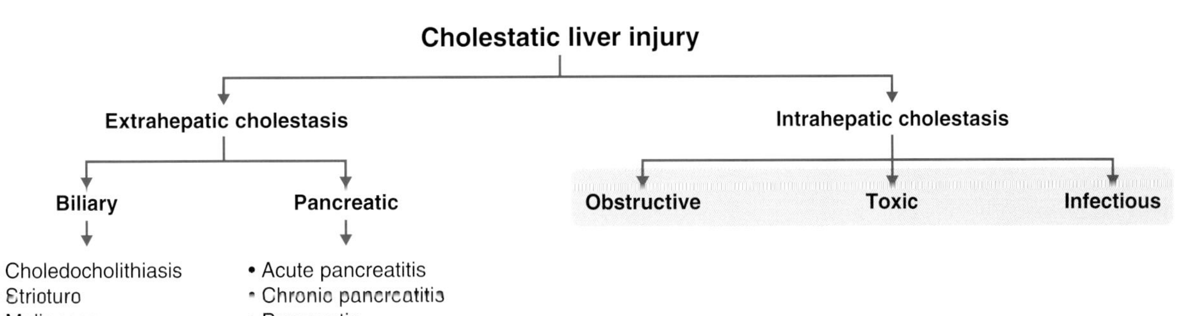


## INTRAHEPATIC CHOLESTASIS RELATED TO OBSTRUCTION

### What are the obstructive causes of intrahepatic cholestasis?

| | |
|---|---|
| **May be associated with elevated serum α-fetoprotein levels.** | Hepatocellular carcinoma. |
| **More common in women, with a 10:1 female-to-male ratio.** | Primary biliary cholangitis (PBC).[2] |
| **A 28-year-old man with ulcerative colitis is found to have elevated serum ALP and GGT levels.** | Primary sclerosing cholangitis. |
| **Obstructive pulmonary disease, pancreatic insufficiency, and infertility.** | Cystic fibrosis. |
| **These conditions commonly affect multiple organs; low-voltage electrocardiogram is a classic cardiac manifestation, and kidney enlargement is a classic renal manifestation.** | Infiltrative disorders (eg, sarcoidosis). |
| **Red blood cells lodged within the hepatic sinusoids.** | Sickle cell anemia. |
| **A patient develops cholestasis after liver transplantation.** | Posttransplant complications. |
| **A patient develops cholestasis after bone marrow transplantation.** | Graft-versus-host disease (GVHD). |

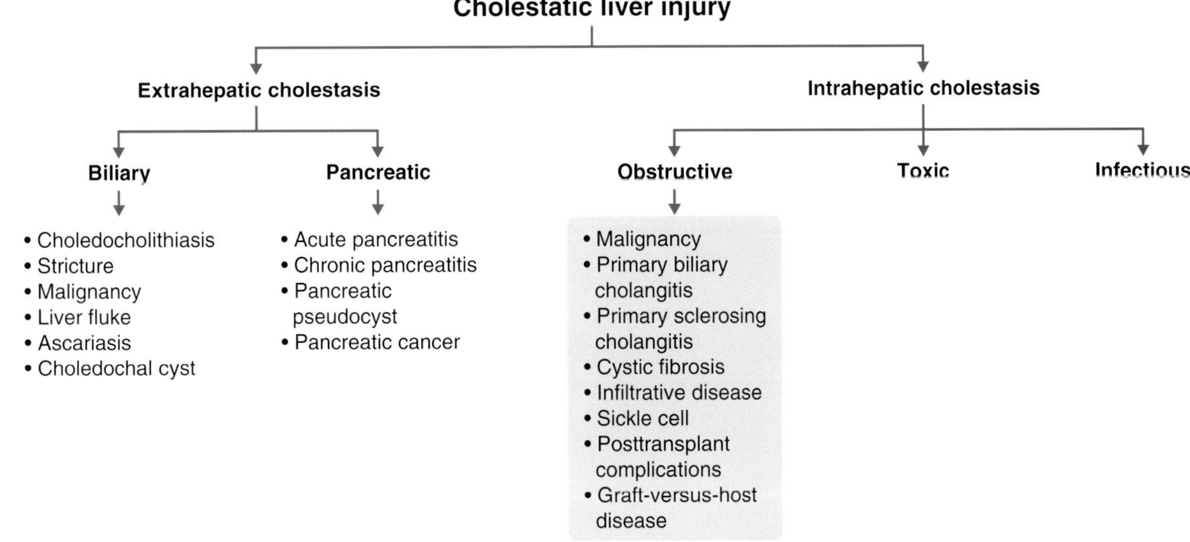

**What are the malignant causes of intrahepatic cholestasis?**

The most common malignant causes of intrahepatic cholestasis include hepatocellular carcinoma, cholangiocarcinoma, lymphoma, and metastases from primary tumors of the gastrointestinal tract (eg, colon), breast, lung, and pancreas.[13,14]

**What serologic test(s) should be obtained to evaluate for primary biliary cholangitis?**

Positive serum antimitochondrial antibody (AMA) is the hallmark of PBC, with sensitivity and specificity that exceed 95%. Additional antibody testing (eg, anti-Sp100 and anti-Gp210) and liver biopsy are required to make the diagnosis in the few patients who are AMA negative. Some patients may have an overlap syndrome, with features of PBC and autoimmune hepatitis. A subset of these patients has clinical features of PBC but a serologic pattern suggestive of autoimmune hepatitis (eg, negative AMA and positive antinuclear antibody, with or without positive anti–smooth muscle antibody).[2,15]

**How is the diagnosis of primary sclerosing cholangitis made?**

PSC is associated with the presence of perinuclear antineutrophil cytoplasmic antibodies (p-ANCA). MRCP is the noninvasive diagnostic study of choice for PSC, and may demonstrate diffuse multifocal stricturing and dilations of the intrahepatic and/or extrahepatic ducts. ERCP has the advantage of offering additional diagnostic capabilities via brushings to rule out cholangiocarcinoma and therapeutic capabilities (eg, biliary dilation and stenting).[2]

**What is the mechanism of intrahepatic cholestasis caused by cystic fibrosis?**

The cystic fibrosis transmembrane regulator (CFTR) protein is found within biliary epithelium and is partly responsible for the water and ion composition of bile. In patients with severe CFTR mutations, increased bile viscosity leads to congestion and obstruction within the intrahepatic bile ducts. Chronic biliary obstruction results in fibrosis and eventually cirrhosis.[16]

**What are the features of hepatic sarcoidosis?**

Most patients with systemic sarcoidosis have hepatic involvement, however the majority are asymptomatic. A cholestatic pattern of liver injury may be the only clue to the diagnosis. CT imaging of the liver may reveal hepatomegaly or multiple hypodense nodular lesions. Histology reveals noncaseating granulomas along the portal tract. However, noncaseating granulomas are not specific for sarcoidosis and other confirmatory features should be sought, such as additional extrahepatic manifestations of sarcoidosis (eg, pulmonary disease). Glucocorticoids are the treatment of choice. *Other infiltrative diseases that cause cholestasis include lymphoma and amyloidosis.*[2,13]

**What are the features of sickle cell intrahepatic cholestasis?**

Sickle cell intrahepatic cholestasis is likely a severe variant of sickle hepatic crisis, which is a syndrome characterized by right upper quadrant abdominal pain, fever, jaundice, leukocytosis, and moderate elevation of ALP. It is caused by hepatic ischemia related to widespread sinusoidal sickling. Patients with sickle cell intrahepatic cholestasis often develop severe jaundice, renal impairment, a bleeding diathesis, and encephalopathy. *A more common cause of cholestasis in patients with sickle cell anemia is choledocholithiasis from pigmented gallstones related to chronic hemolysis.*[17]

**What are the causes of intrahepatic cholestasis after liver transplantation?**

Intrahepatic cholestasis is common after liver transplantation. Early causes (<6 months posttransplant) include ischemia-reperfusion injury, initial graft dysfunction, immunosuppressive medication, infection, and acute cellular rejection. Late causes include hepatic artery thrombosis, chronic rejection, biliary complications (eg, stricture at an anastomotic site), recurrent cholestatic disease (eg, PBC or PSC), recurrent viral hepatitis, and posttransplant lymphoproliferative disorder.[18]

**What are the features of graft-versus-host disease of the liver?**

GVHD occurs following hematopoietic stem cell transplantation when donor T cells identify and attack host antigens as foreign. In the liver, the small bile duct cells are the targets of this immune-mediated attack. It is usually accompanied by GVHD of the skin or gastrointestinal tract resulting in the typical presentation of rash, diarrhea, and elevated ALP.[13]

## INTRAHEPATIC CHOLESTASIS RELATED TO TOXICITY

### What are the toxic causes of intrahepatic cholestasis?

**This iatrogenic cause of liver injury can present with a variety of different biochemical patterns of injury, including hepatocellular, cholestatic, or mixed.**

Medication (ie, drug-induced liver injury).

**Increased estrogen levels likely play a role in the pathogenesis of this condition.**

Intrahepatic cholestasis of pregnancy.[2]

**Associated with mild hepatocellular liver injury (aminotransferase levels typically <300 U/L) with an AST:ALT ratio ≥2:1.**

Alcoholic hepatitis.[19]

**Used to provide nutrition to patients who cannot tolerate enteral nutrition.**

Total parenteral nutrition (TPN).

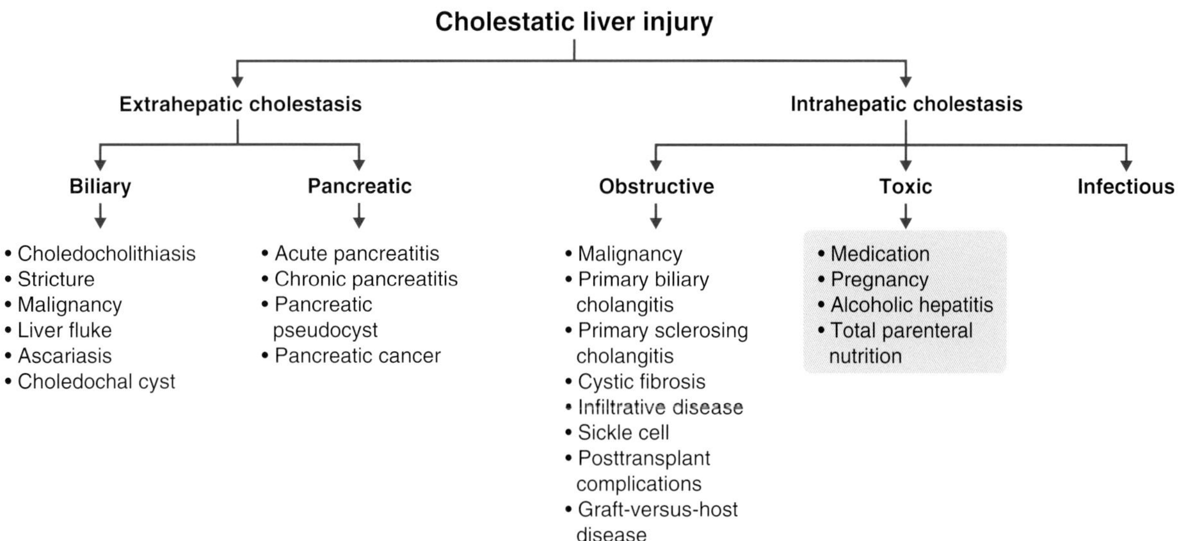


**How common is drug-induced liver injury?**

Drug-induced liver injury is the most common cause of acute liver failure in the industrialized world, responsible for more than one-half of all cases. A detailed history of prescription and nonprescription medications, herbs, supplements, and other substances is a critical part of making the diagnosis. The timing of liver injury after the onset of exposure is widely variable and drug-dependent, ranging from hours to up to a year. Cholestatic injury tends to recover slowly after discontinuation of the offending agent. However, some cases progress to chronic liver disease.[20]

**Why is the serum alkaline phosphatase level of limited diagnostic utility in evaluating for intrahepatic cholestasis of pregnancy?**

Intrahepatic cholestasis of pregnancy typically occurs around 25 to 32 weeks of gestation. Affected women experience pruritis that is usually worse at night. Serum aminotransferases and bilirubin may be elevated. Because the placenta is a source of ALP, serum levels may be elevated in pregnant women even in the absence of cholestasis, limiting its diagnostic value. An elevated serum bile acid level is a better biochemical marker for intrahepatic cholestasis of pregnancy. Resolution after delivery is expected; however, recurrences during subsequent pregnancies are common. Ursodeoxycholic acid can be used to manage symptoms during pregnancy.[2]

**What are the clinical features of alcoholic hepatitis?**

Patients with alcoholic hepatitis have a compatible history of alcohol use, fever, and tender hepatomegaly. Most patients experience modest elevations in aminotransferases (usually <300 U/L), marked hyperbilirubinemia, and variable elevations in ALP (from normal to values in the thousands U/L). *Alcoholic hepatitis is usually classified as a cause of hepatocellular liver injury, but it can be cholestatic in some cases.*[13,19,21]

**In what time frame does cholestasis develop after starting total parenteral nutrition?**

In adults, cholestasis typically occurs several weeks after starting TPN but may occur later. Infusions with high lipid content are more likely to cause cholestasis. Discontinuation of TPN or modification of the infusion formula (eg, reduction in lipid emulsion component) usually results in resolution of cholestasis. However, cholestasis may continue to progress to severe liver disease in a minority of patients.[2]

## INTRAHEPATIC CHOLESTASIS RELATED TO INFECTION

### What are the infectious causes of intrahepatic cholestasis?

**A common cause of cholestasis in the intensive care unit.**

Sepsis.

**Most commonly associated with marked hepatocellular liver injury, often with aminotransferase elevation >50 times the upper limit of normal.**

Viral hepatitis.

**A 58-year-old man who recently emigrated from India presents with fever, right upper quadrant abdominal pain, shortness of breath, and cough and is found to have hepatomegaly and a cholestatic pattern of liver injury.**

Hepatic tuberculosis (TB).

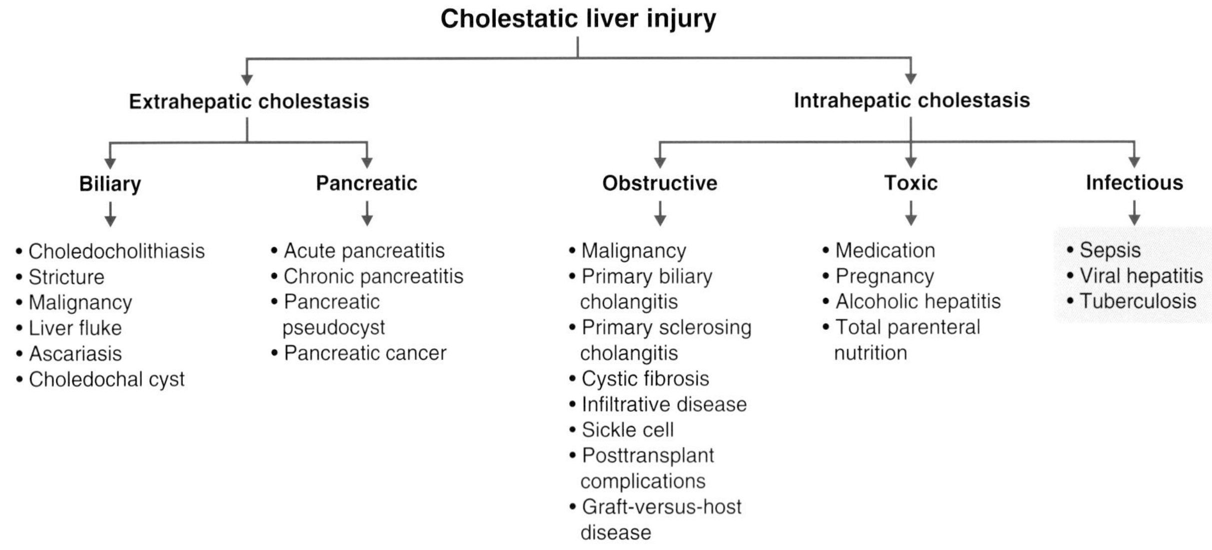


**Which organisms are most commonly associated with the cholestasis of sepsis?**

Cholestasis from sepsis most commonly develops in association with gram-negative organisms and some gram-positive organisms, such as *Staphylococcus aureus* and *Streptococcus pneumoniae*. Other bacteria associated with cholestasis include *Leptospira*, *Clostridium*, and *Borrelia*.[13]

**Is cholestasis an early or late finding in the course of acute viral hepatitis?**

Cholestasis tends to follow the acute phase of viral hepatitis (which is associated with hepatocellular liver injury), usually coinciding with clinical improvement. It most commonly occurs with hepatitis A, acute hepatitis C, and hepatitis E infections. Jaundice may last for up to 6 months, but the vast majority of patients experience complete recovery. *Most cases of acute viral hepatitis are diagnosed during the acute phase of the illness, at which time there is a hepatocellular pattern of liver injury.*[13]

**What diagnostic tests are available for hepatic tuberculosis?**

Hepatic TB should be suspected in any patient with risk factors for TB (eg, homelessness) who presents with hepatomegaly, fever, respiratory symptoms, and cholestatic liver injury. CT scan of the liver can identify findings suggestive of either focal or miliary hepatic TB. The most specific diagnostic test for hepatic TB is liver biopsy with histology (Figure 14-5) and mycobacterial culture. However, sensitivity is poor. Polymerase chain reaction (PCR) for *Mycobacterium tuberculosis* of the biopsy specimen is highly sensitivity and specific.[22]

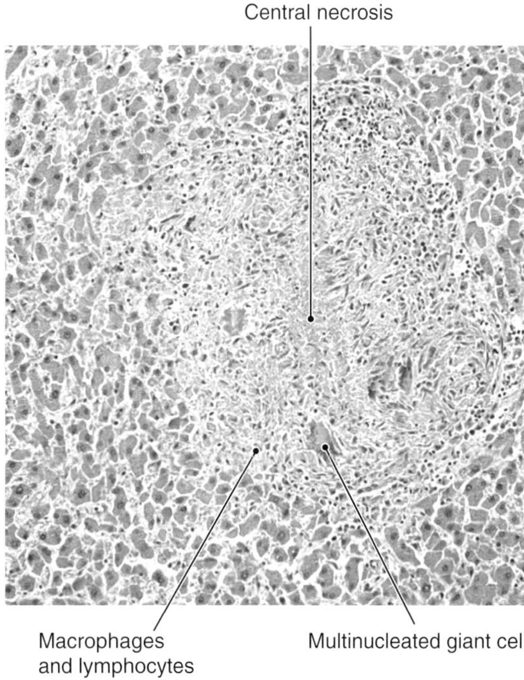


**Figure 14-5.** Hepatic TB. Normal liver cells surround a granuloma, which is comprised of a central core of necrotic tissue and a halo of lymphocytes and macrophages, some of which fuse to form multinucleated giant cells. (From Chowdhury SH, Cozma AI, Chowdhury JH. *Essentials for the Canadian Medical Licensing Exam*. 2nd ed. Philadelphia, PA: Wolters Kluwer Health; 2017.)

## Case Summary

A previously healthy 48-year-old woman presents with chronic fatigue and pruritis and is found to have cholestatic liver injury without evidence of biliary dilation on imaging.

***What is the most likely cause of cholestatic liver injury in this patient?***

Primary biliary cholangitis.

### BONUS QUESTIONS

***What is significant about the transcutaneous abdominal ultrasound results in this case?***

The absence of biliary duct dilation on TUS in this case is suggestive of an intrahepatic cholestatic process. When suspicion for extrahepatic cholestasis remains despite a negative TUS or CT, patients should undergo further diagnostic imaging studies (eg, MRCP, EUS, or ERCP). Otherwise, history and physical examination should direct a workup for intrahepatic cholestasis.[2]

***What is significant about the fatigue and pruritis in this case?***

Fatigue and pruritis are the most common symptoms in patients with chronic intrahepatic cholestasis caused by conditions such as PBC.[2]

***What is significant about the skin findings in this case?***

The skin lesions described over the elbows in this case are consistent with xanthomas, and the lesions around the eyelids (see Figure 14-1) are consistent with xanthelasma. Both of these lesions are suggestive of hyperlipidemia, which is found in most patients with PBC.[15]

***What is the significance of the age and gender of the patient in this case?***

PBC is a condition found primarily in women, with a female-to-male ratio of 10:1. Patients most frequently present in the fifth or sixth decade of life.[2,15]

***What is the next diagnostic step in this case?***

The chronicity of symptoms and absence of biliary dilation on TUS in this case make extrahepatic cholestasis (ie, biliary obstruction) unlikely. The history and physical examination are suggestive of PBC. Serum AMA titer should be checked. AMA is positive in the vast majority of patients with PBC and is associated with specificity >95%. The combination of elevated ALP and positive AMA is diagnostic of PBC. Additional antibody testing (eg, anti-Sp100 and anti-Gp210) and/or liver biopsy are required to make the diagnosis in the few patients who are AMA-negative.[2,15]

***What is the treatment for primary biliary cirrhosis?***

Ursodeoxycholic acid is the treatment of choice for PBC and is capable of halting disease progression, leading to an overall survival rate that is similar to the general population. However, just under one-half of all patients with PBC have an unsatisfactory response to ursodeoxycholic acid. Patients with progressive PBC may develop cirrhosis and portal hypertension, and in some cases require liver transplantation. PBC recurs after transplantation in one-quarter of cases.[15]

## KEY POINTS

- Cholestatic liver injury refers to the predominance of serum ALP elevation compared with serum aminotransferases. Serum bilirubin levels are usually also elevated.
- Diseases of the hepatobiliary system and bone are the most common causes of elevated serum ALP.
- Elevated serum GGT or 5′-NT levels can confirm a hepatobiliary source of ALP elevation.
- Clinical manifestations of cholestasis depend on the underlying cause but include pruritis, fatigue, dark-colored urine, acholic stools, jaundice, and palpable dilation of the gallbladder.
- Cholestasis can be extrahepatic or intrahepatic.
- The presence of dilated biliary ducts on imaging suggests extrahepatic cholestasis.
- Extrahepatic cholestasis occurs as a result of obstruction of the larger bile ducts related to either the pancreas or the biliary system.
- Intrahepatic cholestasis can be obstructive, toxic, or infectious.

## REFERENCES


1. Giannini EG, Testa R, Savarino V. Liver enzyme alteration: a guide for clinicians. *CMAJ*. 2005;172(3):367-379.
2. Siddique A, Kowdley KV. Approach to a patient with elevated serum alkaline phosphatase. *Clin Liver Dis*. 2012;16(2):199-229.
3. Moss DW. Physicochemical and pathophysiological factors in the release of membrane-bound alkaline phosphatase from cells. *Clin Chim Acta*. 1997;257(1):133-140.
4. Schlaeger R, Haux P, Kattermann R. Studies on the mechanism of the increase in serum alkaline phosphatase activity in cholestasis: significance of the hepatic bile acid concentration for the leakage of alkaline phosphatase from rat liver. *Enzyme*. 1982;28(1):3-13.
5. Scharschmidt BF, Goldberg HI, Schmid R. Current concepts in diagnosis. Approach to the patient with cholestatic jaundice. *N Engl J Med*. 1983;308(25):1515-1519.
6. Skellenger ME, Patterson D, Foley NT, Jordan Jr PH. Cholestasis due to compression of the common bile duct by pancreatic pseudocysts. *Am J Surg*. 1983;145(3):343-348.
7. Lim JH. Liver flukes: the malady neglected. *Korean J Radiol*. 2011;12(3):269-279.
8. Sripa B, Kaewkes S, Sithithaworn P, et al. Liver fluke induces cholangiocarcinoma. *PLoS Med*. 2007;4(7):e201.
9. Das AK. Hepatic and biliary ascariasis. *J Glob Infect Dis*. 2014;6(2):65-72.
10. Abou-Saif A, Al-Kawas FH. Complications of gallstone disease: Mirizzi syndrome, cholecystocholedochal fistula, and gallstone ileus. *Am J Gastroenterol*. 2002;97(2):249-254.
11. Crino SF, Scalisi G, Consolo P, et al. Novel endoscopic management for pancreatic pseudocyst with fistula to the common bile duct. *World J Gastrointest Endosc*. 2014;6(12):620-624.
12. Yabar CS, Winter JM. Pancreatic cancer: a review. *Gastroenterol Clin North Am*. 2016;45(3):429-445.
13. Assy N, Jacob G, Spira G, Edoute Y. Diagnostic approach to patients with cholestatic jaundice. *World J Gastroenterol*. 1999;5(3):252-262.
14. Sica GT, Ji H, Ros PR. CT and MR imaging of hepatic metastases. *Am J Roentgenol*. 2000;174(3):691-698.
15. Carey EJ, Ali AH, Lindor KD. Primary biliary cirrhosis. *Lancet*. 2015;386(10003):1565-1575.
16. Strazzabosco M. Transport systems in cholangiocytes: their role in bile formation and cholestasis. *Yale J Biol Med*. 1997;70(4):427-434.
17. Banerjee S, Owen C, Chopra S. Sickle cell hepatopathy. *Hepatology*. 2001;33(5):1021-1028.
18. Corbani A, Burroughs AK. Intrahepatic cholestasis after liver transplantation. *Clin Liver Dis*. 2008;12(1):111-129, ix.
19. Lucey MR, Mathurin P, Morgan TR. Alcoholic hepatitis. *N Engl J Med*. 2009;360(26):2758-2769.
20. Padda MS, Sanchez M, Akhtar AJ, Boyer JL. Drug-induced cholestasis. *Hepatology*. 2011;53(4):1377-1387.
21. Singal AK, Kodali S, Vucovich LA, Darley-Usmar V, Schiano TD. Diagnosis and treatment of alcoholic hepatitis: a systematic review. *Alcohol Clin Exp Res*. 2016;40(7):1390-1402.
22. Hickey AJ, Gounder L, Moosa MY, Drain PK. A systematic review of hepatic tuberculosis with considerations in human immunodeficiency virus co-infection. *BMC Infect Dis*. 2015;15:209.

Chapter 15

# DIARRHEA

## Case: A 58-year-old man with dyspnea

A previously healthy 58-year-old man presents to the clinic with persistent diarrhea over the course of 6 months. The diarrhea is watery, occurs up to 15 times per day, continues during periods of time when he does not eat, and is sometimes associated with abdominal cramping. There is no blood in the stools. He has experienced a weight loss of 20 pounds over this time. He has not experienced night sweats or fever. He complains of intermittent episodes of redness and warmth of his face and neck that last around 5 minutes. Over the past 4 weeks, he has become increasingly short of breath with activity. There has been no recent travel outside of the United States. He does not use any medications, including laxatives. He has not taken antibiotics in years.

The patient is cachectic. The liver is palpable 4 finger widths below the costal margin. Digital rectal examination reveals loose, brown stool. There is a 2/4 decrescendo diastolic murmur that augments with inspiration, best heard over the left upper sternal border.

A fecal leukocyte test is negative. Stool osmotic gap is <50 mOsm/kg. Measurement of 24-hour urinary excretion of 5-hydroxyindoleacetic acid (5-HIAA) is elevated. Cross-sectional imaging of the abdomen shows numerous ring-enhancing hepatic lesions of varying size, some with central necrosis (Figure 15-1A). Whole-body somatostatin-receptor scintigraphy (octreotide scan) is completed (Figure 15-1B).

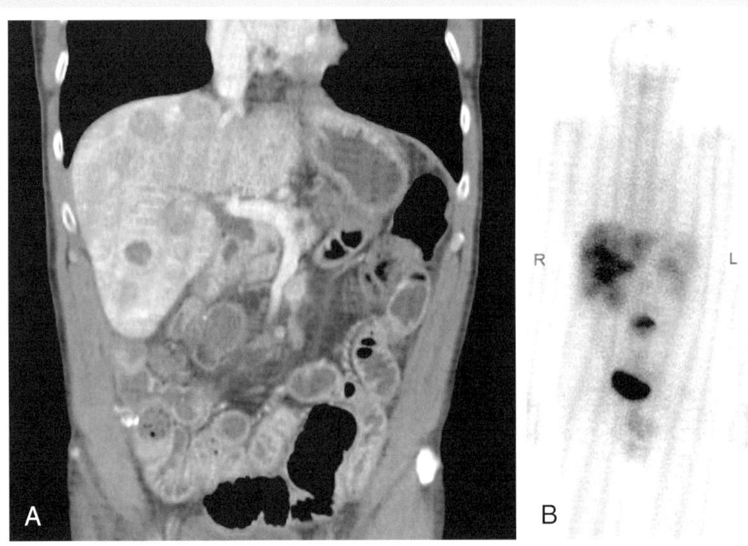


**Figure 15-1.**

***What is the most likely cause of diarrhea in this patient?***

**What is diarrhea?**

Diarrhea describes an increase in water content, volume, or frequency of stool, typically occurring at least 3 times in a 24-hour period. Acute diarrhea lasts ≤14 days; persistent diarrhea lasts >14 days; and chronic diarrhea lasts >30 days. The duration of a diarrheal illness can narrow the differential diagnosis. For example, most cases of acute diarrhea are infectious in nature.[1,2]

**How much fluid normally enters the gastrointestinal (GI) tract in a 24-hour period?**

Each day, approximately 7.5 liters of fluid enters the GI tract via oral ingestion and secretions. Most of this fluid is reabsorbed by the small intestine, leaving about 1.2 liters to enter the colon each day. The colon typically recovers about 1 liter of fluid (with a reserve absorptive capacity of up to 3 L/d), leaving a stool volume of <200 mL/d in healthy individuals. *Large-volume diarrhea is suggestive of a small bowel process.*[3]

**How does the gastrointestinal tract absorb water?**

Absorption of water within the GI tract is coupled with ion transport. Passive and active transport of ions such as sodium, chloride, and bicarbonate in the small and large intestines generate electrochemical gradients that drive the absorption of water. *Diarrhea is often associated with electrolyte disturbances (eg, hypokalemia) and non-anion gap metabolic acidosis.*[3,4]

**What are the 4 general mechanisms of diarrhea?**

Diarrhea can be inflammatory, osmotic, secretory, or related to intestinal dysmotility.

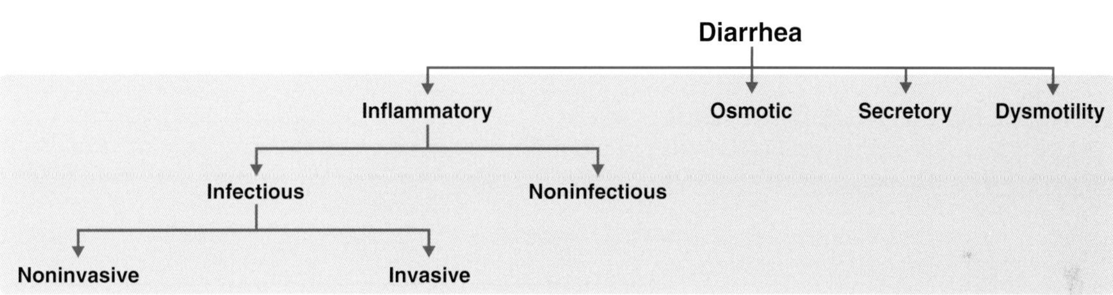


*Most etiologies of diarrhea act through a variety of these mechanisms. For simplicity, entities will be listed under 1 category of the framework in this chapter.*

## INFLAMMATORY DIARRHEA

**What is the fundamental mechanism of inflammatory diarrhea?**

Inflammatory diarrhea occurs when mucosal disruption results in exudation of serum into the intestinal lumen; destruction of the absorptive epithelium also leads to malabsorption.[3,5]

**What historical features can be suggestive of inflammatory diarrhea?**

Inflammatory diarrhea caused by either invasive infections or noninfectious conditions may be associated with abdominal pain, fever, tenesmus, and bloody or mucoid stools. Extraintestinal manifestations (eg, uveitis) may be present in some conditions, such as inflammatory bowel disease (IBD).[1,3]

**What stool study is suggestive of inflammatory diarrhea?**

Inflammatory diarrhea caused by either invasive infections or noninfectious conditions may be associated with the presence of polymorphonuclear leukocytes or leukocyte proteins (eg, calprotectin, lactoferrin) in stool. *Evidence of an inflammatory response is frequently absent in patients with noninvasive infectious diarrhea.*[1]

**What life-threatening complication of inflammatory colitis should be considered in patients with abdominal distention?**

Patients with inflammatory colitis related to either infectious or noninfectious conditions can develop toxic megacolon, a life-threatening complication that presents with abdominal distention and signs of systemic toxicity, such as fever, tachycardia, and delirium. Diagnosis can be confirmed with abdominal imaging (Figure 15-2).[6]

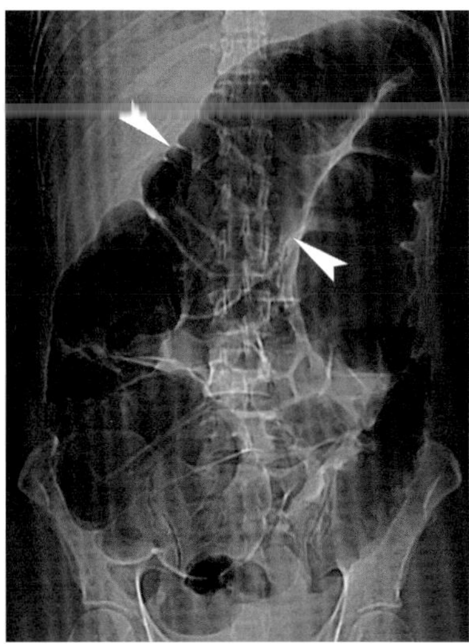

**Figure 15-2.** Upright abdominal radiograph of a patient with ulcerative colitis presenting with fever, abdominal pain, and distention showing marked dilatation of the colon, consistent with toxic megacolon. The transverse colon measures more than 10 cm in diameter (arrowheads). (From Brant WE, Helms C. *Fundamentals of Diagnostic Radiology*. 4th ed. Philadelphia, PA: Lippincott Williams & Wilkins; 2012.)

## NONINVASIVE INFECTIOUS DIARRHEA

**What are the 3 main types of organisms that cause noninvasive infectious diarrhea?**

Noninvasive infectious diarrhea is most commonly caused by viruses, bacteria, or protozoa.

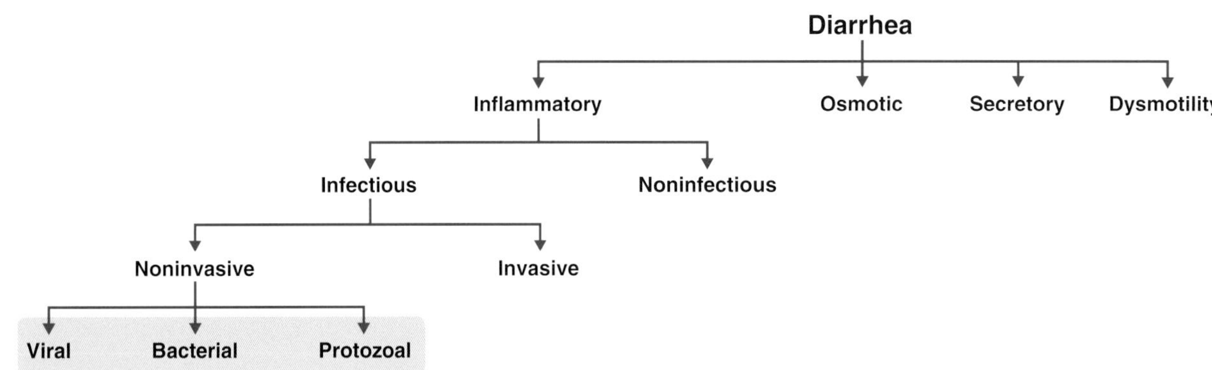


## NONINVASIVE VIRAL DIARRHEA

**How is the diagnosis of viral gastroenteritis made?**

The diagnosis of viral gastroenteritis is usually made on clinical grounds, but a variety of diagnostic stool assays are available, including immune-based assays (eg, enzyme-linked immunosorbent assay) and nucleic acid testing (eg, polymerase chain reaction [PCR]).[2,7]

### What are the causes of noninvasive viral diarrhea?

**This virus is commonly associated with outbreaks of gastroenteritis on cruise ships.**

Norovirus.

**The leading cause of diarrheal illness in infants and toddlers.**

Rotavirus.[2]

**More often associated with respiratory tract infection.**

Adenovirus.

**Named after the Greek word for "star" because of its characteristic appearance on electron microscopy.**

Astrovirus.[8]

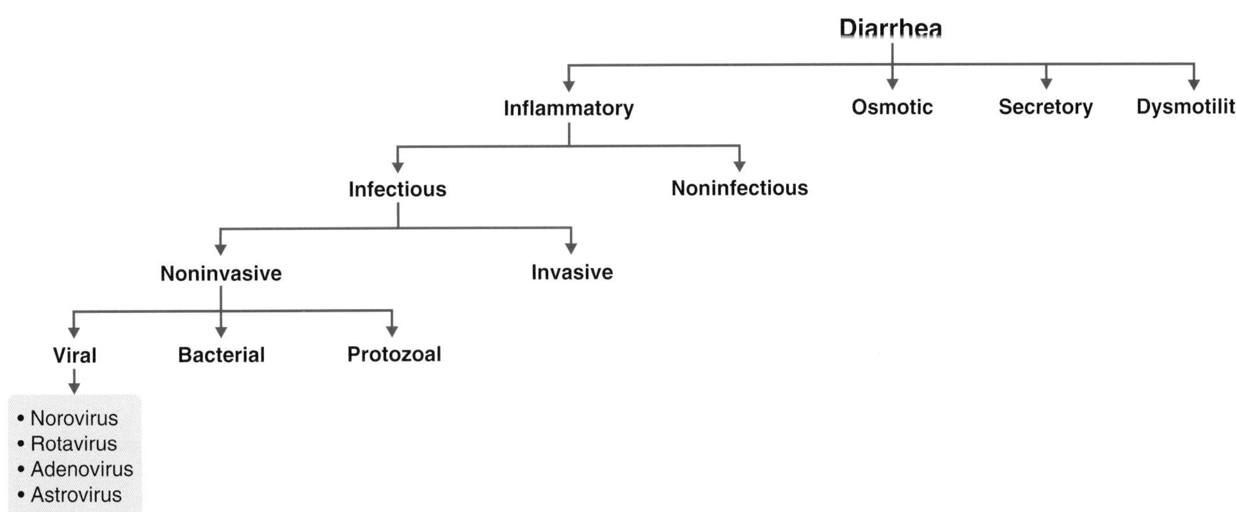


**What are the clinical features of norovirus gastroenteritis?**

Norovirus is the predominant cause of acute infectious diarrhea in adults and older children, and is often responsible for outbreaks in community settings such as recreational camps, cruise ships, and nursing homes. As a result of the large burden of organisms in stool and emesis, and the low inoculum required to cause infection, it is highly contagious. Symptoms begin 12 to 48 hours after exposure. Manifestations include fever, myalgias, headache, vomiting, and voluminous watery diarrhea. The duration of illness is typically 1 to 2 days.[2,7]

**What are the clinical features of rotavirus gastroenteritis?**

Rotavirus is the predominant cause of acute infectious diarrhea in young children but also affects adults. As a result of its ability to survive on environmental surfaces and the low inoculum required for infection, it is highly contagious. When a member of a family becomes infected, around one-half of children and up to one-third of adults in the household will become infected. In temperate climates, infection rates are highest during the winter months. Symptoms begin 1 to 3 days after exposure. Manifestations include fever, vomiting, and voluminous watery diarrhea, frequently requiring hospitalization for rehydration. However, most adults are asymptomatic. The duration of illness is typically 5 to 7 days but may be longer in immunocompromised hosts.[2,7]

**What are the clinical features of enteric adenovirus gastroenteritis?**

Enteric adenoviruses are a common cause of acute infectious diarrhea in infants and young children. Most infected adults are asymptomatic. Symptoms begin 8 to 10 days after exposure, and the duration of illness is typically 5 to 12 days, which is a longer incubation period and duration of illness than other viral causes of diarrhea. Manifestations include fever, vomiting, and prolonged watery diarrhea. Unlike conventional adenovirus serotypes, enteric adenoviruses do not cause nasopharyngitis and keratoconjunctivitis.[2,7]

**What are the clinical features of astrovirus gastroenteritis?**

Astrovirus gastroenteritis primarily affects infants and young children, but outbreaks do occur in adult communities (eg, military recruits, nursing homes for the elderly). Symptoms begin 1 to 2 days after exposure. Manifestations are similar to rotaviral illness but less severe, and watery diarrhea is prominent. The duration of illness is typically 2 to 5 days.[2,7]

## NONINVASIVE BACTERIAL DIARRHEA

| | |
|---|---|
| **How is the diagnosis of noninvasive bacterial gastrointestinal infection made?** | The diagnosis of most noninvasive bacterial GI infections is made clinically, but culture isolation from stool is confirmatory; culture-independent techniques (eg, PCR assays to detect organism-specific toxins) may be useful in some cases. |

### What are the causes of noninvasive bacterial diarrhea?

| | |
|---|---|
| **Antibiotic use commonly precedes infection with this organism.** | *Clostridium difficile.* |
| **A spore-forming gram-positive bacterium that causes foodborne illness, commonly involving meat and poultry.** | *Clostridium perfringens.* |
| **This organism, commonly found on skin, causes foodborne illness via preformed toxins.** | *Staphylococcus aureus.* |
| **Fried rice is the classic source of this bacterium in foodborne illness.** | *Bacillus cereus.* |
| **The most common cause of GI infection among travelers.** | Enterotoxigenic *Escherichia coli* (ETEC).[9] |
| **Another noninvasive strain of *Escherichia coli*.** | Enteropathogenic *Escherichia coli* (EPEC). |
| **A gram-positive, rod-shaped organism that most often affects patients with impaired cell-mediated immunity.** | *Listeria monocytogenes.* |
| **An organism that causes severe secretory diarrhea.** | *Vibrio cholerae.* |
| **A gram-positive, non-acid-fast, periodic acid-Schiff (PAS)–positive bacillus.** | *Tropheryma whipplei.* |

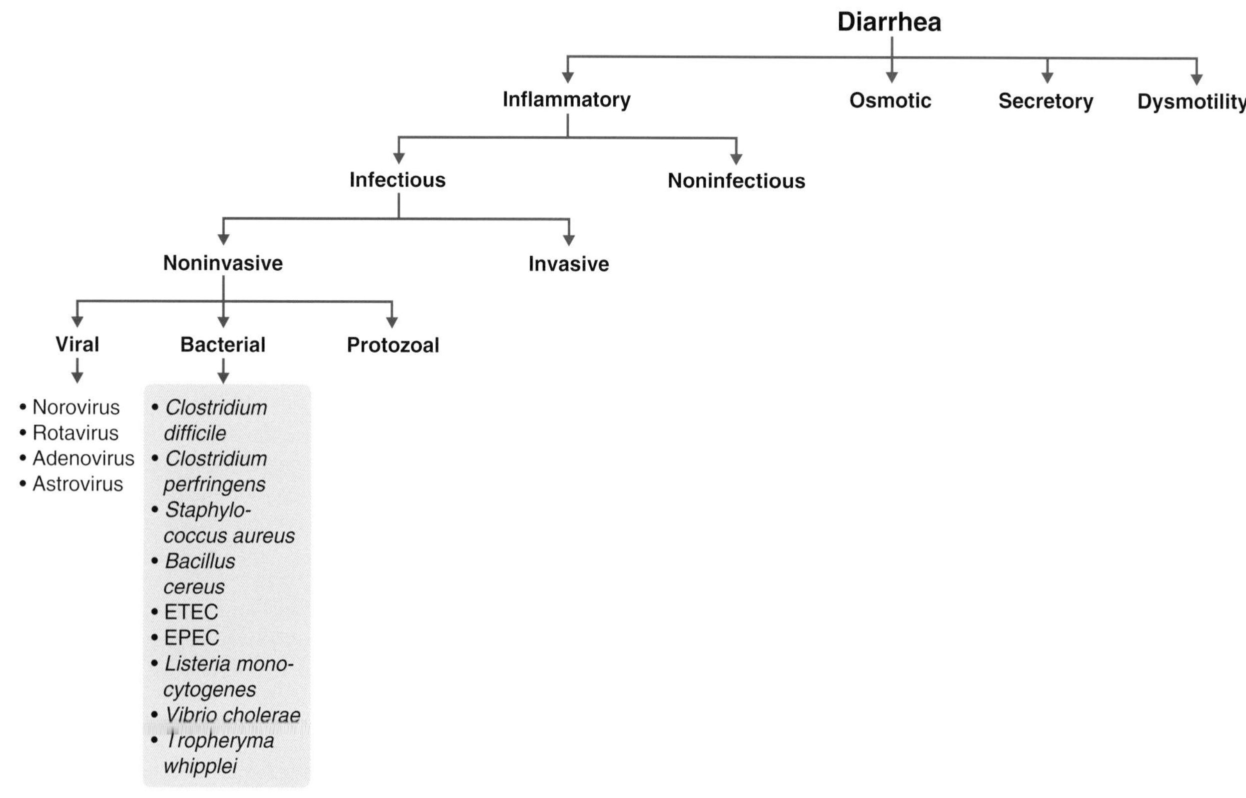

**What are the clinical features of *Clostridium difficile* colitis?**

*Clostridium difficile* colitis follows the disruption of normal intestinal bacterial flora, usually as a result of antibiotic use. Manifestations of *Clostridium difficile* colitis vary widely, from self-limited diarrhea to life-threatening bowel perforation. Severe disease is defined by the presence of leukocytosis ≥15 K/μL or serum creatinine >1.5 mg/dL. Fulminant disease refers to the presence of hypotension or shock, ileus, or megacolon. Additional manifestations of fulminant disease may include delirium, abdominal distention, marked leukocytosis (>35 K/μL), lactic acidosis, and evidence of end-organ failure. Oral vancomycin or oral fidaxomicin is the pharmacologic treatment of choice for non-severe infection, whereas oral vancomycin alone or in combination with parenteral metronidazole should be used for more severe cases. The infection is easily spread from person to person, and contact and isolation precautions should be taken.[10,11]

**What are the clinical features of *Clostridium perfringens* foodborne illness?**

*Clostridium perfringens* is a common cause of foodborne illness. Toxin-mediated symptoms typically appear 8 to 12 hours after ingestion of contaminated food and include intense abdominal cramps and watery diarrhea. The duration of illness is typically <24 hours but can be protracted in the elderly.[12]

**What is the timing of symptom onset after ingestion of food contaminated with *Staphylococcus aureus*?**

Symptoms of staphylococcal foodborne illness can begin as early as one-half hour after ingestion of contaminated food because of the presence of preformed enterotoxins (no incubation period is necessary). Nausea, vomiting, and abdominal cramps usually occur first, sometimes followed by fever and diarrhea.[13]

**What are the clinical features of *Bacillus cereus* foodborne illness?**

*Bacillus cereus* foodborne illness is associated with 2 distinct clinical presentations. The first is marked by vomiting within 30 minutes to a few hours after ingesting contaminated food, sometimes followed by abdominal cramps and diarrhea, with resolution of symptoms in less than 24 hours (similar to staphylococcal food poisoning). The second, referred to as diarrhea-type illness, is marked by watery diarrhea and abdominal cramps 6 to 15 hours after ingesting contaminated food, lasting around 24 hours (similar to *Clostridium perfringens* foodborne illness).[12]

**What are the clinical manifestations of enterotoxigenic *Escherichia coli* gastrointestinal illness?**

ETEC GI illness occurs after ingestion of contaminated food or water and is characterized by rapid onset watery diarrhea with or without abdominal pain, malaise, nausea, and vomiting. It typically occurs in travelers to developing countries, with a peak onset on the second or third day after arrival. The duration of illness is typically 1 to 3 days. A short course (1-3 days) of antibiotics can decrease the duration of illness and may be appropriate in some cases.[9,14]

**What demographic is at highest risk for enteropathogenic *Escherichia coli* gastrointestinal illness?**

Diarrheal illness caused by EPEC predominantly occurs in infants, particularly in developing countries.[9]

**What are the clinical features of *Listeria monocytogenes* gastrointestinal illness?**

*Listeria monocytogenes* is a rare cause of foodborne gastroenteritis in healthy persons, characterized by fever, watery diarrhea, arthromyalgias, and headache. Symptoms begin ≤24 hours after exposure, and the duration of illness is typically 1 to 3 days. It more commonly develops in patients with impaired cell-mediated immunity, such as neonates, pregnant women, elderly persons, and patients on chronic immunosuppressive medication, where it is frequently associated with bacteremia and meningoencephalitis.[15]

**What are the clinical features of *Vibrio cholerae* gastrointestinal illness?**

*Vibrio cholerae* causes toxin-mediated GI disease after ingestion of contaminated water. It is primarily a problem in developing countries with poor sanitation, where it is usually associated with seasonal outbreaks. Infection results in severe secretory diarrhea with a high rate of mortality, particularly in those who are untreated. Aggressive fluid resuscitation is the cornerstone of management.[16]

**What are the clinical features of Whipple disease?**

*Tropheryma whipplei* is a ubiquitous organism and the causative agent of Whipple disease, a chronic illness that develops in a minority of exposed patients. Although it has been described in patients of all ages throughout the world, there is a predilection for middle-aged white men. It often affects multiple systems, producing a variety of clinical features. The manifestations of "classic" Whipple disease are intermittent migratory arthralgias or arthritis, diarrhea, abdominal pain, and weight loss. Neurologic and cardiac involvement can occur as part of classic Whipple disease, or independently without the classic clinical picture. Diagnosis is usually made with small bowel biopsy demonstrating PAS-positive macrophages within the lamina propria. Without treatment with antibiotics, the disease is fatal. Even with treatment, there is a significant chance of recurrence.[17]

## NONINVASIVE PROTOZOAL DIARRHEA

**How is the diagnosis of protozoal gastrointestinal infection made?**

Protozoal GI infections are typically diagnosed via microscopic examination of stool specimens for the presence of ova and parasites. A variety of other methods (eg, PCR) are also available.

### What are the causes of noninvasive protozoal diarrhea?

**A flagellated organism first identified in the stool of its discoverer in the 17th century.**

*Giardia lamblia* (ie, *Giardia duodenalis* or *Giardia intestinalis*).[18]

**These 2 protozoa most commonly affect immunocompromised patients.**

*Cryptosporidium* species and *Cystoisospora belli*.

**This endemic protozoan mostly affects local populations and travelers.**

*Cyclospora cayetanensis*.

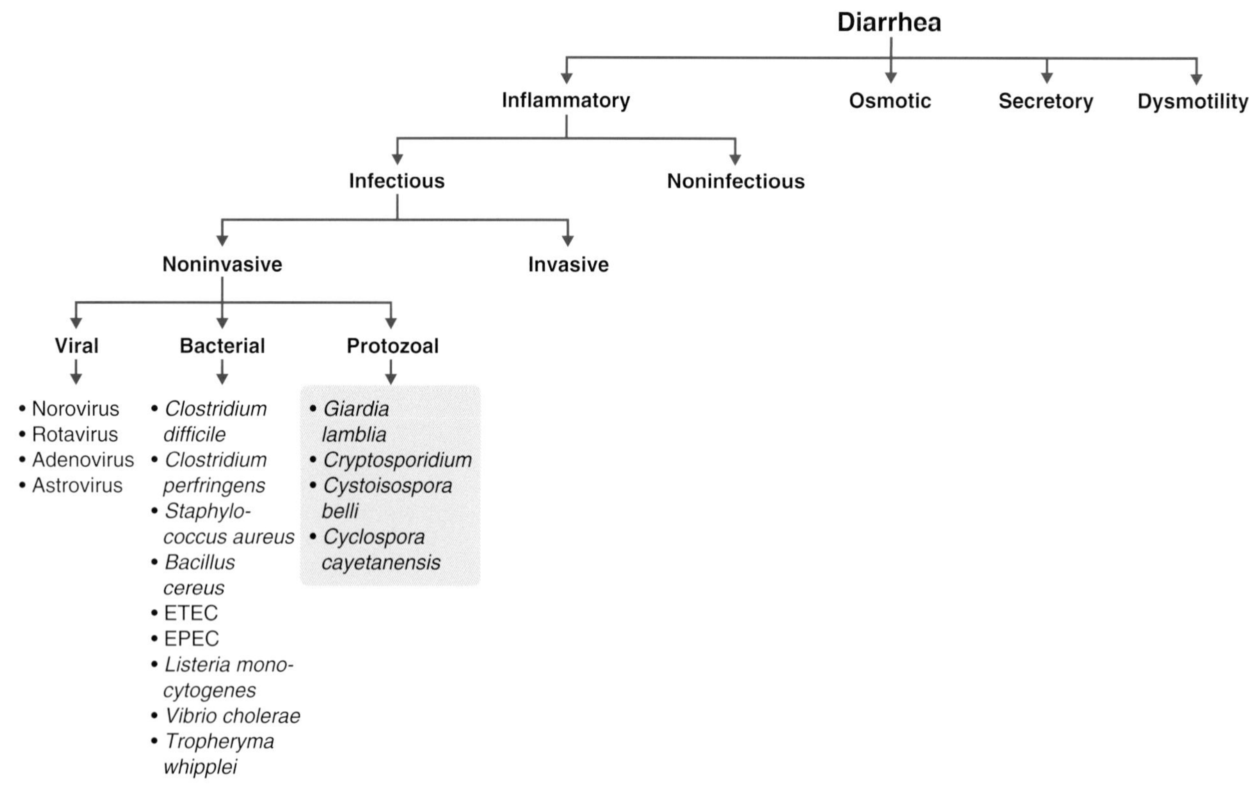

**What are the clinical features of giardiasis?**

Giardiasis is a common cause of diarrhea across the world, acquired by ingesting cysts from contaminated water or food. It affects patients of all ages, with a peak incidence in the late summer and fall. Symptoms begin 7 to 14 days after exposure. Manifestations include diarrhea, malaise, flatulence, foul-smelling and greasy stools, abdominal cramps, bloating, nausea, anorexia, and weight loss. The duration of illness is prolonged, often >14 days. A variety of diagnostic stool assays are available. Treatment options include metronidazole, tinidazole, or nitazoxanide.[18]

**What complication should be considered when a patient with human immunodeficiency virus (HIV) develops cholestatic liver injury during the course of cryptosporidiosis?**

Cryptosporidiosis in patients with HIV infection or acquired immunodeficiency syndrome (AIDS) is typically characterized by chronic diarrhea, foul-smelling and bulky stools, and weight loss. Biliary involvement (eg, sclerosing cholangitis) can occur, particularly when CD4 cell counts are <50/μL, and should be suspected when serum alkaline phosphatase levels become elevated during the course of illness. Suppressing viremia and preventing loss of CD4 cells are the cornerstone of managing cryptosporidiosis in patients with HIV. The antiparasitic agent nitazoxanide may also be beneficial. Procedural intervention may be necessary for biliary complications. In immunocompetent hosts, cryptosporidiosis presents with watery diarrhea with or without abdominal cramps, nausea, vomiting, and fever. The illness is self-limited with a typical duration of 5 to 10 days.[18]

**What are the clinical manifestations of *Cystoisospora* gastrointestinal infection?**

*Cystoisospora* most commonly infects immunocompromised patients. Its clinical course is indistinguishable from that of *Cryptosporidium*. However, unlike *Cryptosporidium*, highly effective treatment is available; patients respond promptly to trimethoprim-sulfamethoxazole.[19]

**What are the clinical features of *Cyclospora* gastrointestinal infection?**

Manifestations of *Cyclospora* infection include low-grade fever, abdominal cramps, diarrhea, anorexia, nausea, flatulence, fatigue, and weight loss. In endemic areas, children and the elderly tend to have more severe presentations, while asymptomatic infections are common in nonelderly adults. In travelers or in individuals affected by outbreaks in nonendemic areas, *Cyclospora* infection is invariably symptomatic and tends to be more severe in HIV or AIDS patients. Symptoms begin around 7 days after exposure, and untreated illness often lasts weeks to months, although is even longer in HIV or AIDS patients. Trimethoprim-sulfamethoxazole is the treatment of choice in any population with symptomatic infection, significantly shortening the duration of illness.[20]

## INVASIVE INFECTIOUS DIARRHEA

**What clinical features are suggestive of invasive infectious diarrhea?**

Invasive infectious diarrhea often presents with abdominal pain, fever, tenesmus, and bloody or mucoid stools. It is frequently associated with extraintestinal manifestations such as inflammatory arthritis and conjunctivitis.[1,3]

**How is the diagnosis of invasive bacterial gastrointestinal infection made?**

The diagnosis of invasive bacterial GI infection is typically made via culture isolation from stool; culture-independent techniques (eg, PCR) may be useful in some cases.

### What are the causes of invasive infectious diarrhea?

**Typhoidal and nontyphoidal subtypes.**

*Salmonella* species.

**A 38-year-old man develops ascending paralysis following a bout of gastroenteritis.**

*Campylobacter* species.

**Invasive strains of *Escherichia coli*.**

Enterohemorrhagic *Escherichia coli* (EHEC) and enteroinvasive *Escherichia coli* (EIEC).

**Discovered at the end of the 19th century in Japan during an investigation of an outbreak of "sekiri" (meaning "red diarrhea").**

*Shigella* species.[21]

**A 43-year-old woman develops diarrhea after consuming raw pork while vacationing in Hawaii.**

*Yersinia* species.

**A protozoan often associated with liver abscesses.**

*Entamoeba histolytica*.

**A previously healthy patient develops abdominal pain and diarrhea 1 day after consuming raw shellfish.**

*Vibrio parahaemolyticus*.

**Most symptomatic and invasive infections from this virus occur in immunocompromised hosts.**

Cytomegalovirus (CMV).

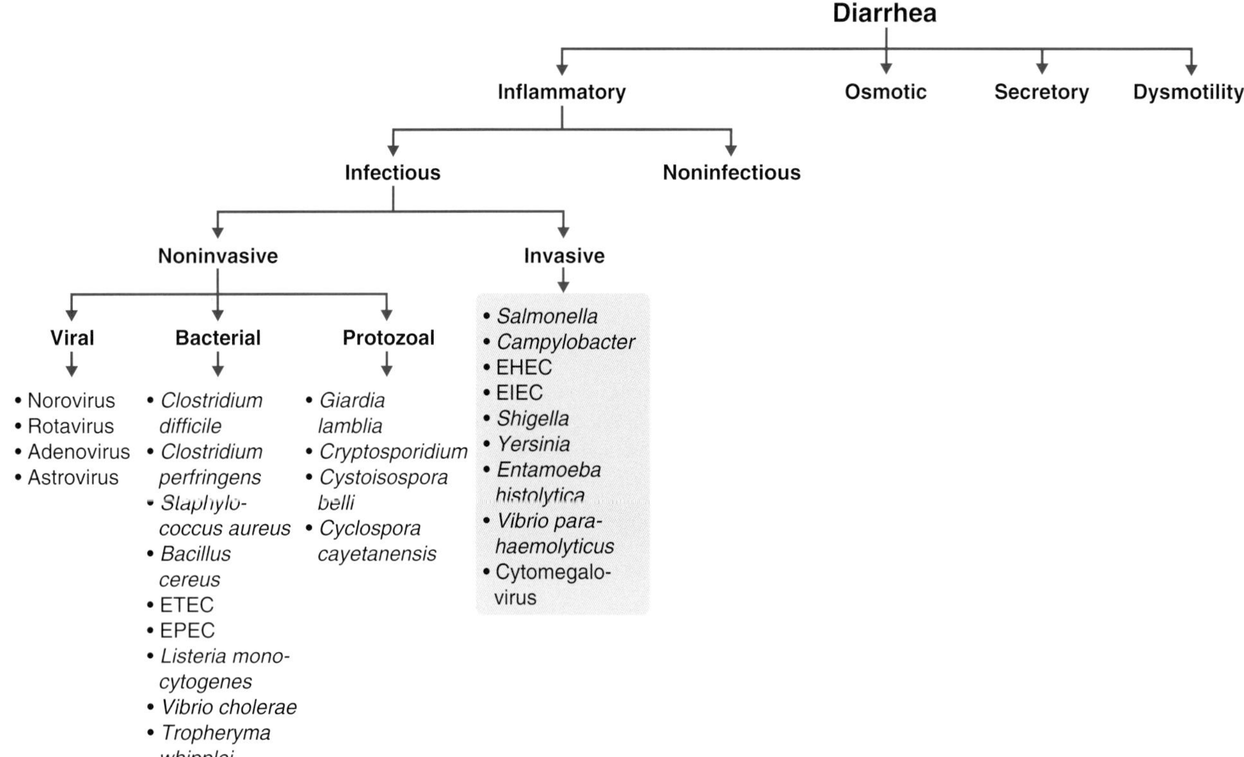


**What are the clinical features of *Salmonella* gastrointestinal infection?**

*Salmonella* species are capable of causing 2 different GI presentations: gastroenteritis and enteric fever (ie, typhoid fever or paratyphoid fever). Gastroenteritis is caused by nontyphoidal *Salmonella* and is one of the most common foodborne illnesses in the world. Manifestations include watery or bloody diarrhea, abdominal pain, nausea and vomiting, headache, and myalgias. Severity is greater in children, elderly, and immunocompromised patients. It is typically self-limited and lasts ≤10 days. Enteric fever collectively refers to typhoid fever (caused by *Salmonella enterica* serovar Typhi) and paratyphoid fever (caused by *Salmonella enterica* serovar Paratyphi), which are clinically indistinguishable. Enteric fever is transmitted via ingestion of contaminated food or water. It is uncommon in the industrialized world. Manifestations include watery or bloody diarrhea (sometimes constipation occurs instead of diarrhea), abdominal pain, headache, and fever. Complications include bradycardia, hepatomegaly, splenomegaly, pancreatitis, hepatitis, cholecystitis, and GI hemorrhage from perforation of Peyer's patches. The duration of illness is weeks to months. Antibiotics are highly effective; however, multidrug resistant strains of *Salmonella enterica* serovars Typhi and Paratyphi are on the rise.[22]

**What are the clinical features of *Campylobacter* gastroenteritis?**

*Campylobacter* gastroenteritis most often develops after ingestion of contaminated food, particularly poultry meat. Infection is common in the developing world; it occurs as outbreaks in the industrialized world. Symptoms begin 1 to 3 days after exposure. Manifestations include watery or bloody diarrhea, fever, weight loss, and abdominal cramps. It is self-limited with an average duration of 6 days. *Campylobacter* gastroenteritis can be associated with various extraintestinal manifestations, including Guillain-Barré syndrome.[23]

**What serious extraintestinal complication can occur in patients with enterohemorrhagic *Escherichia coli* gastrointestinal infection?**

EHEC infection is most often caused by *Escherichia coli* O157:H7, a Shiga toxin–producing invasive organism usually acquired via ingestion of contaminated food or water. Symptoms typically begin 3 days after ingestion but may present up to 12 days later. Early manifestations (within the first 1 to 3 days) include severe abdominal cramping, vomiting, watery diarrhea, and fever. After the initial phase, the diarrhea typically becomes bloody. The most serious complication of EHEC infection is hemolytic uremic syndrome (HUS), which is characterized by the triad of hemolytic anemia, thrombocytopenia, and acute kidney injury. It occurs in up to one-fifth of patients with EHEC infection. Use of antibiotics does not shorten the duration of illness related to EHEC infection, and there is some evidence that suggests it is associated with the development of HUS.[24]

**What are the clinical features of *Shigella* gastroenteritis?**

Shigellosis is most commonly caused by Shiga toxin–producing *Shigella dysenteriae*, transmitted via the fecal-oral route, usually as a result of person-to-person contact or ingestion of contaminated food or water. The vast majority of cases occur in developing countries. In the United States, individuals at highest risk include children in day-care centers, migrant workers, travelers to developing countries, and homosexual men. Symptoms begin 1 to 4 days after exposure, but may present up to 8 days later. Early manifestations (within the first 1 to 2 days) include fever, fatigue, malaise, anorexia, and watery diarrhea. Abdominal cramps, tenesmus, and mucoid and bloody stools follow the initial phase. Intestinal complications (eg, toxic megacolon) and extraintestinal complications (eg, HUS, seizure, reactive arthritis) can occur. In previously healthy individuals, the illness is self-limited, lasting 5 to 7 days. *EIEC illness is closely related to Shigella with indistinguishable clinical manifestations.*[21,25]

**What are the clinical features of *Yersinia* gastroenteritis?**

Yersiniosis is most commonly caused by *Yersinia enterocolitica*, usually acquired via ingestion of contaminated food, particularly undercooked or raw pork. Infections occur worldwide but are most common in European countries, with a predilection for the winter months. Symptoms begin 1 to 11 days after exposure. Typical manifestations include fever, abdominal pain, and watery or bloody diarrhea; nausea, vomiting, and pharyngitis sometimes occur. It can also present with a pseudoappendicular syndrome (a mimic of acute appendicitis), which is more common in children and young adults. Postinfectious complications are more common in adults (particularly Scandinavian women), and include reactive arthritis and erythema nodosum. In uncomplicated cases, yersiniosis is self-limited and typically lasts 5 to 14 days.[26]

**What are the clinical features of *Entamoeba histolytica* gastrointestinal infection?**

Intestinal amebiasis develops after ingestion of contaminated food or water. It occurs worldwide but is more common in developing countries. Infection is often asymptomatic. Clinical manifestations are insidious in onset, typically occurring over weeks, and include cramping abdominal pain, weight loss, and watery or bloody diarrhea. Severe manifestations include necrotizing colitis, toxic megacolon, ameboma (a mass of colonic granulation tissue), and perianal ulceration. Metronidazole is the treatment of choice. Amebic liver abscess is the most common extraintestinal manifestation; it is significantly more common in men than women or children.[27]

**What are the clinical manifestations of *Vibrio parahaemolyticus* gastroenteritis?**

*Vibrio parahaemolyticus* lives in marine or estuarine environments, typically causing gastroenteritis when contaminated seafood is ingested. It is a worldwide disease; in the United States, it occurs in foodborne outbreaks. Symptoms typically begin 17 hours after exposure (range 4-90 hours). Watery or bloody diarrhea is the most frequent symptom and may be accompanied by abdominal cramps, nausea, and vomiting. The illness is self-limited, lasting on average 2.5 days (range 8 hours to 12 days).[28]

**What are the clinical features of cytomegalovirus infection of the gastrointestinal tract?**

CMV infection of the GI tract most often affects immunocompromised patients such as those with HIV infection or AIDS and those on chronic immunosuppressive medication. Although clinical manifestations are more severe in immunocompromised individuals, it does occur in immunocompetent hosts. CMV can affect any part of the GI tract, but the colon is most commonly involved. Manifestations include abdominal pain, fever, weight loss, and watery or bloody diarrhea. Ulcerative and erosive lesions are frequently observed on endoscopic evaluation; biopsy is necessary to confirm the diagnosis. CMV colitis cannot be excluded based on a negative plasma or whole blood PCR test. Patients with symptomatic CMV GI disease should be treated with antiviral therapy.[29,30]

## NONINFECTIOUS INFLAMMATORY DIARRHEA

### What are the causes of noninfectious inflammatory diarrhea?

**Look for extraintestinal manifestations such as erythema nodosum (Figure 15-3).**

Inflammatory bowel disease.

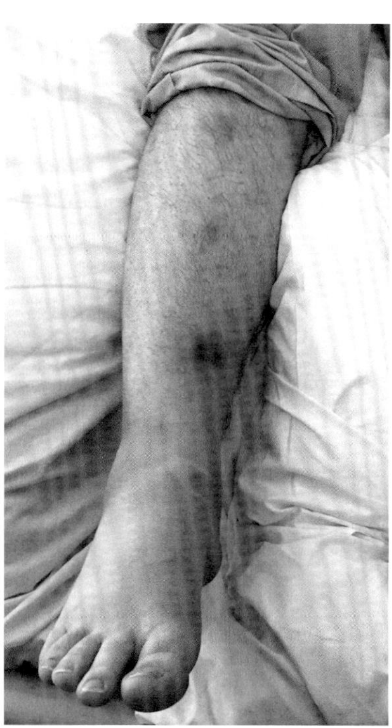

**Figure 15-3.** Erythema nodosum on the lower extremity of a patient with an acute flare of inflammatory bowel disease.

**An 80-year-old woman presents with mild left lower quadrant abdominal pain and bloody diarrhea, and is found to have a blood pressure of 88/55 mm Hg.**

Ischemic colitis.

***Streptococcus bovis* endocarditis.**

Colorectal cancer (CRC).

**Look for tattoo marks around the abdominal area.**

External beam radiation therapy.

**A previously healthy 36-year-old woman presents with several months of nausea and vomiting, diarrhea, and painful neuropathy; her husband recently increased her life insurance policy.**

Arsenic poisoning.

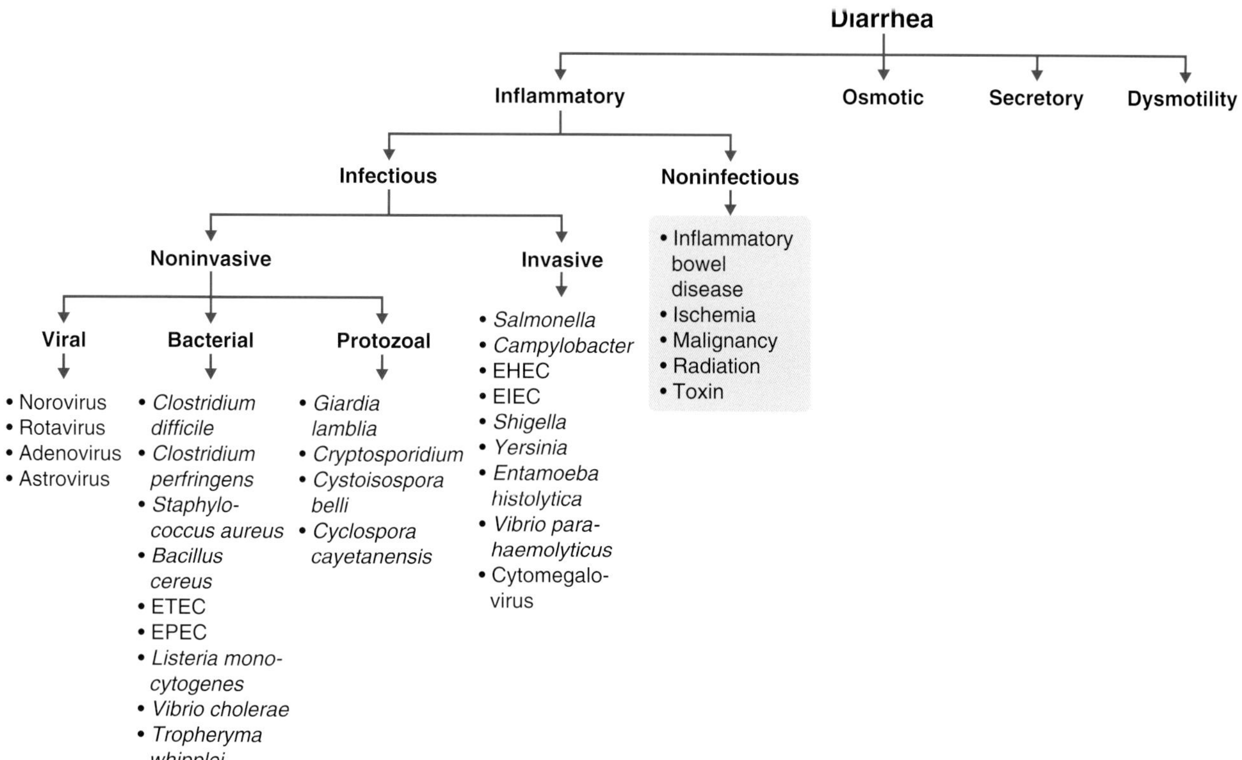


**What must be ruled out in any patient with a history of inflammatory bowel disease who presents with a flare?**

When patients with IBD present with acute symptoms, infectious enterocolitis must be ruled out with stool evaluation. Enteric infection can be found in 10% of these patients, and the most common agent is *Clostridium difficile*.[31]

**What findings on cross-sectional imaging can help distinguish ischemic colitis from other causes of colitis, including infection and inflammatory bowel disease?**

Computed tomography (CT) imaging can be a valuable tool in working up patients with diarrhea, particularly when it is bloody. Intestinal wall thickening and fat stranding on CT imaging are common features of enterocolitis, regardless of underlying etiology. Ischemic colitis is suggested when these changes occur in a vascular or "watershed" distribution (eg, distal transverse colon and distal descending colon) (see Figure 18-3).[32]

**What are the risk factors for colorectal cancer?**

CRC is one of the most common cancers in the world. The lifetime risk of CRC in the average American is 1 in 20. Nonmodifiable risk factors include age, family history of CRC, and IBD. Modifiable risk factors include alcohol use, obesity, smoking, and consuming processed and red meats.[33]

**How long after external beam radiation therapy do patients develop radiation enteropathy?**

Radiation enteropathy is a common side effect of external beam radiation therapy used to treat abdominal and pelvic cancers. Incidence is directly related to the dose of radiation received. Most cases are acute, occurring at the time of or shortly after therapy (within 90 days postradiation), and are generally reversible. However, delayed-onset radiation enteropathy can develop beyond 90 days postradiation (up to decades later) and is typically not reversible.[34]

**What are the characteristics of diarrhea associated with arsenic toxicity?**

Acute arsenic toxicity results in voluminous diarrhea similar to that caused by cholera, except it is bloody. It is described as "bloody rice water" diarrhea. It can result in death from hypovolemic shock. The diarrhea of chronic arsenic toxicity is intermittent and may be associated with vomiting. Arsenic poisoning should be suspected when other characteristic extraintestinal manifestations are present, including dermatologic manifestations (eg, diffuse hyperpigmentation, palmar keratosis) and neurologic manifestations (eg, peripheral neuropathy). *Hair sample analysis can reveal the timeline of arsenic exposure.*[35]

## OSMOTIC DIARRHEA

**What is the fundamental mechanism of osmotic diarrhea?**

Osmotically active particles can accumulate in the intestinal lumen as a result of ingestion of nonabsorbable substances, maldigestion, or malabsorption, generating an osmotic gradient that favors the movement of fluid into the lumen, resulting in diarrhea.[3]

**What historical features are suggestive of osmotic diarrhea?**

The volume of osmotic diarrhea decreases during periods of fasting, including at night. Weight loss and steatorrhea are clues to the presence of maldigestion or malabsorption. Steatorrhea describes greasy, bulky, and malodorous stools that are difficult to flush, often leaving an oil residue on the toilet bowl.[3,36]

**What stool study is suggestive of osmotic diarrhea?**

Osmotic diarrhea is associated with an elevated stool osmotic gap (the difference between measured and calculated osmolality of stool fluid). Stool osmolality can be directly measured, or assumed to be 290 mOsm/kg (similar to serum osmolality). Because stool fluid is normally electroneutral, osmolality is calculated by multiplying the sum of sodium and potassium concentrations of stool fluid by a factor of 2 (to account for the anions). Stool osmotic gap = measured osmolality – (2 × [Na + K]). An osmotic gap >50 mOsm/kg suggests the presence of osmotically active substances in stool fluid. An osmotic gap <50 mOsm/kg suggests a secretory process.[3,37,38]

**In which setting should stool osmolality be directly measured (rather than assumed to be 290 mOsm/kg)?**

When factitious diarrhea is suspected, and there is a possibility that the stool sample has been surreptitiously diluted, stool osmolality should be directly measured. Stool osmolality that is unexpectedly high (eg, >600 mOsm/kg) suggests that the sample was likely an admixture of stool and urine.[5,39]

**Which test is used to investigate osmotic diarrhea related to malabsorption?**

Small intestine malabsorption is suggested by a positive D-xylose absorption test. The patient is given a dose of D-xylose, and its concentrations in serum and urine are subsequently measured. If serum and urine levels of D-xylose are abnormally low, it suggests small intestine malabsorption. False positive results can occur in patients with renal dysfunction and small bowel bacterial overgrowth. Because pancreatic enzymes are not necessary for the absorption of xylose, this test is unreliable for the detection of malabsorption caused by pancreatic insufficiency.[40]

### What are the causes of osmotic diarrhea?

**A patient complains of recurrent diarrhea within a few hours of consuming dairy products.**

Lactose intolerance.

**Used to treat constipation but sometimes abused.**

Laxatives.

**A 23-year-old man complains of watery diarrhea after he eats his favorite sugar-free candy.**

Ingestion of a sugar alcohol (eg, sorbitol).

| | |
|---|---|
| **The small intestine normally contains fewer bacteria than the large intestine.** | Small intestinal bacterial overgrowth. |
| **Villous atrophy is the hallmark histologic finding of this autoimmune condition.** | Celiac disease. |
| **An extrapulmonary sequela of cystic fibrosis.** | Pancreatic exocrine insufficiency. |
| **Look for surgical scars.** | Short bowel syndrome. |
| **Impaired enterohepatic circulation.** | Cholerheic diarrhea. |
| **A disease of the tropics, affecting both indigenous populations and travelers who stay for more than a few weeks.** | Tropical sprue. |

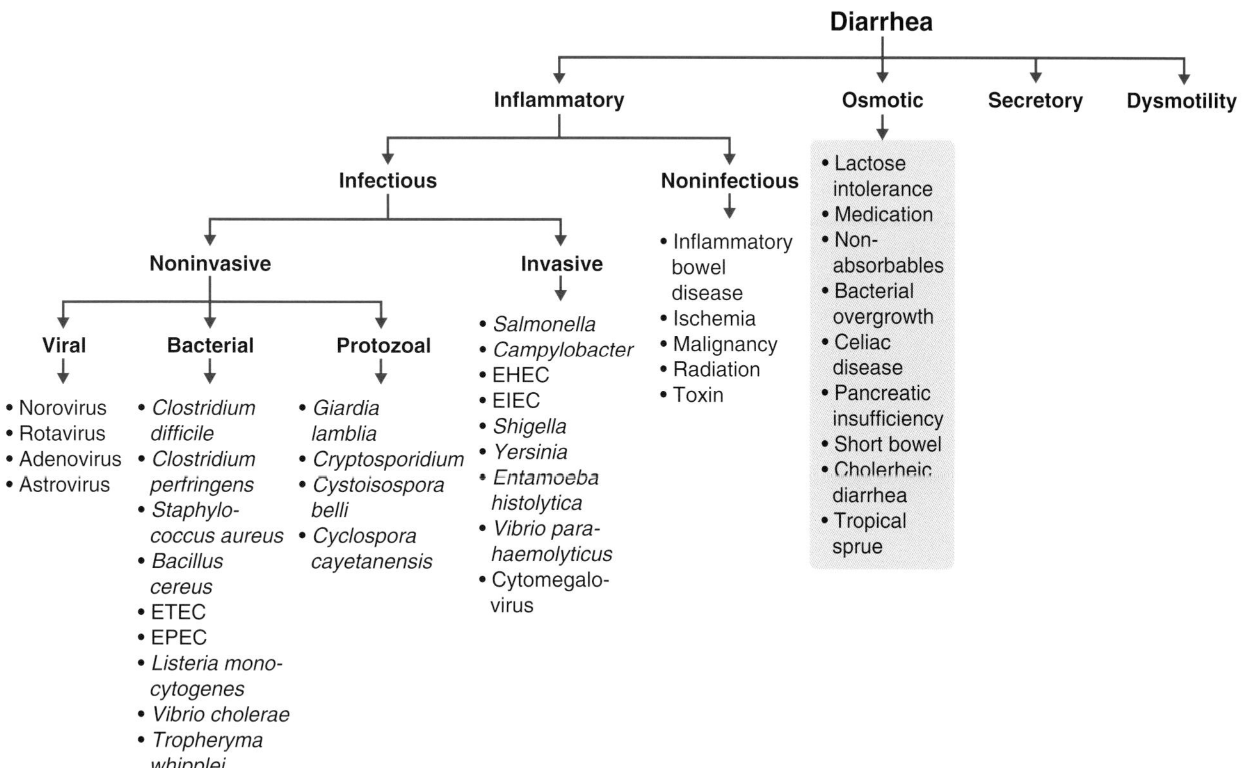


| | |
|---|---|
| **How is lactose intolerance diagnosed?** | Digestion of dietary lactose requires the enzyme lactase-phlorizin hydrolase (ie, lactase), which is present on the apical surface of enterocytes of the small intestine. Lactase hydrolyzes lactose to produce glucose and galactose, which can then be absorbed by intestinal enterocytes. The activity of lactase declines in most individuals after infancy, resulting in lactose malabsorption, but only some will develop symptoms (ie, lactose intolerance). Lactose intolerance occurs when undigested lactose is fermented in the colon, producing symptoms such as abdominal pain, bloating, flatulence, diarrhea, and borborygmi. A presumptive diagnosis can be made in patients with a compatible clinical history. The lactose hydrogen breath test detects the production of hydrogen from lactose fermentation and can confirm the diagnosis in most patients.[41] |
| **What medications can cause osmotic diarrhea?** | Medications that cause osmotic diarrhea include antibiotics (eg, ampicillin, clindamycin), enteral feeding formulas, laxatives (eg, magnesium salts, polyethylene glycol, lactulose), prebiotics, methyldopa, quinidine, propranolol, hydralazine, angiotensin-converting enzyme inhibitors, and procainamide.[5] |

**What sugar alcohols are commonly used as artificial sweeteners?**

Sugar alcohols are often used as artificial sweeteners, including sorbitol, mannitol, xylitol, erythritol, lactitol, maltitol, and glycerol. Sorbitol-containing excipients are included in many pharmaceutical agents. Diarrhea can develop by consuming as little as 10 g/d of sorbitol.[5]

**How is small intestinal bacterial overgrowth managed?**

Small intestinal bacterial overgrowth is associated with a number of underlying conditions, including anatomic abnormalities (eg, small intestinal diverticulosis, strictures in patients with Crohn's disease, surgery) and abnormal small intestinal motility (eg, diabetes, scleroderma, hypothyroidism, amyloidosis, radiation enteritis). The principles of management include treatment of the underlying condition (if possible), eradication of overgrowth with antibiotics, and correction of associated nutritional deficiencies.[42]

**What are the clinical features of celiac disease?**

The most common symptoms of celiac disease are chronic diarrhea, weight loss, and abdominal distention. Other manifestations include iron deficiency, abdominal pain, aphthous stomatitis, aminotransferase elevation, and chronic fatigue. Patients who do not have IgA deficiency (which is associated with celiac disease) should be tested for the presence of serum IgA anti–tissue transglutaminase, which is associated with high sensitivity and specificity. False positives may occur in patients with other autoimmune conditions (eg, type 1 diabetes mellitus). In patients with IgA deficiency, IgG anti–tissue transglutaminase antibodies should be measured instead. Measurement of IgA anti-endomysial antibodies may be helpful in patients with borderline anti–tissue transglutaminase levels or in those who might have false positive results. The diagnosis is definitively established with biopsy of the small intestine.[43]

**What are the causes of pancreatic exocrine insufficiency?**

Pancreatic exocrine insufficiency most commonly occurs as a result of pancreatic parenchymal disease (eg, chronic pancreatitis, cystic fibrosis, necrotizing acute pancreatitis, pancreatic resection), pancreatic duct obstruction (eg, tumor, stricture), or inadequate stimulation of pancreatic enzyme secretion (eg, small bowel resection, celiac disease). The gold standard diagnostic test is 72-hour fecal fat quantification; however, this test is inconvenient. Fecal elastase-1 measurement can be used to make the diagnosis instead. When results are equivocal but clinical suspicion persists, direct tests of pancreatic exocrine function can be performed (eg, pancreatic stimulation with secretin or cerulein).[44]

**What is short bowel syndrome?**

Short bowel syndrome describes malabsorption that occurs after small intestine resection. The normal length of small intestine varies from 275 to 850 cm and is generally longer in men. Malabsorption typically develops when <200 cm of small intestine remains. Common reasons for short bowel syndrome include Crohn's disease, superior mesenteric artery thrombosis, and radiation enteritis. It is more common in women by a ratio of 2:1 likely because, compared to men, women have a shorter length of small intestine.[45]

**What is cholerheic diarrhea?**

Bile acids produced in the liver and secreted into the small intestine are normally reabsorbed in the terminal ileum for reuse (ie, enterohepatic circulation). Cholerheic diarrhea occurs when bile acids are not effectively reabsorbed in the ileum and reach the colon, where their presence leads to diarrhea by stimulating colonic electrolyte and water secretion and increasing colonic motility. Conditions associated with bile acid malabsorption include cholecystectomy, ileal inflammation or resection (usually related to Crohn's disease), small intestinal bacterial overgrowth, and pancreatic insufficiency. Bile acid sequestrants, such as cholestyramine, are an effective treatment option for most patients.[46]

**What type of anemia is found in patients with tropical sprue?**

Tropical sprue is an acquired malabsorptive syndrome endemic to certain regions of the world, including parts of Asia, some Caribbean islands, and parts of Latin America, affecting indigenous populations and travelers. It is thought to be infectious in nature. Patients develop chronic diarrhea, anorexia, weight loss, and megaloblastic anemia from vitamin B12 or folate deficiency, which can be an important clue to the diagnosis. Treatment with tetracycline is highly effective.[47]

## SECRETORY DIARRHEA

**What is the fundamental mechanism of secretory diarrhea?**

Secretory diarrhea occurs as a result of the secretion of excess isotonic fluid into the intestine.[3]

**What historical features can be suggestive of secretory diarrhea?**

The volume of secretory diarrhea, which is typically high, does not change during periods of fasting, including at night. Watery diarrhea is typical; the presence of steatorrhea or blood is unusual.[3]

**What stool study is suggestive of secretory diarrhea?**

A stool osmotic gap <50 mOsm/kg is suggestive of secretory diarrhea.[3,37,38]

### What are the causes of secretory diarrhea?

**A patient develops diarrhea after starting treatment for an acute gout flare.**

Colchicine.

**A neuroendocrine tumor that secretes serotonin.**

Carcinoid.

**A neuroendocrine tumor that secretes gastrin.**

Gastrinoma.

**A neuroendocrine tumor that secretes glucagon.**

Glucagonoma.

**A neuroendocrine tumor that secretes vasoactive intestinal peptide (VIP).**

VIPoma.

**Excess histamine.**

Systemic mastocytosis.

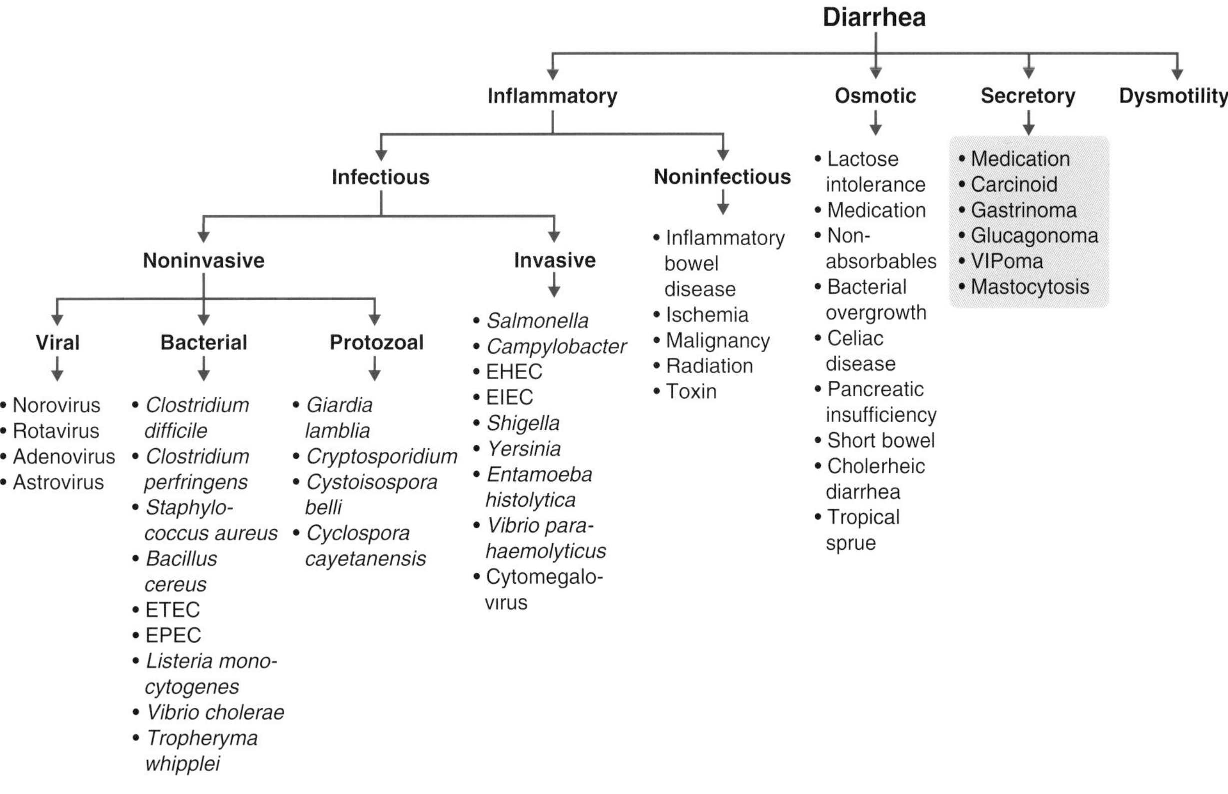


**What medications can cause secretory diarrhea?**

Numerous medications can cause secretory diarrhea, some of which include antibiotics (eg, amoxicillin-clavulanate), laxatives (eg, senna glycoside, bisacodyl), caffeine, digoxin, carbamazepine, calcitonin, cimetidine, chemotherapeutic agents (eg, idarubicin), and metformin.[5]

**What is carcinoid syndrome?**

Carcinoid syndrome occurs when serotonin and other vasoactive substances secreted by neuroendocrine tumors reach the systemic circulation, resulting in characteristic clinical manifestations such as abdominal pain, diarrhea, and episodic facial flushing.[48]

**What are the clinical features of gastrinoma?**

Gastrinomas cause gastric acid hypersecretion, which leads to abdominal pain, gastroesophageal reflux disease, peptic ulcer disease, and chronic diarrhea. Around one-half of gastrinomas are malignant. Diagnostic laboratory tests include fasting serum gastrin level and the secretin stimulation test.[49]

**What are the clinical features of glucagonoma?**

Glucagonomas are associated with glucose intolerance and a skin rash characterized by painful and pruritic erythematous plaques that are well-demarcated and often located in intertriginous areas (necrolytic migratory erythema). Chronic diarrhea is present in some patients. Most glucagonomas are malignant. Elevated plasma glucagon level >1000 pg/mL is diagnostic.[49]

**What are the clinical features of VIPoma?**

VIPomas are associated with intermittent, severe, watery diarrhea, sometimes in excess of 5 L/d, which leads to hypokalemia and metabolic acidosis in most patients. Most VIPomas are malignant. Elevated plasma VIP level is diagnostic. However, VIP secretion is often episodic and may be missed with a single measurement.[49]

**How common are gastrointestinal symptoms in patients with systemic mastocytosis?**

Mastocytosis refers to the proliferation of mast cells within the skin (cutaneous mastocytosis) or extracutaneous tissues (systemic mastocytosis) with or without skin involvement. The vast majority of patients with systemic mastocytosis experience GI symptoms, the most common of which are abdominal pain and diarrhea. In patients with mastocytosis, the release of mast cell mediators can be precipitated by various stimuli, including medication (eg, nonsteroidal anti-inflammatory drugs), alcohol, and stress. Avoiding triggers is a critical part of management; a variety of pharmacologic agents can also be used to treat the GI symptoms of mastocytosis, including antihistamines, cromolyn, antileukotriene drugs (eg, montelukast), and budesonide.[50]

## DIARRHEA RELATED TO INTESTINAL DYSMOTILITY

**What are the mechanisms of diarrhea related to intestinal dysmotility?**

Hypermotility decreases transit time of intestinal contents, preventing reabsorption of fluid in the small intestine and overwhelming the absorptive capacity of the large intestine. Hypomotility is associated with the development of small intestinal bacterial overgrowth.[3]

**What historical features can be suggestive of diarrhea related to dysmotility?**

Intestinal dysmotility often produces small-volume, high-frequency stools. Steatorrhea is common, although the presence of blood suggests an alternative mechanism. Dysmotility is often a symptom of a systemic disease (eg, diabetes mellitus) that can frequently be recognized by the presence of characteristic extraintestinal manifestations.[3]

### What are the causes of diarrhea related to intestinal dysmotility?

**One of the most common GI conditions, present in up to one-fifth of the general population.**

Irritable bowel syndrome (IBS).[51]

**A 34-year-old woman develops diarrhea after starting treatment for myasthenia gravis.**

Acetylcholinesterase inhibitor.

**Gastroparesis is the more typical GI manifestation of this common systemic disease.**

Diabetes mellitus.

**A 36-year-old woman with diarrhea, weight loss, rapid heart rate, and fine tremor.**

Thyrotoxicosis

**A 48-year-old woman with sclerodactyly, Raynaud's phenomenon, and dysphagia.**

Scleroderma (ie, systemic sclerosis).

**A 56-year-old man with weight loss, autonomic dysfunction, nephrotic syndrome, and elevated serum protein gap.**

Amyloidosis.

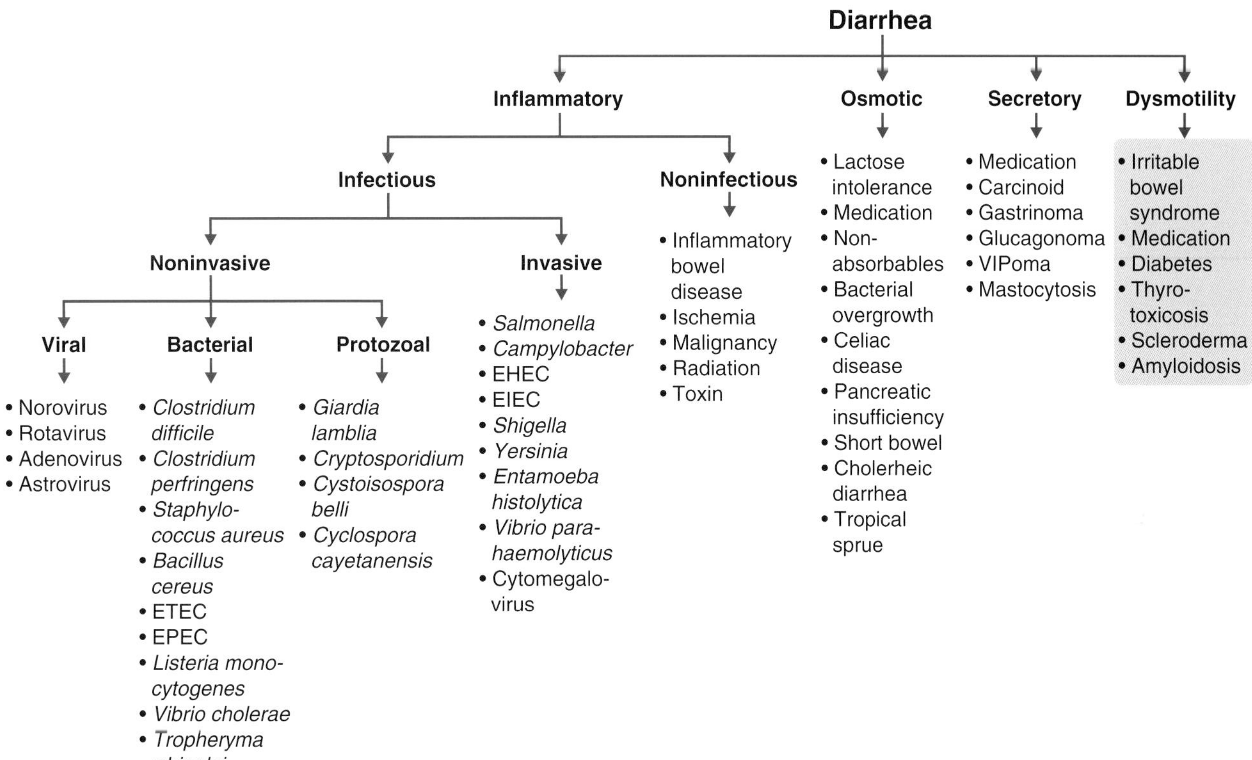


**What is irritable bowel syndrome?**

IBS is a symptom-based condition characterized by abdominal pain and altered bowel habits, including constipation, diarrhea, or both. It is a chronic condition in most patients, but symptoms may vary over time. IBS is somewhat of a diagnosis of exclusion; concerning clinical features should always be investigated to rule out more harmful conditions. Concerning features include the onset of symptoms after 50 years of age, unexplained weight loss, family history of organic GI disease (eg, colon cancer, IBD), GI bleeding, or unexplained iron-deficiency anemia.[51]

**What medications can cause diarrhea related to dysmotility?**

Medications that can cause diarrhea related to dysmotility include acetylcholinesterase inhibitors (eg, pyridostigmine), cholinergics (eg, bethanechol), prokinetic agents (eg, metoclopramide, cisapride), macrolides (eg, erythromycin), and colchicine.[5]

**What are the clinical features of the diarrhea caused by diabetes mellitus?**

Diabetes mellitus more often presents with symptoms and signs of hypomotility, such as gastroparesis. However, diarrhea occurs in up to one-fifth of patients with diabetes as a result of dysmotility, small intestinal bacterial overgrowth, and pancreatic exocrine insufficiency. It is watery or fatty in nature and tends to be intermittent, often separated by periods of normal bowel movements or constipation. It most often occurs in middle-aged diabetics with long-standing and poorly-controlled disease; most patients have concurrent peripheral neuropathy and evidence of autonomic dysfunction elsewhere (eg, bladder dysfunction). Treatment is often unsatisfactory.[52]

**How common is diarrhea in patients with thyrotoxicosis?**

Up to one-quarter of patients with thyrotoxicosis experience diarrhea, which is usually small-volume but high-frequency. Steatorrhea is present in some. Patients with Graves' disease have an increased risk of concurrent celiac disease. In addition to addressing the underlying disease, β-antagonists (eg, propranolol) can be effective in treating the diarrhea of thyrotoxicosis.[53]

**How common is diarrhea in patients with systemic sclerosis?**

The vast majority of patients with systemic sclerosis have GI involvement. Symptoms and signs of hypomotility such as constipation are common. Diarrhea is also common and is mostly the result of small intestinal bacterial overgrowth related to intestinal stasis. Patients often complain of alternating episodes of constipation and diarrhea. Because of anorectal involvement, fecal incontinence is also common in these patients.[54]

**How common is diarrhea in patients with amyloidosis?**

Amyloidosis more often presents with symptoms and signs of hypomotility. However, chronic diarrhea occurs in up to 15% of patients with amyloidosis, as a result of dysmotility, intestinal inflammation, and small intestinal bacterial overgrowth. It can be treated with loperamide or octreotide. Intractable diarrhea is associated with poor survival; less than one-half of patients are alive after 5 years.[55]

## Case Summary

A 58-year-old man presents with chronic voluminous watery diarrhea, weight loss, facial flushing, and dyspnea and is found to have a murmur on examination and numerous lesions of the liver on cross-sectional imaging.

***What is the most likely cause of diarrhea in this patient?***

Carcinoid syndrome.

### BONUS QUESTIONS

***What features in this case are consistent with secretory diarrhea?***

Persistent voluminous watery diarrhea despite fasting is characteristic of secretory diarrhea. The stool osmotic gap <50 mOsm/kg in this case is also consistent with the diagnosis.

***Where are most carcinoid tumors located in the body?***

Carcinoid tumors describe well-differentiated neuroendocrine tumors. Most are located in the GI tract (particularly the small intestine) or lung. Carcinoid syndrome occurs in up to one-half of patients with carcinoid tumors of the GI tract but in only 5% of those with bronchial tumors.[48]

***Why does carcinoid syndrome suggest the presence of liver metastases?***

When carcinoid tumors are limited to the GI tract, vasoactive substances are secreted into the portal circulation and subsequently inactivated by the liver, preventing carcinoid syndrome from developing. When there is hepatic involvement, vasoactive substances are secreted directly into the systemic circulation, which is necessary for the syndrome to develop.[48]

***What are the clinical features of carcinoid syndrome?***

Flushing is the most common manifestation of carcinoid syndrome, occurring in the vast majority of patients. It is intermittent, sudden in onset, typically involves the face and upper trunk, and lasts 5 to 10 minutes. Diarrhea occurs in most patients. Flushing and diarrhea can be triggered by stress, alcohol, and certain foods (eg, chocolate, walnut, banana, pineapple, tomato, plum, avocado). Around one-half of patients experience abdominal pain, particularly after large meals. Other manifestations include wheezing (more common in patients with bronchial tumors), weight loss, and features of right-sided heart failure.[48]

***What is the significance of the heart murmur in this case?***

The vasoactive substances released by carcinoid tumors cause endocardial fibrotic plaques, involving structures such as valves and subvalvular apparati, which become distorted, leading to stenosis, regurgitation, or both. The left-sided valves are spared in the vast majority of cases because the lungs inactivate the vasoactive substances before they reach the left side of the heart. The decrescendo diastolic murmur in this case could be consistent with either aortic or pulmonic regurgitation. However, the presence of Carvallo's sign (murmur intensity increases with inspiration), which is indicative of right-sided valvular lesions, suggests pulmonic regurgitation. *For an audio/video demonstration of Carvallo's sign, see the associated reference.*[56,57]

***What is the most useful initial diagnostic laboratory test for carcinoid syndrome?***

Serotonin secreted by carcinoid tumors is metabolized to 5-HIAA; urinary excretion of 5-HIAA can be measured with a random urine test or a 24-hour urine collection, both of which are associated with excellent sensitivity and specificity (diet must be free of tyramine for >24 hours before urine collection). A positive urinary 5-HIAA test should be followed by measurement of serum chromogranin A and an octreotide scan to confirm the diagnosis and stage the disease. In this case, the octreotide scan shows areas of normal radiotracer uptake (eg, bladder, kidneys, spleen), but there is a focus of increased uptake in the region of the small intestine (the primary tumor site), and multiple globular foci of increased uptake in the liver, which confirms the presence of liver metastases.[48]

***How is carcinoid syndrome managed?***

The symptoms of carcinoid syndrome can be abated in most patients with somatostatin analogues (eg, octreotide), or interferon alfa. Depending on the stage of disease, surgical tumor removal can be offered and is potentially curative.[48]

## KEY POINTS

- Diarrhea describes an increase in water content, volume, or frequency of stools, typically occurring at least 3 times in a 24-hour period.
- Acute diarrhea lasts ≤14 days; persistent diarrhea lasts >14 days; and chronic diarrhea lasts >30 days.
- Diarrhea can be inflammatory, osmotic, secretory, or related to intestinal dysmotility.
- Inflammatory diarrhea can be infectious or noninfectious.
- Infectious diarrhea can be noninvasive or invasive.
- Noninvasive infectious diarrhea can be viral, bacterial, or protozoal.
- Historical features such as exposures (eg, medications, travel history), time course (eg, acute, chronic), and stool characteristics (eg, watery, bloody, fatty) are helpful in determining the etiology of diarrhea.
- Infection is the most common cause of acute diarrhea; chronicity should broaden the investigative focus.
- Inflammatory diarrhea caused by either invasive infections or noninfectious conditions is associated with the presence of polymorphonuclear leukocytes or leukocyte proteins in stool.
- Persistence of diarrhea despite fasting suggests a secretory cause.
- The stool osmotic gap can be helpful in distinguishing between osmotic (gap >50 mOsm/kg) and secretory (gap <50 mOsm/kg) diarrhea.

## REFERENCES


1. Guerrant RL, Van Gilder T, Steiner TS, et al. Practice guidelines for the management of infectious diarrhea. *Clin Infect Dis*. 2001;32(3):331-351.
2. Musher DM, Musher BL. Contagious acute gastrointestinal infections. *N Engl J Med*. 2004;351(23):2417-2427.
3. Camilleri M. Chronic diarrhea: a review on pathophysiology and management for the clinical gastroenterologist. *Clin Gastroenterol Hepatol*. 2004;2(3):198-206.
4. Agarwal R, Afzalpurkar R, Fordtran JS. Pathophysiology of potassium absorption and secretion by the human intestine. *Gastroenterology*. 1994;107(2):548-571.
5. Philip NA, Ahmed N, Pitchumoni CS. Spectrum of drug-induced chronic diarrhea. *J Clin Gastroenterol*. 2017;51(2):111-117.
6. Autenrieth DM, Baumgart DC. Toxic megacolon. *Inflamm Bowel Dis*. 2012;18(3):584-591.
7. Blacklow NR, Greenberg HB. Viral gastroenteritis. *N Engl J Med*. 1991;325(4):252-264.
8. Bosch A, Pinto RM, Guix S. Human astroviruses. *Clin Microbiol Rev*. 2014;27(4):1048-1074.
9. Baron S, ed. *Medical Microbiology*. 4th ed. Galveston, TX: University of Texas Medical Branch at Galveston; 1996.
10. Ong GK, Reidy TJ, Huk MD, Lane FR. Clostridium difficile colitis: a clinical review. *Am J Surg*. 2017;213(3):565-571.
11. McDonald LC, Gerding DN, Johnson S, et al. Clinical practice guidelines for Clostridium difficile infection in adults and children: 2017 update by the Infectious Diseases Society of America (IDSA) and Society for Healthcare Epidemiology of America (SHEA). *Clin Infect Dis*. 2018;66(7):987-994.
12. Le Loir Y, Baron F, Gautier M. *Staphylococcus aureus* and food poisoning. *Genet Mol Res*. 2003;2(1):63-76.
13. Balaban N, Rasooly A. *Staphylococcal* enterotoxins. *Int J Food Microbiol*. 2000;61(1):1-10.
14. Barrett J, Brown M. Travellers' diarrhoea. *BMJ*. 2016;353:i1937.
15. Ooi ST, Lorber B. Gastroenteritis due to *Listeria monocytogenes*. *Clin Infect Dis*. 2005;40(9):1327-1332.
16. Faruque SM, Albert MJ, Mekalanos JJ. Epidemiology, genetics, and ecology of toxigenic *Vibrio cholerae*. *Microbiol Mol Biol Rev*. 1998;62(4):1301-1314.
17. Fenollar F, Puechal X, Raoult D. Whipple's disease. *N Engl J Med*. 2007;356(1):55-66.
18. Huang DB, White AC. An updated review on *Cryptosporidium* and *Giardia*. *Gastroenterol Clin North Am*. 2006;35(2):291-314, viii.
19. Gellin BG, Soave R. Coccidian infections in AIDS. Toxoplasmosis, cryptosporidiosis, and isosporiasis. *Med Clin North Am*. 1992;76(1):205-234.
20. Ortega YR, Sanchez R. Update on *Cyclospora cayetanensis*, a food-borne and waterborne parasite. *Clin Microbiol Rev*. 2010;23(1):218-234.
21. Niyogi SK. Shigellosis. *J Microbiol*. 2005;43(2):133-143.
22. Eng SK, Pusparajah P, Mutalib NS, Ser HL, Chan KG, Lee LH. Salmonella: a review on pathogenesis, epidemiology and antibiotic resistance. *Front Life Sci*. 2015;8(3):284-293.
23. Kaakoush NO, Castano-Rodriguez N, Mitchell HM, Man SM. Global epidemiology of *Campylobacter* infection. *Clin Microbiol Rev*. 2015;28(3):687-720.
24. Page AV, Liles WC. Enterohemorrhagic *Escherichia coli* infections and the hemolytic-uremic syndrome. *Med Clin North Am*. 2013;97(4):681-695, xi
25. Clements A, Young JC, Constantinou N, Frankel G. Infection strategies of enteric pathogenic *Escherichia coli*. *Gut Microb*. 2012;3(2):71-87.
26. Cover TL, Aber RC. *Yersinia enterocolitica*. *N Engl J Med*. 1989;321(1):16-24.
27. Haque R, Huston CD, Hughes M, Houpt E, Petri WA Jr. Amebiasis. *N Engl J Med*. 2003;348(16):1565-1573.
28. Daniels NA, MacKinnon L, Bishop R, et al. *Vibrio parahaemolyticus* infections in the United States, 1973-1998. *J Infect Dis*. 2000;181(5):1661-1666.
29. Chetty R, Roskell DE. Cytomegalovirus infection in the gastrointestinal tract. *J Clin Pathol*. 1994;47(11):968-972.
30. Klauber E, Briski LE, Khatib R. Cytomegalovirus colitis in the immunocompetent host: an overview. *Scand J Infect Dis*. 1998;30(6):559-564.
31. Mylonaki M, Langmead L, Pantes A, Johnson F, Rampton DS. Enteric infection in relapse of inflammatory bowel disease: importance of microbiological examination of stool. *Eur J Gastroenterol Hepatol*. 2004;16(8):775-778.
32. Thoeni RF, Cello JP. CT imaging of colitis. *Radiology*. 2006;240(3):623-638.
33. Johnson CM, Wei C, Ensor JE, et al. Meta-analyses of colorectal cancer risk factors. *Cancer Causes Control*. 2013;24(6):1207-1222.
34. Shadad AK, Sullivan FJ, Martin JD, Egan LJ. Gastrointestinal radiation injury: symptoms, risk factors and mechanisms. *World J Gastroenterol*. 2013;19(2):185-198.
35. Ratnaike RN. Acute and chronic arsenic toxicity. *Postgrad Med J*. 2003;79(933):391-396.
36. Sweetser S. Evaluating the patient with diarrhea: a case based approach. *Mayo Clin Proc*. 2012;87(6):596-602.
37. Eherer AJ, Fordtran JS. Fecal osmotic gap and pH in experimental diarrhea of various causes. *Gastroenterology*. 1992;103(2):545-551.
38. Shiau YF, Feldman GM, Resnick MA, Coff PM. Stool electrolyte and osmolality measurements in the evaluation of diarrheal disorders. *Ann Intern Med*. 1985;102(6):773-775.
39. Topazian M, Binder HJ. Brief report: factitious diarrhea detected by measurement of stool osmolality. *N Engl J Med*. 1994;330(20):1418-1419.
40. Craig RM, Atkinson AJ Jr. D-xylose testing: a review. *Gastroenterology*. 1988;95(1):223-231.
41. Lomer MC, Parkes GC, Sanderson JD. Review article: lactose intolerance in clinical practice–myths and realities. *Aliment Pharmacol Ther*. 2008;27(2):93-103.
42. Quigley EM, Abu-Shanab A. Small intestinal bacterial overgrowth. *Infect Dis Clin North Am*. 2010;24(4):943-959, viii-ix.
43. Fasano A, Catassi C. Clinical practice. Celiac disease. *N Engl J Med*. 2012;367(25):2419-2426.
44. Lindkvist B. Diagnosis and treatment of pancreatic exocrine insufficiency. *World J Gastroenterol*. 2013;19(42):7258-7266.
45. Nightingale J, Woodward JM, Small Bowel and Nutrition Committee of the British Society of Gastroenterology. Guidelines for management of patients with a short bowel. *Gut*. 2006;55 suppl 4:iv1-iv12.
46. Walters JR, Pattni SS. Managing bile acid diarrhoea. *Therap Adv Gastroenterol*. 2010;3(6):349-357.
47. Khokhar N, Gill ML. Tropical sprue: revisited. *J Pak Med Assoc*. 2004;54(3):133-134.
48. Srirajaskanthan R, Shanmugabavan D, Ramage JK. Carcinoid syndrome. *BMJ*. 2010;341:c3941.

49. Milan SA, Yeo CJ. Neuroendocrine tumors of the pancreas. *Curr Opin Oncol*. 2012;24(1):46-55.
50. Ramsay DB, Stephen S, Borum M, Voltaggio L, Doman DB. Mast cells in gastrointestinal disease. *Gastroenterol Hepatol*. 2010;6(12):772-777.
51. Chey WD, Kurlander J, Eswaran S. Irritable bowel syndrome: a clinical review. *JAMA*. 2015;313(9):949-958.
52. Ogbonnaya KI, Arem R. Diabetic diarrhea. Pathophysiology, diagnosis, and management. *Arch Intern Med*. 1990;150(2):262-267.
53. Daher R, Yazbeck T, Jaoude JB, Abboud B. Consequences of dysthyroidism on the digestive tract and viscera. *World J Gastroenterol*. 2009;15(23):2834-2838.
54. Tian XP, Zhang X. Gastrointestinal complications of systemic sclerosis. *World J Gastroenterol*. 2013;19(41):7062-7068.
55. Petre S, Shah IA, Gilani N. Review article: gastrointestinal amyloidosis—clinical features, diagnosis and therapy. *Aliment Pharmacol Ther*. 2008;27(11):1006-1016.
56. Fox DJ, Khattar RS. Carcinoid heart disease: presentation, diagnosis, and management. *Heart*. 2004;90(10):1224-1228.
57. Burgess TE, Mansoor AM. Giant a waves. *BMJ Case Rep*. 2017;2017.

# Chapter 16

# GASTROINTESTINAL BLEEDING

## Case: An 84-year-old woman with hypotension

An 84-year-old woman with coronary artery disease, hypertension, and vascular dementia is admitted to the hospital with abdominal pain and bloody diarrhea. The pain is located over the left lower quadrant and is cramping in quality. It began suddenly 2 days before admission. She subsequently developed bloody diarrhea, prompting evaluation. The patient has a history of dementia and lives with her son, who has noticed that her needs have been increasing over the past few months, particularly owing to forgetfulness and generalized weakness. The patient's son recently left town for an extended period of time on a business trip and left her alone at home for the first time in over a year. She has not had fever, sweats, or chills.

Heart rate is 108 beats per minute, and blood pressure is 92/57 mm Hg. The jugular venous waveform rises above the clavicle only in Trendelenburg position. Abdominal examination is notable for minimal pain to deep palpation of the left lower quadrant. There is no rebound, guarding, or rigidity. Rectal examination reveals the presence of bright red blood in the rectal vault. Cross-sectional imaging of the abdomen shows segmental thickening of the colonic wall involving the splenic flexure (arrows, Figure 16-1).

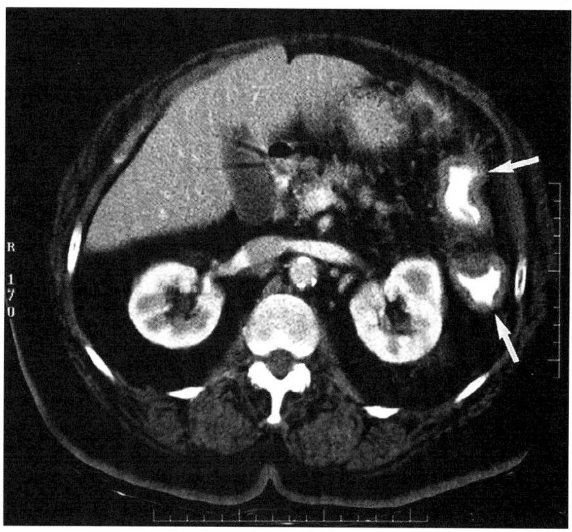

**Figure 16-1.** (From Pope TL, Harris JH. *Harris & Harris' The Radiology of Emergency Medicine*. 5th ed. Philadelphia, PA: Lippincott Williams & Wilkins; 2012.)

***What is the most likely cause of gastrointestinal bleeding in this patient?***

What is gastrointestinal (GI) bleeding?

GI bleeding refers to the extravasation of blood into the lumen of the GI tract. It can be overt (acute) or occult (chronic), and is sometimes obscure. Overt GI bleeding is visible to the naked eye and presents with hematemesis, coffee-ground emesis, melena, or hematochezia. Occult GI bleeding is not visible to the patient or clinician but can be established with a positive stool guaiac test with or without the presence of iron-deficiency anemia. Obscure GI bleeding refers to either overt or occult GI bleeding when a source remains unidentified after upper and lower endoscopy.[1]

What is hematemesis?

Hematemesis refers to vomiting fresh blood, indicative of acute and active GI bleeding.[1]

**What is coffee-ground emesis?**

Coffee-ground emesis refers to vomitus consisting of dark blood that has the appearance of coffee grounds (a result of the oxidation of iron from gastric acid), indicating that the GI bleeding has slowed or stopped.[1]

**What is melena?**

Melena refers to black tarry stool (Figure 16-2).[1]

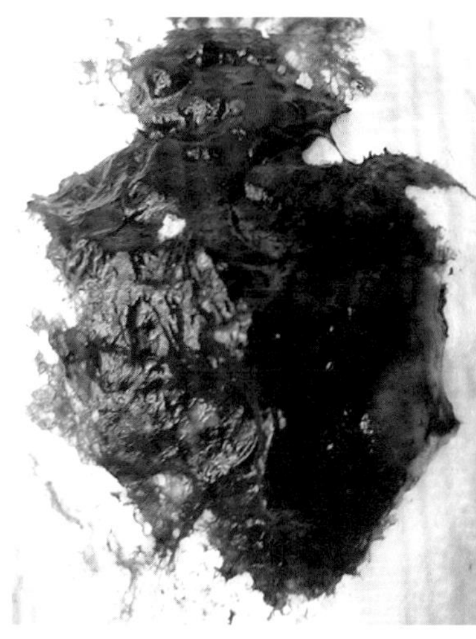

**Figure 16-2.** Characteristic black tarry stool of melena. (From Sherman SC. *Atlas of Clinical Emergency Medicine*. Philadelphia, PA: Wolters Kluwer Health; 2016.)

**What is hematochezia?**

Hematochezia refers to the passage of red or maroon blood from the rectum.[1]

**How common is gastrointestinal bleeding?**

In the industrialized world, GI bleeding is a common clinical problem, resulting in up to 150 hospital admissions per 100,000 persons annually.[1]

**What is the initial management of patients presenting with overt gastrointestinal bleeding?**

Overt GI bleeding can be massive and life-threatening with an overall mortality rate of up to 10%. Before undergoing diagnostic evaluation, hemodynamically unstable patients should be adequately resuscitated with isotonic crystalloid solution (eg, normal saline) and blood products (overaggressive resuscitation may exacerbate bleeding in some cases). Hemoglobin concentration should be followed serially, as a significant drop may not initially be apparent in acute hemorrhage. Blood is typically transfused to maintain hemoglobin concentration ≥7 g/dL (or higher in patients with comorbidities such as coronary artery disease). Additional therapeutic interventions such as endoscopic hemostasis or surgery may be necessary.[1,2]

**What are the 2 anatomic categories of gastrointestinal bleeding?**

Causes of GI bleeding can involve the upper or lower GI tract.

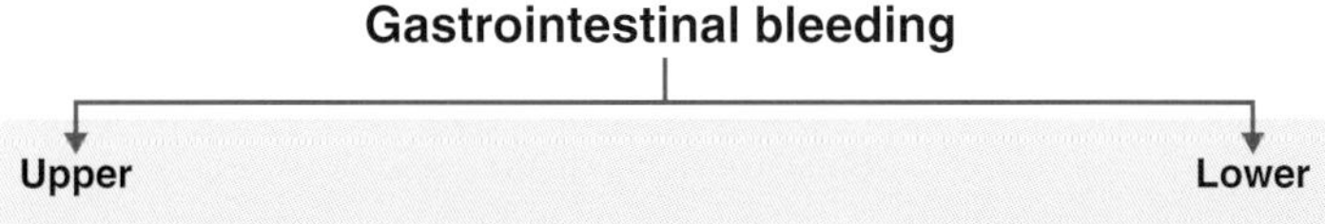


**What anatomic landmark distinguishes the upper and lower gastrointestinal tracts?**

Upper GI bleeding arises from a site above the ligament of Treitz at the duodenojejunal flexure; lower GI bleeding arises from a site below the ligament of Treitz.[1]

**What are the visible characteristics of overt upper and lower gastrointestinal bleeding?**

Overt upper GI bleeding typically presents with hematemesis, coffee-ground emesis, or melena; overt lower GI bleeding typically presents with hematochezia.[1]

**Under what circumstance might upper gastrointestinal bleeding present with hematochezia?**

Upper GI bleeding can present with hematochezia if the rate is brisk.[1]

**Under what circumstance might lower gastrointestinal bleeding present with melena?**

Lower GI bleeding can present with melena if the source is in the small intestine or right colon. The stool may also appear maroon-colored and mixed with blood.[1]

**What investigative modalities are helpful for identifying the source of overt gastrointestinal bleeding?**

The initial diagnostic modality of choice for overt GI bleeding is upper endoscopy or colonoscopy, depending on whether the clinical presentation suggests an upper or lower source. If a source of bleeding is not identified after upper and lower endoscopy (ie, obscure overt GI bleeding), diagnostic modalities such as computed tomography (CT) angiography, catheter angiography, or radionuclide imaging should be considered. Active bleeding must be present for these studies to be useful. Other options for obscure overt GI bleeding in hemodynamically stable patients with low-volume bleeding include push enteroscopy, deep small bowel enteroscopy, and capsule endoscopy.[1]

**How can CT angiography be useful for the detection of gastrointestinal bleeding?**

CT angiography is a noninvasive modality used to identify a source of active GI bleeding in hemodynamically stable patients when endoscopy is nondiagnostic. It requires an arterial bleeding rate ≥0.5 mL/min to be reliable. Under these circumstances, it is associated with excellent sensitivity (86%) and specificity (95%). It has the additional advantage of being able to identify the etiology of bleeding in some cases (eg, tumor). The lack of therapeutic capability is a disadvantage. However, it can be used to direct and plan definitive treatment.[1]

**How can catheter angiography be useful for the detection of gastrointestinal bleeding?**

Catheter angiography is used to identify a source of active GI bleeding when endoscopy is not feasible (eg, hemodynamic instability) or nondiagnostic (eg, bleeding obscures view), particularly when the source is thought to be in the lower GI tract. It requires an arterial bleeding rate ≥0.5-1.5 mL/min to be reliable. Sensitivity is variable, but specificity is close to 100%. Disadvantages include the invasive nature of the study and potential complications. However, it has the advantage of diagnostic and therapeutic capabilities, allowing for the infusion of vasoconstrictive drugs and the performance of embolization.[1]

**How can radionuclide imaging be useful for the detection of gastrointestinal bleeding?**

Radionuclide imaging uses red blood cells that are labeled with a radioactive tracer to detect sites of bleeding. It is the most sensitive diagnostic modality for active GI bleeding, requiring a minimum arterial bleeding rate of only 0.1 mL/min. The main limitation of radionuclide imaging is poor anatomic localization of the site of bleeding.[1]

**What investigative modalities are helpful for identifying the source of occult gastrointestinal bleeding?**

Like overt GI bleeding, the initial diagnostic modalities of choice for occult GI bleeding are upper endoscopy and/or colonoscopy, which together identify the culprit lesion in up to one-half of cases. When initial endoscopic studies fail to identify a source, repeat examinations should be considered. The most common site of obscure occult GI bleeding is the small intestine, which should be evaluated further with capsule endoscopy, push enteroscopy, or deep small bowel enteroscopy (eg, double balloon enteroscopy). CT or magnetic resonance enterography may be considered in some cases, particularly when capsule endoscopy and deep enteroscopy are nondiagnostic.[1]

**How can capsule endoscopy be useful for the detection of gastrointestinal bleeding?**

Capsule endoscopy is a simple, noninvasive modality that evaluates the small intestine in the setting of obscure GI bleeding. A capsule containing a tiny camera is swallowed by the patient and takes photographs of the GI tract as it passes through. It is generally the initial diagnostic modality of choice for the evaluation of obscure occult GI bleeding, identifying the culprit lesion in more than one-half of patients. The main disadvantage of capsule endoscopy is the lack of therapeutic capability.[1]

**How can push enteroscopy and deep enteroscopy be useful for the detection of gastrointestinal bleeding?**

Push enteroscopy can reach as far as the proximal 60 to 80 cm of the jejunum. However, it has largely been replaced by deep enteroscopy, which reaches the distal small bowel. The diagnostic yield of deep enteroscopy is comparable with that of capsule endoscopy, but it is more invasive with higher risk. The therapeutic capabilities of push enteroscopy and deep enteroscopy provide an advantage over capsule endoscopy.[1]

## UPPER GASTROINTESTINAL BLEEDING

**Which biochemical laboratory abnormality can provide a clue to the presence of upper gastrointestinal bleeding?**

Digested blood is a source of urea, which raises the blood urea nitrogen (BUN) level, leading to an increased BUN-to-creatinine ratio in patients with upper GI bleeding.[1]

**Which bedside procedure can confirm the presence of upper gastrointestinal bleeding when it is suspected but not clinically apparent?**

Red blood or coffee-ground aspirate from nasogastric lavage can confirm the presence of upper GI bleeding.

**What is the initial diagnostic modality of choice for upper gastrointestinal bleeding?**

Most causes of upper GI bleeding can be definitively diagnosed with upper endoscopy. It should be performed within 24 hours in most patients with overt bleeding after adequate fluid resuscitation. Endoscopy may also be therapeutic in many cases. Conventional endoscopic techniques used to achieve hemostasis include injection therapy (eg, epinephrine, tissue adhesives), mechanical therapy (eg, clips, band ligation), and thermal therapy, including contact techniques (eg, electrocoagulation, thermocoagulation) and noncontact techniques (eg, argon plasma coagulation, laser photocoagulation). The method of choice depends on the nature of the target lesion.[3]

**What are the anatomic subcategories of upper gastrointestinal bleeding?**

Upper GI bleeding can be esophageal, gastric, or duodenal.

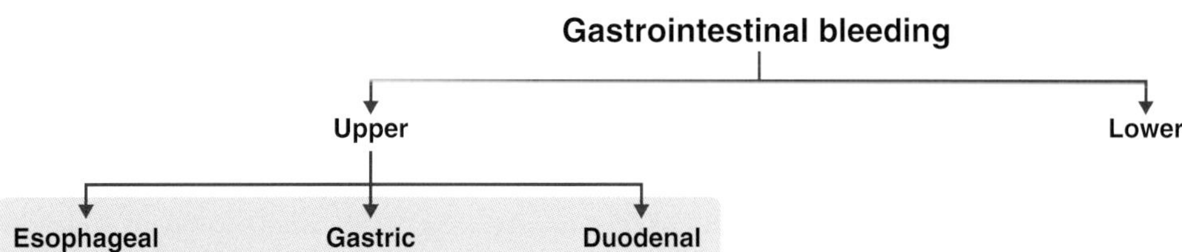


## ESOPHAGEAL CAUSES OF UPPER GASTROINTESTINAL BLEEDING

### What are the esophageal causes of upper gastrointestinal bleeding?

**A 48-year-old man with a history of cirrhosis and portal hypertension presents with acute-onset massive hematemesis.**

Variceal hemorrhage.

**A 54-year-old man with active alcohol abuse presents with hematemesis that began shortly after an episode of heavy retching.**

Mallory-Weiss tear.

**This condition can be caused by a variety of processes, from swallowing pills to infection.**

Esophagitis.

**Risk factors include smoking tobacco, alcohol use, and gastroesophageal reflux disease.**

Esophageal cancer.

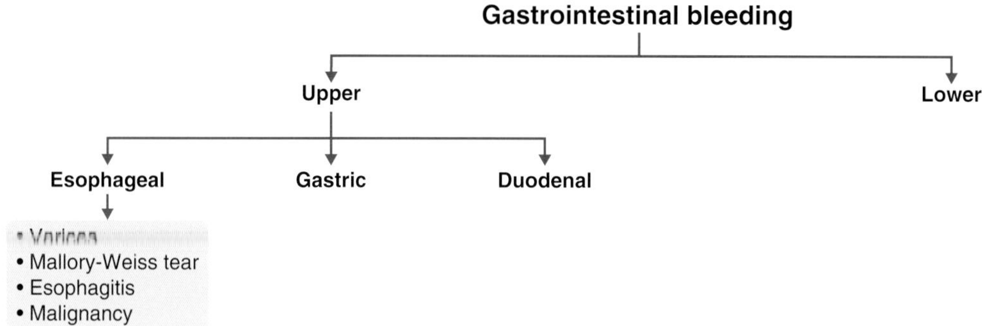


**What is the acute management of esophageal variceal hemorrhage?**

Gastroesophageal varices are portosystemic collaterals that develop as a result of portal hypertension and are present in up to one-half of patients with cirrhosis at the time of diagnosis. Acute esophageal variceal hemorrhage is a life-threatening condition associated with a high mortality rate. It accounts for the vast majority of GI bleeding in cirrhotics. In addition to basic resuscitative measures, patients should be treated with a vasoconstrictor (eg, octreotide) to reduce portal blood flow. In those with cirrhosis, short-term prophylactic antibiotics (eg, ceftriaxone) should be added. Pharmacologic therapy should coincide with endoscopic techniques such as balloon tamponade and band ligation. When bleeding cannot be controlled with the aforementioned strategies, transjugular intrahepatic portosystemic shunt (TIPS) may be helpful. A nonselective β-blocker (eg, propranolol) can help prevent future bleeding.[4]

**What is the acute management of a Mallory-Weiss tear?**

Mallory-Weiss tears account for up to 15% of upper GI bleeding. Most episodes stop spontaneously with rebleeding rates of up to 10%. Hemostasis can be achieved endoscopically with bipolar electrocoagulation, epinephrine injection, clips, or band ligation.[3]

**What are the clinical features of gastrointestinal bleeding caused by esophagitis?**

Esophagitis accounts for approximately 10% of upper GI bleeding; most patients have underlying gastroesophageal reflux disease. It typically presents with hematemesis. Patients tend to experience less hemodynamic instability compared with other causes of upper GI bleeding. Prognosis is excellent overall with a low risk of rebleeding.[5]

**What are the clinical features of gastrointestinal bleeding caused by esophageal cancer?**

Esophageal cancer typically presents with progressive mechanical dysphagia and weight loss. Overt GI bleeding is uncommon. It tends to be occult, presenting with iron-deficiency anemia. However, overt bleeding can occur when a tumor erodes into nearby vascular structures, such as the aorta.[6]

## GASTRIC CAUSES OF UPPER GASTROINTESTINAL BLEEDING

### What are the gastric causes of upper gastrointestinal bleeding?

**Responsible for most cases of upper GI bleeding.**

Peptic ulcer disease (PUD).[3]

**Gastric epithelial cell injury associated with inflammation.**

Gastritis.

**Gastric epithelial cell injury without inflammation.**

Gastropathy.

**A manifestation of portal hypertension.**

Gastric varices.

**A 75-year-old Japanese man with an extensive history of cigarette smoking presents with epigastric abdominal pain, weight loss, and melena.**

Gastric cancer.

**"Watermelon stomach."**

Gastric antral vascular ectasia (GAVE).

**A rare cause of upper GI bleeding, this lesion is characterized by a single large tortuous arteriole in the submucosa of the stomach.**

Dieulafoy's lesion.

**Associated with a hiatal hernia.**

Cameron lesion.

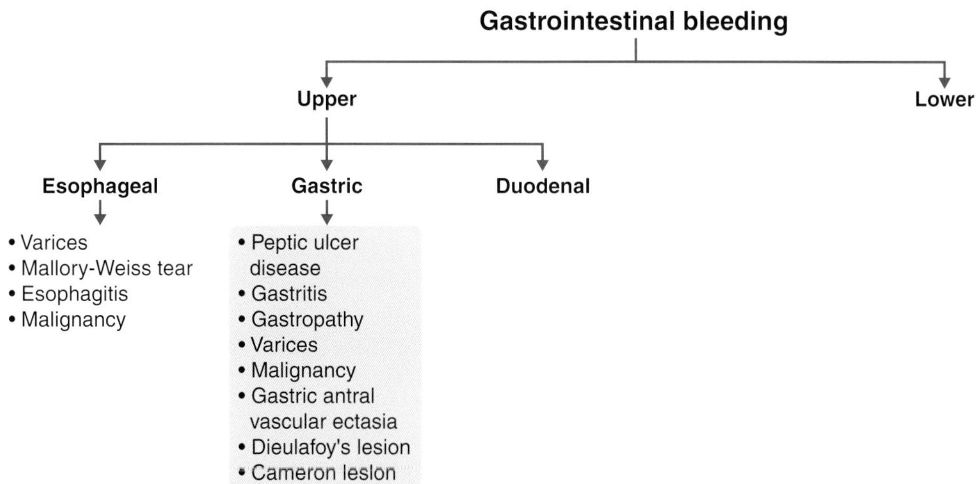


**In addition to the usual resuscitation measures, what is the acute management of gastrointestinal bleeding caused by peptic ulcer disease?**

Intravenous infusion of a proton pump inhibitor should be started immediately in patients suspected of GI bleeding from PUD. Diagnostic endoscopy should be performed within 24 hours in most patients. Endoscopic hemostasis (eg, thermal therapy, epinephrine injection, clips) is indicated for ulcers with active bleeding (eg, spurting or oozing) or nonbleeding visible vessels; it is unnecessary for ulcers with a clean base or flat pigmented spot. After achieving hemostasis, intravenous proton pump inhibitor therapy should be continued for 72 hours before transitioning to an oral agent.[2]

**What common bacterial infection is a leading cause of gastritis?**

*Helicobacter pylori* affects nearly half of the world's population and is associated with conditions such as gastritis, PUD, mucosa-associated lymphoid tissue (MALT) lymphoma, and gastric cancer. Noninvasive options for diagnosing active infection include the urea breath test and stool antigen test. Active infection can also be detected via endoscopic gastric biopsy with histology, culture, polymerase chain reaction, and rapid urease test. Various combinations of antibiotics (eg, clarithromycin and amoxicillin) and antisecretory agents (eg, proton pump inhibitors) are used to treat the infection. Diagnostic tests should be repeated after treatment to confirm eradication.[7]

**What kind of gastropathy is common in patients with cirrhosis?**

Portal hypertensive gastropathy (PHG) is common in patients with cirrhotic and noncirrhotic portal hypertension. The diagnosis is made endoscopically, usually based on characteristic gross appearance of the gastric mucosa (a mosaic-like pattern resembling snake skin). PHG can cause both overt and occult GI bleeding. The treatment for overt bleeding is similar to that of variceal hemorrhage, including a vasoconstrictor (eg, octreotide) and prophylactic antibiotics in patients with cirrhosis. TIPS can be considered in some patients but is usually ineffective. Once the episode has resolved, a nonselective β-blocker (eg, propranolol) can help prevent future bleeding.[8]

**How does the acute management of gastric variceal hemorrhage differ from esophageal hemorrhage?**

Gastric varices are present in one-fifth of patients with cirrhosis, often occurring along with esophageal varices. Management of bleeding gastric varices is similar to that of esophageal varices, except obturation with tissue adhesives (eg, *N*-butyl-2-cyanoacrylate glue) is more effective than ligation for gastric varices. Procedures such as balloon-occluded retrograde transvenous obliteration (BRTO), TIPS, and surgery may be necessary.[4]

**What are the risk factors for gastric adenocarcinoma?**

The strongest risk factor for gastric adenocarcinoma is *Helicobacter pylori* infection; others include cigarette smoking, alcohol use, male sex, a diet rich in salt and lacking in fruits and vegetables, and pernicious anemia.[9]

**What are the clinical differences between gastric antral vascular ectasia and portal hypertensive gastropathy?**

Like PHG, GAVE is diagnosed based on endoscopic appearance. GAVE is characterized by the presence of linear red stripes separated by normal mucosa (resembling a watermelon). It occurs in patients with portal hypertension but, unlike PHG, is also associated with autoimmune and connective tissue diseases, such as atrophic gastritis, systemic sclerosis, and pernicious anemia. Unlike PHG, pharmacologic management (eg, octreotide) is unhelpful in the setting of overt bleeding; endoscopy with argon plasma coagulation is the treatment of choice.[8]

**In addition to the usual resuscitation measures, what is the acute management of gastrointestinal bleeding caused by Dieulafoy's lesions?**

Dieulafoy's lesions are more common in men and account for up to 5% of upper GI bleeding. Often difficult to locate endoscopically, particularly when bleeding has stopped, Dieulafoy's lesions can be a source of obscure GI bleeding. Overt bleeding is often massive and life-threatening. Endoscopic hemostasis using any of a variety of techniques (eg, epinephrine injection with electrocoagulation) is the treatment of choice.[10]

**What are Cameron lesions?**

Cameron lesions describe linear gastric erosions and ulcers within the distal neck of a hiatal hernia, often associated with gastroesophageal reflux disease. The lesions are typically asymptomatic but can cause overt or occult bleeding, the latter of which is more common and may present with iron-deficiency anemia. Diagnosis and management are endoscopic.[11]

## DUODENAL CAUSES OF UPPER GASTROINTESTINAL BLEEDING

### What are the duodenal causes of upper gastrointestinal bleeding?

**A 48-year-old man with months of epigastric abdominal pain that tends to improve after eating presents with melena and light-headedness.**

Peptic ulcer disease.

**Inflammation of the duodenum from any cause.**

Duodenitis.

**Types of vascular anomalies.**

Angiodysplasia (ie, vascular ectasia, arteriovenous malformation, angiectasia) and telangiectasia. *These entities also occur elsewhere in the GI tract.*

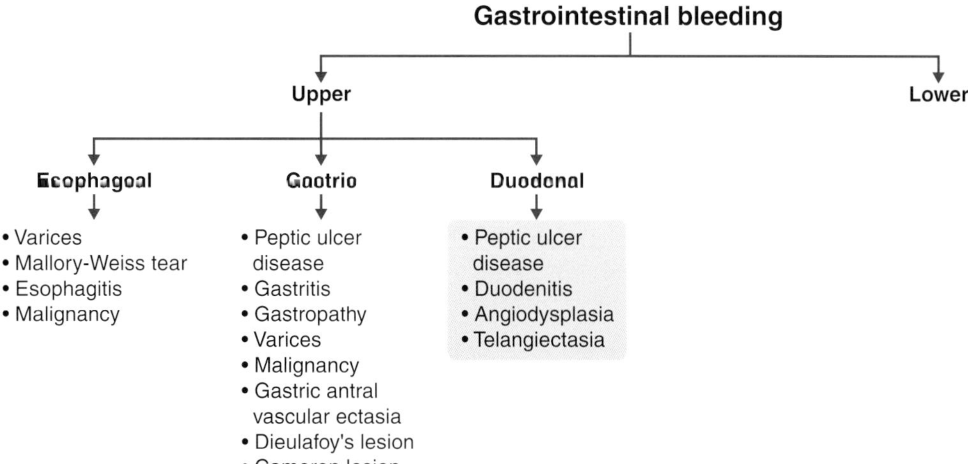


**What are the strongest risk factors for peptic ulcer disease?**

Infection with *Helicobacter pylori* and use of nonsteroidal anti-inflammatory drugs (NSAIDs) are the strongest risk factors for gastric and duodenal ulcers. Duodenal ulcers cause overt GI bleeding more often than gastric ulcers because of proximity to the gastroduodenal artery.

**What are some causes of duodenitis?**

Duodenitis is often identified endoscopically or by imaging. Causes are similar to those of gastritis or gastropathy and include NSAID use, alcohol use, infection (eg, *Helicobacter pylori*), Crohn's disease, celiac disease, and external beam radiation.

**What is angiodysplasia of the gastrointestinal tract?**

Angiodysplasia refers to abnormal, ectatic, dilated, tortuous, and usually small (<10 mm) blood vessels that arise within the mucosal or submucosal layers of the GI tract. It is the most common vascular malformation of the GI tract, typically affecting patients >60 years of age. Lesions can be asymptomatic or result in overt or occult GI bleeding. Endoscopy is the diagnostic and therapeutic modality of choice.[12]

**What hereditary disease is associated with telangiectasias of the gastrointestinal tract?**

Hereditary hemorrhagic telangiectasia (HHT) is frequently associated with telangiectasias of the GI tract. Up to one-third of patients with HHT have experienced overt GI bleeding (hematemesis or melena), most often affecting patients in the fourth or fifth decades of life. Culprit lesions can be treated endoscopically (eg, laser therapy). *Epistaxis is common in patients with HHT and can be confused for GI bleeding when blood is swallowed.*[13]

## LOWER GASTROINTESTINAL BLEEDING

**What is the initial diagnostic modality of choice for lower gastrointestinal bleeding?**

Most causes of lower GI bleeding can be definitively diagnosed with colonoscopy. It should generally be performed within 24 hours in most patients with overt lower GI bleeding after adequate fluid resuscitation. Colonoscopy may also be therapeutic in many cases. Conventional endoscopic techniques used to achieve hemostasis include injection therapy, mechanical therapy, and thermal therapy. The method of choice depends on the nature of the target lesion.[14]

**What are the general subcategories of lower gastrointestinal bleeding?**

Lower GI bleeding can be structural, vascular, or inflammatory.

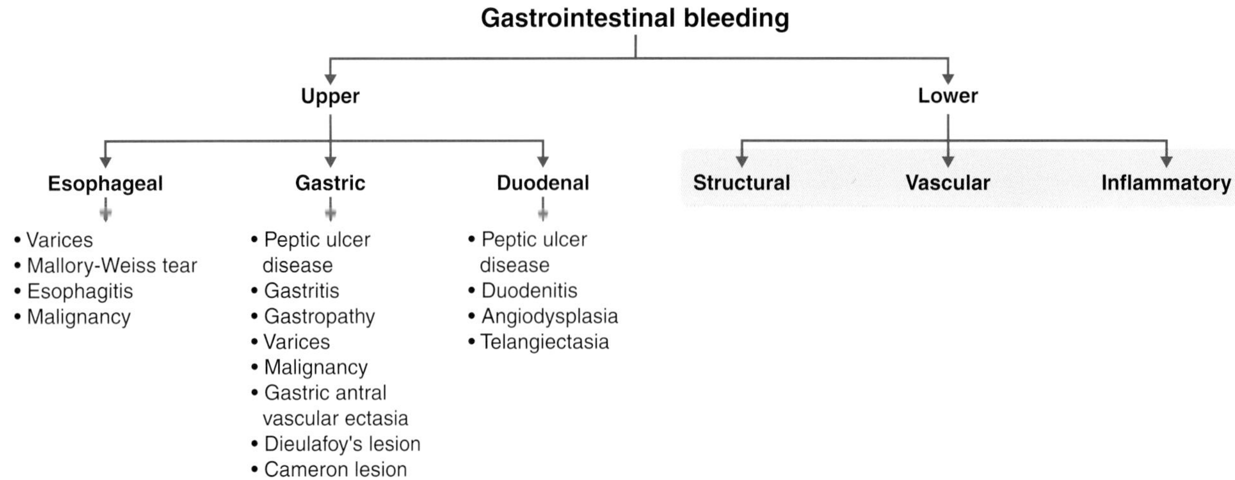


## STRUCTURAL CAUSES OF LOWER GASTROINTESTINAL BLEEDING

### What are the structural causes of lower gastrointestinal bleeding?

**A 28-year-old man with Crohn's disease presents with painful defecation and bright red blood on the toilet paper.**

Anal fissure.

**Older adults with painless hematochezia.**

Diverticulosis.

**These lesions may be benign, premalignant, or malignant.**

Colorectal polyps.

**A 68-year-old woman presents with a change in bowel pattern, iron-deficiency anemia, weight loss, and hematochezia.**

Malignancy.

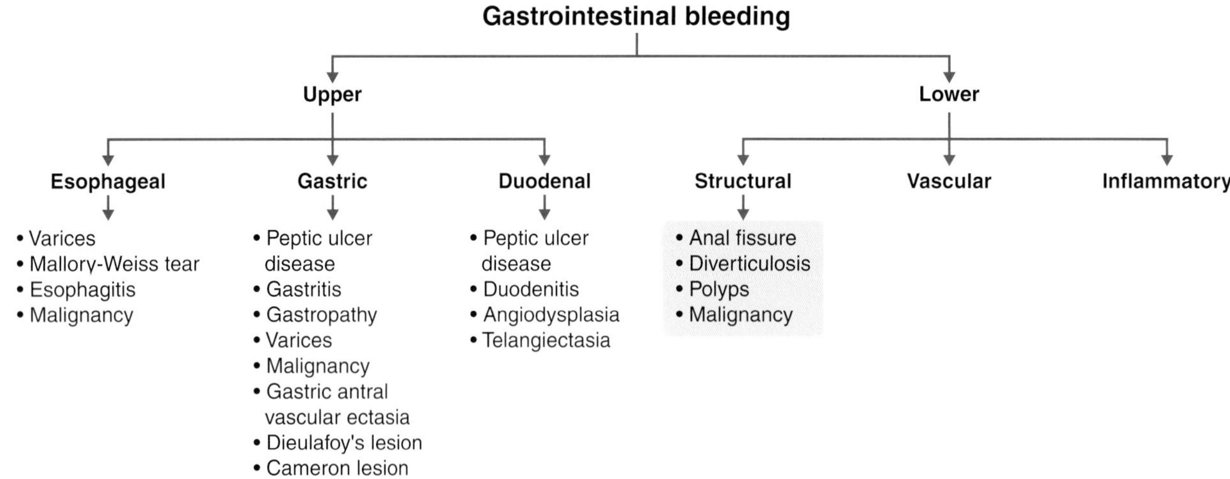


**What are the clinical characteristics of anal fissures?**

An anal fissure is a tear in the mucosa of the anal canal. It typically presents with painful defecation and red blood streaks on the surface of stool or toilet paper. Most fissures occur along the posterior midline; fissures that are not midline suggest an underlying condition such as anal cancer, Crohn's disease, or syphilis. First-line therapies for acute and chronic fissures include increased water and fiber intake, and sitz baths.[15]

**What is the usual treatment for diverticular bleeding?**

Diverticulosis is the most common cause of lower GI bleeding requiring hospitalization. Like most causes of lower GI bleeding, it is typically self-limited. However, endoscopic hemostasis is recommended when active bleeding or stigmata of recent bleeding (eg, visible vessel, clot) are present.[14]

**What should be suspected in a patient who presents with hematochezia after a recent screening colonoscopy?**

Postpolypectomy bleeding accounts for just fewer than 10% of lower GI bleeding. However, incidence is on the rise likely because of the increased use of antiplatelet and anticoagulant medications. Endoscopy can be used to achieve hemostasis.[14]

**What types of gastrointestinal bleeding occur in patients with colorectal cancer?**

Colon cancer most often presents with occult GI bleeding, resulting in anemia and fatigue, but overt GI bleeding occasionally occurs. Lesions in the rectum frequently cause overt hematochezia. Colorectal cancer complicated by GI bleeding usually requires surgical management.[16]

## VASCULAR CAUSES OF LOWER GASTROINTESTINAL BLEEDING

### What are the vascular causes of lower gastrointestinal bleeding?

**A 22-year-old man who is an avid weight lifter presents with intermittent hematochezia.**

Hemorrhoids.

**These acquired lesions are a common source of lower GI bleeding in elderly patients.**

Angiodysplasia.

**A 44-year-old woman with tight, shiny skin, dysphagia, Raynaud's phenomenon, and intermittent hematochezia.**

Telangiectasias associated with systemic sclerosis (ie, scleroderma).

**Benign tumor of vascular origin.**

Hemangioma.

**Consider this malignant vascular tumor in patients with acquired immunodeficiency syndrome (AIDS).**

Kaposi sarcoma.

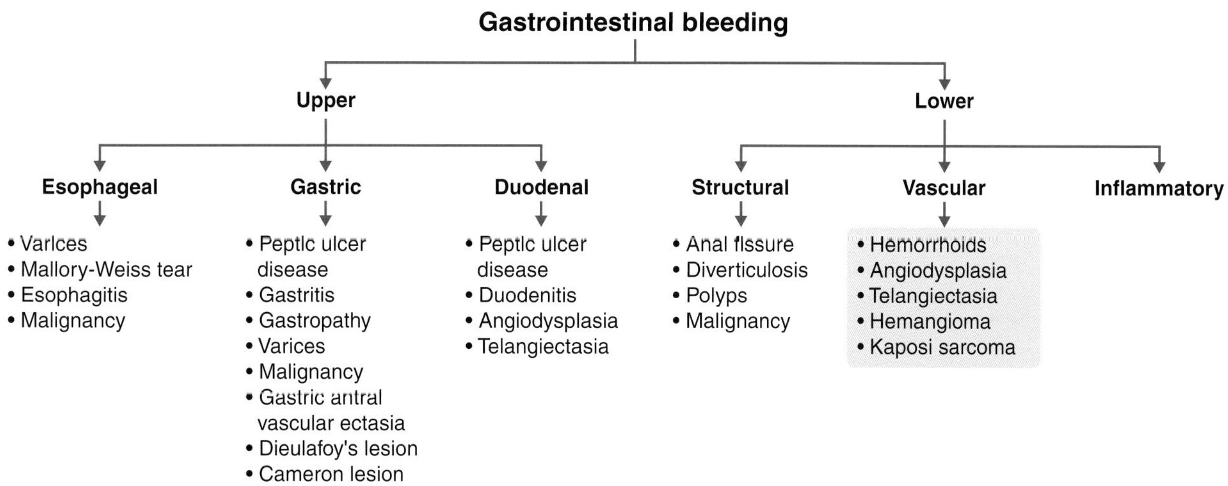


**What is the management of bleeding internal hemorrhoids that are refractory to conservative measures (eg, increased water and fiber intake)?**

Internal hemorrhoids are the second most common cause of lower GI bleeding requiring hospitalization. Rubber band ligation is commonly used to treat bleeding internal hemorrhoids. Complete evaluation of the colon with colonoscopy should be considered, particularly in older patients.[14]

**What conditions are associated with bleeding from angiodysplasia?**

Conditions associated with bleeding from angiodysplasia include aortic stenosis (Heyde's syndrome), von Willebrand disease, and chronic kidney disease. The endoscopic technique of choice to establish hemostasis is argon plasma photocoagulation.[12]

**What are the characteristics of gastrointestinal telangiectasias associated with systemic sclerosis?**

Telangiectasias are the most common vascular anomaly associated with systemic sclerosis and can occur virtually anywhere in the GI tract. Bleeding events are often recurrent and severe, but occult GI bleeding also occurs frequently. Therapeutic options are limited, endoscopic and surgical treatments are associated with variable results.[17]

**What are the characteristics gastrointestinal hemangiomas?**

Hemangiomas are benign vascular tumors that infrequently involve the GI tract. Most patients experience painless and recurrent GI bleeding, usually presenting as large-volume hematochezia. A significant number of patients experience occult bleeding that manifests with iron-deficiency anemia. Diagnosis may be established with various imaging modalities and endoscopy. Treatment options include a variety of endoscopic and surgical techniques, which are often successful.[18]

**What are the characteristics of Kaposi sarcoma of the gastrointestinal tract?**

Kaposi sarcoma is the most common GI malignancy in patients with AIDS. Forms of Kaposi sarcoma also occur in non-HIV populations, such as post-transplant patients on chronic immunosuppressive medication and certain indigenous populations (eg, elderly Eastern European and Mediterranean men). It can affect virtually any part of the GI tract. Most lesions are asymptomatic, however both overt and occult bleeding can occur. The diagnosis is made endoscopically and confirmed with histology.[19]

## INFLAMMATORY CAUSES OF LOWER GASTROINTESTINAL BLEEDING

**How does bleeding manifest in patients with inflammatory causes of lower gastrointestinal bleeding?**

Inflammatory causes of lower GI bleeding often present with bloody diarrhea.[1]

### What are the inflammatory causes of lower gastrointestinal bleeding?

**Often precipitated by hypotension.**

Ischemic colitis.

**Dozens of patrons of a particular fast-food restaurant develop bloody diarrhea.**

Infectious colitis.

**A 26-year-old man presents with chronic abdominal pain, weight loss, and bloody diarrhea and is found to have erythema nodosum (see Figure 15-3).**

Inflammatory bowel disease.

**Related to the treatment for a variety of malignancies, including prostate, cervical, and rectal cancer.**

Radiation coloproctitis.

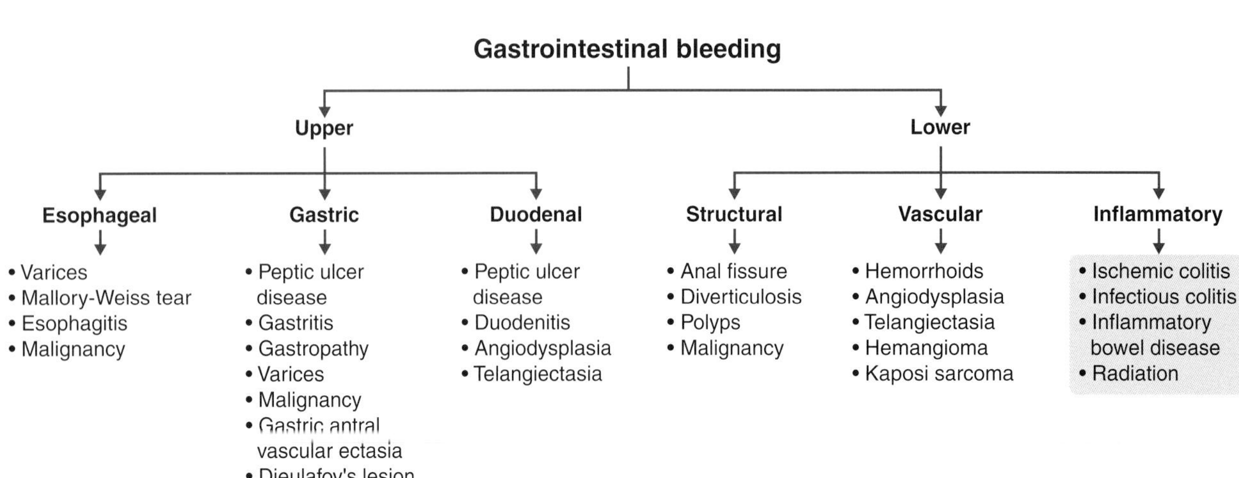

**What findings on plain abdominal radiography can be suggestive of ischemic colitis?**

Abdominal CT imaging is the modality of choice in patients suspected of ischemic colitis. However, a plain abdominal radiograph may be obtained in the general evaluation of abdominal pain. Severe cases of ischemia are associated with findings such as pneumatosis intestinalis and "thumbprinting," which is the result of submucosal edema (Figure 16-3).[20]

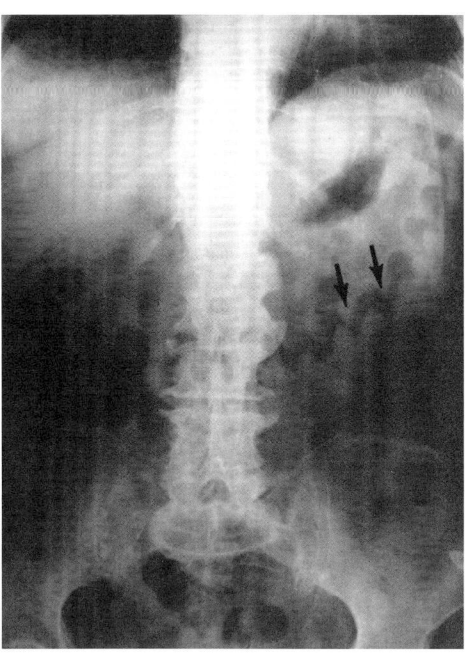

**Figure 16-3.** An abdominal radiograph showing the "thumbprinting" sign (arrows) of ischemic colitis. (From Riddell R, Jain D. *Lewin, Weinstein and Riddell's Gastrointestinal Pathology and its Clinical Implications*. 2nd ed. Philadelphia, PA: Wolters Kluwer Health; 2017.)

**What should be suspected in a patient who develops bloody diarrhea followed by hemolytic anemia, thrombocytopenia, and acute kidney injury?**

Hemolytic uremic syndrome can be a complication of infectious colitis caused by invasive organisms, particularly *Escherichia coli* O157:H7.

**Which type of inflammatory bowel disease is more commonly associated with hematochezia?**

The vast majority of patients with ulcerative colitis experience hematochezia. The clinical features of Crohn's disease are more variable; most often characterized by chronic nonbloody diarrhea with abdominal pain and weight loss. Lower endoscopy with biopsy is diagnostic of both subtypes. Ulcerative colitis involves the rectum and colon, and is characterized by continuous mucosal and submucosal inflammation. Crohn's disease can affect any part of the GI tract and is characterized by noncontinuous transmural inflammation (ie, "skip" lesions). A small proportion of patients have features of both, referred to as "unclassified" inflammatory bowel disease.[21]

**What are the clinical features of radiation coloproctitis?**

The risk of developing coloproctitis after regional external beam radiation therapy correlates with the field size and dose of radiation. Acute coloproctitis presents within 90 days of therapy with symptoms such as diarrhea with or without blood, nausea, cramps, tenesmus, urgency, and mucus discharge. Chronic coloproctitis can present during the acute period but more often presents months to years later. Symptoms are similar to acute coloproctitis but may also include severe bleeding, strictures, fistula formation, bowel obstruction, and perforation. Bleeding complications are addressed endoscopically or surgically.[22]

## Case Summary

An 84-year-old woman with a history of vascular disease presents with left lower quadrant abdominal pain, diarrhea, and hematochezia, in the context of poor oral intake and hypotension, and is found to have colonic inflammation involving the splenic flexure on cross-sectional imaging.

***What is the most likely cause of gastrointestinal bleeding in this patient?***

Ischemic colitis.

BONUS QUESTIONS

***What risk factors for ischemic colitis are present in this case?***

Risk factors for ischemic colitis include increasing age and comorbidities, particularly vascular disease. The patient in this case most likely has atherosclerotic disease of the mesenteric arteries, which makes the colon susceptible to ischemia, particularly when there is an abrupt change in perfusion pressure.[20]

***What features of this case make ischemic colitis more likely than other causes of inflammatory lower gastrointestinal bleeding?***

Abrupt onset of symptoms is characteristic of ischemic colitis; symptoms of infectious colitis or inflammatory bowel disease tend to be more insidious in onset. On cross-sectional imaging, segmental involvement of the GI tract in a vascular or "watershed" distribution—in this case the splenic flexure (see Figure 16-1, arrows)—is suggestive of ischemia.[20]

***What clinical features are suggestive of fulminant gangrenous ischemic colitis?***

Fulminant gangrenous ischemic colitis occurs in a subset of patients with ischemic colitis when there is severe and prolonged ischemia that results in transmural necrosis, leading to complications such as bowel perforation. Physical findings of peritonitis, including rebound tenderness, involuntary guarding, and abdominal rigidity, are suggestive. The identification of peritoneal free air on abdominal imaging provides additional evidence.[20]

***What is the role of endoscopy in the diagnosis of ischemic colitis?***

Lower endoscopy can confirm the diagnosis of ischemic colitis via direct visualization and biopsy and provides an assessment of severity, which has implications on prognosis and treatment. The presence of cyanosis and pseudopolyps are suggestive of transmural ischemia.[20]

***How should the patient in this case be treated?***

Aggressive fluid resuscitation to restore favorable hemodynamics is the cornerstone of managing uncomplicated ischemic colitis. Most patients improve with these measures alone. Complicated cases may require surgical intervention.[20]

## KEY POINTS

- GI bleeding can be overt (acute) or occult (chronic), and is sometimes obscure.
- Overt GI bleeding is visibly evident to the patient or clinician and presents with hematemesis, coffee-ground emesis, melena, or hematochezia.
- Occult GI bleeding is not visibly evident but can be established with a positive stool guaiac test, with or without the presence of iron-deficiency anemia.
- Obscure GI bleeding refers to recurrent GI bleeding (either overt or occult) in which a source remains unidentified after upper and lower endoscopy.
- Patients with overt GI bleeding and hemodynamic instability must be resuscitated with isotonic crystalloid solutions and blood products.
- Causes of GI bleeding can involve the upper or lower GI tract.
- Upper GI bleeding is generally associated with hematemesis, coffee-ground emesis, and/or melena.
- Lower GI bleeding is generally associated with hematochezia.
- Upper or lower endoscopy is the initial diagnostic (and often therapeutic) modality of choice in the setting of GI bleeding.
- Upper GI bleeding can be esophageal, gastric, or duodenal.
- Lower GI bleeding can be structural, vascular, or inflammatory.

## REFERENCES


1. Kim BS, Li BT, Engel A, et al. Diagnosis of gastrointestinal bleeding: a practical guide for clinicians. *World J Gastrointest Pathophysiol*. 2014;5(4):467-478.
2. Laine L, Jensen DM. Management of patients with ulcer bleeding. *Am J Gastroenterol*. 2012;107(3):345-360; quiz 61.
3. Szura M, Pasternak A. Upper non-variceal gastrointestinal bleeding—review the effectiveness of endoscopic hemostasis methods. *World J Gastrointest Endosc*. 2015;7(13):1088-1095.
4. Garcia-Tsao G, Bosch J. Management of varices and variceal hemorrhage in cirrhosis. *N Engl J Med*. 2010;362(9):823-832.
5. Guntipalli P, Chason R, Elliott A, Rockey DC. Upper gastrointestinal bleeding caused by severe esophagitis: a unique clinical syndrome. *Dig Dis Sci*. 2014;59(12):2997-3003.
6. Rustgi AK, El-Serag HB. Esophageal carcinoma. *N Engl J Med*. 2014;371(26):2499-2509.
7. Garza-Gonzalez E, Perez-Perez GI, Maldonado-Garza HJ, Bosques-Padilla FJ. A review of *Helicobacter pylori* diagnosis, treatment, and methods to detect eradication. *World J Gastroenterol*. 2014;20(6):1438-1449.
8. Cubillas R, Rockey DC. Portal hypertensive gastropathy: a review. *Liver Int*. 2010;30(8):1094-1102.
9. Thrumurthy SG, Chaudry MA, Hochhauser D, Mughal M. The diagnosis and management of gastric cancer. *BMJ*. 2013;347:f6367.
10. Chaer RA, Helton WS. Dieulafoy's disease. *J Am Coll Surg*. 2003;196(2):290-296.
11. Kapadia S, Jagroop S, Kumar A. Cameron ulcers: an atypical source for a massive upper gastrointestinal bleed. *World J Gastroenterol*. 2012;18(35):4959-4961.
12. Sami SS, Al-Araji SA, Ragunath K. Review article: gastrointestinal angiodysplasia—pathogenesis, diagnosis and management. *Aliment Pharmacol Ther*. 2014;39(1):15-34.
13. Kjeldsen AD, Kjeldsen J. Gastrointestinal bleeding in patients with hereditary hemorrhagic telangiectasia. *Am J Gastroenterol*. 2000;95(2):415-418.
14. Ghassemi KA, Jensen DM. Lower GI bleeding: epidemiology and management. *Curr Gastroenterol Rep*. 2013;15(7):333.
15. Steele SR, Madoff RD. Systematic review: the treatment of anal fissure. *Aliment Pharmacol Ther*. 2006;24(2):247-257.
16. De Rosa M, Pace U, Rega D, et al. Genetics, diagnosis and management of colorectal cancer (review). *Oncol Rep*. 2015;34(3):1087-1096.
17. Duchini A, Sessoms SL. Gastrointestinal hemorrhage in patients with systemic sclerosis and CREST syndrome. *Am J Gastroenterol*. 1998;93(9):1453-1456.
18. Tan MC, Mutch MG. Hemangiomas of the pelvis. *Clin Colon Rectal Surg*. 2006;19(2):94-101.
19. Arora M, Goldberg EM. Kaposi sarcoma involving the gastrointestinal tract. *Gastroenterol Hepatol*. 2010;6(7):459-462.
20. Trotter JM, Hunt L, Peter MB. Ischaemic colitis. *BMJ*. 2016;355:i6600.
21. Mozdiak E, O'Malley J, Arasaradnam R. Inflammatory bowel disease. *BMJ*. 2015;351:h4416.
22. Do NL, Nagle D, Poylin VY. Radiation proctitis: current strategies in management. *Gastroenterol Res Pract*. 2011;2011:917941.

Chapter 17

# HEPATOCELLULAR LIVER INJURY

## Case: A 37-year-old man with a skin rash

A 37-year-old man with a history of allogeneic stem cell transplantation at 35 years of age for chronic myelogenous leukemia, complicated by cutaneous graft-versus-host disease, is admitted to the hospital with fever, skin rash, and abdominal pain. The patient describes a new skin rash affecting his face, torso, arms, and legs that started 1 week before admission. He has had fever and chills over this time. The development of abdominal pain prompted him to seek medical care. Medications include prednisone 40 mg daily for graft-versus-host disease and trimethoprim/sulfamethoxazole for prophylaxis against *Pneumocystis jirovecii* pneumonia. There have been no recent medication changes, and the patient does not take over-the-counter medications or herbal supplements.

Temperature is 38.6°C. There is scleral icterus. Papular lesions in various stages of healing are observed over the skin of the face, torso, and arms. Some of the lesions are flaccid vesicles that are easily unroofed, revealing serosanguinous fluid; others appear dry and crusted (Figure 17-1A and B). Tender hepatomegaly is present.

Serum alanine aminotransferase (ALT) is 5340 U/L; aspartate aminotransferase (AST), 4325 U/L; alkaline phosphatase (ALP), 252 U/L; total bilirubin, 3.3 mg/dL; and international normalized ratio (INR), 2.8. A skin lesion (arrow, Figure 17-1A) is swabbed for molecular identification of herpes simplex virus, which returns negative.

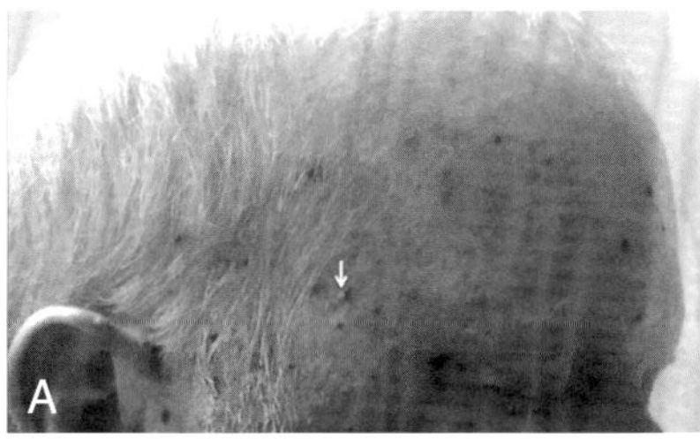

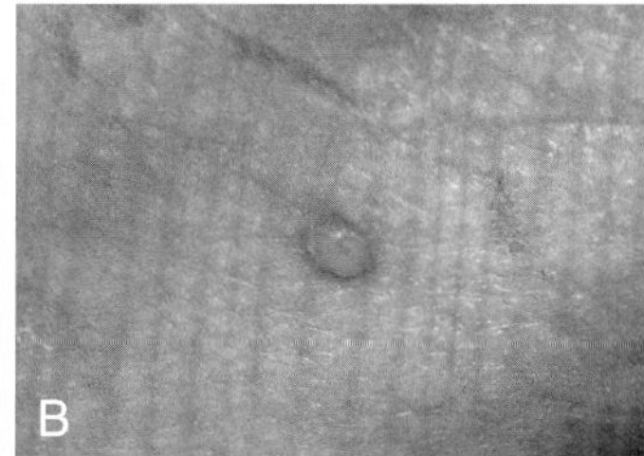


**Figure 17-1.** (Courtesy of Jesse J. Keller, MD.)

***What is the most likely cause of hepatocellular liver injury in this patient?***

**What biochemical laboratory pattern describes hepatocellular liver injury?**

Diseases of the liver produce characteristic biochemical patterns of injury. Distinguishing hepatocellular liver injury from cholestatic liver injury can be helpful in narrowing the differential diagnosis. Hepatocellular liver injury refers to the predominance of serum aminotransferase elevation compared with serum ALP. Serum bilirubin levels may or may not be elevated.[1]

**What are the aminotransferases?**

The aminotransferases, which include AST and ALT, are enzymes that catabolize amino acids, generating products that enter the Krebs cycle. AST and ALT are highly concentrated in the liver and are immediately leaked into the circulation when there is hepatocyte necrosis.[1]

**What are the sources of aminotransferases in the body?**

AST and ALT are present in high concentrations in the liver. AST is also present in the tissues of the heart, skeletal muscle, kidney, and brain, and in red blood cells. There are low levels of ALT in skeletal muscle and kidney. Elevated serum ALT is generally more specific for liver damage than elevated AST.[1]

**What is the definition of an abnormal aminotransferase level?**

An abnormal aminotransferase level is defined by a value that exceeds the upper limit of normal (normal values vary by laboratory). Aminotransferase levels below the lower limit of normal are of no clinical significance.[1]

**How is the normal value range determined for most laboratory tests?**

Generally, the normal range for a given laboratory test is defined as the values within 2 standard deviations of the mean of the general population.

**Using the 2 standard deviation rule, what percentage of healthy patients will have abnormal aminotransferase levels?**

In a normal distribution, 95% of values lie within 2 standard deviations of the mean. This means that 2.5% of healthy individuals will have aminotransferase levels below normal, and 2.5% of healthy individuals will have aminotransferase levels above normal.[1]

**How sensitive is aminotransferase elevation for the presence liver damage?**

Aminotransferase elevation is generally a sensitive marker of liver damage but may not be present in all patients. For example, some patients with chronic hepatitis C infection and others with nonalcoholic fatty liver disease have normal aminotransferase levels despite histologic evidence of liver damage.[1]

**How is the severity of aminotransferase elevation delineated?**

Severity of hepatocellular liver injury is variably defined, but the following thresholds provide a rule of thumb: Serum aminotransferase elevation is considered mild when it is <5 times the upper limit of normal, moderate when 5 to 10 times the upper limit of normal, and marked when >10 times the upper limit of normal. Marked aminotransferase elevation is usually the result of acute liver injury.[1]

**What life-threatening condition can occur in patients with hepatocellular liver injury?**

Acute liver failure is a life-threatening condition that usually occurs in patients without preexisting liver disease and is characterized by biochemical laboratory evidence of acute liver injury and coagulopathy, jaundice, and encephalopathy over a period of days to months. Multiple organ failure and death occur in up to half of cases. In patients with acute liver injury, the risk of acute liver failure is generally low but can be significant in certain circumstances. For example, acute liver failure occurs in approximately 15% of pregnant women with hepatitis E infection.[2,3]

**The causes of hepatocellular liver injury can be separated into which general categories?**

The causes of hepatocellular liver injury can be separated into the following categories: infectious, toxic, vascular, hereditary, and other.

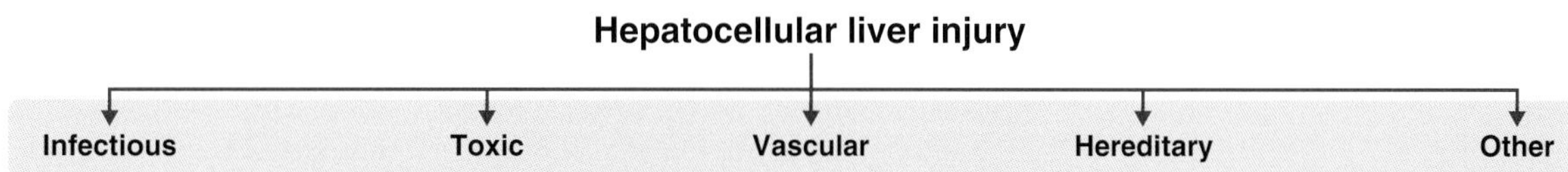


## INFECTIOUS CAUSES OF HEPATOCELLULAR LIVER INJURY

### What are the infectious causes of hepatocellular liver injury?

**A vaccine is available for this virus that is transmitted via the fecal-oral route.**

Hepatitis A virus (HAV).

**A vaccine is not available for this virus that is transmitted via the fecal-oral route.**

Hepatitis E virus (HEV).

**In adult patients, this virus is most commonly acquired through sexual transmission.**

Hepatitis B virus (HBV).

**Often acquired when needles are shared between intravenous drug users.**

Hepatitis C virus (HCV).

**Infection with this virus occurs exclusively in patients with hepatitis B infection.**

Hepatitis D virus (HDV).

**This virus is responsible for causing infectious mononucleosis.**

Epstein-Barr virus (EBV).

**In the immunocompetent host, infection with this virus is typically asymptomatic but can present with a syndrome similar to mononucleosis.**

Cytomegalovirus (CMV).

**Hepatitis caused by these viruses may be associated with characteristic cutaneous lesions.**

Herpes simplex virus (HSV) and varicella-zoster virus (VZV).

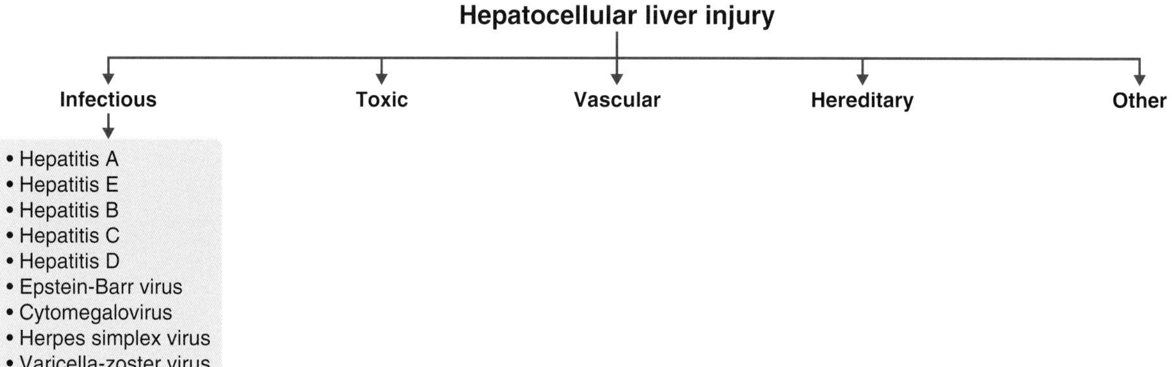


**What are the clinical features of hepatitis A virus infection?**

HAV infection is found worldwide, endemic in areas with poor sanitation. Most infected adults are symptomatic. The preicteric phase is characterized by symptoms that develop 15 to 50 days (mean, 30 days) after exposure and include anorexia, nausea and vomiting, malaise, fever, headache, and abdominal pain. This is followed by the onset of the icteric phase, characterized by dark urine, acholic stools, and jaundice. Aminotransferases are usually markedly elevated, often >1000 U/L. Extrahepatic manifestations can occur (eg, arthralgias). Diagnosis is established by detecting serum immunoglobulin M (IgM) anti-HAV antibodies. The illness is usually self-limited, and the vast majority of patients fully recover within weeks to months.[4]

**What are the clinical features of hepatitis E virus infection?**

HEV infection is found worldwide, endemic in areas with poor sanitation. The incubation period ranges from 20 to 60 days (mean, 40 days). Most patients are asymptomatic. Those with symptoms experience a syndrome similar to that of HAV infection, including the preicteric phase, icteric phase, and potential extrahepatic manifestations. Aminotransferases are usually markedly elevated, often >1000 U/L. There are a variety of diagnostic serum assays, each with variable performance characteristics; a combination of tests may ultimately be needed to confirm the diagnosis. In healthy populations, the illness is usually self-limited, and the vast majority of patients fully recover within weeks to months. However, there is a risk of acute liver failure, particularly in pregnant women.[5]

**What is the natural history of acute hepatitis B virus infection?**

HBV infection is acquired via contact with infected blood or body fluid. In the industrialized world, adults most commonly acquire the infection via sexual contact. Most adults are symptomatic, and clinical manifestations are similar to other forms of acute viral hepatitis. Aminotransferases are usually markedly elevated, often >1000 U/L. In healthy patients, the illness is self-limited in the vast majority of cases. It progresses to acute liver failure in <1% of adults, which is associated with a mortality rate of approximately 80% without liver transplantation. Chronic HBV infection develops in <5% of adult patients.[6]

**What is the natural history of acute hepatitis C virus infection?**

HCV infection is most commonly acquired through blood transfusion or intravenous drug use. Most adults are asymptomatic. Patients who are symptomatic experience a syndrome similar to other causes of acute viral hepatitis. Aminotransferases are usually markedly elevated, often >1000 U/L. Acute HCV infection rarely causes acute liver failure. Although the illness can be self-limited, most patients develop chronic infection.[7]

**What is the natural history of acute hepatitis D virus infection?**

Like HBV, HDV is transmitted via contact with infected blood or body fluid. Infection requires the presence of either acute or chronic HBV infection. Acute coinfection typically results in more severe clinical manifestations compared with acute HBV infection alone, and it is cleared along with HBV in the vast majority of cases. In contrast, superinfection in patients with chronic HBV infection usually results in chronic HDV infection, which is associated with more rapid progression to cirrhosis.[8]

**What are the clinical features of Epstein-Barr virus hepatitis?**

Most healthy patients with EBV infection are asymptomatic, but some experience infectious mononucleosis, which is characterized by the constellation of fever, sore throat, and lymphadenopathy. Mild hepatocellular liver injury is found in most patients with mononucleosis. Serologic tests (eg, heterophile antibody test) are used to establish the diagnosis. Some patients (particularly those who are immunocompromised) develop severe hepatitis. Histologic findings include vacuolization of the hepatocytes and periportal infiltration with lymphocytes and monocytes. Antiviral therapy (eg, ganciclovir) may be effective in severe disease.[9,10]

**What are the clinical features of cytomegalovirus hepatitis?**

Most healthy patients with CMV infection are asymptomatic, but some experience a self-limited mononucleosis-like illness. Immunocompromised patients are at risk for primary infection or reactivation of dormant infection, which can result in tissue-invasive disease, including hepatitis. The spectrum of severity can range from mild to acute liver failure. Definitive diagnosis of CMV hepatitis requires histopathologic identification of characteristic inclusion bodies (ie, Owl's eye appearance) or viral elements by immunohistochemical or molecular techniques. Ganciclovir is the antiviral agent of choice for severe disease.[10-12]

**What are the clinical features of herpes simplex virus hepatitis?**

HSV hepatitis is a life-threatening condition associated with disseminated HSV-1 and HSV-2 infections. It accounts for <10% of viral causes of acute liver failure. Immunocompromised patients and women in the third trimester of pregnancy are at highest risk. Aminotransferases are often 100 to 1000 times the upper limit of normal. In some cases, disseminated HSV involves the skin, producing vesicular or pustular lesions in a generalized distribution, which evolve into dried crusted papules and eventually shallow punched-out ulcers. On clinical examination, lesions are often found in various stages of healing. Diagnosis of HSV hepatitis is based on histopathologic identification of characteristic intranuclear inclusion bodies or viral elements by immunohistochemical or molecular techniques. Intravenous acyclovir is the antiviral agent of choice.[10,12]

**What are the clinical features of varicella-zoster virus hepatitis?**

Immunocompromised patients are at risk for disseminated VZV infection, which typically occurs as a result of reactivation of dormant infection. Hepatic involvement usually leads to acute liver failure. Cutaneous lesions are frequently present, which are clinically indistinguishable from disseminated cutaneous HSV. The diagnosis is confirmed through the identification of VZV from skin lesions or affected organs. Intravenous acyclovir is the antiviral agent of choice.[10]

*Acute viral hepatitis is generally associated with ALT:AST ratio >1.*[13]

## TOXIC CAUSES OF HEPATOCELLULAR LIVER INJURY

### What are the toxic causes of hepatocellular liver injury?

**AST:ALT ratio >2:1.**

Alcohol.

**A 33-year-old woman with depression and prior suicide attempts presents with nausea, vomiting, and marked hepatocellular liver injury.**

Acetaminophen overdose.

**A 22-year-old woman is admitted to the intensive care unit with acute liver failure after a weekend of partying.**

Recreational drug use.

**Patients with a history of repeated blood transfusions are at risk.**

Iron overload (ie, secondary hemochromatosis).

**Makes Mario bigger and faster.**

Mushrooms.

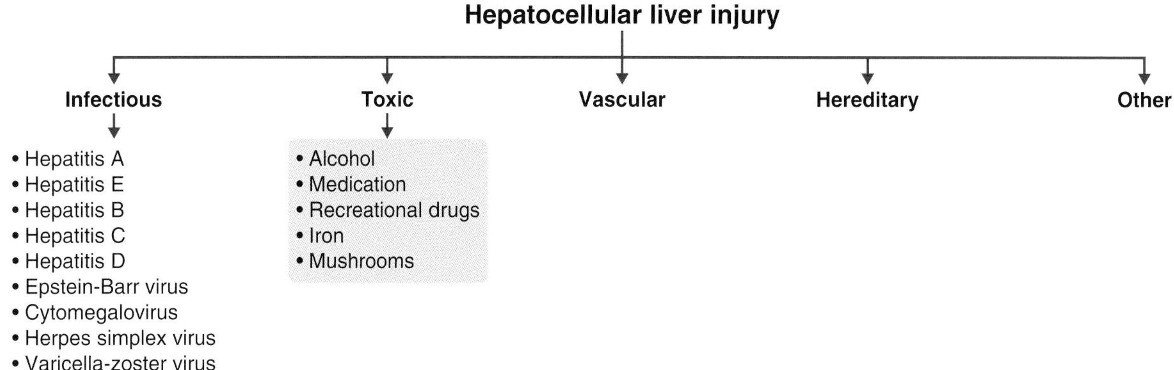


**What are the characteristic biochemical laboratory features of alcoholic hepatitis?**

Alcoholic hepatitis can develop as acute or acute-on-chronic liver injury. Fever, jaundice, and tender hepatomegaly are the hallmarks of the condition. Unlike most causes of toxic hepatitis, aminotransferase levels rarely exceed 300 U/L in alcoholic hepatitis. The AST:ALT ratio is typically >2. Alkaline phosphatase is frequently elevated, and total bilirubin is elevated at least 5-10 times the upper limit of normal, although it can be >10 times the upper limit of normal in some cases. Because of the limited degree of aminotransferase elevation, patients may have a cholestatic pattern of liver injury.[1,14]

**What medications are most commonly implicated in acute liver failure?**

Virtually any medication can lead to liver injury. Acetaminophen is one of the most common causes of acute liver failure, particularly in young previously healthy patients. Other medications that cause acute liver failure with relatively high frequency include isoniazid, propylthiouracil, phenytoin, valproate, nitrofurantoin, and ketoconazole. In patients with hepatocellular liver injury, it is important to carefully review prescription and over-the-counter medications, as well as herbal supplements.[15]

**Which recreational drug frequently causes acute liver failure in the industrialized world?**

The synthetic amphetamine 3,4-methylenedioxymethamphetamine (MDMA, "ecstasy," or "molly") is used as a recreational drug for its euphoric effects. It can cause acute hepatitis and is responsible for a significant proportion of cases of acute liver failure in young patients. There is marked aminotransferase elevation (often >1000 U/L) along with marked hyperbilirubinemia. Management is supportive; transplantation may be necessary in some cases.[16]

**What conditions are associated with secondary hemochromatosis?**

Secondary hemochromatosis can develop as a result of increased intestinal absorption of iron or recurrent blood transfusions. Associated conditions include hemoglobinopathies (eg, sickle cell disease, thalassemia), inherited hemolytic anemia (eg, glucose-6-phosphate dehydrogenase deficiency, hereditary spherocytosis), and myelodysplasia.

**Which species of mushroom is most frequently responsible for acute liver failure and death?**

Known as the "death cap," *Amanita phalloides* is responsible for most cases of acute liver failure caused by mushroom poisoning. Accidental ingestion by amateur mushroom hunters is the most frequent manner of intoxication. Clinical manifestations range from a mild subclinical presentation to acute liver failure. Gastrointestinal symptoms (eg, abdominal pain, vomiting, diarrhea) typically appear 6 to 24 hours after ingestion. This phase is usually followed by a period of apparent clinical improvement before the onset of marked aminotransferase elevation and acute liver failure.[17]

*With the exception of alcoholic hepatitis, toxic causes of acute hepatitis are generally associated with ALT:AST ratio >1.*[13]

## VASCULAR CAUSES OF HEPATOCELLULAR LIVER INJURY

### What are the vascular causes of hepatocellular liver injury?

**A 23-year-old woman is admitted to the hospital with hemorrhagic shock after a motor vehicle accident and is found to have aminotransferase elevation >75 times the upper limit of normal.**

Ischemic hepatitis (ie, shock liver).

**"Nutmeg liver."**

Congestive hepatopathy.

**A 24-year-old woman with factor V Leiden thrombophilia who recently started oral contraceptives presents with acute abdominal pain and hepatocellular liver injury.**

Budd-Chiari syndrome.

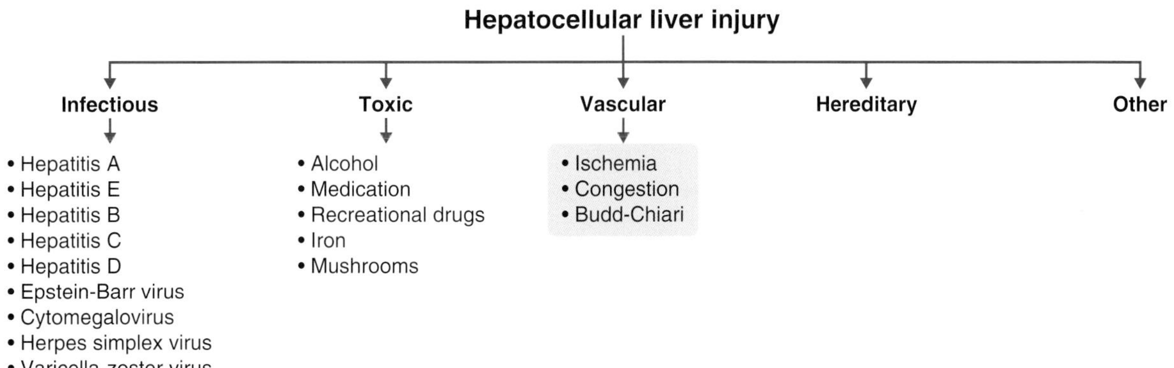


**What are the characteristic biochemical laboratory features of ischemic hepatitis?**

Ischemic hepatitis occurs as a result of inadequate perfusion of the liver. Aminotransferase elevation is marked, often >50 times the upper limit of normal. When hemodynamics are restored, there is often a rapid decrease in aminotransferase levels after the initial peak.[1,14]

**What are the clinical features of congestive hepatopathy?**

Congestive hepatopathy occurs as a result of elevated central venous pressure, most commonly related to cardiomyopathy, pulmonary hypertension, constrictive pericarditis, or valvulopathy (eg, mitral stenosis, tricuspid regurgitation). Manifestations include hepatomegaly, jaundice, peripheral edema, pleural effusions, ascites, and splenomegaly. Mild hyperbilirubinemia (usually <3 mg/dL) is the most common laboratory abnormality; when present, aminotransferase elevation is only mild. Marked aminotransferase elevation in patients with decompensated heart failure is suggestive of ischemic hepatitis.[18]

**What are the biochemical laboratory features of Budd-Chiari syndrome?**

Acute Budd-Chiari syndrome is characterized by abdominal pain, hepatomegaly, ascites, and hepatocellular liver injury that is at least moderate in severity. Acute liver failure is uncommon. In subacute and chronic forms of the disease, aminotransferase levels may be normal or only mildly elevated.[19]

*Vascular causes of acute hepatitis are generally associated with AST:ALT ratio >1.*[13]

## HEREDITARY CAUSES OF HEPATOCELLULAR LIVER INJURY

### What are the hereditary causes of hepatocellular liver injury?

**Men with this condition are usually diagnosed at a younger age than women.**

Hereditary hemochromatosis. *Blood loss from menstruation is protective against iron overload.*

**A 26-year-old man presents with hepatocellular liver injury, hemolytic anemia, delusions, and hallucinations.**

Wilson's disease.

**Associated with emphysema.**

α-1 Antitrypsin deficiency.

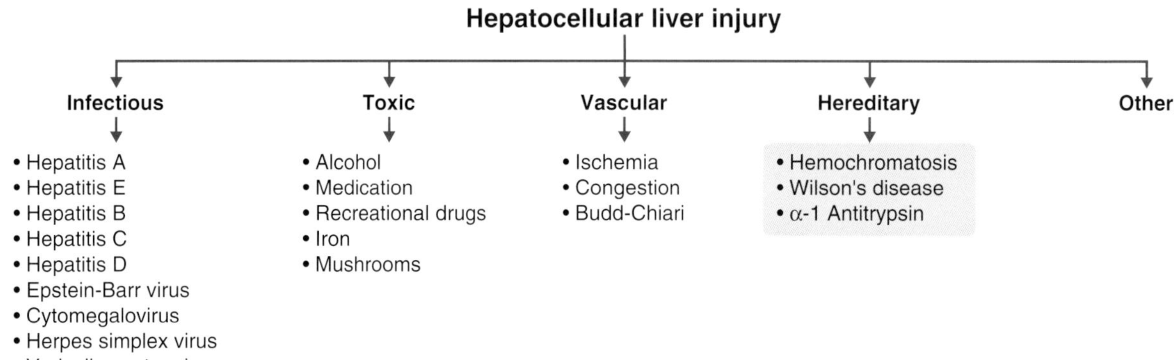


**How sensitive is aminotransferase elevation in patients with hereditary hemochromatosis?**

Hereditary hemochromatosis is an autosomal recessive condition and is common in whites. Aminotransferase levels are typically normal or only mildly increased, even in patients who develop fibrotic liver disease. Elevated aminotransferase levels in these patients should prompt consideration of other causes of hepatocellular liver injury (eg, chronic viral hepatitis).[20]

**What is the spectrum of liver disease in patients with Wilson's disease?**

Wilson's disease is most commonly diagnosed in late childhood or adolescence, but it can present later in life. It should be suspected in patients with hepatocellular liver injury and concomitant hemolytic anemia, with or without psychiatric or neurologic symptoms. There is a wide spectrum of liver involvement, including asymptomatic aminotransferase elevation, acute hepatitis, acute liver failure, and progressive chronic liver disease. Low serum ceruloplasmin levels, elevated 24-hour urine copper excretion, and the presence of Kayser-Fleischer rings (a brown ring around the iris from copper deposition) (Figure 17-2) are consistent with the diagnosis. Liver biopsy is sometimes necessary to confirm the diagnosis.[1,21]

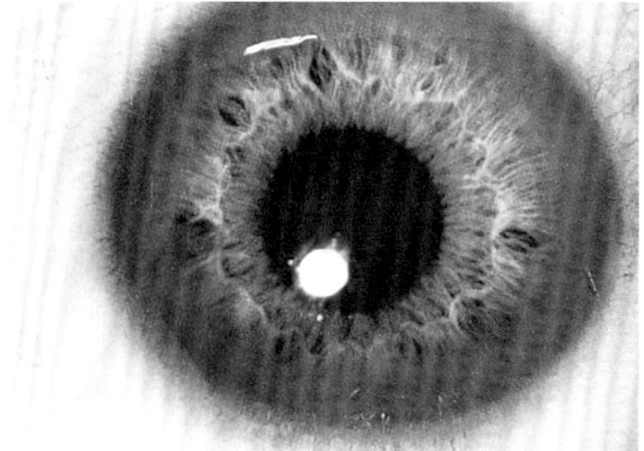

**Figure 17-2.** Brown copper deposition in the periphery of the cornea (Kayser-Fleischer ring) in a patient with Wilson's disease. *Rings are not often this pronounced. Milder cases may not be visible with the naked eye but can be identified with a slit lamp examination.* (From Tasman W, Jaeger E. *The Wills Eye Hospital Atlas of Clinical Ophthalmology*. 2nd ed. Philadelphia, PA: Lippincott Williams & Wilkins; 2001.)

**What is the mechanism of liver injury in the setting of α-1 antitrypsin deficiency?**

α-1 Antitrypsin deficiency is most often diagnosed in childhood, but in adults it may present with pulmonary or hepatic manifestations. The mechanisms of lung and liver disease differ. Increased proteolytic activity in the lung leads to the development of emphysema. In contrast, liver disease is the result of intrahepatic accumulation of abnormally folded α-1 antitrypsin protein. Aminotransferase elevation is mild in most patients. The diagnosis can be confirmed with low serum α-1 antitrypsin levels and phenotype or genotype determination.[22]

*Hereditary causes of acute hepatitis are generally associated with ALT:AST ratio >1.*[13]

## OTHER CAUSES OF HEPATOCELLULAR LIVER INJURY

### What are the other causes of hepatocellular liver injury?

**Associated with the metabolic syndrome.**

Nonalcoholic fatty liver disease (NAFLD).

**A middle-aged woman with a history of Graves' disease presents with marked hepatocellular liver injury and is found to have an elevated serum protein gap, positive antinuclear antibody, and positive anti–smooth muscle antibody.**

Autoimmune hepatitis.

**Cholestatic liver injury eventually predominates in patients with this condition.**

Acute biliary obstruction.

**Pregnancy.**

HELLP syndrome.

**Hepatocellular liver injury and elevated tissue transglutaminase antibodies.**

Celiac disease.

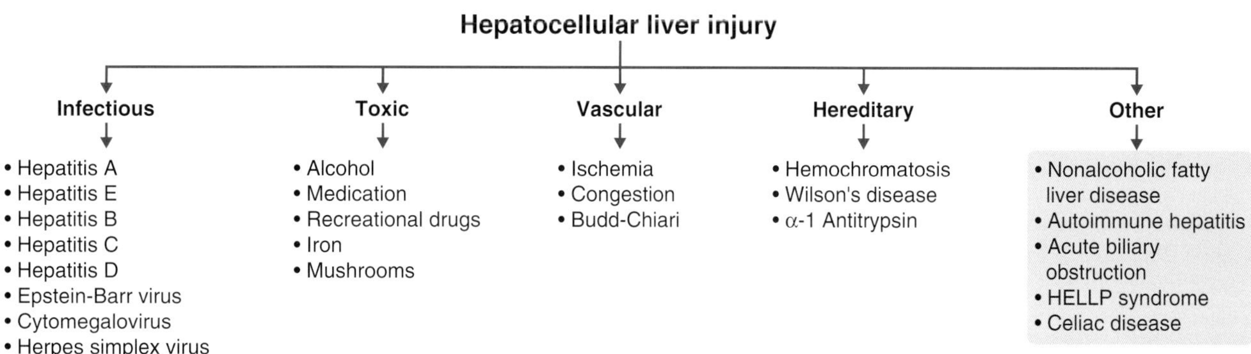


**What are the clinical features of nonalcoholic fatty liver disease?**

NAFLD is the most common cause of hepatocellular liver injury in the industrialized world. Most patients are asymptomatic or have nonspecific symptoms and the diagnosis is suspected because of mild aminotransferase elevation. There is no specific blood test for NAFLD, and it is a diagnosis of exclusion. Liver biopsy can distinguish between simple steatosis (nonalcoholic fatty liver) and steatohepatitis (nonalcoholic steatohepatitis) with or without fibrosis.[1]

**What are the clinical features of autoimmune hepatitis?**

Autoimmune hepatitis occurs globally in patients of various ages and ethnicities but is most common in women. It generally causes chronic and progressive hepatitis but may follow a fluctuating course with periods of increased or decreased disease activity. Presentation can vary from subclinical with mild hepatocellular liver injury, to acute liver failure with aminotransferases >1000 U/L. Some cases are characterized by a cholestatic pattern of liver injury. An elevated serum protein gap can be a clue to the diagnosis. The presence of serum antinuclear and anti–smooth muscle antibodies is characteristic. Immunosuppressive medication (eg, prednisone with or without azathioprine) is the cornerstone of treatment.[23]

**What are the biochemical laboratory features of acute biliary obstruction?**

Although biliary obstruction will eventually cause a cholestatic pattern of liver injury, a hepatocellular pattern occurs early on. Aminotransferases are usually moderately elevated with an associated hyperbilirubinemia. The early hepatocellular predominance is explained by the fact that the aminotransferases are immediately leaked into the circulation upon hepatocyte necrosis. In contrast, ALP is synthesized in response to cholestasis and accumulating bile salts, which requires more time.[1]

**What is HELLP syndrome?**

HELLP is an acronym that stands for Hemolysis, Elevated Liver enzymes, and Low Platelets. It is a syndrome that develops in pregnant women, usually between the 27th and 37th gestational weeks. The pathogenesis of HELLP syndrome is unclear but it may be a severe variant of preeclampsia. Aminotransferase elevation >2 times the upper limit of normal is required for the diagnosis. The presence of either AST >150 U/L or ALT >100 U/L is associated with a higher risk of serious maternal morbidity.[24]

**How common is celiac disease in patients with unexplained hepatocellular liver injury?**

Hepatocellular liver injury may be the only manifestation of celiac disease. Patients with unexplained hepatocellular liver injury should be tested for celiac disease, which is present in up to 10% of cases.[1]

*These "other" causes of hepatitis are generally associated with ALT:AST ratio >1.*[13]

## Case Summary

A 37-year-old immunocompromised man presents with fever and abdominal pain and is found to have diffuse cutaneous vesicular lesions and marked hepatocellular liver injury.

***What is the most likely cause of hepatocellular liver injury in this patient?***

Disseminated varicella-zoster virus infection.

### BONUS QUESTIONS

***Is the severity of aminotransferase elevation helpful in establishing the cause of hepatocellular liver injury?***

In patients with hepatocellular liver injury, the degree of aminotransferase elevation can be helpful in narrowing the differential diagnosis. Marked aminotransferase elevation (>10 times the upper limit of normal) is usually the result of acute liver injury, which may be caused by viral infection, drug toxicity (especially acetaminophen), ischemic hepatitis, autoimmune hepatitis, mushroom toxicity, or Wilson's disease.[1]

***What historical information makes disseminated varicella-zoster virus an important consideration in this case?***

Disseminated VZV is significantly more common in immunocompromised patients. It typically manifests with cutaneous lesions with or without visceral involvement (eg, hepatitis, pneumonitis, encephalitis). Visceral involvement may precede the development of cutaneous lesions in some cases. Disseminated VZV is the most frequent late infection of bone marrow transplantation recipients, and concurrent graft-versus-host disease is a major risk factor.[25]

| | |
|---|---|
| ***What other infectious cause of hepatocellular liver injury can present with similar cutaneous lesions?*** | Disseminated VZV and HSV infections can both present with cutaneous vesicular lesions in a generalized distribution that are clinically indistinguishable from one another. To discriminate between HSV and VZV infection, the lesions can be swabbed and tested using molecular (eg, polymerase chain reaction) or immunohistochemical (eg, immunofluorescence) techniques. In this case, molecular testing for HSV was negative, making VZV the most likely diagnosis (testing for VZV should be performed to confirm the diagnosis).[10] |
| ***Should graft-versus-host disease of the liver be considered in this case?*** | Graft-versus-host disease of the liver should be considered in this case, particularly given the presence of cutaneous graft-versus-host disease. However, the pattern of liver injury is typically cholestatic, not hepatocellular (see chapter 14, Cholestatic Liver Injury). |
| ***How should the patient in this case be treated?*** | Disseminated VZV with visceral involvement is associated with a high mortality rate. Prompt administration of intravenous acyclovir is associated with improved outcomes.[10,26] |

## KEY POINTS

- Hepatocellular liver injury refers to the predominance of aminotransferase elevation compared with ALP. Serum bilirubin levels may or may not be elevated.
- Aminotransferase elevation is mild when it is <5 times the upper limit of normal, moderate when it is 5 to 10 times the upper limit, and marked when it is >10 times the upper limit.
- The causes of hepatocellular liver injury can be separated into the following categories: infectious, toxic, vascular, hereditary, and other.
- In patients with hepatocellular liver injury, the degree of aminotransferase elevation and the ratio between AST and ALT levels can help narrow the differential diagnosis.
- Marked aminotransferase elevation is usually the result of acute liver injury, which may be caused by acute viral infection, drug toxicity (especially acetaminophen), ischemic hepatitis, autoimmune hepatitis, mushroom toxicity, or Wilson's disease.

## REFERENCES


1. Giannini EG, Testa R, Savarino V. Liver enzyme alteration: a guide for clinicians. *CMAJ*. 2005;172(3):367-379.
2. Bernal W, Wendon J. Acute liver failure. *N Engl J Med*. 2013;369(26):2525-2534.
3. Ryder SD, Beckingham IJ. ABC of diseases of liver, pancreas, and biliary system: acute hepatitis. *BMJ*. 2001;322(7279):151-153.
4. Cuthbert JA. Hepatitis A: old and new. *Clin Microbiol Rev*. 2001;14(1):38-58.
5. Hartl J, Wehmeyer MH, Pischke S. Acute hepatitis E: two sides of the same coin. *Viruses*. 2016;8(11).
6. Trepo C, Chan HL, Lok A. Hepatitis B virus infection. *Lancet*. 2014;384(9959):2053-2063.
7. Kamal SM. Acute hepatitis C: a systematic review. *Am J Gastroenterol*. 2008;103(5):1283-1297; quiz 98.
8. Hughes SA, Wedemeyer H, Harrison PM. Hepatitis delta virus. *Lancet*. 2011;378(9785):73-85.
9. Crum NF. Epstein Barr virus hepatitis: case series and review. *South Med J*. 2006;99(5):544-547.
10. Gallegos-Orozco JF, Rakela-Brodner J. Hepatitis viruses: not always what it seems to be. *Rev Med Chil*. 2010;138(10):1302-1311.
11. Kotton CN, Kumar D, Caliendo AM, et al. Updated international consensus guidelines on the management of cytomegalovirus in solid-organ transplantation. *Transplantation*. 2013;96(4):333-360.
12. Norvell JP, Blei AT, Jovanovic BD, Levitsky J. Herpes simplex virus hepatitis: an analysis of the published literature and institutional cases. *Liver Transpl*. 2007;13(10):1428-1434.
13. Kwo PY, Cohen SM, Lim JK. ACG Clinical Guideline: evaluation of abnormal liver chemistries. *Am J Gastroenterol*. 2017;112(1):18-35.
14. Lucey MR, Mathurin P, Morgan TR. Alcoholic hepatitis. *N Engl J Med*. 2009;360(26):2758-2769.
15. Russo MW, Galanko JA, Shrestha R, Fried MW, Watkins P. Liver transplantation for acute liver failure from drug induced liver injury in the United States. *Liver Transpl*. 2004;10(8):1018-1023.
16. Andreu V, Mas A, Bruguera M, et al. Ecstasy: a common cause of severe acute hepatotoxicity. *J Hepatol*. 1998;29(3):394-397.
17. Erden A, Esmeray K, Karagoz H, et al. Acute liver failure caused by mushroom poisoning: a case report and review of the literature. *Int Med Case Rep J*. 2013;6:85-90.
18. Kavoliuniene A, Vaitiekiene A, Cesnaite G. Congestive hepatopathy and hypoxic hepatitis in heart failure: a cardiologist's point of view. *Int J Cardiol*. 2013;166(3):554-558.

19. Menon KV, Shah V, Kamath PS. The Budd-Chiari syndrome. *N Engl J Med*. 2004;350(6):578-585.
20. Adams PC, Speechley M, Barton JC, McLaren CE, McLaren GD, Eckfeldt JH. Probability of C282Y homozygosity decreases as liver transaminase activities increase in participants with hyperferritinemia in the hemochromatosis and iron overload screening study. *Hepatology*. 2012;55(6):1722-1726.
21. Das SK, Ray K. Wilson's disease: an update. *Nat Clin Pract Neurol*. 2006;2(9):482-493.
22. Dawwas MF, Davies SE, Griffiths WJ, Lomas DA, Alexander GJ. Prevalence and risk factors for liver involvement in individuals with PiZZ-related lung disease. *Am J Respir Crit Care Med*. 2013;187(5):502-508.
23. Krawitt EL. Autoimmune hepatitis. *N Engl J Med*. 2006;354(1):54-66.
24. Haram K, Svendsen E, Abildgaard U. The HELLP syndrome: clinical issues and management. A review. *BMC Pregnancy Childbirth*. 2009;9:8.
25. Locksley RM, Flournoy N, Sullivan KM, Meyers JD. Infection with varicella zoster virus after marrow transplantation. *J Infect Dis*. 1985;152(6):1172-1181.
26. Miller GG, Dummer JS. Herpes simplex and varicella zoster viruses: forgotten but not gone. *Am J Transplant*. 2007;7(4):741-747.

Chapter 18

# INTESTINAL ISCHEMIA

## Case: A 44-year-old man with testicular pain

A 44-year-old man with a history of hypertension presents to the emergency department with acute-on-chronic abdominal pain. Symptoms began 1 year ago with the onset of diffuse abdominal pain that worsens shortly after meals. He has been eating less frequently and has experienced weight loss of 50 pounds over this time. On the day of presentation, the abdominal pain became severe and unrelenting. Additional history is notable for chronic testicular soreness.

Temperature is 38.5°C, heart rate is 125 beats per minute, and blood pressure is 148/93 mm Hg. The patient is diaphoretic and appears uncomfortable. The abdomen is mildly tender to palpation; there is no guarding, rebound, or rigidity. Livedo reticularis is present over the lower extremities.

Peripheral white blood cell count is 16 K/μL with 92% neutrophils, blood lactate is 12 mmol/L, and serum alkaline phosphatase is 280 U/L. Hepatitis B surface antigen is negative. Cross-sectional imaging of the abdomen reveals segmental small bowel wall thickening, pneumatosis intestinalis, and portal vein gas. Conventional mesenteric angiography is shown in Figure 18-1.

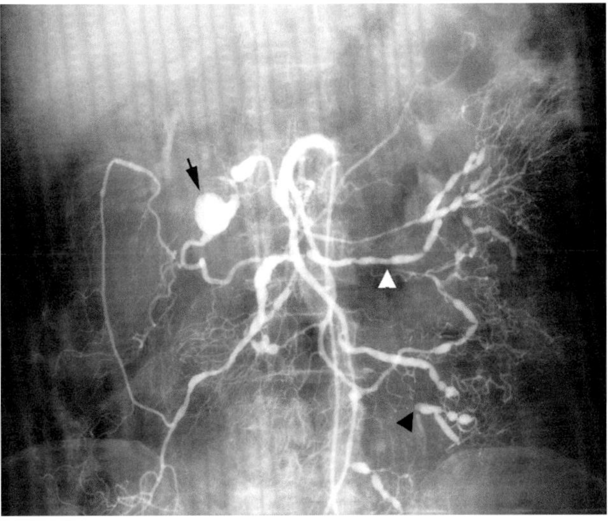

**Figure 18-1.** (From Stanson AW, Friese JL, Johnson CM, et al. Polyarteritis nodosa: spectrum of angiographic findings. *Radiographics*. 2001;21:151-159, with permission.)

***What is the most likely underlying cause of intestinal ischemia in this patient?***

What is intestinal ischemia?

Intestinal ischemia occurs when oxygen and nutrient delivery to intestinal tissue is insufficient to meet metabolic demand, which can lead to necrosis and perforation. Its effects are usually limited in location to either the small or large intestine.

What are the 2 main types of intestinal ischemia?

Mesenteric ischemia and ischemic colitis are the 2 main types of intestinal ischemia.

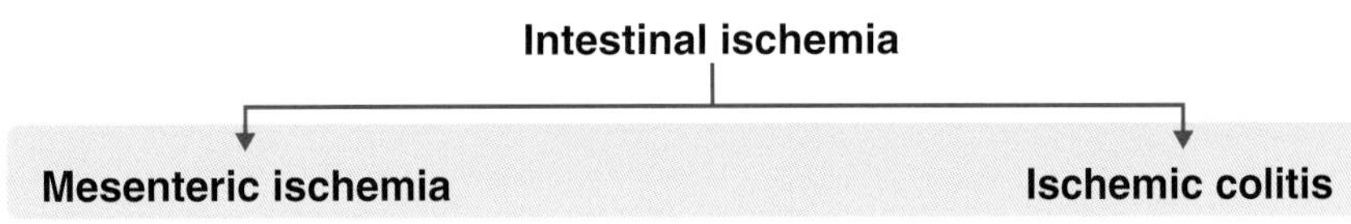

**Which parts of the gastrointestinal (GI) tract are affected by mesenteric ischemia and ischemic colitis?**

Mesenteric ischemia refers to involvement of the small intestine; ischemic colitis refers to involvement of the large intestine.

## MESENTERIC ISCHEMIA

**Which blood vessels supply the small intestine?**

The entire small intestine except the proximal portion of the duodenum is supplied by the superior mesenteric artery (SMA), which arises directly from the aorta. An extensive collateral network (the arcades) protects the small intestine from ischemia related to hypoperfusion (Figure 18-2).[1]

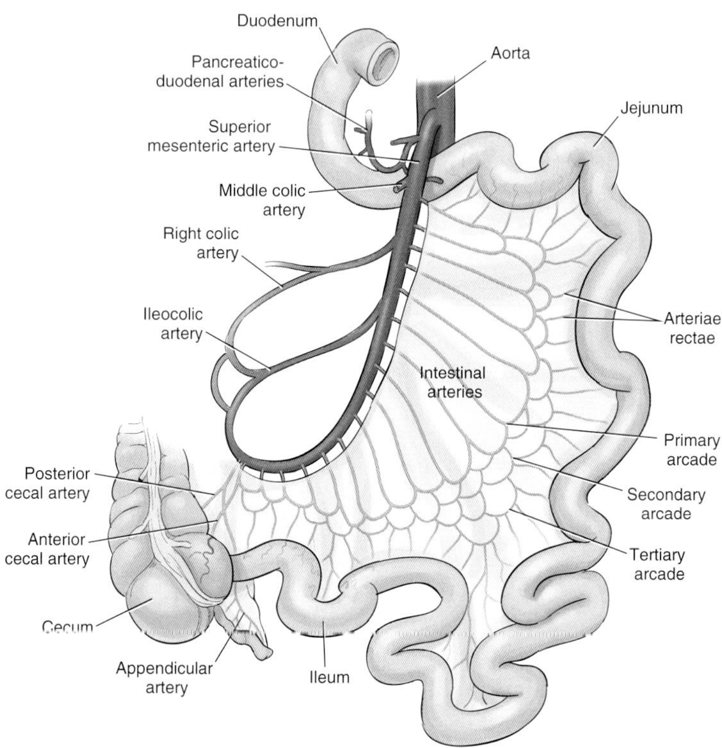


**Figure 18-2.** Blood supply of the small intestine. (From Jones HW, Rock JA. *Te Linde's Operative Gynecology*. 11th ed. Philadelphia, PA: Wolters Kluwer; 2015.)

**What are the 2 subtypes of mesenteric ischemia?**

Mesenteric ischemia can be acute or chronic.

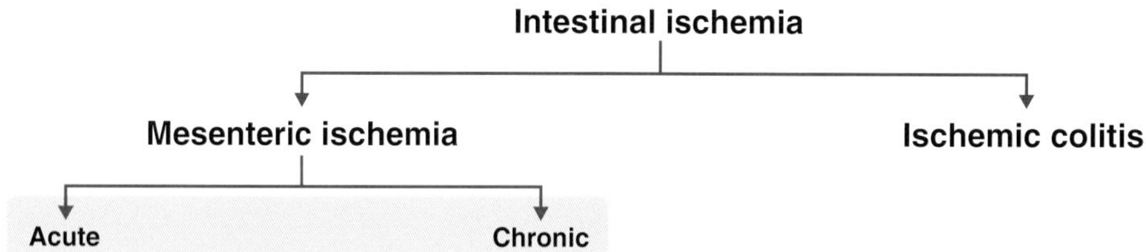


## ACUTE MESENTERIC ISCHEMIA

**What are the symptoms of acute mesenteric ischemia?**

Abdominal pain is present in most cases of acute mesenteric ischemia. Other symptoms may include nausea, vomiting, delirium (particularly in the elderly), and bloody diarrhea.[2,3]

**What are the physical findings of acute mesenteric ischemia?**

Patients with acute mesenteric ischemia often report pain that is out of proportion to the findings on physical examination. The clinical findings of acute mesenteric ischemia can be subtle and nonspecific early on. However, when transmural infarction results in bowel perforation, overt findings may include fever, tachycardia, hypotension, abdominal distention, decreased or absent bowel sounds, and signs of peritonitis such as abdominal wall rigidity, rebound tenderness, and guarding.[2]

**Which biochemical laboratory abnormalities are associated with acute mesenteric ischemia?**

Biochemical derangements of acute mesenteric ischemia may include leukocytosis with neutrophilia, metabolic acidosis, and elevated lactate, amylase, phosphate, and alkaline phosphatase levels (*recall from chapter 14, Cholestatic Liver Injury, that alkaline phosphatase is present in intestinal tissue*).[2]

**What is the role of conventional radiography in the diagnosis of acute mesenteric ischemia?**

Plain abdominal radiography demonstrates nonspecific findings early in the course of acute mesenteric ischemia, including intestinal dilation, thickened bowel loops, thickened folds, and air-fluid levels. More specific findings can be identified in advanced cases, including thumbprinting from interstitial edema (see Figure 16-3), pneumatosis intestinalis from gas-forming bacteria in the bowel wall, portal vein pneumatosis from gas-forming bacteria in the portal vein, and pneumoperitoneum from bowel perforation (identified by the presence of air under the diaphragm in the upright film).[2]

**What is the role of computed tomography (CT) imaging in the diagnosis of acute mesenteric ischemia?**

CT imaging is more sensitive than conventional radiography in demonstrating findings suggestive of acute mesenteric ischemia, including thumbprinting, pneumatosis intestinalis, portal vein pneumatosis, segmental bowel wall thickening in a vascular distribution, and pneumoperitoneum. CT imaging may occasionally identify the underlying cause of intestinal ischemia (eg, arterial occlusion). It is also useful in excluding other causes of abdominal pain.[2]

**What is the role of CT angiography in the diagnosis of acute mesenteric ischemia?**

CT angiography is the study of choice for diagnosing acute mesenteric ischemia. It provides information about the underlying cause (eg, thrombosis vs embolism) as well as location, which is helpful for procedural planning. Magnetic resonance angiography may also be used.[3]

**What is the role of conventional angiography in the diagnosis of acute mesenteric ischemia?**

Conventional angiography has been supplanted by CT angiography as the diagnostic study of choice for acute mesenteric ischemia. However, conventional angiography still has a role in diagnosis when CT angiography is equivocal. It is also used as a therapeutic modality when combined with endovascular techniques such as thrombolysis, thrombectomy, angioplasty with or without stenting, and administration of vasodilators.[3]

**What is the prognosis of acute mesenteric ischemia?**

Acute mesenteric ischemia is a life-threatening condition, associated with a mortality rate of up to 80%.[3]

**What are the 2 general mechanisms of acute mesenteric ischemia?**

Acute mesenteric ischemia can be caused by occlusive or nonocclusive mechanisms.

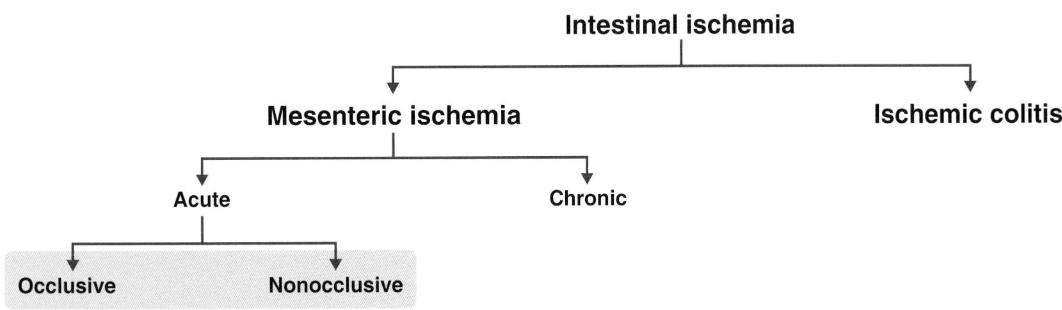


**Are nonocclusive or occlusive causes of acute mesenteric ischemia more common?**

Occlusive causes of mesenteric ischemia are most frequent, accounting for up to two-thirds of cases.[2]

## OCCLUSIVE CAUSES OF ACUTE MESENTERIC ISCHEMIA

### What are the occlusive causes of acute mesenteric ischemia?

Look for an irregularly irregular heart rhythm on examination.

Arterial embolism related to atrial fibrillation.

Older patients with a history of atherosclerotic disease.

Arterial thrombosis.

A 28-year-old woman with factor V Leiden thrombophilia who recently started oral contraceptives presents with acute abdominal pain, fever, elevated blood lactate, and segmental small bowel wall thickening on cross-sectional imaging.

Venous thrombosis.

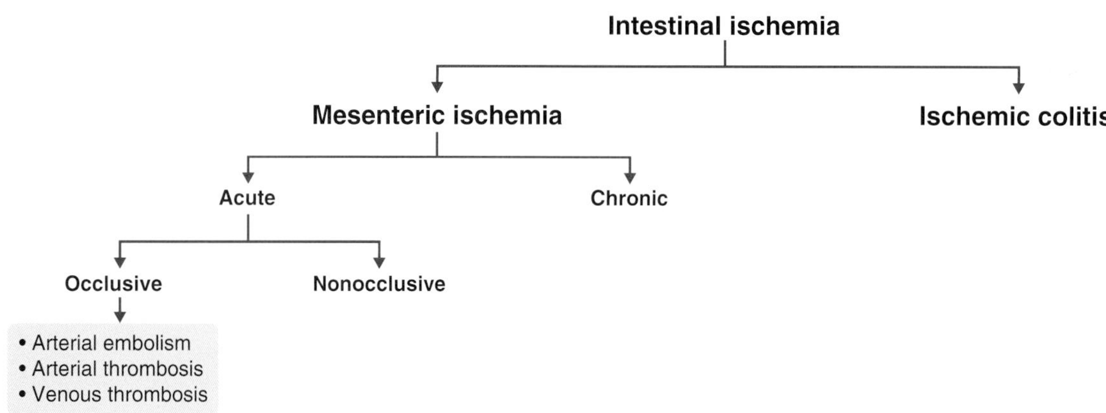


What are the characteristics of mesenteric artery embolism?

Arterial embolism accounts for most cases of acute mesenteric ischemia. Compared with the inferior mesenteric artery (IMA), the SMA is anatomically more susceptible to embolic events because it has a larger diameter and narrower takeoff angle from the aorta. Patients typically have a history of prior embolic events, most often involving the brain, kidneys, or lower extremities. Sources of emboli include the heart (from the left atrium, left ventricle, or valves) and proximal aorta (from an ulcerated atherosclerotic plaque or thrombosed aortic aneurysm). Atrial fibrillation is present in most patients with acute mesenteric ischemia related to arterial embolism; anticoagulation in these patients markedly reduces risk of future events.[2]

What are the characteristics of mesenteric artery thrombosis?

Patients with mesenteric artery thrombosis tend to be older than those with emboli. There is usually widespread atherosclerotic disease, with a history of coronary artery disease, cerebrovascular disease, or peripheral artery disease. Acute thrombosis develops within stenotic arteries during periods of sluggish blood flow. Less common causes of mesenteric artery thrombosis include underlying thrombophilia (eg, antiphospholipid antibody syndrome), vasculitis (eg, Behçet's disease), aortic or mesenteric artery aneurysm or dissection, and blunt abdominal trauma. Clinical manifestations tend to be less severe and slower in onset compared with those in patients with emboli, because preexisting atherosclerotic disease leads to the development of a protective network of collateral circulation.[2]

**What are the causes of acute mesenteric vein thrombosis?**

Acute mesenteric vein thrombosis most often involves the superior mesenteric vein. Most cases are related to underlying thrombophilia, including protein C deficiency, protein S deficiency, factor V Leiden thrombophilia, antithrombin III deficiency, malignancy, and antiphospholipid antibody syndrome. Patients often have a history of deep vein thrombosis. Other causes include hyperviscosity syndromes (eg, polycythemia vera), trauma, localized infection (eg, diverticulitis), localized inflammation (eg, acute pancreatitis), and portal hypertension. Most patients respond favorably to systemic anticoagulation and treatment of the associated condition.[2,3]

## NONOCCLUSIVE CAUSES OF ACUTE MESENTERIC ISCHEMIA

### What are the nonocclusive causes of acute mesenteric ischemia?

**A 58-year-old woman presents with crushing substernal chest pain and subsequently develops hypotension, cool extremities, severe abdominal pain, and elevated blood lactate.**

Cardiogenic shock.

**A 24-year-old man presents with sudden-onset severe abdominal pain, fever, tachycardia, and elevated blood lactate shortly after using cocaine.**

Mesenteric vasospasm.

**A 54-year-old man with an abdominal wall hernia presents with sudden onset intense abdominal pain.**

Extrinsic vessel compression related to a strangulated intestinal hernia.

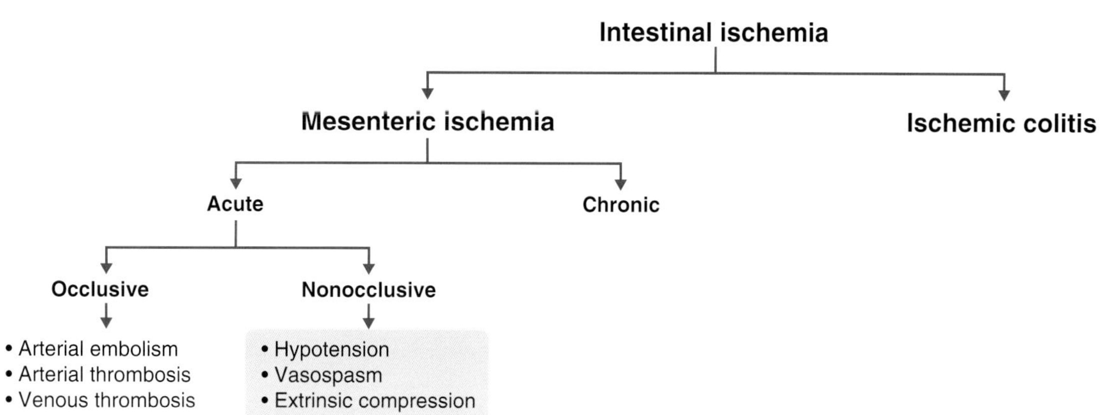


**What is the compensatory capacity of the small intestine when there is reduction in systemic blood flow?**

A compensatory increase in oxygen extraction allows the small intestine to tolerate up to a 75% reduction in blood flow for up to 12 hours.[4]

**What are the causes of hypotension or vasospasm that can lead to acute mesenteric ischemia?**

Nonocclusive acute mesenteric ischemia most often occurs as a result of systemic hypotension related to cardiogenic shock, hypovolemic shock, septic shock, anaphylactic shock, hemodialysis, or intraoperative cardiopulmonary bypass. Mesenteric arterial vasospasm is often superimposed on systemic hypotension as a compensatory mechanism to maintain blood flow to the vital organs at the expense of the intestines. It can also occur independently as a result of cocaine or methamphetamine abuse and the actions of vasoconstrictive medications (eg, digoxin, $\alpha$-adrenergic agonists).[2,5]

**What are the causes of acute extrinsic mesenteric artery compression?**

Extrinsic mesenteric artery compression can occur as a result of strangulated intestinal hernia, volvulus, and hematoma from blunt abdominal trauma.[2]

## CHRONIC MESENTERIC ISCHEMIA

**What is the epidemiology of chronic mesenteric ischemia?**

Chronic mesenteric ischemia is more common in women and in patients older than 60 years. Patients tend to have a smoking history and other risk factors for vascular disease.[6]

**What are the symptoms of chronic mesenteric ischemia?**

Symptoms of chronic mesenteric ischemia are gradual in onset and include postprandial abdominal pain (known as "intestinal angina"), nausea, vomiting, early satiety, diarrhea or constipation, and weight loss. The abdominal pain typically occurs 30 to 60 minutes after eating, resulting in sitophobia: the fear of eating food.[3,6]

**What abnormal physical finding might be present on auscultation of the abdomen in patients with chronic mesenteric ischemia?**

A bruit might be present on auscultation of the abdomen in patients with chronic mesenteric ischemia.

**Which imaging modalities are useful for diagnosing chronic mesenteric ischemia?**

Calcifications of the mesenteric vasculature can often be demonstrated on conventional abdominal radiography or CT imaging. Duplex ultrasonography of the mesenteric vessels is associated with high sensitivity and specificity for the presence of proximal mesenteric artery stenosis, the most common site of involvement. CT angiography has excellent operating characteristics for the diagnosis of chronic mesenteric ischemia and is better at evaluating the distal vessels compared to ultrasonagraphy.[3]

**What are the indications for revascularization in patients with chronic mesenteric ischemia related to atherosclerosis?**

Revascularization is indicated in symptomatic patients with documented severe mesenteric vessel stenosis. The goal of treatment is to prevent progression to acute mesenteric ischemia and bowel infarction. Endovascular repair with angioplasty and stenting is most often used. Although it is successful at resolving symptoms in the vast majority of patients, restenosis is common.[3,7]

### What are the causes of chronic mesenteric ischemia?

**Responsible for the overwhelming majority of cases of chronic mesenteric ischemia.**

Atherosclerotic disease.[6,7]

**Microaneurysms may be present on mesenteric angiography.**

Vasculitis.

**A cause of secondary hypertension in young women.**

Fibromuscular dysplasia.

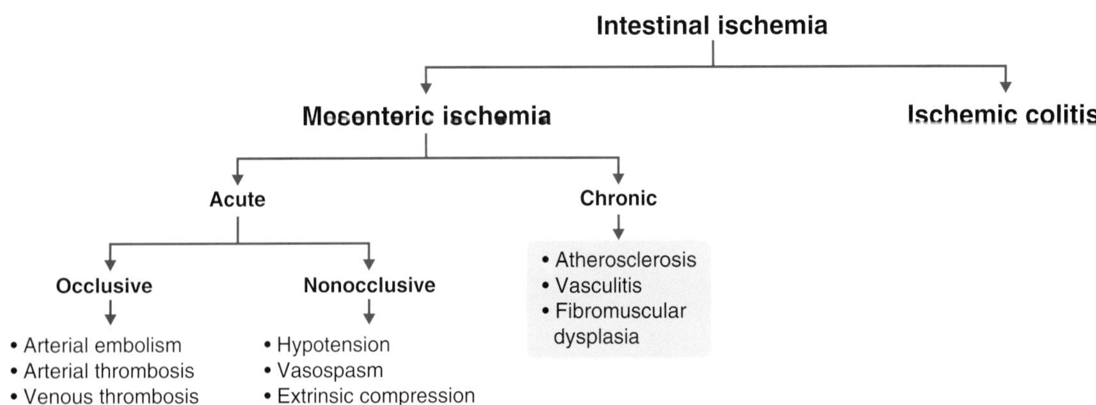


**What are the risk factors for atherosclerosis of the mesenteric vessels?**

Risk factors for atherosclerosis of the mesenteric vessels include older age, smoking history, chronic hypertension, diabetes mellitus, and hypercholesterolemia. Because of the development of extensive collateral circulation, only a small proportion of patients with mesenteric atherosclerosis experience symptoms.[6,7]

**Which systemic vasculitides can involve the mesenteric vessels and cause chronic mesenteric ischemia?**

The systemic vasculitides cause <5% of cases of chronic mesenteric ischemia. The most frequent offenders include polyarteritis nodosa (PAN), granulomatosis with polyangiitis (GPA, or Wegener's granulomatosis), eosinophilic granulomatosis with polyangiitis (EGPA, or Churg-Strauss syndrome), microscopic polyangiitis, Henoch-Schönlein purpura, and Takayasu arteritis. GI involvement occurs less commonly with giant cell arteritis, Behçet's disease, and vasculitis associated with systemic disease (eg, rheumatoid arthritis). Chronic inflammation causes arterial wall thickening with resultant stenoses and occlusions. Immunosuppression is the cornerstone of management; revascularization may be necessary in some cases.[8,9]

**How often does fibromuscular dysplasia involve the gastrointestinal tract?**

GI involvement occurs in around 10% of patients with fibromuscular dysplasia, but symptomatic disease is rare. The renal arteries are the most common sites of involvement, leading to secondary hypertension. The vessels take on a "string of beads" appearance on angiography (see Figure 39-2).[10]

*Other rare causes of chronic mesenteric ischemia include thromboangiitis obliterans, median arcuate ligament syndrome, external beam radiation therapy, and retroperitoneal fibrosis.*

## ISCHEMIC COLITIS

**Which blood vessels supply the large intestine?**

The SMA supplies the ascending colon and proximal two-thirds of the transverse colon (ileocolic, right colic, and middle colic branches); the IMA, which also arises directly from the aorta, supplies the remainder of the colon (left colic and sigmoid branches) (Figure 18-3).[1]

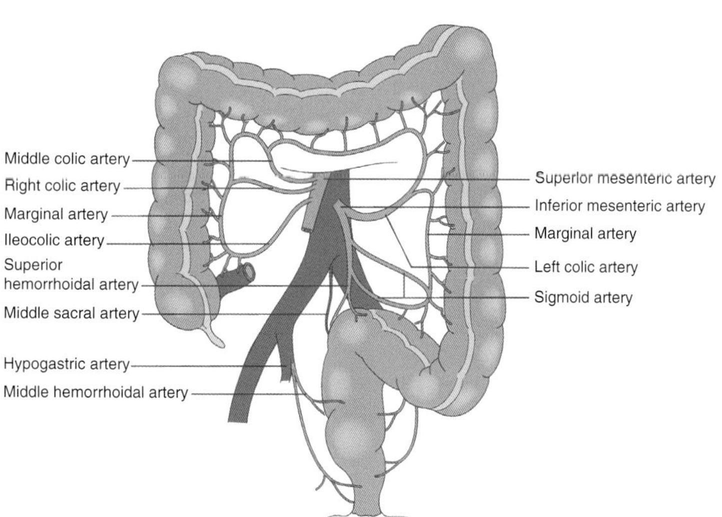


**Figure 18-3.** Blood supply of the large intestine. (From Mulholland MW, Lillemoe KD, Doherty GM, Maier RV, Simeone DM, Upchurch GR, eds. *Greenfield's Surgery: Scientific Principles & Practice*. 5th ed. Philadelphia, PA: Lippincott Williams & Wilkins; 2011.)

**What natural mechanism protects the large intestine from ischemic injury related to hypoperfusion?**

A network of collateral circulation protects the large intestine from ischemic injury related to hypoperfusion. The marginal artery of Drummond, which gives rise to the vasa recta, receives blood from the terminal portions of each colic artery and therefore receives blood from both the SMA and the IMA (see Figure 18-3). The meandering mesenteric artery, when present, is an additional potential connection between the SMA and IMA systems.[1]

**Which regions of the colon, known as the watershed areas, have more limited collateral circulation and are therefore susceptible to ischemic injury?**

There is limited collateral circulation to the splenic flexure, right colon, and rectosigmoid junction, making those areas vulnerable to ischemic injury when perfusion is compromised.[1,5]

**What is the epidemiology of ischemic colitis?**

Ischemic colitis is the most common form of intestinal ischemia, accounting for more than one-half of all cases. It is a disease of the elderly, with the vast majority of patients older than 60 years of age. Most have a positive history or risk factors for vascular disease including chronic hypertension, diabetes mellitus, and hypercholesterolemia.[1,5]

**What are the symptoms of ischemic colitis?**

The most frequent symptom of ischemic colitis is sudden-onset mild crampy abdominal pain, usually involving the left lower quadrant. Pain is followed by tenesmus and the passage of bloody stool within 24 hours. Other symptoms may include nausea, vomiting, abdominal distention, and anorexia.[1,5]

**What are the physical findings of ischemic colitis?**

Physical findings of ischemic colitis may include mild to moderate tenderness over the affected segments of colon; when bowel perforation is present, there are signs of peritonitis.[1]

**Which biochemical laboratory abnormalities are associated with ischemic colitis?**

Biochemical derangements of ischemic colitis are often subtle, but advanced disease may be associated with peripheral leukocytosis with neutrophilia, metabolic acidosis, and elevated blood lactate and amylase levels.[1]

**What is the role of imaging in the diagnosis of ischemic colitis?**

As with mesenteric ischemia, conventional radiography and CT imaging in patients with ischemic colitis can demonstrate evidence of intestinal ischemia and bowel perforation. CT imaging findings suggestive of ischemic colitis include segmental bowel wall thickening in a vascular distribution, thumbprinting, pneumatosis intestinalis, portal vein pneumatosis, and pneumoperitoneum (when there is bowel perforation). CT imaging is also useful in excluding other causes of abdominal pain. Unlike mesenteric ischemia, the role of CT angiography is limited in patients with ischemic colitis.[1,5]

**What is the role of endoscopy in the diagnosis of ischemic colitis?**

Colonoscopy is the most sensitive and specific diagnostic modality for ischemic colitis when performed within 48 hours. Visual inspection of the colonic mucosa can confirm the presence of colitis. Histopathology can differentiate ischemic colitis from infectious or inflammatory colitis. Colonoscopy must be performed with caution in these patients, as it carries risks of exacerbating ischemia and causing perforation.[1]

**What is the prognosis of ischemic colitis?**

Most cases of ischemic colitis are mild and do not result in bowel necrosis and perforation (ie, nongangrenous colitis). In such cases, most patients recover with supportive management. Long-term complications can include the formation of colonic stenoses or strictures and the development of chronic colitis from irreversible ischemic injury, which is characterized by chronic diarrhea, rectal bleeding, and weight loss. Cases of ischemic colitis complicated by bowel necrosis and perforation (ie, gangrenous colitis) are managed surgically and are associated with significant mortality.[1]

**What are the 2 general mechanisms of ischemic colitis?**

Ischemic colitis can be caused by nonocclusive or occlusive mechanisms.

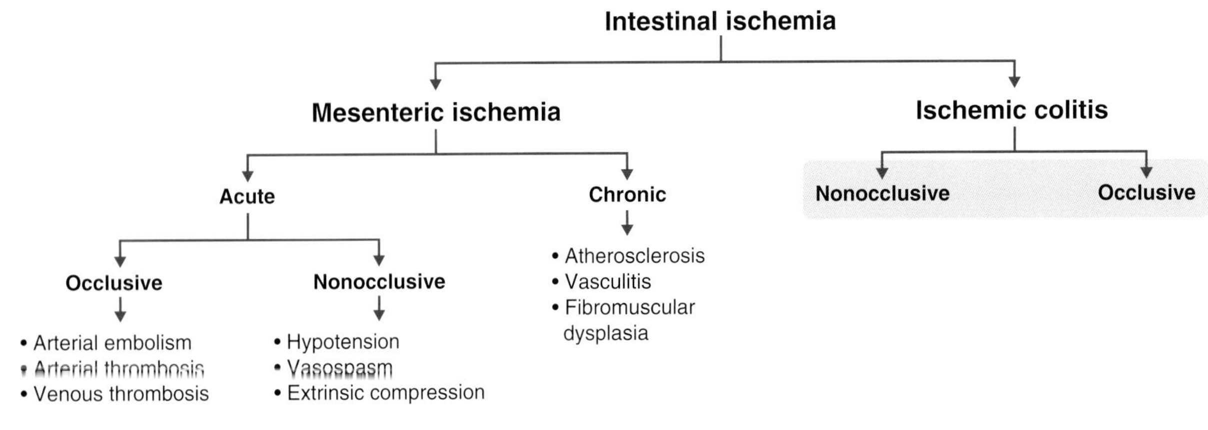

**Are nonocclusive or occlusive causes of ischemic colitis more common?**

Nonocclusive causes of ischemic colitis are responsible for the vast majority of cases.[1]

## NONOCCLUSIVE CAUSES OF ISCHEMIC COLITIS

**Which regions of the colon are most commonly affected by nonocclusive ischemic colitis?**

The splenic flexure, right colon, and rectosigmoid areas (ie, watershed regions) are vulnerable to ischemic injury related to hypoperfusion.[1,5]

### What are the nonocclusive causes of ischemic colitis?

**Responsible for the vast majority of cases of ischemic colitis.**

Hypotension.

**A patient with septic shock develops abdominal pain and bloody diarrhea shortly after starting treatment with norepinephrine.**

Vasospasm.

**Mechanical bowel obstruction may also be present.**

Extrinsic compression.

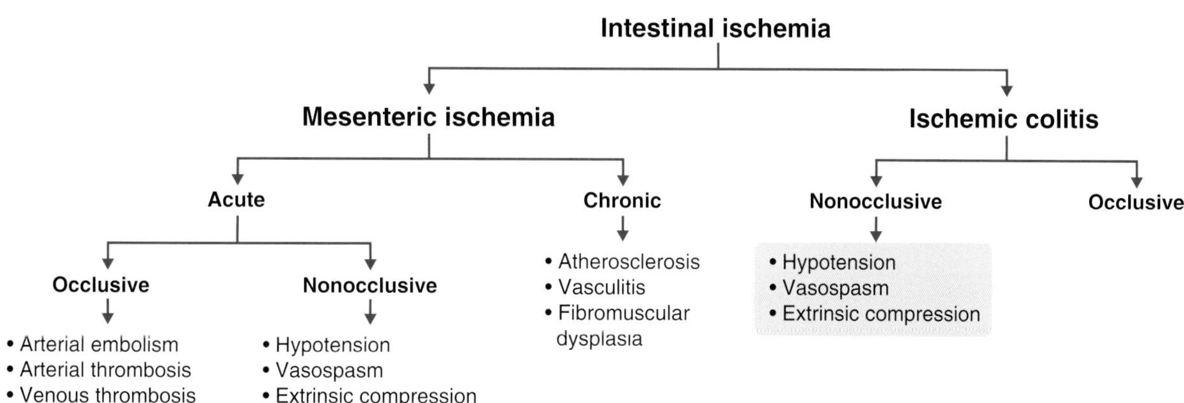


**Why is the large intestine more susceptible to hypotension and vasospasm compared with the small intestine?**

Compared with the rest of the GI tract, the large intestine receives less blood flow. In addition, the colonic microvasculature plexus is less developed and buried within a thicker wall. These features make it more vulnerable to the hypoperfusion associated with hypotension and vasospasm. Common causes of hypotension that lead to ischemic colitis include dehydration, heart failure, hemorrhage, and sepsis. It has also been reported in patients after strenuous physical activity, such as long distance running or bicycling.[5]

**Which etiology should be suspected in younger patients without vascular disease who present with ischemic colitis?**

Vasospasm related to cocaine or methamphetamine use should be suspected when ischemic colitis occurs in younger patients without risk factors for vascular disease.

**What are the causes of ischemic colitis related to extrinsic blood vessel compression?**

Ischemic colitis related to extrinsic blood vessel compression can occur as a result of diverticulitis, volvulus, tumor, adhesions, or intestinal prolapse.[5]

## OCCLUSIVE CAUSES OF ISCHEMIC COLITIS

**Does occlusive ischemic colitis most frequently involve the watershed regions of the colon?**

Unlike the nonocclusive causes of ischemic colitis, which predominantly affect the watershed regions of the colon, occlusive causes of ischemic colitis affect the regions of the colon supplied by the occluded vessel.

## What are the occlusive causes of ischemic colitis?

A common cause of acute mesenteric ischemia; this event rarely involves the IMA because of its small diameter.

Arterial embolism.

Sluggish blood flow can lead to this occlusive cause of ischemic colitis.

Arterial thrombosis.

A patient with nephrotic syndrome develops ischemic colitis.

Venous thrombosis.

A 68-year-old man develops evidence of ischemic colitis after endovascular repair of a ruptured abdominal aortic aneurysm.

Iatrogenic (eg, aortoiliac instrumentation or surgery).

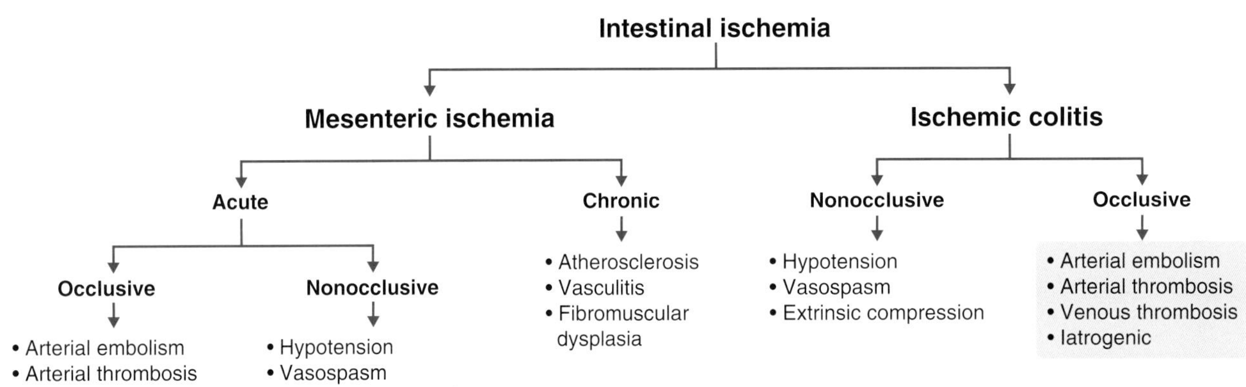


What is the most frequent source of embolic ischemic colitis?

Cardiac sources of embolism (eg, atrial fibrillation, endocarditis, dilated cardiomyopathy) are present in a significant proportion of patients with ischemic colitis. In some cases, anticoagulation may be helpful in preventing future cardioembolic events.[11]

What patients are at highest risk for ischemic colitis related to thrombosis of the inferior mesenteric artery?

Most cases of IMA thrombosis are related to atherosclerotic disease. The SMA provides a rich collateral blood supply to the left colon, allowing most healthy patients to tolerate acute IMA occlusion without severe clinical sequelae. However, patients with inborn deficiencies of the collateral network or atherosclerotic disease of the SMA are at risk for ischemic colitis related to IMA thrombosis.[12]

How often is the colon involved in cases of mesenteric vein thrombosis?

Ischemic colitis occurs in up to 15% of patients with mesenteric vein thrombosis; it usually involves the proximal colon and occurs along with small intestine involvement. Colonic involvement is associated with increased mortality. Anticoagulation is the cornerstone of management; surgical intervention may be necessary in some cases.[13]

What are the mechanisms of occlusive ischemic colitis related to aortoiliac instrumentation or surgery?

Ischemic colitis can develop after aortoiliac instrumentation or surgery as a result of IMA ligation, "jailing" of the IMA after stent placement, embolic events, or vascular compression with surgical instruments. Hemodynamic instability during or after surgery can also contribute to colonic ischemia. It typically presents 1 to 2 days after the procedure.[1]

## Case Summary

A 44-year-old man with chronic abdominal pain, sitophobia, weight loss, and testicular pain presents with sudden-onset severe abdominal pain and is found to have evidence of systemic toxicity, hypertension, livedo reticularis, elevated blood lactate, and abnormal abdominal imaging.

***What is the most likely underlying cause of intestinal ischemia in this patient?***

Vasculitis.

### BONUS QUESTIONS

***What types of intestinal ischemia are present in this case?***

This case describes features of both chronic mesenteric ischemia and acute mesenteric ischemia. The chronic postprandial pain, sitophobia, and weight loss are indicative of chronic mesenteric ischemia. Acute mesenteric ischemia is suggested by the sudden increase in severity of pain, evidence of systemic toxicity, elevated blood lactate, elevated serum alkaline phosphatase, and evidence of small bowel ischemia on cross-sectional imaging.

***What significant findings are present on conventional mesenteric angiography in this case?***

The mesenteric angiogram in this case (see Figure 18-1) demonstrates multiple abnormalities of the SMA, including fusiform aneurysms (white arrowhead), a large saccular aneurysm (arrow), and occlusive lesions (black arrowhead).

***What type of vasculitis does the patient in this case most likely have?***

Weight loss, testicular pain, livedo reticularis, elevated diastolic blood pressure, and the presence of medium-vessel microaneurysms on angiography are highly suggestive of PAN. The diagnosis can be confirmed with small bowel biopsy demonstrating focal, segmental panmural necrotizing inflammation of medium- or small-sized arteries.[14]

***What is the mechanism of chronic mesenteric ischemia related to vasculitis?***

The chronic inflammation of vasculitis causes thickening of the vessel wall and intimal proliferation, leading to luminal narrowing and inadequate perfusion during times of increased metabolic demand.

***What is the mechanism of acute mesenteric ischemia related to vasculitis?***

The combination of vessel inflammation and sluggish blood flow related to luminal narrowing can result in acute thrombosis. One-third of cases of PAN with GI involvement present with acute mesenteric ischemia.[14]

***What acute interventions should be offered to the patient in this case?***

In patients with acute mesenteric ischemia related to arterial occlusion, endovascular techniques such as thrombolysis, thrombectomy, embolectomy, angioplasty with or without stenting, and administration of vasodilators can be used to restore perfusion. In some cases, open surgical therapy is required, using techniques such as embolectomy, thrombectomy, arterial bypass, and administration of local intra-arterial thrombolytic agents. Intestine that is not viable after revascularization should be resected.[3]

***What Is the relevance of the negative hepatitis B virus serologies in this case?***

PAN can be associated with chronic hepatitis B infection. Antiviral therapy is the focus of treatment for PAN associated with hepatitis B. Patients who do not respond to antiviral therapy or have severe manifestations of PAN may require immunosuppressive therapy.[14]

***What is the initial pharmacologic treatment of choice for polyarteritis nodosa with major organ involvement?***

In patients with PAN and major organ involvement (eg, GI tract), the combination of glucocorticoids and cyclophosphamide has been shown to improve survival and is the cornerstone of initial pharmacologic management.[14,15]

## KEY POINTS

- Intestinal ischemia occurs when oxygen delivery to intestinal tissue is incapable of meeting metabolic demand, which can lead to necrosis and perforation.
- Abdominal pain is the most common symptom in patients with intestinal ischemia.
- Mesenteric ischemia refers to involvement of the small intestine; ischemic colitis refers to involvement of the large intestine.
- Acute mesenteric ischemia is most commonly caused by arterial embolism or thrombosis, often resulting in bowel necrosis that can be life-threatening.
- Chronic mesenteric ischemia (intestinal angina) is most commonly caused by atherosclerotic disease and is characterized by chronic postprandial abdominal pain, sitophobia, and weight loss.
- Ischemic colitis is a disease of the elderly, most commonly caused by nonocclusive mechanisms such as hypotension or vasospasm.

## REFERENCES

1. Sun MY, Maykel JA. Ischemic colitis. *Clin Colon Rectal Surg*. 2007;20(1):5-12.
2. Cappell MS. Intestinal (mesenteric) vasculopathy. I. Acute superior mesenteric arteriopathy and venopathy. *Gastroenterol Clin North Am*. 1998;27(4):783-825, vi.
3. Clair DG, Beach JM. Mesenteric ischemia. *N Engl J Med*. 2016;374(10):959-968.
4. Boley SJ. Circulatory responses to acute reduction of superior mesenteric arterial flow. *Physiologist*. 1969;12:180.
5. Tendler DA. Acute intestinal ischemia and infarction. *Semin Gastrointest Dis*. 2003;14(2):66-76.
6. Keese M, Schmitz-Rixen T, Schmandra T. Chronic mesenteric ischemia: time to remember open revascularization. *World J Gastroenterol*. 2013;19(9):1333-1337.
7. Hohenwalter EJ. Chronic mesenteric ischemia: diagnosis and treatment. *Semin Intervent Radiol*. 2009;26(4):345-351.
8. Rits Y, Oderich GS, Bower TC, et al. Interventions for mesenteric vasculitis. *J Vasc Surg*. 2010;51(2):392-400 e2.
9. Salvarani C, Calamia KT, Crowson CS, et al. Localized vasculitis of the gastrointestinal tract: a case series. *Rheumatology*. 2010;49(7): 1326-1335.
10. Senadhi V. A rare cause of chronic mesenteric ischemia from fibromuscular dysplasia: a case report. *J Med Case Rep*. 2010;4:373.
11. Hourmand-Ollivier I, Bouin M, Saloux E, et al. Cardiac sources of embolism should be routinely screened in ischemic colitis. *Am J Gastroenterol*. 2003;98(7):1573-1577.
12. Karmody AM, Jordan FR, Zaman SN. Left colon gangrene after acute inferior mesenteric artery occlusion. *Arch Surg*. 1976;111(9): 972-975.
13. Abu-Daff S, Abu-Daff N, Al-Shahed M. Mesenteric venous thrombosis and factors associated with mortality: a statistical analysis with five-year follow-up. *J Gastrointest Surg*. 2009;13(7):1245-1250.
14. De Virgilio A, Greco A, Magliulo G, et al. Polyarteritis nodosa: a contemporary overview. *Autoimmun Rev*. 2016;15(6):564-570.
15. Leib ES, Restivo C, Paulus HE. Immunosuppressive and corticosteroid therapy of polyarteritis nodosa. *Am J Med*. 1979;67(6):941-947.

# SECTION 6

# General Internal Medicine

## Chapter 19

# DELIRIUM

### Case: A 27-year-old man with flushed skin

A 27-year-old man is brought to the emergency department by law enforcement after he was found undressed and wandering the streets. He became agitated when confronted and had to be forcefully restrained. The patient's wife is at his side and reports that he was previously healthy except for seasonal allergies. He takes no prescription medications but has been consuming escalating quantities of over-the-counter allergy medication over the past few weeks. According to his wife, he has taken "handfuls" of pills daily over the past few days.

Temperature is 38.6°C, and heart rate is 125 beats per minute. There is generalized skin flushing. The patient is looking about the room without any clear focus of attention, frequently picking at his body and nearby bedsheets. He is disoriented and unable to follow 2-step commands. He is unable to state the days of the week backward. Bowel sounds are decreased. A photograph of the patient in a well-lit room is shown in Figure 19-1.

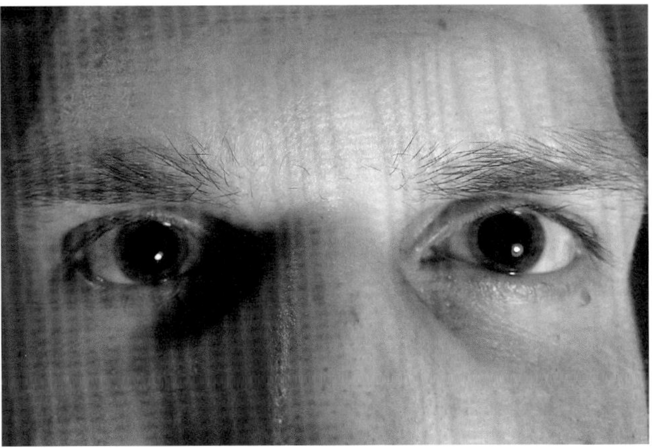

**Figure 19-1.** (Courtesy of Ross Passo, MD.)

***What is the most likely diagnosis in this patient?***

**What is delirium?**

Delirium is a clinical diagnosis, defined as an acute disturbance in attention and awareness (lasting hours to days), accompanied by an additional disturbance in cognition (ie, memory, orientation, language, visuospatial ability, or perception). There must be evidence that the disturbance is caused by a medical condition, withdrawal or intoxication from medication or illicit substances, is not better explained by a preexistent neurocognitive disorder, and is not occurring in the context of a severely reduced level of arousal (eg, coma).[1,2]

**How can attention be evaluated on examination?**

Inattention is the neurocognitive hallmark of delirium. It can be observed simply by taking a history from a patient. It may manifest as tangential speech, fragmentary flow of ideas, or inability to follow complex commands. Asking the patient to repeat successively longer random strings of digits is one way to actively assess attention. The average adult can repeat a string of 5 to 7 digits without failing; inability to achieve this target is indicative of inattention. More formal neuropsychological testing may be helpful.[3]

**In addition to cognitive disturbances, what other clinical features are common in patients with delirium?**

Patients with delirium often experience fluctuating symptoms over the course of the day and may even appear lucid at times. Disturbances in perception (eg, visual hallucinations), the sleep-wake cycle, psychomotor activity (ie, hypoactivity or hyperactivity), emotional control, and behavior regulation are common.[4]

**What is altered mental status?**

Unlike delirium, the term "altered mental status" is nonspecific and poorly defined. It is generally used to indicate a change in cognitive function or level of consciousness. Other nonspecific and poorly defined terms often used interchangeably with delirium include encephalopathy and acute confusional state.[5]

**What is encephalitis?**

Encephalitis refers to inflammation of the brain that may result in delirium and other characteristic clinical manifestations depending on the affected location (eg, limbic system, brainstem). Encephalitis is most often infectious in nature but can also occur as a result of noninfectious inflammatory conditions (eg, autoimmune encephalitis).[6]

**What is limbic encephalitis?**

Limbic encephalitis refers to a particular clinical syndrome that occurs as a result of inflammation of the limbic system. It is most often caused by autoimmune or paraneoplastic syndromes. Characteristic clinical features include rapid-onset confusion, working memory deficits, mood changes, and seizure.[6]

**In a patient with psychosis, when should causes other than delirium be suspected?**

Causes of psychosis other than delirium (eg, drug-induced psychosis, schizophrenia, bipolar mania) should be considered when patients experience auditory hallucinations, delusions, and disorganized thoughts and behaviors, but relatively preserved alertness and memory.[7]

**How common is delirium in hospitalized patients?**

Delirium is a common disorder in the hospital setting, developing in up to one-third of patients. It is particularly common in patients ≥65 years of age, developing in up to one-half of those hospitalized.[4,8]

**What predisposing factors increase the risk of delirium in hospitalized patients?**

Predisposing factors that increase risk of delirium in hospitalized patients include older age, dementia, cognitive impairment, depression, alcohol abuse, functional impairment, sensory impairment (eg, visual, auditory), history of delirium, and history of stroke.[4]

**What is the role of neuroimaging in patients with delirium?**

Neuroimaging (eg, computed tomography and magnetic resonance imaging) is normal in the vast majority of patients with delirium, limiting its diagnostic yield. However, neuroimaging should be obtained in select patients with delirium, such as those with focal neurologic findings, to evaluate for etiologies such as stroke, intracranial hemorrhage (ICH), and brain abscess.[4]

**What is the role of electroencephalography (EEG) in patients with delirium?**

Delirium is associated with the characteristic EEG pattern of diffuse slowing, with poor organization of background rhythm; certain etiologies of delirium may have other distinctive features (eg, herpes simplex encephalitis is associated with lateralized periodic discharges). However, EEG is not routinely obtained in the evaluation of delirium. In select cases when the diagnosis is uncertain, EEG can be useful in differentiating organic disease from functional or psychiatric disorders, and in identifying occult seizures.[4]

**What is the role of lumbar puncture in patients with delirium?**

Evaluation of cerebrospinal fluid (CSF) should be considered in select patients with delirium who are suspected of having conditions such as meningitis, encephalitis, or subarachnoid hemorrhage.[4]

**What are the principles of managing delirium?**

Other than addressing the underlying cause(s), management of delirium includes minimizing centrally acting medications (eg, narcotics and anticholinergics), maximizing presence of and interaction with friends and family, decreasing sleep-wake disturbance, adequately treating pain, and maintaining a quiet environment.[4]

**When are pharmacologic agents useful in the management of delirium?**

Medications, such as antipsychotic agents, should be considered in delirious patients with severe agitation who exhibit behavior that may be harmful to themselves or others, and in those with distressing psychotic symptoms.[4]

**The causes of delirium can be separated into which general categories?**

The causes of delirium can be separated into the following categories: neurologic, toxic, metabolic, infectious, and other.

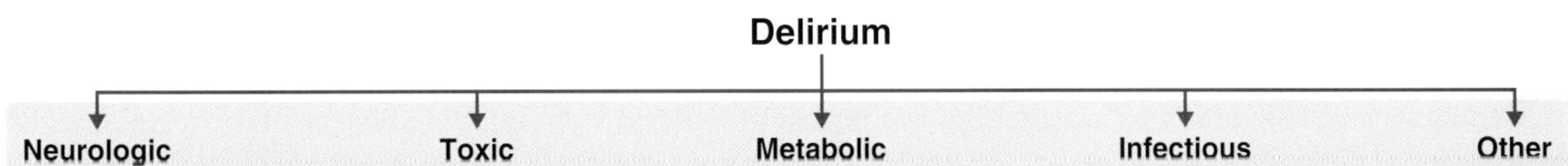


## NEUROLOGIC CAUSES OF DELIRIUM

### What are the neurologic causes of delirium?

**A 78-year-old man with a history of atrial fibrillation presents with confusion and left-sided hemiparesis.**

Stroke.

**EEG can confirm the diagnosis.**

Seizure.

**A high school running back presents to the student health center with persistent disorientation after sustaining a hard hit to the head during a recent football game.**

Concussion.

**An acute complication of traumatic brain injury (TBI) that can be diagnosed with neuroimaging or evaluation of CSF.**

Intracranial hemorrhage.

**Astrocytoma, oligodendroglioma, and ependymoma.**

Brain tumor.

**Enlarged ventricles on neuroimaging.**

Hydrocephalus.

**Blood vessel wall inflammation.**

Central nervous system (CNS) vasculitis, including primary angiitis of the central nervous system (PACNS), systemic vasculitis (eg, Behçet's disease), and vasculitis associated with systemic disease (eg, systemic lupus erythematosus).

**Noninfectious causes of encephalitis.**

Immune-mediated encephalitis, including paraneoplastic encephalitis, autoimmune encephalitis, Hashimoto's encephalitis, acute disseminated encephalomyelitis, Bickerstaff's brainstem encephalitis, and IgG4-related disease.

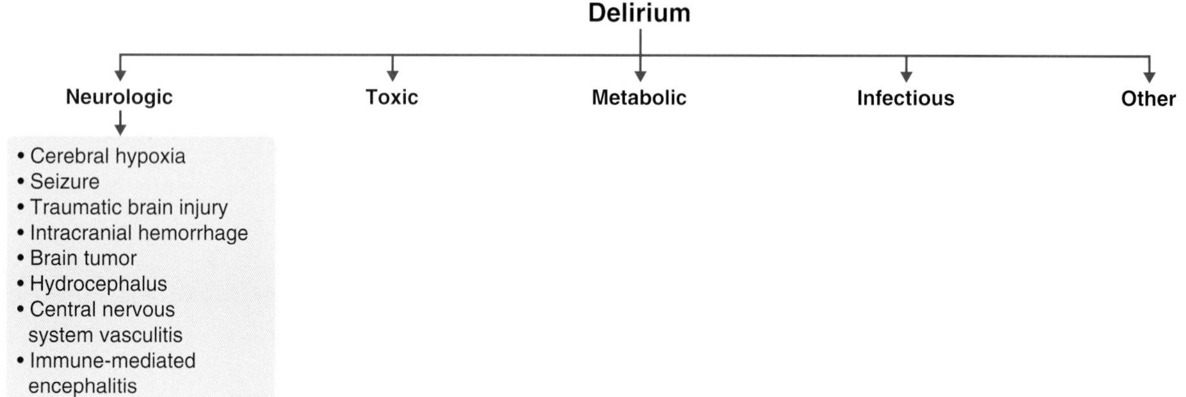


**What are the causes of cerebral hypoxia?**

Causes of cerebral hypoxia include stroke, hypoxemia from any cause (eg, pneumonia), systemic hypotension from any cause (eg, myocardial infarction), severe anemia from any cause (eg, autoimmune hemolytic anemia), and toxins (eg, carbon monoxide).

**What is the significance of delirium in patients with acute stroke?**

Delirium occurs in up to one-third of patients admitted to the hospital with acute stroke. It is associated with increased duration of hospitalization, poorer functional outcomes, and increased mortality. The 12-month mortality is 5 times higher in patients with poststroke delirium than in stroke patients without delirium.[9]

**How long does postseizure delirium typically last?**

Delirium can be challenging to distinguish from seizure, particularly focal seizure with impairment of consciousness and nonconvulsive status epilepticus. Many of the causes and clinical features overlap, however delirium tends to be more gradual in onset. EEG can often be helpful in distinguishing the 2 conditions. True postseizure delirium usually resolves within hours of the event but can last for days in some cases.[7]

**What are the characteristics of delirium in patients with traumatic brain injury?**

Delirium is common in patients hospitalized for TBI, usually developing within the first day of the trauma. Although most manifestations resolve within a few days, agitation and disruption of the sleep-wake cycle tend to last longer.[10]

**Which type of intracranial hemorrhage tends to affect elderly patients, often presenting weeks after minor trauma?**

Chronic subdural hematoma is a common cause of cognitive impairment in the elderly. It describes the presence of blood in the subdural space, usually caused by minor trauma. Gait disturbance, limb weakness, headache, and delirium are common features, typically progressing over a period of days to weeks. Noncontrast CT imaging of the head is diagnostic. Bleeding diatheses should be corrected when possible; most symptomatic patients require surgical management.[11]

**Are neurocognitive symptoms more typical of primary or metastatic brain tumors?**

Metastatic tumors, which account for up to one-quarter of all brain tumors, tend to involve more areas of the brain compared with primary tumors, which increases the likelihood of neurocognitive symptoms.[12]

**What is the classic triad of normal pressure hydrocephalus (NPH)?**

NPH is a disease of older adults characterized by the triad of gait disturbance, urinary incontinence, and cognitive deficits. The early neurocognitive symptoms of NPH include psychomotor slowing and impaired attention, executive, and visuospatial function. Neuroimaging reveals enlarged cerebral ventricles (Figure 19-2). Timely diagnosis and treatment with CSF shunting procedures (eg, ventriculoperitoneal shunt placement) can lead to resolution of symptoms. *Although it is usually categorized as a reversible dementia, NPH should be considered in the differential diagnosis of delirium.*[13]

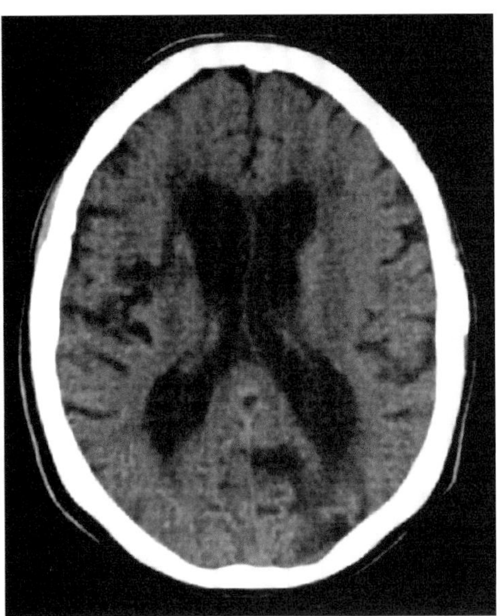

**Figure 19-2.** Computed tomography imaging of the brain reveals bilateral ventricular enlargement in a patient with normal pressure hydrocephalus. (From Garcia MJ. *Noninvasive Cardiovascular Imaging: A Multimodality Approach*. Philadelphia, PA: Lippincott Williams & Wilkins; 2010.)

**How common is delirium in patients with primary angiitis of the central nervous system?**

Delirium occurs in one-half of patients with PACNS at the time of presentation. Other frequent manifestations include headache and focal neurologic findings. CSF analysis reveals pleocytosis or elevated protein in most patients. Neuroimaging, including cerebral angiography, and brain biopsy are often needed to make the diagnosis.[14]

**What is autoimmune encephalitis?**

Autoimmune encephalitis refers to a group of disorders that cause encephalitis, often in association with antibodies to neuronal cell-surface or synaptic proteins. Anti-*N*-methyl-D-aspartate (anti-NMDA) receptor encephalitis is the most well-described type of autoimmune encephalitis. It predominantly affects women and patients under 45 years of age. Presenting symptoms include abnormal behavior, psychosis, speech dysfunction, dyskinesia, memory deficits, autonomic instability, decreased level of consciousness, and seizure. CSF is abnormal in most patients and will often demonstrate a moderate lymphocytic pleocytosis with normal or mildly increased protein concentration. CSF-specific oligoclonal bands are present in most patients. The detection of anti-NMDA receptor antibodies, which are present in the vast majority of affected patients, confirms the diagnosis.[6,15]

**What is paraneoplastic encephalitis?**

Paraneoplastic encephalitis refers to encephalitis caused by a distant underlying malignancy. It typically manifests as limbic or brainstem encephalitis. It can be associated with a variety of malignancies, but small cell lung cancer is responsible for most cases. The onset of neurologic symptoms precedes the diagnosis of cancer in most patients. Characteristic antibodies (eg, anti-Hu) can be found in the serum and CSF of affected patients.[16]

## TOXIC CAUSES OF DELIRIUM

### What are the toxic causes of delirium?

**One of the most common causes of delirium, particularly in the elderly.**

Medication.

**This substance can cause delirium through a variety of mechanisms, including intoxication, withdrawal, and associated vitamin deficiencies.**

Alcohol.

**After becoming confused at a party, a 22-year-old woman is taken to the emergency department.**

Recreational drug use.

**Said Voltaire, "A dish of mushrooms changed the destiny of Europe."**

*Amanita phalloides* (ie, the "death cap" mushroom).[17]

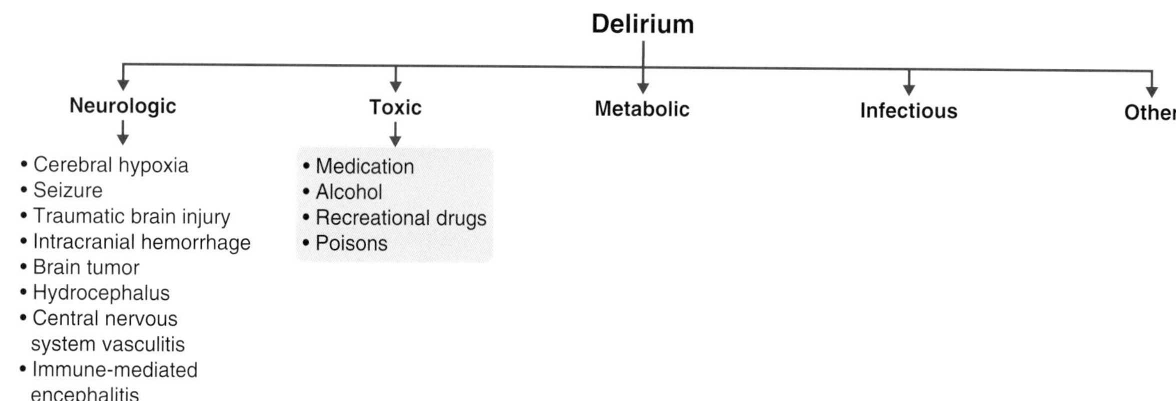


**Which medications can cause delirium?**

Numerous medications can cause delirium. The most frequent culprits include sedative hypnotics (eg, benzodiazepines), analgesics (eg, narcotics), and anticholinergics (eg, antihistamines, which are available over-the-counter). Other delirium-producing medications include anticonvulsants (eg, barbiturates), muscle relaxants, glucocorticoids, tricyclic antidepressants, antiemetics (eg, scopolamine), digoxin, lithium, and fluoroquinolones. Keys to identifying and treating medication-induced delirium include a thorough review of the medication list (including over-the-counter and herbal substances), reviewing for possible adverse interactions between medications (eg, serotonin syndrome), and recognizing the potential for altered pharmacokinetics (eg, renal or hepatic impairment). *It is important to be aware that delirium may be part of a withdrawal syndrome, particularly involving sedative, hypnotic, and anxiolytic substances.*[18]

**What is delirium tremens?**

Delirium can be caused by both alcohol intoxication and withdrawal. Delirium tremens is a life-threatening manifestation of alcohol withdrawal, characterized by rapid onset disturbances in attention and cognition, sometimes with hallucinations and extreme autonomic hyperactivity (eg, fever, tachycardia, hypertension). Onset is typically 72 hours after the appearance of alcohol withdrawal symptoms and lasts for several days. It is most often treated with benzodiazepines.[19]

**Which recreational drugs can cause delirium?**

Virtually any recreational drug can cause delirium. Common culprits include amphetamines (eg, methamphetamine and 3,4-methylenedioxymethamphetamine [MDMA]), cocaine, heroin, γ-hydroxybutyric acid (GHB), benzodiazepines, ketamine, phencyclidine (PCP), lysergic acid diethylamide (LSD), and psilocybin (mushrooms). *It is important to be aware that delirium may be part of a withdrawal syndrome, particularly involving sedative, hypnotic, and anxiolytic substances.*[3]

Which poison should be suspected in a patient with delirium and cherry-red lips?

The presence of cherry-red lips can be a clue to the diagnosis of carbon monoxide poisoning. Other poisons that can cause delirium include methanol, ethylene glycol, pesticides (eg, organophosphates), cyanide, mushrooms (particularly *Amanita phalloides*), and *Datura stramonium* (jimson weed).[3]

## METABOLIC CAUSES OF DELIRIUM

### What are the metabolic causes of delirium?

Associated with elevated blood ammonia levels.

Hepatic encephalopathy.

Auscultation of the heart reveals the presence of a scratchy sound with 3 components.

Uremia.

A 22-year-old woman with type 1 diabetes mellitus (hemoglobin A1C of 5.8%) presents with confusion and somnolence.

Hypoglycemia.

A 66-year-old man with type 2 diabetes mellitus (hemoglobin A1C of 13.8%) presents with confusion and dehydration.

Hyperosmolar hyperglycemic state.

A 28-year-old woman with anorexia nervosa is admitted to the hospital and develops delirium 2 days after being started on parenteral nutrition.

Electrolyte disturbances caused by refeeding syndrome.

A 60-year-old man with chronic alcohol use is admitted with confusion and ataxia, which acutely worsen after he is given a meal.

Wernicke's encephalopathy (thiamine deficiency).

A 66-year-old man with severe chronic obstructive pulmonary disease is admitted to the hospital with confusion, obtundation, and poor air movement.

Hypercarbia.

Endocrinopathies.

Thyroid disease (both hyperthyroidism and hypothyroidism) and Cushing's syndrome.

Osborn waves on the electrocardiogram (Figure 19-3).

Hypothermia.

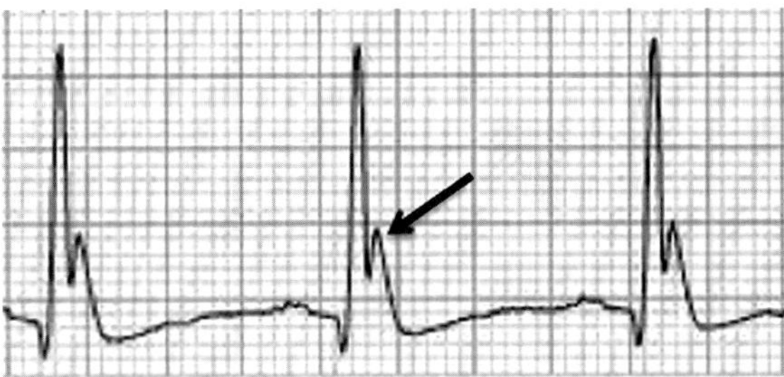

**Figure 19-3.** An electrocardiogram demonstrating prominent Osborn waves (arrow) in a patient with hypothermia.

A 32-year-old woman with schizophrenia presents with fever, muscle rigidity, autonomic lability, and delirium after a recent increase in haloperidol dose.

Hyperthermia caused by neuroleptic malignant syndrome.

GENERAL INTERNAL MEDICINE

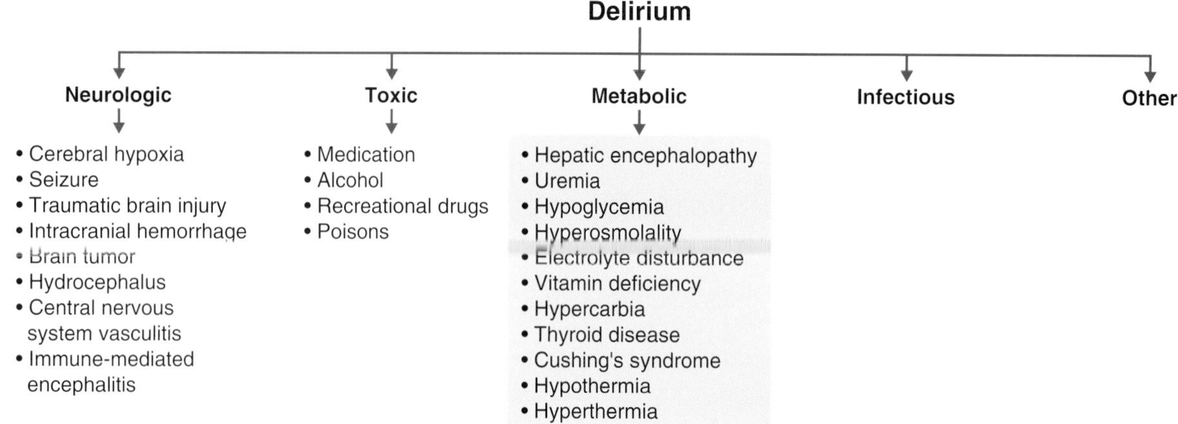


**What is considered first-line pharmacologic treatment for hepatic encephalopathy?**

First-line pharmacologic treatment for hepatic encephalopathy is a nonabsorbable disaccharide (eg, lactulose). It should be dosed to achieve 2 to 4 semisoft bowel movements per day. Colonic bacteria metabolize these disaccharides, which creates an acidic environment that is hostile to the intestinal bacteria that produce ammonia. This acidic environment also facilitates the conversion of ammonia to a nonabsorbable form ($NH_3 \rightarrow NH_4^+$), essentially trapping it in the colon for excretion. These effects combine to decrease the amount of ammonia entering the circulation.[20]

**In addition to uremia, what is another major mechanism by which end-stage renal disease contributes to the development and persistence of delirium?**

Decreased renal clearance of medications and metabolites can lead to toxicity at doses that were previously therapeutic. A thorough review of the medication list is important in any patient with reduced renal function; medications should be removed or dosed accordingly.

**What is the threshold blood glucose level at which neurocognitive impairment develops?**

Normal metabolism in the brain relies on an adequate concentration of glucose in blood. In healthy research subjects with insulin induced hypoglycemia, cognitive impairment begins to occur when blood glucose levels drop to about 50 mg/dL. Neuroglycopenic manifestations include confusion, tiredness, speaking difficulties, headache, inability to concentrate, behavioral changes, seizure, and coma. The vast majority of cases of hypoglycemia occur as an unintentional result of the pharmacologic treatment for diabetes mellitus. Other causes of hypoglycemia include medications (eg, β-blockers), toxins (eg, ethanol), adrenal insufficiency, intense exercise, insulinoma, critical illness (eg, liver failure), and surreptitious insulin use.[21]

**What are the principal mechanisms of neurocognitive dysfunction in patients with hyperosmolality?**

Plasma hypertonicity leads to fluid shift from the intracellular fluid compartment to the extracellular fluid compartment, with resultant neuronal dehydration and dysfunction. Osmotic diuresis may also lead to electrolyte disturbances that contribute to neurocognitive dysfunction.[22]

**Which electrolyte disturbances can cause delirium?**

Electrolyte disturbances most frequently associated with delirium include hyponatremia, hypernatremia, hypercalcemia, hypocalcemia, and hypomagnesemia. The likelihood of neurocognitive impairment from an electrolyte disturbance depends on the severity of the disturbance and its rate of development.[3]

**Which vitamin deficiencies can cause delirium?**

Delirium can be caused by deficiencies in thiamine, vitamin B12, folate, and niacin.[3]

**What are the mechanisms of delirium in patients with hypercarbia?**

Hypercarbia causes delirium through a variety of mechanisms. First, it increases intracranial pressure via its vasodilatory effect on cerebral vasculature. Second, it leads to CSF and brain tissue acidosis, which further increases cerebral blood flow and intracranial pressure. Finally, hypercarbia causes systemic hypoxemia, which can lead to cerebral hypoxia. Mechanical ventilation is the treatment of choice for hypercarbia complicated by delirium.[23]

**What are the neurocognitive features of hypothyroidism?**

Neurocognitive manifestations occur frequently in patients with hypothyroidism and are sometimes the earliest and most prominent expressions of the condition. Early symptoms include inattention, memory deficits, and mental slowness; later symptoms include delusions and hallucinations. Early recognition and treatment may reverse the cognitive effects of hypothyroidism; however, deficits may persist in some cases.[24]

**How common is neurocognitive impairment in patients with Cushing's syndrome?**

Neurocognitive impairment occurs in most patients with Cushing's syndrome, including deficits in memory, attention, and concentration. Treatment for Cushing's syndrome ameliorates these symptoms in most patients; however, symptoms may be irreversible or slow to improve, particularly in the elderly.[25]

**What are the neurocognitive manifestations of hypothermia?**

Hypothermia (core temperature <35°C) can occur when the thermoregulatory actions of the body are either overwhelmed by exposure to a cold environment or impaired as a result of a variety of medical conditions, such as stroke, alcohol ingestion, hypothyroidism, or sepsis. Older patients are particularly susceptible to hypothermia. Confusion and memory impairment are among the earliest neurocognitive manifestations. With progression, patients develop apathy, impaired judgment (eg, paradoxical undressing), and dysarthria. If hypothermia progresses, consciousness is ultimately lost.[26]

**What are the neurocognitive manifestations of hyperthermia?**

Hyperthermia can be caused by infectious and noninfectious etiologies, such as heat stroke and medications. Neurocognitive manifestations include impairment in attention, memory, reasoning, problem solving, comprehension, and consciousness. These deficits resolve in most patients. However, some are left with permanent changes in attention, memory, or personality.[27]

## INFECTIOUS CAUSES OF DELIRIUM

### What are the infectious causes of delirium?

**Delirium may be the only clinical manifestation of this common infection, particularly in the elderly.**

Urinary tract infection.

**Purulent cough and fever.**

Pneumonia.

**Any infection with signs of systemic toxicity.**

Sepsis.

**Neck stiffness, photophobia, and headache.**

Meningitis.

**Most commonly viral in nature, this CNS infection is usually associated with pleocytosis.**

Encephalitis.

**This CNS infection may present with focal neurologic findings.**

Brain abscess.

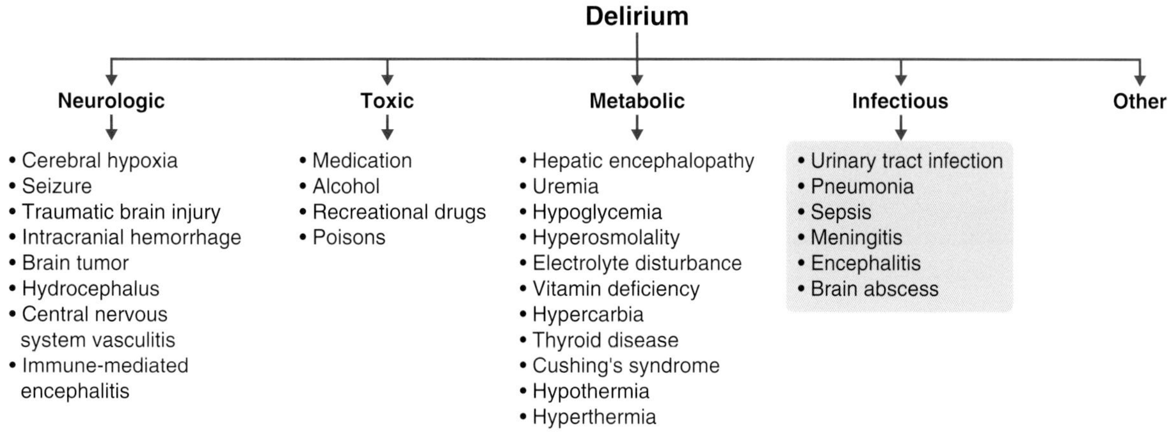

**Which class of antibiotics, commonly used to treat urinary tract infection, should be avoided in older patients who are at risk for delirium?**

Fluoroquinolones can cause delirium and should generally be avoided in patients with risk factors, including advanced age.[18]

**How is the prognosis of elderly patients with pneumonia affected by the presence of delirium?**

The presence of delirium in elderly patients with pneumonia increases the risk of in-hospital mortality by a factor of 6. This is approximately equivalent to the increased risk associated with the presence of underlying chronic obstructive pulmonary disease in patients with pneumonia.[28]

**What is sepsis-induced delirium?**

Delirium due to sepsis is caused by the systemic inflammatory response to infection originating outside of the central nervous system. It is present in up to one-quarter of septic patients and may even precede the typical features of sepsis. The presence of delirium in septic patients doubles the rate of mortality.[29]

**Is meningitis or encephalitis more likely to present with neurocognitive dysfunction early in the course of illness?**

Compared with meningitis, encephalitis is more likely to be associated with neurocognitive dysfunction early in the course of illness. Viruses are responsible for most cases of encephalitis but must be distinguished from immune-mediated processes (eg, autoimmune encephalitis). Neuroimaging and CSF evaluation are key investigations in patients with encephalitis. Importantly, normal CSF findings (including the absence of pleocytosis) are present in up to 10% of patients with viral encephalitis.[30]

**What are the most common symptoms reported by patients with brain abscess?**

Headache is the most frequent symptom reported by patients with brain abscess. Fever, delirium, focal neurologic findings, and nausea and vomiting are also common manifestations. The classic triad of fever, headache, and focal neurologic findings is present in less than one-half of patients. Neuroimaging is key to the diagnosis.[31]

## OTHER CAUSES OF DELIRIUM

### What are the other causes of delirium?

**A common occurrence in hospitalized patients owing to a noisy environment, constant interruptions, artificial light, pain, and underlying illness.**

Insomnia.

**Acute headache, confusion, and papilledema in a patient with an S4 gallop and the presence of left ventricular hypertrophy on electrocardiogram.**

Hypertensive encephalopathy.

**Headache, vision changes, delirium, and the presence of cerebral edema predominantly involving the white matter of the posterior regions of the brain.**

Posterior reversible encephalopathy syndrome (PRES).

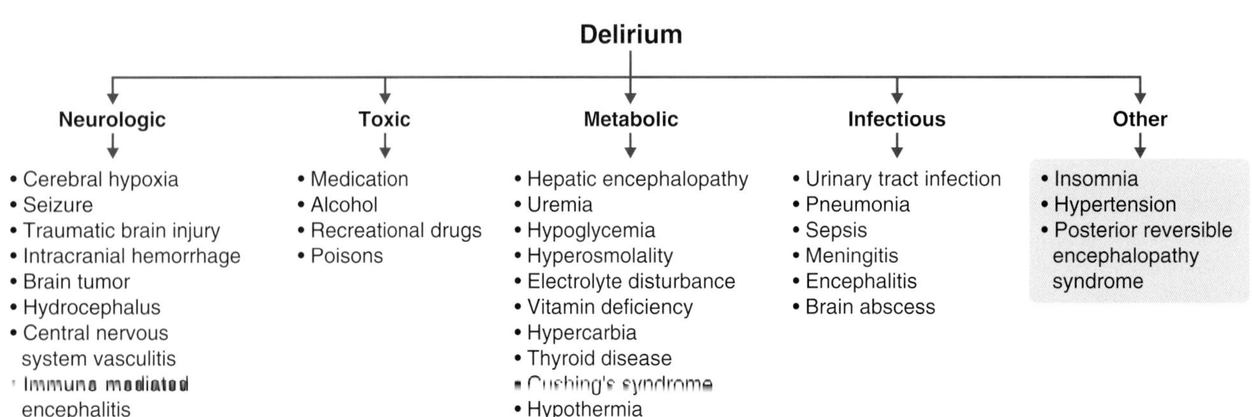

**Which pharmacologic agent may be helpful in preventing insomnia and delirium in hospitalized patients?**

Melatonin or melatonin agonists (eg, ramelteon) may be useful in the prevention and treatment of delirium in hospitalized patients. Ramelteon is well-tolerated and, unlike other pharmacologic sleep aids, is not associated with cognitive impairment, withdrawal symptoms, rebound insomnia, or potential abuse.[32]

**What is hypertensive encephalopathy?**

Hypertensive encephalopathy occurs when systemic hypertension overwhelms the autoregulatory capacity of the cerebral vasculature, resulting in hyperperfusion, cerebral edema, and delirium. Common manifestations include lethargy, confusion, headache, visual disturbance, and seizure. Neuroimaging may reveal the presence of cerebral edema predominantly involving the white matter of the parietal and occipital regions, a finding consistent with PRES.[33]

**What is posterior reversible encephalopathy syndrome?**

PRES describes the development of neurocognitive dysfunction in association with cerebral edema that develops as a result of endothelial dysfunction, typically involving the posterior brain regions (Figure 19-4). It most often arises when there are pronounced fluctuations in systemic blood pressure, particularly abrupt and severe elevations. Other associated conditions include renal failure, use of cytotoxic medications, autoimmune disorders (eg, systemic lupus erythematosus), and preeclampsia or eclampsia. Treatment is aimed at the precipitating condition. Most patients fully recover within 1 week.[34]

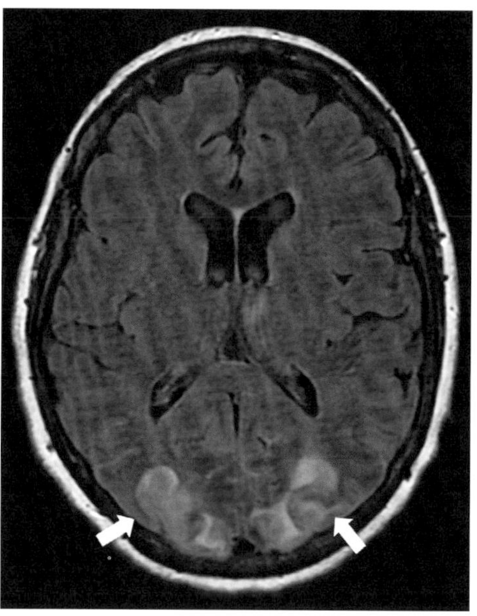

**Figure 19-4.** Brain MRI shows symmetric patchy areas of cortical and subcortical abnormal signal in the parieto-occipital lobes corresponding to vasogenic edema (arrows), findings characteristic of PRES. (From Sanelli PC, Schaefer P, Loevner LA. *Neuroimaging: The Essentials*. Philadelphia, PA: Wolters Kluwer Health; 2016.)

## Case Summary

A 27-year-old man presents with agitation after ingesting large quantities of over-the-counter allergy medication and is found to have delirium, fever, tachycardia, and abnormal skin and eye findings.

***What is the most likely diagnosis in this patient?***

Anticholinergic syndrome.

## BONUS QUESTIONS

| | |
|---|---|
| ***What is anticholinergic syndrome?*** | Anticholinergic syndrome is a toxidrome resulting from the inhibition of neurotransmission at muscarinic acetylcholine receptors sites, which are located both centrally (ie, within the CNS) and peripherally (eg, within the heart, gastrointestinal tract, and sweat glands).[35,36] |
| ***What are the clinical manifestations of anticholinergic syndrome?*** | Anticholinergic syndrome includes manifestations related to both central and peripheral muscarinic receptor blockade. Inhibition of the receptors located in the CNS can result in delirium, psychosis, hallucinations, seizure, and coma. Inhibition of the peripheral receptors can result in hyperthermia, tachycardia, anhidrosis, dry mucous membranes, skin flushing (vasodilation), mydriasis, decreased bowel sounds, and urinary retention.[35,36] |
| ***What findings are present in the photograph of the patient in this case?*** | Mydriasis and skin flushing can be appreciated in the photograph of the patient in this case (see Figure 19-1), both of which are signs of anticholinergic toxicity. |
| ***Which classes of medications are capable of causing anticholinergic syndrome?*** | Classes of medications with anticholinergic properties include antihistamines, tricyclic antidepressants, antipsychotics, antidiarrheals, antiemetics, antiparkinsonian agents, antispasmodics, bronchodilators, mydriatics, and skeletal muscle relaxants. Poisons such as *Datura stramonium* (jimson weed) are also capable of causing anticholinergic syndrome.[35,36] |
| ***How is the diagnosis of anticholinergic syndrome made?*** | Anticholinergic syndrome is a clinical diagnosis. A compatible history, including exposure to medications or other substances with anticholinergic properties, must be sought from family or friends. Laboratory investigation is often fruitless, as many anticholinergic agents are not detected on toxicology screens and results are slow to return.[36] |
| ***What is the management of anticholinergic syndrome?*** | Supportive management is the cornerstone of treatment for anticholinergic syndrome. Depending on the degree of agitation, sedatives such as benzodiazepines may also be needed. Physostigmine prevents the degradation of acetylcholine and can be used as an antidote; however, it can cause serious side effects, including seizure and cardiac dysrhythmia, so its use must be carefully considered.[36] |

## KEY POINTS

- Delirium is a clinical diagnosis caused by one or more underlying medical conditions, characterized by a disturbance in attention and awareness, along with additional disturbances in cognition.
- Additional features of delirium include fluctuating disturbances involving perception, the sleep-wake cycle, psychomotor activity, emotional control, and behavior regulation.
- Risk factors for delirium include older age, dementia, cognitive impairment, history of delirium, functional impairment, sensory impairment, history of stroke, alcohol abuse, and depression.
- The causes of delirium can be separated into the following categories: neurologic, toxic, metabolic, infectious, and other.
- History and physical examination are fundamental to determining the cause(s) of delirium. Neuroimaging, lumbar puncture, and EEG can be helpful in some cases.
- Treatment for delirium hinges on the identification and reversal of the underlying medical condition(s).
- Other basic tenets of treating delirium include minimizing centrally acting medications (eg, narcotics), maximizing presence of family, avoiding sleep-wake disturbances, adequately treating pain, and maintaining a quiet environment.
- Pharmacologic treatment (eg, antipsychotic agents) should be considered in patients with severe agitation who exhibit behavior that may be harmful to themselves or others, and in those with distressing psychotic symptoms.

## REFERENCES

1. American Psychiatric Association. *Diagnostic and Statistical Manual of Mental Disorders*. 5th ed. Washington, DC: American Psychiatric Publishing; 2013.
2. European Delirium Association, American Delirium Society. The DSM-5 criteria, level of arousal and delirium diagnosis: inclusiveness is safer. *BMC Med*. 2014;12:141.
3. Longo DL, Fauci AS, Kasper DL, Hauser SL, Jameson JL, Loscalzo J, eds. *Harrison's Principles of Internal Medicine*. 18th ed. New York, NY: McGraw-Hill; 2012.
4. Inouye SK, Westendorp RG, Saczynski JS. Delirium in elderly people. *Lancet*. 2014;383(9920):911-922.
5. Douglas VC, Josephson SA. Altered mental status. *Continuum*. 2011;17(5 Neurologic Consultation in the Hospital):967-983.
6. Graus F, Titulaer MJ, Balu R, et al. A clinical approach to diagnosis of autoimmune encephalitis. *Lancet Neurol*. 2016;15(4):391-404.
7. Kaplan PW. Delirium and epilepsy. *Dialogues Clin Neurosci*. 2003;5(2):187-200.
8. Siddiqi N, House AO, Holmes JD. Occurrence and outcome of delirium in medical in-patients: a systematic literature review. *Age Ageing*. 2006;35(4):350-364.
9. Shi Q, Presutti R, Selchen D, Saposnik G. Delirium in acute stroke: a systematic review and meta-analysis. *Stroke*. 2012;43(3):645-649.
10. Maneewong J, Maneeton B, Maneeton N, et al. Delirium after a traumatic brain injury: predictors and symptom patterns. *Neuropsychiatr Dis Treat*. 2017;13:459-465.
11. Kolias AG, Chari A, Santarius T, Hutchinson PJ. Chronic subdural haematoma: modern management and emerging therapies. *Nat Rev Neurol*. 2014;10(10):570-578.
12. Madhusoodanan S, Ting MB, Farah T, Ugur U. Psychiatric aspects of brain tumors: a review. *World J Psychiatry*. 2015;5(3):273-285.
13. Nassar BR, Lippa CF. Idiopathic normal pressure hydrocephalus: a review for general practitioners. *Gerontol Geriatr Med*. 2016;2:2333721416643702.
14. Salvarani C, Brown RD Jr, Calamia KT, et al. Primary central nervous system vasculitis: analysis of 101 patients. *Ann Neurol*. 2007;62(5):442-451.
15. Dalmau J, Lancaster E, Martinez-Hernandez E, Rosenfeld MR, Balice-Gordon R. Clinical experience and laboratory investigations in patients with anti-NMDAR encephalitis. *Lancet Neurol*. 2011;10(1):63-74.
16. Sillevis Smitt P, Grefkens J, de Leeuw B, et al. Survival and outcome in 73 anti-Hu positive patients with paraneoplastic encephalomyelitis/sensory neuronopathy. *J Neurol*. 2002;249(6):745-753.
17. Wasson RG. *The Death of Claudius, or Mushrooms for Murderers*. Botanical Museum Leaflets, Harvard University. 1972;23(3):101-128.
18. Alagiakrishnan K, Wiens CA. An approach to drug induced delirium in the elderly. *Postgrad Med J*. 2004;80(945):388-393.
19. Schuckit MA. Recognition and management of withdrawal delirium (delirium tremens). *N Engl J Med*. 2014;371(22):2109-2113.
20. Sharma P, Sharma BC. Disaccharides in the treatment of hepatic encephalopathy. *Metab Brain Dis*. 2013;28(2):313-320.
21. Service FJ. Hypoglycemic disorders. *N Engl J Med*. 1995;332(17):1144-1152.
22. Maccario M. Neurological dysfunction associated with nonketotic hyperglycemia. *Arch Neurol*. 1968;19(5):525-534.
23. Scala R. Hypercapnic encephalopathy syndrome: a new frontier for non-invasive ventilation? *Respir Med*. 2011;105(8):1109-1117.
24. Heinrich TW, Grahm G. Hypothyroidism presenting as psychosis: myxedema madness revisited. *Prim Care Companion J Clin Psychiatry*. 2003;5(6):260-266.
25. Starkman MN. Neuropsychiatric findings in Cushing syndrome and exogenous glucocorticoid administration. *Endocrinol Metab Clin North Am*. 2013;42(3):477-488.
26. Mallet ML. Pathophysiology of accidental hypothermia. *QJM*. 2002;95(12):775-785.
27. Walter EJ, Carraretto M. The neurological and cognitive consequences of hyperthermia. *Crit Care*. 2016;20(1):199.
28. Pieralli F, Vannucchi V, Mancini A, et al. Delirium is a predictor of in-hospital mortality in elderly patients with community acquired pneumonia. *Intern Emerg Med*. 2014;9(2):195-200.
29. Zampieri FG, Park M, Machado FS, Azevedo LC. Sepsis-associated encephalopathy: not just delirium. *Clinics*. 2011;66(10):1825-1831.
30. Tunkel AR, Glaser CA, Bloch KC, et al. The management of encephalitis: clinical practice guidelines by the Infectious Diseases Society of America. *Clin Infect Dis*. 2008;47(3):303-327.
31. Patel K, Clifford DB. Bacterial brain abscess. *Neurohospitalist*. 2014;4(4):196-204.
32. Chakraborti D, Tampi DJ, Tampi RR. Melatonin and melatonin agonist for delirium in the elderly patients. *Am J Alzheimers Dis Other Demen*. 2015;30(2):119-129.
33. Vaughan CJ, Delanty N. Hypertensive emergencies. *Lancet*. 2000;356(9227):411-417.
34. Fugate JE, Rabinstein AA. Posterior reversible encephalopathy syndrome: clinical and radiological manifestations, pathophysiology, and outstanding questions. *Lancet Neurol*. 2015;14(9):914-925.
35. Corallo CE, Whitfield A, Wu A. Anticholinergic syndrome following an unintentional overdose of scopolamine. *Ther Clin Risk Manag*. 2009;5(5):719-723.
36. Dart RC, ed. *Medical Toxicology*. 3rd ed. Philadelphia, PA: Lippincott Williams & Wilkins; 2004.

Chapter 20

# DYSPNEA

## Case: A 71-year-old woman with facial edema

A 71-year-old woman with a history of chronic obstructive pulmonary disease (COPD) is admitted to the hospital with progressive shortness of breath. She is a former smoker with a 60-pack-year history. Recent spirometry shows forced expiratory volume in 1 second ($FEV_1$) of 55% of predicted. At baseline, she can walk 4 to 5 city blocks before needing to stop to catch her breath. Over the past few weeks she has noticed a marked decrease in her functional capacity, now becoming short of breath with minimal exertion. Over the same period of time she has developed nonproductive cough, swelling of the arms and face, and unintentional weight loss of 15 pounds.

Heart rate is 106 beats per minute, and respiratory rate is 28 breaths per minute. Jugular venous pressure (JVP) is 14 cm $H_2O$, and the external jugular vein is engorged. There is edema of the face, neck, and upper extremities. Photographs of the patient are shown in Figure 20-1A and B. The patient is asked to elevate her arms above her head, which is followed 30 seconds later by the onset of facial plethora.

A chest radiograph shows a left apical mass.

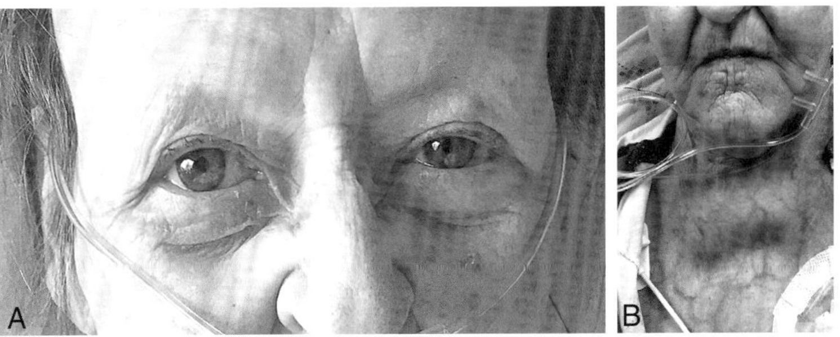


**Figure 20-1.**

***What is the most likely diagnosis in this patient?***

**What is dyspnea?**

Dyspnea is the subjective experience of breathing discomfort or breathlessness. Patients perceive dyspnea in a variety of ways, including increased work or effort of breathing, tightness, and air hunger (ie, unsatisfying inspiration), often occurring together. Dyspnea on exertion is considered abnormal when it occurs at a level of activity that is usually well tolerated.[1,2]

**How is breathing regulated?**

Respiratory drive is controlled by the respiratory centers in the brainstem, which are regulated by various central and peripheral sensory inputs. Examples of sensory inputs include central chemoreceptors, peripheral chemoreceptors, pulmonary stretch receptors, pulmonary C-fibers, and peripheral proprioceptors and metaboreceptors (Figure 20-2). Afferent information from the respiratory centers produces the sensation of dyspnea when an increase in respiratory drive is not satisfied (afferent/efferent mismatch).[1,3,4]

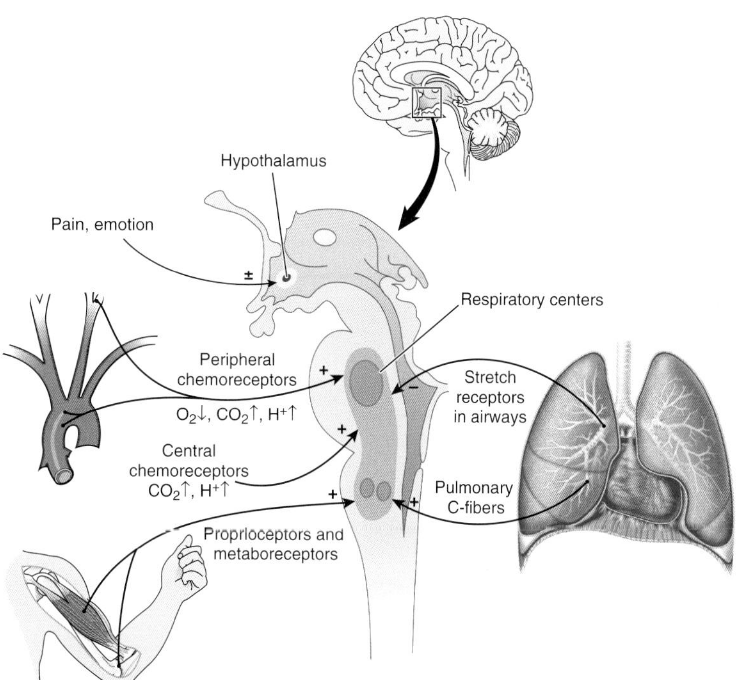


**Figure 20-2.** Regulation of respiration. Respiratory drive is dependent on information from various sensory inputs. + indicates increased respiration; – indicates decreased respiration; ± means that response may vary with circumstances. (From Taylor JJ. *Memmler's Structure and Function of the Human Body*. 10th ed. Philadelphia, PA: Wolters Kluwer Health; 2013.)

**What are the differences between dyspnea, tachypnea, and hyperventilation?**

Dyspnea is strictly a sensation that can only be experienced and reported by a patient, whereas tachypnea and hyperventilation are objective and measurable, and may or may not be associated with dyspnea. Tachypnea describes an increase in respiratory rate above normal. Hyperventilation describes an increase in minute ventilation relative to metabolic demand.[2]

**Which 2 organ systems are responsible for most causes of dyspnea?**

Most causes of dyspnea are related to the heart or the lungs.

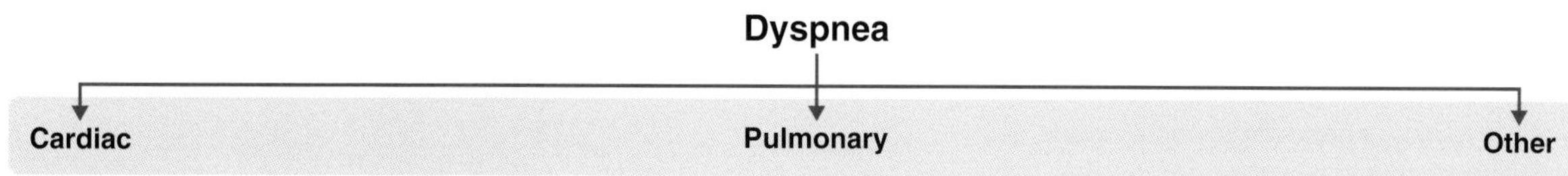


**What are the roles of the heart and lungs in cellular respiration?**

Aerobic respiration requires the exchange of oxygen and other nutrients for carbon dioxide and other waste products. The lungs are the sites of oxygen and carbon dioxide exchange, whereas the heart provides the means of delivery. Dyspnea is most often the result of failure of one or both of these systems.[3]

## CARDIAC CAUSES OF DYSPNEA

**What are the mechanisms of dyspnea related to heart disease?**

The mechanisms of dyspnea in patients with heart disease are diverse, and there is extensive overlap with the pulmonary system. Aerobic respiration depends on the delivery of deoxygenated blood to the lungs and oxygenated blood to the peripheral tissues. These demands increase during exercise: when the heart is unable to adequately respond, metabolic derangements such as tissue acidosis develop, which stimulate the respiratory centers via local metaboreceptors. Additionally, pulmonary congestion related to elevated left atrial pressure directly stimulates local vascular and interstitial receptors (eg, C-fibers, also called juxtapulmonary or J-receptors), which prompt the respiratory centers to increase respiratory drive (see Figure 20-2). Acute pulmonary edema is the most dramatic manifestation of pulmonary congestion, which impairs gas exchange and may trigger bronchoconstriction (known as cardiac asthma).[1,2,5]

**What formula describes oxygen delivery ($Do_2$) to the tissues?**

Oxygen delivery to the tissues is a function of the oxygen content of arterial blood ($Cao_2$) and cardiac output (CO).[6]

$$Do_2\ (\text{mL/min}) = Cao_2\ (\text{mL/L}) \times CO\ (\text{L/min})$$

**What are the main determinants of cardiac output?**

Cardiac output to the peripheral tissues is equal to the forward stroke volume (SV) of the left ventricle per beat multiplied by heart rate (HR).[3]

$$CO = SV \times HR$$

### What are the cardiac causes of dyspnea?

**Electrocardiograms and event monitors are often helpful in diagnosing this group of conditions.**

Cardiac dysrhythmia.

**A 48-year-old woman with hypertension and diabetes mellitus presents with chronic exertional dyspnea; an exercise stress echocardiogram demonstrates inducible wall motion abnormalities.**

Myocardial ischemia (angina equivalent).

**A disease of heart muscle that can be caused by a variety of conditions, such as myocardial ischemia, toxins (eg, alcohol), valvular disease, long-standing hypertension, myocarditis, and chronic tachyarrhythmia.**

Cardiomyopathy.

**A 72-year-old man presents with exertional dyspnea and is found to have a late-peaking crescendo-decrescendo systolic murmur best heard over the right upper sternal border with radiation to the clavicle.**

Aortic stenosis.

**Pulsus paradoxus in a patient with an enlarged cardiac silhouette on chest radiograph.**

Cardiac tamponade.

**Elevated JVP with Kussmaul's sign (a rise in JVP with inspiration) and Friedreich's sign (a sharp and deep Y descent of the jugular venous waveform).**

Constrictive pericarditis.

**Most often caused by viral infection, this condition results in dilated cardiomyopathy in some patients.**

Myocarditis.

**Impaired venous return to the heart from the upper body.**

Superior vena cava (SVC) syndrome.

**May be diagnosed using echocardiography with agitated saline contrast.**

Intracardiac shunt.

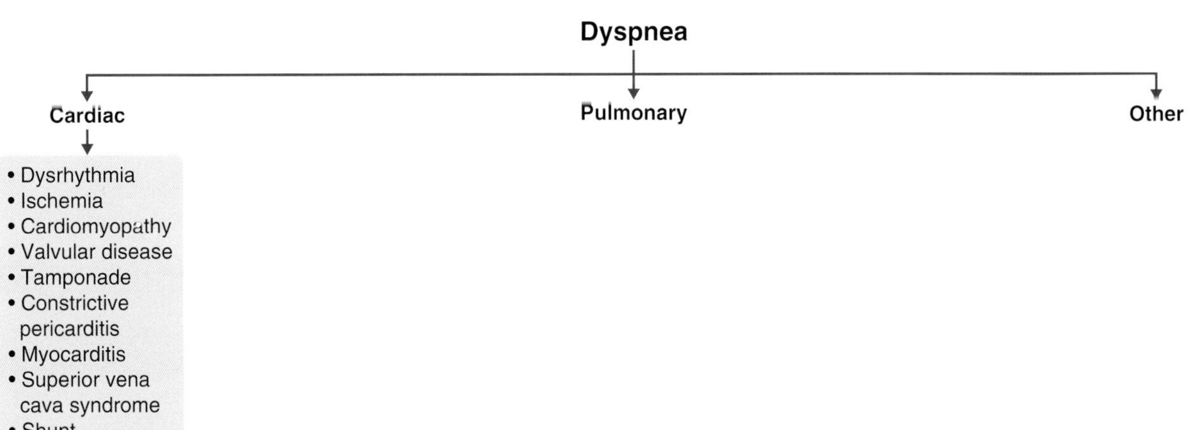


**Which cardiac dysrhythmia might present with exertional dyspnea and the electrocardiographic presence of dropped QRS complexes in an unpredictable pattern?**

Second-degree atrioventricular (AV) block is characterized electrocardiographically by the presence of both conducted beats (ie, P wave followed by an associated QRS complex) and nonconducted (or dropped) beats (ie, P wave not followed by an associated QRS complex). Mobitz II second-degree AV block, which is often symptomatic, is defined by the presence of nonconducted beats that do not occur in a predictable pattern (see Figure 3-4). Exercise typically worsens conduction in the setting of Mobitz II second-degree AV block.[7]

**What is an angina equivalent?**

Chronic stable angina describes chest or arm discomfort that is reproducible with physical exertion or emotional stress, and is relieved promptly (in <5 minutes) with rest or the use of sublingual nitroglycerin. Some patients (particularly women, the elderly, and diabetics) may experience other symptoms that are associated with exertion or stress, and are relieved with rest or sublingual nitroglycerin. These symptoms should be considered equivalent to angina. Exertional dyspnea is the most common angina equivalent symptom; others include isolated discomfort in the jaw, neck, ear, arm, shoulder, back, or epigastric region, nausea, vomiting, diaphoresis, and unexplained fatigue. *Patients with acute coronary syndrome (eg, non-ST elevation myocardial infarction) may also present with angina equivalent symptoms.*[8]

**What are the characteristics of dyspnea in patients with cardiomyopathy who develop heart failure?**

Patients with heart failure frequently complain of dyspnea on exertion, orthopnea, and paroxysmal nocturnal dyspnea. Orthopnea describes dyspnea that occurs in the recumbent position. Paroxysmal nocturnal dyspnea describes dyspnea that awakens the patient from sleep, typically after 1 or 2 hours, and often abates in the upright position.[2]

**What are the mechanisms of dyspnea in patients with aortic stenosis?**

Aortic stenosis is typically asymptomatic until it becomes severe. Exertional dyspnea is one of the most common symptoms in patients with severe aortic stenosis. It occurs when concentric left ventricular hypertrophy leads to elevated end-diastolic pressure with associated pulmonary venous hypertension, reduced cardiac output from diastolic dysfunction, or myocardial ischemia from increased oxygen demand and reduced coronary flow reserve even in the absence of coronary artery disease (dyspnea in this context is an angina equivalent). Once overt systolic heart failure develops, mean survival is 2 years in patients who do not receive treatment.[9,10]

GENERAL INTERNAL MEDICINE

**What is cardiac tamponade?**

Cardiac tamponade describes a reduction in cardiac output as a consequence of compression from pericardial fluid, pus, blood, or gas, either alone or in combination (see Figure 5-2). Virtually any cause of pericarditis can result in cardiac tamponade. Dyspnea on exertion is a common symptom in patients with tamponade physiology, typically progressing to air hunger at rest. Orthopnea is occasionally present. Intravenous fluids can be beneficial to the hypovolemic patient with cardiac tamponade; however, definitive treatment requires urgent evacuation of the pericardial space.[11]

**What are the most common causes of constrictive pericarditis in the industrialized world?**

Constrictive pericarditis can develop following virtually any cause of acute pericarditis. The most common causes in the industrialized world include infectious pericarditis (most often viral), cardiac or pericardial surgery, and external beam radiation to the mediastinum. Dyspnea becomes more prominent at higher central diastolic pressures (ie, >15 mm Hg). Orthopnea is occasionally present.[12]

**What symptoms are associated with myocarditis?**

Myocarditis is associated with a wide spectrum of clinical presentations, from asymptomatic disease to fulminant heart failure. Dyspnea and chest pain are among the most common presenting complaints. Some patients experience complete recovery, whereas others develop chronic dilated cardiomyopathy and progressive heart failure, necessitating transplantation.[13]

**What is superior vena cava syndrome?**

SVC syndrome occurs when obstruction of the SVC results in impaired cardiac filling, giving rise to a constellation of characteristic symptoms and signs. Dyspnea is one of the most frequent symptoms; orthopnea occurs in around one-half of patients. Distended neck veins, distended superficial chest veins, and edema of the face, neck, and arms are among the most common signs.[14]

**What is the mechanism of dyspnea in patients with right-to-left intracardiac shunt?**

Significant right-to-left intracardiac shunt causes hypoxemia that is sensed by central and peripheral chemoreceptors and relayed to the respiratory centers in the brainstem, which respond by increasing respiratory drive (see Figure 20-2). Because hypoxemia caused by anatomic shunt cannot be corrected with increased ventilation, afferent/efferent mismatch sensed by the respiratory centers results in dyspnea.

## PULMONARY CAUSES OF DYSPNEA

**What are the mechanisms of dyspnea related to pulmonary disease?**

Aerobic respiration depends on the exchange of carbon dioxide and oxygen in the lungs. When this function is impaired, patients may develop hypercarbia or hypoxemia. These metabolic derangements are sensed by the central and peripheral chemoreceptors, which then provide stimulatory feedback to the respiratory centers. If the lungs are unable to satisfy the central demand for improved gas exchange, then the patient will experience dyspnea. In addition, some pulmonary diseases (eg, pulmonary edema) activate local receptors (eg, pulmonary C-fibers), which stimulate the respiratory centers and may contribute to the sensation of dyspnea (see Figure 20-2).

**What are the determinants of effective gas exchange in the lungs?**

Gas exchange in the lungs is determined by the balance between pulmonary ventilation (V) and capillary blood flow (Q). A perfect match between ventilation and perfusion (ie, V/Q of 1) is the reference point for defining normal and abnormal gas exchange in the lungs. Dead space occurs when there is excess alveolar ventilation relative to pulmonary capillary perfusion (ie, V/Q >1). Shunt occurs when there is excess pulmonary capillary perfusion relative to alveolar ventilation (ie, V/Q <1) (see Figure 46-6).[6]

**The pulmonary causes of dyspnea can be separated into which anatomic subcategories?**

The pulmonary causes of dyspnea can be separated into the following subcategories: airway, parenchyma, vasculature, and pleura.

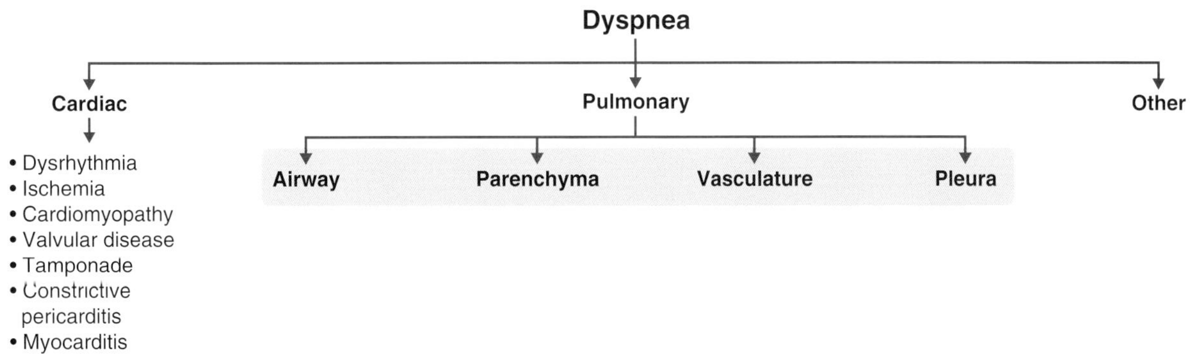




## DYSPNEA RELATED TO THE AIRWAY

### What are the causes of dyspnea related to the airway?

Self-limited inflammation of the large airways. — Acute bronchitis.

A 63-year-old man with an extensive smoking history requires hospitalization at least once per year for episodes of increased cough with sputum production and dyspnea. — Chronic obstructive pulmonary disease.

A 26-year-old man experiences episodes of dyspnea, chest tightness, and wheezing triggered by cold air, dust, and perfume. — Asthma.

Airway dilation and thickening on chest imaging (Figure 20-3). — Bronchiectasis.

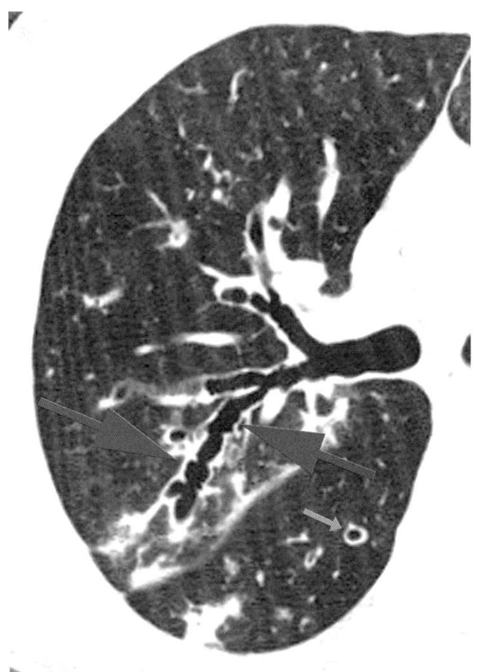

**Figure 20-3.** Bronchiectasis in a patient with cystic fibrosis. A dilated bronchus in the right upper lobe (large arrows) shows a lack of tapering. The signet ring sign (small arrow) describes the cross-sectional appearance of a dilated bronchus compared with the pulmonary artery branch that accompanies it (these structures are normally the same size). (From Webb WR, Higgins CB. *Thoracic Imaging Pulmonary and Cardiovascular Radiology*. 3rd ed. Philadelphia, PA: Wolters Kluwer Health; 2017.)

**A 36-year-old man develops acute dyspnea, stridor, and hives during dinner at a seafood restaurant.**

Anaphylaxis.

**Dynamic airway collapse on expiratory chest imaging.**

Tracheomalacia.

**Acute upper airway obstruction that may be visible on chest imaging.**

Foreign body aspiration.

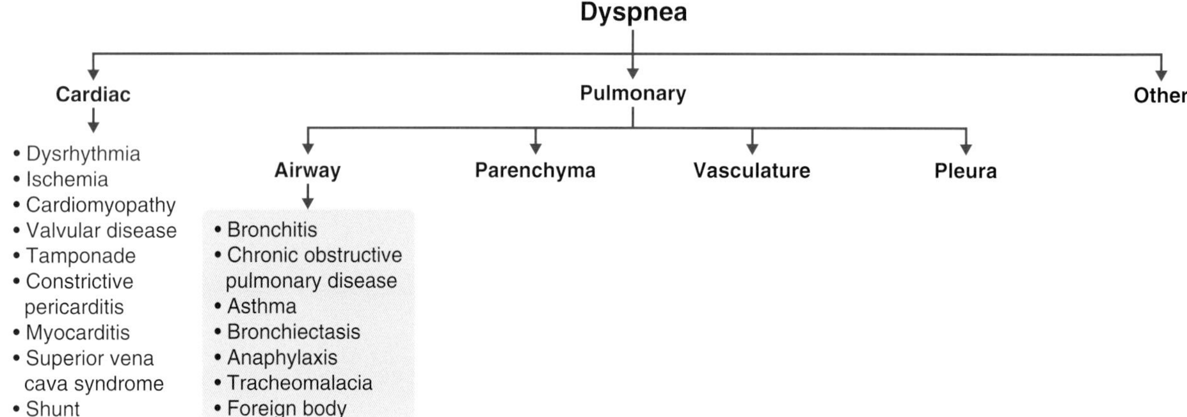


**What causes acute bronchitis in adults?**

Acute bronchitis is most often caused by viral infection. Cough is the predominant symptom and can be either productive or nonproductive. Dyspnea and wheezing may also be present. The condition is self-limited but often protracted, with a mean duration of about 24 days. Treatment is supportive in most cases. Antimicrobial agents may be useful in select circumstances, such as influenza and *Bordetella pertussis* infections. Airway irritants such as smoke can also cause acute bronchitis.[15]

**What is the pharmacologic treatment for acute exacerbations of chronic obstructive pulmonary disease?**

Exacerbations of COPD are characterized by periods of increased dyspnea and cough with sputum production. Common triggers include viral or bacterial lower respiratory tract infection, heart failure, pulmonary embolism (PE), nonadherence to inhaler therapy, and inhalation of irritants such as tobacco smoke or particles. Exacerbations that are severe enough to require hospitalization are typically treated with inhaled short-acting bronchodilators (eg, albuterol) and systemic glucocorticoids (eg, prednisone) with or without antibiotics (eg, doxycycline).[16]

**What is the key spirometric finding in patients with asthma?**

Asthma is associated with reversible airway obstruction on spirometric testing. Reversibility is the key feature that distinguishes asthma from COPD and other causes of obstructive lung disease.

**What are the clinical manifestations of bronchiectasis?**

The vast majority of patients with bronchiectasis have chronic cough productive of sputum that is thick and mucoid. Dyspnea occurs in most patients. Common physical findings include rales, wheezing, and rhonchi. Patients with acute exacerbations of bronchiectasis experience fever and increased dyspnea, wheezing, cough, and sputum production. Antibiotics are the mainstay of treatment. Sputum culture can be helpful in guiding therapy.[17]

**What is the pharmacologic treatment of choice for anaphylaxis?**

Anaphylaxis is a life-threatening systemic hypersensitivity reaction that typically develops within 5 to 30 minutes of antigen exposure. Pulmonary manifestations occur as a result of bronchospasm and include dyspnea, wheezing, cough, and chest tightness. Securing the airway is critical, sometimes requiring intubation. Intramuscular epinephrine should be administered to all patients suspected of having anaphylaxis. It relieves respiratory distress by inducing bronchodilation, with an onset of action of 3 to 5 minutes.[18]

What are the most common causes of tracheomalacia in adults?

Tracheomalacia refers to weakness of the tracheal wall such that it is softer and susceptible to collapse, particularly on expiration. Tracheobronchomalacia refers to the combination of tracheal and mainstem bronchial involvement, whereas bronchomalacia refers to isolated involvement of the mainstem bronchi. The most common acquired causes in adults include tracheostomy and intubation with an endobronchial tube. Chronic inflammation from inhaled irritants such as tobacco smoke is an important risk factor. Symptoms most often include dyspnea, cough (described as "barking" in quality), sputum production, and hemoptysis.[19]

Which lung is most often affected by the aspiration of foreign material?

The right mainstem bronchus is wider and more vertically oriented than the left, making the right lung more susceptible to foreign body aspiration. Men aspirate foreign bodies more frequently than women. Common symptoms include dyspnea, wheezing, and cough; some patients may present with acute respiratory failure. Flexible bronchoscopy is both diagnostic and therapeutic.[20]

## DYSPNEA RELATED TO THE PULMONARY PARENCHYMA

### What are the causes of dyspnea related to the pulmonary parenchyma?

Fever and purulent cough, with focal rales and egophony on auscultation of the lung.

Pneumonia.

Chest radiography typically demonstrates bilateral ground glass opacities, vascular indistinctness, and septal thickening in the periphery.

Pulmonary edema.

This condition can be associated with decreased chest excursion on the affected side with inspiratory rales that clear after deep breathing or cough.

Atelectasis.[21]

A 72-year-old woman with an extensive smoking history presents with chronic dyspnea and is found to have flattened diaphragms and hyperlucency of the lower lungs on chest radiograph (Figure 20-4).

Emphysema (a subtype of COPD).

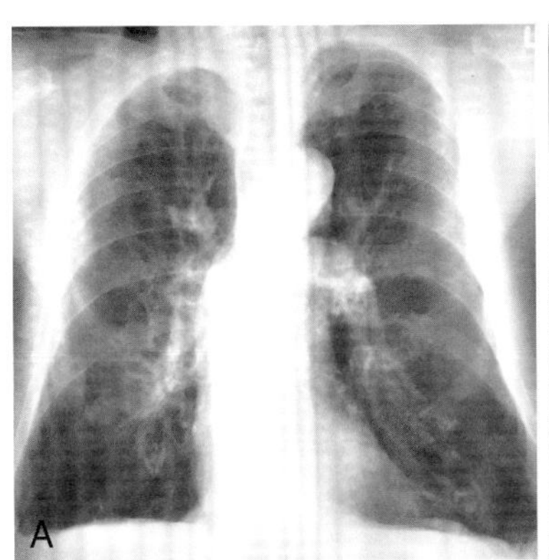


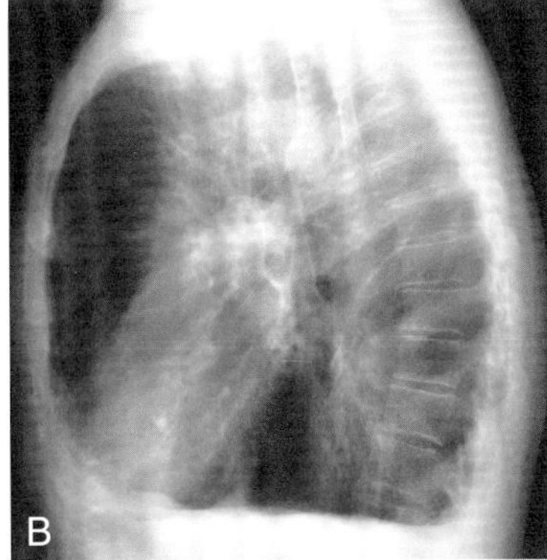


**Figure 20-4.** Posteroanterior (A) and lateral (B) chest radiographs of a patient with emphysema show flattening of the diaphragm with blunting of the costophrenic angles, hyperlucency in the lower lungs, increased retrosternal lucency, increased anteroposterior diameter of the chest, and enlarged central pulmonary arteries. (From Collins J, Stern EJ. *Chest Radiology: The Essentials*. Philadelphia, PA: Wolters Kluwer Health. 2015.)

A 65-year-old man with COPD and active cigarette use presents with weight loss, dyspnea, and hemoptysis.

Lung cancer.

**Digital clubbing and bilateral fine end-inspiratory rales on auscultation of the chest.**

Interstitial lung disease (ILD) (eg, idiopathic pulmonary fibrosis).

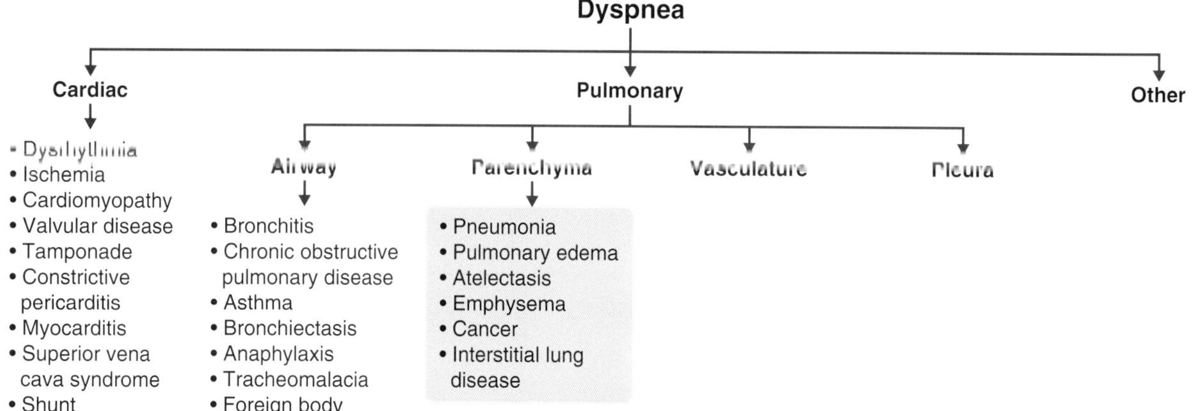


**How can tactile fremitus aid in the diagnosis of pneumonia?**

Dullness to percussion is typical over an area of consolidated lung but also occurs over a pleural effusion. Tactile fremitus can be helpful in distinguishing between the 2 conditions. Tactile fremitus is increased over an area of consolidation, whereas it is decreased (often absent) over an effusion. *The area of compressed lung just above an effusion is sometimes associated with a thin band of increased tactile fremitus and other signs of consolidation.*[22]

**What are the mechanisms of dyspnea in patients with pulmonary edema?**

Pulmonary edema may be caused by left heart failure (ie, cardiogenic), or injury to the endothelial and epithelial barriers (ie, noncardiogenic). It leads to impaired gas exchange in the form of physiological shunt and activation of local interstitial receptors (C-fibers) that stimulate the respiratory centers (see Figure 20-2).[2,23]

**Which group of hospitalized patients is at high risk for atelectasis?**

Atelectasis is common in postoperative patients and can lead to dyspnea, cough, tachypnea, hypoxemia, and even acute respiratory failure. Early ambulation, breathing exercises, and incentive spirometry may be helpful in the prevention and treatment of atelectasis in this population.[21]

**What are the key pulmonary function test findings in patients with emphysema?**

COPD describes chronic airflow limitation, typically as a result of small airway disease and parenchymal destruction. Airway disease predominates in some patients producing the chronic bronchitis phenotype (the "blue bloater"), whereas in others parenchymal destruction predominates producing the emphysema phenotype (the "pink puffer"). Pulmonary function studies differ between the two. Both are associated with decreased $FEV_1$ and decreased ratio between $FEV_1$ and forced vital capacity (FVC). Emphysema is additionally associated with increased total lung capacity (mostly as a result of increased residual volume) and decreased diffusing capacity for carbon monoxide (DLCO).[24]

**How common is dyspnea in patients with lung cancer?**

Dyspnea is common in all stages of lung cancer. It is distressing to patients and interferes with activities of daily living. Mechanisms are diverse, including direct tumor invasion, associated pleural effusion, PE, anemia, and treatment-related complications (eg, radiation pneumonitis).[25]

**What are the key pulmonary function test findings in patients with interstitial lung disease?**

ILD is a restrictive lung disease. Spirometry demonstrates decreased $FEV_1$ with a preserved or increased $FEV_1$/FVC ratio; total lung capacity is decreased; and DLCO is decreased.

## DYSPNEA RELATED TO THE PULMONARY VASCULATURE

### What are the causes of dyspnea related to the pulmonary vasculature?

**A 68-year-old woman with pancreatic cancer develops new dyspnea and hemoptysis; electrocardiogram demonstrates sinus tachycardia, T-wave inversions in leads $V_1$-$V_3$, and right axis deviation.**

Pulmonary embolism.

**Loud and palpable P2 in a patient with ILD.**

Pulmonary hypertension.

**A 44-year-old woman with a history of chronic sinusitis presents with dyspnea and hemoptysis and is found to have hematuria and acute kidney injury with dysmorphic red blood cells (see Figure 34-4) and red blood cell casts on urine sediment analysis.**

Granulomatosis with polyangiitis (GPA, or Wegener's granulomatosis).

**A patient with hereditary hemorrhagic telangiectasia develops dyspnea and hypoxemia that does not correct with 100% inhaled oxygen.**

Pulmonary arteriovenous malformation.

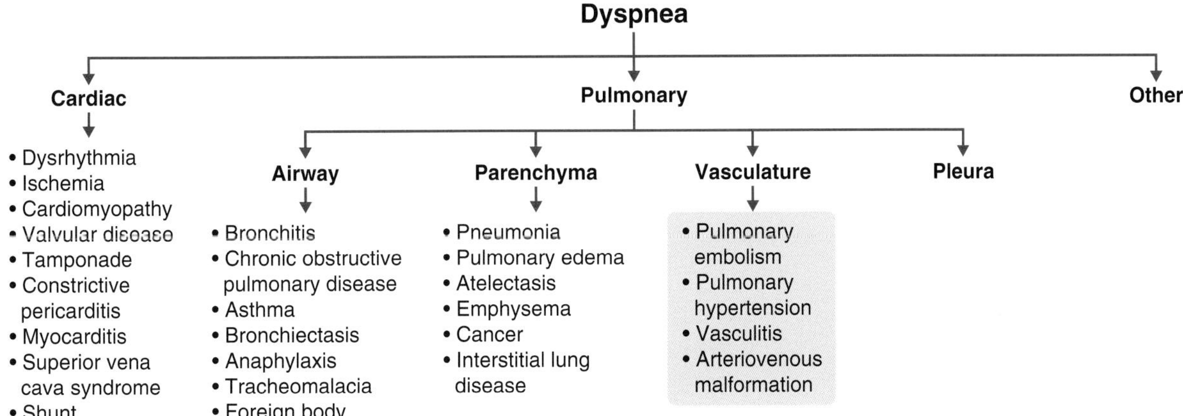


What are the characteristics of dyspnea related to pulmonary embolism?

Most patients with PE experience acute dyspnea on exertion or at rest. Onset is typically rapid, within seconds to hours. Orthopnea is frequently present. The vast majority of patients have either dyspnea or tachypnea on presentation. Other common symptoms include pleuritic chest pain, cough, and hemoptysis.[26]

What are the mechanisms of dyspnea in pulmonary hypertension?

Dyspnea on exertion is a common symptom of pulmonary hypertension. Mechanisms include impaired gas exchange related to increased dead space and decreased DLCO, stimulation of local vascular receptors (eg, C-fibers), opening of a right-to-left intracardiac shunt, and right heart failure (ie, cor pulmonale).[27]

Which systemic vasculitides are most often associated with pulmonary-renal syndrome?

Diffuse alveolar hemorrhage (DAH) is a life-threatening condition that typically presents with dyspnea, cough, and hemoptysis. Pulmonary-renal syndrome refers to the combination of DAH and glomerulonephritis. It is most frequently caused by the antineutrophil cytoplasmic antibody (ANCA)–associated small vessel vasculitides (eg, microscopic polyangiitis), antiglomerular basement membrane disease, or vasculitis associated with systemic disease, particularly systemic lupus erythematosus.[28]

**What condition should be suspected in a cirrhotic patient who develops dyspnea that worsens in the upright position and improves while lying flat?**

Hepatopulmonary syndrome describes the development of pulmonary arteriovenous malformations at the lung bases in patients with advanced liver disease. The upright position augments blood flow to the lung bases, which increases shunt fraction, whereas the supine position decreases shunt fraction. This physiology causes dyspnea in the upright position (platypnea), as well as arterial desaturation (orthodeoxia), both of which improve with recumbency.

## DYSPNEA RELATED TO THE PLEURA

### What are the causes of dyspnea related to the pleura?

**Dullness to percussion of the chest with decreased tactile fremitus.**

Pleural effusion.

**Hyperresonance to percussion of one side of the chest.**

Pneumothorax.

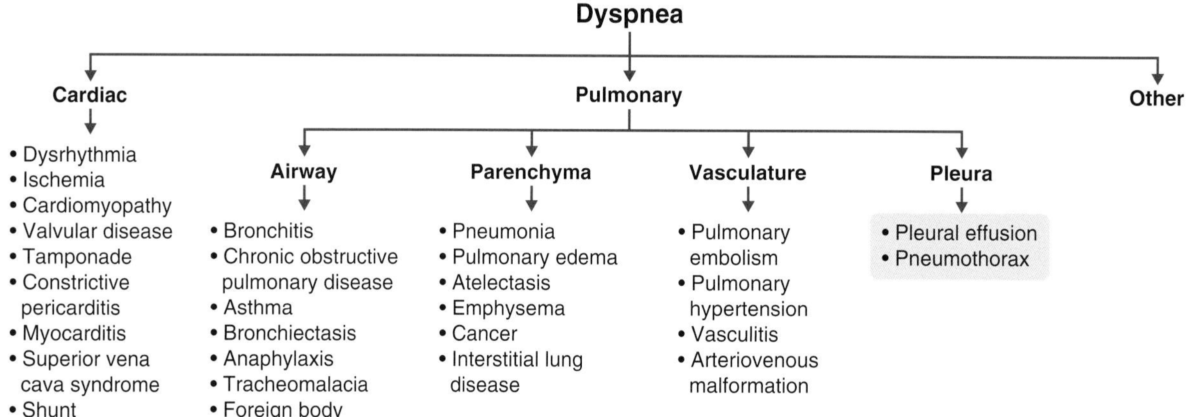


**What is the treatment for the dyspnea associated with pleural effusion?**

Treatment strategies for pleural effusions depend on the size, nature of the fluid, and symptom burden. For example, small to moderate size transudative pleural effusions caused by heart failure are often responsive to diuretic therapy. Large and symptomatic malignant pleural effusions, on the other hand, are generally best managed with drainage (ie, thoracentesis) along with treatment for the underlying malignancy (if possible). Patients often experience immediate relief when large pleural effusions are drained.

**Which patients are at highest risk for spontaneous pneumothorax?**

Pneumothorax describes the presence of air in the pleural space (see Figure 24-3). Symptoms include dyspnea and chest pain, the severity of which is generally proportional to the size of the pneumothorax. Primary spontaneous pneumothorax occurs in patients without underlying lung disease. The prototypical patient is a tall, thin male between 10 and 30 years of age who actively smokes or has a history of smoking. Secondary spontaneous pneumothorax occurs in patients with underlying lung disease (eg, COPD, cystic fibrosis).[29]

## DYSPNEA RELATED TO OTHER CAUSES

### What are the other causes of dyspnea?

**A young woman with agoraphobia suffers from recurrent episodes of dyspnea and chest pain.**

Panic attack.

**Conjunctival pallor.**

Anemia.

**A traveling soccer team unexpectedly loses to a weaker home team in La Paz, Bolivia, a city that is 3600 m above sea level.**

Reduced partial pressure of inspired oxygen ($P_IO_2$) caused by high altitude.

**A 38-year-old woman presents with double vision and drooping eyelids that are more noticeable at the end of the day, and is found to have a mediastinal mass.**

Myasthenia gravis (associated with thymoma).

**Respiratory compensation.**

Metabolic acidosis.

**Women are at risk.**

Pregnancy.

**An endocrinopathy.**

Thyrotoxicosis.

**Associated with a sedentary lifestyle or prolonged hospitalization.**

Deconditioning.

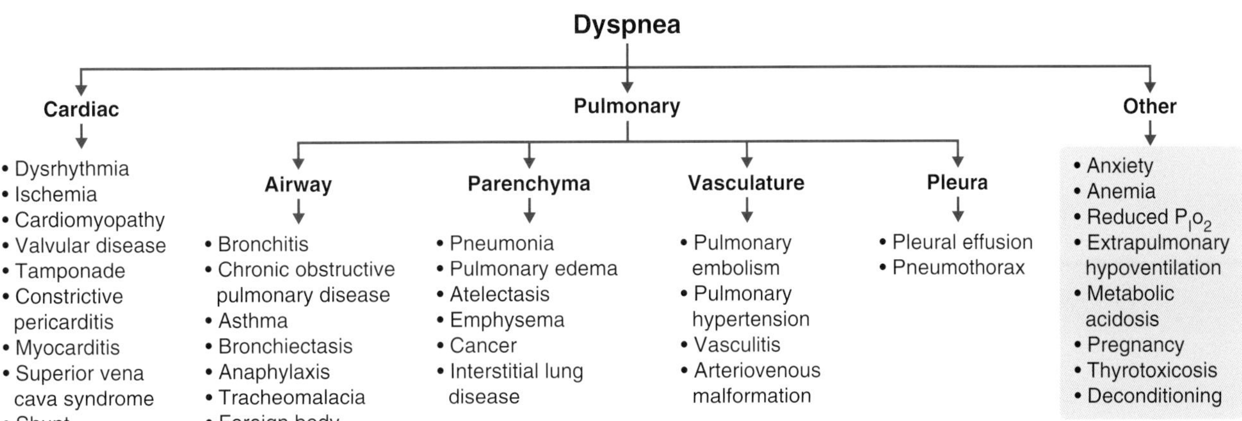


**Is there an association between cardiopulmonary disease and anxiety?**

Patients with underlying cardiopulmonary disease, particularly obstructive lung disease, experience a high rate of anxiety, which can exacerbate existing chronic dyspnea. It is important to identify anxiety and panic disorders in this population, as treatment can improve functional status and quality of life. Options for patients with respiratory disease include nonpharmacologic and limited pharmacologic (eg, selective serotonin reuptake inhibitors, buspirone) treatment. Benzodiazepines and other respiratory depressants should generally be avoided unless patients are receiving hospice care.[30]

**What is the mechanism of dyspnea in patients with anemia?**

Hemoglobin concentration is one of the key determinants of the oxygen content in arterial blood (see chapter 46, Hypoxemia). Anemia causes impaired oxygen delivery to the tissues, resulting in metabolic derangements such as tissue acidosis, which stimulate the respiratory centers via local metaboreceptors (see Figure 20-2).[1]

**What life-threatening condition should be considered in a climber who develops dyspnea and pink frothy sputum at the summit of a mountain?**

High-altitude pulmonary edema (HAPE) is a life-threatening condition that most commonly develops within 2 to 4 days of ascending 2500 m or more above sea level. It is responsible for the majority of deaths related to high altitude. Slow ascent to allow for acclimatization is the most effective way to prevent HAPE; nifedipine is the pharmacologic agent of choice for prevention. If it develops, patients should be treated with supplemental oxygen, advised to rest, and immediately evacuated to lower altitudes in severe cases.[31]

**What extrapulmonary causes of hypoventilation are associated with dyspnea?**

Extrapulmonary causes of hypoventilation associated with dyspnea include obesity, ascites, neuromuscular diseases (eg, amyotrophic lateral sclerosis, myasthenia gravis, Guillain-Barré syndrome), and chest wall deformities (eg, pectus excavatum).

**In a patient with pure metabolic acidosis and serum bicarbonate ($HCO_3^-$) concentration of 10 mEq/L, what is the expected partial pressure of carbon dioxide ($Paco_2$) after respiratory compensation?**

Metabolic acidosis generates a compensatory increase in ventilation with a target $Paco_2$ lower than the normal 40 mm Hg in arterial blood. Winters' formula can be used to calculate the expected $Paco_2$: predicted $Paco_2 = (1.5 \times [HCO_3^-]) + 8 \pm 2$.

In a patient with normal lung function and a serum $HCO_3^-$ of 10 mEq/L, predicted $Paco_2 = (1.5 \times 10) + 8 \pm 2 = 23 \pm 2$ mm Hg.[32]

**When does dyspnea occur during the course of a normal pregnancy?**

Dyspnea is a common feature of normal pregnancy. It can begin in the first trimester and occurs in most patients by the end of the second trimester. A variety of mechanisms are involved, including an increase in respiratory drive mediated by estrogen and progesterone.[33]

**What is the mechanism of dyspnea in patients with thyrotoxicosis?**

Patients with thyrotoxicosis frequently experience dyspnea, particularly with exertion. It occurs as a result of exaggerated central respiratory drive in response to hypercapnia and hypoxemia. Severity correlates with the degree of thyrotoxicosis. β-Blocker therapy is often effective at mitigating dyspnea until euthyroidism can be achieved. Other mechanisms of dyspnea in patients with thyrotoxicosis include respiratory muscle weakness and pulmonary hypertension, both of which are reversible with management of thyrotoxicosis.[34,35]

**What is the mechanism of dyspnea in patients with deconditioning?**

Deconditioned muscles generate increased metabolic byproducts during exercise that stimulate the respiratory centers via local metaboreceptors (see Figure 20-2). Patients with cardiopulmonary disease and chronic dyspnea are at risk for becoming sedentary and developing deconditioning, which can worsen symptoms. Pulmonary rehabilitation and exercise training can be helpful.[1]

## Case Summary

A 71-year-old woman with an extensive smoking history presents with progressive dyspnea and weight loss, and is found to have elevated JVP, dilated superficial veins on the chest, an abnormal cranial nerve examination, and an apical mass on chest imaging.

***What is the most likely diagnosis in this patient?***

Superior vena cava syndrome.

### BONUS QUESTIONS

***What features in this case are suggestive of superior vena cava syndrome?***

The patient in this case has classic symptoms of SVC syndrome, including facial and neck swelling, dyspnea, and cough. Physical findings suggestive of SVC syndrome in this case include elevated JVP, dilated superficial veins of the chest (see Figure 20-1B), edema of the face, neck, and upper extremities, and the onset of facial plethora after raising the arms above the head (Pemberton's sign).

***What are the causes of superior vena cava syndrome?***

Most cases of SVC syndrome in the industrialized world are related to intrathoracic malignancy (eg, lung cancer, mediastinal lymphoma); other causes include SVC stenosis or thrombosis (usually caused by intravascular devices), goiter, aortic aneurysm, and fibrosing mediastinitis.[14]

***Which cranial nerve abnormalities are evident in Figure 20-1A?***

Ptosis and miosis of the left eye are demonstrated in Figure 20-1A.

***What is the significance of the combination of ptosis and miosis in this case?***

The combination of ptosis and miosis in this case is suggestive of Horner's syndrome, which describes a constellation of findings caused by disruption of the sympathetic innervation of the eye (anhidrosis rounds out the classic triad). The sympathetic neurons originate in the hypothalamus, descend into the cervical spinal cord, travel across the pulmonary apex, and travel up the wall of the internal carotid artery before joining the ophthalmic division of the trigeminal nerve. Disruption of the sympathetic neurons at any point along this pathway will result in ipsilateral Horner's syndrome.[36]

| | |
|---|---|
| ***What is the most likely cause of superior vena cava obstruction and Horner's syndrome in this case?*** | The smoking history, weight loss, and apical mass on chest imaging in this case suggest an apical lung tumor (Pancoast tumor), which is likely causing external compression of the SVC as well as disruption of the sympathetic neurons that travel across the pulmonary apex. |
| ***What is the treatment for superior vena cava syndrome related to lung cancer?*** | Symptoms of SVC syndrome related to extrinsic compression from lung cancer generally improve with chemotherapy and local radiation. If there is associated SVC thrombosis, anticoagulation should be started. Endovascular revascularization techniques (eg, stenting) or open surgical procedures may also be considered.[14] |

## KEY POINTS

- Dyspnea is the subjective experience of breathing discomfort or breathlessness.
- Breathing is regulated by the respiratory centers in the brainstem, which receive information from various sensory inputs, including chemoreceptors, mechanoreceptors, and metaboreceptors.
- The causes of dyspnea can be separated into the following categories: cardiac, pulmonary, and other.
- Most causes of dyspnea are related to the heart and/or the lungs.
- Pulmonary causes of dyspnea can be separated into the following anatomic subcategories: airway, parenchyma, vasculature, and pleura.

GENERAL INTERNAL MEDICINE

## REFERENCES


1. Parshall MB, Schwartzstein RM, Adams L, et al. An official American Thoracic Society statement: update on the mechanisms, assessment, and management of dyspnea. *Am J Respir Crit Care Med.* 2012;185(4):435-452.
2. Walker HK, Hall WD, Hurst JW, eds. *Clinical Methods: The History, Physical, and Laboratory Examinations.* 3rd ed. Boston: Butterworths; 1990.
3. Berne RML, Levy MN. *Physiology.* 4th ed. St. Louis, MO: Mosby, Inc.; 1998.
4. Burki NK, Lee LY. Mechanisms of dyspnea. *Chest.* 2010;138(5):1196-1201.
5. Witte KK, Clark AL. Why does chronic heart failure cause breathlessness and fatigue? *Prog Cardiovasc Dis.* 2007;49(5):366-384.
6. Marino PL. *The ICU Book.* 3rd ed. Philadelphia, PA: Lippincott Williams & Wilkins—a Wolters Kluwer business; 2007.
7. Merideth J, Pruitt RD. Cardiac arrhythmias. 5. Disturbances in cardiac conduction and their management. *Circulation.* 1973;47(5):1098-1107.
8. Anderson JL, Adams CD, Antman EM, et al. 2011 ACCF/AHA focused update incorporated into the ACC/AHA 2007 guidelines for the management of patients with unstable angina/non-ST-elevation myocardial infarction: a report of the American College of Cardiology Foundation/American Heart Association Task Force on practice guidelines. *Circulation.* 2011;123(18):e426-e579.
9. Maganti K, Rigolin VH, Sarano ME, Bonow RO. Valvular heart disease: diagnosis and management. *Mayo Clin Proc.* 2010;85(5):483-500.
10. Ross Jr J, Braunwald E. Aortic stenosis. *Circulation.* 1968;38(1 suppl):61-67.
11. Spodick DH. *The Pericardium*: A Comprehensive Textbook. New York, NY: Marcel Dekker, Inc.; 1997.
12. Schwefer M, Aschenbach R, Heidemann J, Mey C, Lapp H. Constrictive pericarditis, still a diagnostic challenge: comprehensive review of clinical management. *Eur J Cardio Thorac Surg.* 2009;36(3):502-510.
13. Schultz JC, Hilliard AA, Cooper Jr LT, Rihal CS. Diagnosis and treatment of viral myocarditis. *Mayo Clin Proc.* 2009;84(11):1001-1009.
14. Cheng S. Superior vena cava syndrome: a contemporary review of a historic disease. *Cardiol Rev.* 2009;17(1):16-23.
15. Wenzel RP, Fowler AA, 3rd. Clinical practice. Acute bronchitis. *N Engl J Med.* 2006;355(20):2125-2130.
16. Decramer M, Janssens W, Miravitlles M. Chronic obstructive pulmonary disease. *Lancet.* 2012;379(9823):1341-1351.
17. Barker AF. Bronchiectasis. *N Engl J Med.* 2002;346(18):1383-1393.
18. Arnold JJ, Williams PM. Anaphylaxis: recognition and management. *Am Fam Physician.* 2011;84(10):1111-1118.
19. Carden KA, Boiselle PM, Waltz DA, Ernst A. Tracheomalacia and tracheobronchomalacia in children and adults: an in-depth review. *Chest.* 2005;127(3):984-1005.
20. Sehgal IS, Dhooria S, Ram B, et al. Foreign body inhalation in the adult population: experience of 25,998 bronchoscopies and systematic review of the literature. *Respir Care.* 2015;60(10):1438-1448.
21. Restrepo RD, Braverman J. Current challenges in the recognition, prevention and treatment of perioperative pulmonary atelectasis. *Expert Rev Respir Med.* 2015;9(1):97-107.
22. Sapira JD. *The Art & Science of Bedside Diagnosis.* Baltimore, MD: Urban & Schwarzenberg, Inc.; 1990.
23. Murray JF. Pulmonary edema: pathophysiology and diagnosis. *Int J Tuberc Lung Dis.* 2011;15(2):155-160, i.
24. Ranu H, Wilde M, Madden B. Pulmonary function tests. *Ulster Med J.* 2011;80(2):84-90.
25. Williams AC, Grant M, Tiep B, Kim JY, Hayter J. Dyspnea management in early stage lung cancer: a palliative perspective. *J Hosp Palliat Nurs.* 2012;14(5):341-342.
26. Stein PD, Beemath A, Matta F, et al. Clinical characteristics of patients with acute pulmonary embolism: data from PIOPED II. *Am J Med.* 2007;120(10):871-879.

27. Sajkov D, Petrovsky N, Palange P. Management of dyspnea in advanced pulmonary arterial hypertension. *Curr Opin Support Palliat Care*. 2010;4(2):76-84.
28. McCabe C, Jones Q, Nikolopoulou A, Wathen C, Luqmani R. Pulmonary-renal syndromes: an update for respiratory physicians. *Respir Med*. 2011;105(10):1413-1421.
29. Choi WI. Pneumothorax. *Tuberc Respir Dis*. 2014;76(3):99-104.
30. Smoller JW, Pollack MH, Otto MW, Rosenbaum JF, Kradin RL. Panic anxiety, dyspnea, and respiratory disease. Theoretical and clinical considerations. *Am J Respir Crit Care Med*. 1996;154(1):6-17.
31. Bhagi S, Srivastava S, Singh SB. High-altitude pulmonary edema: review. *J Occup Health*. 2014;56(4):235-243.
32. Albert MS, Dell RB, Winters RW. Quantitative displacement of acid-base equilibrium in metabolic acidosis. *Ann Intern Med*. 1967;66(2):312-322.
33. Lee SY, Chien DK, Huang CH, Shih SC, Lee WC, Chang WH. Dyspnea in pregnancy. *Taiwan J Obstet Gynecol*. 2017;56(4):432-436.
34. Small D, Gibbons W, Levy RD, de Lucas P, Gregory W, Cosio MG. Exertional dyspnea and ventilation in hyperthyroidism. *Chest*. 1992;101(5):1268-1273.
35. Thurnheer R, Jenni R, Russi EW, Greminger P, Speich R. Hyperthyroidism and pulmonary hypertension. *J Intern Med*. 1997;242(2):185-188.
36. Kanagalingam S, Miller NR. Horner syndrome: clinical perspectives. *Eye Brain*. 2015;7:35-46.

Chapter 21

# FEVER OF UNKNOWN ORIGIN

## Case: A 37-year-old man with oral ulcers

A previously healthy 37-year-old Syrian man is evaluated in the clinic for fever and joint pain. Approximately 8 weeks ago, he experienced a self-limited illness characterized by fever, abdominal pain, and diarrhea. He recovered to his usual state of good health but 2 weeks later developed intermittent fever that coincided with right knee discomfort. He was evaluated in the clinic and found to have a temperature of 38.4°C with warmth and swelling of the right knee. Urinalysis, blood cultures, and chest radiograph were unrevealing. The symptoms in the right knee eventually resolved, but intermittent fever persisted. Another visit to the clinic was nondiagnostic. A few days later, he developed pain and swelling of the left knee. He also complains of occasional burning when he urinates, and bilateral eye discomfort without vision changes. Family history is notable for a first-degree relative with ulcerative colitis and ankylosing spondylitis.

Temperature is 38.6°C. There is mild bilateral conjunctival erythema. There are painless ulcerative lesions of the oral mucosa (Figure 21-1A). The left knee is warm with a large effusion (Figure 21-1B). The insertion sites of the Achilles tendons are erythematous and tender to palpation. There are no genital ulcers.

Synovial fluid analysis from left knee arthrocentesis is notable for a white blood cell count of 6134/μL (67% neutrophils) with a negative Gram stain and culture. Synovial fluid polymerase chain reaction (PCR) for *Neisseria gonorrhoeae* is negative. Tests for serum antinuclear antibody, rheumatoid factor, and anti–cyclic citrullinated peptide antibody are negative. Urine PCR studies for *Chlamydia trachomatis* and *Neisseria gonorrhoeae* are negative.

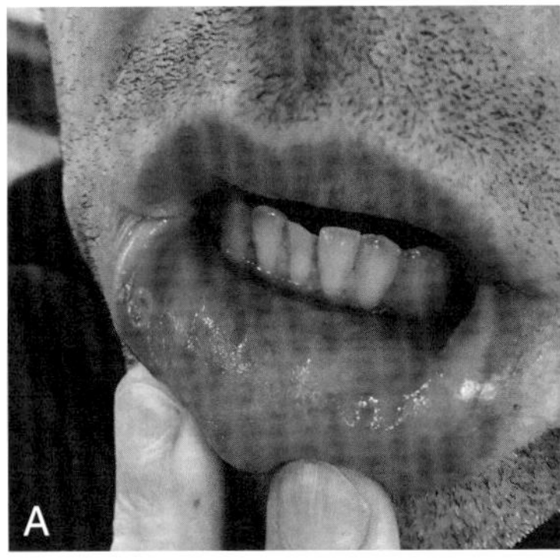


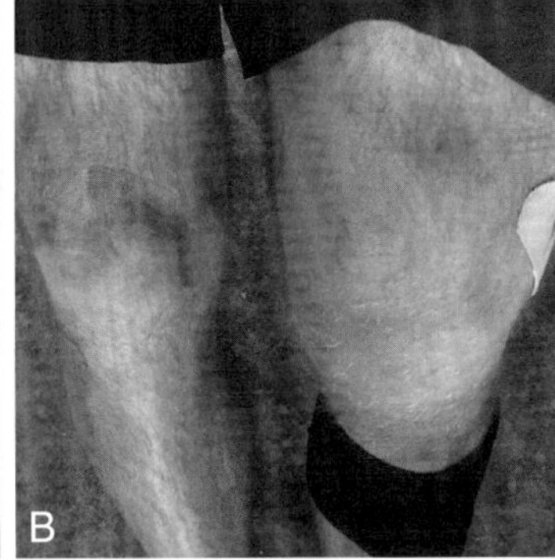


**Figure 21-1.**

***What is the most likely diagnosis in this patient?***

What is fever of unknown origin (FUO)?

FUO is classically defined as an illness lasting longer than 3 weeks, with measured temperature >38.3°C on several occasions, and failure to reach a diagnosis despite 1 week of inpatient investigation. Modifications have been made to this definition to incorporate more modern styles of practice, adjusting the minimum duration of investigation to 3 days in the hospital or 3 outpatient visits.[1-3]

How common is fever of unknown origin?

Fever is a ubiquitous problem that occurs in virtually all patients at some point during life. True FUO is uncommon; for example in 1 community hospital setting in the United States, it was present in approximately 1 out of every 75 cases that involved infectious disease specialists. Although FUO occurs infrequently, it is associated with a heavy burden: most hospitalized patients remain in-house for prolonged periods of time (often weeks to months) and undergo considerable diagnostic testing.[4]

**The causes of fever of unknown origin can be separated into which general categories?**

The causes of FUO can be separated into the following categories: infectious, noninfectious inflammatory, malignant, and other.

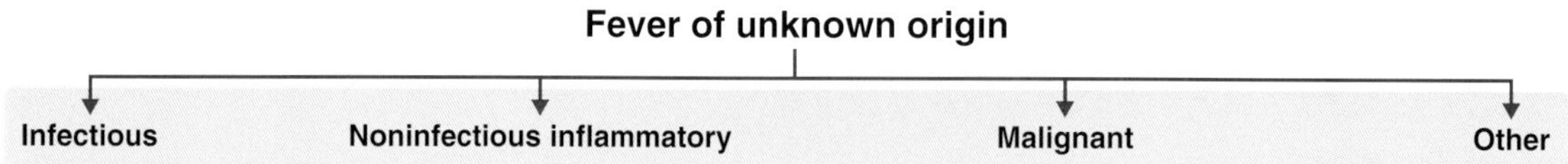


**What is the relative prevalence of each category of fever of unknown origin?**

The causes of FUO have evolved over time, and the prevalence of each category depends on host and geographic factors. In the modern industrialized world, infection accounts for approximately 25% of cases; noninfectious inflammatory conditions account for 25%; malignancy, 15%; and the remainder consist of miscellaneous or idiopathic causes (most cases in this group remain undiagnosed). *FUO is more likely to be caused by an atypical presentation of a common disease than a typical presentation of a rare disease.*[1,5,6]

**What is the prognosis of fever of unknown origin?**

The prognosis of FUO depends on the underlying cause. The prognosis of idiopathic FUO is excellent; most cases resolve spontaneously within a few weeks. Infectious causes of FUO are also generally associated with a favorable prognosis; most patients survive without significant morbidity. Patients with noninfectious inflammatory causes of FUO are most likely to experience persistent morbidity. The highest mortality rates are associated with FUO due to malignancy; the majority of patients are dead within 5 years.[4,6]

## INFECTIOUS CAUSES OF FEVER OF UNKNOWN ORIGIN

**What historical information is important to obtain when considering infectious causes of fever of unknown origin?**

Types of historical information pertinent to infectious causes of FUO include demographic (eg, country of origin), medical (eg, history of diverticulitis, recent dental procedures or antibiotic use, blood transfusion, presence of indwelling foreign material), and social (eg, sexual and drug behaviors; travel history; sick contacts; and zoonotic, recreational, dietary, and occupational exposures).[2]

### What are the infectious causes of fever of unknown origin?

**A 73-year-old man with a history of diverticulitis, including a recent bout 6 weeks ago that was treated with oral antibiotics, presents with several weeks of fever and is found to have focal tenderness to palpation over the left lower quadrant of the abdomen.**

Intra-abdominal abscess.

**A 47-year-old woman who emigrated from Iran to the United States presents with FUO and is found to have cholestatic liver injury, normal chest radiograph, and computed tomography (CT) imaging of the abdomen demonstrating hepatomegaly and multiple low-density micronodules throughout the liver.**

Miliary tuberculosis (TB).

**A 62-year-old man, who recently completed an empiric course of antibiotics for fever 6 weeks after a dental cleaning, now presents with persistent fever, weight loss, and night sweats and is found to have negative blood cultures. Careful physical examination reveals a decrescendo diastolic murmur heard best over the third intercostal space of the left sternal border.**

Culture-negative endocarditis.

**This infection is typically acquired via contiguous spread or hematogenous seeding.**

Osteomyelitis.

**Antibiotics are not helpful for this type of infection.**

Viral infection.

**A 42-year-old man presents with fever, headache, myalgias, conjunctival suffusion (Figure 21-2), acute kidney injury, moderate hepatocellular liver injury, hyponatremia, and thrombocytopenia a few weeks after windsurfing on the Columbia River, a fresh water source.**

Leptospirosis.

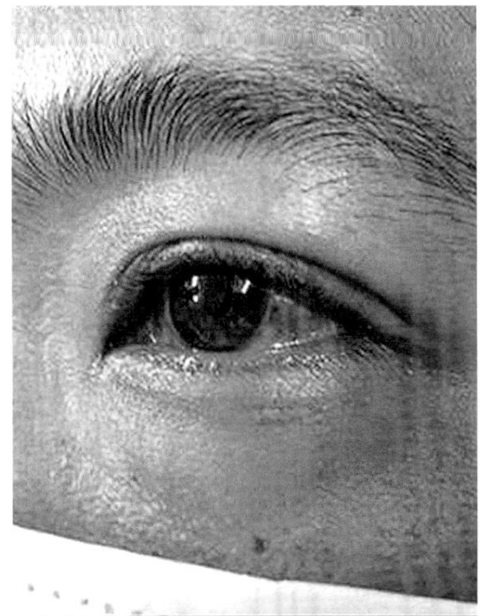

**Figure 21-2.** Conjunctival suffusion with subconjunctival hemorrhage is suggestive of leptospirosis. (Reprinted with permission from Lin CY, Chiu NC, Lee CM. Leptospirosis after typhoon. *Am J Trop Med Hyg*. 2012;86:187. Copyright © 2012 by The American Society of Tropical Medicine and Hygiene.)



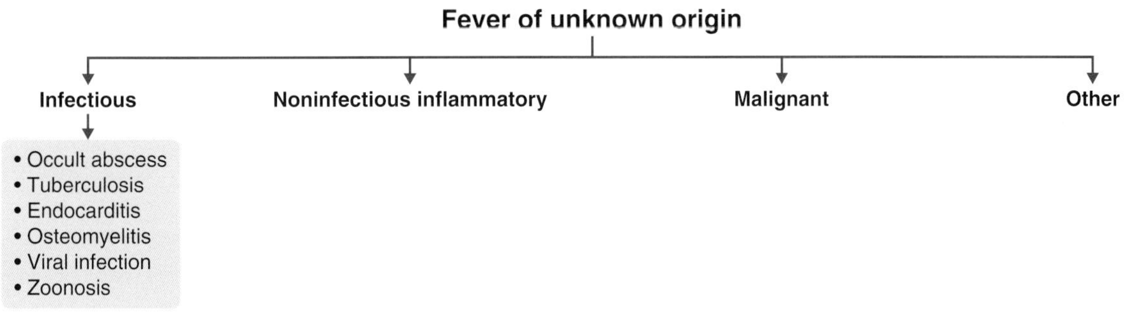


**What are the characteristics of fever of unknown origin caused by intra-abdominal abscess?**

Intra-abdominal abscess is the most common infectious cause of FUO in the industrialized world. Commonly affected sites include the liver, spleen, and intraperitoneal cavity. Most patients have a compatible history, such as biliary disease, diverticulitis, appendicitis, or Crohn's disease. Tenderness on examination is typically present; however, elderly patients tend to have more subtle symptoms and signs, which can result in a protracted course. CT imaging of the abdomen has a high diagnostic yield and should be one of the first studies performed in patients with FUO, particularly with a suggestive history or examination. Dental, renal, and perinephric abscess are other common sources of occult infection in patients with FUO.[5-7]

**Under what circumstances is infection with *Mycobacterium tuberculosis* most likely to go undetected?**

Forms of TB most likely to present with FUO include extrapulmonary disease (eg, hepatic TB) without clear localizing features, miliary disease without the characteristic pattern on chest radiography, and pulmonary disease in patients with compromised immune systems (chest radiography may be normal in patients with acquired immunodeficiency syndrome). Key investigations include imaging to evaluate for subtle pulmonary or extrapulmonary disease, tuberculin skin testing or blood interferon-$\gamma$ release assay, studies to identify *Mycobacterium tuberculosis* in samples from sputum or bronchoscopy with bronchoalveolar lavage (eg, smear, culture, PCR), and histopathologic evaluation of involved tissue (eg, lung, liver, bone marrow).[7,8]

**Under what circumstances is endocarditis most likely to present with negative blood cultures?**

Culture-negative endocarditis can occur with typical pathogens (eg, *Streptococcus* species) when antibiotics have been administered before culture is obtained. It can also occur with atypical organisms that do not grow in routine culture media, such as *Bartonella* species, *Brucella* species, *Coxiella burnetii*, *Abiotrophia defectiva*, *Granulicatella* species, *Tropheryma whipplei*, and fungi. The HACEK organisms (*Haemophilus* species, *Aggregatibacter* species, *Cardiobacterium hominis*, *Eikenella corrodens*, and *Kingella* species) will grow in culture if given sufficient time. Key investigations to evaluate for culture-negative endocarditis include careful physical examination (eg, cardiovascular, fundoscopic), special culturing techniques, serologic tests (eg, *Coxiella*), molecular techniques (eg, PCR), and echocardiography.[7,9]

**What is the most common site of osteomyelitis in patients presenting with fever of unknown origin?**

The spine is the most common site of osteomyelitis in patients presenting with FUO. Local discomfort may be minimal. Magnetic resonance imaging (MRI) of the spine is helpful for identification. Infected joint prostheses are also a frequent source of osteomyelitis in patients with FUO, highlighting the importance of identifying the presence of foreign material in the body.[5,10]

**What are the most common viral causes of fever of unknown origin?**

Viral infections most frequently implicated in cases of FUO include cytomegalovirus (CMV), Epstein-Barr virus (EBV), and human immunodeficiency virus (HIV). These viruses can produce a protracted mononucleosis-like illness. One-quarter of immunocompetent patients with CMV infection have fever longer than 3 weeks. Key investigations include peripheral white blood cell count with differential, peripheral blood smear, liver biochemical tests, serologic tests, and molecular techniques.[5,10]

**Which zoonotic infection should be suspected in a previously healthy 18-year-old patient with a pet cat who presents with fever of unknown origin and tender regional lymphadenopathy?**

Infection with *Bartonella henselae* is an important cause of FUO in immunocompetent and immunocompromised patients. It is transmitted via a scratch or bite from an infected cat, or a bite from an infected cat flea. Classic cat scratch disease (fever and regional lymphadenopathy lasting <7 days) is the most common clinical manifestation. However, when presenting as FUO, cat scratch disease can occur with or without regional lymphadenopathy. The diagnosis is usually made with serologic or molecular techniques. A number of zoonotic infections can present with FUO, including borreliosis, bartonellosis, Rocky Mountain spotted fever, Q fever, ehrlichiosis, tularemia, leptospirosis, and brucellosis.[11,12]

## NONINFECTIOUS INFLAMMATORY CAUSES OF FEVER OF UNKNOWN ORIGIN

**What historical information is important to obtain when considering noninfectious inflammatory causes of fever of unknown origin?**

Historical information pertinent to noninfectious inflammatory causes of FUO include a history of recent illness (eg, gastroenteritis), morning stiffness lasting >1 hour, prominent arthralgias or myalgias, ocular symptoms, recurrent or persistent skin rash, change in bowel patterns, response to glucocorticoid therapy during the course of illness, and familial disorders. *Because noninfectious inflammatory conditions often result in systemic manifestations, a thorough review of systems is important.*[7]

## What are the noninfectious inflammatory causes of fever of unknown origin?

Dramatic elevation in serum ferritin, often >2000 ng/mL.

Adult-onset Still's disease (AOSD).[13]

Classically presents with symmetric polyarticular inflammatory arthritis, most often involving the wrist, metacarpophalangeal, and proximal interphalangeal joints.

Rheumatoid arthritis (RA).

A 32-year-old woman with several weeks of intermittent fever, pancytopenia, and low serum complement levels.

Systemic lupus erythematosus (SLE).

A 29-year-old man with multiple recent sexual partners presents with fever and sterile inflammatory arthritis of the right knee several weeks after being treated for dysuria with urethral discharge.

Reactive arthritis.

Bilateral hilar lymphadenopathy on chest imaging.

Sarcoidosis.

A 47-year-old man with chronic hepatitis B infection, testicular pain, and livedo reticularis.

Polyarteritis nodosa.

Associated with giant cell arteritis (GCA).

Polymyalgia rheumatica (PMR).

Colonoscopy is necessary for diagnosis.

Inflammatory bowel disease (IBD).

A 34-year-old Lebanese man has experienced recurrent episodes of fever, abdominal pain, and inflammatory arthritis since he was 8 years of age.

Familial Mediterranean fever (FMF).

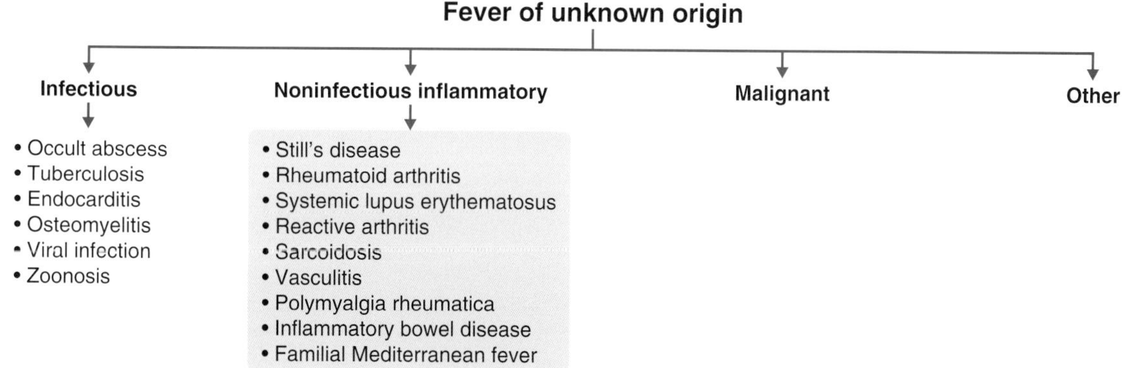


What is adult-onset Still's disease?

AOSD is a systemic inflammatory disorder of unknown etiology. It occurs worldwide and is associated with a bimodal age distribution with peaks between the ages 15 to 25 years and 36 to 46 years. Typical clinical manifestations include fever, nonsuppurative pharyngitis, arthralgias/arthritis, and a transient, evanescent, salmon-colored macular or maculopapular skin rash. The fever is usually high (temperature ≥39°C) and quotidian (recurring daily) or double quotidian (2 peaks daily). The rash often appears when the patient is febrile and disappears during afebrile periods. AOSD presents as FUO in up to 10% of patients. Markedly elevated serum ferritin levels (often >2000 ng/mL) are characteristic. Glucocorticoids are generally first-line treatment.[13,14]

**What diagnostic studies are helpful in evaluating for rheumatoid arthritis in patients with fever of unknown origin?**

In patients with FUO, the presence of serum rheumatoid factor or anti–cyclic citrullinated peptide antibodies can be suggestive of RA. Radiographs of the hands and feet may reveal joint space narrowing and erosions of the bone (Figure 21-3).[14]

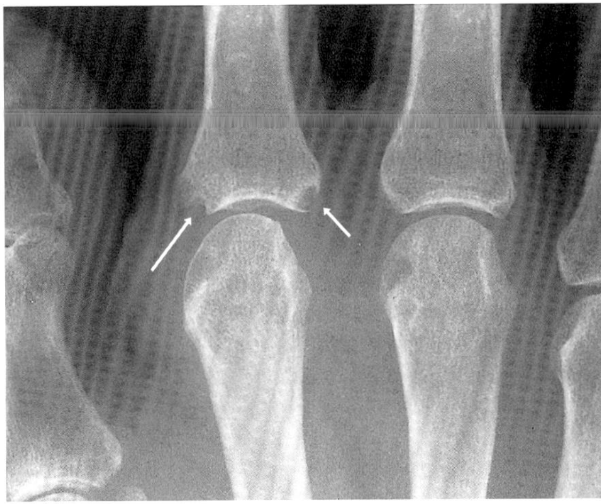

**Figure 21-3.** Bone erosions (arrows) at the metacarpophalangeal joints in a patient with rheumatoid arthritis. (From Greenspan A. *Orthopedic Imaging: A Practical Approach*. 5th ed. Philadelphia, PA: Lippincott Williams & Wilkins; 2011.)

**Which laboratory studies are helpful in evaluating for systemic lupus erythematosus in patients with fever of unknown origin?**

In patients with FUO, the presence of leukopenia, serum antinuclear antibodies (ANA), double-stranded DNA antibodies, or low serum complement levels can be suggestive of SLE. *There is a significant false positive ANA rate in the general FUO population.*[11,14]

**Which general types of infection are most often associated with reactive arthritis?**

Infections of the genitourinary and gastrointestinal tracts are most frequently associated with the development of reactive arthritis.[15]

**What diagnostic studies are helpful in evaluating for sarcoidosis in patients with fever of unknown origin?**

The presence of hilar lymphadenopathy on chest imaging (Figure 21-4) or granulomas on histopathologic evaluation of involved tissue (eg, lymph node, liver) can be suggestive of sarcoidosis. In general, excisional lymph node biopsy is associated with higher yield compared with needle aspiration. The posterior cervical, epitrochlear, supraclavicular, hilar, mediastinal, and retroperitoneal lymph nodes are most likely to provide a diagnosis in patients with FUO. The anterior cervical, axillary, and inguinal nodes are more likely to yield nonspecific information.[2,14]

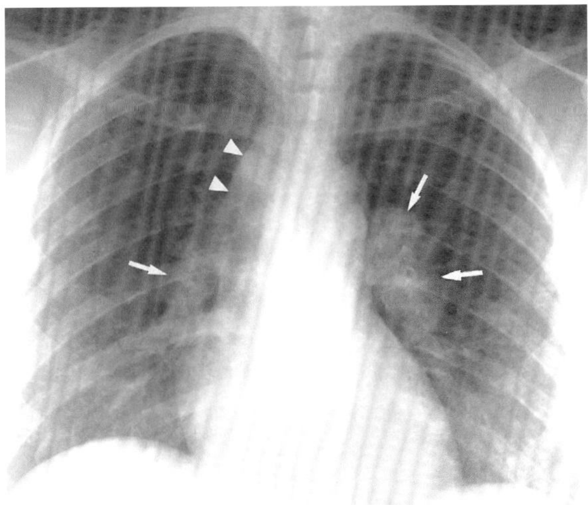

**Figure 21-4.** Posteroanterior (PA) chest radiograph showing right paratracheal (arrowheads) and bilateral hilar (arrows) lymphadenopathy, classic for sarcoidosis. (From Collins J, Stern EJ. *Chest Radiology: The Essentials*. 3rd ed. Philadelphia, PA: Wolters Kluwer Health; 2015.)

**What type of systemic vasculitis is a frequent cause of fever of unknown origin in elderly patients?**

GCA accounts for almost one-fifth of cases of FUO in the elderly. Clinical manifestations include headache, jaw claudication, fever, and elevated erythrocyte sedimentation rate. The temporal artery may be tender, thickened, or nodular on examination (see Figure 50-2). Temporal artery biopsy can confirm the diagnosis. Glucocorticoids are the treatment of choice.[7]

**What test can confirm the diagnosis of polymyalgia rheumatica?**

There is no confirmatory diagnostic test for PMR; it is strictly a clinical diagnosis. PMR is closely associated with GCA (it most often occurs in isolation but develops in a significant proportion of patients with GCA). Clinical manifestations include pain and stiffness in the muscles of the neck, shoulders, lower back, hips, and thighs. There is often a dramatic response to glucocorticoid therapy.[7]

**Which type of inflammatory bowel disease is most likely to present with fever of uknown origin?**

FUO is a rare presentation of IBD and has been reported mostly in patients with ulcerative colitis. Fever is present in almost one-half of patients with ulcerative colitis at the time of presentation. It is often low-grade and may have been present for weeks or longer without having been recognized. Colonoscopy with or without nuclear medicine imaging (eg, labeled leukocyte scintigraphy, positron emission tomography) can be helpful in identifying atypical cases of IBD presenting with FUO. Nuclear medicine imaging is often used to direct the colonoscopic evaluation.[16]

**What is familial Mediterranean fever?**

FMF is an autosomal recessive hereditary disease that predominantly affects ethnic groups near the Mediterranean Sea, particularly Arabs, Armenians, Turks, North Africans, and Jews. Symptoms include periodic attacks of fever and serositis (eg, peritonitis, pleuritis, synovitis) with or without painful erysipelas-like erythema of the lower extremities. The first attack occurs before 10 years of age in most patients, and before 20 years of age in the vast majority of patients. Attacks tend to last 1 to 4 days. Symptom-free intervals are highly variable, even within the same individual, and may be as short as days or as long as years. Colchicine is the treatment of choice. Family history is key to identifying FMF.[7,17]

## MALIGNANT CAUSES OF FEVER OF UNKNOWN ORIGIN

**What historical information is important to obtain when considering malignant causes of fever of unknown origin?**

Information pertinent to malignant causes of FUO includes a history of malignancy and significant weight loss (>2 lbs/wk) with anorexia.[14]

**What is the most common cause of fever of unknown origin in patients with known malignancy?**

Infection is responsible for most cases of FUO in patients with known malignancy. The malignancy itself is responsible for fever in just under one-half of cases.[18]

### What are the malignant causes of fever of unknown origin?

**Two general types of hematologic malignancies.**

Lymphoma and leukemia.

**Often associated with macrocytosis.**

Myelodysplastic syndrome (MDS).

**The biopsy of a hepatic mass stains positive for human epidermal growth factor receptor 2 (HER2).**

Metastatic breast cancer.

**A 63-year-old man with an extensive smoking history presents with intermittent fever and is found to have hematuria and polycythemia.**

Renal cell carcinoma.

**A 64-year-old man with *Streptococcus gallolyticus* (formerly *Streptococcus bovis*) endocarditis.**

Colon cancer.

**Occurs in patients with cirrhosis.**

Hepatocellular carcinoma (HCC).

**Tumor plop.**

Atrial myxoma.

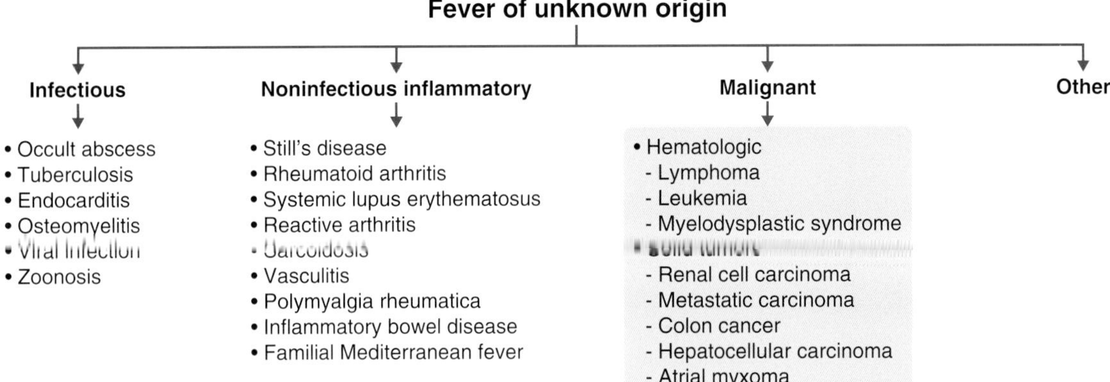


**What are the characteristics of lymphoma presenting with fever of unknown origin?**

Lymphoma accounts for around one-quarter of the malignant causes of FUO. The presence of lymphadenopathy, splenomegaly, and elevated serum lactate dehydrogenase levels can be suggestive. Physical examination, cross-sectional imaging of the chest, abdomen, and pelvis, and bone marrow examination can often identify sites of involvement. However, in patients with FUO, lymphoma may occur exclusively in non-nodal locations (eg, blood vessel lumina [ie, intravascular lymphoma], central nervous system, spleen, liver, bone marrow). Lymphoma presenting with FUO is generally associated with rapid progression and poor prognosis.[7,18]

**Is fever of unknown origin more commonly associated with acute or chronic leukemia?**

FUO is more common in patients with acute leukemia (often the nonlymphocytic types). It is rare in patients with chronic leukemia, most often occurring after Richter transformation to lymphoma. In patients with acute leukemia presenting with FUO, peripheral blood smear is frequently unrevealing (ie, aleukemic leukemia) and bone marrow examination is necessary to establish the diagnosis.[5,19]

**What are the characteristics of myelodysplastic syndrome presenting with fever of unknown origin?**

The myelodysplastic syndromes comprise a group of disorders characterized by abnormal proliferation and differentiation of the hematopoietic stem cell, resulting in ineffective hematopoiesis. MDS typically occurs in patients >50 years of age. Most patients are asymptomatic or present with manifestations related to at least 1 peripheral blood cytopenia (anemia, thrombocytopenia, neutropenia). In a minority of cases, fever is the dominant and presenting feature. Peripheral blood smear evaluation may provide diagnostic clues, including macrocytosis (Figure 21-5), anisocytosis, poikilocytosis, nucleated red blood cells, acanthocytosis, hypogranulation and hyposegmentation of the neutrophils, and hypogranularity or hypergranularity and enlargement of the platelets. Bone marrow examination is necessary to establish the diagnosis.[5]

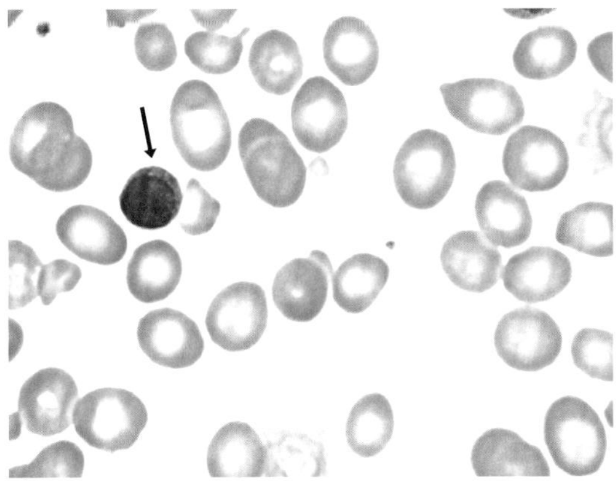

**Figure 21-5.** Oval macrocytes demonstrated on peripheral blood smear. A red blood cell is typically similar in size to the nucleus of a resting lymphocyte (arrow). The presence of oval macrocytes may indicate megaloblastic anemia or myelodysplastic syndrome. (From Pereira I, George TI, Arber DA. *Atlas of Peripheral Blood: The Primary Diagnostic Tool*. Philadelphia, PA: Wolters Kluwer Health; 2013.)

**What are the characteristics of renal cell carcinoma presenting with fever of unknown origin?**

Renal cell carcinoma most often presents with weight loss and fatigue, but fever is part of the presentation in up to 15% of cases. Microscopic hematuria and peripheral erythrocytosis (secondary to increased erythropoietin production by the tumor) may provide clues. Other causes of fever and renal mass include renal abscess, renal tuberculosis, xanthogranulomatous pyelonephritis, and renal malakoplakia.[5,7,20]

**What is the most frequent site of metastasis in patients with metastatic carcinoma presenting with fever of unknown origin?**

The liver is the most frequent site of metastasis in patients with metastatic carcinoma presenting with FUO. Other sites include the bone, lung, adrenal glands, and abdominal lymph nodes. Cross-sectional imaging and tissue biopsy are usually necessary to make the diagnosis.[3,18]

**How often does colon cancer present with fever?**

Colon cancer infrequently presents with fever, although when it does, fever is due to infection in around one-half of cases. Bacteremia from *Streptococcus gallolyticus*, *Escherichia coli*, and *Clostridium septicum* can lead to endocarditis or prosthesis infection. Colonoscopy is the diagnostic study of choice.[18]

**Which laboratory test can be helpful in patients at risk for hepatocellular carcinoma?**

Although serum α-fetoprotein (AFP) can be elevated in benign liver conditions, it is often found in higher concentration in patients with HCC (typically >500 ng/mL), and can be a useful test in patients with FUO who are at risk for HCC.[21]

**How common is fever in patients with atrial myxoma?**

Fever is present in around one-third of patients with atrial myxoma. Other manifestations include syncope, heart failure, peripheral or pulmonary emboli, weight loss, myalgias, arthralgias, and rash. Some cases are associated with an extra heart sound (tumor plop), which most often occurs in early diastole. Echocardiography can confirm the diagnosis.[5,7]

## OTHER CAUSES OF FEVER OF UNKNOWN ORIGIN

### What are the other causes of fever of unknown origin?

**A careful medication review, including over-the-counter and herbal substances, is a key component in the evaluation of FUO.**

Drug fever.

**Consider this condition in patients with Virchow's triad.**

Venous thromboembolism (ie, deep vein thrombosis, pulmonary embolism [PE]).

**Often associated with tender hepatomegaly and jaundice.**

Alcoholic hepatitis.

**A 32-year-old female nurse presents with complaints of intermittent fever with temperature up to 41°C for several weeks; she appears well on physical examination.**

Factitious disorder.

**A previously healthy 29-year-old man presents with recurrent daily fever several weeks after sustaining abdominal trauma and is found to have anemia.**

Intra-abdominal hematoma.

**A young woman who recently gave birth complains of anterior neck discomfort, heat intolerance, and palpitations.**

Postpartum thyroiditis.

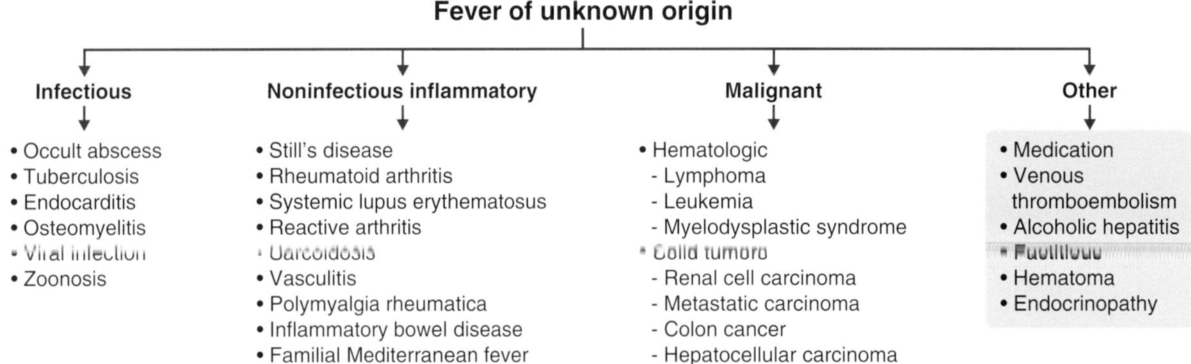


**What are the characteristics of drug fever?**

Numerous medications can cause fever, including some that are used to treat fever (eg, nonsteroidal anti-inflammatory drugs [NSAIDs], antibiotics). Fever usually occurs several weeks after initiating the medication but can present at any point. Peripheral eosinophilia or skin rash are present in around one-fifth of patients, and can be important clues to the diagnosis. Fever usually resolves within 2 days of stopping the causative agent.[5,7]

**How common is fever in patients with pulmonary embolism?**

Fever occurs in around one-half of patients with acute PE. Temperature is typically <39°C, and fever resolves a few days after therapy is initiated. However, fever can persist for weeks, usually when recurrent emboli go undetected and untreated. Pulmonary symptoms can be absent or unimpressive in some cases, leading to a protracted course.[5]

**Which laboratory feature is helpful in identifying alcoholic hepatitis?**

Alcoholic patients may be hesitant to disclose a history of alcohol use. Confirming the presence of ethanol in serum or urine samples may be helpful; however, alcohol consumption is often stopped days or weeks before patients present with alcoholic hepatitis. Leukocytosis is frequently present, but this is nonspecific, particularly in patients with FUO. A more specific feature is a mild to moderate elevation of aminotransferases, with an AST:ALT ratio >2:1.[5]

**What are the main clues to the presence of factitious fever?**

Factitious fever most often occurs in young women who work or have previously worked in health care. Patients often appear well on examination; however, there may be signs of self-mutilation or injection. Other clues include markedly elevated temperatures (>41°C) with the absence of associated tachycardia or diaphoresis, and rapid defervescence.[5]

**What are the characteristics of hematoma presenting with fever of unknown origin?**

Hematoma can cause fever when it occurs in an enclosed space, usually the abdominal cavity or retroperitoneal space. It can also occur in patients with aortic dissection, usually preceded by a transient episode of chest, back, or abdominal pain. Cross-sectional imaging is a key diagnostic modality to identify the presence of a hematoma. In some cases, fever is caused by secondary infection.[5,7]

**What are the endocrinologic causes of fever of unknown origin?**

Thyrotoxicosis is the most frequent endocrinologic cause of FUO. Other endocrinologic causes of FUO include adrenal insufficiency and pheochromocytoma.[5]

## Case Summary

A 37-year-old Syrian man presents with a prolonged clinical course of intermittent fever, migratory inflammatory arthritis, and painless oral ulcers following a diarrheal illness.

***What is the most likely diagnosis in this patient?***

Reactive arthritis.

### BONUS QUESTIONS

***What is reactive arthritis?***

Reactive arthritis is one of the seronegative spondyloarthritides and is characterized by a sterile, asymmetric inflammatory mono- or oligoarthritis that develops 1 to 4 weeks following infection elsewhere in the body (usually gastrointestinal or genitourinary infections). The inciting infection can be asymptomatic in some cases. The classic triad of postinfectious arthritis, conjunctivitis, and nongonococcal urethritis (ie, Reiter's syndrome) represents a subtype of reactive arthritis. In many cases, postinfectious arthritis occurs in isolation or with only 1 of the other 2 extra-articular features. Other extra-articular manifestations of reactive arthritis include tendinitis, bursitis, anterior uveitis, erythema nodosum, and circinate balanitis.[15,22]

***Reactive arthritis is most likely to develop after infections with what organisms?***

Organisms most often associated with reactive arthritis include *Chlamydia trachomatis*, *Yersinia* species, *Salmonella enterica*, *Campylobacter* species, *Shigella* species, and *Clostridium difficile*. It can also develop following infection with other organisms, such as *Escherichia coli* and *Chlamydia pneumoniae*.[15,22,23]

***What is the epidemiology of reactive arthritis?***

Reactive arthritis occurs worldwide, with an annual incidence in some populations of up to 30 per 100,000. It occurs most frequently in young adults 20 to 40 years of age. Compared with women, men are more likely to develop and experience a severe course of reactive arthritis related to *Chlamydia trachomatis* urethritis.[15,22]

***What features in this case are suggestive of reactive arthritis?***

In this case, the development of migratory, asymmetric, sterile inflammatory oligoarthritis affecting the larger joints of the lower extremities following a gastrointestinal illness is characteristic of reactive arthritis. As a young adult, the patient in this case fits the epidemiologic profile. The presence of extra-articular manifestations, including enthesitis, conjunctivitis, urethritis, oral ulcers, and the absence of serologic evidence of RA are also consistent with the diagnosis. The patient in this case should undergo an ophthalmologic examination to evaluate for uveitis.[22]

***What is the significance of the patient's Syrian ancestry in this case?***

The Syrian ancestry of the patient in this case should bring FMF and Behçet's disease into consideration. Although FMF is relatively more common in Syrians, it would be unusual for the first attack to occur after 20 years of age, and there is no family history of FMF in this patient. Genetic testing to evaluate for FMF may be helpful in this case. Behçet's disease is also known as "Silk Road disease" and should be considered in any patient of Syrian descent who presents with FUO, particularly given the presence of oral ulcers. However, the oral ulcers of Behçet's disease are typically painful. The pathergy test to evaluate for Behçet's disease may be helpful in this case.[17,24]

***What is the relevance of the family history in this case?***

The spondyloarthritides, including reactive arthritis and ankylosing spondylitis (present in a first-degree relative in this case), are associated with human leukocyte antigen B27 (HLA-B27). HLA-B27 positive patients tend to experience more severe arthritis with a protracted course.[22]

***What is the treatment for reactive arthritis?***

Cases of reactive arthritis in which there is ongoing infection (eg, *Chlamydia trachomatis* urethritis) require treatment with antibiotics. NSAIDs are first-line treatment for arthritis. Some patients may also benefit from intra-articular glucocorticoids. Patients who do not respond to NSAIDs may benefit from systemic glucocorticoids. Disease-modifying antirheumatic drugs (eg, sulfasalazine) may be necessary in some cases. Patients with extra-articular manifestations may benefit from additional therapy (eg, topical glucocorticoids for uveitis).[15,22]

***What is the prognosis of reactive arthritis?***

Most patients with reactive arthritis fully recover within 2 to 6 months. However, up to one-fifth of patients experience chronic disease, defined by the persistence of symptoms beyond 6 months. Some of these patients may later develop features of other spondyloarthritides.[15]

## KEY POINTS

- FUO is defined as an illness lasting longer than 3 weeks, with measured temperature >38.3°C on several occasions, and failure to reach a diagnosis despite thorough investigation.
- The causes of FUO can be separated into the following categories: infectious, noninfectious inflammatory, malignant, and other.
- Relative prevalence of the causes of FUO depends on host and geographic factors. In the modern industrialized world, infections account for 25% of cases; noninfectious inflammatory conditions, 25%; malignancy, 15%; and miscellaneous or idiopathic causes make up the remaining cases.
- History and physical examination are critically important for directing the diagnostic workup in patients with FUO.
- Diagnostic studies that may be helpful in identifying the cause of FUO include various laboratory studies (eg, serologies), imaging studies (eg, cross-sectional imaging), endoscopic studies (eg, colonoscopy), and histopathologic studies (eg, lymph node biopsy).
- Treatment and prognosis of FUO depend on the underlying cause. Prognosis is excellent in patients with idiopathic FUO but poor in those with malignant FUO.

## REFERENCES


1. Longo DL, Fauci AS, Kasper DL, Hauser SL, Jameson JL, Loscalzo J, eds. *Harrison's Principles of Internal Medicine*. 18th ed. New York, NY: McGraw-Hill; 2012.
2. Hayakawa K, Ramasamy B, Chandrasekar PH. Fever of unknown origin: an evidence-based review. *Am J Med Sci*. 2012;344(4):307-316.
3. Petersdorf RG, Beeson PB. Fever of unexplained origin: report on 100 cases. *Medicine (Baltim)*. 1961;40:1-30.
4. Kazanjian PH. Fever of unknown origin: review of 86 patients treated in community hospitals. *Clin Infect Dis*. 1992;15(6):968-973.
5. Hirschmann JV. Fever of unknown origin in adults. *Clin Infect Dis*. 1997;24(3):291-300; quiz 1-2.
6. Mourad O, Palda V, Detsky AS. A comprehensive evidence based approach to fever of unknown origin. *Arch Intern Med*. 2003;163(5):545-551.
7. Arnow PM, Flaherty JP. Fever of unknown origin. *Lancet*. 1997;350(9077):575-580.
8. Greenberg SD, Frager D, Suster B, Walker S, Stavropoulos C, Rothpearl A. Active pulmonary tuberculosis in patients with AIDS: spectrum of radiographic findings (including a normal appearance). *Radiology*. 1994;193(1):115-119.
9. Baddour LM, Wilson WR, Bayer AS, et al. Infective endocarditis in adults: diagnosis, antimicrobial therapy, and management of complications:a scientific statement for healthcare professionals from the American Heart Association. *Circulation*. 2015;132(15):1435-1486.
10. Alavi SM, Nadimi M, Zamani GA. Changing pattern of infectious etiology of fever of unknown origin (FUO) in adult patients in Ahvaz, Iran. *Caspian J Intern Med*. 2013;4(3):722-726.
11. Bleeker-Rovers CP, Vos FJ, de Kleijn EM, et al. A prospective multicenter study on fever of unknown origin: the yield of a structured diagnostic protocol. *Medicine*. 2007;86(1):26-38.
12. Tsukahara M, Tsuneoka H, Iino H, Murano I, Takahashi H, Uchida M. Bartonella henselae infection as a cause of fever of unknown origin. *J Clin Microbiol*. 2000;38(5):1990-1991.
13. Gopalarathinam R, Orlowsky E, Kesavalu R, Yelaminchili S. Adult onset Still's disease: a review on diagnostic workup and treatment options. *Case Rep Rheumatol*. 2016;2016:6502373.
14. Cunha BA, Lortholary O, Cunha CB. Fever of unknown origin: a clinical approach. *Am J Med*. 2015;128(10):1138 e1-1138 e15.
15. Kim PS, Klausmeier TL, Orr DP. Reactive arthritis: a review. *J Adolesc Health*. 2009;44(4):309-315.

16. Voukelatou P, Sfendouraki E, Karianos T, et al. Ulcerative colitis activity presenting as fever of unknown origin, in a patient with longstanding disease under continuous treatment with mesalazine. *Case Rep Med*. 2016;2016:4396256.
17. Sari I, Birlik M, Kasifoglu T. Familial Mediterranean fever: an updated review. *Eur J Rheumatol*. 2014;1(1):21-33.
18. Loizidou A, Aoun M, Klastersky J. Fever of unknown origin in cancer patients. *Crit Rev Oncol Hematol*. 2016;101:125-130.
19. Cunha BA, Mohan S, Parchuri S. Fever of unknown origin: chronic lymphatic leukemia versus lymphoma (Richter's transformation). *Heart Lung*. 2005;34(6):437-441.
20. Chandrankunnel J, Cunha BA, Petelin A, Katz D. Fever of unknown origin (FUO) and a renal mass: renal cell carcinoma, renal tuberculosis, renal malakoplakia, or xanthogranulomatous pyelonephritis? *Heart Lung*. 2012;41(6):606-609.
21. Wu JT. Serum alpha-fetoprotein and its lectin reactivity in liver diseases: a review. *Ann Clin Lab Sci*. 1990;20(2):98-105.
22. Hannu T. Reactive arthritis. *Best Pract Res Clin Rheumatol*. 2011;25(3):347-357.
23. Townes JM. Reactive arthritis after enteric infections in the United States: the problem of definition. *Clin Infect Dis*. 2010;50(2):247-254.
24. Sakane T, Takeno M, Suzuki N, Inaba G. Behcet's disease. *N Engl J Med*. 1999;341(17):1284-1291.

Chapter 22

# HYPOTENSION

## Case: A 48-year-old man with cool extremities

A 48-year-old man with a history of hypertension and insulin-dependent type 2 diabetes mellitus is admitted to the hospital with episodes of increasing chest discomfort over the course of a few days. The pain is located in the center of the chest with radiation to the jaw. It is pressure-like in quality. It had been intermittent for a few days but is now constant. He is also short of breath and feels light-headed. He smokes 1 pack of cigarettes per day but denies any significant alcohol use. His father died of a myocardial infarction (MI) at 52 years of age.

Heart rate is 144 beats per minute, blood pressure is 70/40 mm Hg (similar in all extremities), respiratory rate is 36 breaths per minute, and hemoglobin oxygen saturation by pulse oximetry is 88% on 4 L supplemental oxygen. Jugular venous pressure (JVP) is 16 cm $H_2O$. An extra heart sound is heard just after S2 with the bell of the stethoscope over the apex. There are bilateral late inspiratory rales. The extremities are cool to the touch, and the peripheral pulses are weak.

Electrocardiogram (ECG) is shown in Figure 22-1.

Chest radiograph shows bilateral patchy ground glass opacities with bilateral pleural effusions.

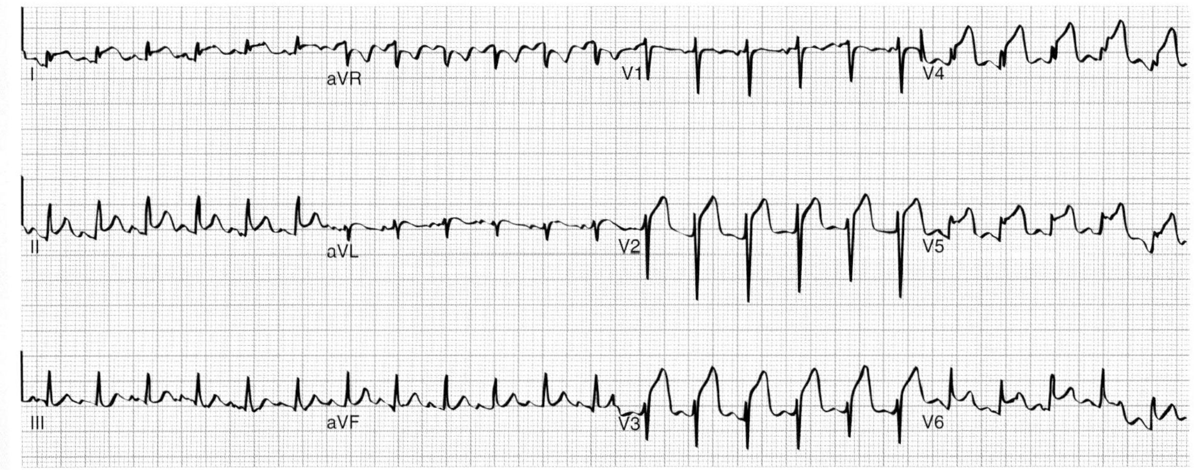


**Figure 22-1.** (From Woods SL, Froelicher ES, Motzer SA, Bridges EJ. *Cardiac Nursing*. 6th ed. Philadelphia, PA: Wolters Kluwer Health; 2010.)

***What is the most likely cause of hypotension in this patient?***

**What is the relationship between arterial blood pressure, cardiac output (CO), and systemic vascular resistance (SVR)?**

Mean arterial pressure (MAP) is the product of cardiac output and systemic vascular resistance.[1]

MAP = CO × SVR

**What are the main determinants of cardiac output?**

Cardiac output is equal to the forward stroke volume (SV) of the left ventricle per beat multiplied by heart rate (HR).

CO = SV × HR

In the setting of hypotension, neurally-mediated compensatory increases in heart rate and stroke volume will occur.[2]

**How is blood pressure regulated?**

Moment-to-moment control of blood pressure is regulated by the neurally-mediated baroreceptors found in the carotid sinus and aortic arch. Long-term control of blood pressure is primarily regulated via the hormonally-mediated renin-angiotensin-aldosterone system (Figure 22-2).[3]

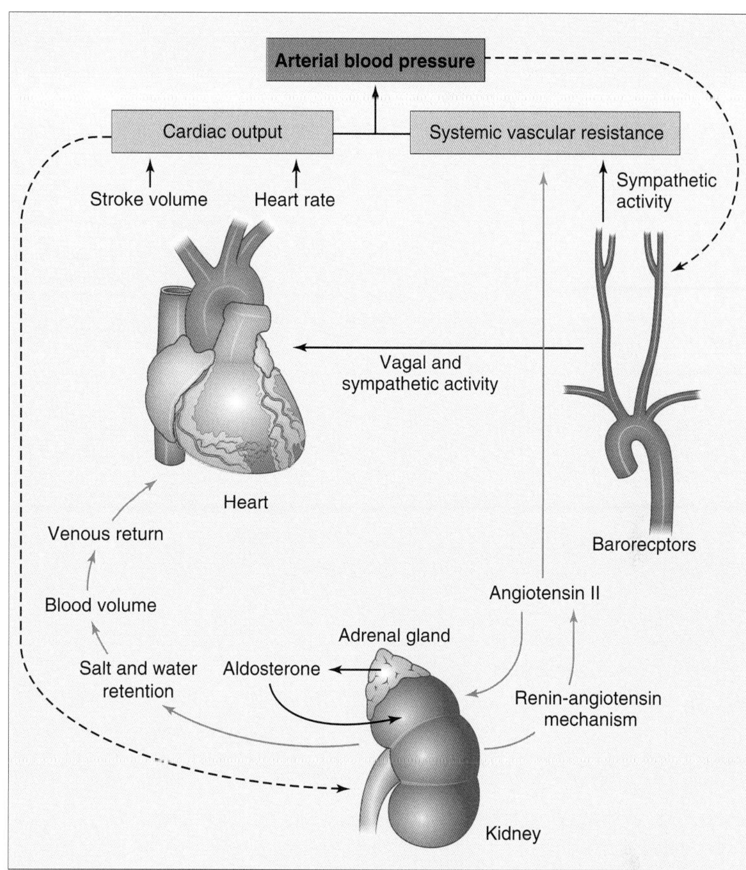


**Figure 22-2.** Mechanisms of blood pressure regulation. Dashed lines represent stimulation of blood pressure regulation. Solid lines represent response to stimulation of kidneys and baroreceptors. (From Porth CM. *Essentials of Pathophysiology: Concepts of Altered Health States*. Philadelphia, PA: Lippincott Williams & Wilkins; 2003.)

**How is blood pressure measured?**

Blood pressure is usually measured indirectly by using a stethoscope and a sphygmomanometer. It can be measured directly by cannulating a peripheral artery, which is the method of choice in patients with significant hemodynamic compromise.[1]

**What conditions optimize the indirect measurement of blood pressure?**

Korotkoff sounds, used to measure blood pressure, are low pitched and are best appreciated in a quiet room using the bell of the stethoscope. The size of the bladder on the sphygmomanometer can affect the accuracy of blood pressure measurements. The length of the bladder should be ≥80% of the circumference of the upper arm, and the width should be ≥40% of the circumference of the upper arm. Bladders that are too large result in falsely low blood pressure readings, whereas bladders that are too small result in falsely elevated blood pressure readings.[1]

**What are the symptoms of hypotension?**

Symptoms of hypotension may include light-headedness, dizziness on sitting up or standing (ie, orthostasis), syncope, dyspnea, blurry vision, malaise, and confusion.

**What are the physical findings of hypotension?**

In addition to low arterial blood pressure, physical findings of hypotension may include positive orthostatic vital signs, cool or warm extremities (depending on the underlying cause), and diminished peripheral pulses.

**What is hypotensive shock?**

Hypotensive shock occurs when tissue oxygenation is inadequate for the demands of aerobic metabolism. In adults, it is typically associated with acute systolic arterial pressure <90 mm Hg or MAP <70 mm Hg (these thresholds may be higher in patients with chronic hypertension). Clinical manifestations include cutaneous changes (eg, cool, clammy, cyanotic skin), decreased urine output, and delirium. Lactate levels in blood are elevated due to increased generation of lactate from a cellular shift to anaerobic metabolism, and decreased clearance related to impaired liver function.[1,4]

**What are the 4 general mechanisms of hypotension?**

Hypotension can be hypovolemic, cardiogenic, distributive, or obstructive.

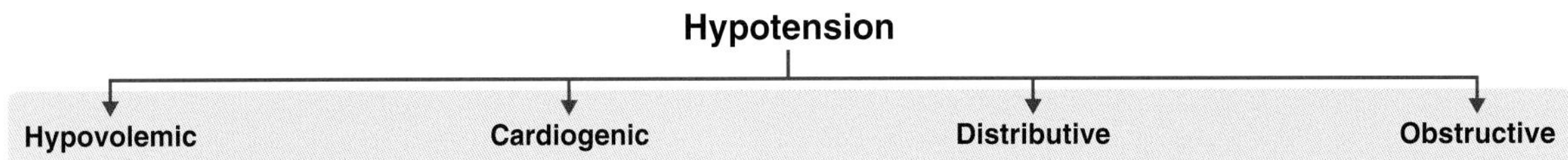


**What is the relative prevalence of each category of hypotension in patients with shock?**

Among patients with shock in the industrialized world, distributive hypotension causes approximately 65% of cases (among which sepsis is by far the most frequent etiology). Hypovolemic hypotension and cardiogenic hypotension account for around 15% of cases each, and <5% are due to obstructive hypotension.[4]

## HYPOVOLEMIC HYPOTENSION

**What are the fundamental pathophysiologic mechanisms of low blood pressure in hypovolemic hypotension?**

Hypovolemic hypotension occurs as a result of decreased hydrostatic pressure within blood vessels, and decreased cardiac preload with an associated decrease in cardiac output.

**In the setting of hypovolemic shock, are the extremities typically warm or cool to the touch?**

Hypovolemic shock is typically associated with cool extremities. This reflects the compensatory increase in SVR that aims to shunt blood to the vital organs.

**Which of the following patterns of jugular venous pressure, cardiac output, and systemic vascular resistance are characteristic of hypovolemic hypotension?**

| | JVP | CO | SVR |
|---|---|---|---|
| A | ↑ | ↓ | ↑ |
| B | ↓ | ↑ | ↓ |
| C | ↓ | ↓ | ↑ |

Hypovolemic hypotension is characterized by decreased JVP (primary issue), decreased CO, and increased SVR (answer C).[1]

**Why is it important to use isotonic fluid when resuscitating patients with hypovolemic hypotension?**

Isotonic solutions (eg, crystalloids, colloids) are more effective at expanding intravascular fluid volume compared with hypotonic solutions. The infusion of isotonic fluid does not generate a tonicity gradient between the extracellular and intracellular fluid compartments. Therefore, the infusate will remain within the extracellular compartment; one-fourth of which consists of the intravascular space. In contrast, hypotonic solutions generate a tonicity gradient favoring redistribution of infusate into the intracellular compartment. For example, if 1 L of free water is infused, only one-third of it will remain in the extracellular compartment and only one-twelfth in the intravascular space (Figure 22-3).

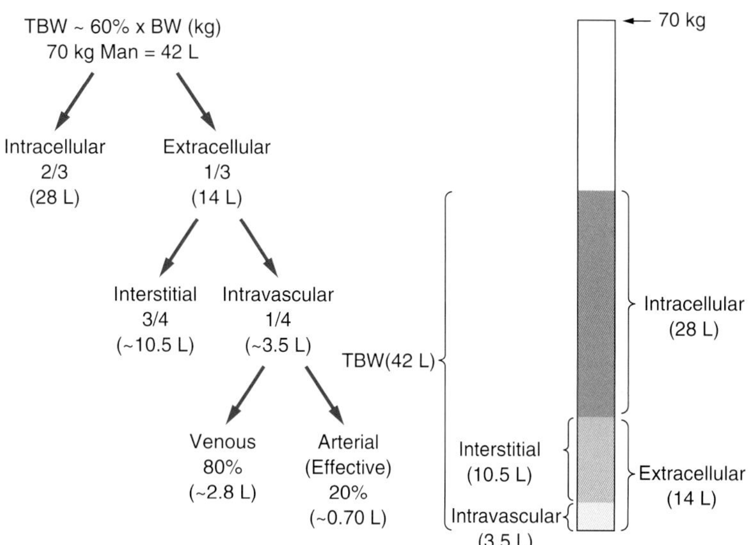


**Figure 22-3.** Approximate relationships of body water compartments to total body weight. Total body water (TBW) is approximately 60% of body weight (BW) in the average 70-kg man. The majority of water is distributed within the intracellular compartment, whereas a relatively small amount is distributed within the intravascular space. (From Rennke HG, Denker BM. *Renal Pathophysiology: The Essentials.* 4th ed. Philadelphia, PA: Lippincott Williams & Wilkins; 2014.)

## What are the causes of hypovolemic hypotension?

**Common in elderly patients who live alone.**

Poor oral intake.

**Often encountered in trauma patients.**

Hemorrhagic shock.

**Polyuria.**

Renal salt wasting (eg, diuretic use).

**True isotonic extracellular fluid loss.**

Gastrointestinal losses (eg, diarrhea, vomiting).

**Massive fluid loss through the skin.**

Severe burn injury.

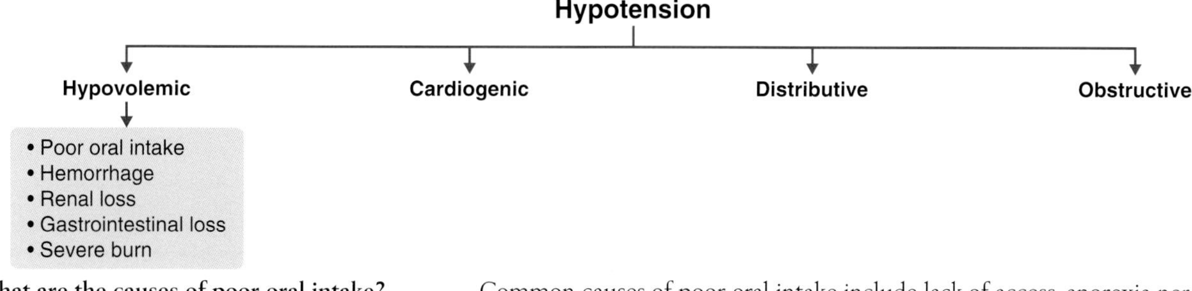


**What are the causes of poor oral intake?**

Common causes of poor oral intake include lack of access, anorexia nervosa, loss of appetite, early satiety, intestinal obstruction, socioeconomic factors, delirium, mental health disorders, and sitophobia from chronic mesenteric ischemia. In some cases, the patient readily provides a history of poor oral intake, but in other cases, it must be inferred or gathered from family members.

GENERAL INTERNAL MEDICINE

**Which areas of the body can hide large amounts of blood?**

Extensive bleeding can occur within the retroperitoneal space, pelvis, or thigh without significant physical findings. A history of trauma, predisposing factors (eg, anticoagulation use, liver disease), or the presence of anemia may provide clues. *Acute blood loss may not initially result in decreased hemoglobin concentration*. Imaging studies are key to making the diagnosis. In patients with hemorrhagic shock, resuscitation with crystalloid solutions or packed red blood cells (RBC) can worsen or induce coagulopathy because of a dilutional effect on coagulation proteins and platelets. To prevent this, massive resuscitation should include the administration of fresh frozen plasma and platelets (aiming for a 1:1:1 ratio of plasma:platelets:RBCs as a general rule of thumb). *Metabolic alkalosis and hypocalcemia can also develop in these patients as a result of the citrate present in blood products.*[5,6]

**Which laboratory test indicates that volume depletion may be related to renal salt wasting?**

Extrarenal causes of volume depletion are associated with urine sodium concentration <20 mEq/L. In contrast, volume depletion related to renal salt wasting (eg, primary adrenal insufficiency, diuretic use) tends to be associated with relatively higher urine sodium concentrations (>20-30 mEq/L).[7-9]

**What is the significance of true isotonic extracellular fluid loss?**

Loss of extracellular fluid that is hypotonic relative to intracellular fluid (eg, pure water) will generate a tonicity gradient between the extracellular and intracellular compartments, which favors the movement of water into the extracellular compartment, thereby restoring some extracellular fluid volume. In contrast, loss of extracellular fluid that is isotonic relative to intracellular fluid (eg, gastrointestinal loss) does not generate a tonicity gradient between the extracellular and intracellular compartments, and there is no resultant restoration of extracellular fluid volume from the intracellular space. Therefore, extracellular isotonic fluid loss tends to be associated with more severe clinical manifestations.[10]

**Which validated formula is useful for guiding fluid replacement in the setting of severe burns?**

The Parkland formula can guide fluid replacement in burn victims, using the patient's body weight (in kg) and the estimated percentage of body surface area burned. During the initial 24 hours, crystalloid should be given at a rate of 4 mL/kg/% burn (for adults).[11]

## CARDIOGENIC HYPOTENSION

**What is the fundamental pathophysiologic mechanism of low blood pressure in cardiogenic hypotension?**

Cardiogenic hypotension occurs as a result of pump failure with an associated decrease in cardiac output.

**In the setting of cardiogenic shock, are the extremities typically warm or cool to the touch?**

Cardiogenic shock is typically associated with cool extremities. This reflects the compensatory increase in SVR that aims to shunt blood to the vital organs. However, when MI is the cause of cardiogenic shock, there is a subset of patients who develop systemic inflammatory response syndrome (SIRS), causing decreased SVR and warm extremities.[12]

**Which of the following patterns of jugular venous pressure, cardiac output, and systemic vascular resistance is characteristic of cardiogenic shock?**

| | JVP | CO | SVR |
|---|---|---|---|
| A | ↑ | ↓ | ↑ |
| B | ↓ | ↑ | ↓ |
| C | ↓ | ↓ | ↑ |

Cardiogenic shock is characterized by increased JVP, decreased CO (primary issue), and increased SVR (answer A).[1]

## What are the causes of cardiogenic hypotension?

**Diseases of heart muscle that generally result in concentric or eccentric hypertrophy.**

Cardiomyopathy (see chapter 4, Heart Failure).

**Sometimes associated with palpitations.**

Dysrhythmia.

**A 52-year-old man with an extensive smoking history presents with chest pain and hypotension and is found to have 2 mm ST-segment elevation in leads II, III, and aVF on ECG.**

Acute inferior ST-elevation myocardial infarction.

**A 27-year-old man with Marfan syndrome presents with syncope and is found to have hypotension with a wide pulse pressure, a III/IV decrescendo diastolic murmur, de Musset sign (to-and-fro head bob), and Traube sign (a "pistol-shot" sound heard with the stethoscope over the femoral artery).**

Acute aortic regurgitation.

**Sudden development of pulmonary hypertension.**

Acute pulmonary embolism (PE).

**Functionally similar to aortic stenosis, but the valve itself may not be the culprit.**

Left ventricular outflow tract obstruction.

**A previously healthy 33-year-old woman presents with months of progressive dyspnea on exertion and is found to have elevated JVP, a right ventricular heave, and a loud pulmonic component of the second heart sound.**

Primary pulmonary hypertension.



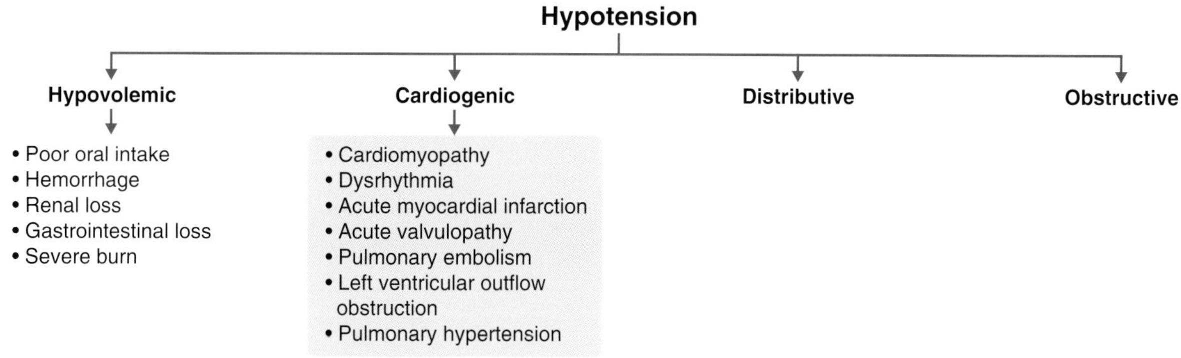


**What class of medications can be used to directly increase cardiac output in patients with cardiogenic shock?**

Inotropic agents (eg, dobutamine) can increase myocardial contractility and are useful in the management of cardiogenic shock. Additional support with vasopressor agents (eg, norepinephrine) may also be helpful. Mechanical support with intra-aortic balloon counterpulsation (ie, intra-aortic balloon pump) may be necessary to maintain coronary and peripheral perfusion in select cases of cardiogenic shock. Intra-aortic balloon counterpulsation increases diastolic pressure via diastolic balloon inflation, and augments left ventricular performance by decreasing afterload via systolic balloon deflation.[13]

**What is the immediate treatment of choice for atrial fibrillation associated with hypotension?**

Atrial fibrillation with hemodynamic compromise (eg, hypotension or decompensated heart failure) should be treated with immediate synchronized cardioversion using direct current (DC) electric shocks. Patients should be premedicated with sedatives and narcotics when possible, as electrical cardioversion is traumatic and painful.[7]

**What additional therapies should be used in patients with cardiogenic shock related to acute myocardial infarction?**

In addition to hemodynamic support with inotropes and vasopressors, pharmacologic management of cardiogenic shock related to acute MI includes antiplatelet and antithrombotic therapy. Survival in patients with cardiogenic shock related to MI is improved with early reperfusion, particularly revascularization, whether percutaneous (ie, percutaneous coronary intervention) or surgical (ie, coronary artery bypass grafting). Thrombolytic therapy, although less effective than revascularization, should be given when revascularization is unavailable or significantly delayed. Mechanical support with an intra-aortic balloon pump can be helpful in select patients. In some cases, left ventricular assist devices or extracorporeal life support should be considered.[13]

**Which valvulopathies are associated with cardiogenic shock?**

Cardiogenic shock can occur as a result of acute-onset severe aortic or mitral regurgitation. Because left ventricular adaptation has not had time to develop, the hemodynamic consequences of acute regurgitant valvular lesions are more severe than those of chronic valvular regurgitation. Causes of acute-onset aortic regurgitation include infective endocarditis with leaflet perforation, type A aortic dissection, blunt trauma, prosthetic valve dysfunction, and iatrogenic injury (eg, valve injury during cardiac catheterization). Causes of acute-onset mitral regurgitation include infective endocarditis with leaflet perforation, chordal rupture related to myxomatous degeneration, papillary muscle rupture from MI, acute cardiomyopathy (ie, functional mitral regurgitation), acute rheumatic fever, prosthetic valve dysfunction, and iatrogenic injury.[14]

**What is the treatment for acute pulmonary embolism with hemodynamic compromise?**

Patients with acute PE that are hypotensive should receive support with intravenous fluids and vasopressors. In patients without a contraindication, systemic thrombolytic therapy should be administered. Embolectomy (either surgical or catheter-based) may be considered when there is contraindication to, or failure of, thrombolytics.[15]

**Where are the 3 general sites of left ventricular outflow tract obstruction?**

The general sites of left ventricular outflow tract obstruction are subvalvular (eg, hypertrophic obstructive cardiomyopathy), valvular (eg, aortic stenosis), and supravalvular (eg, coarctation of aorta). *Coarctation of the aorta typically results in hypertension of the upper extremities, with normal or low blood pressure in the lower extremities.*

**What physical findings are associated with pulmonary hypertension?**

The physical findings of pulmonary hypertension include sinus tachycardia, elevated JVP, right ventricular heave, right ventricular gallop, loud pulmonic component of the second heart sound (P2), ascites, and peripheral edema. The presence of clear lungs can help differentiate right-sided heart failure from acute left-sided heart failure.[16]

## DISTRIBUTIVE HYPOTENSION

**What is the fundamental pathophysiologic mechanism of low blood pressure in distributive hypotension?**

Distributive hypotension occurs as a result of pathologic peripheral vasodilation with an associated decrease in SVR.

**In the setting of distributive shock, are the extremities usually warm or cool to the touch?**

Distributive shock is typically associated with warm extremities, a reflection of the decrease in SVR that is characteristic of this condition.

**Which of the following patterns of jugular venous pressure, cardiac output, and systemic vascular resistance is characteristic of distributive shock?**

|  | JVP | CO | SVR |
|---|---|---|---|
| A | ↑ | ↓ | ↑ |
| B | ↓ | ↑ | ↓ |
| C | ↓ | ↓ | ↑ |

Distributive shock is characterized by decreased JVP, increased CO, and decreased SVR (primary issue) (answer B).[1]

## What are the causes of distributive hypotension?

A 55-year-old woman presents with dyspnea and purulent cough and is found to have a temperature of 39.2°C, heart rate of 132 beats per minute, blood pressure of 88/55 mm Hg, and leukocytosis of 18 K/μL.

Sepsis caused by pneumonia.

A 42-year-old man with a history of alcohol abuse presents with nausea and postprandial epigastric abdominal pain that radiates to the back.

Acute pancreatitis.

A 43-year-old man with a history of hypertension and poor medication adherence is admitted to the hospital for an elective procedure and unexpectedly becomes hypotensive before the procedure.

Medication. *Patients with poor medication adherence are often mistakenly diagnosed with refractory hypertension and prescribed unnecessary antihypertensive medications. These patients are at risk for becoming hypotensive in the hospital setting when home medications are reliably administered.*

Hypotension accompanied by bronchoconstriction and an urticarial eruption.

Anaphylaxis.

Hyperpigmentation, hyponatremia, and hyperkalemia.

Primary adrenal insufficiency.

Sudden loss of autonomic tone as a result of spinal cord injury.

Neurogenic shock.

A 76-year-old man with a history of Parkinson's disease presents with months of light-headedness and is found to have a blood pressure of 188/105 mm Hg supine that drops to 90/50 mm Hg on standing, with no appreciable change in heart rate.

Dysautonomia.

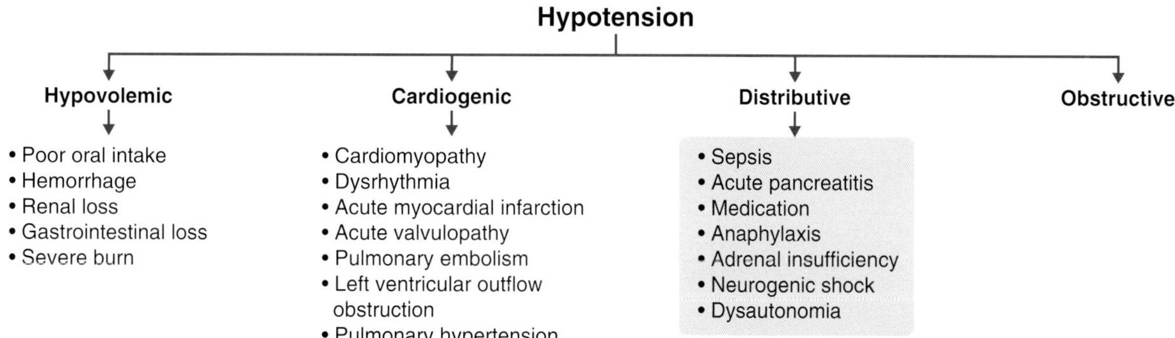


What are the general principles of treating septic shock?

Sepsis accounts for the vast majority of cases of distributive shock. The principles of treatment include administering supplemental oxygen to increase oxygen delivery to the tissues (mechanical ventilation may be necessary), isotonic intravenous fluids (eg, crystalloid), broad-spectrum antibiotics, and vasopressors if necessary. The placement of an arterial catheter to monitor arterial blood pressure and sample blood, and the insertion of a central venous catheter to monitor hemodynamics and administer fluids and vasoactive medications, are important steps in the management of septic shock.[4]

What is the underlying mechanism of hypotension in patients with acute pancreatitis?

The mechanism of hypotension in patients with acute pancreatitis is incompletely understood but is related in part to a systemic inflammatory response syndrome that causes vasodilation. Up to one-fifth of patients with acute pancreatitis develop severe disease with systemic inflammatory response. Hypotension is associated with a higher risk of death. Aggressive fluid resuscitation is an important part of management.[17]

**What medications can cause hypotension?**

Medications most commonly associated with hypotension (particularly orthostatic hypotension) include diuretics, sedatives, centrally acting adrenergic blockers, peripherally acting adrenergic blockers, vasodilators, β-blockers, and nitrates.[18]

**What is the initial pharmacologic treatment for anaphylaxis?**

The cornerstone of pharmacologic management of anaphylaxis is the administration of epinephrine (generally at a dose between 0.3-0.5 mg in adults, depending on weight). Intramuscular injection is the preferred route, and the optimal site of injection is the vastus lateralis muscle. Epinephrine can be lifesaving for patients with anaphylaxis, and there is no alternative agent. Adjunctive medications include antihistamines, glucocorticoids, and bronchodilators.[19]

**What is the initial treatment for adrenal crisis?**

Adrenal crisis in adult patients should be treated with fluid resuscitation and parenteral hydrocortisone. An initial injection of a 100 mg bolus of hydrocortisone should be followed by 200 mg daily (eg, 50 mg every 6 hours). If hydrocortisone is unavailable, prednisolone can be used instead. Identifying and addressing the underlying trigger of adrenal crisis is also important for management.[20]

**What is neurogenic shock?**

Neurogenic shock describes the development of hypotension following disruption of sympathetic pathways in patients with severe spinal cord lesions at the level of T-6 or higher. Intravenous fluids and vasopressor support to achieve a minimum MAP of 85 mm Hg may be helpful in preventing secondary ischemic injury to the spinal cord. However, vasopressors must be used cautiously in trauma patients because of the risk of increasing intracranial pressure. Bradycardia is often present in patients with neurogenic shock, particularly when the higher levels of the cervical cord are involved. Pharmacologic management (eg, atropine) and temporary pacing may be necessary in these patients to improve hemodynamics.[21]

**What are the general principles of treatment for hypotension associated with dysautonomia?**

Hypotension related to dysautonomia can be challenging to treat. Nonpharmacologic strategies include avoiding sudden postural changes, increasing daily salt and water intake, and using compression stockings. Pharmacologic agents can be used to increase blood volume (eg, fludrocortisone) and peripheral vasoconstriction (eg, midodrine).[22]

## OBSTRUCTIVE HYPOTENSION

**What is the fundamental mechanism of low blood pressure in obstructive hypotension?**

Obstructive hypotension occurs as a result of decreased cardiac filling with an associated decrease in both preload and cardiac output.

**In the setting of obstructive shock, are the extremities typically warm or cool to the touch?**

Obstructive shock is typically associated with cool extremities. This reflects the compensatory increase in SVR that aims to shunt blood to the vital organs.

**Which of the following patterns of jugular venous pressure, cardiac output, and systemic vascular resistance is characteristic of obstructive shock?**

| | JVP | CO | SVR |
|---|---|---|---|
| A | ↑ | ↓ | ↑ |
| B | ↓ | ↑ | ↓ |
| C | ↓ | ↓ | ↑ |

Obstructive shock is characterized by increased JVP (primary issue), decreased CO, and increased SVR (answer A).

### What are the causes of obstructive hypotension?

**An acutely enlarged cardiac silhouette on chest radiograph.**

Cardiac tamponade.

**Tracheal deviation on chest radiograph.**

Tension pneumothorax (see Figure 24-3).

**Kussmaul's sign and a pericardial knock.**

Constrictive pericarditis.

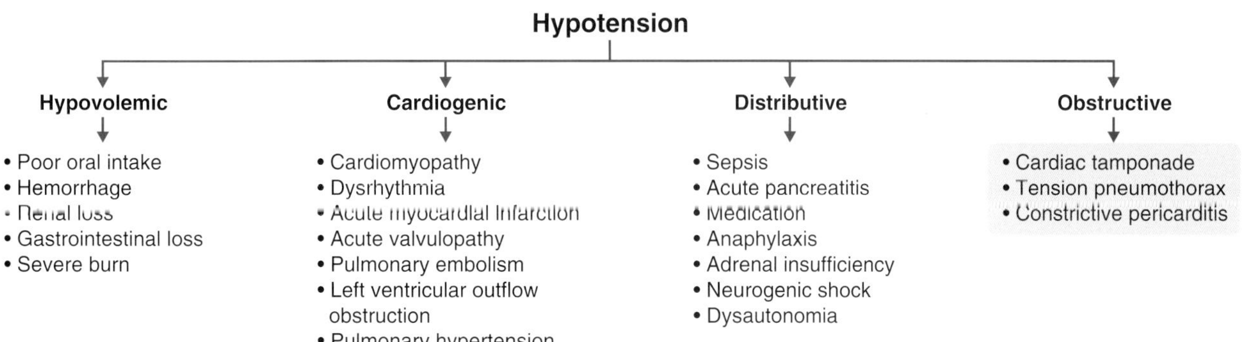


**What are the physical findings of cardiac tamponade?**

Physical findings of cardiac tamponade include tachycardia, hypotension, elevated JVP, muffled heart sounds, and pulsus paradoxus (>10 mm Hg drop in systolic blood pressure with inspiration).

**What is the acute treatment for tension pneumothorax?**

Tension pneumothorax develops in approximately 1 out of 20 patients who experience major trauma. It is a life-threatening condition that requires emergency decompression. The initial technique of choice is needle thoracostomy on the affected side, in which a 14-G catheter of sufficient length is advanced into the second rib space in the midclavicular line using a "catheter-over-needle" approach. When placement is successful, there will be a rush of air out of the chest with an immediate improvement in clinical status.[23]

**How can a pericardial knock be differentiated from an S3 gallop?**

The pericardial knock is an early diastolic sound thought to be the consequence of the sudden arrest of ventricular filling that occurs when noncompliant pericardium halts ventricular relaxation. It is higher pitched and occurs closer in proximity to S2 compared with the S3 gallop. Chest imaging can provide clues to the diagnosis of constrictive pericarditis (Figure 22-4).[24]

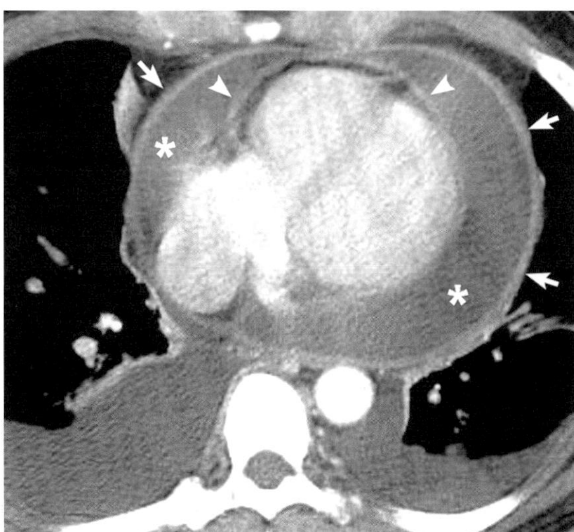

**Figure 22-4.** Contrast-enhanced computed tomography imaging at the midventricular level shows thickening and enhancement of both the visceral (arrowheads) and parietal (arrows) pericardium associated with a large pericardial effusion (asterisks). The combination of a pericardial effusion and constrictive pericarditis is known as effusive-constrictive pericarditis. (From Webb WR, Higgins CB. *Thoracic Imaging Pulmonary and Cardiovascular Radiology*. 3rd ed. Philadelphia, PA: Wolters Kluwer Health; 2017.)

## Case Summary

A 48-year-old man presents with chest pain and severe hypotension, and is found to have elevated JVP, an extra heart sound, diffuse inspiratory rales on auscultation of the lungs, cold extremities, and an abnormal ECG.

***What is the most likely cause of hypotension in this patient?***

Cardiogenic shock.

BONUS QUESTIONS

***What is the most likely cause of cardiogenic shock in this case?***

Acute MI is the most common cause of cardiogenic shock in the industrialized world. An acute MI is likely in this case given the electrocardiographic presence of ST elevation in anterolateral leads I, aVL, and $V_{2-6}$ (see Figure 22-1) in the setting of a compatible clinical syndrome.[13]

***What is the extra heart sound in this case?***

Heart sounds that occur near S2 include split S2, S3 gallop, opening snap, pericardial knock, and tumor plop. The extra sound in this case is most likely an S3 gallop based on location, pitch, and clinical history. S3 gallops are common in the setting of cardiogenic shock (S4 gallops are also common in the context of acute ischemia).[16,24]

***Which physical finding in this case helps rule out hypovolemic hypotension?***

The presence of elevated JVP in this case rules out hypovolemia.

***Which physical findings in this case make distributive hypotension unlikely?***

Elevated JVP before fluid resuscitation would be an unexpected finding in patients with distributive shock. Furthermore, the presence of cool extremities in this case indicates increased SVR, which is discordant with the pathophysiology of distributive shock.

***Which physical finding in this case makes obstructive hypotension unlikely?***

The bilateral inspiratory rales in this case most likely represent acute cardiogenic pulmonary edema from left-sided heart failure. Patients with obstructive hypotension have signs of right-sided heart failure (eg, elevated JVP), but the lungs are typically clear because left-sided cardiac filling pressures are not elevated.

***What general treatment strategies should be used in this case?***

The patient in this case should be treated with inotropic and vasopressor support as needed and evaluated for an intra-aortic balloon pump. For the acute MI, antiplatelet and antithrombotic therapy should be provided. Revascularization via percutaneous coronary intervention or coronary artery bypass grafting should be pursued as soon as possible. If revascularization is not available, fibrinolytic therapy should be given instead.[13]

## KEY POINTS

- Symptoms of hypotension include light-headedness, orthostasis, syncope, dyspnea, blurry vision, malaise, and confusion.
- Physical findings of hypotension include low arterial blood pressure, positive orthostatic vital signs, cool or warm extremities (depending on the underlying cause), and diminished peripheral pulses.
- Hypotensive shock occurs when tissue oxygenation is inadequate for the demands of aerobic metabolism.
- Hypotension can be hypovolemic, cardiogenic, distributive, or obstructive.
- Hypovolemic hypotension is characterized by decreased JVP (primary issue), decreased CO, and increased SVR.
- Cardiogenic hypotension is characterized by increased JVP, decreased CO (primary issue), and increased SVR.
- Distributive hypotension is characterized by decreased JVP, increased CO, and decreased SVR (primary issue).
- Obstructive hypotension is characterized by increased JVP (primary issue), decreased CO, and increased SVR.

## REFERENCES


1. Marino PL. *The ICU Book*. 3rd ed. Philadelphia, PA: Lippincott Williams & Wilkins—A Wolters Kluwer Business; 2007.
2. Mangrum JM, DiMarco JP. The evaluation and management of bradycardia. *N Engl J Med*. 2000;342(10):703-709.
3. Berne RML, Levy MN. *Physiology*. 4th ed. St. Louis, MO: Mosby, Inc.; 1998.
4. Vincent JL, De Backer D. Circulatory shock. *N Engl J Med*. 2013;369(18):1726-1734.
5. Gutierrez G, Reines HD, Wulf-Gutierrez ME. Clinical review: hemorrhagic shock. *Crit Care*. 2004;8(5):373-381.
6. Holcomb JB, Wade CE, Michalek JE, et al. Increased plasma and platelet to red blood cell ratios improves outcome in 466 massively transfused civilian trauma patients. *Ann Surg*. 2008;248(3):447-458.
7. Chung HM, Kluge R, Schrier RW, Anderson RJ. Clinical assessment of extracellular fluid volume in hyponatremia. *Am J Med*. 1987;83(5):905-908.
8. Schrier RW. Body water homeostasis: clinical disorders of urinary dilution and concentration. *J Am Soc Nephrol*. 2006;17(7):1820-1832.
9. Longo DL, Fauci AS, Kasper DL, Hauser SL, Jameson JL, Loscalzo J, eds. *Harrison's Principles of Internal Medicine*. 18th ed. New York, NY: McGraw-Hill; 2012.
10. Bhave G, Neilson EG. Volume depletion versus dehydration: how understanding the difference can guide therapy. *Am J Kidney Dis*. 2011;58(2):302-309.
11. Baxter CR, Shires T. Physiological response to crystalloid resuscitation of severe burns. *Ann N Y Acad Sci*. 1968;150(3):874-894.
12. Kohsaka S, Menon V, Lowe AM, et al. Systemic inflammatory response syndrome after acute myocardial infarction complicated by cardiogenic shock. *Arch Intern Med*. 2005;165(14):1643-1650.
13. Reynolds HR, Hochman JS. Cardiogenic shock: current concepts and improving outcomes. *Circulation*. 2008;117(5):686-697.
14. Mokadam NA, Stout KK, Verrier ED. Management of acute regurgitation in left-sided cardiac valves. *Tex Heart Inst J*. 2011;38(1):9-19.
15. Torbicki A, Perrier A, Konstantinides S, et al. Guidelines on the diagnosis and management of acute pulmonary embolism: the task force for the diagnosis and management of acute pulmonary embolism of the european society of cardiology (ESC). *Eur Heart J*. 2008;29(18):2276-2315.
16. Alpert JS, Becker RC. Cardiogenic shock: elements of etiology, diagnosis, and therapy. *Clin Cardiol*. 1993;16(3):182-190.
17. Garcia M, Calvo JJ. Cardiocirculatory pathophysiological mechanisms in severe acute pancreatitis. *World J Gastrointest Pharmacol Ther*. 2010;1(1):9-14.
18. Sathyapalan T, Aye MM, Atkin SL. Postural hypotension. *BMJ*. 2011;342:d3128.
19. Dhami S, Panesar SS, Roberts G, et al. Management of anaphylaxis: a systematic review. *Allergy*. 2014;69(2):168-175
20. Bornstein SR, Allolio B, Arlt W, et al. Diagnosis and treatment of primary adrenal insufficiency: an Endocrine Society Clinical Practice Guideline. *J Clin Endocrinol Metab*. 2016;101(2):364-389.
21. Jia X, Kowalski RG, Sciubba DM, Geocadin RG. Critical care of traumatic spinal cord injury. *J Intensive Care Med*. 2013;28(1):12-23.
22. Ziemssen T, Reichmann H. Treatment of dysautonomia in extrapyramidal disorders. *Ther Adv Neurol Disord*. 2010;3(1):53-67.
23. Aho JM, Thiels CA, El Khatib MM, et al. Needle thoracostomy: clinical effectiveness is improved using a longer angiocatheter. *J Trauma Acute Care Surg*. 2016;80(2):272-277.
24. Marriott HJL. *Bedside Cardiac Diagnosis*. Philadelphia, PA: Lippincott Company; 1993

Chapter 23

# PERIPHERAL EDEMA

## Case: A 47-year-old woman with palmar erythema

A 47-year-old woman presents to the emergency department with progressive swelling of the legs over the past few months. Over the same period of time she has also experienced an increase in abdominal girth and a weight gain of 30 pounds. She reports drinking 2 bottles (1.5 L) of wine daily for the past 20 years.

Blood pressure is 98/57 mm Hg. Jugular venous pressure (JVP) is 8 cm $H_2O$. Fingernails on both hands demonstrate white-colored opacification involving the majority of the nail bed except the distal end where a strip of normal pink tissue remains. There are dilated superficial veins radiating from the umbilicus. The abdomen is symmetrically distended with dullness over the flanks. There is marked edema of the lower extremities. An indentation appears in the skin after pressure is applied over the tibia. There is no edema of the upper extremities. Photographs of the patient are shown in Figure 23-1.

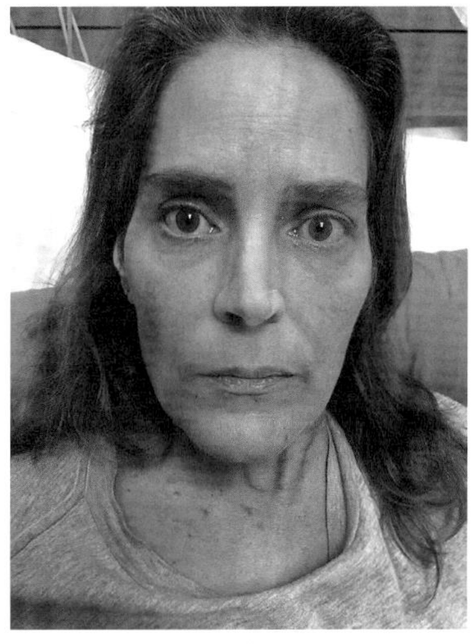

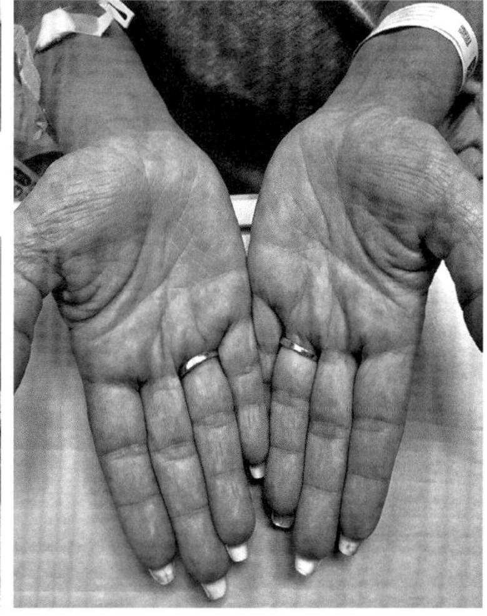

**Figure 23-1.**

***What are the most likely cause(s) of peripheral edema in this patient?***

What is edema?

Edema describes the presence of excess fluid within the interstitial space of the body. Peripheral edema involves the visible tissues (eg, extremities, sacral area, face, tongue, scrotum). Examples of nonperipheral edema include cerebral edema, pulmonary edema, pleural effusion, and ascites. Peripheral and nonperipheral edema may occur together, depending on the underlying condition.

What is pitting edema?

Pitting edema is characterized by the presence of a temporary indentation in the skin after firm pressure is applied to it. The severity of pitting edema can generally be graded on a scale from 1+ (mild) to 4+ (severe). A more precise way to grade pitting edema is to measure the depth of indentation over a bony prominence in millimeters.

**What is dependent edema?**

Dependent edema accumulates in the lower regions of the peripheral tissues due to gravity, such as the distal lower extremities in patients who are ambulatory, and the sacral area in patients who are bedbound. Dependent edema can be present in a localized (eg, unilateral upper extremity) or generalized distribution.

**What is generalized edema?**

Generalized edema (ie, anasarca) accumulates throughout the peripheral tissues, including gravity-dependent and gravity-independent regions. There is a dependent component to generalized edema, with more fluid accumulating in the gravity-dependent regions of the body. Generalized edema is frequently associated with pleural effusions and ascites.

**How is total body water distributed?**

Two-thirds of total body water is distributed within the intracellular fluid compartment, and one-third is within the extracellular fluid compartment. The extracellular compartment can be further divided into the intravascular (one-fourth) and interstitial (three-fourths) spaces (see Figure 22-3).[1]

**What factors regulate fluid balance between the intravascular and interstitial spaces?**

The movement of fluid between the intravascular and interstitial spaces is regulated by the interplay between hydrostatic pressures, oncotic pressures, capillary permeability, and the lymphatic system (Figure 23-2). The lymphatic system is responsible for returning net fluid efflux and filtered proteins from the interstitial space to the intravascular space. Lymphatic insufficiency causes proteins to accumulate within the interstitial space, increasing its oncotic pressure.[1,2]

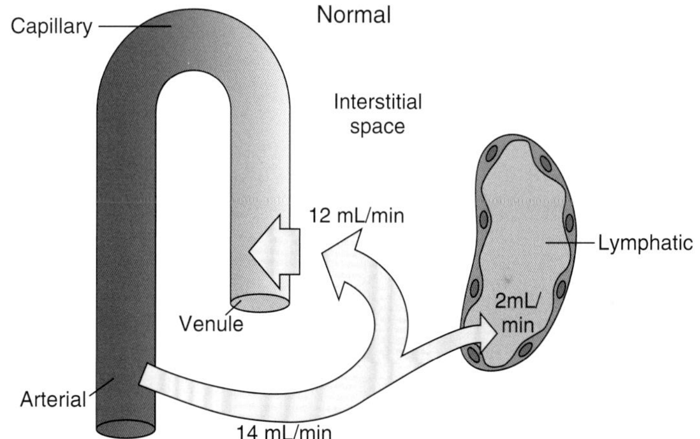


**Figure 23-2.** The differential between hydrostatic and oncotic pressures at the arterial end of the capillary bed favors the movement of fluid into the interstitial space. The differential at the venous end of the capillary bed favors the reabsorption of most fluid back into the intravascular space. The lymphatic system reabsorbs fluid and proteins from the interstitial space. (Adapted from Rubin R, Strayer DS. *Rubin's Pathology: Clinicopathologic Foundations of Medicine*. 5th ed. Philadelphia, PA: Lippincott Williams & Wilkins; 2008.)

**What are the 4 general mechanisms of edema formation?**

Fluid accumulation within the interstitial space (ie, edema) can occur as a result of increased capillary hydrostatic pressure, decreased capillary oncotic pressure, increased interstitial oncotic pressure, or increased capillary permeability.

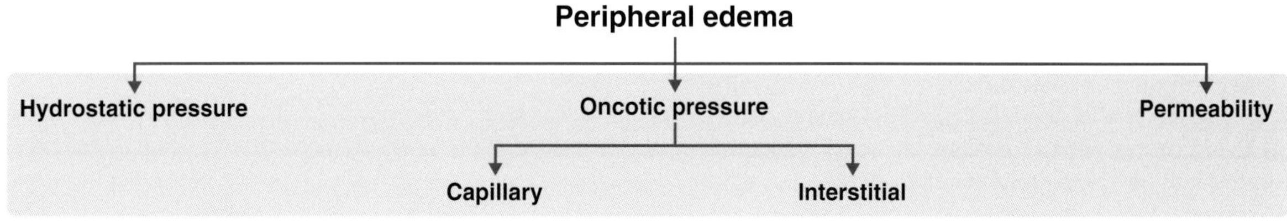

## PERIPHERAL EDEMA RELATED TO INCREASED CAPILLARY HYDROSTATIC PRESSURE

**How does capillary hydrostatic pressure cause peripheral edema?**

An increase in capillary hydrostatic pressure, which opposes capillary oncotic pressure and interstitial hydrostatic pressure, will lead to net efflux of fluid from the capillaries into the interstitial space. Edema forms when the maximal drainage capacity of the lymphatic system is exceeded (Figure 23-3A).

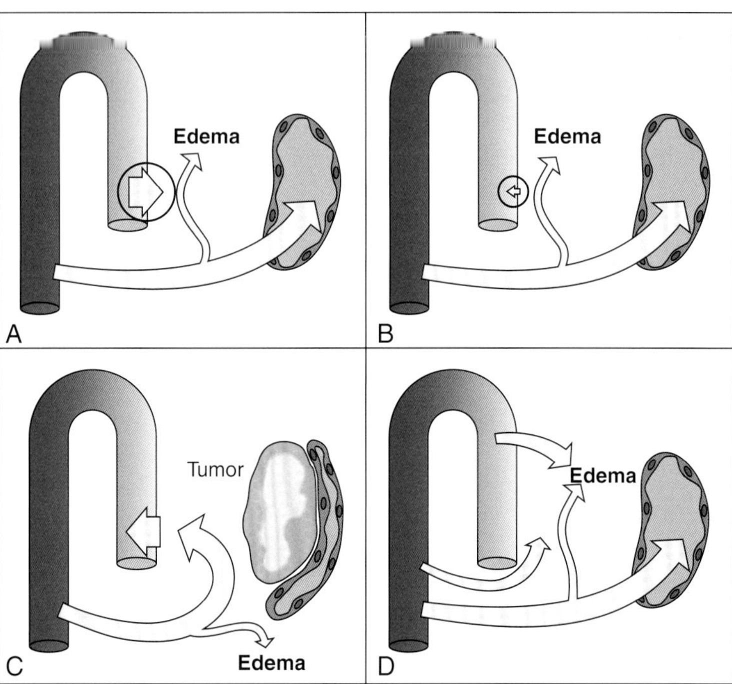


**Figure 23-3.** Mechanisms of edema formation. A, Increased capillary hydrostatic pressure. B, Decreased capillary oncotic pressure. C, Increased interstitial oncotic pressure. D, Increased capillary permeability. (Adapted from Rubin R, Strayer DS. *Rubin's Pathology: Clinicopathologic Foundations of Medicine*. 5th ed. Philadelphia, PA: Lippincott Williams & Wilkins; 2008.)

**Does systemic arterial hypertension cause peripheral edema?**

Systemic arterial hypertension does not cause peripheral edema because local autoregulation involving precapillary sphincters prevents arterial pressures from being directly transmitted to the capillary bed.[1]

**What are the general characteristics of peripheral edema caused by increased capillary hydrostatic pressure?**

Increased capillary hydrostatic pressure generally results in localized, dependent, pitting peripheral edema. It can be unilateral or bilateral depending on the underlying cause.

### What are the causes of peripheral edema related to increased capillary hydrostatic pressure?

**A 56-year-old man with a history of obstructive sleep apnea presents with elevated JVP, ascites, and peripheral edema.**

Right-sided heart failure.

**In addition to peripheral edema, other physical findings might include asterixis and a pericardial friction rub.**

Renal failure.

**Look for spider angiomas on the chest.**

Cirrhosis.

**A 55-year-old cancer patient develops acute onset unilateral lower extremity pain, erythema, and edema.**

Deep vein thrombosis (DVT).

**Advanced disease is associated with ulcerations around the medial malleoli.**

Chronic venous insufficiency.

**Affects women of reproductive age.**

Pregnancy.

**Iatrogenic peripheral edema.**

Medication.

**Pancoast tumor.**

Superior vena cava (SVC) syndrome.

**Elevated JVP, Kussmaul's sign, and an extra heart sound in early diastole best heard with the diaphragm of the stethoscope.**

Constrictive pericarditis.

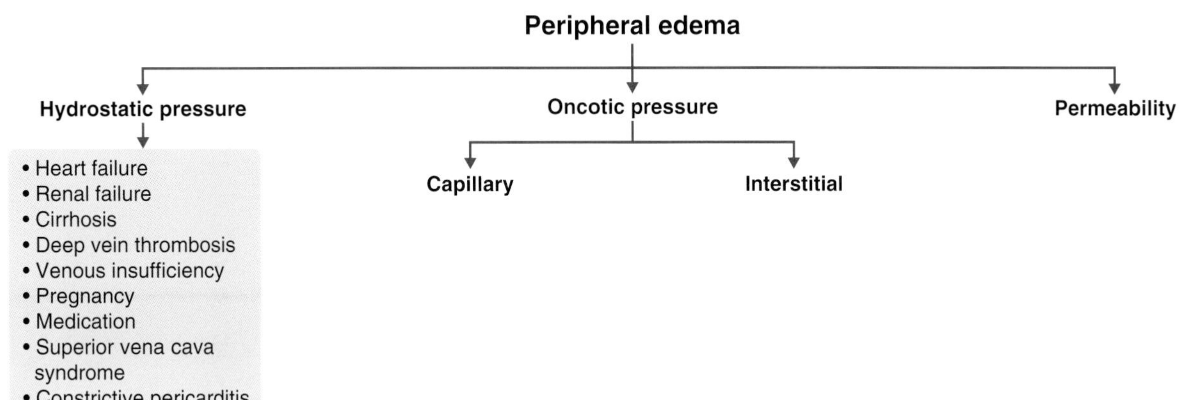




**What are the characteristics of peripheral edema caused by heart failure?**

Heart failure causes peripheral edema as a result of increased capillary hydrostatic pressure. In addition, ineffective arterial volume leads to renal retention of sodium and water, which contributes further to edema formation, usually involving the lower extremities. The edema is typically bilateral, symmetric, dependent, pitting, gradual in onset, and can be associated with ascites. Pulmonary edema or pleural effusions may be present in patients with left-sided heart failure. Diuretics, and dietary restriction of sodium and fluid are the mainstays of treatment. In some patients, bowel wall edema can limit diuretic medication absorption, necessitating use of the parenteral route.[1]

**What are the principles of managing hypervolemia in patients with renal failure?**

The characteristics of peripheral edema caused by renal failure parallel those of right-sided heart failure. Dietary restriction and fluid removal via hemodialysis or peritoneal dialysis are the cornerstones of treating hypervolemia and maintaining fluid balance in these patients. For those with severe manifestations of hypervolemia (eg, pulmonary edema), plasma ultrafiltration can be used to remove several liters of fluid per day.

**What are the characteristics of peripheral edema caused by cirrhosis?**

Most fluid retention in patients with cirrhosis manifests as ascites, although peripheral edema tends to become prominent as the disease progresses. The edema is typically bilateral, symmetric, dependent, pitting, gradual in onset, and usually involves the lower extremities.[1]

**What are the characteristics of peripheral edema caused by deep vein thrombosis?**

The peripheral edema of DVT is typically unilateral, dependent, pitting, acute in onset, and often associated with pain and erythema. Compression Doppler ultrasonography is the diagnostic modality of choice. Anticoagulation is used to prevent complications in patients with proximal DVT (at or proximal to the level of the popliteal vein) and in some patients with distal DVT. In select patients with severe disease, thrombolytic therapy (eg, catheter-directed thrombolysis) can be considered. In patients with bilateral lower extremity edema, thrombosis of the inferior vena cava should be considered.[3]

**What is chronic venous insufficiency?**

Chronic venous insufficiency occurs when dysfunction of the venous system of the lower extremities leads to venous hypertension. This process most commonly develops as a result of venous valvular incompetence related to previous clinical or occult DVTs. Clinical sequelae include pain, edema, and skin changes such as telangiectasias, varicosities, hemosiderosis-related hyperpigmentation, lipodermatosclerosis (a fibrotic process involving the dermis and subcutaneous fat), and ulcerations (typically near the medial malleoli) (Figure 23-4). The edema is dependent and gradual in onset, and usually asymmetric although it can be unilateral or bilateral. Early in the course of the disease, it is soft and pitting but may become more resistant to palpation as it progresses. Compression stockings are first-line treatment.[1,4]

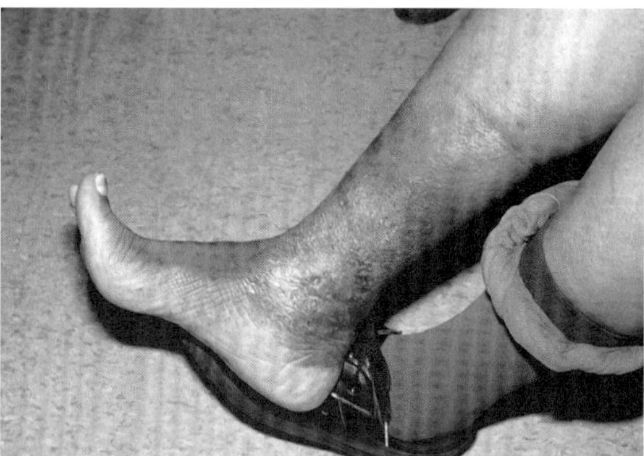

**Figure 23-4.** Hemosiderosis and an early ulceration near the medial malleolus (classic location) in a patient with chronic venous insufficiency. (From Goodheart HP. *Goodheart's Same-Site Differential Diagnosis: A Rapid Method of Diagnosing and Treating Common Skin Disorders*. Philadelphia, PA: Lippincott Williams & Wilkins; 2011.)

**How common is peripheral edema during pregnancy?**

Most pregnancies are complicated by peripheral edema, which occurs in the lower extremities in one-half of cases. Mechanisms of edema in pregnancy include increased plasma volume and sodium retention, decreased plasma protein concentration, and increased capillary hydrostatic pressure from mechanical compression of the internal vena cava and iliac veins.[1]

**Which medications are most commonly associated with peripheral edema?**

Medications most often associated with peripheral edema include dihydropyridine calcium channel blockers (eg, amlodipine), direct vasodilators (eg, hydralazine), and nonsteroidal anti-inflammatory drugs (eg, ibuprofen).[1,5]

**Where does peripheral edema occur in patients with superior vena cava syndrome?**

Peripheral edema caused by SVC syndrome involves the face, neck, and upper extremities. Arm involvement tends to be bilateral, symmetric, dependent, and pitting.[6]

**What physical finding is useful for differentiating constrictive pericarditis from cirrhosis in patients presenting with ascites and peripheral edema?**

The clinical presentation of constrictive pericarditis can be similar to that of cirrhosis, including hepatic congestion, ascites, and peripheral edema. Elevated JVP is indicative of a cardiac condition, and in patients with constriction, the JVP typically increases with inspiration, a finding known as Kussmaul's sign. *For a video of Kussmaul's sign, see the associated reference.*[7]

## PERIPHERAL EDEMA RELATED TO DECREASED CAPILLARY ONCOTIC PRESSURE

**How does capillary oncotic pressure cause peripheral edema?**

Capillary oncotic pressure opposes capillary hydrostatic pressure and interstitial oncotic pressure to maintain fluid within the capillaries and promote reabsorption of interstitial fluid at the venous end of the capillary bed. A decrease in capillary oncotic pressure will lead to net efflux of fluid from the capillaries to the interstitial space (see Figure 23-3B).

**What generates capillary oncotic pressure?**

Plasma proteins, primarily albumin, generate capillary oncotic pressure. Plasma albumin concentration <2 g/dL is associated with peripheral edema.[1,8]

**What are the general characteristics of peripheral edema caused by decreased capillary oncotic pressure?**

Decreased capillary oncotic pressure usually results in generalized, dependent, pitting peripheral edema. It is frequently associated with ascites and pleural effusions, but the presence of pulmonary edema suggests an alternative or additional disorder.[9]

## What are the causes of peripheral edema related to decreased capillary oncotic pressure?

**These conditions result in decreased protein synthesis.**

Liver disease and malnutrition.

**These conditions result in abnormal protein loss from the body.**

Nephrotic syndrome and protein-losing enteropathy.

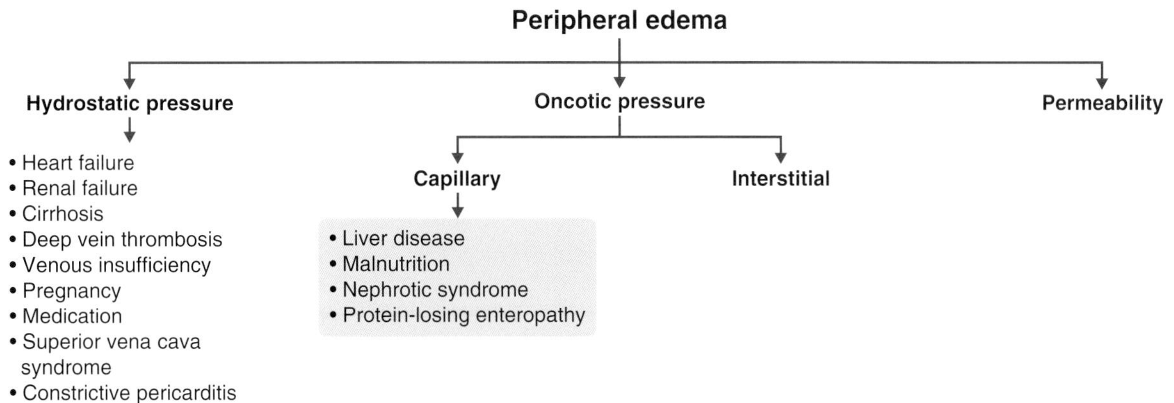


**How much albumin is synthesized per day?**

The liver is the only site of albumin synthesis. A healthy liver generates approximately 15 g of albumin daily. It can increase production by 2- to 3-fold when necessary. Decreased serum albumin concentration in patients with liver disease correlates with poorer prognosis. The fingernails can provide a clue to the presence of liver disease (Figure 23-5).[10,11]

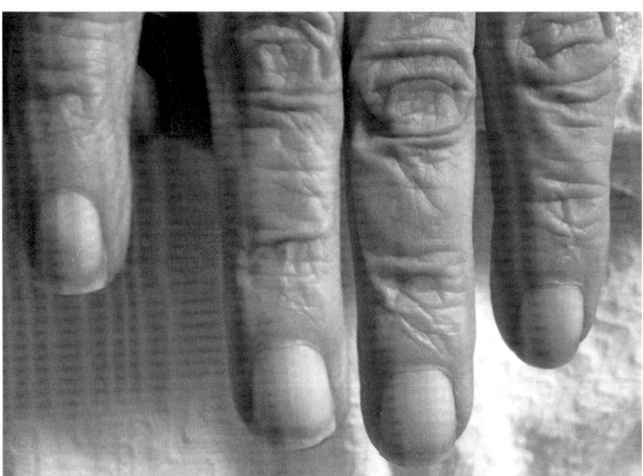

**Figure 23-5.** Terry's nails describes white-colored opacification of most of the nail bed, sparing a narrow 1 to 2 mm band of normal pink to brown tissue at the distal end. It is a sign of systemic disease (eg, cirrhosis).

**What are the physical findings of protein-calorie malnutrition?**

Protein-calorie malnutrition results in atrophy of muscle and fat, and peripheral edema. Clues to the presence of muscle atrophy include hollowed temples and rib protrusion in the pectoralis muscle area. Atrophy of the temporalis muscle is particularly informative because other muscles in the body (eg, quadriceps) may atrophy as a result of disuse, independent of nutritional status. Signs of subcutaneous fat atrophy include hollowed appearance and dark circles in the orbital region, marked intercostal depressions, and prominent iliac crests. Kwashiorkor is a pediatric condition caused by severe protein-calorie malnutrition and is characterized by dermatitis, protuberant abdomen, thinning hair, and peripheral edema (see Figure 13-4).[12,13]

**What are the characteristic urinary findings of nephrotic syndrome?**

Nephrotic syndrome is characterized by proteinuria of at least 3.5 g/d. A minority of patients may also experience microscopic hematuria, but the urine sediment is typically bland. The peripheral edema of nephrotic syndrome is usually generalized, dependent, and pitting.[14]

**What is the initial test of choice to evaluate for protein-losing enteropathy?**

The initial diagnostic test of choice for protein-losing enteropathy is measurement of fecal clearance of α-1 antitrypsin, which is elevated in affected patients. Characteristic clinical manifestations include peripheral edema, ascites, pleural effusions, and pericardial effusion.[15]

## PERIPHERAL EDEMA RELATED TO INCREASED INTERSTITIAL ONCOTIC PRESSURE

**How does increased interstitial oncotic pressure cause peripheral edema?**

Interstitial oncotic pressure opposes capillary oncotic pressure and interstitial hydrostatic pressure to draw fluid into the interstitial space and prevent its reabsorption at the venous end of the capillary bed. An increase in interstitial oncotic pressure will lead to net efflux of fluid from the capillaries to the interstitial space (see Figure 23-3C).

**What generates interstitial oncotic pressure?**

Interstitial oncotic pressure is primarily generated by glycosaminoglycans (ie, mucopolysaccharides) and filtered proteins (eg, albumin), the concentrations of which are influenced by capillary wall protein permeability and the rate of lymphatic clearance.[1]

**What are the general characteristics of peripheral edema caused by increased interstitial oncotic pressure?**

Increased interstitial oncotic pressure generally results in localized, dependent, nonpitting peripheral edema. It can be unilateral or bilateral, depending on the underlying cause.

### What are the causes of peripheral edema related to increased interstitial oncotic pressure?

**The most common causes of this condition are malignancy (in the industrialized world) and infection (worldwide).**

Lymphedema.[1]

**A 45-year-old woman presents with weight gain, constipation, dry hair, bradycardia, and bilateral nonpitting lower extremity edema.**

Myxedema.

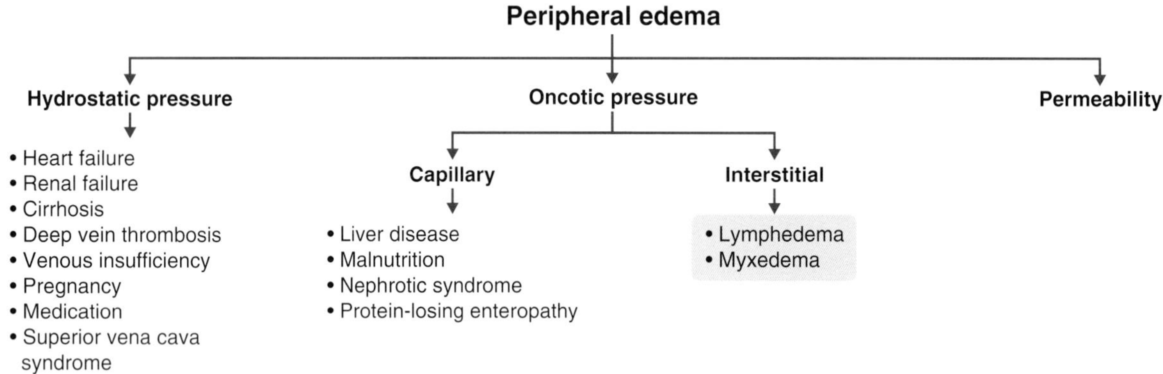


**Why does lymphatic obstruction cause an increase in interstitial oncotic pressure?**

Lymphatic obstruction leads to retention of protein-rich fluid in the interstitium, generating an increase in interstitial oncotic pressure. The most common causes include malignant obstruction (eg, lymphoma), iatrogenesis (surgery involving lymphatics, radiation treatment), and infection (eg, filariasis). The peripheral edema occurs on the ipsilateral side and is usually dependent. Pitting occurs early in the course of the disease. Over time the skin becomes thickened and darkened, and may develop warty projections (ie, lymphostatic verrucosis). Treatment options, including diuretics, are usually unsuccessful. *Lipedema refers to abnormal deposition of fatty substances in the subcutaneous tissues that results in soft tissue swelling, which is frequently mistaken for lymphedema. It predominates in women and almost always involves the lower extremities (but usually spares the feet).*[1,5,16]

**What are the characteristics of myxedema?**

Myxedema can develop in the setting of hypothyroidism or hyperthyroidism but is more common in the former. Hypothyroidism causes increased capillary permeability and decreased lymphatic clearance, leading to the accumulation of glycosaminoglycans and albumin in the interstitial space. This generates nonpitting peripheral edema that most often involves the lower extremities but may become generalized or involve nondependent areas, such as the eyelids, face, or dorsum of the hands. A particular type of myxedema occurs in patients with Graves' disease, called Graves' dermopathy. It results from an inflammatory-mediated accumulation of glycosaminoglycans in the interstitial space. It develops over the pretibial region in the vast majority of cases (ie, pretibial myxedema) and is characterized by bilateral, asymmetric, nondependent, nonpitting, painless, often discolored (yellow-brown to erythematous) nodules and plaques. Over time the lesions may coalesce to produce symmetric involvement of the pretibial regions, which become thickened and hardened, taking on a peau d'orange (orange peel) appearance and texture (Figure 23-6).[1,17–19]

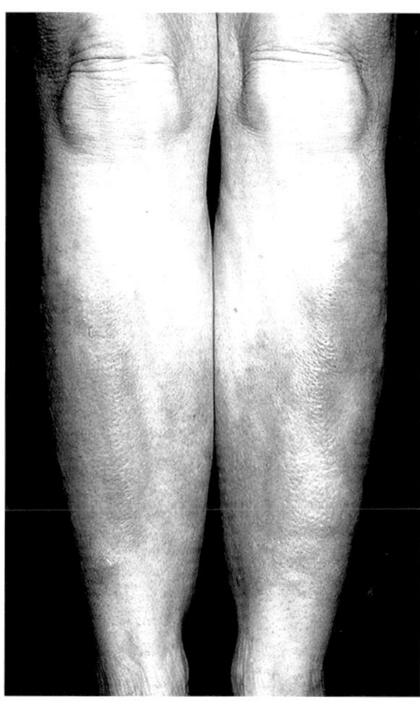

**Figure 23-6.** Graves' dermopathy (ie, pretibial myxedema). There are erythematous plaques in the pretibial region. Note the peau d'orange (orange peel) appearance in some areas. (From Goodheart HP. *Goodheart's Same-Site Differential Diagnosis: A Rapid Method of Diagnosing and Treating Common Skin Disorders*. Philadelphia, PA: Lippincott Williams & Wilkins; 2011.)

## PERIPHERAL EDEMA RELATED TO INCREASED CAPILLARY PERMEABILITY

**How does increased capillary permeability cause peripheral edema?**

The capillary membrane maintains fluid within the intravascular space and prevents equilibration of large proteins between the intravascular and interstitial spaces, which would diminish the oncotic pressure gradient that inhibits the movement of fluid out of the capillaries. An increase in permeability leads to net efflux of fluid and proteins from the capillaries to the interstitial space (see Figure 23-3D).

**What are the general characteristics of peripheral edema caused by increased capillary permeability?**

Increased capillary permeability can be associated with a variety of phenotypes, including pitting or nonpitting peripheral edema that is localized or generalized depending on the underlying etiology.

## What are the causes of peripheral edema related to increased capillary permeability?

**Local cytokine release.**

Local inflammation.

**A 29-year-old pregnant woman in the 35th week of gestation develops hypertension, proteinuria, and peripheral edema.**

Preeclampsia.

**A 46-year-old man with hypertension develops swelling of the tongue, lips, and hands after starting a new antihypertensive medication.**

Angioedema caused by use of an angiotensin-converting enzyme inhibitor.

**A 28-year-old woman with unexplained episodes of edema involving the hands, legs, and abdomen despite a thorough diagnostic investigation.**

Idiopathic edema.

**A rare disorder characterized by episodes of hypotension, hemoconcentration, and peripheral edema.**

Systemic capillary leak syndrome.

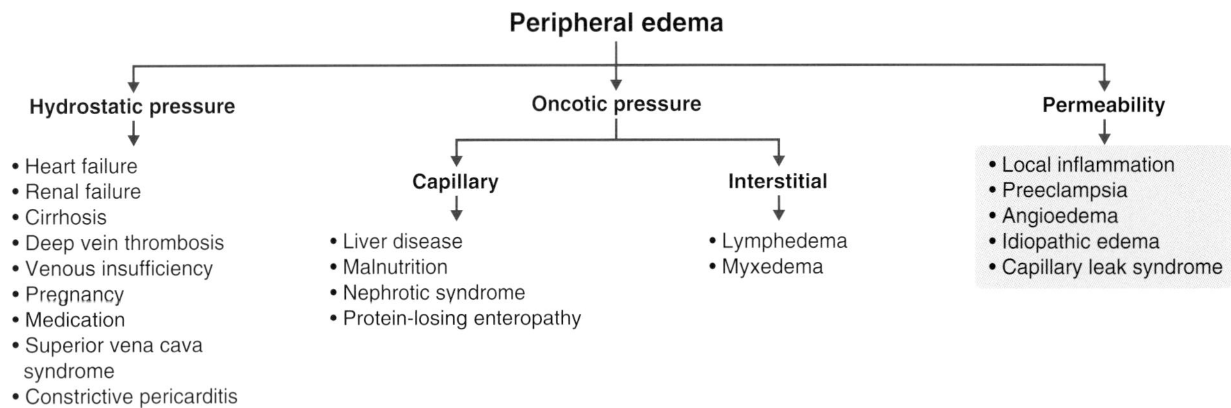


**What causes of local inflammation can result in edema?**

Peripheral edema can occur as a result of trauma, stinging insects (eg, bees, wasps), infection (eg, cellulitis), or burn injury. It is typically localized and nonpitting. History is key in making the diagnosis. In trauma patients, limb pain, paresthesias, tense edema, and rising serum creatine kinase levels suggests acute compartment syndrome, a surgical emergency.

**What are the characteristics of peripheral edema caused by preeclampsia?**

The combination of hypoalbuminemia and endothelial dysfunction with increased capillary permeability causes peripheral edema in patients with preeclampsia. It tends to involve the lower extremities and may be accompanied by pulmonary and cerebral edema. Management depends on severity and gestational age. Clinical manifestations typically resolve within hours of delivery.[20]

**What are the characteristics of angioedema?**

Angioedema results in localized, nondependent, and nonpitting peripheral edema, most often involving the face (eg, lips, tongue, periorbital region), hands, feet, or genitalia. Increased capillary permeability is usually mediated by histamine or bradykinin. Common causes include allergies (eg, food, venom), medications (eg, angiotensin-converting enzyme inhibitors, nonsteroidal anti-inflammatory drugs), and environmental triggers (eg, cold urticaria, exercise-induced anaphylaxis).[21]

What are the characteristics of idiopathic edema?

Idiopathic edema most commonly affects menstruating women in the third and fourth decades of life. It is periodic in nature but not clearly associated with the menstrual cycle. Edema develops in the upright position as the day progresses, most often affecting the lower extremities, face, and hands. Patients frequently misuse diuretics or laxatives in an effort to treat the condition. Idiopathic edema is different than premenstrual edema, which occurs in most women in the days before the onset of menses and resolves with menses.[1,5,22]

What is systemic capillary leak syndrome?

Systemic capillary leak syndrome is a rare and life-threatening disorder that typically affects middle-aged adults. It is characterized by episodes of rapid-onset generalized edema and hypovolemic shock associated with manifestations of hemoconcentration (eg, elevated hematocrit) and hypoalbuminemia without albuminuria. The edema may be pitting or nonpitting. The pathogenesis of increased capillary permeability in this condition is not known. A monoclonal gammopathy is present in most patients.[23]



## Case Summary

A 47-year-old woman with chronic heavy alcohol use presents with increasing abdominal girth, weight gain, and lower extremity edema.

***What are the most likely cause(s) of peripheral edema in this patient?***

Cirrhosis with or without hypoalbuminemia.

BONUS QUESTIONS

***What are the characteristics of the peripheral edema described in this case?***

The peripheral edema in this case is localized to the lower extremities, dependent, and pitting, suggesting that the underlying cause is related to increased capillary hydrostatic pressure. The bilateral location makes DVT unlikely, further narrowing the differential diagnosis.

***What is the significance of the fingernail findings in this case?***

Terry's nails describes white-colored opacification of most of the nail bed, sparing a narrow 1 to 2 mm band of normal pink to brown tissue at the distal end (see Figure 23-5). The opacification results in disappearance of the lunula. Terry's nails are a sign of systemic disease, such as cirrhosis, chronic heart failure, and chronic kidney disease.[24]

***What is the significance of the jugular venous pressure in this case?***

Right-sided heart failure and constrictive pericarditis can mimic the presentation of cirrhosis. The normal JVP in this case indicates that cardiac and renal causes of increased capillary hydrostatic pressure are unlikely.

***What are the relevant physical findings in Figure 23-1?***

Figure 23-1 demonstrates jaundice, scleral icterus, palmar erythema, and spider angiomas on the chest, all of which are associated with advanced liver disease. Palmar erythema describes erythema of the thenar and hypothenar eminences of the hands with central pallor. Spider angiomas are cutaneous vascular lesions that most often appear on the upper trunk. There is a central arteriole from which small branching vessels radiate. The lesion will blanch with pressure and fill from the central arteriole outward. Other stigmata of advanced liver disease include ascites, caput medusae (tortuous superficial veins that radiate from the umbilicus), and gynecomastia in men. The hollowed temples and orbital regions suggest malnutrition; hypoalbuminemia from the combination of liver disease and malnutrition is likely in this case.[25]

***What is the most likely cause of liver disease in this case?***

The history of chronic heavy alcohol use by the patient in this case is suggestive of alcoholic liver disease; the presence of Terry's nails and stigmata of advanced liver disease suggest progression to cirrhosis (Laennec's cirrhosis). The risk of developing cirrhosis becomes significant with chronic consumption of >30 g of alcohol per day (a 750-mL bottle of wine contains 75 g of alcohol); risk rises proportionally with intake greater than 30 g. Even in patients with a history compatible with Laennec's cirrhosis, other common etiologies of cirrhosis (eg, chronic hepatitis B or C virus infection) should be ruled out.[26,27]

***How is the diagnosis of cirrhosis made?***

Liver biopsy is the gold standard for diagnosing cirrhosis but is seldom required. The diagnosis is most often made clinically based on characteristic history, examination, biochemical laboratory data (eg, hypoalbuminemia, elevated prothrombin time), and imaging data (eg, evidence of liver nodularity, signs of portal hypertension).[28]

***What are the treatment options for the peripheral edema in this case?***

Conservative nonpharmacologic management of peripheral edema in cirrhotics includes dietary sodium restriction, leg elevation, and compression stockings. Diuretic therapy is often necessary. The combination of spironolactone and furosemide is particularly effective, usually starting at 100 mg and 40 mg, respectively. The spironolactone:furosemide dosing ratio of 50:20 mg is used to maintain serum potassium (at these doses, the potassium-wasting effect of furosemide is counterbalanced by the potassium-sparing effect of spironolactone). Unlike some patients with heart failure who experience impaired absorption related to bowel wall edema, the bioavailability of oral diuretics is usually preserved in cirrhotics.[1,29,30]

## KEY POINTS

- Peripheral edema describes the presence of excess fluid in the interstitial space.
- The movement of fluid between the intravascular and interstitial spaces is regulated by the interplay between hydrostatic pressures, oncotic pressures, capillary permeability, and the lymphatic system.
- Peripheral edema can be caused by increased capillary hydrostatic pressure, decreased capillary oncotic pressure, increased interstitial oncotic pressure, or increased capillary permeability.
- Lymphatic insufficiency leads to the accumulation of proteins within the interstitial space, increasing its oncotic pressure.
- Increased capillary hydrostatic pressure generally results in localized, dependent, pitting peripheral edema. It can be unilateral or bilateral, depending on the underlying cause.
- Decreased capillary oncotic pressure usually results in generalized, dependent, pitting peripheral edema. It is frequently associated with ascites and pleural effusions.
- Increased interstitial oncotic pressure generally results in localized, dependent, nonpitting peripheral edema. It can be unilateral or bilateral, depending on the underlying cause.
- Increased capillary permeability can be associated with a variety of phenotypes, including pitting or nonpitting peripheral edema with a localized or generalized distribution, depending on the underlying etiology.

## REFERENCES


1. Cho S, Atwood JE. Peripheral edema. *Am J Med*. 2002;113(7):580-586.
2. Warren AG, Brorson H, Borud LJ, Slavin SA. Lymphedema: a comprehensive review. *Ann Plast Surg*. 2007;59(4):464-472.
3. Kesieme E, Kesieme C, Jebbin N, Irekpita E, Dongo A. Deep vein thrombosis: a clinical review. *J Blood Med*. 2011;2:59-69.
4. Eberhardt RT, Raffetto JD. Chronic venous insufficiency. *Circulation*. 2014;130(4):333-346.
5. Ely JW, Osheroff JA, Chambliss ML, Ebell MH. Approach to leg edema of unclear etiology. *J Am Board Fam Med*. 2006;19(2):148-160.
6. Cheng S. Superior vena cava syndrome: a contemporary review of a historic disease. *Cardiol Rev*. 2009;17(1):16-23.
7. Mansoor AM, Karlapudi SP. Images in clinical medicine. Kussmaul's sign. *N Engl J Med*. 2015;372(2):e3.
8. Weisberg HF. Osmotic pressure of the serum proteins. *Ann Clin Lab Sci*. 1978;8(2):155-164.
9. Zarins CK, Rice CL, Peters RM, Virgilio RW. Lymph and pulmonary response to isobaric reduction in plasma oncotic pressure in baboons. *Circ Res*. 1978;43(6):925-930.
10. Limdi JK, Hyde GM. Evaluation of abnormal liver function tests. *Postgrad Med J*. 2003;79(932):307-312.
11. Nicholson JP, Wolmarans MR, Park GR. The role of albumin in critical illness. *Br J Anaesth*. 2000;85(4):599-610.
12. Bharadwaj S, Ginoya S, Tandon P, et al. Malnutrition: laboratory markers vs nutritional assessment. *Gastroenterol Rep (Oxf)*. 2016;4(4):272-280.
13. Tierney EP, Sage RJ, Shwayder T. Kwashiorkor from a severe dietary restriction in an 8-month infant in suburban Detroit, Michigan: case report and review of the literature. *Int J Dermatol*. 2010;49(5):500-506.
14. Hull RP, Goldsmith DJ. Nephrotic syndrome in adults. *BMJ*. 2008;336(7654):1185-1189.
15. Umar SB, DiBaise JK. Protein-losing enteropathy: case illustrations and clinical review. *Am J Gastroenterol*. 2010;105(1):43-49; quiz 50.
16. Forner-Cordero I, Szolnoky G, Forner-Cordero A, Kemeny L. Lipedema: an overview of its clinical manifestations, diagnosis and treatment of the disproportional fatty deposition syndrome – systematic review. *Clin Obes*. 2012;2(3-4):86-95.
17. Doshi DN, Blyumin ML, Kimball AB. Cutaneous manifestations of thyroid disease. *Clin Dermatol*. 2008;26(3):283-287.

18. Parving HH, Hansen JM, Nielsen SL, Rossing N, Munck O, Lassen NA. Mechanisms of edema formation in myxedema–increased protein extravasation and relatively slow lymphatic drainage. *N Engl J Med*. 1979;301(9):460-465.
19. Wolff K, Johnson RA, Saavedra AP. *Fitzpatrick's Color Atlas and Synopsis of Clinical Dermatology*. 7th ed. United States of America: The McGraw-Hill Companies, Inc.; 2013.
20. Uzan J, Carbonnel M, Piconne O, Asmar R, Ayoubi JM. Pre-eclampsia: pathophysiology, diagnosis, and management. *Vasc Health Risk Manag*. 2011;7:467-474.
21. Kaplan AP. Angioedema. *World Allergy Organ J*. 2008;1(6):103-113.
22. Coleman M, Horwith M, Brown JL. Idiopathic edema. Studies demonstrating protein-leaking angiopathy. *Am J Med*. 1970;49(1):106-113.
23. Kapoor P, Greipp PT, Schaefer EW, et al. Idiopathic systemic capillary leak syndrome (Clarkson's disease): the Mayo clinic experience. *Mayo Clin Proc*. 2010;85(10):905-912.
24. Witkowska AB, Jasterzbski TJ, Schwartz RA. Terry's nails: a sign of systemic disease. *Indian J Dermatol*. 2017;62(3):309-311.
25. Karnath B. Stigmata of chronic liver disease. *Hosp Physician*. 2003;39(14):14-16, 28.
26. Bellentani S, Saccoccio G, Costa G, et al. Drinking habits as cofactors of risk for alcohol induced liver damage. The Dionysos Study Group. *Gut*. 1997;41(6):845-850.
27. Lucey MR, Mathurin P, Morgan TR. Alcoholic hepatitis. *N Engl J Med*. 2009;360(26):2758-2769.
28. Tsochatzis EA, Bosch J, Burroughs AK. Liver cirrhosis. *Lancet*. 2014;383(9930):1749-1761.
29. Fogel MR, Sawhney VK, Neal EA, Miller RG, Knauer CM, Gregory PB. Diuresis in the ascitic patient: a randomized controlled trial of three regimens. *J Clin Gastroenterol*. 1981;3(suppl 1):73-80.
30. Sawhney VK, Gregory PB, Swezey SE, Blaschke TF. Furosemide disposition in cirrhotic patients. *Gastroenterology*. 1981;81(6):1012-1016.

Chapter 24

# SYNCOPE

## Case: A 64-year-old man with an enlarged cardiac silhouette

A 64-year-old man with a history of metastatic renal cell carcinoma presents to the emergency department with dyspnea and light-headedness. Symptoms have progressed over the course of a week and culminated in an episode of lost consciousness on the day of presentation. He denies any chest pain or palpitations. His wife witnessed the episode and did not observe any seizure-like activity. He was unconscious for approximately 30 seconds and did not appear to be confused on arousal. The patient was diagnosed with metastatic renal cell carcinoma 10 months ago and has been treated with cytoreductive nephrectomy and a tyrosine kinase inhibitor. Despite therapy, recent imaging revealed enlarging lymphadenopathy and new bone lesions.

Heart rate is 104 beats per minute, and blood pressure is 98/61 mm Hg. Jugular venous pressure is elevated to 16 cm $H_2O$ with an attenuated Y descent. Heart sounds are distant. Lungs are clear. Electrocardiogram shows low voltage and sinus tachycardia.

Chest radiograph is shown in Figure 24-1A (for comparison, imaging from 2 weeks prior is shown in Figure 24-1B).

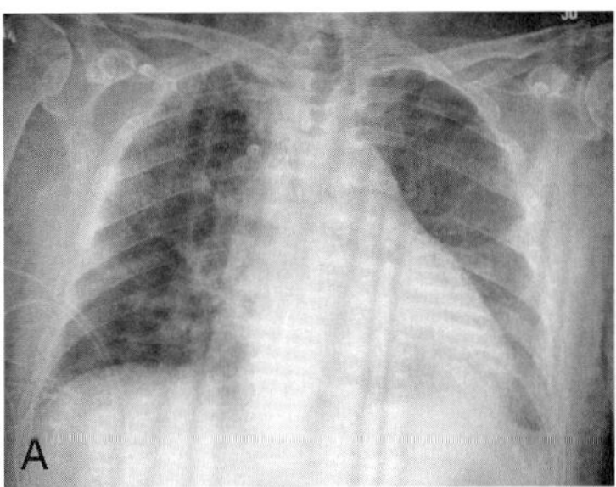

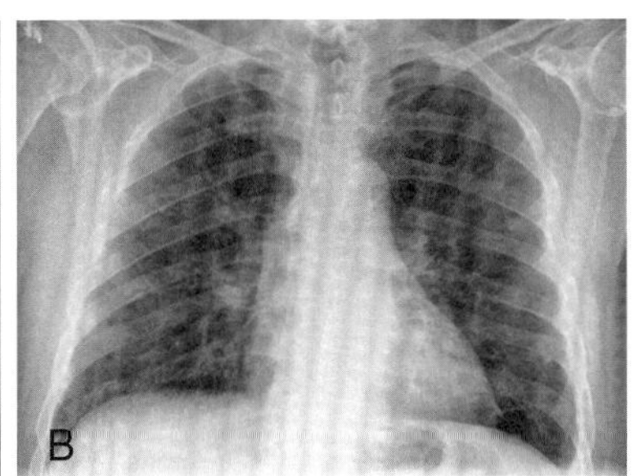


**Figure 24-1.**

***What is the most likely cause of syncope in this patient?***

What is syncope?

Syncope is the transient loss of consciousness resulting from cerebral hypoxia, with spontaneous revival. *Conditions that cause loss of consciousness through other mechanisms will be included within the framework of this chapter.*[1]

What is the hemodynamic mechanism of most causes of cerebral hypoxia?

Cerebral hypoxia most often occurs as a result of decreased cerebral blood flow.

How common is syncope?

Syncope occurs in one-third of individuals in the general population at some point in life. First-time episodes of syncope follow a bimodal distribution, with peaks at ages 20 and 80 years. In the industrialized world, syncope accounts for 1% of emergency department visits. Around one-third of those patients are subsequently admitted to the hospital.[1]

What is the prognosis of syncope?

The prognosis of syncope varies widely based on the underlying cause, from benign (eg, vasovagal syncope) to life-threatening (eg, cardiac tamponade).

The causes of syncope can be separated into which general categories?

The causes of syncope can be separated into the following categories: cardiovascular, neurocardiogenic, neurologic, and other.

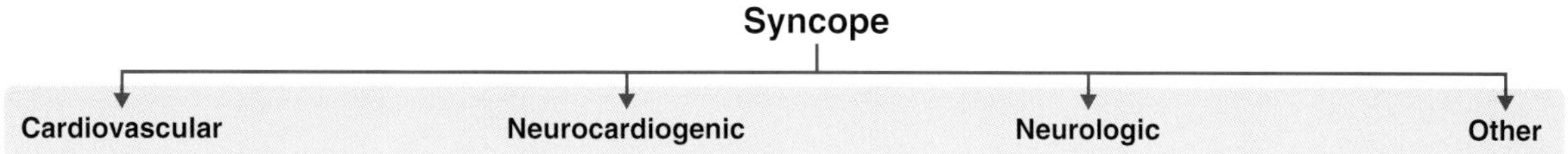


## CARDIOVASCULAR CAUSES OF SYNCOPE

What is the mechanism of most cardiovascular causes of syncope?

Cardiovascular syncope generally occurs as a result of decreased cardiac output (CO).

What are the main determinants of cardiac output?

Cardiac output is equal to the forward stroke volume (SV) of the left ventricle per beat multiplied by heart rate (HR).[2]

$$CO = SV \times HR$$

### What are the cardiovascular causes of syncope?

Low central venous pressure, low cardiac output, and elevated systemic vascular resistance.

Hypovolemia.

An episode of syncope is preceded by palpitations.

Dysrhythmia.

Pulsus alternans and cold extremities.

Heart failure.

Levine's sign.

Acute myocardial infarction (MI).

A 60-year-old woman from Germany presents with leg swelling and syncope the day after arriving in Portland, Oregon, to visit her son.

Pulmonary embolism (PE).

These conditions are associated with murmurs on cardiac auscultation.

Valvular lesions and left ventricular outflow tract obstruction (eg, hypertrophic obstructive cardiomyopathy [HOCM]).

Tearing chest pain associated with blood pressure of 185/110 mm Hg in one arm and 90/60 mm Hg in the other arm.

Aortic dissection.

A strong pulsation is palpated over the left second intercostal space of the chest.

Pulmonary hypertension.

Elevated central venous pressure, low cardiac output, and muffled heart sounds.

Cardiac tamponade.

A young woman with Takayasu arteritis complains of recurrent episodes of syncope when she does upper arm exercises.

Subclavian steal syndrome.

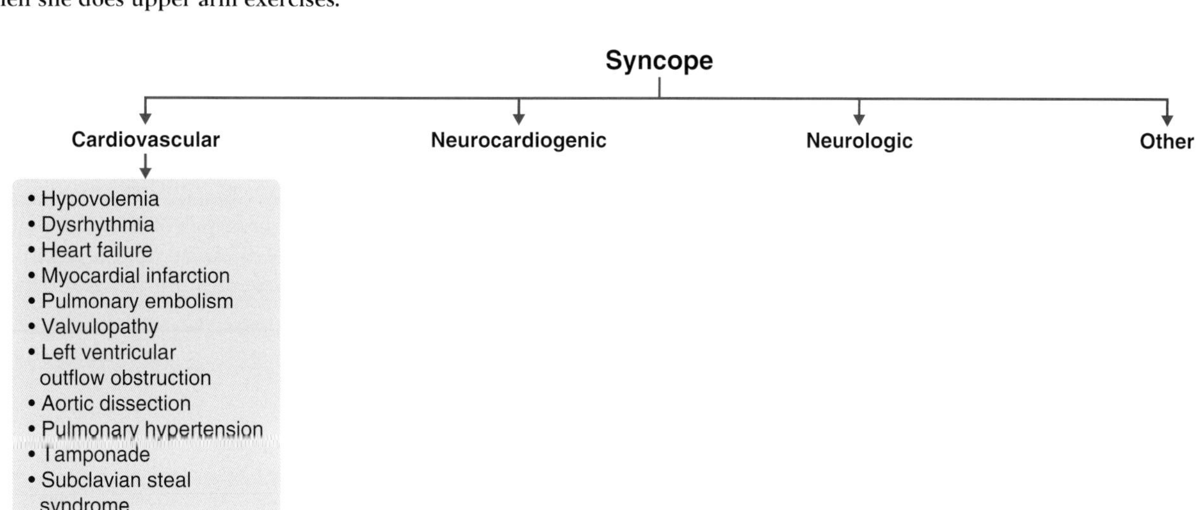

**What are the causes of hypovolemia?**

Hypovolemic hypotension can occur as a result of poor oral intake, gastrointestinal fluid loss (eg, diarrhea, vomiting), renal loss (eg, diuretic use, primary adrenal insufficiency), hemorrhage, burns, or insensible loss (eg, excessive perspiration).

**What is the treatment for heart block associated with syncope?**

In cases of symptomatic heart block (eg, third-degree AV block), urgent pharmacologic treatment (eg, atropine) or temporary cardiac pacing should be pursued. Unless a reversible cause can be addressed, placement of a permanent pacemaker is usually necessary.[3,4]

**Which class of medications can be used to directly increase cardiac output in patients with cardiogenic shock?**

Inotropic agents (eg, dobutamine) can increase myocardial contractility and are useful for treating cardiogenic shock. Additional support with vasopressor agents (eg, norepinephrine) may also be helpful. Mechanical support with intra-aortic balloon counterpulsation (ie, intra-aortic balloon pump) may be beneficial in select patients with cardiogenic shock. It improves coronary and peripheral perfusion by increasing diastolic pressure via diastolic balloon inflation, and augments left ventricular performance by decreasing afterload via systolic balloon deflation.[5]

**What widely available treatment should be given immediately to patients who present with hypotension or syncope in the setting of a right ventricular infarction?**

Patients with right ventricular infarction are particularly sensitive to inadequate preload. Intravenous crystalloid fluid should be given to patients with hemodynamic instability to increase preload and right ventricular contractility. If optimization of preload does not improve hemodynamics, inotropic support (eg, dobutamine) can be effective. Agents that decrease preload (eg, nitrates, diuretics) should be avoided. Early coronary reperfusion (eg, percutaneous coronary intervention) improves right ventricular performance and survival.[6]

**What is the treatment for acute pulmonary embolism complicated by hemodynamic instability?**

Patients with acute PE complicated by hemodynamic instability should receive support with intravenous fluids and vasopressors. In patients without contraindications, systemic thrombolytic therapy should be administered. Embolectomy (surgical or catheter-based) may be considered when there is contraindication to, or failure of, thrombolytics.[7]

**Which valvular lesion most frequently causes syncope?**

Syncope is one of the classic clinical manifestations of severe aortic stenosis. The other common manifestations include chest pain and dyspnea. Without treatment, the mean survival in patients with syncope caused by severe aortic stenosis is 3 years.[8]

**What classes of medications can precipitate syncope in patients with hypertrophic obstructive cardiomyopathy?**

Pharmacologic agents that may increase outflow obstruction in patients with HOCM include diuretics (via volume depletion), vasodilators (via decreased preload), and inotropic agents (via decreased left ventricular end-diastolic volume as a result of increased contractility).[9]

**What are the risk factors for aortic dissection?**

Risk factors for aortic dissection include male sex, age in the 60s and 70s, hypertension, prior cardiac surgery (especially aortic valve repair), bicuspid aortic valve, and Marfan syndrome.[10]

**Which echocardiographic measurement is used to assess pulmonary arterial pressure?**

Echocardiography can estimate right ventricular systolic pressure, which can be used as a surrogate for pulmonary arterial pressure. Calculating the right ventricular systolic pressure requires an estimate of right atrial pressure and the presence of tricuspid regurgitation. Based on the estimated right atrial pressure (P) and the measured velocity (V) of the regurgitant jet, the simplified Bernoulli equation ($\Delta P = 4V^2$) can be used to calculate the difference between right ventricular systolic pressure and estimated right atrial pressure.[11]

**What blood pressure finding is associated with cardiac tamponade?**

Cardiac tamponade is associated with pulsus paradoxus, which is a drop in systolic blood pressure ≥10 mm Hg during inspiration. To measure the pulsus, the cuff should be inflated above the highest systolic pressure. The patient should breath naturally. The cuff is then slowly deflated until the first Korotkoff sounds are heard (pressure A). These sounds will be appreciable during expiration only, when systolic arterial pressure is highest and able to overcome the cuff pressure. The cuff should be deflated further until the Korotkoff sounds are appreciable during both expiration and inspiration (pressure B). The difference between pressures A and B is the value of the pulsus.[12]

**What is subclavian steal syndrome?**

Subclavian steal syndrome describes retrograde blood flow in the vertebral artery as a result of a hemodynamically significant proximal narrowing of the ipsilateral subclavian artery. When the pressure distal to the site of stenosis falls below the pressure of the contralateral vertebral and internal carotid arteries there will be flow reversal down the ipsilateral vertebral artery, "stealing" blood from the cerebral circulation (Figure 24-2). When perfusion to the posterior brain is significantly compromised, symptoms such as light-headedness and syncope may appear. Upper arm activity can precipitate symptoms by increasing blood flow to the arm. Atherosclerosis is the most common cause of subclavian stenosis. Other causes should be considered in younger patients with subclavian steal syndrome, including large vessel vasculitis, thoracic outlet syndrome, and postsurgical stenosis (eg, after aortic coarctation repair).[13]

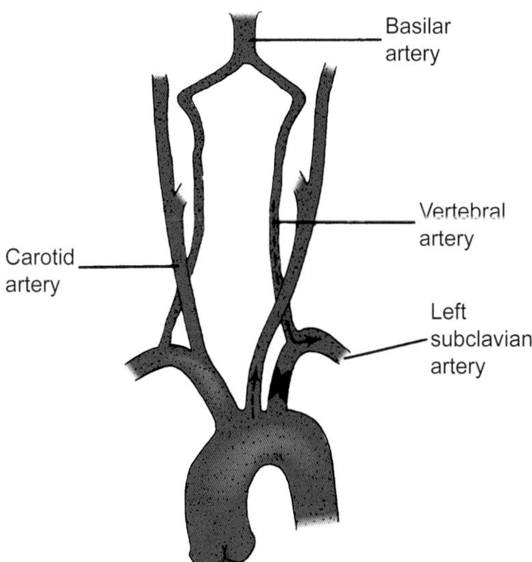


**Figure 24-2.** Subclavian steal syndrome. Proximal occlusion of the left subclavian artery causes retrograde blood flow through the left vertebral artery, "stealing" blood from the basilar circulation and causing transient dizziness and syncope with arm exercise. (From Lawrence PF, Bell RM, Dayton MT. *Essentials of General Surgery*. 5th ed. Philadelphia, PA: Lippincott Williams & Wilkins; 2013.)

## NEUROCARDIOGENIC CAUSES OF SYNCOPE

**What is neurocardiogenic syncope?**

Neurocardiogenic syncope occurs as a result of either a neurally mediated reflex that results in bradycardia and vasodilation, or impairment of the normal neurally mediated compensatory reflex that maintains blood pressure. Neurocardiogenic syncope is sometimes called "reflex" syncope.[14]

### What are the neurocardiogenic causes of syncope?

**A young boy passes out at the sight of a needle before receiving a vaccine.**

Vasovagal syncope.

**A previously healthy 40-year-old woman experiences recurrent episodes of syncope that only occur in the restroom.**

Situational syncope.

**A 66-year-old man complains when his wife asks him to shave because sometimes it causes him to pass out.**

Carotid hypersensitivity.

**Labile blood pressure in the elderly.**

Dysautonomia.

**This form of autonomic dysfunction is most commonly seen in children and young adults.**

Postural orthostatic tachycardia syndrome (POTS).

**A consequence of spinal trauma.**

Neurogenic shock.

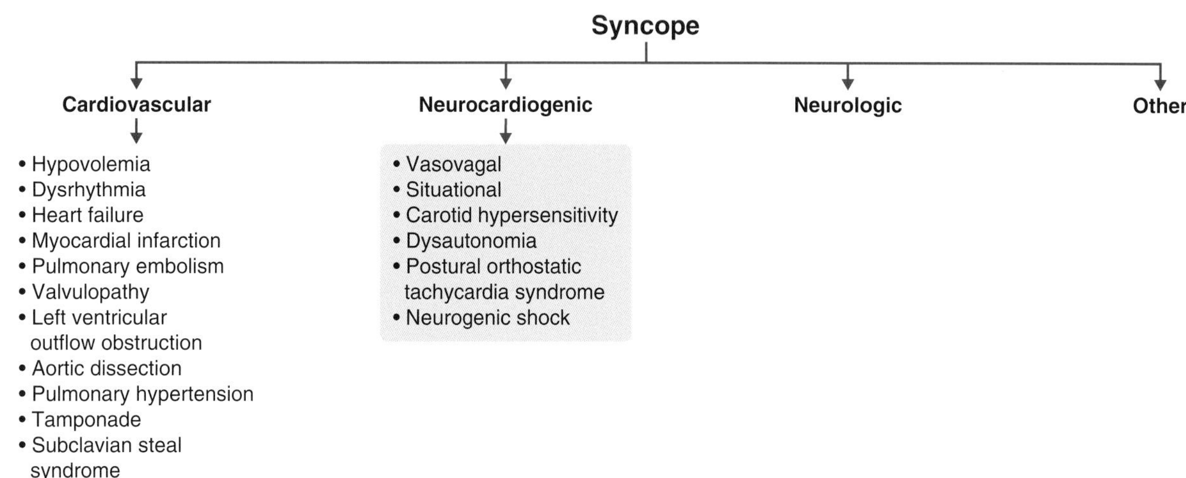


**How common is vasovagal syncope?**

Vasovagal syncope is the most common cause of syncope in the general population, accounting for around one-quarter of syncopal events. Clues to the presence of vasovagal syncope include onset during the teenage years, a family history of similar episodes, and association with emotional events.[15,16]

**What are the scenarios in which situational syncope occurs?**

Situational syncope can occur with coughing, swallowing, laughing, micturition, or defecation. First-line therapy is avoidance of known triggers when possible.[14]

**What is the mechanism of carotid hypersensitivity?**

Syncope may occur when bradycardia and hypotension develop as a result of an exaggerated response to mechanical stimulation of the baroreceptors within the carotid sinus. It is rare in patients under 40 years of age; prevalence increases with age and cardiovascular comorbidities. In addition to shaving, it may also occur with rotation or turning of the head or use of tight collars or neckwear. Carotid sinus massage (for 5-10 seconds) can be diagnostic when it results in >50 mm Hg reduction in systolic blood pressure or a ventricular pause of ≥3 seconds.[14]

**In patients with dysautonomia, what pattern of blood pressure and heart rate changes occur with tilt table testing?**

In patients with dysautonomia, tilt table testing results in a drop in blood pressure with little change in heart rate. This pattern distinguishes dysautonomia from orthostatic hypotension, a common cause of syncope, in which there is a compensatory increase in heart rate when blood pressure drops (except in patients receiving negative chronotropic therapy; eg, β-blockers).[17]

**What patient demographic is most commonly affected by postural orthostatic tachycardia syndrome?**

POTS overwhelmingly affects young women. The pathophysiology of POTS has not been fully elucidated. In addition to orthostatic symptoms, patients often experience other autonomic abnormalities (eg, hyperhidrosis), fatigue, migraine headache, and sleep abnormalities. Tilt table testing typically results in an exaggerated increase in heart rate. Pharmacologic agents that may be effective in treating symptoms of this condition include β-blockers, fludrocortisone, midodrine, and selective serotonin reuptake inhibitors.[18]

**What type of cardiac dysrhythmia frequently develops in patients with neurogenic shock?**

Patients with neurogenic shock typically exhibit hypotension with bradycardia, particularly when the higher levels of the cervical cord are involved. Pharmacologic management (eg, atropine) or temporary pacing may be necessary in these patients to improve hemodynamics.[19]

## NEUROLOGIC CAUSES OF SYNCOPE

### What are the neurologic causes of syncope?

**Loss of consciousness associated with uncontrollable myoclonic jerking.**

Seizure.

**This condition must be considered in any diabetic patient presenting with syncope.**

Neuroglycopenia (hypoglycemia).

**Loss of consciousness associated with focal neurologic symptoms or signs.**

Transient ischemic attack (TIA) or stroke.

**A 78-year-old man loses consciousness when attempting to change a light bulb in his kitchen ceiling.**

Vertebrobasilar insufficiency.

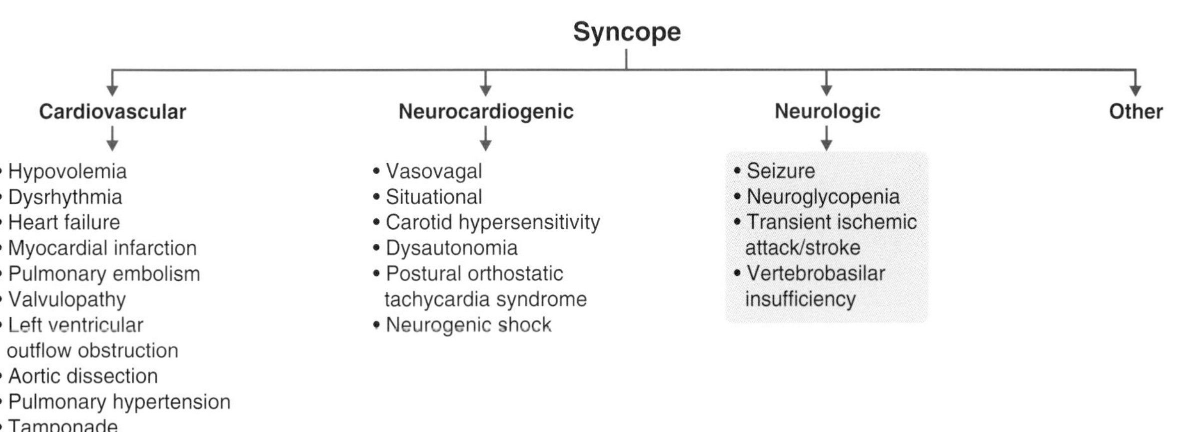


**What historical features can help distinguish seizure from true syncope (related to decreased cerebral blood flow)?**

Compared with true syncope, features that favor seizure include a sense of déjà vu or jamais vu preceding an episode, evidence of tongue biting, witnessed head turning or posturing during an episode, and a postictal state. The absence of sweating, a history of light-headedness, or orthostatic position changes further support the diagnosis.[20]

**What are the symptoms and signs of neuroglycopenia?**

Manifestations of neuroglycopenia range from behavioral changes, fatigue, and confusion to seizure and syncope. Hypoglycemia should be treated urgently with the ingestion of carbohydrates if possible, or the administration of parenteral glucagon or glucose. Reversal of hypoglycemia results in complete recovery in most cases. However, severe and prolonged hypoglycemia can result in brain death.[21]

**What additional symptoms and signs are present in patients with syncope related to transient ischemic attack or stroke?**

Patients with syncope related to TIA or stroke tend to have concurrent neurologic manifestations associated with compromise of the posterior circulation, including vertigo (most common), ataxia, paresthesia, diplopia, nausea or vomiting, dysarthria, headache, dysphagia, and paresis. The prototypical patient is an older man with a history of hypertension and ischemic heart disease.[22]

**Why would the act of changing a light bulb precipitate syncope in patients with vertebrobasilar insufficiency?**

In patients with vertebrobasilar insufficiency, turning the head upward creates external mechanical forces on the already-compromised vertebrobasilar arteries, which result in further decreases in cerebral blood flow. Syncope results when there is poor perfusion to the reticular activating system, located in the paramedian tegmentum of the upper brain stem.[23]

GENERAL INTERNAL MEDICINE

## OTHER CAUSES OF SYNCOPE

### What are the other causes of syncope?

**A 76-year-old man experiences light-headedness and syncope after starting treatment for benign prostatic hyperplasia.**

α-Blocker medication.

**In these conditions, oxygen delivery to the brain is compromised even in the setting of normal blood flow.**

Hypoxemia and anemia.

**Low carbon dioxide levels in arterial blood.**

Hyperventilation.

**Hyperresonance to percussion on one side of the chest.**

Tension pneumothorax.

**Think of this condition in patients with a mental health disorder in whom an etiology of recurrent syncope-like episodes cannot be determined.**

Psychogenic pseudosyncope.

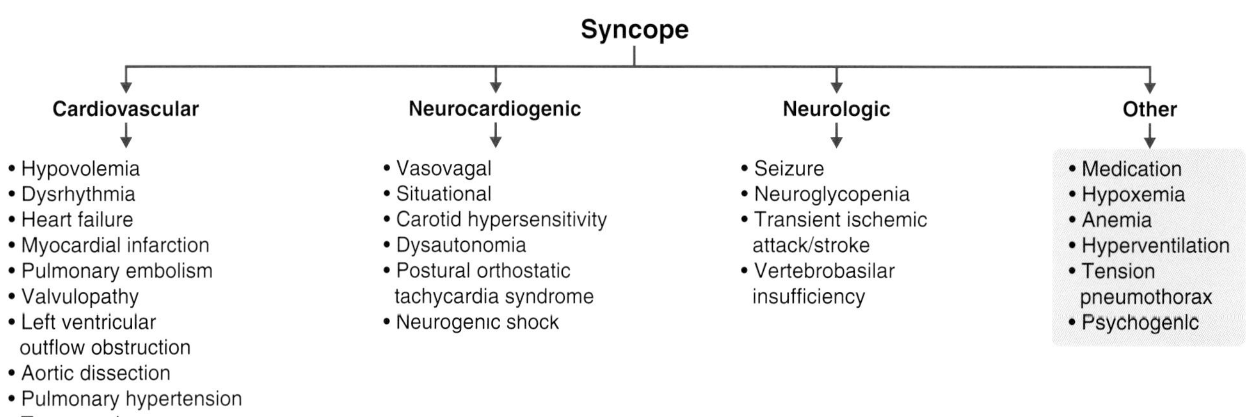


**What medications most often cause or precipitate syncope?**

Diuretics and nitrates are the medications most strongly associated with syncope; others include sedatives, centrally acting α-adrenergic blockers, peripherally acting α-adrenergic blockers, vasodilators, and β-blockers.[24,25]

**What formula describes the effects of hypoxemia and anemia on the delivery of oxygen to the tissues?**

The significance of anemia and hypoxemia can be demonstrated in the formula that describes the delivery of oxygen ($DO_2$) to the tissues:

$$DO_2 = [1.34 \times Hb \times Sao_2 + (0.003 \times Pao_2)] \times CO$$

*In the above formula, 1.34 is the oxygen-binding capacity of hemoglobin (mL $O_2$/g of Hb), Hb is the hemoglobin concentration in blood (g/dL), $Sao_2$ is the fraction of oxygenated hemoglobin in arterial blood, 0.003 is the solubility coefficient of $O_2$ in blood (mL $O_2$/100 mL blood/mm Hg $Pao_2$), $Pao_2$ is the partial pressure of oxygen in arterial blood (mm Hg), and CO is cardiac output (L/min).*[26]

**What is the mechanism of syncope related to hyperventilation?**

Hyperventilation leads to hypocapnia, which causes cerebral vasoconstriction and an associated decrease in cerebral blood flow. For every 1 mm Hg drop in $Paco_2$, there is a 2% decrease in cerebral blood flow.[27]

**What is the mechanism of syncope related to tension pneumothorax?**

Tension pneumothorax compresses the heart and other mediastinal structures, impeding venous return and decreasing cardiac output (Figure 24-3). Emergency needle thoracostomy is the treatment of choice.

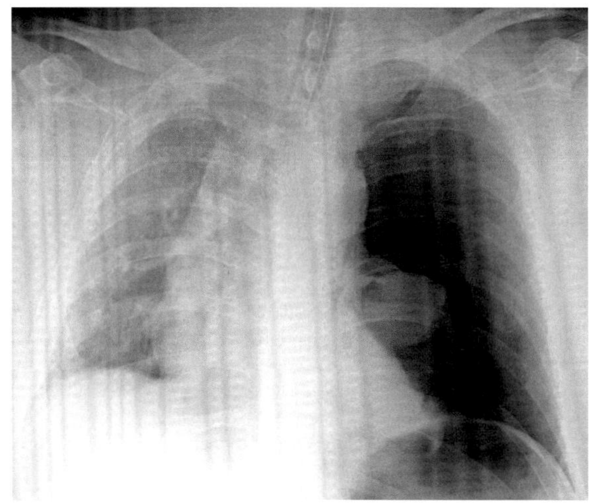

**Figure 24-3.** AP supine chest radiograph of a 35-year-old man involved in a motor vehicle accident shows a large left pneumothorax, collapse of the left lung, depressed left hemidiaphragm, and rightward shift of the mediastinum. The findings suggest a tension pneumothorax, which requires immediate decompression. (From Collins J, Stern EJ. *Chest Radiology: The Essentials*. Philadelphia, PA: Wolters Kluwer Health; 2015.)

**What is psychogenic pseudosyncope?**

Psychogenic pseudosyncope is a type of conversion disorder characterized by the appearance of syncope in the absence of true loss of consciousness. The absence of seizure-like body movement differentiates it from psychogenic nonepileptic seizures. The prototypical patient is a young woman with increasingly frequent episodes over a period of several months. Patients often experience prodromal symptoms such as light-headedness, palpitations, chest pain, dyspnea, and tingling. During episodes, the eyes are often closed, in contrast to patients with true syncope. History is key to making the diagnosis. However, head-up tilt testing, electroencephalography, and transcranial Doppler ultrasonography can confirm the absence of cerebral hypoperfusion or other hemodynamic derangements characteristic of syncope (eg, hypotension, bradycardia) during an episode.[28]

## Case Summary

A 64-year-old man with a history of metastatic renal cell carcinoma presents with syncope and is found to have tachycardia, hypotension, elevated jugular venous pressure, muffled heart sounds, low-voltage ECG, and an abnormal chest radiograph.

***What is the most likely cause of syncope in this patient?***

Cardiac tamponade.

### BONUS QUESTIONS

***What is the most likely explanation for the pericardial effusion in this case?***

The pericardial effusion in this case is most likely malignant, related to metastatic renal cell carcinoma.

***What are the electrocardiographic features of cardiac tamponade?***

Sinus tachycardia is the most common electrocardiographic manifestation of cardiac tamponade. More specific findings include reduced voltage and electrical alternans (alternating amplitude of the QRS complex).[12]

***What relevant finding is present on the chest radiograph in this case?***

The chest radiograph in this case (see Figure 24-1A) shows an enlarged cardiac silhouette, consistent with pericardial effusion. For the cardiac silhouette to increase, effusions must be large, typically >250 mL. Significantly smaller effusions can be detected by echocardiography.[12]

GENERAL INTERNAL MEDICINE

| | |
|---|---|
| ***Why is the enlarged cardiac silhouette in this case more likely caused by a pericardial effusion than cardiomegaly?*** | When compared to the historical chest radiograph (see Figure 24-1B), the recent chest radiograph (see Figure 24-1A) in this case indicates an acute or subacute process that is more consistent with pericardial effusion, as cardiomegaly generally develops over a longer period of time. Furthermore, clear lungs would not be expected in patients with recent development of cardiomegaly and congestive heart failure. |
| ***What is the mechanism of syncope in the setting of cardiac tamponade?*** | In patients with cardiac tamponade, external cardiac restraint causes underfilling of the left ventricle, which leads to decreased cardiac output. The amount of pericardial fluid required to become hemodynamically significant depends on the rate of accumulation and the compliance of the pericardium. Acute pericardial effusion can result in tamponade with as little as 200 mL of fluid or even less in patients with thickened or scarred pericardium (ie, effusive-constrictive pericarditis). Effusions over 1L in size may not be hemodynamically significant if the rate of accumulation is slow.[12] |
| ***What is the mechanism of pulsus paradoxus?*** | Pulsus paradoxus is the decrease in systolic blood pressure of 10 mm Hg or greater during inspiration. It occurs as a result of ventricular interdependence. During inspiration, intrathoracic pressure falls, which leads to increased filling of the right ventricle. Normally, the right ventricle can accommodate this increase by expanding outward. However, in the setting of external cardiac restraint, outward expansion of the right ventricle becomes limited. Instead, the interventricular septum bows toward the left ventricle, impairing left ventricular filling and resulting in a decrease in cardiac output and blood pressure.[12] |
| ***What are the treatment strategies for cardiac tamponade?*** | Patients with cardiac tamponade and concomitant hypovolemia benefit from intravenous fluid administration. However, definitive treatment for cardiac tamponade is urgent evacuation of the pericardial space.[12] |

## KEY POINTS

- Syncope is the transient loss of consciousness resulting from cerebral hypoxia, with spontaneous revival.
- Syncope is a common problem in the general population, with a variety of underlying causes that range from benign to life-threatening.
- Syncope most often occurs as a result of decreased cerebral blood flow. Anemia and hypoxemia are examples of conditions that can cause syncope without compromised cerebral blood flow.
- The causes of syncope can be separated into the following categories: cardiovascular, neurocardiogenic, neurologic, and other.
- Cardiovascular syncope generally occurs as a result of decreased cardiac output.
- Neurocardiogenic syncope occurs as a result of either a neurally mediated reflex that results in bradycardia and vasodilation, or impairment of the normal neurally mediated compensatory reflex that maintains blood pressure.

## REFERENCES


1. Saklani P, Krahn A, Klein G. Syncope. *Circulation*. 2013;127(12):1330-1339.
2. Mangrum JM, DiMarco JP. The evaluation and management of bradycardia. *N Engl J Med*. 2000;342(10):703-709.
3. Merideth J, Pruitt RD. Cardiac arrhythmias. 5. Disturbances in cardiac conduction and their management. *Circulation*. 1973;47(5):1098-1107.
4. Vogler J, Breithardt G, Eckardt L. Bradyarrhythmias and conduction blocks. *Rev Esp Cardiol (Engl Ed)*. 2012;65(7):656-667.
5. Reynolds HR, Hochman JS. Cardiogenic shock: current concepts and improving outcomes. *Circulation*. 2008;117(5):686-697.
6. Ondrus T, Kanovsky J, Novotny T, Andrsova I, Spinar J, Kala P. Right ventricular myocardial infarction: from pathophysiology to prognosis. *Exp Clin Cardiol*. 2013;18(1):27-30.
7. Torbicki A, Perrier A, Konstantinides S, et al. Guidelines on the diagnosis and management of acute pulmonary embolism: the Task Force for the Diagnosis and Management of Acute Pulmonary Embolism of the European Society of Cardiology (ESC). *Eur Heart J*. 2008;29(18):2276-2315.
8. Ross J Jr, Braunwald E. Aortic stenosis. *Circulation*. 1968;38(1 suppl):61-67.
9. Nishimura RA, Holmes DR Jr. Clinical practice. Hypertrophic obstructive cardiomyopathy. *N Engl J Med*. 2004;350(13):1320-1327.
10. Criado FJ. Aortic dissection: a 250-year perspective. *Tex Heart Inst J*. 2011;38(6):694-700.
11. Yock PG, Popp RL. Noninvasive estimation of right ventricular systolic pressure by Doppler ultrasound in patients with tricuspid regurgitation. *Circulation*. 1984;70(4):657-662.

12. Spodick DH. *The Pericardium: A Comprehensive Textbook*. New York, NY: Marcel Dekker, Inc.; 1997.
13. Potter BJ, Pinto DS. Subclavian steal syndrome. *Circulation*. 2014;129(22):2320-2323.
14. Chen-Scarabelli C, Scarabelli TM. Neurocardiogenic syncope. *BMJ*. 2004;329(7461):336-341.
15. Mathias CJ, Deguchi K, Schatz I. Observations on recurrent syncope and presyncope in 641 patients. *Lancet*. 2001;357(9253):348-353.
16. Soteriades ES, Evans JC, Larson MG, et al. Incidence and prognosis of syncope. *N Engl J Med*. 2002;347(12):878-885.
17. Grubb BP. Neurocardiogenic syncope and related disorders of orthostatic intolerance. *Circulation*. 2005;111(22):2997-3006.
18. Thieben MJ, Sandroni P, Sletten DM, et al. Postural orthostatic tachycardia syndrome: the Mayo clinic experience. *Mayo Clin Proc*. 2007;82(3):308-313.
19. Jia X, Kowalski RG, Sciubba DM, Geocadin RG. Critical care of traumatic spinal cord injury. *J Intensive Care Med*. 2013;28(1):12-23.
20. Sheldon R, Rose S, Ritchie D, et al. Historical criteria that distinguish syncope from seizures. *J Am Coll Cardiol*. 2002;40(1):142-148.
21. Cryer PE, Axelrod L, Grossman AB, et al. Evaluation and management of adult hypoglycemic disorders: an Endocrine Society Clinical Practice Guideline. *J Clin Endocrinol Metab*. 2009;94(3):709-728.
22. Davidson E, Rotenbeg Z, Fuchs J, Weinberger I, Agmon J. Transient ischemic attack-related syncope. *Clin Cardiol*. 1991;14(2):141-144.
23. Savitz SI, Caplan LR. Vertebrobasilar disease. *N Engl J Med*. 2005;352(25):2618-2626.
24. Mussi C, Ungar A, Salvioli G, et al. Orthostatic hypotension as cause of syncope in patients older than 65 years admitted to emergency departments for transient loss of consciousness. *J Gerontol A Biol Sci Med Sci*. 2009;64(7):801-806.
25. Sathyapalan T, Aye MM, Atkin SL. Postural hypotension. *BMJ*. 2011;342:d3128.
26. Marino PL. *The ICU Book*. 3rd ed. Philadelphia, PA: Lippincott Williams & Wilkins—a Wolters Kluwer business; 2007.
27. Raichle ME, Plum F. Hyperventilation and cerebral blood flow. *Stroke*. 1972;3(5):566-575.
28. Raj V, Rowe AA, Fleisch SB, Paranjape SY, Arain AM, Nicolson SE. Psychogenic pseudosyncope: diagnosis and management. *Auton Neurosci*. 2014;184:66-72.

SECTION 7

# Hematology

## Chapter 25

# ANEMIA

### Case: A 41-year-old man with pleuritic chest pain

A 41-year-old military veteran with a history of traumatic brain injury complicated by ataxia and frequent falls presents to the emergency department with lethargy. He has been fatigued ever since sustaining a mechanical ground-level fall a few days ago. He also describes progressive shortness of breath and left-sided chest pain with inspiration.

Heart rate is 122 beats per minute, and blood pressure is 108/74 mm Hg supine (which drops to 94/63 mm Hg on standing). The skin and mucous membranes are pale; the patient's hand is shown below the examiner's hand in Figure 25-1A. There is a 2/6 early-peaking crescendo-decrescendo systolic murmur best heard over the base of the heart. There is dullness to percussion over the left hemithorax with decreased tactile fremitus and no audible breath sounds.

Hemoglobin (Hb) is 6.2 mg/dL (there is no recent baseline for comparison) with a mean corpuscular volume (MCV) of 97 fL. Corrected reticulocyte count is 21%. Total serum bilirubin, haptoglobin, and lactate dehydrogenase (LDH) levels are within normal limits. Peripheral blood smear shows many reticulocytes.

Chest radiograph is shown in Figure 25-1B.

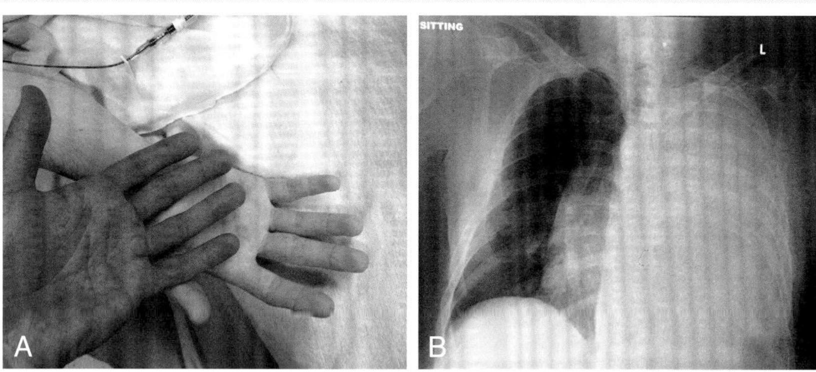


**Figure 25-1.**

***What is the most likely cause of anemia in this patient?***

**What is anemia?**

Anemia is defined by a reduced absolute quantity of circulating red blood cells (RBCs) in the setting of normal plasma volume. It can be identified and measured with several laboratory tests, including hemoglobin concentration, hematocrit, or RBC count. In practice, hemoglobin concentration and hematocrit are most commonly used. Hematocrit is the percentage of packed blood containing intact RBCs after it has been spun in a centrifuge. *The hematocrit is approximately 3 times the value of the hemoglobin concentration.*[1]

**Are hemoglobin concentration, hematocrit, and red blood cell count always congruent in anemic patients?**

In the setting of anemia, hemoglobin concentration, hematocrit, and RBC count usually decrease in parallel. In patients with profound microcytic anemia, such as thalassemia, the RBC count may be unexpectedly increased, a clue to the diagnosis.[2]

**What is the role of the red blood cell in aerobic metabolism?**

Aerobic metabolism requires that oxygen and nutrients be exchanged for carbon dioxide and other waste products. RBCs carry oxygen from the lungs to metabolizing tissues, and carbon dioxide from the tissues back to the lungs where it is eliminated. Hemoglobin is the molecule found inside RBCs that allows for the transport of oxygen and carbon dioxide.[3]

**Which formula describes the effects of anemia on tissue oxygenation?**

The effect of anemia on tissue oxygenation is demonstrated in the formula that defines the oxygen content of arterial blood ($Cao_2$):

$$Cao_2 = 1.34 \times [Hb] \times Sao_2 + (0.003 \times Pao_2)$$

*In the above formula, 1.34 is the oxygen-binding capacity of hemoglobin (mL $O_2$/g of Hb), [Hb] is the hemoglobin concentration in blood (g/dL), $Sao_2$ is the fraction of oxygenated hemoglobin in arterial blood, 0.003 is the solubility coefficient of $O_2$ in blood (mL $O_2$/100 mL blood/mm Hg $Pao_2$), and $Pao_2$ is the partial pressure of oxygen in arterial blood (mm Hg).*[3]

A 50% reduction in hemoglobin concentration (from 14 g/dL → 7 g/dL) results in a 50% reduction in $Cao_2$, whereas a similar 50% reduction in $Pao_2$ (from 90 mm Hg → 45 mm Hg) results in only a 20% decrease in $Cao_2$.

**What is normal hemoglobin concentration?**

Normal hemoglobin concentration varies by sex, age, race, and environmental factors (eg, altitude). The lower limit of normal in young white men (ages 20-59 years) is 13.7 g/dL; in older white men (>60 years), it is 13.2 g/dL; in white women of all ages, it is 12.2 g/dL. These values are 0.5 to 1 g/dL lower in blacks. Pregnancy lowers the threshold by an additional 0.5 to 1 g/dL. *Around 5% of normal individuals in these populations will have hemoglobin concentrations below these thresholds.*[4,5]

**How is the severity of anemia defined?**

Severity of anemia is variably defined (and dependent on factors such as sex, age, and race); however, the following thresholds provide a rule of thumb: Hemoglobin ≥9.5 g/dL is mild; hemoglobin 8 to 9.4 is moderate; hemoglobin <8 g/dL is severe.[6]

**How is red blood cell production regulated?**

The average RBC has a life span of 120 days; production of new RBCs (erythropoiesis) replaces approximately 1% of circulating RBCs on a daily basis. Erythropoiesis normally occurs within the bone marrow and is stimulated by the hormone erythropoietin (EPO), which is produced and secreted primarily by the kidney. Impaired oxygen delivery to the kidney as a result of either anemia or hypoxemia (or rarely, decreased blood flow from renal artery stenosis) provides the stimulus for EPO production (Figure 25-2).[7,8]

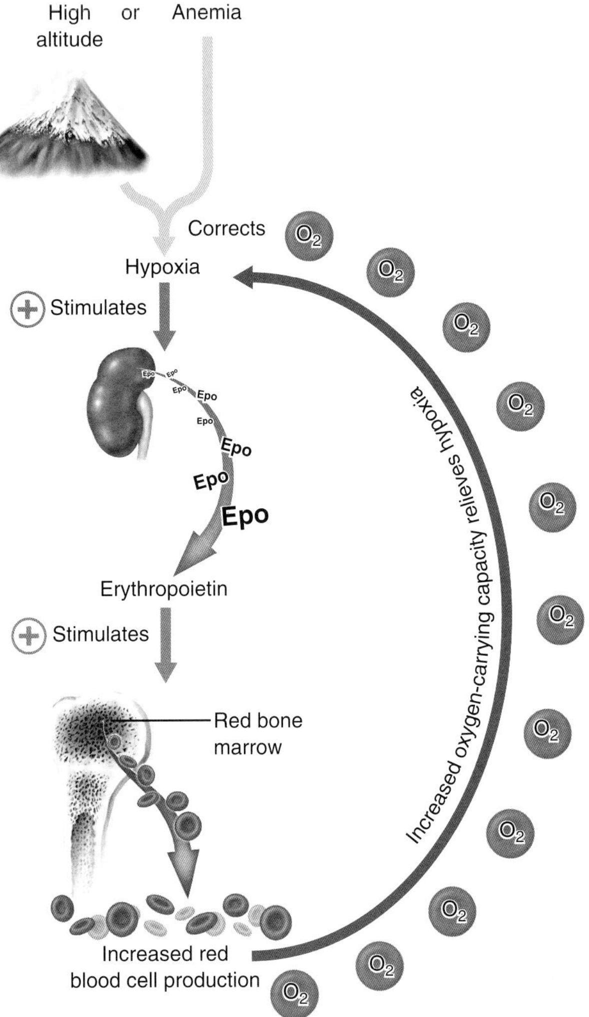


**Figure 25-2.** Impaired oxygen delivery to the kidney triggers EPO production, which increases the oxygen carrying capacity of blood by stimulating erythropoiesis. The negative feedback loop is completed when the increase in oxygen carrying capacity improves oxygen delivery to the kidney, reducing EPO production. (Adapted with permission from McConnell TH, Hull KL. *Human Form, Human Function: Essentials of Anatomy and Physiology*. Philadelphia, PA: Lippincott Williams & Wilkins; 2011.)

**What conditions may lead to elevated baseline hemoglobin concentration?**

Baseline hemoglobin concentration in an individual may be elevated as a compensatory response to chronic smoking, high altitude, or other medical conditions that lead to chronic hypoxemia (eg, chronic obstructive pulmonary disease). New laboratory values should be compared with recent baseline values if possible.

**Which acute conditions can affect the laboratory evaluation of anemia?**

The RBC count, hemoglobin concentration, and hematocrit can be influenced by plasma volume. These laboratory values may be falsely elevated by hypovolemia and falsely lowered by hypervolemia. Acute and congruent changes involving all 3 blood cells of the complete blood count (white blood cells, RBCs, and platelets) can provide a clue to the presence of hemoconcentration or hemodilution. New laboratory values should be compared with recent baseline values if possible. Causes of hemodilution include intravenous fluid administration, heart failure, renal failure, and pregnancy.

**How common is anemia?**

Anemia affects up to one-third of the world's population and is often associated with significant morbidity and mortality. Compared with men, prevalence is higher in women, particularly during pregnancy.[1,5]

**What are some of the physiologic adaptations that occur as a result of anemia?**

Physiologic adaptations to anemia begin after a period of days to weeks, and include increased cardiac output (from increased stoke volume and heart rate); increased 2,3-biphosphoglycerate (2,3-BPG) production, which shifts the oxygen-hemoglobin dissociation curve to the right; decreased systemic vascular resistance; and increased coronary and cerebral blood flow.[7,9]

**What are the symptoms of anemia?**

The clinical features of anemia depend on the severity, chronicity, and rate of onset. Mild anemia is frequently asymptomatic, but may be incidentally diagnosed on routine laboratory measurement. When gradual in onset, even severe anemia can remain subtle as a result of physiologic adaptation. Symptoms of anemia may include fatigue, loss of stamina, and dyspnea.[7]

**What are the physical findings of anemia?**

Physical findings of anemia may include tachycardia, wide pulse pressure, forceful heartbeat, strong peripheral pulses, systolic flow murmur, and pallor of the mucous membranes and skin—particularly in locations where vessels are close to the surface (eg, palmar creases and nail beds).[7]

**What are the red blood cell indices?**

The RBC indices are part of a routine complete blood count (CBC) and include the MCV in femtoliters, mean cell hemoglobin (MCH) in picograms per cell, and the mean cell hemoglobin concentration (MCHC) in grams per deciliter. Characteristic changes to the MCV occur with certain causes of anemia, making it valuable in narrowing the differential diagnosis. Low MCH/MCHC is referred to as hypochromia, which is consistent with impaired hemoglobin synthesis.[7]

**What are the 3 general categories of anemia based on mean corpuscular volume?**

Anemia can be microcytic, normocytic, or macrocytic.

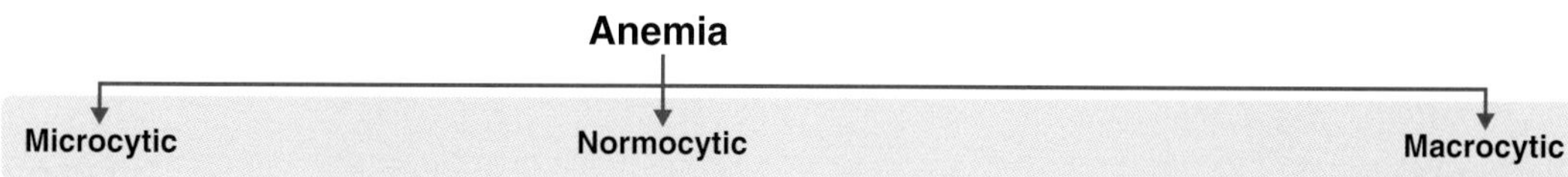

**How is mean corpuscular volume determined?**

MCV can be calculated using data from the CBC or by reviewing the peripheral blood smear. An automated blood cell counter calculates it as follows:

MCV (fL) = [hematocrit (percent) × 10]/[RBC count ($10^6/\mu L$)]

Although the calculation is highly accurate, the peripheral blood smear is more sensitive to changes in MCV (Figure 25-3). Microcytosis is defined by an MCV <80 fL; macrocytosis is defined by an MCV >100 fL.[10]

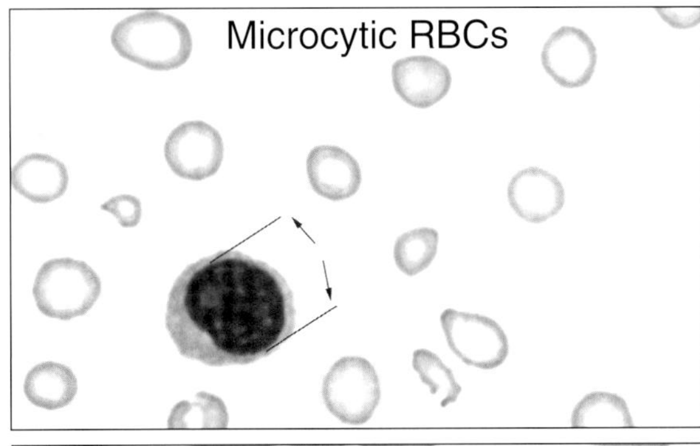


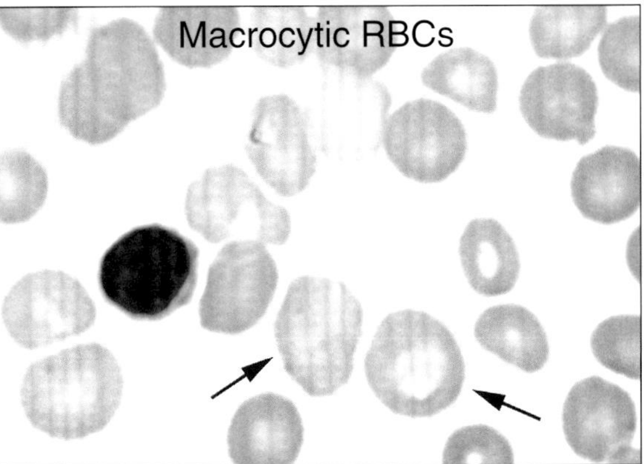


**Figure 25-3.** Peripheral blood smears demonstrating changes in RBC size. Normal RBCs are approximately the same size as the nuclei of small lymphocytes (8 μm in diameter). The top panel shows numerous microcytic RBCs that are significantly smaller than the diameter of the lymphocyte nucleus (indicated by the lines and arrows). The microcytic cells are also hypochromic, with a large region of central pallor and just a thin peripheral rim that is hemoglobinized. The bottom panel demonstrates macrocytic RBCs (arrows). The one on the left is a polychromatophilic RBC (prematurely released reticulocyte). (From Weksler BB, Schechter GP, Ely SA. *Wintrobe's Atlas of Clinical Hematology*. 2nd ed. Philadelphia, PA: Wolters Kluwer; 2018.)

## MICROCYTIC ANEMIA

### What are the causes of microcytic anemia?

**A previously healthy 28-year-old woman presents with fatigue and is found to have mild microcytic anemia with a serum ferritin of 7 ng/mL.**

Iron deficiency.

**A 28-year-old Greek man with microcytic anemia and codocytes (ie, target cells) on peripheral blood smear.**

Thalassemia.

**Ring around the nucleus.**

Sideroblastic anemia.

**Analysis of Ludwig van Beethoven's hair and bones supports the theory that this condition may have been responsible for his death, possibly related to chronic consumption of adulterated wine.**

Lead poisoning. *Lead was often used illegally during Beethoven's era to improve the taste of inexpensive wine.*[11,12]

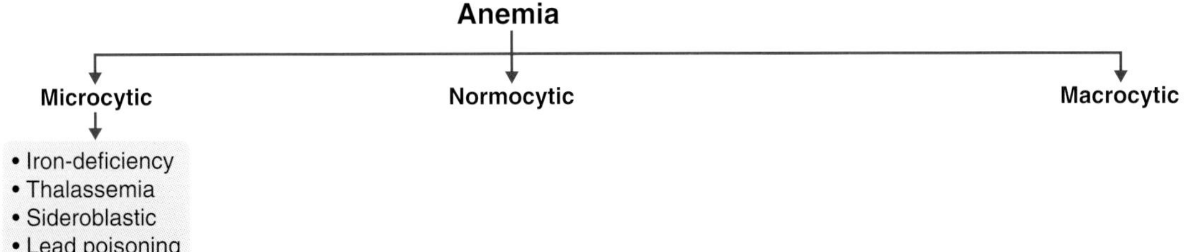


**What is the most powerful noninvasive test to evaluate for iron-deficiency anemia?**

Iron-deficiency anemia is the most common cause of anemia worldwide. Causes include insufficient intake (eg, malnutrition), decreased absorption (eg, celiac disease), chronic blood loss (eg, inflammatory bowel disease), and increased demand (eg, pregnancy). Initial laboratory clues to the diagnosis include microcytosis and hypochromia. Serum ferritin is the single most powerful noninvasive test to evaluate for iron-deficiency anemia. Baseline ferritin values decline with age. Values may be increased in the presence of chronic kidney disease, liver disease, or inflammatory conditions (eg, infection, rheumatoid arthritis, malignancy). However in any patient, a serum ferritin value <15 ng/mL confirms the diagnosis of iron deficiency, while a value of >100 ng/mL rules it out. Values between 15 and 100 require additional consideration, and other laboratory tests may be helpful, including the ratio of serum iron to total iron-binding capacity (ie, transferrin saturation).[5,13,14]

**What is thalassemia?**

Thalassemia refers to a group of inherited conditions that result in decreased or absent synthesis of 1 of the 2 polypeptide chains ($\alpha$ or $\beta$) that constitute the adult hemoglobin molecule (hemoglobin A, $\alpha_2/\beta_2$). The inheritance pattern is autosomal recessive, and there are a variety of genotypes. Clinical severity ranges from asymptomatic disease (eg, $\alpha$- thalassemia minor, $\beta$-thalassemia minor) to the presence of hepatosplenomegaly and chronic transfusion-dependent hemolytic anemia (eg, $\beta$-thalassemia major). Most patients with thalassemia have at least some degree of anemia, microcytosis, and hypochromia. Increased RBC count may be a clue to the diagnosis. In addition to hypochromic microcytosis, the peripheral blood smear may demonstrate poikilocytes (abnormal variation in RBC shape) such as target cells and teardrop-shaped RBCs (Figure 25-4), basophilic stippling, and nucleated RBCs (see Figure 27-5). Hemoglobin evaluation (separation and measurement of the hemoglobin fractions) or genetic testing can confirm the diagnosis.[15]

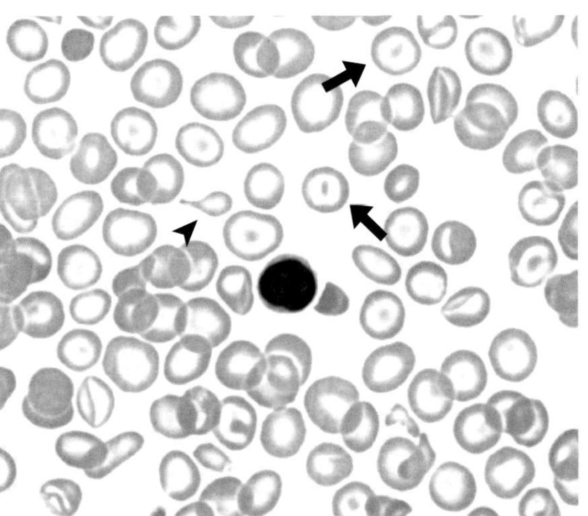

**Figure 25-4.** Peripheral blood smear from a patient with $\beta$-thalassemia minor demonstrating hypochromic microcytosis, target cells (arrows), and teardrop-shaped RBCs (arrowhead). (From Weksler BB, Schechter GP, Ely SA. *Wintrobe's Atlas of Clinical Hematology*. 2nd ed. Philadelphia, PA: Wolters Kluwer; 2018.)

HEMATOLOGY

**What is sideroblastic anemia?**

Sideroblastic anemia refers to a group of inherited and acquired conditions characterized by impaired heme biosynthesis and the distinctive presence of ring sideroblasts (RBC precursors with excessive mitochondrial iron accumulation) in the bone marrow. Acquired sideroblastic anemias are significantly more common than the hereditary varieties; underlying etiologies include toxins (eg, alcohol), medication (eg, isoniazid), nutritional deficiencies (eg, copper deficiency), and myelodysplastic syndromes. Sideroblastic anemias tend to produce hemoglobin in the 4 to 10 g/dL range. The peripheral blood smear typically demonstrates hypochromic microcytosis, although normocytosis and macrocytosis are both possible, and basophilic stippling is occasionally seen.[16]

**What characteristic finding may be present on peripheral blood smear in patients with lead poisoning?**

In addition to hypochromic microcytosis, the peripheral blood smear in patients with lead poisoning may reveal basophilic stippling: visible inclusions of ribosomes that appear as small dots in the periphery of RBCs (see Figure 41-5). Lead toxicity causes anemia because it inhibits heme biosynthesis and increases the fragility of RBCs, resulting in hemolysis.[12]

## NORMOCYTIC ANEMIA

**What laboratory test is helpful in subcategorizing the causes of normocytic anemia?**

The reticulocyte count of blood can determine whether normocytic anemia is hypoproliferative (low or normal reticulocyte count) or hyperproliferative (elevated reticulocyte count).

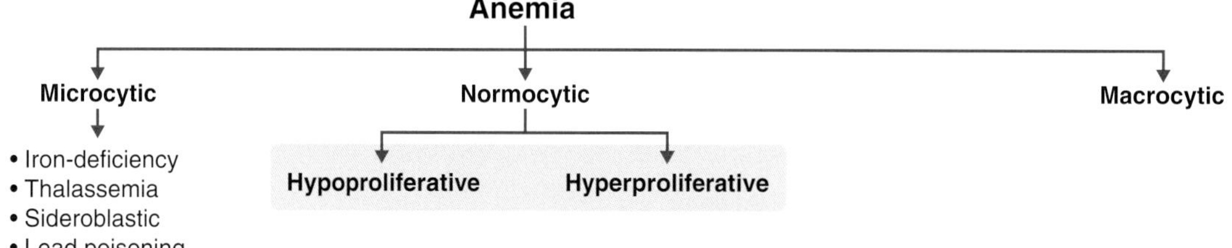


**What are reticulocytes?**

Reticulocytes are immature RBCs that are produced in bone marrow, released into the bloodstream, and mature into RBCs within 24 to 36 hours. Reticulocytes are larger than mature RBCs (see Figure 25-3). *If the reticulocyte count is significantly elevated, it can tip the balance toward macrocytosis.*[7]

**What does the reticulocyte count indicate about the function of the bone marrow?**

The normal reticulocyte count is 1% to 2%, a reflection of normal daily RBC turnover. In the setting of anemia, an increase in reticulocyte count suggests that the bone marrow is responding appropriately by increasing production of RBCs; a reticulocyte count <2% (even if it is in the "normal" range) suggests that the bone marrow is not responding appropriately. To use the reticulocyte count as an index of RBC production, it must be corrected for anemia (ie, corrected reticulocyte count).[7]

## NORMOCYTIC, HYPOPROLIFERATIVE ANEMIA

### What are the causes of normocytic, hypoproliferative anemia?

**A 56-year-old woman with diabetes and chronic osteomyelitis of the left great toe develops moderate, normocytic anemia over a period of several months.**

Anemia of inflammation (ie, anemia of chronic disease).

**The bone marrow cannot produce red blood cells without a stimulus.**

Insufficient erythropoietin from chronic kidney disease (CKD).

**Weight gain, constipation, dry skin, and depression.**

Hypothyroidism.

**A group of conditions that usually cause pancytopenia.**

Bone marrow failure.

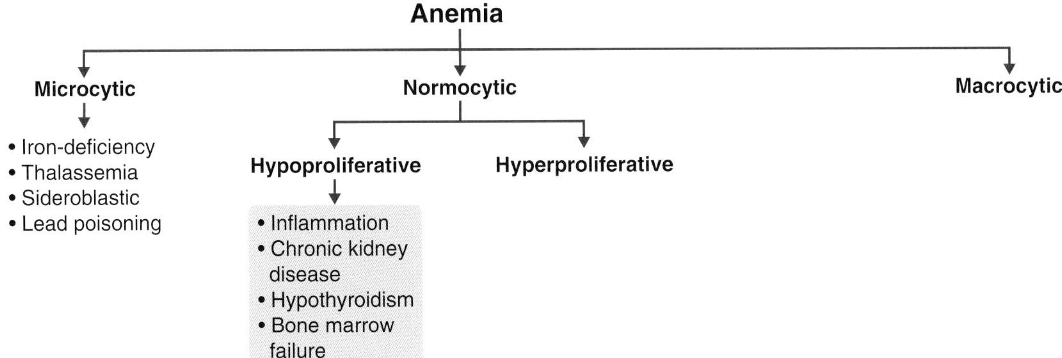


**What are the characteristics of anemia of inflammation?**

Anemia can occur as a result of acute or chronic inflammation through a variety of mechanisms, including changes in iron homeostasis (eg, limited iron availability for erythropoiesis), impaired proliferation and differentiation of erythroid progenitor cells, decreased production of and response to EPO, and shortened life span of RBCs. Anemia of inflammation is typically mild to moderate in severity, normochromic, and normocytic. Serum iron and transferrin saturation are both reduced. Serum ferritin is normal or increased. *Anemia of inflammation can sometimes present with mild microcytosis.*[6]

**What are the characteristics of anemia of chronic kidney disease?**

Anemia of CKD mainly occurs as a result of EPO deficiency. It is typically normochromic and normocytic, with an incidence and severity proportional to the degree of underlying kidney disease. When hemoglobin targets are modest (eg, 10-11.5 g/dL), treatment with erythropoiesis-stimulating agents (eg, darbepoetin) is associated with improved symptoms from anemia, improved quality of life, and decreased need for blood transfusions. However, higher hemoglobin targets (>13 g/dL) are associated with adverse outcomes, including stroke and hypertension.[17]

**What are the characteristics of anemia of hypothyroidism?**

Anemia occurs in almost one-half of patients with overt or subclinical hypothyroidism and is frequently the presenting manifestation. It is typically normochromic and normocytic, with a severity proportional to the degree of hypothyroidism. Mechanisms include marrow hypoproliferation from thyroid hormone deficiency, and decreased EPO production as a result of reduced oxygen requirements associated with the hypothyroid state. Iron deficiency is associated with hypothyroidism as a result of decreased gastrointestinal iron absorption and menorrhagia in women. Pernicious anemia is 20 times more common in patients with hypothyroidism and can result in vitamin B12 deficiency. These associated conditions can give rise to microcytic and macrocytic anemias in patients with hypothyroidism.[18,19]

**What is bone marrow failure?**

Bone marrow failure refers to a group of inherited and acquired conditions characterized by intrinsic dysfunction of hematopoiesis, usually resulting in pancytopenia. Causes of acquired bone marrow failure include aplastic anemia and infiltrative conditions (eg, leukemia, myelofibrosis) (see chapter 27, Pancytopenia). Pure red cell aplasia is a type of inherited or acquired bone marrow failure that presents with isolated anemia. Associated conditions include infection (eg, parvovirus B19), hematologic malignancies (eg, large granular lymphocyte leukemia), thymoma, medications (eg, phenytoin), and collagen vascular diseases (eg, systemic lupus erythematosus). The anemia is typically moderate to severe, normochromic, and normocytic, with a profound reticulocytopenia. Bone marrow is typically normocellular or hypocellular with a selective decrease or absence of erythroblasts.[20]

## NORMOCYTIC, HYPERPROLIFERATIVE ANEMIA

### What are the causes of normocytic, hyperproliferative anemia?

**A 48-year-old man who has been taking ibuprofen regularly for the past month for low back pain presents with acute-onset hematemesis, black stools, light-headedness, and hypotension.**

Gastrointestinal bleeding caused by peptic ulcer disease.

**A 29-year-old man presents with jaundice, dark urine, and normocytic anemia after starting trimethoprim-sulfamethoxazole for a soft tissue infection.**

Hemolytic anemia from glucose-6-phosphate dehydrogenase (G6PD) deficiency.

**May be palpable on physical examination.**

Splenomegaly.

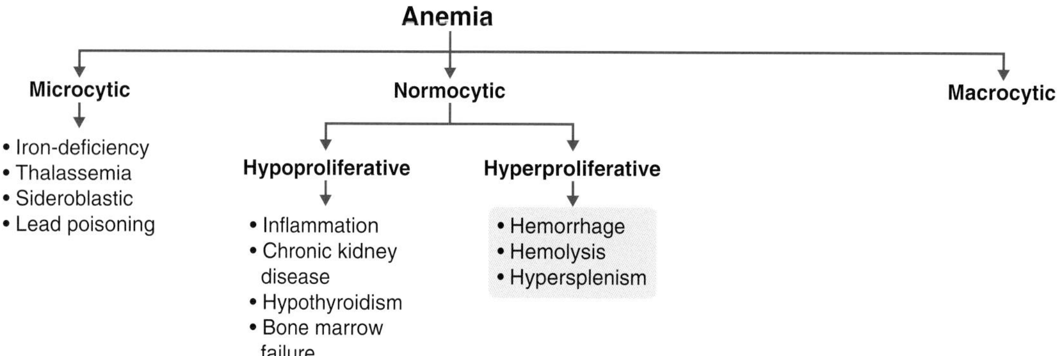


**What are the characteristics of anemia caused by acute hemorrhage?**

The effects of hypovolemia, including hypotension and decreased organ perfusion, dominate the clinical picture of acute blood loss anemia. Healthy young adult men in the third decade of life have approximately 6 L of total blood volume, which decreases to around 5 L by the seventh decade of life. Acute blood loss of up to 30% of total blood volume can manifest tachycardia and tachypnea, however blood pressure is typically normal or only mildly decreased. Acute blood loss >30% of total blood volume causes orthostatic hypotension that may progress to hypotensive shock, and is frequently associated with dyspnea, diaphoresis, cold and clammy skin, decreased urine output, and delayed capillary refill. *Acute blood loss may not initially result in decreased hemoglobin concentration. Chronic blood loss anemia may gradually deplete iron stores and result in microcytic iron-deficiency anemia.*[7,21]

**What are the laboratory features of hemolytic anemia?**

Hemolytic anemia is typically characterized by hyperproliferative anemia associated with evidence of RBC destruction, such as increased serum indirect bilirubin, increased serum aspartate aminotransferase, increased serum LDH, increased free serum hemoglobin, decreased serum haptoglobin, hemoglobinuria, and increased urine and stool urobilinogen. The pattern of laboratory abnormalities depends on whether hemolysis is intravascular or extravascular (see chapter 26, Hemolytic Anemia). The peripheral blood smear may demonstrate evidence of hemolysis (eg, reticulocytosis, polychromasia, nucleated RBCs) and other features suggestive of certain causes of hemolytic anemia (eg, schistocytes, spherocytes, bite cells). *Hemolysis may be associated with macrocytic anemia because reticulocytes are larger than mature RBCs.*[7,10]

**How does splenomegaly cause anemia?**

Splenomegaly and associated hypersplenism cause decreased hemoglobin concentration via 3 main mechanisms. First, there is an increased rate of RBC destruction (ie, hemolysis) within the enlarged spleen. Second, there is sequestration of RBCs; massively enlarged spleens are capable of sequestering as much as one-third of the total RBC mass. Third, splenomegaly causes an increase in plasma volume, resulting in a dilutional effect that decreases hemoglobin concentration. Splenomegaly is considered massive when it reaches the iliac crest, crosses the abdominal midline, or weighs more than 1500 g. The most common causes of massive splenomegaly include hematologic disorders (eg, chronic myeloid leukemia, primary myelofibrosis, polycythemia vera, indolent lymphoma, hairy cell leukemia, β-thalassemia major), infections (eg, visceral leishmaniasis [kala-azar], malaria), and infiltrative diseases (eg, Gaucher disease).[22,23]

## MACROCYTIC ANEMIA

**What are the 2 subcategories of macrocytic anemia?**

Macrocytic anemia can be megaloblastic or nonmegaloblastic.

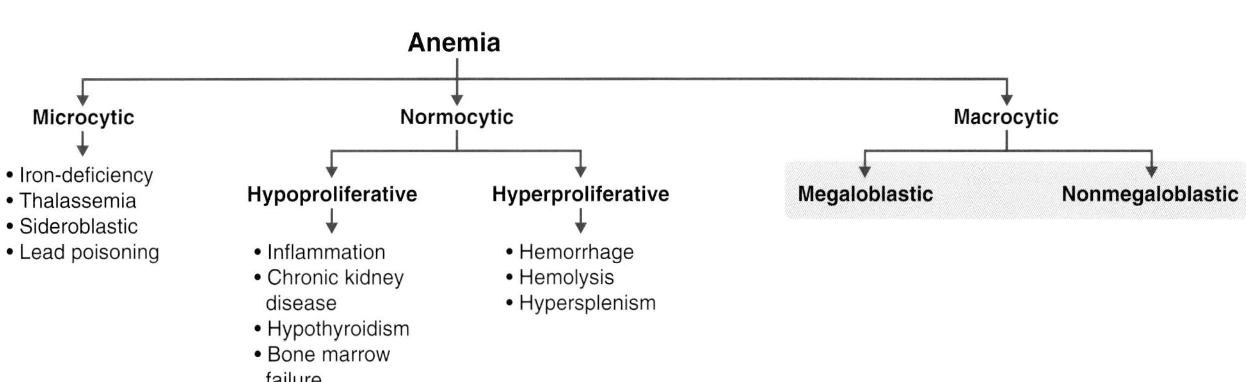


**What is megaloblastic anemia?**

Megaloblastic anemia occurs as a result of impaired deoxyribonucleic acid (DNA) synthesis that interferes with RBC proliferation and maturation. It is associated with characteristic features on peripheral blood smear and bone marrow aspirate. The impaired DNA synthesis of megaloblastic anemia affects all developing blood cells, often resulting in pancytopenia. Intramedullary lysis of erythroid progenitors can result in manifestations such as jaundice and elevated serum LDH levels.[10]

HEMATOLOGY

**What are the features of megaloblastic anemia on peripheral blood smear?**

The peripheral blood smear of megaloblastic anemia is characterized by the presence of large (MCV often >115 fL) and oval-shaped RBCs (macro-ovalocytes), hypersegmented neutrophils, anisocytosis (abnormal variation in RBC size), and poikilocytosis (eg, teardrop-shaped RBCs) (Figure 25-5). With the exception of myelodysplasia, nonmegaloblastic causes of macrocytosis generally result in round macrocytes.[10]

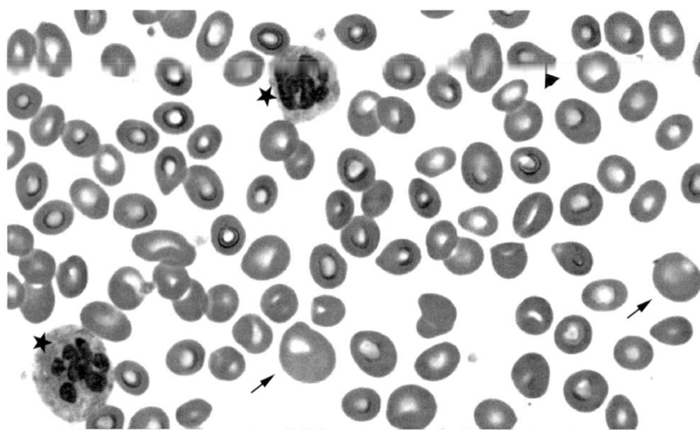

**Figure 25-5.** Peripheral blood smear from a patient with megaloblastic anemia due to vitamin B12 deficiency demonstrating many macro-ovalocytes (arrows) with anisocytosis, hypersegmented neutrophils (stars), and teardrop-shaped RBCs (arrowhead). Neutrophils are considered hypersegmented when more than 5% have 5 or more lobes, or when there are occasional neutrophils with 6 or more lobes. (From Weksler BB, Schechter GP, Ely SA. *Wintrobe's Atlas of Clinical Hematology*. 2nd ed. Philadelphia, PA: Wolters Kluwer; 2018.)

**What are the features of megaloblastic anemia on bone marrow evaluation?**

Megaloblastic anemia is associated with marrow hypercellularity and evidence of abnormal proliferation and maturation of multiple myeloid cell lines, including large, oval-shaped erythroblasts that contain a characteristic finely stippled, lacy nuclear chromatin pattern surrounded by normal-appearing cytoplasm (ie, nuclear-cytoplasmic dissociation). Such progenitor cells are referred to as "megaloblasts." Nonmegaloblastic conditions such as myelodysplasia and leukemia may be associated with "megaloblastic-like" abnormalities of the bone marrow, but can usually be distinguished with careful examination.[10,24]

## MEGALOBLASTIC ANEMIA

### What are the causes of megaloblastic anemia?

**A 68-year-old woman with Hashimoto's thyroiditis and vitiligo develops macrocytic anemia and ataxia.**

Vitamin B12 deficiency caused by pernicious anemia.

**Green leafy vegetables are an important part of a healthy diet.**

Folate deficiency.

**A patient with Wilson's disease who is taking more than the recommended doses of penicillamine and zinc acetate develops megaloblastic anemia and ataxia, and is found to have a positive Romberg test with brisk knee reflexes and absent ankle reflexes.**

Copper deficiency related to excess penicillamine (a copper-chelating agent) and zinc.

**A 23-year-old woman presents with megaloblastic anemia and admits to regularly tampering with whipped cream canisters to get high.**

Nitrous oxide inhalation (called "whippets").

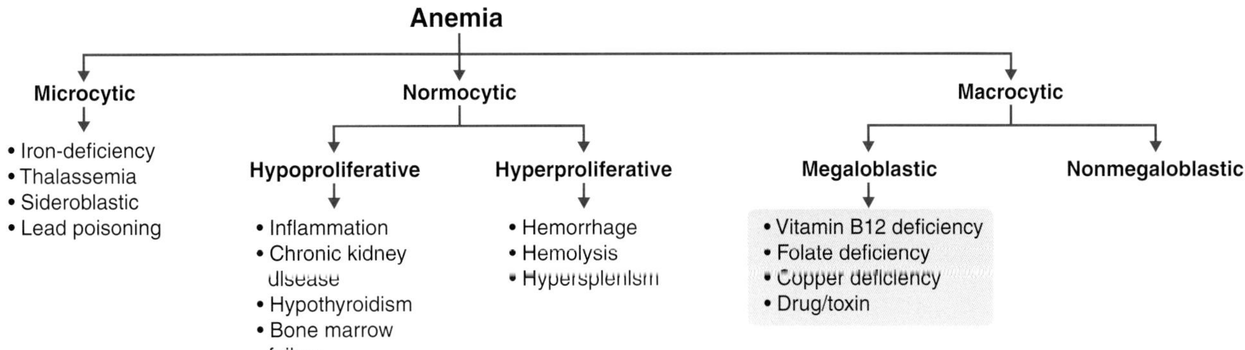


**What are the nonhematologic features of vitamin B12 deficiency?**

In addition to megaloblastic anemia, vitamin B12 deficiency often causes myeloneuropathy, the combination of spinal cord disease and peripheral neuropathy. The earliest clinical manifestations include ataxia and paresthesias in the extremities; other features include sensory loss, lower limb weakness, spasticity, hyperreflexia and/or hyporeflexia (eg, brisk patellar reflex with diminished Achilles reflex), cognitive impairment, and vision loss.[25]

**What serum laboratory tests can be helpful in diagnosing and differentiating megaloblastic anemia related to vitamin B12 and folate deficiency?**

In the context of a compatible clinical condition, plasma homocysteine and methylmalonic acid can be useful in the diagnosis of megaloblastic anemia. In patients with vitamin B12 deficiency, both metabolites are typically elevated, whereas in patients with folate deficiency, only homocysteine is elevated.[10]

**How common is folate deficiency in the industrialized world?**

Folate deficiency is rare in countries that fortify food with folic acid. However, some patients may have predisposing conditions that lead to folate deficiency, including poor nutritional intake (eg, eating disorders), gastrointestinal disease (eg, bariatric surgery), chronic alcohol use, chronic hemolysis (eg, sickle cell anemia), and conditions with high cellular turnover (eg, exfoliative dermatitis). In such patients it may be necessary to provide long-term prophylactic folic acid supplementation.[10]

**What are the risk factors for copper deficiency?**

Conditions that predispose patients to developing copper deficiency include gastrectomy, use of copper-chelating agents (eg, penicillamine), excessive zinc intake (due to zinc's interference with copper absorption in the small intestine), gastrointestinal disease (eg, inflammatory bowel disease), and chronic enteral or parenteral nutrition with insufficient copper supplementation.[25]

**What are the general mechanisms of megaloblastic anemia related to drugs or toxins?**

Drugs and toxins cause megaloblastic anemia by impairing either the cellular availability or use of vitamin B12 or folic acid. Nitrous oxide blocks the conversion of vitamin B12 from the reduced to the oxidized form, leading to impaired DNA synthesis. The list of drugs and toxins that can cause or contribute to megaloblastic anemia is extensive; some of the common ones include alcohol, immunomodulators (eg, azathioprine, mycophenolate), antineoplastic agents (eg, methotrexate, hydroxyurea), antimicrobial agents (eg, tetracyclines, penicillins, trimethoprim), antiseizure agents (eg, phenytoin), allopurinol, colchicine, metformin, and proton-pump inhibitors. *Medications that affect DNA synthesis (eg, hydroxyurea, azathioprine) can cause macrocytosis with or without megaloblastic changes.*[24,26]

## NONMEGALOBLASTIC MACROCYTIC ANEMIA

### What are the causes of nonmegaloblastic macrocytic anemia?

**Patients who consume this toxin in excess are also at risk for folate deficiency and liver disease.**

Alcohol.

**A 48-year-old woman with a history of chronic hepatitis C infection presents with jaundice, multiple spider angiomas on the chest, and mild, macrocytic anemia.**

Liver disease.

HEMATOLOGY

**A hematopoietic disease of the elderly.**

Myelodysplasia.

**A high percentage of immature RBCs.**

Reticulocytosis.

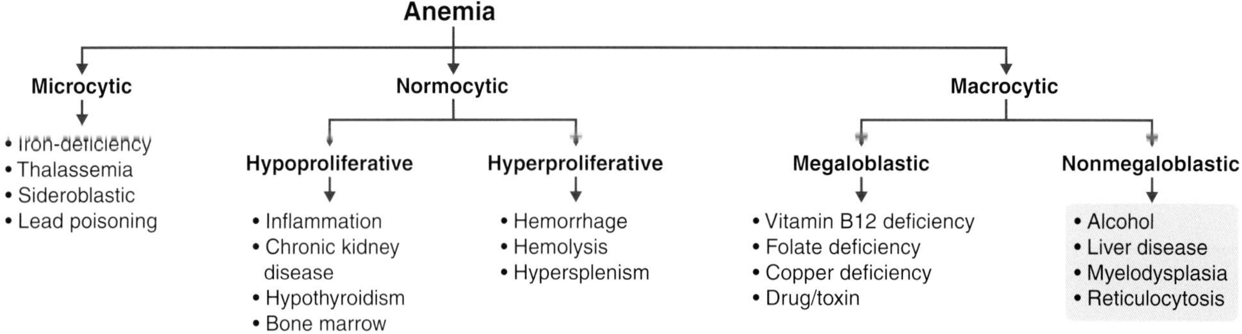


**How severe is the macrocytosis of alcoholism?**

Macrocytosis without anemia can occur with regular consumption of 30 to 40 g of alcohol (half a bottle of wine) daily, particularly in women. Anemia eventually develops, especially in patients with higher alcohol consumption (eg, >80 g/d). The mechanism of alcohol-related macrocytosis is unknown. The macrocytes are round, and the degree of severity is typically modest; the vast majority of cases are associated with MCV <110 fL when concomitant liver disease or megaloblastic anemia is absent.[26,27]

**What are the characteristics of the macrocytosis associated with liver disease?**

Patients with macrocytosis related to liver disease virtually always have stigmata of advanced liver disease on examination (eg, jaundice, spider angiomas) and abnormal liver function tests (eg, aminotransferase elevation). Concomitant thrombocytopenia and/or leukopenia is common. The round macrocytosis of nonalcoholic liver disease is typically modest with an average MCV of 105 fL; the average MCV of alcoholic liver disease is higher at 108 fL. The peripheral blood smear may also demonstrate target cells or acanthocytes (including spur cells) (Figure 25-6).[27]

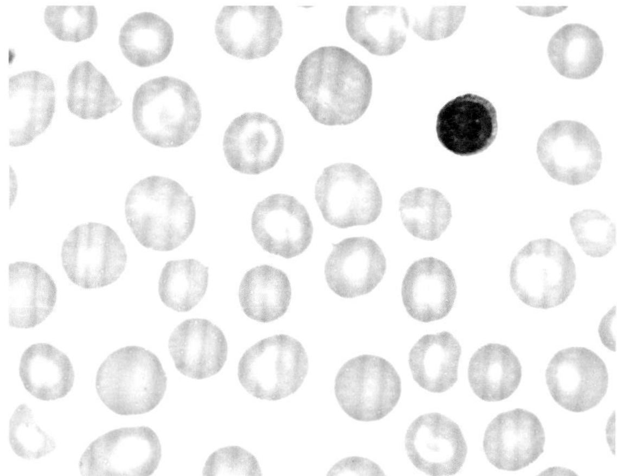

**Figure 25-6.** Peripheral blood smear from a patient with alcoholic liver disease demonstrating round macrocytosis and target cells. (From Pereira I, George TI, Arber DA. *Atlas of Peripheral Blood: The Primary Diagnostic Tool*. Philadelphia, PA: Wolters Kluwer Health; 2012.)

**Why is myelodysplasia sometimes confused for megaloblastic anemia?**

Both myelodysplasia and B12 deficiency are diseases of the elderly and often present with pancytopenia. Myelodysplasia is associated with megaloblastic-like changes of the bone marrow that can be confused for megaloblastic anemia. Careful examination is needed to make the distinction.[10]

**What degree of reticulocytosis is associated with macrocytosis?**

The vast majority of cases of macrocytosis caused by reticulocytosis feature a reticulocyte count ≥10%. Most cases are related to hemolytic anemia (eg, sickle cell anemia).[27]

**What are other causes of nonmegaloblastic macrocytosis?**

Other causes of nonmegaloblastic macrocytosis include pregnancy, hypothyroidism, aplastic anemia, pure red cell aplasia, acute leukemia, and multiple myeloma.[10,26]

## Case Summary

A 41-year-old man presents with fatigue and dyspnea following a mechanical fall and is found to have severe normocytic anemia with an elevated reticulocyte count, and complete opacification of the left hemithorax on chest imaging.

***What is the most likely cause of anemia in this patient?***

Hemothorax.

### BONUS QUESTIONS

***What is the most likely cause of the heart murmur in this case?***

The heart murmur in this case is likely a physiologic flow murmur related to the high output state of anemia. Other physical findings of anemia include tachycardia, wide pulse pressure, forceful heartbeat, strong peripheral pulses, and pallor of the mucous membranes and skin (see Figure 25-1A).[7]

***What physical findings suggest the presence of a pleural effusion?***

Physical findings of a pleural effusion include decreased inspiratory expansion of the chest wall on the affected side, dullness to percussion, decreased tactile fremitus, and reduced breath sounds over the effusion. *Lung consolidation may also present with dullness to percussion, however tactile fremitus is usually increased.*

***What are the causes of complete hemithorax opacification?***

In addition to pleural effusion, complete opacification of the hemithorax can occur as a result of lobar atelectasis from mucus plugging or endobronchial tumor. The direction of the trachea on the chest radiograph can help distinguish these conditions. Tracheal deviation toward the opacified hemithorax suggests volume loss over that area (ie, atelectasis); tracheal deviation away from the opacified hemithorax suggests a volume-occupying process (eg, pleural effusion). In this case, there is tracheal deviation away from the opacified hemithorax (see Figure 25-1B), consistent with pleural effusion.

***What is the most likely cause of the pleural effusion in this case?***

Given the associated severe anemia, the effusion in this case is most likely a hemothorax. An intercostal artery may have been disrupted by a rib fracture sustained during the ground-level fall. Hemothorax is confirmed when the pleural fluid hematocrit level is greater than half that of blood. An estimate of the hematocrit of the fluid can be obtained by dividing the RBC count by 100,000 (eg, RBC count of 1,000,000 = hematocrit of 10).[28]

| | |
|---|---|
| ***What are the causes of hemothorax?*** | Hemothorax is most often the result of chest trauma, including iatrogenesis (eg, cardiopulmonary surgery). Spontaneous hemothorax is less common but can occur in the context of anticoagulation therapy, tumors (eg, schwannoma, pleural metastases), rupture of pleural adhesions, pulmonary infarction, rupture of aneurysmatic thoracic arteries, rupture of pulmonary vascular malformations (eg, in patients with hereditary hemorrhagic telangiectasia), and thoracic endometriosis. Retention of blood in the pleural space can lead to chronic fibrothorax, trapped lung, impaired lung function, and infection.[29] |
| ***How should the hemothorax in this case be managed?*** | In most cases, hemothorax should be treated with insertion of a large bore (≥28 French) chest tube to drain the blood and allow for re-expansion of the lung. A chest radiograph should be repeated after thoracostomy to identify the position of the chest tube, identify any intrathoracic pathology, and confirm that the blood has been fully drained. Intrapleural fibrinolytic therapy may be necessary to break down residual blood clots and pleural adhesions. In order to maintain hemodynamic stability, a surgical approach may be necessary in patients with high rates of active bleeding that require repeated blood transfusions.[29] |

## KEY POINTS

- Anemia is defined by a reduced absolute quantity of circulating RBCs.
- Normal hemoglobin concentration varies by sex, age, race, and other environmental factors.
- The clinical features of anemia depend on severity, chronicity, and rate of onset.
- Symptoms of anemia include fatigue, loss of stamina, and dyspnea.
- Physical findings of anemia include tachycardia, wide pulse pressure, forceful heartbeat, strong peripheral pulses, systolic flow murmur, and pallor of the mucous membranes and skin.
- Anemia can be microcytic, normocytic, or macrocytic.
- The reticulocyte count determines whether normocytic anemia is hypoproliferative (reticulocyte count decreased or inappropriately normal) or hyperproliferative (reticulocyte count increased).
- Macrocytic anemia can be megaloblastic or nonmegaloblastic.
- Anemia of inflammation is usually associated with normocytic anemia but is sometimes associated with mild microcytosis.
- Reticulocytosis can be associated with either normocytic or macrocytic anemia.

## REFERENCES


1. Sankaran VG, Weiss MJ. Anemia: progress in molecular mechanisms and therapies. *Nat Med.* 2015;21(3):221-230.
2. Schriever HG. Red cell indices in thalassemia minor. *Ann Clin Lab Sci.* 1974;4(5):339-342.
3. Marino PL. *The ICU Book.* 3rd ed. Philadelphia, PA: Lippincott Williams & Wilkins; 2007.
4. Beutler E, Waalen J. The definition of anemia: what is the lower limit of normal of the blood hemoglobin concentration? *Blood.* 2006;107(5):1747-1750.
5. Lopez A, Cacoub P, Macdougall IC, Peyrin-Biroulet L. Iron deficiency anaemia. *Lancet.* 2016;387(10021):907-916.
6. Weiss G, Goodnough LT. Anemia of chronic disease. *N Engl J Med.* 2005;352(10):1011-1023.
7. Longo DL, Fauci AS, Kasper DL, Hauser SL, Jameson JL, Loscalzo J, eds. *Harrison's Principles of Internal Medicine.* 18th ed. New York, NY: McGraw-Hill; 2012.
8. Shemin D, Rittenberg D. The life span of the human red blood cell. *J Biol Chem.* 1946;166(2):627-636.
9. Hebert PC, Van der Linden P, Biro G, Hu LQ. Physiologic aspects of anemia. *Crit Care Clin.* 2004;20(2):187-212.
10. Aslinia F, Mazza JJ, Yale SH. Megaloblastic anemia and other causes of macrocytosis. *Clin Med Res.* 2006;4(3):236-241.
11. Stevens MH, Jacobsen T, Crofts AK. Lead and the deafness of Ludwig van Beethoven. *Laryngoscope.* 2013;123(11):2854-2858.
12. Wani AL, Ara A, Usmani JA. Lead toxicity: a review. *Interdiscip Toxicol.* 2015;8(2):55-64.
13. Camaschella C. Iron-deficiency anemia. *N Engl J Med.* 2015;372(19):1832-1843.
14. Guyatt GH, Oxman AD, Ali M, Willan A, McIlroy W, Patterson C. Laboratory diagnosis of iron-deficiency anemia: an overview. *J Gen Intern Med.* 1992;7(2):145-153.
15. Peters M, Heijboer H, Smiers F, Giordano PC. Diagnosis and management of thalassaemia. *BMJ.* 2012;344:e228.
16. Alcindor T, Bridges KR. Sideroblastic anaemias. *Br J Haematol.* 2002;116(4):733-743.
17. Kalantar-Zadeh K, Aronoff GR. Hemoglobin variability in anemia of chronic kidney disease. *J Am Soc Nephrol.* 2009;20(3):479-487.

18. Antonijevic N, Nesovic M, Trbojevic B, Milosevic R. Anemia in hypothyroidism. *Med Pregl*. 1999;52(3-5):136-140.
19. Erdogan M, Kosenli A, Ganidagli S, Kulaksizoglu M. Characteristics of anemia in subclinical and overt hypothyroid patients. *Endocr J*. 2012;59(3):213-220.
20. Leguit RJ, van den Tweel JG. The pathology of bone marrow failure. *Histopathology*. 2010;57(5):655-670.
21. Davy KP, Seals DR. Total blood volume in healthy young and older men. *J Appl Physiol (1985)*. 1994;76(5):2059-2062.
22. Hess CE, Ayers CR, Sandusky WR, Carpenter MA, Wetzel RA, Mohler DN. Mechanism of dilutional anemia in massive splenomegaly. *Blood*. 1976;47(4):629-644.
23. Paz YMHL, Gonzalez-Estrada A, Alraies MC. Massive splenomegaly. *BMJ Case Rep*. 2013;2013.
24. Hesdorffer CS, Longo DL. Drug-induced megaloblastic anemia. *N Engl J Med*. 2015;373(17):1649-1658.
25. Garg RK, Malhotra HS, Kumar N. Approach to a case of myeloneuropathy. *Ann Indian Acad Neurol*. 2016;19(2):183-187.
26. Hoffbrand V, Provan D. ABC of clinical haematology. Macrocytic anaemias. *BMJ*. 1997;314(7078):430-433.
27. Savage DG, Ogundipe A, Allen RH, Stabler SP, Lindenbaum J. Etiology and diagnostic evaluation of macrocytosis. *Am J Med Sci*. 2000;319(6):343-352.
28. Light RW. *Pleural Diseases*. 5th ed. Philadelphia, PA: Lippincott Williams & Wilkins; 2007.
29. Boersma WG, Stigt JA, Smit HJ. Treatment of haemothorax. *Respir Med*. 2010;104(11):1583-1587.

Chapter 26

# HEMOLYTIC ANEMIA

## Case: A 31-year-old woman with dark urine

A previously healthy 31-year-old woman presents to the emergency department with several days of fatigue, dyspnea, and dark tea-colored urine. The symptoms developed during a trip to Denver for an Ultimate Frisbee tournament. A few days before the trip, she went rafting on the Snake River in Oregon, where she was bitten by a spider but reports no other significant exposures. She consumed a bowl of fresh fava beans a day before the symptoms began. She has not recently taken any medications or supplements.

Heart rate is 105 beats per minute. There is generalized jaundice and scleral icterus. There is conjunctival pallor. No organomegaly is appreciated.

Hemoglobin is 6.9 g/dL, mean corpuscular volume (MCV) is 98 fL, and total bilirubin is 7.5 mg/dL with an indirect fraction of 7 mg/dL. The corrected reticulocyte count is 13%, lactate dehydrogenase (LDH) is 687 U/L, and haptoglobin is not detectable. The direct antiglobulin (Coombs) test is negative. Peripheral blood smear is shown in Figure 26-1.

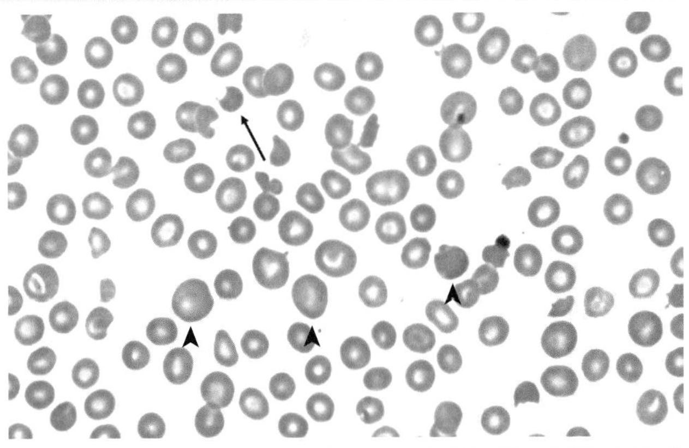

**Figure 26-1.** (Courtesy of Michael J. Cascio, MD.)

***What is the most likely cause of hemolytic anemia in this patient?***

What is hemolytic anemia?

Hemolysis describes premature destruction of red blood cells (RBCs), leading to a decrease in the average life span of the cells in circulation. Hemolytic anemia occurs when hemolysis outpaces bone marrow production.

What is the average life span of a red blood cell?

The average RBC has a life span of approximately 120 days; production of new RBCs (erythropoiesis) replaces 1% of circulating RBCs on a daily basis. Erythropoiesis normally occurs within the bone marrow and is stimulated by the hormone erythropoietin (EPO), which is produced and secreted primarily by the kidney (see Figure 25-2).[1–3]

Where does hemolysis occur within the body?

Hemolysis can be intravascular, extravascular, or both. Intravascular hemolysis occurs when RBC damage is severe enough to cause immediate lysis of cells within the intravascular space, which releases free hemoglobin into the bloodstream. Less severe RBC damage prompts the reticuloendothelial macrophages of the spleen and liver to remove the affected cells, generating unconjugated bilirubin from the breakdown of hemoglobin. *Disorders of ineffective hematopoiesis, such as megaloblastic anemia, can lead to premature intramedullary lysis of erythroid progenitors, mimicking hemolytic anemia.*[4]

**What are the symptoms of hemolytic anemia?**

The clinical features of hemolytic anemia depend on severity, chronicity, rate of onset, and location of hemolysis (intravascular or extravascular). Symptoms may include fatigue, loss of stamina, and dyspnea. Dark, "cola-colored" urine can indicate intravascular or severe extravascular hemolysis, red-colored urine can indicate rapid intravascular hemolysis, and flank pain can be present in abrupt-onset hemolysis.[3,4]

**What are the mechanisms of discolored urine in patients with hemolytic anemia?**

Intravascular and severe extravascular hemolysis results in the release of free hemoglobin into the bloodstream. It is oxidized to the darkly pigmented methemoglobin, which is filtered into urine, turning it a dark cola color. In cases of rapid intravascular hemolysis, fresh nonoxidized hemoglobin, which is bright red in color, is filtered into urine, giving it a reddish appearance. *A common misconception is that bilirubin is the cause of the dark urine of hemolytic anemia (the unconjugated bilirubin generated by extravascular hemolysis is water-insoluble and is not filtered into urine).*

**What are the physical findings of hemolytic anemia?**

Physical findings of hemolytic anemia may include fever, tachycardia, wide pulse pressure, forceful heartbeat, strong peripheral pulses, systolic flow murmur, pallor of the mucous membranes and skin (particularly in the palmar creases and nail beds where vessels are close to the skin), and jaundice and splenomegaly (in extravascular hemolysis).[3,4]

**What are the laboratory features of hemolytic anemia?**

Hemolytic anemia is typically a normocytic or macrocytic hyperproliferative anemia associated with evidence of RBC destruction such as increased excretion of urobilinogen in urine and stool, increased serum aspartate aminotransferase, increased serum indirect bilirubin (particularly in extravascular hemolysis), as well as increased serum LDH and decreased serum haptoglobin (particularly in intravascular hemolysis). When intravascular hemolysis is predominant or extravascular hemolysis is severe, there is increased free serum hemoglobin and hemoglobinuria (giving rise to cola-colored or red-colored urine). In hemolysis that is predominantly intravascular, serum bilirubin may be normal because only extravascular hemolysis involves the breakdown of hemoglobin into unconjugated bilirubin within reticuloendothelial macrophages. The peripheral blood smear may demonstrate evidence of hemolysis (eg, reticulocytosis, polychromasia, nucleated RBCs) and other features suggestive of certain causes of hemolytic anemia (eg, schistocytes, spherocytes, bite cells).[3,5]

**What are the clinical sequelae of chronic hemolysis?**

Chronic hemolysis can lead to the development of folate deficiency, cholelithiasis with pigmented gallstones, splenomegaly, leg ulcers, and pulmonary hypertension.[4]

**What are the 2 general ways in which patients develop hemolytic anemia?**

Hemolytic anemia can be inherited or acquired.

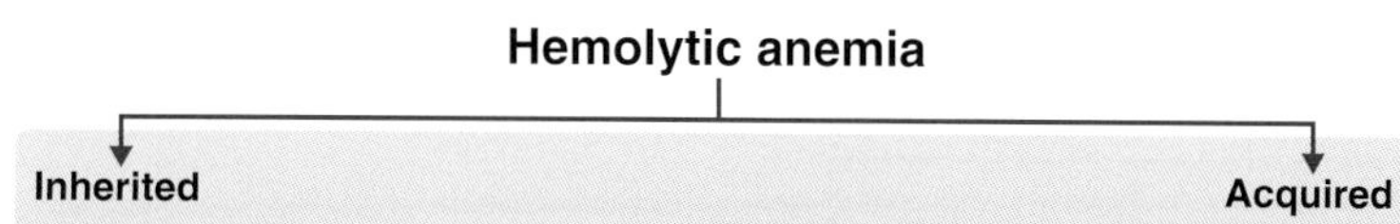


**What historical clues can help differentiate inherited and acquired causes of hemolytic anemia?**

Patients with inherited hemolytic anemia are more likely to present at a younger age and may have a positive family history. However, a family history is not always present when the inheritance pattern is recessive or when the patient has a de novo mutation. Additionally, children frequently acquire hemolytic anemia (eg, hemolytic uremic syndrome [HUS]), and some inherited conditions do not present until adulthood.[3]

## INHERITED HEMOLYTIC ANEMIA

**What are the subcategories of inherited hemolytic anemia based on the structural components of red blood cells?**

Inherited hemolytic anemia can be caused by defects that involve hemoglobin, intracellular enzymes, or the membrane-cytoskeleton complex.

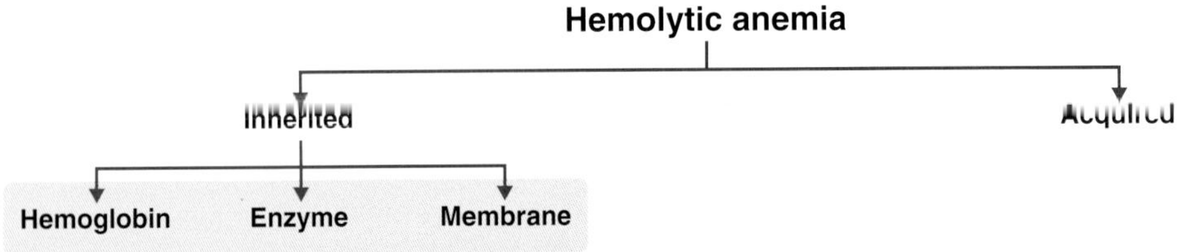


## INHERITED HEMOLYTIC ANEMIA RELATED TO HEMOGLOBIN DEFECTS

**What is hemoglobin?**

Hemoglobin is a molecule found in high concentrations inside RBCs and is responsible for carrying oxygen from the lungs to the rest of the tissues in the body. Hemoglobin A, which is composed of 2 $\alpha$ and 2 $\beta$ subunits, is the main form of hemoglobin in normal adults. Each subunit of hemoglobin contains a heme moiety made up of a porphyrin ring with an iron atom at its center, which allows for the binding of oxygen.[3]

**What is hemoglobinopathy?**

The hemoglobinopathies are a group of disorders characterized by defects in hemoglobin structure, function, or production. Solubility, reversible oxygen binding, and other important properties of hemoglobin may be deranged in hemoglobinopathies, leading to damaged RBCs and hemolysis.[3]

### What are the inherited hemoglobinopathies?

**The prevalence of this disease, caused by a missense mutation, is highest in regions of the world with current or past history of endemic malaria.**

Sickle cell anemia.

**This disease, found largely in Mediterranean and Southeast Asian populations, typically results in chronic microcytic anemia.**

Thalassemia.

**The allele that causes this hemoglobinopathy is sometimes found in combination with other abnormal alleles such as hemoglobin S.**

Hemoglobin C disease.

**There are numerous known variants, usually caused by amino acid substitutions.**

Unstable hemoglobin.

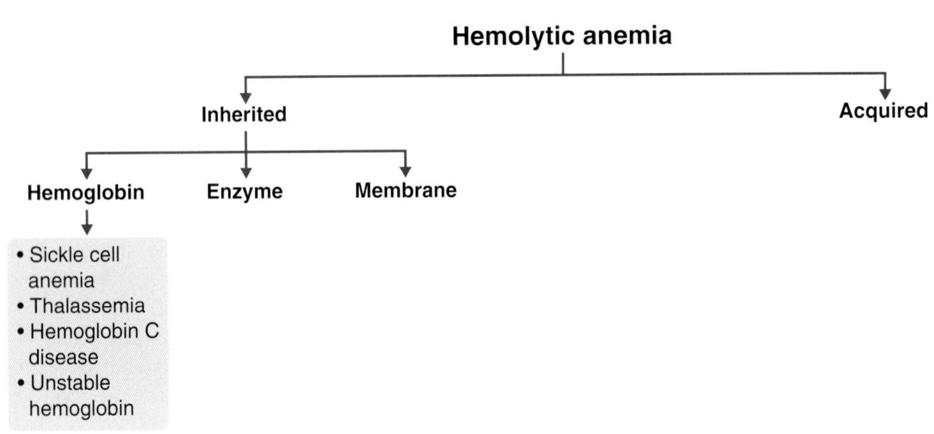

**What are the clinical features of sickle cell anemia?**

Sickle cell anemia is most often diagnosed in childhood. The mutated hemoglobin molecules are prone to polymerization, which distorts the shape of the RBC. Hemolysis occurs because the sickled RBCs are destroyed in the spleen. In addition to hemolytic anemia, clinical manifestations include vaso-occlusive events, acute chest syndrome, hip osteonecrosis, stroke, leg ulcers, priapism, myocardial infarction, and pulmonary hypertension. The peripheral blood smear demonstrates sickled cells (Figure 26-2). The diagnosis can be confirmed when hemoglobin electrophoresis demonstrates an excess of hemoglobin S.[4]

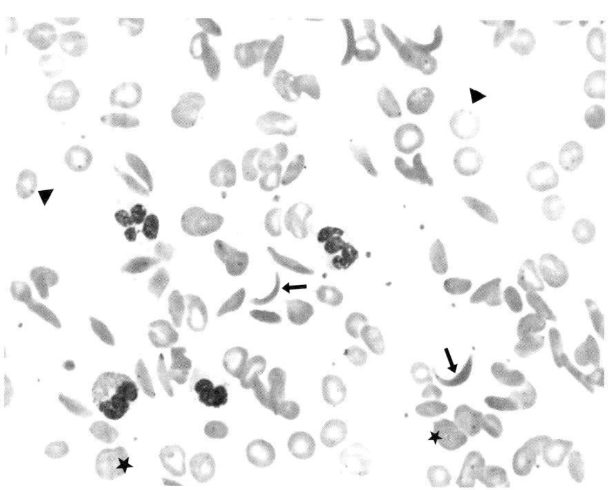

**Figure 26-2.** Sickle cells (drepanocytes) are crescent-shaped red cells with pointed ends on either side (arrows). Polychromatic RBCs (stars) and Howell-Jolly bodies (arrowheads) are also present, the latter of which indicate hyposplenism, a common complication of sickle cell disease. (From Pereira I, George TI, Arber DA. *Atlas of Peripheral Blood: The Primary Diagnostic Tool*. Philadelphia, PA: Wolters Kluwer Health; 2012.)

**What basic laboratory finding can provide a clue to the diagnosis of thalassemia?**

Most patients with thalassemia have at least some degree of anemia, microcytosis, and hypochromia. Hemolytic anemia occurs when the spleen detects and destroys abnormal RBCs. An increased RBC count in the face of decreased hemoglobin concentration and hematocrit may be a clue to the diagnosis of thalassemia. In addition to hypochromic microcytosis, the peripheral blood smear may demonstrate poikilocytes such as target cells and teardrop-shaped RBCs (see Figure 25-4), basophilic stippling, and nucleated RBCs. Hemoglobin evaluation (separation and measurement of the hemoglobin fractions) and genetic testing can confirm the diagnosis.[6]

**What are the characteristics of hemoglobin C disease?**

The hemoglobin C allele is protective against malaria and is found most frequently in patients from West Africa. The clinical features of homozygous hemoglobin C disease are generally benign. Most patients experience mild hemolytic anemia, and splenomegaly is found in more than one-half of patients. Peripheral blood smear may demonstrate target cells, spherocytes, and rod-shaped cells containing hemoglobin C crystals. In contrast to homozygotes, patients with hemoglobin SC disease (the combination of sickle cell trait and hemoglobin C trait) tend to have moderate to severe disease.[7,8]

**What peripheral blood smear finding is characteristic of the unstable hemoglobins?**

The unstable hemoglobins occur as a result of a variety of amino acid substitutions that reduce solubility or increase susceptibility to oxidation, resulting in the precipitation of hemoglobin and the formation of inclusion bodies that damage the RBC membrane. The inclusion bodies of denatured hemoglobin are called Heinz bodies and may be detected on the peripheral blood smear with special staining. When the spleen removes these inclusions, the cellular membranes become damaged, resulting in shortened survival with both extravascular and intravascular hemolysis.[3,4]

## INHERITED HEMOLYTIC ANEMIA RELATED TO INTRACELLULAR ENZYME DEFECTS

**What are the primary roles of the red blood cell enzymes?**

The 2 main functions of the RBC enzymes are the production of energy and the prevention of oxidative damage to hemoglobin and other proteins. Both processes are important for the maintenance of RBC organization, shape, structure, and survival.[3,4]

### What are the inherited red blood cell enzyme defects?

**A 33-year-old Syrian man develops jaundice and hemolytic anemia after eating warmed fūl (fava beans) mixed with olive oil, lemon juice, and garlic.**

Glucose 6 phosphate dehydrogenase (G6PD) deficiency.

**This condition involves the enzyme that catalyzes the final step in glycolysis.**

Pyruvate kinase deficiency.

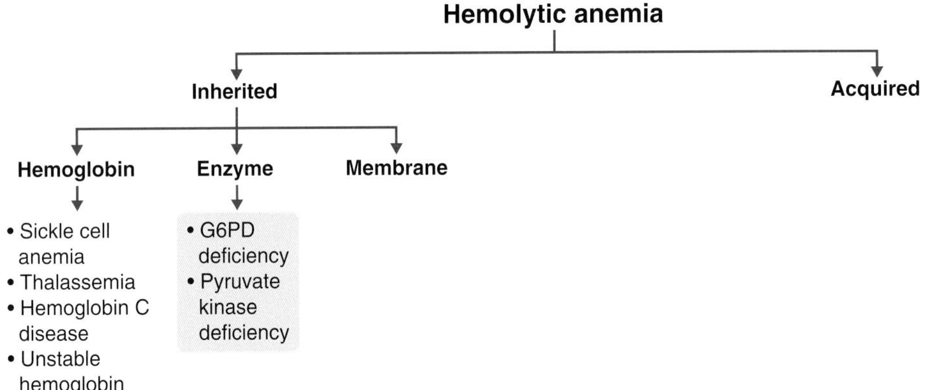


**What peripheral smear findings are associated with G6PD deficiency during an episode of acute hemolysis?**

Peripheral smear findings associated with the hemolysis of G6PD deficiency include anisocytosis (abnormal variation in RBC size), polychromasia, irregularly contracted cells (which are hyperchromic-like spherocytes but can be distinguished by an irregular outline), Heinz bodies, and characteristic poikilocytes, including blister cells or "hemighosts" (Figure 26-3) and bite cells (cells that appear as if a semicircular bite has been taken from them, which occurs when the spleen removes Heinz bodies).

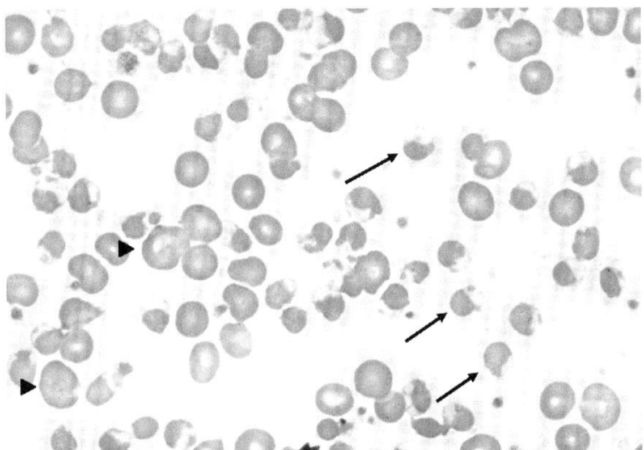

**Figure 26-3.** Peripheral blood smear from a patient with acute hemolysis related to G6PD deficiency, demonstrating blister cells (arrows) and polychromatic RBCs (arrowheads). Blister cells appear as if hemoglobin has been pushed to one side of the cell and are usually only present when hemolysis is brisk.[1] (Courtesy of Michael J. Cascio, MD.)

**What are the clinical features of pyruvate kinase deficiency?**

Pyruvate kinase deficiency is an uncommon disorder but is the most frequent defect of the glycolytic pathway. The degree of hemolysis between patients is highly variable, including some who are virtually asymptomatic and others who require regular blood transfusions. Hemolysis is mostly extravascular. Peripheral smear findings are nonspecific (eg, polychromasia, reticulocytosis). Splenectomy may be beneficial in patients with severe disease.[3,4]

## INHERITED HEMOLYTIC ANEMIA RELATED TO CELL MEMBRANE DEFECTS

**What are the main functions of the red blood cell membrane?**

The RBC membrane is designed to allow for a high degree of deformability, which is necessary for the cell to squeeze through microscopic structures; it is also responsible for maintaining cellular water balance. Defects in the RBC membrane may lead to the loss of cellular elasticity or dehydration or overhydration, shortening the life span of the cell.

### What are the inherited cell membrane defects?

**The peripheral smear findings of this condition could also be consistent with autoimmune hemolytic anemia.**

Hereditary spherocytosis.

**Also known as ovalocytosis, this disease confers some resistance against malaria.**

Hereditary elliptocytosis.

**Two conditions of abnormal red blood cell hydration.**

Hereditary stomatocytosis and hereditary xerocytosis.

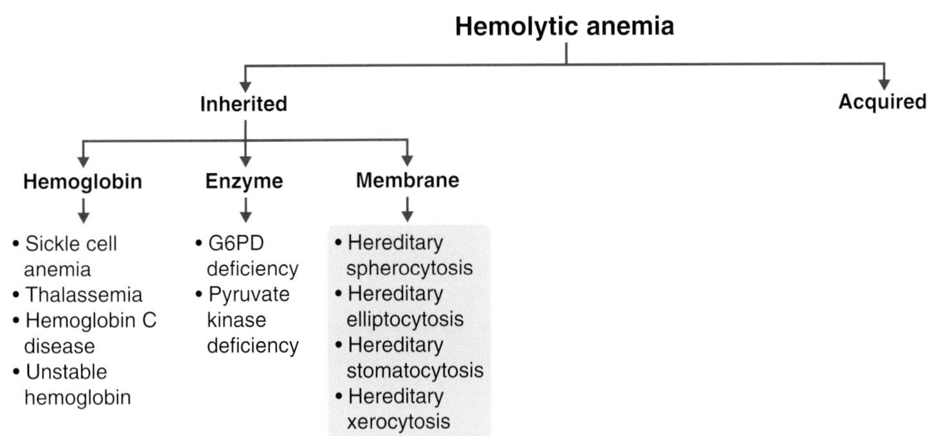


**What are the clinical features of hereditary spherocytosis?**

Hereditary spherocytosis is associated with a wide spectrum of disease, from severe hemolytic anemia starting in infancy to largely asymptomatic cases that present in adulthood. Presenting manifestations in adults may include jaundice, splenomegaly, or gallstones. Hereditary spherocytosis is one of the few conditions associated with an increased mean corpuscular hemoglobin concentration (MCHC), which may be a clue to the diagnosis. Spherocytes are the characteristic finding on peripheral blood smear; these cells are smaller than normal RBCs and lack central pallor. Osmotic fragility testing may be helpful. The condition is definitively diagnosed with molecular testing.[3]

**What are the clinical features of hereditary elliptocytosis?**

Hereditary elliptocytosis is clinically similar to hereditary spherocytosis with a wide range of disease severity. Elliptocytes are the characteristic finding on peripheral blood smear; these cells are elliptic or oval in shape (smaller than the oval macrocytes of megaloblastic anemia and myelodysplasia) (Figure 26-4).[3]

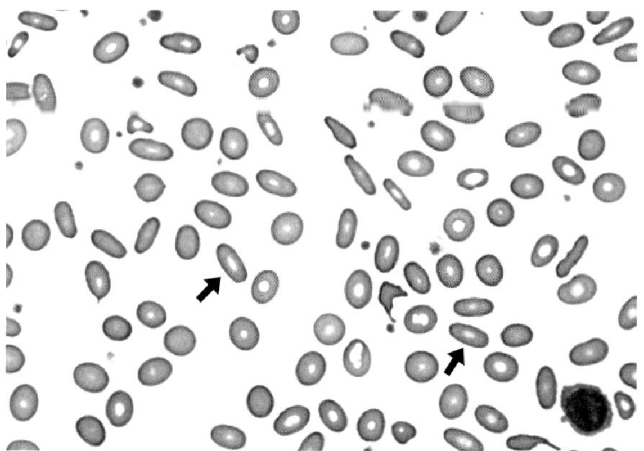

**Figure 26-4.** Peripheral blood smear demonstrating elliptocytes (arrows). Elliptocytes are elongated with rounded edges (as opposed to the sharp edges of sickle cells). (From Weksler BB, Schechter GP, Ely SA. *Wintrobe's Atlas of Clinical Hematology*. 2nd ed. Philadelphia, PA: Wolters Kluwer; 2018.)

**What are the differences between hereditary stomatocytosis and hereditary xerocytosis?**

Hereditary stomatocytosis and hereditary xerocytosis are both autosomal dominant conditions of abnormal RBC water content, thought to be driven by cation transport disturbances. Hereditary stomatocytosis describes RBC overhydration, which results in decreased MCHC and the presence of stomatocytes (RBCs with slit-like central pallor) on peripheral blood smear. Hereditary xerocytosis describes RBC dehydration, which results in increased MCHC and the presence of xerocytes (dense RBCs with marked hyperchromia) on peripheral blood smear. Osmotic fragility is increased in hereditary stomatocytosis but decreased in hereditary xerocytosis. Clinical severity is variable for both disorders. Splenectomy should be avoided in both conditions, as it increases the risk of thromboembolic complications.[3,4]

## ACQUIRED HEMOLYTIC ANEMIA

**What are the 4 mechanisms of acquired hemolytic anemia?**

Acquired hemolytic anemia can be immunologic, toxic, traumatic, or infectious.

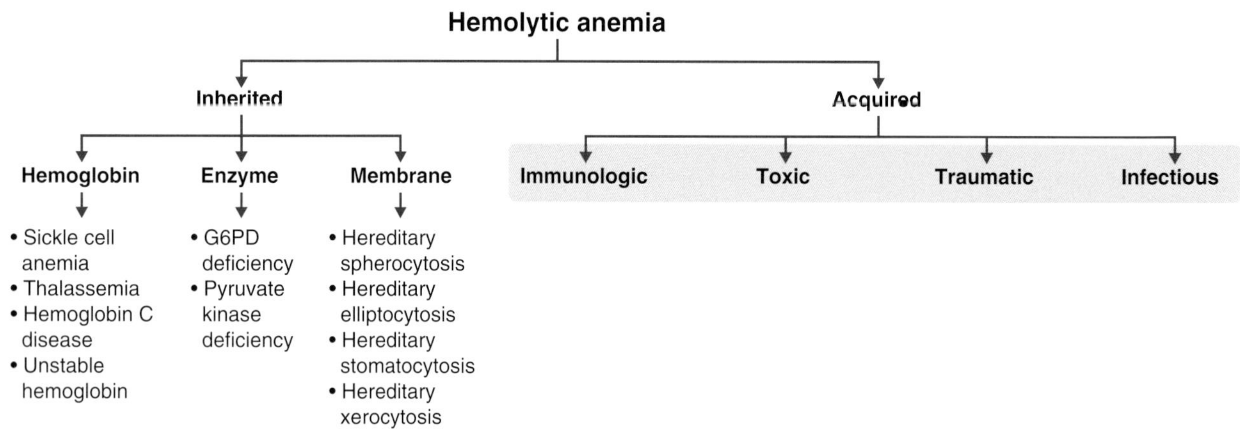

## IMMUNOLOGIC CAUSES OF ACQUIRED HEMOLYTIC ANEMIA

### What are the immunologic causes of acquired hemolytic anemia?

Spherocytosis and a positive direct Coombs test.

Autoimmune hemolytic anemia (AIHA).

History of multiple blood transfusions.

Alloimmune hemolytic anemia (eg, delayed hemolytic transfusion reaction).

A 44-year-old woman who is hospitalized for pyelonephritis develops jaundice and anemia after starting ceftriaxone.

Drug-induced immune hemolytic anemia.

A condition in which the largest lymphatic organ in the body becomes more active.

Hypersplenism.

Examples include acanthocytes (including spur cells) and echinocytes (burr cells).

Acquired erythrocyte membrane defects.

A 35-year-old man with several months of fatigue and episodes of red-colored urine that is most pronounced in the morning presents with acute abdominal pain and is found to have anemia, undetectable haptoglobin, and mesenteric vein thrombosis.

Paroxysmal nocturnal hemoglobinuria (PNH).

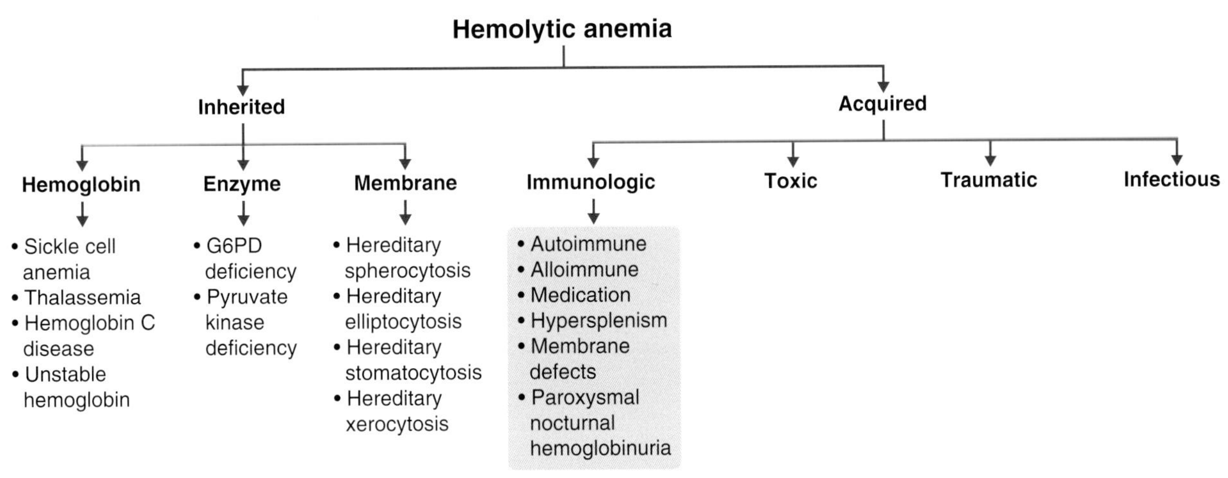


HEMATOLOGY

**What are the clinical features of autoimmune hemolytic anemia?**

AIHA is the most common acquired hemolytic anemia in countries where malaria is not endemic. It occurs when antibodies react with antigens on the surface of RBCs. It can be primary or secondary (eg, systemic lupus erythematosus, medication). Warm AIHA is associated with IgG antibodies, which react with RBC surface antigens at body temperature, causing extravascular hemolysis. Cold AIHA is associated with IgM antibodies, which are capable of fixing complement, resulting in intravascular hemolysis. AIHA is often abrupt in onset and may result in severe anemia, jaundice, and splenomegaly. Spherocytes, which are also seen in hereditary spherocytosis, are the characteristic sign on peripheral blood smear (Figure 26-5).

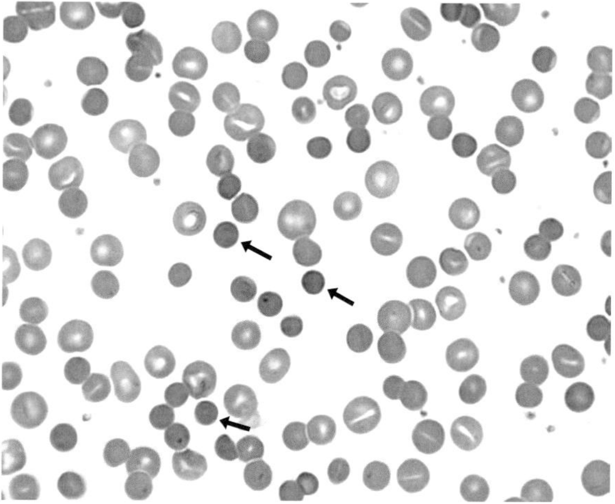

**Figure 26-5.** Peripheral blood smear from a patient with autoimmune hemolytic anemia demonstrating numerous spherocytes (arrows), small round RBCs lacking central pallor, and many polychromatic RBCs. (From Weksler BB, Schechter GP, Ely SA. *Wintrobe's Atlas of Clinical Hematology*. 2nd ed. Philadelphia, PA: Wolters Kluwer; 2018.)

**What is the most devastating type of alloimmune hemolytic anemia?**

Alloantibodies (antibodies directed against foreign antigens) can develop after pregnancy or exposure to blood transfusions. Most often, these alloantibodies are of the IgG class and result in delayed-onset mild extravascular hemolytic anemia. One of the most dramatic examples of alloimmunity is the acute hemolytic transfusion reaction, which occurs with transfusion of ABO-incompatible blood. Naturally occurring ABO alloantibodies are typically of the IgM class, which are capable of fixing complement and causing rapid-onset massive intravascular hemolysis of the foreign RBCs, which can lead to disseminated intravascular coagulation, renal failure, hypotensive shock, and death.[3]

**What medications are most frequently implicated in drug-induced immune-mediated hemolytic anemia?**

Medications can cause hemolytic anemia in a number of ways, such as triggering AIHA (eg, methyldopa), thrombotic microangiopathy (eg, quinine), and oxidative hemolysis, particularly in patients with G6PD deficiency (eg, dapsone). Medications can also cause an immune-mediated hemolytic anemia by coating the RBCs, which are subsequently targeted by drug-dependent antibodies. These antibodies are usually of the IgG class and cause extravascular hemolysis. Antibiotics are the most commonly implicated agents; including cefotetan, ceftriaxone, and piperacillin. The Coombs test is positive in the majority of these patients. Hemolytic anemia resolves quickly after discontinuation of the drug. Future exposures tend to trigger more severe hemolytic anemia.[9]

**What are the features of hemolytic anemia related to hypersplenism?**

Hypersplenism occurs as a result of splenomegaly and describes excessive sequestration and destruction of RBCs. The ensuing hemolytic anemia is typically mild and associated with other cytopenias.[4]

**What is spur cell anemia?**

Acanthocytes are dense and contracted RBCs with irregularly spaced "thorny" projections on the surface (echinocytes are similar, but the projections are longer, more numerous, and more evenly distributed around the periphery of the cell). These cells form in patients with advanced liver disease as a result of an increase in cholesterol content and cholesterol-to-phospholipid ratio of the cell membrane. Acanthocytes evolve into spur cells that are eventually destroyed by the spleen, resulting in extravascular hemolysis of moderate to severe degree.[10]

**What are the clinical features of paroxysmal nocturnal hemoglobinuria?**

PNH is a rare but life-threatening disease that affects men and women equally, and is most frequently diagnosed in the fourth decade of life. A somatic mutation causes deficient production of RBC membrane proteins, leaving cells vulnerable to complement-mediated destruction (particularly in the setting of infectious or inflammatory stimuli). Intravascular hemolysis results in hemoglobinuria that is most pronounced in the morning, a hallmark of the disease. Other common clinical manifestations include venous thrombosis and pancytopenia.[3,4]

## TOXIC CAUSES OF ACQUIRED HEMOLYTIC ANEMIA

### What are the toxic causes of acquired hemolytic anemia?

**Hemolytic anemia, chocolate-colored blood, and hemoglobin oxygen saturation of 85% by pulse oximetry.**

Dapsone toxicity.

**Associated with microcytic anemia and basophilic stippling on the peripheral blood smear.**

Lead poisoning.

**Reptiles and invertebrates.**

Snake bites, spider bites, and bee and wasp stings.

**Liver disease, Kayser-Fleischer rings (see Figure 17-2), and hemolytic anemia.**

Wilson's disease.

**The "gift of the Borgias."**

Arsenic poisoning.[11]

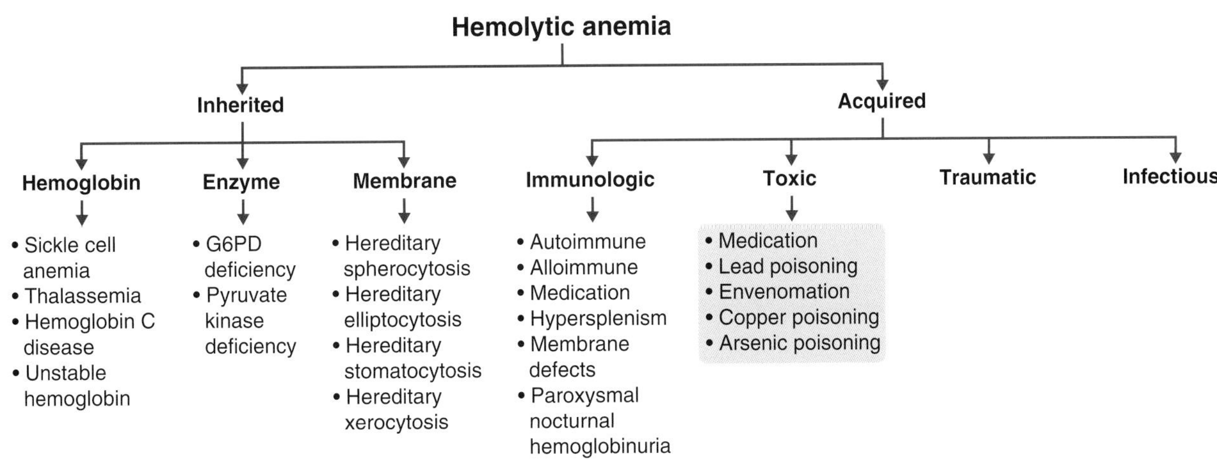


**Which medications can cause oxidative hemolysis even in patients without G6PD deficiency?**

Some medications such as nitrates, chlorates, methylene blue, dapsone, and cisplatin are capable of causing oxidative hemolysis even in the absence of G6PD deficiency.[3]

HEMATOLOGY

**What is the mechanism of hemolytic anemia related to lead toxicity?**

Lead poisoning is associated with an acquired deficiency of erythrocyte pyrimidine 5′-nucleotidase (P5′N-1), an enzyme involved in nucleotide metabolism, which causes hemolytic anemia by an unknown mechanism. Hereditary P5′N-1 deficiency also occurs but is rare. The hemolytic anemia associated with lead poisoning is mild to moderate, and may occur along with abdominal pain and peripheral edema. Basophilic stippling is the characteristic finding on peripheral blood smear (see Figure 41-5).[12]

**Where is the brown recluse spider (*Loxosceles reclusa*) endemic in the United States?**

The brown recluse spider is endemic to the mid-Southern and Southwestern United States. It is the most common cause of morbidity related to spider envenomation. Severe hemolytic anemia tends to develop within a week of envenomation, including features of both intravascular and extravascular hemolysis. Management is supportive, with resolution occurring over a period of several weeks.[13]

**How common is hemolytic anemia in patients with Wilson's disease?**

Wilson's disease is a rare inherited disorder that results in the accumulation of copper to toxic levels, often manifesting with liver and neurologic disease. Hemolytic anemia develops in approximately 10% of cases, usually when liver disease is advanced and hepatocellular necrosis results in the release of copper into the bloodstream. Both intravascular and extravascular hemolysis may occur. The combination of elevated serum copper and low serum ceruloplasmin is consistent with hemolysis related to Wilson's disease, whereas both are typically low in Wilson's disease without hemolysis. Prognosis is poor when Wilson's disease is not recognized and treated.[14]

**What are the features of acute arsenic poisoning?**

Arsenic exposure usually occurs as a result of unintentional arsine gas inhalation (eg, in industrial electronics manufacturing), or arsenic ingestion from contaminated food or drinks. Intoxication can be acute or chronic. Intravascular hemolysis occurs within 2 to 24 hours of acute exposure and is often accompanied by gastrointestinal sequelae (eg, abdominal pain, nausea, vomiting), and neurologic sequelae (eg, peripheral neuropathy, seizure, coma). Total urine arsenic level is most commonly used to make the diagnosis. Hair and nail analysis may also be useful. Plasmapheresis may be beneficial in patients with hemolytic anemia.[10,15]

## TRAUMATIC CAUSES OF ACQUIRED HEMOLYTIC ANEMIA

**What peripheral smear finding is characteristic of traumatic causes of hemolytic anemia?**

The presence of schistocytes on peripheral blood smear is the telltale sign of hemolytic anemia related to trauma. Schistocytes are fragmented RBCs that take the form of crescents, helmets, triangles, or microspheres. Hemolytic anemia related to intravascular RBC fragmentation is referred to as microangiopathic hemolytic anemia (MAHA).[10]

### What are the causes of microangiopathic hemolytic anemia?

**Hemolytic anemia, thrombocytopenia, acute kidney injury, fever, and delirium.**

Thrombotic thrombocytopenic purpura (TTP).

**Iatrogenic.**

Intravascular hardware.

**A previously healthy 24-year-old man who is training for an upcoming marathon complains of episodes of red-colored urine.**

Mechanical "march" hemoglobinuria.

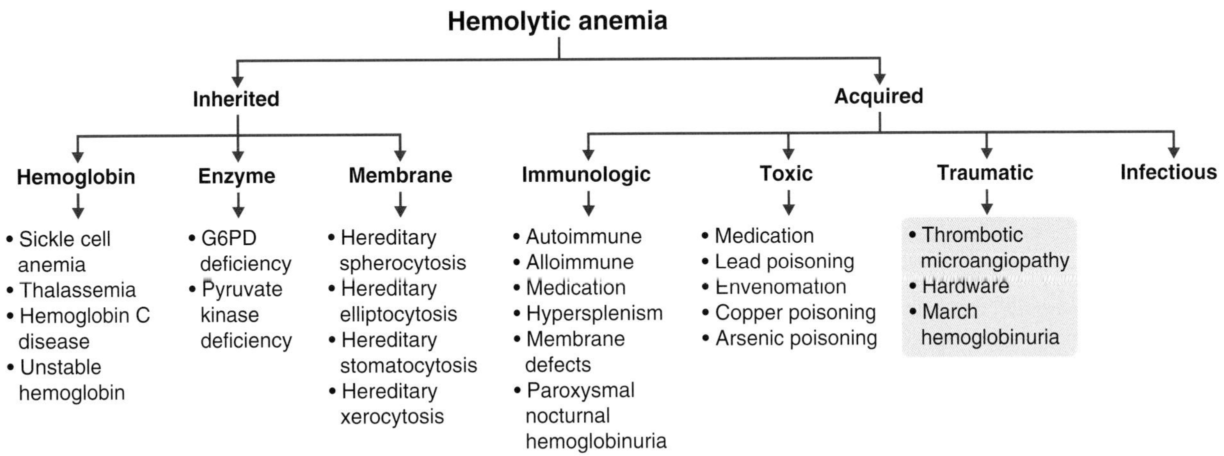


**What is thrombotic microangiopathy (TMA)?**

TMA refers to a diverse group of conditions with characteristic endothelial and blood vessel wall abnormalities associated with arteriolar and capillary thrombosis, leading to MAHA, thrombocytopenia, and organ damage. The primary syndromes of TMA include TTP, HUS (most often caused by Shiga toxin–producing *Escherichia coli* O157:H7), and drug-induced TMA. Thrombotic microangiopathy can also occur as a result of a variety of systemic conditions, including disseminated intravascular coagulation (DIC), severe hypertension, HELLP syndrome (hemolysis, elevated liver enzymes, low platelets), systemic infection (eg, human immunodeficiency virus), malignancy, autoimmune disorders (eg, systemic lupus erythematosus, antiphospholipid syndrome), severe vitamin B12 deficiency, and hematopoietic stem cell or organ transplantation.[16]

**What are some examples of hardware that can cause mechanical hemolysis?**

Prosthetic heart valves, patches for septal defects, ventricular assist devices (eg, left ventricular assist device [LVAD]), and transjugular intrahepatic portosystemic shunt (TIPS) may cause mechanical hemolysis. The presence of turbulent blood flow is generally necessary to cause RBC fragmentation (eg, mitral regurgitation in a patient with a prosthetic mitral valve).[10]

**What are the features of march hemoglobinuria?**

March hemoglobinuria describes mechanical trauma to RBCs caused by repetitive forceful contact of the body with hard surfaces, resulting in mild self-limited episodes of hemolytic anemia. It most often occurs in young men who run competitively but may also be precipitated by activities such as marching, drumming, and karate. Intravascular hemolysis results in red- or cola-colored urine immediately after exercise, which resolves within a few hours. Chronic recurrent hemoglobinuria can lead to iron-deficiency anemia in these patients.[10]

## INFECTIOUS CAUSES OF ACQUIRED HEMOLYTIC ANEMIA

**What are the general mechanisms of hemolysis caused by infection?**

Infectious agents can cause hemolysis via direct invasion of RBCs or through a variety of indirect mechanisms, including immune-mediated destruction, toxin-mediated destruction, hypersplenism, and trauma-mediated destruction (ie, MAHA).[17]

### What are the infectious causes of acquired hemolytic anemia?

**A 25-year-old woman presents with fever, malaise, and hemolytic anemia after a recent trip to the Ivory Coast.**

Malaria.

**Bloody diarrhea, hemolytic anemia, and acute kidney injury.**

Enterohemorrhagic *Escherichia coli* (EHEC).

**An anaerobic gram-positive rod.**

*Clostridium perfringens*.

**Atypical pneumonia.**

*Mycoplasma pneumoniae*.

**This organism is associated with community-acquired pneumonia and meningitis.**

*Haemophilus influenzae* type B.

**A tick-borne disease.**

Babesiosis.

**In 1865, a medical student named Carrión developed fatal hemolytic anemia after inoculating himself with this organism.**

*Bartonella bacilliformis* (Carrión's disease or Oroya fever).[17]

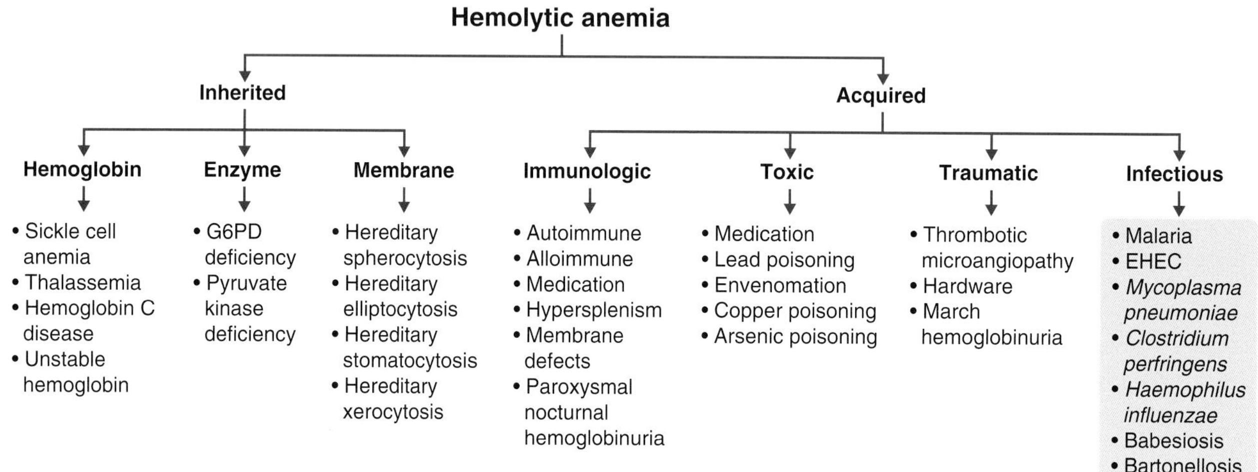


**What are the features of the hemolytic anemia caused by malaria?**

Malaria is a mosquito-borne disease and the most common cause of hemolytic anemia in endemic countries. Four different species are capable of causing disease in humans. *Plasmodia falciparum* is responsible for most cases in Africa and Southeast Asia, while *Plasmodia vivax* is the most frequent culprit in Central America and India. Hemolytic anemia is most often a result of splenic destruction of infected RBCs. However, acute severe intravascular hemolysis (known as blackwater fever) can occur and may be precipitated by certain medications (eg, quinine). Diagnosis of malaria can be made by direct visualization of the parasites using thin and thick blood smears.[10]

**What is the mechanism of hemolysis caused by infection with enterohemorrhagic *Escherichia coli*?**

HUS is the most serious complication of EHEC infection. It is most often caused by serotype O157:H7 and is characterized by the triad of hemolytic anemia, thrombocytopenia, and acute kidney injury. Use of antibiotics does not shorten the duration of EHEC infection, and evidence suggests antibiotics may precipitate HUS in these patients.[18]

**What is the mechanism of hemolysis caused by infection with *Mycoplasma pneumoniae*?**

In more than one-half of cases, *Mycoplasma pneumoniae* infection is associated with cold agglutinins (IgM immunoglobulins) that attack RBCs, fix complement, and cause intravascular hemolysis. These antibodies develop during the first 7 to 10 days of infection, peak after a few weeks, and persist for a few months. Most cases of hemolysis are not severe.[17]

**What is the prognosis of patients with hemolytic anemia related to *Clostridium perfringens*?**

*Clostridium perfringens* bacteremia is complicated by toxin-mediated severe intravascular hemolysis in up to 15% of cases. Mortality rate is approximately 75% with a median time to death of 10 hours. Survival is improved in cases where both penicillin and clindamycin are used instead of monotherapy and in patients who undergo surgical debridement of an infected focus. Hyperbaric oxygen therapy may also be effective, as *Clostridium* species lack superoxide dismutase and cannot survive in oxygen-rich environments.[19]

**What is the mechanism of hemolysis caused by infection with *Haemophilus influenzae* type B?**

Severe hemolysis is a rare complication of invasive *Haemophilus influenzae* B infection. It occurs when the capsular polysaccharide is released from the organism and binds to the surface of RBCs, which later becomes the target of immune-mediated destruction, with ensuing extravascular hemolysis and complement-mediated intravascular hemolysis.[17]

**What finding on peripheral blood smear is pathognomonic for babesiosis?**

Like malaria, *Babesia* parasites directly invade RBCs and alter structure and function, leading to splenic sequestration and destruction. Peripheral blood smear examination may reveal intracellular organisms. Although uncommon, the presence of tetrads of merozoites that resemble a "Maltese cross" is pathognomonic for babesiosis (Figure 26-6).[3,17]

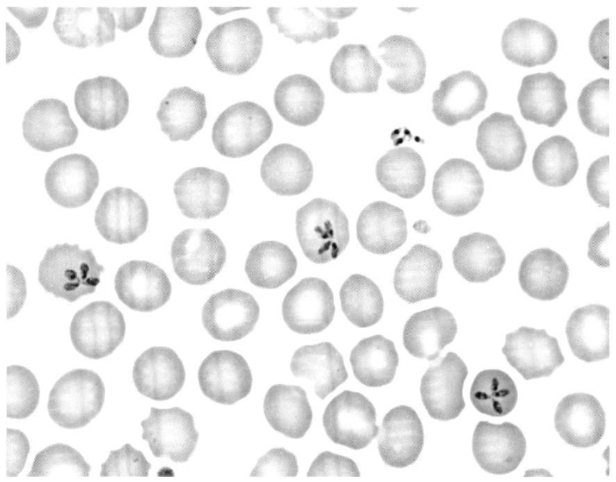

**Figure 26-6.** Although the *Babesia* species can demonstrate ring forms and be confused with *Plasmodia falciparum*, the presence of the "Maltese cross," comprised of tetrads of *Babesia* merozoites, can be a distinguishing feature. (From Pereira I, George TI, Arber DA. *Atlas of Peripheral Blood: The Primary Diagnostic Tool.* Philadelphia, PA: Wolters Kluwer Health; 2012.)

**What are the features of *Bartonella bacilliformis* infection?**

*Bartonella bacilliformis* is endemic to Peru, Ecuador, and Colombia and is transmitted via sand fly bite. The organisms directly invade RBCs, usually resulting in acute-onset intravascular and extravascular hemolysis with severe and life-threatening anemia. The peripheral blood smear may reveal intraerythrocytic bacilli.[3,17]

## Case Summary

A previously healthy 31-year-old woman presents with fatigue, dyspnea, and dark tea-colored urine and is found to have hemolytic anemia in the setting of a spider bite and ingestion of fava beans.

***What is the most likely cause of hemolytic anemia in this patient?***

Glucose-6-phosphate dehydrogenase deficiency.

BONUS QUESTIONS

***How common is G6PD deficiency?***

G6PD deficiency is the most frequent RBC enzyme defect, occurring in up to one-fifth of the general population in some regions. It is most common in patients from Africa, the Mediterranean region, Southeast Asia, and Oceania, where it is relatively protective against malaria. Inheritance is X-linked, but heterozygous females can be affected to the same degree as hemizygous males because of the phenomenon of X-chromosome inactivation.[3]

***Why does G6PD deficiency cause hemolytic anemia?***

G6PD is an enzyme found in RBCs that is important in producing reduced nicotinamide adenine dinucleotide phosphate (NADPH), which acts to stabilize several antioxidant compounds within the RBC. When G6PD is deficient, RBCs are susceptible to oxidative stress, which results in premature lysis. The vast majority of patients are asymptomatic. However, patients can experience acute episodes of moderate to severe intravascular and extravascular hemolytic anemia when exposed to oxidative agents (such as fava beans via direct ingestion of beans or exposure to pollen from the fava plant), infections, or medications (eg, sulfamethoxazole).[3]

***Why does ingestion of fava beans cause hemolytic anemia in patients with G6PD deficiency?***

Divicine and isouramil are thought to be the components of fava beans responsible for the increase in RBC oxidant stress. Not all G6PD-deficient individuals experience favism. *It is said that Greek mathematician and philosopher Pythagoras, when chased by his enemies, chose certain death over fleeing through a field of fava beans.*[20]

***What features of this case are suggestive of G6PD deficiency?***

Features of this case consistent with G6PD deficiency include the dark tea-colored urine, which suggests intravascular hemolysis, the recent exposure to fava beans, and the presence of a bite cell on the peripheral blood smear (see Figure 26-1, arrow). Reticulocytes are also present (see Figure 26-1, arrowheads).

***Why is the peripheral blood smear important in the investigation of G6PD deficiency?***

For a number of reasons, the peripheral blood smear is important in the diagnosis of G6PD deficiency, particularly during an acute attack of hemolytic anemia. First, the results of a peripheral blood smear evaluation return sooner than the G6PD activity assay. Second, G6PD activity may be normal during acute episodes. For example, in heterozygous women, acute hemolysis preferentially involves abnormal RBCs, leaving a higher proportion of normal cells in circulation, leading to a falsely normal assay.[21]

***What is the relevance of the spider bite in this case?***

Envenomation by the brown recluse spider can cause hemolytic anemia. However, in this case, that possibility is unlikely because the brown recluse is not endemic to Oregon.

***How is G6PD deficiency managed?***

The treatment for acute hemolytic anemia associated with G6PD deficiency is mostly supportive, but can include blood transfusions if clinically indicated. Diagnosis and prevention of future episodes are important for long-term management. Patients should be given a list of typical triggers with advice to avoid exposure when possible.[3]

## KEY POINTS

- Hemolysis is the premature destruction of RBCs; hemolytic anemia occurs when hemolysis outpaces bone marrow production.
- The symptoms of hemolytic anemia include fatigue, loss of stamina, and dyspnea. Dark cola-colored urine can indicate intravascular or severe extravascular hemolysis, red-colored urine can indicate rapid intravascular hemolysis, and flank pain can be present in abrupt-onset hemolysis.
- Physical findings of hemolytic anemia include fever, tachycardia, wide pulse pressure, forceful heartbeat, strong peripheral pulses, systolic flow murmur, pallor of the mucous membranes and skin, and jaundice and splenomegaly (in extravascular hemolysis).
- Hemolytic anemia is typically a normocytic or macrocytic hyperproliferative anemia associated with evidence of RBC destruction (eg, elevated serum LDH).
- Hemoglobinemia and hemoglobinuria are the biochemical hallmarks of intravascular hemolysis.
- The peripheral blood smear is an important diagnostic study in patients with hemolytic anemia and can be suggestive of specific etiologies.
- Hemolytic anemia can be inherited or acquired.
- Inherited hemolytic anemia can be caused by defects that involve hemoglobin, intracellular enzymes, or the membrane-cytoskeleton complex.
- Acquired hemolytic anemia can be immunologic, toxic, traumatic, or infectious.

## REFERENCES


1. Eadie GS, Brown IW Jr. The potential life span and ultimate survival of fresh red blood cells in normal healthy recipients as studied by simultaneous Cr51 tagging and differential hemolysis. *J Clin Invest*. 1955;34(4):629-636.
2. Shemin D, Rittenberg D. The life span of the human red blood cell. *J Biol Chem*. 1946;166(2):627-636.
3. Longo DL, Fauci AS, Kasper DL, Hauser SL, Jameson JL, Loscalzo J, eds. *Harrison's Principles of Internal Medicine*. 18th ed. New York, NY: McGraw-Hill; 2012.
4. Guillaud C, Loustau V, Michel M. Hemolytic anemia in adults: main causes and diagnostic procedures. *Expert Rev Hematol*. 2012;5(2):229-241.
5. Aslinia F, Mazza JJ, Yale SH. Megaloblastic anemia and other causes of macrocytosis. *Clin Med Res*. 2006;4(3):236-241.
6. Peters M, Heijboer H, Smiers F, Giordano PC. Diagnosis and management of thalassaemia. *BMJ*. 2012;344:e228.
7. Fairhurst RM, Casella JF. Images in clinical medicine. Homozygous hemoglobin C disease. *N Engl J Med*. 2004;350(26):e24.
8. Nagel RL, Fabry ME, Steinberg MH. The paradox of hemoglobin SC disease. *Blood Rev*. 2003;17(3):167-178.
9. Garratty G. Drug-induced immune hemolytic anemia. *Hematology Am Soc Hematol Educ Program*. 2009:73-79.
10. Greer JP, Foerster J, Rodgers GM, et al, eds. *Wintrobe's Clinical Hematology*. 12th ed. Philadelphia, PA: Lippincott Williams & Wilkins, A Wolters Kluwer Business; 2009.
11. Meek WJ. The gentle art of poisoning. *J Am Med Assoc*. 1955;158(4):335-339.
12. Valentine WN, Paglia DE, Fink K, Madokoro G. Lead poisoning: association with hemolytic anemia, basophilic stippling, erythrocyte pyrimidine 5'-nucleotidase deficiency, and intraerythrocytic accumulation of pyrimidines. *J Clin Invest*. 1976;58(4):926-932.
13. McDade J, Aygun B, Ware RE. Brown recluse spider (Loxosceles reclusa) envenomation leading to acute hemolytic anemia in six adolescents. *J Pediatr*. 2010;156(1):155-157.
14. Walshe JM. The acute haemolytic syndrome in Wilson's disease–a review of 22 patients. *QJM*. 2013;106(11):1003-1008.
15. Lee JJ, Kim YK, Cho SH, et al. Hemolytic anemia as a sequela of arsenic intoxication following long-term ingestion of traditional Chinese medicine. *J Korean Med Sci*. 2004;19(1):127-129.
16. George JN, Nester CM. Syndromes of thrombotic microangiopathy. *N Engl J Med*. 2014;371(7):654-666.
17. McCullough J. RBCs as targets of infection. *Hematology Am Soc Hematol Educ Program*. 2014;2014(1):404-409.
18. Page AV, Liles WC. Enterohemorrhagic *Escherichia coli* infections and the hemolytic-uremic syndrome. *Med Clin North Am*. 2013;97(4):681-695, xi.
19. Simon TG, Bradley J, Jones A, Carino G. Massive intravascular hemolysis from Clostridium perfringens septicemia: a review. *J Intensive Care Med*. 2014;29(6):327-333.
20. Beutler E. Glucose-6-phosphate dehydrogenase deficiency: a historical perspective. *Blood*. 2008;111(1):16-24.
21. Bain BJ. Diagnosis from the blood smear. *N Engl J Med*. 2005;353(5):498-507.

Chapter 27

# PANCYTOPENIA

## Case: A 34-year-old man with easy bruising

A 34-year-old man presents with several weeks of fatigue, dyspnea, and easy bruising. The patient grew up in Belarus, near its southeastern border with Ukraine, before moving to Oregon at 14 years of age. He has not recently traveled outside of the Pacific Northwest. He does not take any prescription or over-the-counter medications or supplements. He does not use illicit drugs.

The patient is afebrile with a heart rate of 96 beats per minute. There is conjunctival pallor. No lymphadenopathy or organomegaly is appreciated.

Peripheral white blood cell (WBC) count is 2.1 K/μL, hemoglobin is 7.6 g/dL, mean corpuscular volume (MCV) is 93 fL, and platelet count is 28 K/μL. Plasma methylmalonic acid and homocysteine levels are within normal limits. Human immunodeficiency virus (HIV) antibodies are not detected in the serum. Peripheral blood smear demonstrates leukopenia, thrombocytopenia, and anemia with reticulocytopenia. Bone marrow aspirate shows hypocellularity with normal cellular morphology. A core biopsy of the bone marrow with hematoxylin and eosin staining is shown in Figure 27-1.

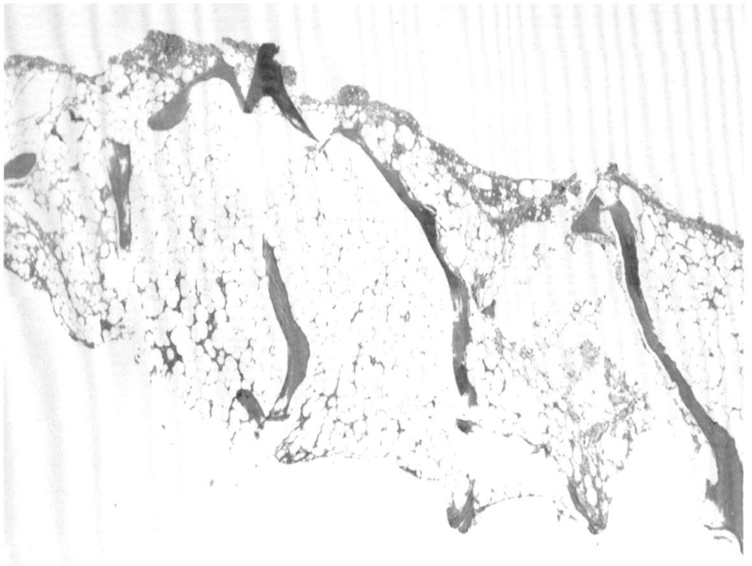

**Figure 27-1.**

***What is the most likely cause of pancytopenia in this patient?***

**What is pancytopenia?**

Pancytopenia describes the simultaneous presence of leukopenia, anemia, and thrombocytopenia.

**Where are blood cells produced?**

Hematopoietic stem cells found within bone marrow give rise to myeloid and lymphoid progenitor cells. These cells further differentiate into WBCs, red blood cells (RBCs), and platelets (Figure 27-2). These cells are eventually cleared by the reticuloendothelial system. WBCs survive for hours to years, depending on type; RBCs survive for 120 days; and platelets survive for 9 days.[1-3]

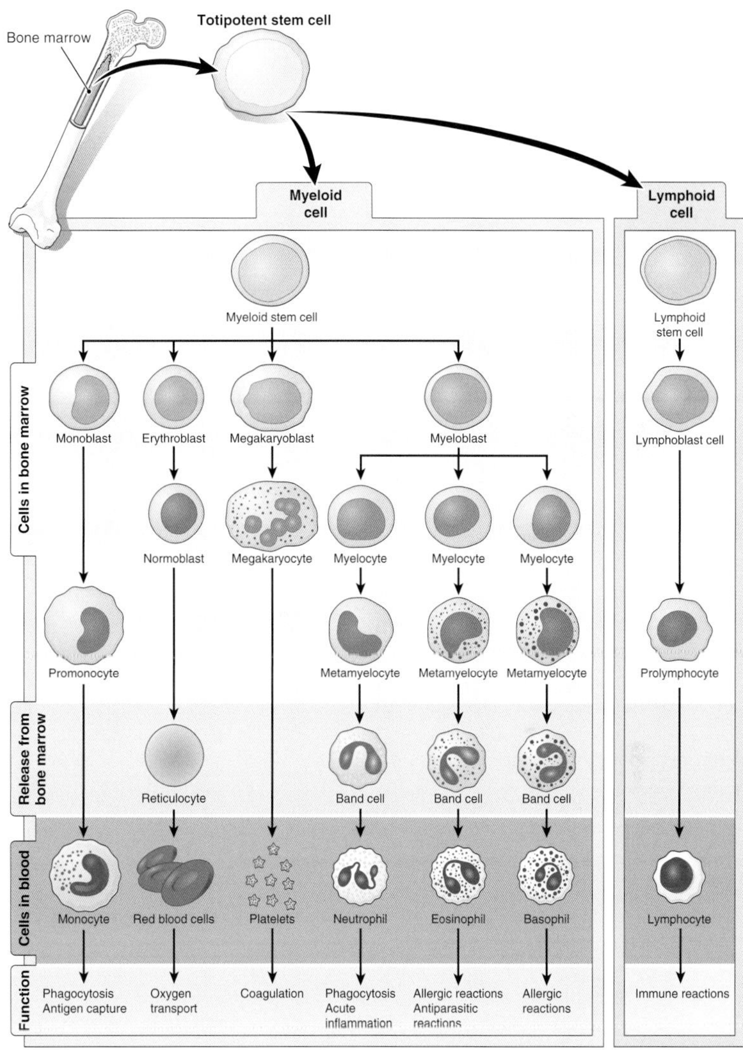


**Figure 27-2.** Hematopoiesis. (From Mc Connell TH. *The Nature of Disease Pathology for the Health Professions*. 2nd ed. Philadelphia: Lippincott Williams & Wilkins; 2007.)

**What are the symptoms of pancytopenia?**

Symptoms of pancytopenia occur as a result of the individual cytopenias (usually anemia and thrombocytopenia) and may include generalized weakness (most common), dyspnea, chills, weight loss, easy bruising, and easy or prolonged bleeding. Patients may also report frequent infections (eg, upper respiratory tract infection).[4]

**What are the physical findings of pancytopenia?**

Physical findings of pancytopenia occur as a result of the individual cytopenias (usually anemia and thrombocytopenia) and may include fever, pallor (most common), splenomegaly, hepatomegaly, jaundice, petechial rash, and lymphadenopathy.[4]

**What is the role of the peripheral blood smear in the investigation of pancytopenia?**

The peripheral blood smear can confirm the presence of pancytopenia and may identify a specific underlying etiology based on cell morphology (eg, megaloblastosis in patients with vitamin B12 deficiency, blast cells in patients with acute leukemia).

**What is the role of bone marrow evaluation in the investigation of pancytopenia?**

Bone marrow aspiration and biopsy are not always necessary in patients with pancytopenia, such as when the underlying etiology is strongly suggested by the history, physical examination, and other laboratory studies, and a primary bone marrow disorder is not suspected (eg, pancytopenia in a patient who recently received cytotoxic chemotherapy). However, when the underlying etiology remains elusive or the pancytopenia is persistent, a bone marrow examination is often helpful. The aspirate may demonstrate abnormal cellular morphology not evident on peripheral blood smear, and the biopsy can determine bone marrow cellularity (hypocellular, normocellular, hypercellular) (Figure 27-3) and identify infiltrative processes (eg, fibrosis).[5,6]

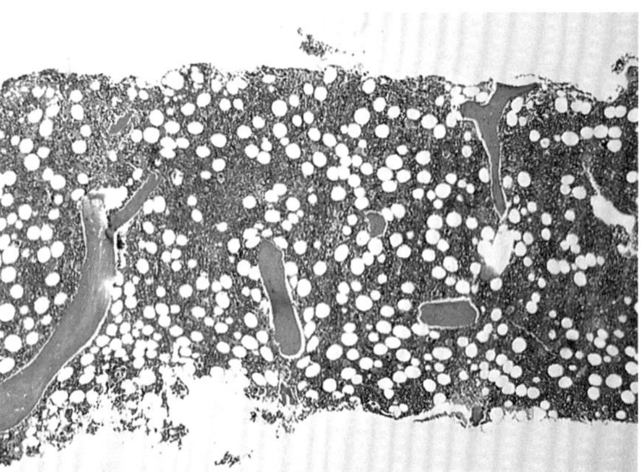

**Figure 27-3.** Bone marrow biopsy from an otherwise healthy 60-year-old man demonstrates normal cellularity (40%-50%). (From McClatchey KD. *Clinical Laboratory Medicine*. 2nd ed. Philadelphia: Lippincott Williams & Wilkins; 2002.)

**What are the general mechanisms of pancytopenia?**

Pancytopenia can develop as a result of bone marrow hypoplasia (ie, hypocellularity), ineffective hematopoiesis, bone marrow infiltration, or hypersplenism.

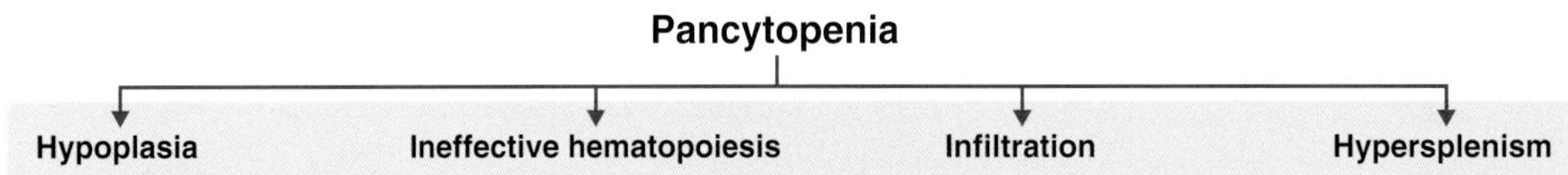


## PANCYTOPENIA RELATED TO BONE MARROW HYPOPLASIA

**What is bone marrow hypoplasia?**

Hypoplastic bone marrow describes an abnormally low proportion of hematopoietic stem cells in the absence of an infiltrative process such as myelofibrosis. The cells are replaced by adipose tissue. Normal bone marrow cellularity in adults ranges from 40% to 60%, with a slight decrease in the elderly. Bone marrow cellularity can be established with biopsy (see Figure 27-3).[7]

*Aplastic anemia is defined as the combination of pancytopenia and bone marrow hypoplasia. However, acute and transient causes of pancytopenia and bone marrow hypoplasia (eg, cytotoxic chemotherapy) are generally not referred to as aplastic anemia. If the cytopenias and hypoplasia are not reversible, then acquired aplastic anemia is an appropriate description.*

## What are the causes of bone marrow hypoplasia?

**A 41-year-old woman develops pancytopenia after starting therapy for a condition characterized by weight loss, heat intolerance, and tremor.**

Antithyroid medication (eg, methimazole, propylthiouracil) for hyperthyroidism.

**A 56-year-old man with recent-onset hair loss, peripheral neuropathy, and pancytopenia has had recurrent hospital admissions for abdominal pain, vomiting, diarrhea, and delirium, which seem to occur only after consuming meals prepared by his wife.**

Arsenic poisoning.

**A 46-year-old man presents with fever, symmetric polyarticular inflammatory arthritis, pancytopenia, and bone marrow biopsy showing giant pronormoblasts with inclusions.**

Parvovirus B19 infection.

**Women of reproductive age.**

Pregnancy.

**Hemolysis, pancytopenia, and thrombosis.**

Paroxysmal nocturnal hemoglobinuria (PNH).

**Congenital.**

Inherited aplastic anemia.

**Failure to identify a cause of acquired bone marrow hypoplasia and pancytopenia despite a complete workup.**

Idiopathic aplastic anemia.

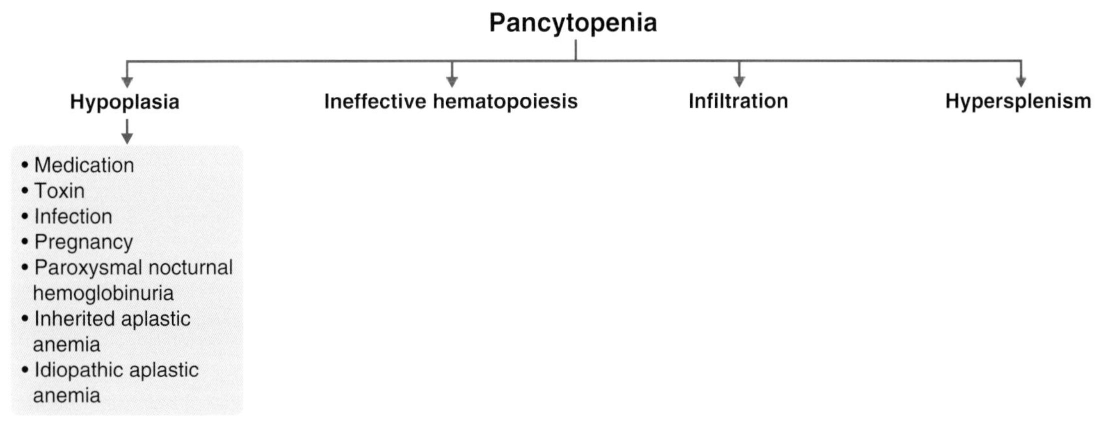


HEMATOLOGY

**Which medications are associated with bone marrow hypoplasia and pancytopenia?**

Numerous medications are associated with bone marrow hypoplasia and pancytopenia, including antibiotics (eg, chloramphenicol), chemotherapeutic agents (eg, doxorubicin), antithyroid agents (eg, methimazole), nonsteroidal anti-inflammatory drugs (eg, indomethacin), anticonvulsants (eg, carbamazepine), and lithium. In some cases the nature of the hypoplasia is transient, resolving within days to weeks of withdrawing the offending agent. However, in other cases, the hypoplasia may persist, resulting in acquired aplastic anemia.[8,9]

**Which toxins are associated with bone marrow hypoplasia and pancytopenia?**

Toxic causes of bone marrow hypoplasia and pancytopenia include alcohol, radiation exposure (both iatrogenic and environmental), benzene, arsenic, and insecticides. Alcohol-related pancytopenia is typically reversed by reducing or abstaining from alcohol consumption. Heavy alcohol consumption is also associated with folate deficiency (ie, megaloblastic anemia) and liver disease with splenomegaly, which may contribute to pancytopenia. Other toxic causes of marrow hypoplasia and pancytopenia may persist despite removal of the toxin, resulting in acquired aplastic anemia.[9,10]

**Which infections are associated with bone marrow hypoplasia and pancytopenia?**

Overwhelming bacterial sepsis is associated with pancytopenia. The mechanisms are multifactorial, including bone marrow hypoplasia from the infection itself, medications used to treat the infection (eg, antimicrobials), and disseminated intravascular coagulation. Other infectious agents associated with bone marrow hypoplasia include seronegative hepatitis (possibly an infectious agent that has yet to be identified), Epstein-Barr virus, cytomegalovirus, HIV, parvovirus B19, miliary tuberculosis (TB), dengue virus, and leptospirosis. Infection can also cause pancytopenia by triggering the life threatening hemophagocytic lymphohistiocytosis (HLH) syndrome. In these patients, bone marrow examination may demonstrate hemophagocytosis.[9,11]

**What are the characteristics of bone marrow hypoplasia related to pregnancy?**

Bone marrow hypoplasia and pancytopenia can develop at any point during pregnancy, and are typically progressive before resolving after abortion or delivery. Patients with true aplastic anemia are more likely to suffer relapse during pregnancy. Supportive care is the mainstay of treatment for these patients; transfusion with blood products (eg, platelets) may be necessary. Cyclosporine is safe during pregnancy and should be considered for patients who require frequent transfusions.[12]

**What is the relationship between paroxysmal nocturnal hemoglobinuria and aplastic anemia?**

A significant portion of patients with PNH will develop bone marrow hypoplasia and pancytopenia. Conversely, up to one-half of patients with acquired aplastic anemia have small PNH clones that can be detected by flow cytometry of peripheral blood. Over time, these clones can remain stable, progress, or regress in size. Clinically significant clones may lead to the manifestations of "classic" PNH, which consists of clinical or laboratory evidence of intravascular hemolysis. The treatment for aplastic anemia is not affected by the presence of PNH.[9,12]

**What are the inherited causes of aplastic anemia?**

Aplastic anemia is associated with several rare genetic disorders, including Fanconi anemia, dyskeratosis congenita, Shwachman-Diamond syndrome, and congenital amegakaryocytic thrombocytopenia. Inherited aplastic anemia is usually diagnosed in childhood but sometimes presents in adulthood. It is important to consider these conditions in any adult newly diagnosed with aplastic anemia. Family history and observation of extrahematopoietic abnormalities can provide clues to an underlying genetic condition (eg, short stature, skin hyper/hypopigmentation, and skeletal abnormalities are suggestive of Fanconi anemia) (Figure 27-4).[9,12]

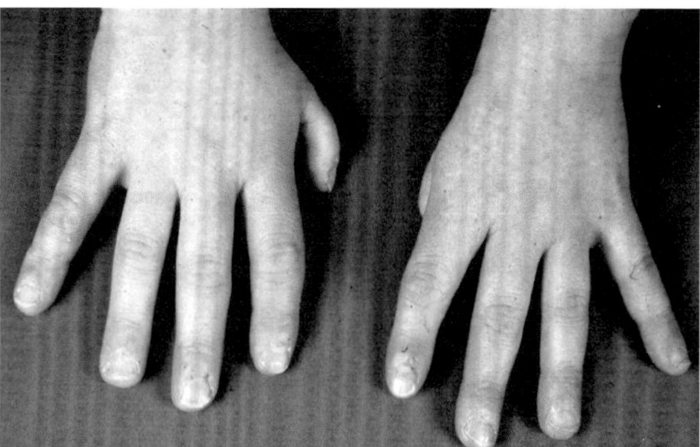

**Figure 27-4.** Hands of a patient with Fanconi anemia. Bilateral thumb hypoplasia is present. Other features include skin pigmentation changes, short stature, upper limb abnormalities, renal malformations, ophthalmologic problems, hypogonadism, and cardiac malformations. (Courtesy of Dr. I. Quirt.)

**What proportion of aplastic anemia cases are idiopathic?**

Most cases of aplastic anemia are idiopathic in nature. Patients with bone marrow hypoplasia and pancytopenia must undergo a thorough workup to rule out alternative causes before a diagnosis of idiopathic aplastic anemia is given.[12]

## PANCYTOPENIA RELATED TO INEFFECTIVE HEMATOPOIESIS

**What is ineffective hematopoiesis?**

Ineffective hematopoiesis describes the failure to produce mature blood cells as a result of dysfunctional progenitor cells, despite the presence of normo- or hypercellular bone marrow.

### What are the causes of ineffective hematopoiesis?

**A 43-year-old woman who follows a strict vegan diet presents with ataxia, peripheral neuropathy, and pancytopenia with oval macrocytosis and hypersegmented neutrophils on the peripheral blood smear.**

Vitamin B12 deficiency.

**Usually a disease of the elderly, associated with macrocytosis.**

Myelodysplasia.

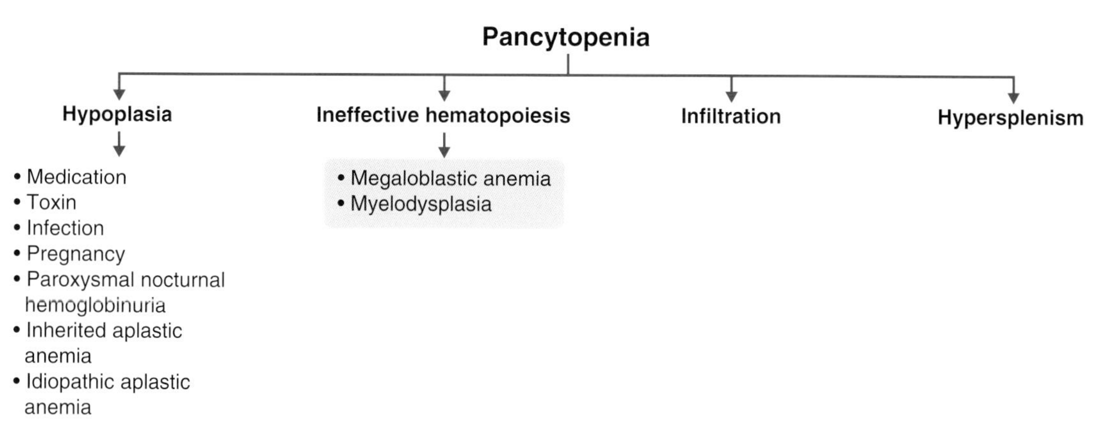


**What are the causes of megaloblastic anemia?**

Megaloblastic anemia may be caused by vitamin B12 deficiency, folate deficiency, copper deficiency, and drugs or toxins. It is the most common cause of pancytopenia in the developing world. Peripheral blood smear usually has characteristic features (see Figure 25-5). Bone marrow aspiration and biopsy demonstrate hypercellularity with evidence of abnormal proliferation and maturation of multiple myeloid cell lines, including large, oval-shaped erythroblasts that contain a characteristic finely stippled, lacy nuclear chromatin pattern surrounded by normal-appearing cytoplasm (known as nuclear-cytoplasmic dissociation).[9,13]

**What are the features of pancytopenia caused by myelodysplasia?**

Myelodysplastic syndrome refers to a group of conditions characterized by bone marrow failure as a result of abnormal cellular maturation. Cytopenias may occur individually or in combination, usually starting with anemia. Pancytopenia is more likely to be a feature of high-grade myelodysplastic syndromes. Bone marrow failure is typically progressive, and may evolve to acute myeloid leukemia. The bone marrow is normo- or hypercellular in most patients with myelodysplasia, however one-fifth of cases present with bone marrow hypoplasia that may be difficult to distinguish from aplastic anemia.[9,14]

## PANCYTOPENIA RELATED TO BONE MARROW INFILTRATION

**What is bone marrow infiltration?**

Bone marrow infiltration describes the replacement of hematopoietic stem cells with nonadipose tissue. This leads to hematopoiesis that occurs outside of the bone marrow (ie, extramedullary hematopoiesis) in locations such as the liver and spleen, which causes hepatosplenomegaly. Extramedullary hematopoiesis is associated with characteristic peripheral blood smear findings, including teardrop-shaped RBCs and leukoerythroblastosis (ie, nucleated RBCs and immature WBCs) (Figure 27-5).

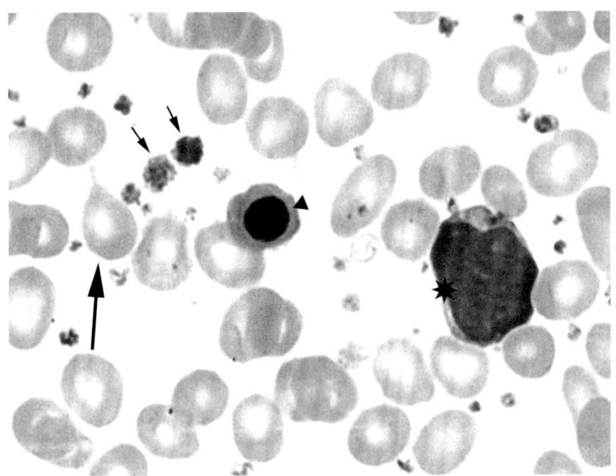

**Figure 27-5.** Peripheral blood smear from a patient with myelofibrosis demonstrating characteristic findings, including teardrop-shaped RBCs (arrow), nucleated RBCs (arrowhead), large platelets (small arrows), and immature WBCs (asterisk). (From Greer JP, Arber DA. *Wintrobe's Clinical Hematology*. 13th ed. Philadelphia, PA: Lippincott Williams and Wilkins; 2014.)

### What are the causes of bone marrow infiltration?

**Blasts on peripheral blood smear.**

Acute leukemia.

**A 39-year-old man from India with a history of HIV presents with fever, dyspnea, and weight loss, and is found to have pancytopenia and innumerable tiny densities throughout the lungs on chest imaging.**

Miliary TB.

**Attempted aspiration of the bone marrow results in a "dry" tap.**

Myelofibrosis.

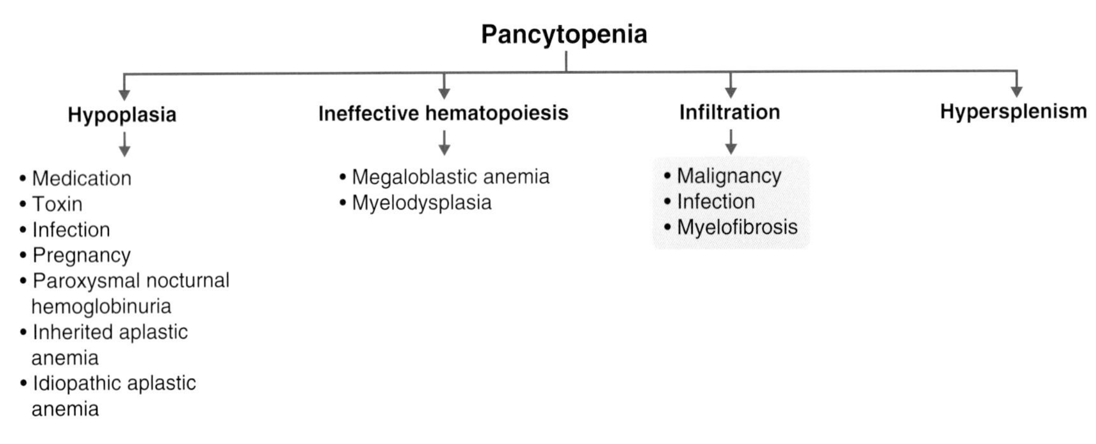

**Which malignancies can cause pancytopenia?**

Acute myeloid leukemia is among the most common causes of pancytopenia in adults. The bone marrow is hypercellular and replaced with blasts, and the peripheral blood smear may also show blasts. Other malignancies associated with pancytopenia include non-Hodgkin's lymphoma, chronic leukemia (most often hairy cell leukemia), multiple myeloma, and nonhematologic malignancies that metastasize to the bone marrow.[9]

**What are the features of pancytopenia caused by miliary tuberculosis?**

Pancytopenia develops in a minority of patients with miliary TB, usually occurring in those with HIV. Common clinical manifestations include fever, respiratory distress, splenomegaly, and lymphadenopathy. Classic miliary nodules are frequently present on chest imaging. Bone marrow biopsy is associated with a high diagnostic yield and typically demonstrates caseating granulomas. Pancytopenia in patients with miliary TB is associated with a poor prognosis even with treatment. Other infections that can invade the bone marrow and cause pancytopenia include fungi and brucellosis.[15,16]

**What is myelofibrosis?**

Fibrosis of the bone marrow can develop as a primary process (primary myelofibrosis) or secondary process (myelophthisis). Conditions that are most often associated with myelophthisis include mycobacterial infection, fungal infection, HIV, sarcoidosis, invading malignancy, lysosomal storage disorders, and external beam radiation therapy. Bone marrow aspiration is often unsuccessful (producing a "dry" tap). On biopsy, the bone marrow is initially hypercellular before becoming hypocellular with increased reticulin or collagen fibrosis.[14]

## PANCYTOPENIA RELATED TO HYPERSPLENISM

**What is hypersplenism?**

Hypersplenism is characterized by splenomegaly and one or more peripheral cytopenias in the setting of normo- or hypercellular bone marrow. When hypersplenism is the sole driver of pancytopenia, splenectomy is often curative. Splenomegaly is frequently associated with conditions that cause pancytopenia independently (eg, myelofibrosis) and may contribute to the severity of the cytopenias.[14]

**What are the mechanisms of pancytopenia related to splenomegaly?**

Pancytopenia in patients with splenomegaly occurs via a variety of mechanisms, including sequestration of blood cells within the spleen, premature destruction of blood cells, and an increase in plasma volume (which can cause pancytopenia via hemodilution). Massive spleens are capable of sequestering up to 90% of peripheral platelets, 65% of granulocytes, and 30% of RBCs.[9,17]

### What are the causes of hypersplenism?

**A 54-year-old man with a history of chronic hepatitis C infection develops jaundice, spider angiomas, ascites, and pancytopenia.**

Cirrhosis.

**Splenomegaly, diffuse lymphadenopathy, and elevated serum lactate dehydrogenase.**

Lymphoma.

**A parasitic infection endemic to some parts of the world that usually presents with months of fatigue, fever, weight loss, and splenomegaly.**

Visceral leishmaniasis (kala-azar).

**A 46-year-old woman with polyarticular inflammatory arthritis, neutropenia, and splenomegaly.**

Felty syndrome (ie, neutropenia and splenomegaly in patients with rheumatoid arthritis).

**An inborn error of metabolism characterized by the accumulation of glucocerebroside within macrophage lysosomes.**

Gaucher disease.

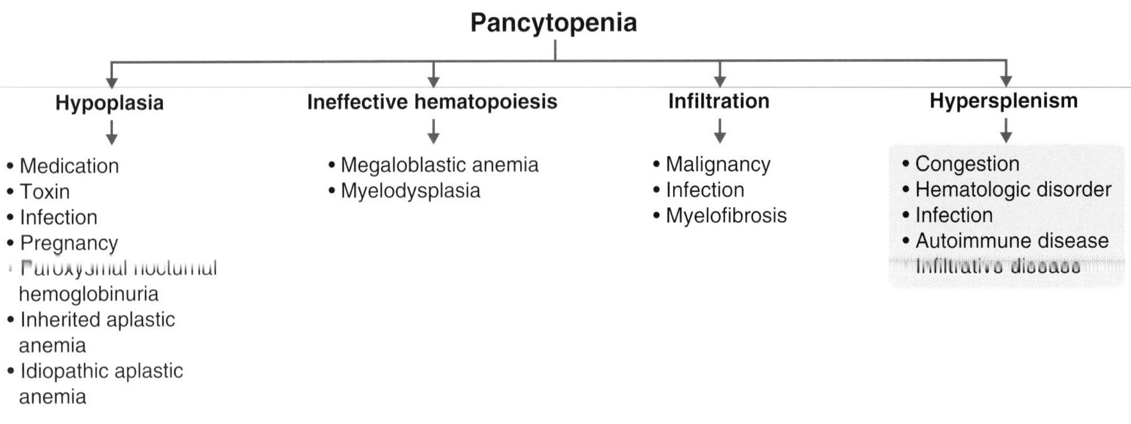


**What are the causes of congestive splenomegaly?**

Congestive splenomegaly can develop with any cause of portal hypertension, including constrictive pericarditis, right-sided heart failure, hepatic vein obstruction, liver disease, portal vein obstruction, and splenic vein obstruction.[18]

**Which hematologic disorders are associated with splenomegaly?**

Hematologic disorders associated with splenomegaly include primary myelofibrosis, chronic leukemia, indolent lymphoma, polycythemia vera, hairy cell leukemia, and thalassemia.[18]

**Which infections are associated with splenomegaly?**

Splenomegaly can be associated with viral infection (eg, Epstein-Barr virus, cytomegalovirus, viral hepatitis, HIV), bacterial infection (eg, endocarditis, enteric fever, TB, brucellosis), parasitic infection (eg, malaria, visceral leishmaniasis, schistosomiasis), and fungal infection (eg, histoplasmosis).[18]

**Which autoimmune diseases are associated with splenomegaly?**

Autoimmune diseases associated with splenomegaly include systemic lupus erythematosus, rheumatoid arthritis (part of the triad of Felty syndrome), and sarcoidosis.[18]

**Which infiltrative diseases are associated with splenomegaly?**

Infiltrative diseases associated with splenomegaly include Gaucher disease, Niemann-Pick disease, amyloidosis, and hemophagocytic lymphohistiocytosis.[18]

## Case Summary

A 34-year-old man presents with fatigue, dyspnea, and easy bruising and is found to have pancytopenia with an abnormal bone marrow examination.

***What is the most likely cause of pancytopenia in this patient?***

Aplastic anemia.

### BONUS QUESTIONS

***What significant finding is present on the bone marrow biopsy in this case?***

The bone marrow biopsy in this case (see Figure 27-1) demonstrates hypocellularity with only small areas containing maturing cells; the majority of the bone marrow is made up of adipose tissue. Normal bone marrow cellularity depends on age; in adults it is 40% to 60% with a slight decrease in the elderly.[7]

***What is aplastic anemia?***

Aplastic anemia is a type of bone marrow failure characterized by the combination of bone marrow hypoplasia and pancytopenia in the absence of an infiltrative process. It is a rare disease with an incidence of 2 to 3 per million in the industrialized world. Distribution is biphasic, with peaks at 10 to 25 years and >60 years of age. Disease severity is based on the degree of bone marrow hypocellularity and peripheral cytopenias.[12]

***What are the causes of acquired aplastic anemia?***

Acquired aplastic anemia describes any form of secondary bone marrow hypoplasia and pancytopenia that does not resolve after removal of the inciting agent. In most cases, aplastic anemia develops in the absence of an identifiable inciting agent (ie, idiopathic aplastic anemia). The pathogenesis of idiopathic aplastic anemia is not known, but there is evidence suggesting it is immune-mediated.[12]

***What definitive treatment options are available for aplastic anemia?***

Untreated severe aplastic anemia is associated with a 1-year mortality rate >80%. First-line definitive treatment options include immunosuppressive therapy (eg, antithymocyte globulin, cyclosporine, glucocorticoids) and allogeneic hematopoietic stem cell transplantation. The initial therapy of choice depends on patient-specific factors (eg, age, comorbidities, donor availability, preference), and disease-specific factors (eg, severity). Other treatment options such as blood transfusions are supportive and aim to improve quality of life.[12,19]

***What important historical event occurred in the 1980s near the Belarusian border with Ukraine?***

The Chernobyl disaster of 1986 resulted in the release of massive amounts of radioactive particles into the atmosphere over a large geographical area. Beginning in the 1990s the incidence of thyroid cancer dramatically increased in children exposed to radiation from the Chernobyl disaster. At this time, there is no data to suggest that the Chernobyl disaster has impacted the incidence of aplastic anemia. However, it is possible that a relationship between the two is established in the future.[20,21]

## KEY POINTS

- Pancytopenia describes the simultaneous presence of leukopenia, anemia, and thrombocytopenia.
- Mature blood cells are developed in the bone marrow and eventually cleared by the reticuloendothelial system.
- Symptoms of pancytopenia include generalized weakness, dyspnea, chills, weight loss, easy bruising, and easy or prolonged bleeding.
- Physical findings of pancytopenia include fever, pallor, splenomegaly, hepatomegaly, jaundice, petechial rash, and lymphadenopathy.
- Pancytopenia can develop as a result of bone marrow hypoplasia, ineffective hematopoiesis, bone marrow infiltration, or hypersplenism.
- Bone marrow hypoplasia describes an abnormally low proportion of hematopoietic stem cells in the absence of an infiltrative process.
- Some causes of hypoplasia can be anticipated and are reversible (eg, cytotoxic chemotherapy).
- Irreversible hypoplasia is referred to as aplastic anemia. It can be inherited or acquired.
- Ineffective hematopoiesis is the failure to produce mature blood cells as a result of dysfunctional progenitor cells, despite the presence of normo- or hypercellular bone marrow.
- Bone marrow infiltration describes the replacement of hematopoietic stem cells with nonadipose tissue, leading to extramedullary hematopoiesis.
- Hypersplenism is characterized by splenomegaly and peripheral cytopenia(s) in the setting of normo- or hypercellular bone marrow.



## REFERENCES


1. Eadie GS, Brown IW Jr. The potential life span and ultimate survival of fresh red blood cells in normal healthy recipients as studied by simultaneous Cr51 tagging and differential hemolysis. *J Clin Invest*. 1955;34(4):629-636.
2. Leeksma CH, Cohen JA. Determination of the life of human blood platelets using labelled diisopropylfluorophosphanate. *Nature*. 1955;175(4456):552-553.
3. Shemin D, Rittenberg D. The life span of the human red blood cell. *J Biol Chem*. 1946;166(2):627-636.
4. Gayathri BN, Rao KS. Pancytopenia: a clinico hematological study. *J Lab Physicians*. 2011;3(1):15-20.
5. Devitt KA, Lunde JH, Lewis MR. New onset pancytopenia in adults: a review of underlying pathologies and their associated clinical and laboratory findings. *Leuk Lymphoma*. 2014;55(5):1099-1105.

6. Weinzierl EP, Arber DA. Bone marrow evaluation in new-onset pancytopenia. *Hum Pathol.* 2013;44(6):1154-1164.
7. Al-Adhadh AN, Cavill I. Assessment of cellularity in bone marrow fragments. *J Clin Pathol.* 1983;36(2):176-179.
8. Laboratory studies in drug-induced pancytopenia. *Br Med J.* 1980;280(6212):429-430.
9. Weinzierl EP, Arber DA. The differential diagnosis and bone marrow evaluation of new-onset pancytopenia. *Am J Clin Pathol.* 2013;139(1):9-29.
10. Nakao S, Harada M, Kondo K, Mizushima N, Matsuda T. Reversible bone marrow hypoplasia induced by alcohol. *Am J Hematol.* 1991;37(2):120-123.
11. Jain A, Naniwadekar M. An etiological reappraisal of pancytopenia – largest series reported to date from a single tertiary care teaching hospital. *BMC Hematol.* 2013;13(1):10.
12. Killick SB, Bown N, Cavenagh J, et al. Guidelines for the diagnosis and management of adult aplastic anaemia. *Br J Haematol.* 2016;172(2):187-207.
13. Aslinia F, Mazza JJ, Yale SH. Megaloblastic anemia and other causes of macrocytosis. *Clin Med Res.* 2006;4(3):236-241.
14. Longo DL, Fauci AS, Kasper DL, Hauser SL, Jameson JL, Loscalzo J, eds. *Harrison's Principles of Internal Medicine.* 18th ed. New York, NY: McGraw-Hill; 2012.
15. Achi HV, Ahui BJ, Anon JC, Kouassi BA, Dje-Bi H, Kininlman H. Pancytopenia: a severe complication of miliary tuberculosis. *Rev Mal Respir.* 2013;30(1):33-37.
16. Maartens G, Willcox PA, Benatar SR. Miliary tuberculosis: rapid diagnosis, hematologic abnormalities, and outcome in 109 treated adults. *Am J Med.* 1990;89(3):291-296.
17. Hess CE, Ayers CR, Sandusky WR, Carpenter MA, Wetzel RA, Mohler DN. Mechanism of dilutional anemia in massive splenomegaly. *Blood.* 1976;47(4):629-644.
18. Elmakki. Hypersplenism: review article. *J Biol Agric Healthc.* 2012;2(10).
19. Young NS. Aplastic anaemia. *Lancet.* 1995;346(8969):228-232.
20. Hatch M, Ron E, Bouville A, Zablotska L, Howe G. The Chernobyl disaster: cancer following the accident at the Chernobyl nuclear power plant. *Epidemiol Rev.* 2005;27:56-66.
21. Reiners C. Radioactivity and thyroid cancer. *Hormones (Athens).* 2009;8(3):185-191.

Chapter 28

# PLATELET DISORDERS

## Case: A 39-year-old man with fever and skin rash

A previously healthy 39-year-old man presents to the emergency department with fatigue and malaise over the past 5 days. He also complains of a skin rash on his lower extremities and intermittent fever. He began bleeding from his gums on the day of presentation. When his wife noticed confusion, she brought him to the emergency department.

Temperature is 37.7°C. There is scleral icterus and subconjunctival pallor. There are innumerable 0.5 to 12 mm non-blanching erythematous macules on the lower extremities. Splenomegaly is not appreciated.

Peripheral white blood cell count is 8 K/μL, hemoglobin is 6.2 g/dL, and platelet count is 6 K/μL. The corrected reticulocyte count is 18% (reference range 0.5%-1.5%) and the immature platelet fraction is 22% (reference range 1%-7.5%). Serum creatinine is 2.6 mg/dL and total bilirubin is 3.1 mg/dL with an indirect component of 2.8 mg/dL. Peripheral blood smear is shown in Figure 28-1.

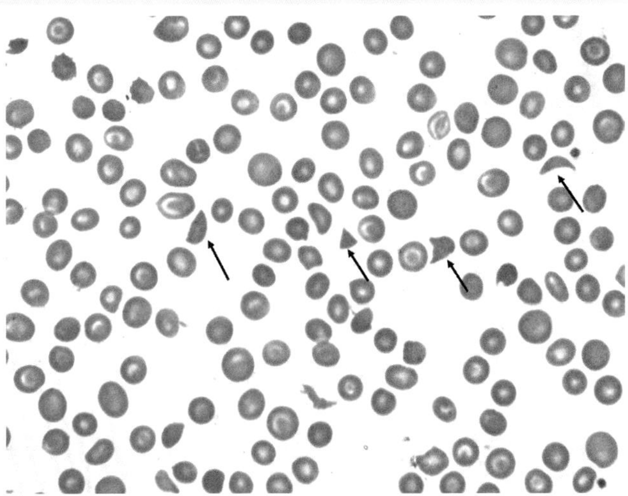

**Figure 28-1.** (Courtesy of Michael J. Cascio, MD.)

***What is the most likely cause of thrombocytopenia in this patient?***

**How is platelet production normally regulated?**

Platelets are generated from megakaryocytes, which are produced in the bone marrow via the myeloid progenitor cells (see Figure 27-2). The principal regulator of platelet production is the hormone thrombopoietin, which is synthesized in the liver. Under normal circumstances, decreases in platelet and megakaryocyte mass stimulate the production of thrombopoietin. The average platelet survives for 9 days before being removed by the reticuloendothelial system.[1,2]

**What is the primary function of platelets?**

Platelets are important for maintaining the integrity of the vascular system. When there is injury to a blood vessel, endothelial cells release von Willebrand factor (VWF), which facilitates platelet adherence to the exposed collagen matrix. Bound platelets become activated and secrete adenosine diphosphate (ADP) and thromboxane $A_2$. These substances promote further platelet aggregation and the formation of a platelet plug, achieving primary hemostasis (Figure 28-2). The coagulation cascade produces fibrin that reinforces the developing thrombus.[3]

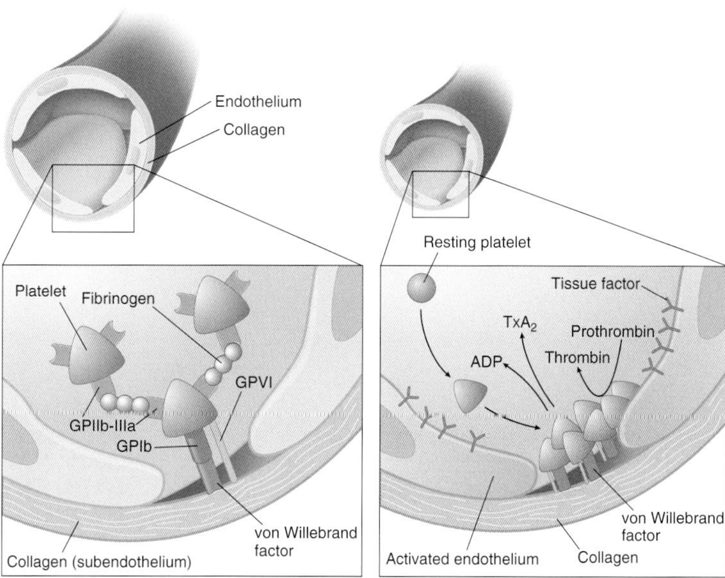


**Figure 28-2.** Platelet adhesion, secretion, and aggregation. Von Willebrand factor mediates platelet adhesion to the subendothelium by binding to both exposed subendothelial collagen and the platelet membrane glycoprotein Ib (GPIb). Platelet adhesion also occurs directly through platelet membrane collagen receptors, such as GPVI. Platelet adhesion leads to platelet activation and secretion of soluble platelet factors, including ADP and thromboxane $A_2$ ($TxA_2$), which facilitate platelet recruitment and aggregation. Platelet aggregation occurs when fibrinogen cross-links platelets by binding to GPIIb-IIIa receptors on platelet membranes.

**What are the clinical manifestations of platelet disorders?**

Clinical manifestations of platelet disorders may include easy bruising, excessive bleeding, and petechial or purpuric rash. Bleeding tends to occur in the skin and mucosa (eg, gums, nasal mucosa). In contrast, coagulation disorders tend to present with ecchymoses or hemarthrosis. Some conditions may affect both platelets and the coagulation cascade (eg, von Willebrand disease), resulting in a mixed clinical picture.[3]

**What are petechiae and purpura?**

Petechiae and purpura are the result of extravasation of blood from the vasculature into the skin or mucosa, usually occurring in the dependent regions of the body. Petechiae are pinpoint hemorrhages ≤2 mm in size, purpura are 2 mm to 1 cm in size, and ecchymoses are >1 cm in size. These lesions do not blanch with pressure.[3]

**Which laboratory tests can be used to detect platelet disorders?**

A complete blood count (CBC), peripheral blood smear, prothrombin time/international normalized ratio (PT/INR), and activated partial thromboplastin time (aPTT) are helpful in the initial evaluation of patients with a suspected bleeding disorder. The PT/INR and aPTT are helpful in identifying coagulation defects. Bleeding time is the classic diagnostic test used to identify dysfunctional platelets but has largely been replaced by instruments that measure platelet-dependent coagulation under flow conditions, such as the Platelet Function Analyzer (PFA-100). Some conditions may affect both platelets and the coagulation cascade, resulting in a mixed laboratory picture.[2,4]

**What are the 2 general categories of platelet disorders?**

Platelet disorders can be qualitative or quantitative.

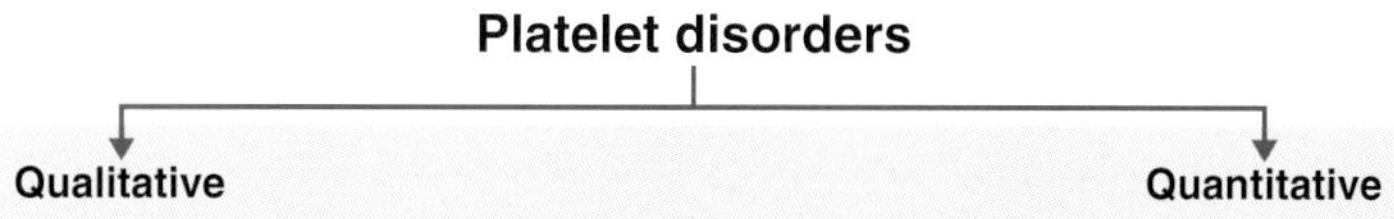


**What is the difference between qualitative and quantitative platelet disorders?**

In qualitative platelet disorders, platelets are normal in number but abnormal in function. In quantitative platelet disorders, platelets are normal in function but abnormal in number.

**Which laboratory tests are helpful in determining whether platelet dysfunction is qualitative or quantitative?**

The CBC and peripheral smear are useful for identifying a quantitative platelet disorder. If the platelet count is normal, then the bleeding time or PFA-100 can be used to identify a qualitative disorder.

## QUALITATIVE PLATELET DISORDERS

**What are the 3 mechanisms of qualitative platelet disorders?**

Qualitative platelet disorders can occur as a result of impaired platelet adhesion, impaired platelet secretion, or impaired platelet aggregation.

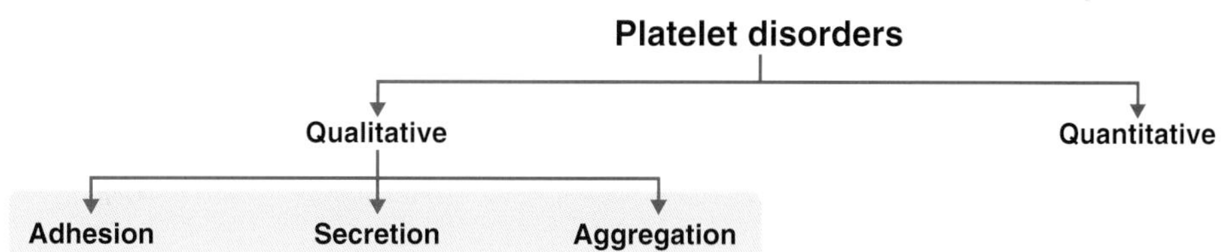


HEMATOLOGY

## DISORDERS OF PLATELET ADHESION

**Which proteins are most important for platelet adhesion?**

Platelet adhesion to subendothelial collagen is dependent on normal quantity and function of glycoprotein Ib (GPIb), VWF, and other specific platelet membrane collagen receptors such as glycoprotein VI (GPVI) (see Figure 28-2).[2]

### What are the causes of impaired platelet adhesion?

**The most common inherited bleeding disorder.**

Von Willebrand disease (VWD).

**Defective binding of VWF to platelets.**

Bernard-Soulier syndrome (BSS).

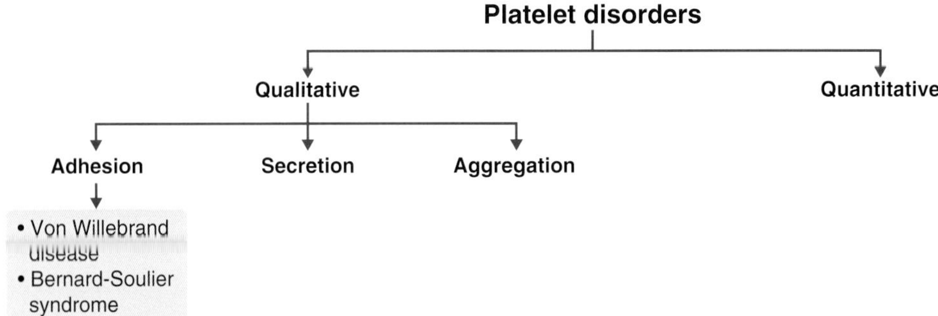


**What is von Willebrand disease?**

VWD is an inherited condition that occurs as a result of quantitative (types 1 and 3) or qualitative (type 2) defects of VWF, a protein necessary for platelet adhesion. The disease is relatively common in the general population with a prevalence of approximately 1%, but most cases are asymptomatic. VWD can also be acquired such as from lymphoproliferative disorders (eg, multiple myeloma) and cardiovascular conditions (eg, aortic stenosis). Hematomas, menorrhagia, and bleeding from minor trauma are the most common manifestations in adults. Other clues include excessive bleeding after surgery or dental procedures. Because VWF serves as a carrier protein for factor VIII, some patients with VWD have low levels of factor VIII activity, resulting in manifestations of hemophilia, including hemarthrosis and prolonged aPTT. Treatment for VWD may be necessary in the setting of clinical bleeding or prophylaxis for surgery. The goal is to normalize VWF and factor VIII levels exogenously with factor concentrate, or endogenously with desmopressin (1-deamino-8-D-arginine vasopressin [DDAVP]), which stimulates release of VWF from the Weibel-Palade bodies of endothelial cells.[5,6]

**What peripheral blood smear finding is characteristic of Bernard-Soulier syndrome?**

BSS is a rare autosomal recessive disorder that results in impaired platelet adhesion because of a congenital absence or dysfunction of GPIb. It typically presents early in life with bleeding manifestations that vary from mild to severe. Thrombocytopenia is variably present in patients with BSS. Giant platelets on peripheral blood smear is a hallmark feature (Figure 28-3). The diagnosis may be confirmed with platelet aggregation studies or flow cytometry.[7]

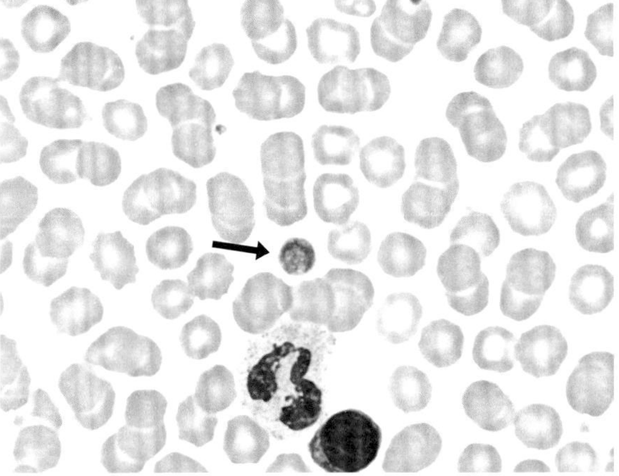

**Figure 28-3.** Giant platelet (arrow) in a patient with Bernard-Soulier syndrome. (From Pereira I, George TI, Arber DA. *Atlas of Peripheral Blood: The Primary Diagnostic Tool.* Philadelphia, PA: Wolters Kluwer Health; 2012.)

## DISORDERS OF PLATELET SECRETION

**What is the role of platelet secretion in hemostasis?**

Platelet adhesion stimulates platelet activation and secretion of substances, such as ADP and thromboxane $A_2$, that promote platelet aggregation and the formation of a platelet plug (see Figure 28-2).

## What are the causes of impaired platelet secretion?

**Iatrogenic.**

Medication.

**A patient with chronic kidney disease presents with new encephalopathy and has a pericardial friction rub.**

Uremia.

**Look for electrocardiographic Osborn waves (ie, J waves) (see Figure 19-3).**

Hypothermia.

**A rare autosomal recessive condition associated with oculocutaneous albinism, recurrent pyogenic infections, bleeding diathesis, neurologic disease (eg, ataxia), and large cytoplasmic granules in neutrophils and other granulocytes.**

Chédiak-Higashi syndrome.[7]

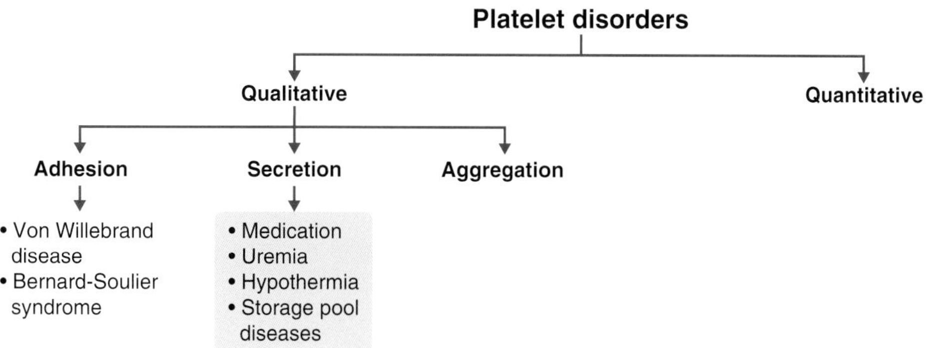


**Which class of medication impairs platelet secretion?**

Nonsteroidal anti-inflammatory drugs (eg, aspirin), which are among the most commonly used medications in the world, impair platelet secretion by inhibiting cyclooxygenase enzymes that catalyze the generation of thromboxane $A_2$ from arachidonic acid.[2]

**What are the features of uremic bleeding diathesis?**

Uremic patients may experience platelet dysfunction that results in benign manifestations such as ecchymoses, epistaxis, and bleeding gums, although serious complications such as overt gastrointestinal bleeding, hemorrhagic pericarditis, and intracranial hemorrhage may occur. Mechanisms are multifactorial, and include impaired platelet secretion, adhesion, and aggregation. DDAVP can be useful in treating platelet dysfunction in uremic patients, particularly before surgical procedures.[8]

**What clinical settings can facilitate hypothermia-induced platelet dysfunction?**

Hypothermia-induced platelet dysfunction may occur in the setting of metabolic disorders (eg, hypothyroidism, hypoglycemia, adrenal insufficiency), disturbed thermoregulation (eg, intracranial tumor), therapeutic interventions (eg, for cardiopulmonary bypass surgery or cardiac arrest from ventricular fibrillation), and environmental cold exposure. In addition to platelet dysfunction, hypothermia also causes platelet sequestration in the liver and spleen, resulting in thrombocytopenia. Platelet dysfunction and sequestration reverse on rewarming.[9,10]

**What are the storage pool diseases?**

The storage pool diseases are a heterogeneous group of conditions characterized by the abnormal presence or function of intracytoplasmic platelet granules involved in platelet secretion, usually resulting in mild to moderate bleeding diathesis. Conditions include gray platelet syndrome, Quebec platelet disorder, Hermansky-Pudlak syndrome, and Chédiak-Higashi syndrome.[7]

HEMATOLOGY

## DISORDERS OF PLATELET AGGREGATION

**Which proteins are most important for platelet aggregation?**

Platelet aggregation is dependent on normal platelet adhesion, activation, and secretion, and the normal quantity and function of GPIIb-IIIa (ie, integrin $\alpha IIb\beta 3$) and fibrinogen (see Figure 28-2).

### What are the causes of impaired platelet aggregation?

**A 48-year-old man with coronary artery disease presents with recurrent epistaxis after recent drug-eluting stent placement.**

Antiplatelet medication (eg, clopidogrel).

**Defective platelet-platelet binding in the setting of normal GPIIb-IIIa.**

Fibrinogen disorders.

**Defective platelet-platelet binding in the setting of normal fibrinogen.**

Glanzmann's thrombasthenia.

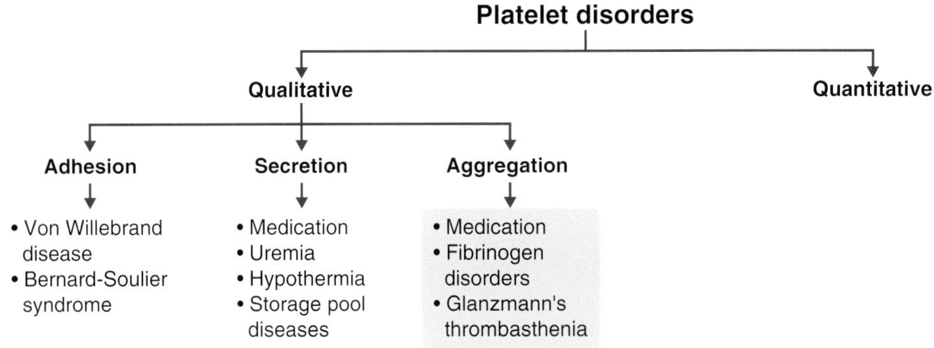


**What is the mechanism of clopidogrel-induced platelet dysfunction?**

ADP receptor inhibitors such as clopidogrel impair platelet function by blocking ADP-mediated platelet aggregation. Other medications that affect platelet aggregation include GPIIb/IIIa inhibitors (eg, abciximab).[2]

**What are the fibrinogen disorders?**

Fibrinogen disorders result from either quantitative abnormalities (eg, afibrinogenemia, hypofibrinogenemia) or qualitative abnormalities (eg, dysfibrinogenemia). These disorders may be inherited or acquired from conditions such as liver disease, disseminated intravascular coagulation (DIC), or malignancy (eg, renal cell carcinoma). Clinical manifestations may include bleeding, thrombosis, or both. Patients with fibrinogen disorders often have prolonged PT/INR and aPTT assays. More specific diagnostic studies include serum fibrinogen activity level and thrombin time. Additional confirmatory tests include thrombin activity-antigen ratio, thrombin time, 1:1 mixing study, fibrinogen electrophoresis, and fibrinogen gene analysis.[11]

**What is the inheritance pattern of Glanzmann's thrombasthenia?**

Glanzmann's thrombasthenia is a rare autosomal recessive disorder that occurs as a result of quantitative and/or qualitative abnormalities of the platelet glycoprotein GPIIb-IIIa. Manifestations of bleeding include purpura, epistaxis, gingival bleeding, and menorrhagia. The severity and frequency of bleeding events are variable. Prognosis is excellent for most adult patients. However, life-threatening bleeding can occur, particularly in association with trauma or other diseases (eg, cancer).[12]

## QUANTITATIVE PLATELET DISORDERS

**What is a normal peripheral platelet count?**

Thrombocytopenia describes a platelet count in the lower 2.5th percentile of the normal platelet count distribution. Traditionally, the lower limit of normal platelet count has been defined as 150 K/μL. However, counts between 100 and 150 K/μL may be considered normal if stable for >6 months.[13]

**What is pseudothrombocytopenia?**

Pseudothrombocytopenia is a laboratory artifact that occurs when the additive agent ethylenediaminetetraacetic acid (EDTA) triggers in vitro platelet clumping, generating a spuriously low platelet count as measured by the automated counter. Approximately 0.1% of the general population has EDTA-dependent antiplatelet antibodies that induce clumping. Review of the peripheral blood smear or use of a non-EDTA additive in these patients will provide an accurate platelet count.[14]

**What are the clinical manifestations of thrombocytopenia?**

Patients with platelet counts >50 K/μL are generally asymptomatic; counts 30 to 50 K/μL may be associated with easy bruising; counts 10 to 30 K/μL may be associated with spontaneous bruising, spontaneous mucosal bleeding (eg, epistaxis), and prolonged bleeding after trauma; and counts <10 K/μL may be associated with spontaneous intracranial hemorrhage.[15,16]

**What are the 2 general mechanisms of thrombocytopenia?**

Thrombocytopenia can occur as a result of decreased platelet production or increased platelet destruction.

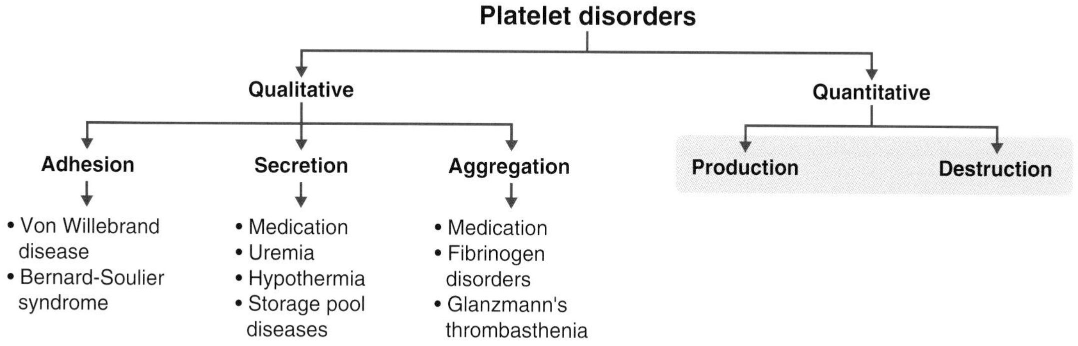


**What laboratory test may be helpful in distinguishing between impaired platelet production and increased destruction?**

The immature platelet fraction (ie, reticulated platelets) of peripheral blood may be helpful in determining whether thrombocytopenia is related to decreased production (immature platelet fraction is low or normal) or increased destruction (immature platelet fraction is elevated).

**What are immature platelets?**

Immature platelets refer to platelets that have recently been released from the bone marrow. These platelets contain more ribonucleic acid (RNA) than mature platelets and can be measured by modern hematology analyzers. The immature platelet fraction reflects the megakaryopoietic activity of the bone marrow. In the setting of thrombocytopenia caused by peripheral destruction, healthy bone marrow responds by increasing megakaryopoiesis, which is reflected by an elevated immature platelet fraction. A fraction that is low or within normal limits suggests that the bone marrow is not responding appropriately (ie, impaired platelet production).[17]

## DECREASED PLATELET PRODUCTION

### What are the causes of decreased platelet production?

**A 42-year-old intravenous drug user presents with fatigue, jaundice, spider angiomas on the chest, symmetric abdominal distension, lower extremity edema, elevated prothrombin time, and thrombocytopenia.**

Liver disease caused by chronic hepatitis C virus infection.

**A decrease in the proportion of bone marrow hematopoietic cells in the absence of an infiltrative process.**

Bone marrow hypoplasia.

HEMATOLOGY

**A patient with a history of gastric bypass surgery develops peripheral neuropathy, pancytopenia, and hypersegmented neutrophils on peripheral blood smear.**

Megaloblastic anemia.

**The peripheral blood smear demonstrates teardrop-shaped red blood cells, nucleated red blood cells, and immature white blood cells.**

Bone marrow infiltration.

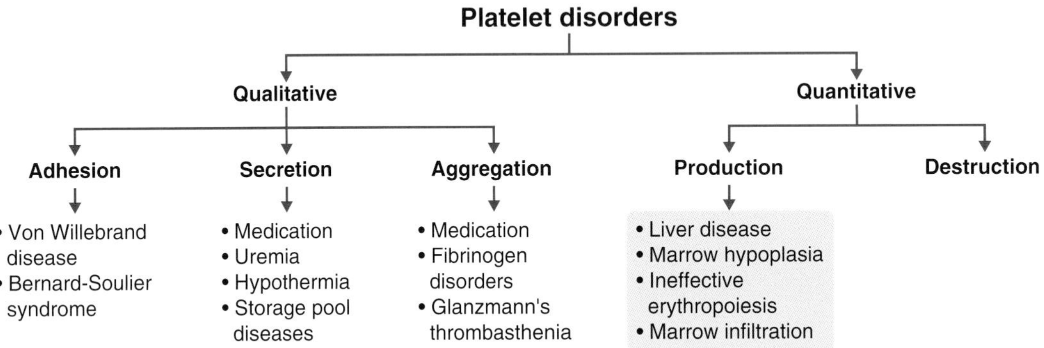


**What is the mechanism of decreased platelet production related to liver disease?**

The liver produces thrombopoietin, which stimulates the production and differentiation of megakaryocytes into platelets.[2]

**What are the causes of bone marrow hypoplasia?**

Bone marrow hypoplasia can be transient or permanent, the latter of which is referred to as aplastic anemia. It is usually associated with pancytopenia. Causes of bone marrow hypoplasia include medications (eg, linezolid), toxins (eg, alcohol), infections (eg, parvovirus B19), and pregnancy. Most cases of aplastic anemia are idiopathic.[18,19]

**What are the causes of ineffective erythropoiesis?**

Ineffective erythropoiesis describes the failure to produce mature blood cells as a result of dysfunctional progenitor cells, despite the presence of normo- or hypercellular bone marrow. It is often associated with pancytopenia. Causes include megaloblastic anemia and myelodysplasia.[19]

**What are the causes of bone marrow infiltration?**

Bone marrow infiltration describes the replacement of hematopoietic stem cells. It is usually associated with pancytopenia. Causes include malignancy (eg, acute leukemia), infection (eg, tuberculosis), and myelofibrosis. Bone marrow infiltration leads to extramedullary hematopoiesis, which is associated with characteristic peripheral blood smear findings, including giant platelets (see Figure 27-5).[19]

## INCREASED PLATELET DESTRUCTION

### What are the causes of increased platelet destruction?

**Increased activity at the normal site of platelet elimination from the body.**

Hypersplenism.

**A previously healthy 38-year-old man presents with bleeding gums and bruising after an upper respiratory infection and is found to have a platelet count of 8 K/μL.**

Immune thrombocytopenic purpura (ITP).

**Hemolytic anemia, thrombocytopenia, and schistocytes on peripheral blood smear.**

Thrombotic microangiopathy (TMA).

**Iatrogenic.**

Heparin-induced thrombocytopenia (HIT).

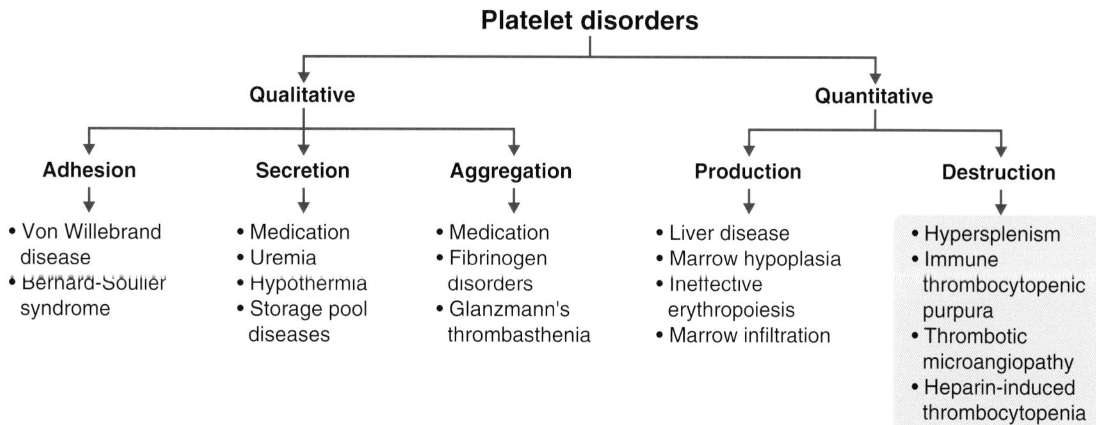


**What is hypersplenism?**

Hypersplenism refers to the combination of splenomegaly, peripheral cytopenia(s), and normo- or hypercellular bone marrow. Massive spleens are capable of sequestering up to 90% of the peripheral platelet mass. Partial splenic embolization can be helpful in treating the thrombocytopenia of hypersplenism. The success of the procedure depends on the extent of embolization (embolization <50% is associated with relapse, while embolization >70% is associated with higher complication rates).[2,19-21]

**What is immune thrombocytopenic purpura?**

ITP is an acquired disorder characterized by autoantibody-mediated platelet destruction that results in thrombocytopenia. It can be either primary, or secondary to a variety of conditions (eg, systemic lupus erythematosus). In adults, incidence follows a bimodal distribution with peaks in young adults and the elderly. Cases may be triggered by antecedent infection, particularly when viral. Clinical manifestations are variable, but can include severe and life-threatening thrombocytopenia. In adults, ITP is usually a chronic condition. Treatment is generally reserved for patients with platelet counts <30 K/μL or those with active bleeding. Glucocorticoids are first-line therapy. Other options include intravenous immune globulin (IVIG), anti-Rh immune globulin (in patients who are Rh-positive), rituximab, thrombopoietin receptor agonists, and splenectomy.[22]

**What is the difference between thrombotic microangiopathy and microangiopathic hemolytic anemia (MAHA)?**

MAHA refers to any cause of intravascular red blood cell fragmentation that results in hemolytic anemia, and generates schistocytes that can be identified on the peripheral blood smear. TMA refers to a group of conditions with characteristic endothelial and blood vessel wall abnormalities associated with arteriolar and capillary thrombosis, which results in MAHA, thrombocytopenia, and organ damage.[23]

**What are the clinical manifestations of heparin-induced thrombocytopenia?**

HIT is characterized by a decrease in platelet count by more than half after exposure to heparin. It usually occurs 5 to 10 days after exposure, but in cases of reexposure (particularly within 30 days) it can occur sooner (rapid-onset HIT). It can also develop up to 3 weeks after heparin has been discontinued (delayed-onset HIT). Unlike most causes of thrombocytopenia in which bleeding dominates the clinical presentation, patients with HIT experience thrombotic complications related to a hypercoagulable state, such as deep vein thrombosis, pulmonary embolism, peripheral arterial thrombosis, and stroke. A high index of suspicion is required to recognize delayed-onset HIT because heparin exposure is relatively remote.[24]

## Case Summary

A previously healthy 39-year-old man presents with fever and confusion and is found to have a dependent petechial and purpuric skin rash, severe thrombocytopenia, renal dysfunction, and evidence of hemolytic anemia with an abnormal peripheral blood smear.

***What is the most likely cause of thrombocytopenia in this patient?***

Thrombotic thrombocytopenic purpura (TTP).

### BONUS QUESTIONS

***What abnormality is present on the peripheral blood smear in this case?***

The peripheral blood smear in this case demonstrates schistocytes, which are fragmented red blood cells that take the form of triangles, helmets, and crescents (see Figure 28-1, arrows). Schistocytes are a marker of traumatic intravascular red blood cell fragmentation (ie, MAHA), occurring in conditions such as TMA, mechanical lysis (eg, from a mechanical heart valve), and march hemoglobinuria.[25]

***What is thrombotic thrombocytopenic purpura?***

TTP is a form of TMA. It occurs when there is functional deficiency of the metalloprotease known as ADAMTS13 (**a d**isintegrin **a**nd **m**etalloproteinase with a **t**hrombo**s**pondin type 1 motif, member **13**). ADAMTS13 is responsible for cleaving large multimers of VWF. Uncleaved VWF leads to increased platelet aggregation on the endothelial surface and microthrombi formation. ADAMTS13 activity <10% is specific for TTP.[26]

***What causes thrombotic thrombocytopenic purpura?***

TTP can be inherited or acquired, the latter of which is far more common and often associated with autoantibodies that inhibit ADAMTS13. One-half of acquired TTP cases are associated with an underlying systemic condition, including bacterial infection, autoimmune disease (eg, systemic lupus erythematosus), pregnancy, drugs (eg, clopidogrel), human immunodeficiency virus infection, pancreatitis, malignancy, and organ transplantation. One-half of cases remain idiopathic.[26]

***What clinical features in this case suggest the diagnosis of thrombotic thrombocytopenic purpura?***

The clinical pentad of TTP consists of fever, thrombocytopenia, MAHA, neurologic manifestations, and renal insufficiency, most of which are present in this case. The complete pentad is present in <10% of patients with acute TTP. The most reliable clinical findings are severe thrombocytopenia (usually <30 K/μL) with associated bleeding manifestations (eg, petechiae), MAHA with schistocytes on the peripheral blood smear, and neurologic manifestations (eg, confusion, headache, stroke, seizure, coma). Other common manifestations include myocardial ischemia and mesenteric ischemia.[26]

***What other conditions should be considered in this case?***

Other forms of TMA should be considered in this case. Primary TMA syndromes include TTP, HUS, and drug-induced TMA. Secondary TMA syndromes occur as a result of a variety of underlying conditions, including DIC, severe hypertension, HELLP syndrome (**h**emolysis, **e**levated **l**iver enzymes, **l**ow **p**latelet count), systemic infection (eg, human immunodeficiency virus), systemic malignancy, autoimmune disorders (eg, systemic lupus erythematosus, antiphospholipid syndrome), severe vitamin B12 deficiency, and hematopoietic stem cell or organ transplantation.[23]

| | |
|---|---|
| ***How should acquired thrombotic thrombocytopenic purpura be treated?*** | Therapeutic plasma exchange to clear the blood of autoantibodies against ADAMTS13 is first-line therapy for acquired TTP. It should be performed daily until there is improvement and stabilization of platelet counts, and resolution of hemolysis and end-organ dysfunction. Glucocorticoids and rituximab are often initiated in parallel with plasma exchange.[26] |
| ***What is the prognosis of thrombotic thrombocytopenic purpura?*** | With prompt recognition and initiation of therapy, the average survival rate after an initial episode of TTP approaches 90%. However, a significant proportion of survivors suffer persistent morbidity such as neurocognitive deficits, arterial hypertension, and major depression. Almost one-half of patients with acquired TTP experience at least 1 relapse.[26] |

## KEY POINTS

- Platelets are produced in the bone marrow and destroyed in the reticuloendothelial system after circulating for about 9 days.
- Platelets are important for maintaining the integrity of the vascular system and achieving primary hemostasis.
- Clinical manifestations of platelet disorders include easy bruising, excessive bleeding, and petechial or purpuric rash.
- Bleeding time and modern platelet analyzers may be helpful in identifying a platelet disorder.
- Platelet disorders can be qualitative or quantitative.
- Qualitative platelet disorders can occur as a result of impaired platelet adhesion, impaired platelet secretion, or impaired platelet aggregation.
- Thrombocytopenia can occur as a result of decreased platelet production or increased platelet destruction.
- The immature platelet fraction may be helpful in determining whether thrombocytopenia is related to decreased platelet production (immature platelet fraction is low or normal) or increased destruction (immature platelet fraction is elevated).

HEMATOLOGY

## REFERENCES


1. Leeksma CH, Cohen JA. Determination of the life of human blood platelets using labelled diisopropylfluorophosphanate. *Nature*. 1955;175(4456):552-553.
2. Longo DL, Fauci AS, Kasper DL, Hauser SL, Jameson JL, Loscalzo J, eds. *Harrison's Principles of Internal Medicine*. 18th ed. New York, NY: McGraw-Hill; 2012.
3. Leung AK, Chan KW. Evaluating the child with purpura. *Am Fam Physician*. 2001;64(3):419-428.
4. Francis J, Francis D, Larson L, Helms E, Garcia M. Can the Platelet Function Analyzer (PFA)-100 test substitute for the template bleeding time in routine clinical practice? *Platelets*. 1999;10(2–3):132-136.
5. Federici AB, Rand JH, Bucciarelli P, et al. Acquired von Willebrand syndrome: data from an international registry. *Thromb Haemost*. 2000;84(2):345-349.
6. Leebeek FW, Eikenboom JC. Von Willebrand's disease. *N Engl J Med*. 2016;375(21):2067-2080.
7. D'Andrea G, Chetta M, Margaglione M. Inherited platelet disorders: thrombocytopenias and thrombocytopathies. *Blood Transfus*. 2009;7(4):278-292.
8. Boccardo P, Remuzzi G, Galbusera M. Platelet dysfunction in renal failure. *Semin Thromb Hemost*. 2004;30(5):579-589.
9. Michelson AD, MacGregor H, Barnard MR, Kestin AS, Rohrer MJ, Valeri CR. Reversible inhibition of human platelet activation by hypothermia in vivo and in vitro. *Thromb Haemost*. 1994;71(5):633-640.
10. Van Poucke S, Stevens K, Marcus AE, Lance M. Hypothermia: effects on platelet function and hemostasis. *Thromb J*. 2014;12(1):31.
11. Cunningham MT, Brandt JT, Laposata M, Olson JD. Laboratory diagnosis of dysfibrinogenemia. *Arch Pathol Lab Med*. 2002;126(4):499-505.
12. Nurden AT. Glanzmann thrombasthenia. *Orphanet J Rare Dis*. 2006;1:10.
13. Stasi R. How to approach thrombocytopenia. *Hematology Am Soc Hematol Educ Program*. 2012;2012:191-197.
14. Vicari A, Banfi G, Bonini PA. EDTA-dependent pseudothrombocytopaenia: a 12-month epidemiological study. *Scand J Clin Lab Invest*. 1988;48(6):537-542.

15. McMillan R. Therapy for adults with refractory chronic immune thrombocytopenic purpura. *Ann Intern Med*. 1997;126(4):307-314.
16. Thachil J, Fitzmaurice D. Thrombocytopenia in an adult. *BMJ*. 2013;346:f3407.
17. Hoffmann JJ. Reticulated platelets: analytical aspects and clinical utility. *Clin Chem Lab Med*. 2014;52(8):1107-1117.
18. Laboratory studies in drug-induced pancytopenia. *Br Med J*. 1980;280(6212):429-430.
19. Weinzierl EP, Arber DA. The differential diagnosis and bone marrow evaluation of new-onset pancytopenia. *Am J Clin Pathol*. 2013;139(1):9-29.
20. Hanafiah M, Shahizon AM, Low SF, Shahrina MH. Severe thrombocytopenia due to hypersplenism treated with partial splenic embolisation. *BMJ Case Rep*. 2013;2013.
21. Paz YMHL, Gonzalez-Estrada A, Alraies MC. Massive splenomegaly. *BMJ Case Rep*. 2013;2013.
22. Lambert MP, Gernsheimer TB. Clinical updates in adult immune thrombocytopenia. *Blood*. 2017;129(21):2829-2835.
23. George JN, Nester CM. Syndromes of thrombotic microangiopathy. *N Engl J Med*. 2014;371(7):654-666.
24. Greinacher A. Clinical practice. Heparin-induced thrombocytopenia. *N Engl J Med*. 2015;373(3):252-261.
25. Greer JP, Foerster J, Rodgers GM, et al, eds. *Wintrobe's Clinical Hematology*. 12th ed. Philadelphia, PA: Lippincott Williams & Wilkins, A Wolters Kluwer Business; 2009.
26. Joly BS, Coppo P, Veyradier A. Thrombotic thrombocytopenic purpura. *Blood*. 2017;129(21):2836-2846.

# SECTION 8

# Infectious Diseases

## Chapter 29

## ENDOCARDITIS

### Case: A 31-year-old man with pulsating nail beds

A 31-year-old man with active intravenous methamphetamine use is admitted to the hospital for evaluation of dyspnea. The patient reports a 1 week history of fever and drenching night sweats. Over the past few days, he has developed progressive shortness of breath. He describes difficulty lying flat and has been waking up in the middle of the night gasping for air.

Temperature is 39.2°C, heart rate is 106 beats per minute, and blood pressure is 110/38 mm Hg. The patient's head is moving in a to-and-fro manner. Jugular venous pressure (JVP) is 18 cm $H_2O$. The carotid and radial pulses are bounding. There is alternating flushing and blanching of the nail beds in concert with the cardiac cycle. There is a 3/6 early-peaking crescendo-decrescendo systolic murmur best heard over the right upper sternal border as well as a 3/4 decrescendo diastolic murmur best heard over the third intercostal space of the left sternal border. There are tender erythematous nodules on the thenar and hypothenar eminences (Figure 29-1A) and the pulps of the fingertips (Figure 29-1B).

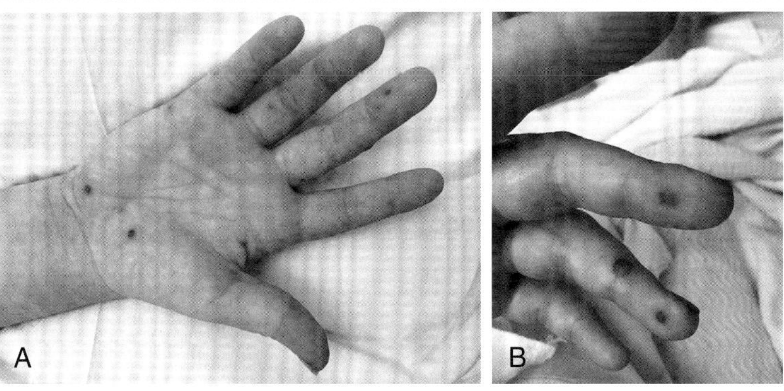


**Figure 29-1.**

***What is the most likely underlying diagnosis in this patient?***

**What is endocarditis?**

Endocarditis refers to inflammation of the innermost layer of the heart (endocardium), usually involving the heart valves.

**What are the 2 general categories of endocarditis?**

Endocarditis can be noninfective or infective.

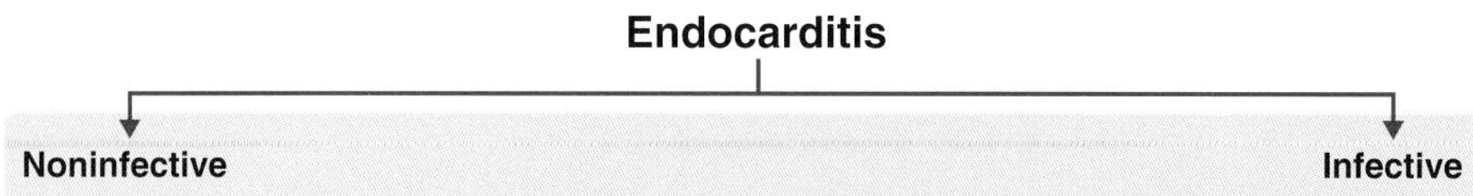


**What is the relative prevalence of noninfective endocarditis compared with that of infective endocarditis (IE)?**

The overwhelming majority of cases of endocarditis are infectious in nature. The annual incidence of IE in the industrialized world is 3 to 10 cases per 100,000 persons. Noninfective endocarditis is comparatively rare, representing <5% of cases.[1-3]

## NONINFECTIVE ENDOCARDITIS

**What is noninfective endocarditis?**

Noninfective endocarditis refers to the presence of sterile vegetations (primarily composed of platelets and fibrin) on the endocardium, most frequently involving the heart valves. It develops in association with a variety of conditions, including inflammatory and hypercoagulable states. Nonbacterial thrombotic endocarditis (NBTE), previously known as marantic endocarditis, is the umbrella term that refers to all forms of noninfective endocarditis regardless of size or location of the vegetation, previous health of the involved valve, or underlying cause.[4,5]

**Which heart valves are most frequently involved in nonbacterial thrombotic endocarditis?**

NBTE may affect both normal and previously damaged heart valves. The mitral valve is most commonly involved (two-thirds of cases) followed by the aortic valve (one-third of cases). NBTE may involve both the mitral and aortic valves in some cases.[1,4,6]

**What are the clinical manifestations of nonbacterial thrombotic endocarditis?**

NBTE tends to be clinically indolent until an advanced complication occurs, such as embolization or valvular dysfunction. Embolic events are common in patients with NBTE; nearly one-half of patients experience a systemic embolic event, often at the time of presentation. Cerebral, coronary, renal, and mesenteric circulations are most frequently involved, with manifestations that include focal neurologic deficits, vision changes, memory loss, pain in the extremities or flank, and acute abdomen. Patients present with valvular destruction or heart failure less frequently; murmurs are only appreciated in around one-quarter of cases.[1,4-6]

**What are the treatment options for nonbacterial thrombotic endocarditis?**

In addition to addressing the underlying cause, anticoagulation is the cornerstone of therapy for NBTE. Oral vitamin K antagonists (eg, warfarin) may not be as effective as low-molecular-weight heparin. Surgical intervention can be considered for some patients, such as those with severe valvular dysfunction or recurrent embolic events. Unlike patients with IE who typically undergo valve replacement, preservation of the affected valve is often possible in patients with NBTE.[1]

### What are the causes of nonbacterial thrombotic endocarditis?

**A 68-year-old man with an extensive smoking history presents with night sweats, weight loss, and hemoptysis.**

Lung cancer.

**A 36-year-old woman with malar rash, generalized lymphadenopathy, and pancytopenia.**

Systemic lupus erythematosus (SLE).

**Ironically categorized under noninfective endocarditis.**

Infection.

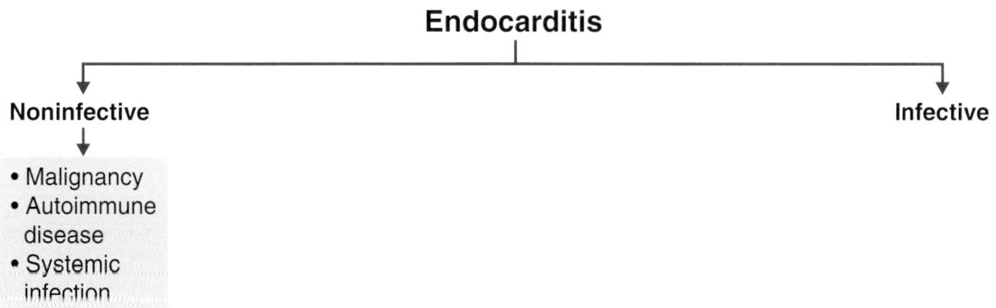


**Which malignancies are most often associated with nonbacterial thrombotic endocarditis?**

NBTE tends to develop in patients with advanced and metastatic malignancy, sometimes in association with disseminated intravascular coagulation. On autopsy, valvular distortion is minimal, suggesting that there is limited time between developing NBTE and death in cancer patients. Malignancies most frequently associated with NBTE include mucin-secreting adenocarcinomas of the lung, ovary, biliary system, pancreas, and stomach. Adenocarcinomas of the lung and ovary represent around one-half of cases.[1,4]

**Which autoimmune conditions are associated with nonbacterial thrombotic endocarditis?**

NBTE can be associated with SLE (including Libman-Sacks endocarditis), antiphospholipid syndrome (primary or secondary), rheumatic heart disease, and rheumatoid arthritis. These patients tend to have more significant valvulopathy (ie, regurgitant lesions) than patients with malignancy-associated NBTE because a comparatively longer clinical course allows for its development. Libman-Sacks endocarditis is a subtype of NBTE that occurs in patients with SLE, particularly in those with antiphospholipid syndrome. The vegetations of Libman-Sacks endocarditis are histologically distinct and tend to form on the ventricular aspect of the posterior mitral leaflet, although clinical manifestations are similar to other causes of NBTE.[4,7]

**What infections are associated with nonbacterial thrombotic endocarditis?**

NBTE can be associated with acute infectious conditions, such as sepsis and pneumonia, and chronic infectious conditions, such as tuberculosis, osteomyelitis, and chronic pyelonephritis. *It is important to note that the vegetations of infectious NBTE are sterile.*[6]

## INFECTIVE ENDOCARDITIS

**What is infective endocarditis?**

IE refers to the presence of endocardial vegetations composed primarily of platelets, fibrin, and microorganisms, most often involving the heart valves. Despite frequent episodes of transient bacteremia related to daily activities, such as chewing and tooth brushing, healthy endothelium is resistant to infection. However, damaged endothelium is susceptible to the direct adherence of microorganisms, leading to subsequent infection, or the development of microthrombi that later become infected. Endothelial damage may develop as a result of degenerative valvular lesions (eg, mitral valve prolapse), trauma from the impact of high-velocity blood jet due to turbulent blood flow (eg, aortic stenosis), or direct trauma from electrodes or catheters.[3,8]

**Which heart valves are most frequently involved in infective endocarditis?**

IE most often involves the left-sided heart valves. This is thought to occur for 3 main reasons: (1) there is more turbulent blood flow on the left side of the heart as a result of higher pressures, predisposing the aortic and mitral valves to endothelial injury; (2) higher oxygen content of arterial blood is supportive of bacterial growth; and (3) a higher proportion of congenital and acquired predisposing heart conditions are left-sided. Intravenous drug users often develop endothelial injury involving the tricuspid valve as a result of repeated intravenous injections of solid particles, predisposing this population to right-sided endocarditis.[3,9]

**What are the symptoms of infective endocarditis?**

Symptoms of IE may include chills, anorexia, weight loss, dyspnea, and flank pain.[10]

**What are the physical findings of infective endocarditis?**

Physical findings of IE may include fever (in up to 90% of patients), heart murmur (in up to 85% of patients), signs of heart failure (eg, elevated JVP, gallop), splenomegaly, petechiae, splinter hemorrhages (Figure 29-2), Osler's nodes (tender erythematous or violaceous subcutaneous nodules on the thenar and hypothenar eminences and pulps of fingers and toes), Janeway lesions (nontender erythematous or hemorrhagic macular lesions on the palms and soles) (Figure 29-3), Roth spots (retinal hemorrhages with a central pallor) on fundoscopic examination (Figure 29-4), and focal lung findings (in patients with right-sided IE). Systemic emboli may lead to other physical findings (eg, focal neurologic deficits).[8,10]

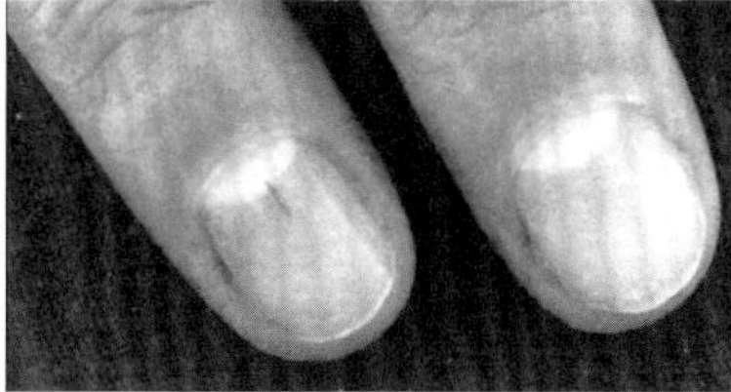

**Figure 29-2.** Splinter hemorrhage in a patient with infective endocarditis. (From Stoller JK, Nielsen C, Buccola J, Brateanu A. *The Cleveland Clinic Foundation Intensive Review of Internal Medicine*. 6th ed. Philadelphia, PA: Wolters Kluwer Health; 2014.)

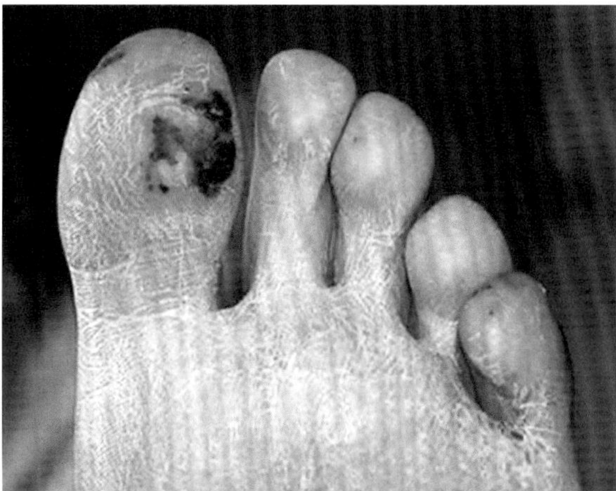

**Figure 29-3.** Janeway lesions in a patient with infective endocarditis. (From Positano RG, DiGiovanni CW, Borer JS, Trepal MJ. *Systemic Disease Manifestations in the Foot, Ankle, and Lower Extremity*. Philadelphia, PA: Wolters Kluwer; 2017.)

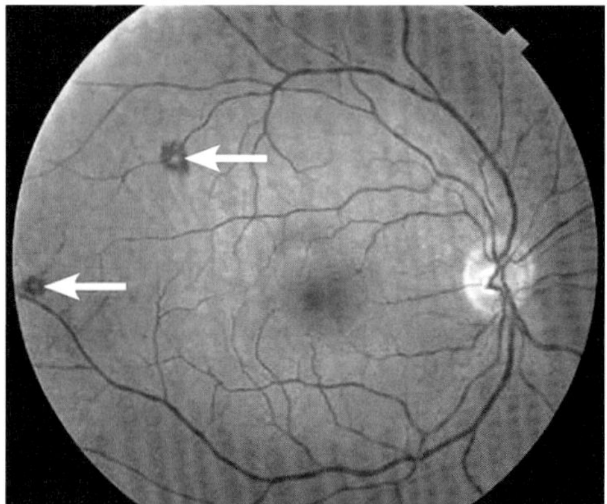

**Figure 29-4.** Roth spots (arrows) in a patient with infective endocarditis. (Reprinted with permission from Hess RL. Roth spots in native valve endocarditis. *J Am Osteopath Assoc*. 2013;113(11):863. doi:10.7556/jaoa.2013.063.)

**What clinical manifestations are unique to right-sided infective endocarditis?**

In addition to the clinical manifestations shared with left-sided IE (eg, chills, fever, murmur), patients with right-sided IE may experience cough and pleuritic chest pain, and develop focal pulmonary findings on examination (eg, signs of consolidation or pleural effusion), which are related to cardiopulmonary septic emboli. In the absence of a right-to-left shunt, right-sided IE is not associated with systemic emboli or peripheral stigmata (eg, Janeway lesions). Signs of right-sided heart failure (eg, elevated JVP, peripheral edema) are more common in patients with right-sided IE.[11]

**How is the diagnosis of infective endocarditis established?**

The diagnosis of IE can be definitively made with histologic and microbiologic examination of vegetations. However, a diagnostic tool, known as the Duke criteria, incorporates clinical, laboratory, and echocardiographic findings to identify the likelihood of IE (Table 29-1). The diagnosis is established with a specificity of 99% when any of the following are present: (1) 2 major criteria; (2) 1 major criterion and 3 minor criteria; (3) 5 minor criteria.

**Table 29-1** Modified Duke Criteria for Infective Endocarditis[12-14]

| Major Criteria | Minor Criteria |
|---|---|
| 1. Positive blood cultures for IE.<br>A. Two separate blood cultures positive for an organism typical for IE, or<br>B. Persistently positive blood cultures with an organism less typical for IE.[a] | 1. Predisposition: predisposing heart condition or IV drug use.<br>2. Fever: temperature ≥38.0°C (100.4°F).<br>3. Vascular phenomena: major arterial emboli, septic pulmonary infarcts, mycotic aneurysms, intracranial hemorrhage, conjunctival hemorrhages, and Janeway lesions. |
| 2. Evidence of endocardial involvement.<br>A. Positive echocardiogram for IE.<br>i. Oscillating intracardiac mass; or<br>ii. Abscess; or<br>iii. New partial dehiscence of prosthetic valve; or<br>B. New valvular regurgitation by physical examination (ie, murmur consistent with valvular regurgitation).[b] | 4. Immunologic phenomena: glomerulonephritis, Osler's nodes, Roth spots, and positive rheumatoid factor.<br>5. Microbiologic evidence: positive blood culture not meeting major criterion or serologic evidence of active infection with an organism consistent with IE. |

[a]Persistently positive blood cultures is defined as recovery of a microorganism from at least 2 blood cultures drawn more than 12 hours apart, or all of 3, or a majority of 4 or more separate blood cultures (with first and last drawn at least 1 h apart).
[b]An isolated regurgitant lesion on echocardiography must be considered carefully, as mechanism is often difficult to determine and clinically insignificant valvular regurgitation is common in the general population.

**How is echocardiography useful in the diagnosis of infective endocarditis?**

In accordance with the Duke criteria (see Table 29-1), echocardiography can be diagnostic of IE when it identifies a vegetation, perivalvular abscess, or new dehiscence of a prosthetic valve. It can be suggestive of IE if there is evidence of valvular destruction, prolapse, aneurysm, or perforation, or rupture of the chordae tendineae or papillary muscle. Isolated valvular regurgitation on echocardiography must be considered carefully, as mechanism is often difficult to determine and clinically insignificant valvular regurgitation is common in the general population. Sequelae of endocarditis, such as valvular regurgitation and left ventricular dysfunction, can be monitored with echocardiography.[15]

**What are the general principles of therapy for infective endocarditis?**

The goal of treatment for IE is eradication of infection. The antimicrobial agents of choice depend on the specific organism(s) involved, however prolonged parenteral bactericidal therapy is generally necessary. It is recommended that 3 sets of blood cultures be drawn 1 hour apart before the administration of antibiotics. The recovery rate of blood cultures is reduced by up to 40% when antimicrobial agents are administered before blood culture collection. Surgical intervention may be necessary in some cases of IE, particularly when there are complications.[2,10]

**What are the complications of infective endocarditis?**

Heart failure is the most common complication of IE, occurring in over one-half of all cases. It typically occurs as a result of valvular dysfunction, developing more frequently in patients with aortic valve involvement. Systemic embolism occurs in up to one-half of patients with IE, most often involving the central nervous system, spleen, kidneys, lungs, and liver. Risk is highest earlier in the course of the disease (within 2 weeks of diagnosis), when vegetations are large (>10 mm), and when the mitral valve is involved. Risk decreases after initiation of antimicrobial therapy. Septic emboli may cause secondary infection in the blood vessel wall, resulting in the formation of a mycotic aneurysm. Intracardiac abscess develops in less than one-half of patients with IE but is more common in those with prosthetic valve endocarditis, and those with native aortic valve disease.[3,8,16]

**What is the prognosis of infective endocarditis?**

The prognosis of IE depends on many factors such as the infecting organism, site of infection, and clinical circumstances including patient-related factors and the presence of complications. However, the overall in-hospital mortality rate of IE approaches 25%; 5-year mortality is approximately 40%. Survivors should continue to be monitored for relapse or reinfection, and progressive valvulopathy.[3,8]

**What are the 3 general subcategories of infective endocarditis?**

IE can be separated into the following subcategories: native valve endocarditis (NVE), prosthetic valve endocarditis (PVE), and IE related to intravenous drug use (IVDU).

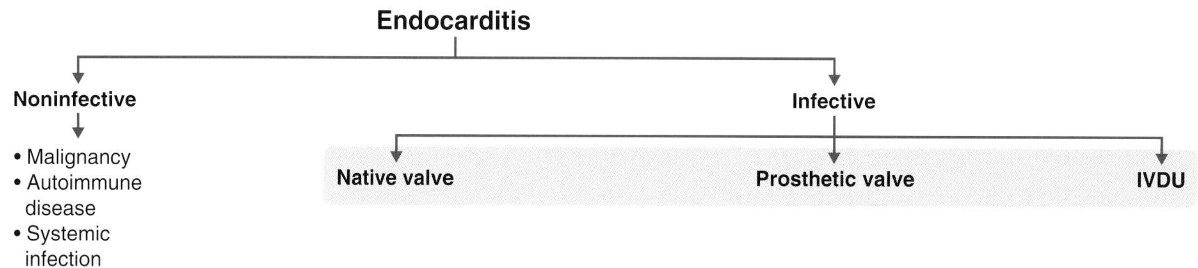


## NATIVE VALVE INFECTIVE ENDOCARDITIS

**How sensitive is echocardiography in identifying lesions that are diagnostic of native valve endocarditis?**

The sensitivity of transthoracic echocardiography (TTE) in identifying vegetations in NVE is approximately 75%; sensitivity improves to 90% with transesophageal echocardiography (TEE). The sensitivity of TTE in identifying a perivalvular abscess in NVE is approximately 50%; sensitivity improves to 90% with TEE.[15]

**What are the 2 subtypes of native valve endocarditis based on clinical course?**

NVE can follow an acute or subacute clinical course.

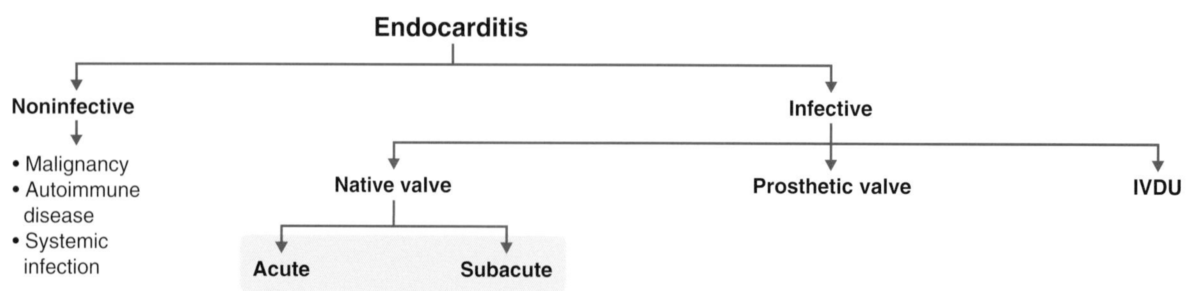

**What are the clinical differences between acute and subacute infective endocarditis?**

Acute IE manifests suddenly (ie, within days) as a fulminant illness with rapid destruction of cardiac structures, hematogenous seeding of extracardiac sites, and progression to death within weeks if left untreated. In contrast, subacute IE tends to be more indolent with nonspecific symptoms (eg, night sweats, weight loss), causing slow damage to cardiac structures and rare extracardiac metastases. Subacute IE is associated with a more favorable prognosis. *The classic clinical manifestations of IE (eg, Osler's nodes) are more common in patients with subacute IE; such manifestations tend to be more limited in patients with acute IE, particularly right-sided disease in IV drug users.*[2,14]

## ACUTE NATIVE VALVE INFECTIVE ENDOCARDITIS

### What are the causes of acute native valve endocarditis?

**Gram-positive cocci in clusters.**

*Staphylococcus aureus.*

**Gram-positive cocci in chains.**

Non–viridans streptococci.

**A coagulase-negative species of *Staphylococcus.***

*Staphylococcus lugdunensis.*

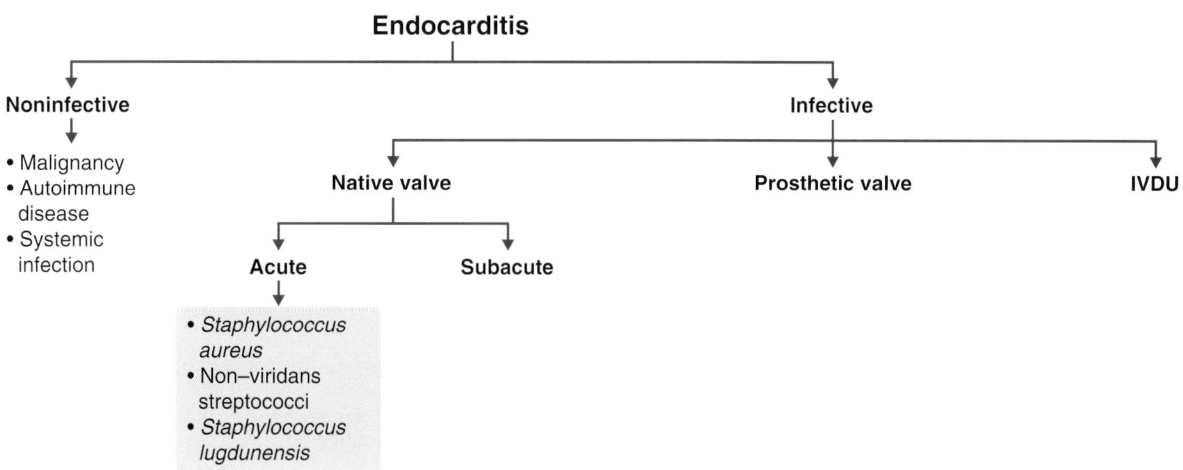


**What is the treatment of choice for native valve endocarditis caused by *Staphylococcus aureus*?**

*Staphylococcus aureus* is the most common cause of acute NVE in the industrialized world. Resistance to oxacillin or methicillin (ie, methicillin-resistant *Staphylococcus aureus* [MRSA]) is on the rise, even in patients without risk factors (eg, health care exposure). *Staphylococcus aureus* IE in non-IV drug users typically involves the left-side of the heart (eg, aortic and mitral valves). The treatment of choice for uncomplicated methicillin-sensitive *Staphylococcus aureus* (MSSA) NVE is intravenous nafcillin or oxacillin for 6 weeks. For uncomplicated MRSA NVE, the agent of choice is vancomycin.[2]

**Which non–viridans streptococcal species cause acute native valve endocarditis?**

Streptococcal species are a frequent cause of IE; however, most cases are caused by viridans streptococci and are subacute in presentation. Non–viridans streptococcal species are capable of causing acute IE. These species include groups A, B, C, F, and G streptococci, and *Streptococcus pneumoniae*. Alcoholism is the most common risk factor for *Streptococcus pneumoniae* IE, which is present in nearly one-third of cases. Pneumonia and meningitis may also be present, forming the classic triad. The treatment of choice for non–viridans streptococcal NVE is penicillin or ceftriaxone for 4 to 6 weeks. Gentamycin may be added for the first 2 weeks in patients with infection caused by serogroups B, C, F, and G.[2,17]

**What is the prognosis of native valve endocarditis caused by *Staphylococcus lugdunensis*?**

Traditionally associated with PVE, coagulase-negative staphylococci are emerging as important causes of NVE, particularly in the health care setting. In contrast with the subacute course characteristic of NVE caused by other coagulase-negative staphylococci, *Staphylococcus lugdunensis* IE tends to be particularly aggressive and is associated with a high rate of perivalvular abscess formation, peripheral emboli, and mortality (similar to *Staphylococcus aureus* IE). Patients should be treated with standard regimens based on in vitro susceptibility patterns.[8,18]

## SUBACUTE NATIVE VALVE INFECTIVE ENDOCARDITIS

### What are the causes of subacute native valve endocarditis?

**Part of normal oral flora, this group of organisms has historically caused most cases of subacute NVE.**

Viridans streptococci.

**Once classified as a streptococcal species.**

Enterococci.

**IE caused by this organism often occurs in patients with abnormalities of the colon.**

*Streptococcus gallolyticus* (formerly *Streptococcus bovis*).

**Traditionally a source of PVE, this organism is becoming a more common cause of subacute NVE.**

*Staphylococcus epidermidis.*

**A group of organisms that require additional time to grow in the laboratory.**

HACEK organisms: ***H**aemophilus* species, ***A**ggregatibacter* species, ***C**ardiobacterium hominis*, ***E**ikenella corrodens*, and ***K**ingella* species.

**Culture may not reveal an organism in up to 10% of cases of IE.**

Culture-negative IE.[2]

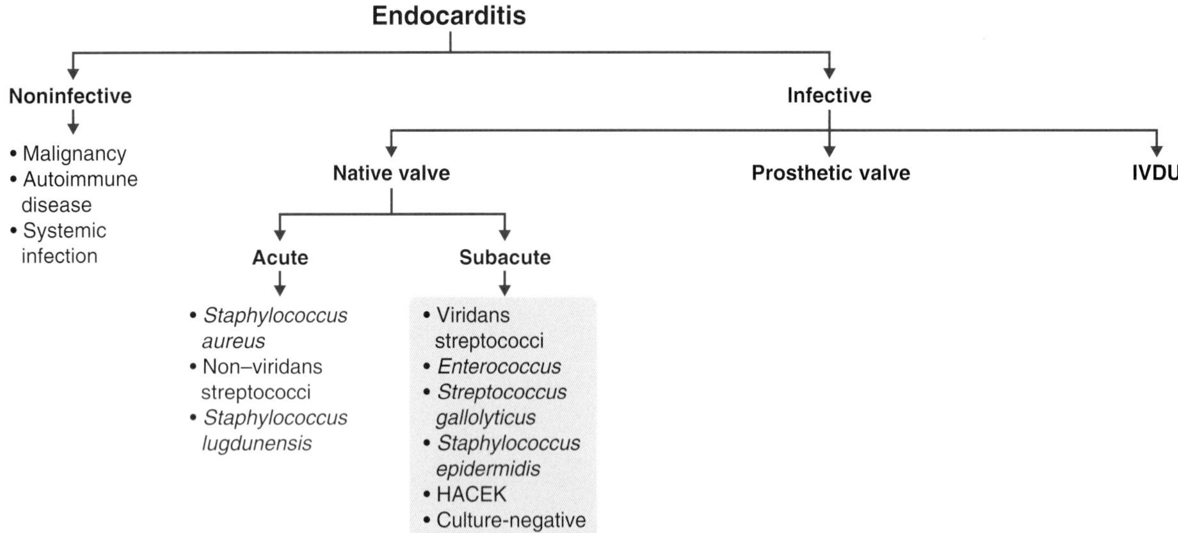


**Which of the viridans streptococci are most commonly associated with native valve endocarditis?**

Viridans streptococci are commensals of the oral, gastrointestinal, and urogenital tract. The species that most often cause subacute NVE are *Streptococcus sanguis*, *Streptococcus mitis*, *Streptococcus salivarius*, and *Streptococcus mutans*. Most strains are highly susceptible to penicillin, and cure rates approach 100% in uncomplicated cases after 4 weeks of IV therapy.[2,8]

**What are the typical sources of enterococcal endocarditis?**

Enterococci account for around 10% of all cases of IE. The vast majority of cases are caused by *Enterococcus faecalis*, with the remainder caused by *Enterococcus faecium*. Sources of these organisms include the gastrointestinal and genitourinary tracts. Susceptibility testing is important in cases of enterococcal IE. In susceptible strains, optimal therapy for enterococcal NVE includes penicillin, ampicillin, or vancomycin in combination with either gentamicin or streptomycin for 4 to 6 weeks. Alternative regimens may be necessary in patients with resistant strains or impaired renal function (eg, ampicillin plus ceftriaxone). *Enterococcal IE may have an acute presentation.*[2]

**Which diagnostic procedure should be considered for patients with *Streptococcus gallolyticus* endocarditis?**

In patients with *Streptococcus gallolyticus* endocarditis, colonoscopy should be performed to evaluate for ulcerative lesions of the colon caused by underlying conditions such malignancy or inflammatory bowel disease. Like viridans streptococci, most strains of *Streptococcus gallolyticus* are highly susceptible to penicillin, and cure rates approach 100% in uncomplicated cases after 4 weeks of IV therapy.[2]

**What are the features of *Staphylococcus epidermidis* native valve endocarditis?**

Coagulase-negative staphylococci are part of the normal skin flora. These organisms are responsible for an increasing proportion of cases of NVE, particularly *Staphylococcus epidermidis*. Extensive contact with health care is an important risk factor. Despite the subacute presentation, coagulase-negative staphylococci NVE is associated with high rates of perivalvular abscess formation, heart failure, and death. Most strains are methicillin resistant and must be treated similar to MRSA (eg, vancomycin).[2,8,19]

**How common is community-acquired native valve endocarditis related to HACEK organisms?**

The HACEK organisms account for up to 10% of cases of community-acquired NVE in patients who do not use IV drugs. Growth of these organisms is slow in standard blood culture media, and identification requires prolonged incubation. The treatment of choice is ceftriaxone for 4 weeks.[2]

**What is culture-negative endocarditis?**

Culture-negative endocarditis refers to IE in which an organism is not identified by blood culture. It may occur for a variety of reasons, including inadequate microbiological techniques, infection with fastidious or noncultivable organisms, or administration of antimicrobial agents before collecting blood cultures. In some cases, blood culture yield may return after several days without antibiotics. Organisms that are associated with negative blood cultures include *Streptococcus* species in which antibiotics have been administered before culture acquisition, *Abiotrophia* and *Granulicatella* species (formerly known as nutritionally variant streptococci), *Coxiella burnetii*, *Bartonella* species, *Brucella* species, *Legionella* species, *Tropheryma whipplei*, and fungi. Other microbiological techniques (eg, serologies) may be helpful. Empiric antimicrobial therapy to cover all likely pathogens is necessary in patients with culture-negative endocarditis.[2]

## PROSTHETIC VALVE INFECTIVE ENDOCARDITIS

**How common is prosthetic valve endocarditis?**

PVE accounts for up to one-third of all cases of IE. It is associated with a higher mortality rate than NVE.[20]

**Which type of prosthetic valve (mechanical or bioprosthetic) is more likely to become infected?**

In the first year after surgery, mechanical valves are more likely than bioprosthetic valves to become infected, but at 5 years, there is no difference in risk.[21]

**How sensitive is echocardiography in identifying lesions that are diagnostic of prosthetic valve endocarditis?**

In patients with PVE, the sensitivity of TTE in identifying vegetations, a perivalvular abscess, or dehiscence of the prosthetic valve is around 25%; sensitivity improves to 90% with TEE.[15,22]

**What are the 2 subtypes of prosthetic valve endocarditis based on the timing of onset?**

PVE can occur in the early or late period following valve replacement surgery.

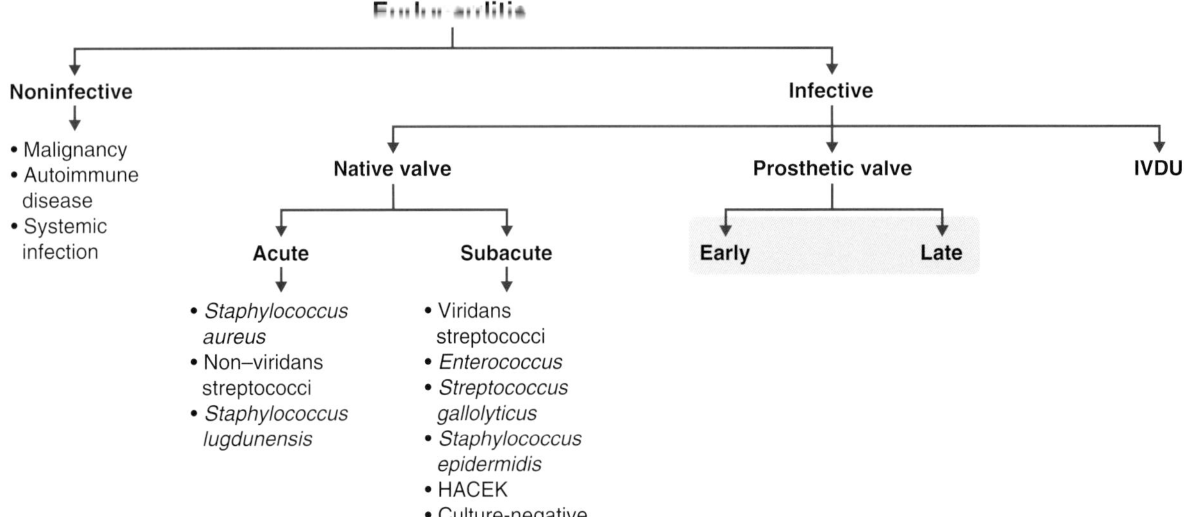


**What time course is generally used to define early versus late prosthetic valve endocarditis?**

PVE is considered early when it occurs within 2 months of valve replacement surgery (less common); late PVE occurs >12 months after surgery (more common). This dichotomy is helpful because the organisms associated with each subtype are distinctive. *When PVE occurs between 2 and 12 months after surgery, it is referred to as intermediate and can be caused by organisms associated with both early and late PVE.*[14,20]

**What are the general microbiological differences between early and late prosthetic valve endocarditis?**

The organisms of early PVE tend to be nosocomial in nature, whereas the organisms of late PVE tend to mirror the community-acquired organisms found in patients with NVE.

## EARLY PROSTHETIC VALVE INFECTIVE ENDOCARDITIS

### What are the causes of early prosthetic valve endocarditis?

**PVE caused by this organism has recently been on the rise and is now considered the most common cause of early PVE.**

*Staphylococcus aureus.*[20]

**Traditionally, this organism had been considered the most common cause of early PVE.**

*Staphylococcus epidermidis.*

**PVE caused by these organisms may be associated with infection of the genitourinary or non–oral gastrointestinal tract.**

Non-HACEK gram-negative bacilli.

**Nonbacterial organisms.**

Fungi.

**Commonly assumed to be a contaminant when isolated from blood cultures.**

Diphtheroids (ie, *Corynebacterium* species).

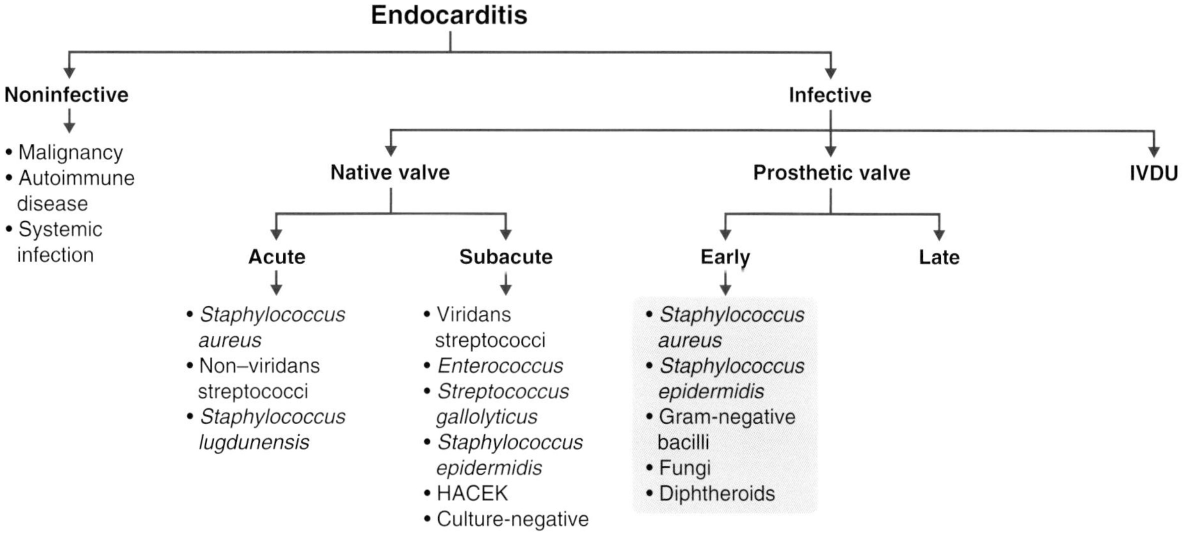

**Endocarditis**

- **Noninfective**
  - Malignancy
  - Autoimmune disease
  - Systemic infection
- **Infective**
  - **Native valve**
    - **Acute**
      - *Staphylococcus aureus*
      - Non–viridans streptococci
      - *Staphylococcus lugdunensis*
    - **Subacute**
      - Viridans streptococci
      - *Enterococcus*
      - *Streptococcus gallolyticus*
      - *Staphylococcus epidermidis*
      - HACEK
      - Culture-negative
  - **Prosthetic valve**
    - **Early**
      - *Staphylococcus aureus*
      - *Staphylococcus epidermidis*
      - Gram-negative bacilli
      - Fungi
      - Diphtheroids
    - **Late**
  - **IVDU**

**What is the optimal antibiotic therapy for prosthetic valve endocarditis caused by *Staphylococcus aureus*?**

PVE caused by *Staphylococcus aureus* is associated with a high mortality rate, and combination antibiotics are recommended. For MSSA PVE, triple-drug therapy is preferred, including nafcillin or oxacillin plus rifampin for at least 6 weeks with gentamycin for the first 2 weeks. For MRSA PVE, the synthetic penicillin should be replaced with vancomycin.[2]

**What are the features of prosthetic valve endocarditis caused by *Staphylococcus epidermidis*?**

Coagulase-negative staphylococcus PVE is almost always caused by *Staphylococcus epidermidis*. It tends to be aggressive with an acute presentation similar to that of *Staphylococcus aureus*, with high rates of complications such as perivalvular abscess, heart failure, and peripheral metastases.[20,21]

**Which non-HACEK gram-negative bacilli are associated with prosthetic valve endocarditis?**

Among the non-HACEK gram-negative bacilli, *Escherichia coli* and *Pseudomonas aeruginosa* are most frequently associated with PVE. Others include *Klebsiella* species, *Serratia* species, and *Proteus* species. Most cases are associated with health care exposure, and organisms are frequently resistant to multiple antibiotics. The combination of a β-lactam agent (eg, penicillin, cephalosporin, carbapenem) with either an aminoglycoside or fluoroquinolone for 6 weeks is a reasonable option. Despite combined medical and surgical approaches, in-hospital mortality rates are high (approximately 25%).[2,23]

**Which fungus is most frequently associated with prosthetic valve endocarditis?**

*Candida* species cause most cases of fungal PVE. Complications such as systemic embolization and perivalvular abscess occur frequently. Optimal antimicrobial treatment consists of amphotericin B with or without flucytosine for at least 6 weeks followed by chronic suppression with fluconazole. Combination medical and surgical therapy is required in most cases; however, despite treatment, more than one-half of patients die. *Candida is also associated with late PVE.*[24]

**What are the features of prosthetic valve endocarditis caused by diphtheroids?**

The diphtheroids are part of normal skin flora and are frequent contaminants of blood cultures. However, these organisms cause up to 10% of early PVE cases and just fewer than 5% of late PVE cases. The isolation of diphtheroids in blood cultures often requires prolonged incubation, but the Gram stain can be revealing (gram-positive bacilli). Complications such as perivalvular abscess, valvular dysfunction, and heart failure are common. Based on susceptibility data, penicillin in combination with gentamycin, or vancomycin alone may be used. A significant proportion of cases require the combination of medical and surgical treatment. Despite therapy, mortality rates are high at about 40%.[25,26]

## LATE PROSTHETIC VALVE INFECTIVE ENDOCARDITIS

### What are the causes of late prosthetic valve endocarditis?

**These organisms, which are part of normal oral flora, are a leading cause of subacute NVE.**

Viridans streptococci.

**The most common cause of acute NVE.**

*Staphylococcus aureus.*

**A common cause of early PVE; this organism has a predilection for hardware.**

*Staphylococcus epidermidis.*

**Formerly classified as group D *Streptococcus.***

*Enterococcus.*

***Streptococcus pyogenes* belongs to this group of organisms.**

Non–viridans streptococci (groups A, B, C, F, and G streptococci, and *Streptococcus pneumoniae*).

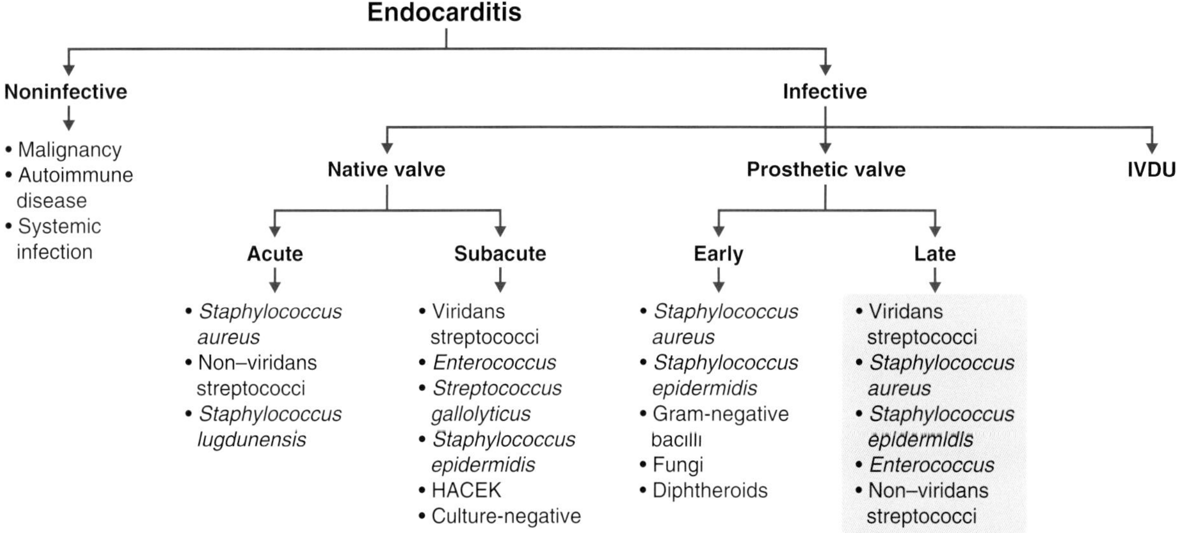


**What is the treatment for prosthetic valve endocarditis caused by viridans streptococci?**

Viridans streptococcal PVE is almost always late-onset. Treatment of choice includes penicillin or ceftriaxone for 6 weeks with or without gentamycin for the first 2 weeks; penicillin-resistant strains should be treated with penicillin or ceftriaxone plus gentamycin for 6 weeks.[2,20]

**How often does *Staphylococcus aureus* cause late prosthetic valve endocarditis?**

*Staphylococcus aureus* frequently causes both early and late PVE; in some populations, it is the most common cause of both. It is a virulent organism with a high rate of complications such as perivalvular abscess, purulent pericarditis, and peripheral metastases.[20]

**What is the optimal antibiotic therapy for prosthetic valve endocarditis caused by *Staphylococcus epidermidis*?**

The antimicrobial regimen used to treat PVE caused by *Staphylococcus epidermidis* is the same as for PVE caused by *Staphylococcus aureus.* For methicillin-sensitive strains, triple-drug therapy is preferred, including nafcillin or oxacillin plus rifampin for at least 6 weeks with gentamycin for the first 2 weeks. For methicillin-resistant strains, the synthetic penicillin should be replaced with vancomycin.[2]

**What is the optimal antibiotic therapy for patients with prosthetic valve endocarditis caused by *Enterococcus* species?**

*Enterococcus* species cause approximately 10% of cases of late PVE. Medical treatment for enterococcal PVE and NVE is the same: in susceptible strains, optimal therapy includes penicillin, ampicillin, or vancomycin in combination with either gentamicin or streptomycin. Duration of treatment should be extended to at least 6 weeks. Alternative regimens may be necessary in patients with resistant strains or impaired renal function.[2]

**How often do non–viridans streptococci cause late prosthetic valve endocarditis?**

Non–viridans streptococci cause approximately 10% of late PVE. Medical treatment for non–viridans streptococcus PVE and NVE is the same, although the duration of therapy for PVE is increased to at least 6 weeks.[2,20]

*Similar to subacute NVE, HACEK organisms and culture-negative endocarditis can also cause late PVE.*

## INFECTIVE ENDOCARDITIS RELATED TO INTRAVENOUS DRUG USE

**Which heart valves are most frequently infected in intravenous drug users?**

Native or prosthetic valves may be infected in IV drug users. These patients often develop endothelial injury involving the tricuspid valve as a result of repeated IV injections of solid particles, resulting in a predisposition for right-sided endocarditis. The affected valve is the tricuspid in 50% of cases; the mitral and aortic valves in 20% of cases each, and multiple valves are involved in 10% of cases. The pulmonic valve is rarely involved. The type of IV drug used may influence the site that is affected (eg, tricuspid valve disease is more frequent in heroin users compared with those who use other IV drugs).[9,11,27,28]

**What physical findings are common in patients with right-sided endocarditis from intravenous drug use?**

Fever is common in IE involving either side of the heart. Evidence of right-sided heart failure (eg, elevated JVP, peripheral edema) caused by tricuspid regurgitation is common in patients with endocarditis related to IV drug use. Tricuspid regurgitation may be associated with a holosystolic murmur best heard over the left lower sternal border that may augment with inspiration (Carvallo's sign). There may also be CV fusion in the jugular venous waveform, which is known as Lancisi's sign. *For videos of Carvallo's sign and Lancisi's sign, see the associated references.*[11,29,30]

**What are the manifestations of embolic events in patients with right-sided endocarditis?**

Embolic events in patients with right-sided endocarditis typically affect the lungs, manifesting as multiple peripheral-based consolidations that are often cavitary on imaging (Figure 29-5). These patients may complain of dyspnea, chest pain, and cough. In patients with right-to-left shunt, systemic embolic phenomena can occur.[31]

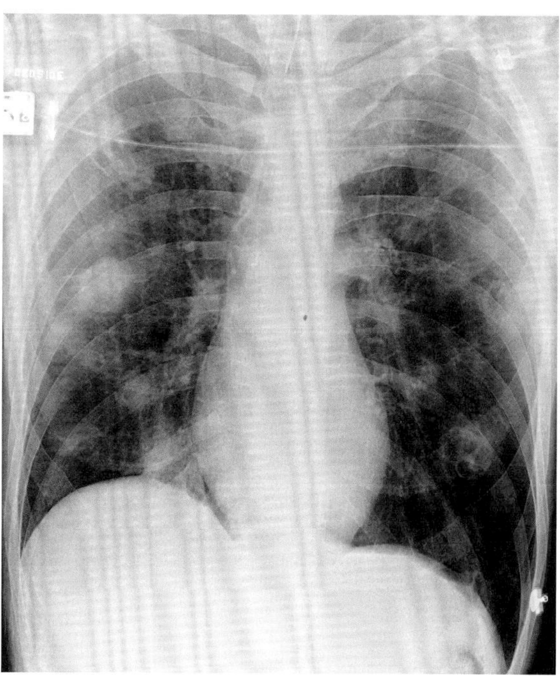

**Figure 29-5.** Multiple septic pulmonary emboli demonstrated on chest imaging in a patient with right-sided infective endocarditis. Note the presence of cavitation in some of the lesions. (From Muller NL, Franquet T, Lee KS, Silva CIS. *Imaging of Pulmonary Infections*. Philadelphia, PA: Lippincott Williams & Wilkins; 2007.)

**What is the optimal treatment for endocarditis related to intravenous drug use?**

The antimicrobial treatment for IE among IV drug users depends on the organism(s) and site of involvement. Duration of therapy is 4 to 6 weeks in most cases, however in select groups a 2-week treatment course may be effective. Surgical intervention may be beneficial in some patients, such as those with refractory heart failure, persistent infection, perivalvular abscess, conduction abnormalities, or prosthetic valve involvement. However, surgical intervention in these patients must be considered carefully given the significant risk of recidivism. Right-sided IE is associated with a favorable prognosis (with mortality <10%).[31,32]

## What are the causes of infective endocarditis related to intravenous drug use?

**This organism is responsible for more than one-half of cases of IE in IV drug users.**

*Staphylococcus aureus*.[14]

***Streptococcus mitis* is an organism within this group.**

Viridans streptococci.

**This genus contains over 15 species, but only 2 are commonly associated with endocarditis.**

*Enterococcus*.[2]

**May be seen in patients who contaminate needles, inoculate injection sites with saliva (via skin or needle licking), or use their teeth to crush tablets before injection.**

*Eikenella corrodens* (a HACEK organism).[31]

**Infection with this group of organisms is often considered a "stand-alone" indication for surgery.**

Fungi.[2]

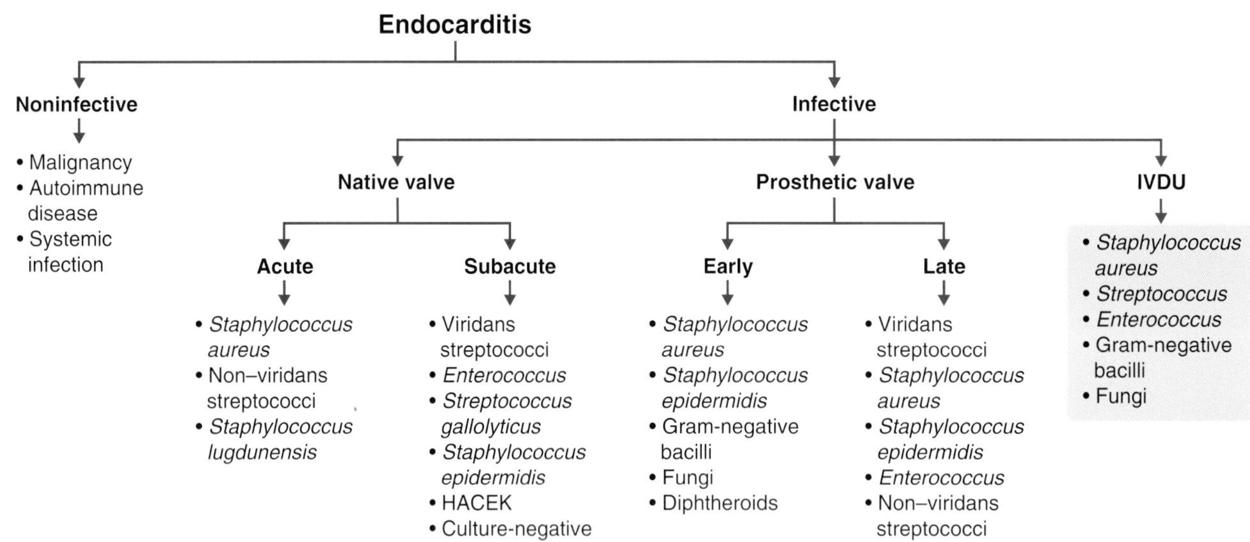


**Which heart valves are most frequently involved in intravenous drug users with *Staphylococcus aureus* infective endocarditis?**

Most cases of *Staphylococcus aureus* IE in IV drug users involve the tricuspid valve. Cases are frequently complicated by extracardiac infection, such as pneumonia, soft tissue abscess, septic arthritis, and osteomyelitis. Nafcillin or oxacillin is the agent of choice for MSSA, whereas vancomycin is the agent of choice for MRSA.[14,31-33]

**Which heart valves are most frequently infected in intravenous drug users with viridans streptococcal infective endocarditis?**

The vast majority of cases of viridans streptococcal IE in IV drug users are left-sided. Penicillin is the agent of choice.[14,31,32]

**Which heart valves are most frequently infected in intravenous drug users with enterococcal infective endocarditis?**

The vast majority of cases of enterococcal IE in IV drug users are left-sided.[14,31]

**Which gram-negative bacilli are associated with infective endocarditis among intravenous drug users?**

IV drug use is a risk factor for IE caused by gram-negative bacilli, most frequently *Pseudomonas aeruginosa* and *Escherichia coli*. Others include the HACEK organisms, *Serratia marcescens*, and *Proteus mirabilis*. The use of tap water or toilet water in drug preparation is a risk factor for infection with *Pseudomonas aeruginosa*. Gram-negative IE among IV drug users is associated with a less favorable prognosis compared with IE caused by more typical organisms in this population.[2,32,34]

**Which fungi are associated with infective endocarditis among intravenous drug users?**

*Candida* and *Aspergillus* species cause most cases of fungal endocarditis among IV drug users. *Candida albicans* is far more common, and is associated with positive blood cultures; *Aspergillus* endocarditis rarely produces positive blood cultures. Treatment almost always requires the combination of parenteral antifungal therapy and surgery. Fungal IE among IV drug users is associated with a less favorable prognosis compared with IE caused by more typical organisms in this population.[2,13]

*Polymicrobial IE is more common among IV drug users, typically involves the tricuspid valve, and is associated with a poor prognosis.*[31]

## Case Summary

A 31-year-old man with a history of IVDU presents with acute-onset fever and dyspnea and is found to have elevated JVP, several heart murmurs, and a variety of other abnormal physical findings.

***What is the most likely underlying diagnosis in this patient?***

Infective endocarditis.

### BONUS QUESTIONS

***Which general categories of infective endocarditis apply to this case?***

This case describes acute left-sided NVE in an IV drug user. Categorizing endocarditis can be helpful in determining the most likely underlying organisms and guiding treatment.

***What clinical findings in this case are suggestive of infective endocarditis?***

This case meets 1 major Duke criterion (new valvular regurgitation by physical examination) and 3 minor criteria (predisposition [IVDU], fever, and immunologic phenomena) (see Table 29-1).

***What is the significance of the heart murmurs in this case?***

The heart murmurs described in this case are consistent with aortic regurgitation. The murmur of aortic regurgitation typically begins early in diastole, is decrescendo in shape, and is best heard over the third intercostal space of the left sternal border (Erb's point). There is often an associated systolic ejection murmur that occurs as the regurgitant bolus of blood generates turbulence on its way back through the aortic valve (technically a flow murmur). Aortic regurgitation may be associated with a low-pitched, "blubbering," mid-to-late diastolic murmur heard over the apex, known as the Austin Flint murmur. The mechanism is thought to be distortion and early closure of the anterior leaflet of the mitral valve caused by the regurgitant aortic jet, resulting in functional mitral stenosis. *For a video demonstrating the mechanism of the Austin Flint murmur, see the associated reference.*[35,36]

***What is the significance of the nail bed pulsation in this case?***

Nail bed pulsation, known as Quincke's pulse, is a sign of aortic regurgitation. Regurgitant blood flow into a dilated left ventricle during diastole leads to a decrease in diastolic pressure and a consequent increase in stroke volume, resulting in blanching and flushing, respectively, of the nail bed. *For a video of Quincke's pulse, see the associated reference.*[37]

***What is the significance of the head bob in this case?***

The to-and-fro head bob, known as de Musset sign, is a sign of aortic regurgitation. Regurgitant blood flow into the left ventricle during diastole leads to an increase in stroke volume, the force of which causes the head to jolt back with each heartbeat.[35]

***What is the significance of the skin finding demonstrated in Figure 29-1?***

The painful erythematous nodules demonstrated in Figure 29-1, known as Osler's nodes, are immunologic phenomena that occur in patients with IE. Peripheral manifestations such as these are more common in patients with subacute IE but can occur in acute cases (such as this one).[2]

***Which organisms are most often associated with infective endocarditis related to intravenous drug use?***

IE related to IVDU is most often caused by *Staphylococcus aureus*, viridans streptococci, and *Enterococcus* infections. Empiric coverage of these organisms while awaiting blood culture results would be a reasonable approach in this case. The possibility of infection with gram-negative bacilli or fungi should always be considered in IV drug users. Given the evidence of severe aortic regurgitation and heart failure, this patient should also be evaluated for aortic valve replacement.[16]

## KEY POINTS

- Endocarditis refers to inflammation of the endocardium, usually involving the heart valves.
- Endocarditis can be noninfective or infective.
- Nonbacterial thrombotic endocarditis refers to the presence of sterile vegetations on the endocardium that develop in association with a variety of inflammatory or hypercoagulable conditions.
- NBTE most often presents with embolic phenomena. Anticoagulation is the cornerstone of medical management.
- Infective endocarditis is a clinical diagnosis based on history, physical examination, laboratory data, and imaging (echocardiography).
- IE can be separated into the following subcategories: NVE, PVE, and IE related to IV drug use.
- NVE can follow an acute or subacute clinical course.
- *Staphylococcus aureus* is the most common cause of acute NVE.
- Viridans streptococci is the most common cause of subacute NVE.
- PVE can occur in the early period (<2 months) or late period (>12 months) following valve replacement surgery.
- Early PVE is most commonly caused by *Staphylococcus aureus* and *Staphylococcus epidermidis*.
- Late PVE is most commonly caused by viridans streptococci.
- IE related to IVDU is most commonly caused by *Staphylococcus aureus*.
- The tricuspid valve is most frequently involved in IE associated with IVDU, but left-sided involvement is also common.

## REFERENCES


1. Aryana A, Esterbrooks DJ, Morris PC. Nonbacterial thrombotic endocarditis with recurrent embolic events as manifestation of ovarian neoplasm. *J Gen Intern Med*. 2006;21(12):C12-C15.
2. Baddour LM, Wilson WR, Bayer AS, et al. Infective endocarditis in adults: diagnosis, antimicrobial therapy, and management of complications: a scientific statement for healthcare professionals from the American Heart Association. *Circulation*. 2015;132(15):1435-1486.
3. Hoen B, Duval X. Clinical practice. Infective endocarditis. *N Engl J Med*. 2013;368(15):1425-1433.
4. Eiken PW, Edwards WD, Tazelaar HD, McBane RD, Zehr KJ. Surgical pathology of nonbacterial thrombotic endocarditis in 30 patients, 1985-2000. *Mayo Clin Proc*. 2001;76(12):1204-1212.
5. Liu J, Frishman WH. Nonbacterial thrombotic endocarditis: pathogenesis, diagnosis, and management. *Cardiol Rev*. 2016;24(5):244-247.
6. Llenas-Garcia J, Guerra-Vales JM, Montes-Moreno S, Lopez-Rios F, Castelbon-Fernandez FJ, Chimeno-Garcia J. Nonbacterial thrombotic endocarditis: clinicopathologic study of a necropsy series. *Rev Esp Cardiol*. 2007;60(5):493-500.
7. Moyssakis I, Tektonidou MG, Vasilliou VA, Samarkos M, Votteas V, Moutsopoulos HM. Libman-Sacks endocarditis in systemic lupus erythematosus: prevalence, associations, and evolution. *Am J Med*. 2007;120(7):636-642.
8. Cahill TJ, Prendergast BD. Infective endocarditis. *Lancet*. 2016;387(10021):882-893.
9. Frontera JA, Gradon JD. Right-side endocarditis in injection drug users: review of proposed mechanisms of pathogenesis. *Clin Infect Dis*. 2000;30(2):374-379.
10. Beynon RP, Bahl VK, Prendergast BD. Infective endocarditis. *BMJ*. 2006;333(7563):334-339.
11. Ashley E, Niebauer J. *Cardiology Explained*. London: Remedica; 2004.
12. Durack DT, Lukes AS, Bright DK. New criteria for diagnosis of infective endocarditis: utilization of specific echocardiographic findings. Duke Endocarditis Service. *Am J Med*. 1994;96(3):200-209.

13. Li JS, Sexton DJ, Mick N, et al. Proposed modifications to the Duke criteria for the diagnosis of infective endocarditis. *Clin Infect Dis*. 2000;30(4):633-638.
14. Longo DL, Fauci AS, Kasper DL, Hauser SL, Jameson JL, Loscalzo J, eds. *Harrison's Principles of Internal Medicine*. 18th ed. New York, NY: McGraw-Hill; 2012.
15. Habib G, Badano L, Tribouilloy C, et al. Recommendations for the practice of echocardiography in infective endocarditis. *Eur J Echocardiogr*. 2010;11(2):202-219.
16. McDonald JR. Acute infective endocarditis. *Infect Dis Clin North Am*. 2009;23(3):643-664.
17. Aronin SI, Mukherjee SK, West JC, Cooney EL. Review of pneumococcal endocarditis in adults in the penicillin era. *Clin Infect Dis*. 1998;26(1):165-171.
18. Anguera I, Del Rio A, Miro JM, et al. Staphylococcus lugdunensis infective endocarditis: description of 10 cases and analysis of native valve, prosthetic valve, and pacemaker lead endocarditis clinical profiles. *Heart*. 2005;91(2):e10.
19. Chu VH, Woods CW, Miro JM, et al. Emergence of coagulase-negative staphylococci as a cause of native valve endocarditis. *Clin Infect Dis*. 2008;46(2):232-242.
20. Lee JH, Burner KD, Fealey ME, et al. Prosthetic valve endocarditis: clinicopathological correlates in 122 surgical specimens from 116 patients (1985-2004). *Cardiovasc Pathol*. 2011;20(1):26-35.
21. Bashore TM, Cabell C, Fowler V Jr. Update on infective endocarditis. *Curr Probl Cardiol*. 2006;31(4):274-352.
22. Morguet AJ, Werner GS, Andreas S, Kreuzer H. Diagnostic value of transesophageal compared with transthoracic echocardiography in suspected prosthetic valve endocarditis. *Herz*. 1995;20(6):390-398.
23. Morpeth S, Murdoch D, Cabell CH, et al. Non-HACEK gram-negative bacillus endocarditis. *Ann Intern Med*. 2007;147(12):829-835.
24. Boland JM, Chung HH, Robberts FJ, et al. Fungal prosthetic valve endocarditis: Mayo Clinic experience with a clinicopathological analysis. *Mycoses*. 2011;54(4):354-360.
25. Belmares J, Detterline S, Pak JB, Parada JP. Corynebacterium endocarditis species-specific risk factors and outcomes. *BMC Infect Dis*. 2007;7:4.
26. Murray BE, Karchmer AW, Moellering RC Jr. Diphtheroid prosthetic valve endocarditis. A study of clinical features and infecting organisms. *Am J Med*. 1980;69(6):838-848.
27. Mathew J, Addai T, Anand A, Morrobel A, Maheshwari P, Freels S. Clinical features, site of involvement, bacteriologic findings, and outcome of infective endocarditis in intravenous drug users. *Arch Intern Med*. 1995;155(15):1641-1648.
28. Sousa C, Botelho C, Rodrigues D, Azeredo J, Oliveira R. Infective endocarditis in intravenous drug abusers: an update. *Eur J Clin Microbiol Infect Dis*. 2012;31(11):2905-2910.
29. Burgess TE, Mansoor AM. Giant a waves. *BMJ Case Rep*. 2017;2017.
30. Mansoor AM, Mansoor SE. Images in clinical medicine. Lancisi's sign. *N Engl J Med*. 2016;374(2):e2.
31. Colville T, Sharma V, Albouaini K. Infective endocarditis in intravenous drug users: a review article. *Postgrad Med J*. 2016;92(1084):105-111.
32. Ji Y, Kujtan L, Kershner D. Acute endocarditis in intravenous drug users: a case report and literature review. *J Community Hosp Intern Med Perspect*. 2012;2(1).
33. Ortiz-Bautista C, Lopez J, Garcia-Granja PE, et al. Current profile of infective endocarditis in intravenous drug users: the prognostic relevance of the valves involved. *Int J Cardiol*. 2015;187:472-474.
34. Kaushik KS, Kapila K, Praharaj AK. Shooting up: the interface of microbial infections and drug abuse. *J Med Microbiol*. 2011;60(Pt 4):408-422.
35. Marriott HJL. *Bedside Cardiac Diagnosis*. Philadelphia, PA: Lippincott; 1993.
36. Weir RA, Dargie HJ. Images in clinical medicine. Austin flint murmur. *N Engl J Med*. 2008;359(10):e11.
37. Mansoor AM, Mansoor SE. Images in clinical medicine. Quincke's pulse. *N Engl J Med*. 2013;369(7):e8.

Chapter 30

# MENINGITIS

## Case: A 34-year-old man with agitated delirium

A 34-year-old man with a history of type 1 diabetes mellitus complicated by end-stage renal disease, status post kidney transplantation from an unrelated donor, is admitted to the hospital with several hours of headache, confusion, and agitation. Medications include prednisone, tacrolimus, and mycophenolate mofetil.

Temperature is 37.8°C, and heart rate is 112 beats per minute. The patient is agitated and disoriented. Neck pain and stiffness are present. Cross-sectional imaging of the head is unremarkable. Lumbar puncture (LP) is performed, and the cerebrospinal fluid (CSF) appears reddish in color. The intensity of the color remains consistent with subsequent sampling; vials 1 (left) and 4 (right) are identical in appearance (Figure 30-1).

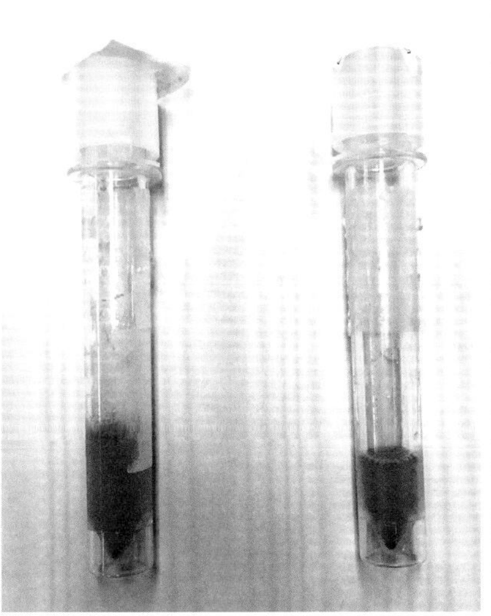

**Figure 30-1.** (Courtesy of Avital O'Glasser, MD, Carlton Scharman, MD, and Danielle M. Taylor.)

CSF studies are shown below:

| Appearance | Opening Pressure (cm $H_2O$) | WBC/μL | Glucose (mg/dL) | Total Protein (mg/dL) |
|---|---|---|---|---|
| Bloody | 14 | 512 (92% lymphocytes) | 63 | 88 |

Magnetic resonance imaging (MRI) of the brain demonstrates abnormal signal involving the left medial temporal lobe.

***What is the most likely diagnosis in this patient?***

**What is meningitis?**

Meningitis refers to inflammation of the meninges associated with an abnormal increase in the number of white blood cells (WBCs) in the CSF (known as pleocytosis).[1]

**What are the symptoms of meningitis?**

Depending on the underlying cause, meningitis can present as an acute fulminant illness with rapid progression within hours, a subacute illness progressing over a period of days, or a chronic illness progressing over months. The spectrum of clinical manifestations depends on the underlying cause, but symptoms may include headache, neck stiffness, neck pain, lethargy, nausea, vomiting, photophobia, phonophobia, and confusion (which is usually not prominent in the initial course of the illness).[2]

**What are the physical findings of meningitis?**

Physical findings of meningitis depend on the underlying cause, but may include fever, nuchal rigidity, positive Kernig's sign (pain and resistance on extension of the knee starting with the hip and knee flexed at 90°), positive Brudziński's sign (reflex flexion of the hips and knees on passive flexion of the neck with the patient in the supine position), papilledema, and other signs of increased intracranial pressure (eg, sixth nerve palsy). Some physical findings may be specific to underlying organisms (eg, the maculopapular and petechial skin rash of meningococcemia).[2,3]

**What is the difference between meningitis and encephalitis?**

Encephalitis is inflammation of the brain parenchyma—usually caused by a viral infection—and is clinically associated with neurologic dysfunction early in the course of the illness. Pleocytosis is often present in patients with encephalitis but may be absent in some cases.[4]

**What is meningoencephalitis?**

The term meningoencephalitis refers to cases in which there are clinical features of both meningitis and encephalitis; viral infection is a frequent cause.[1]

**What are the 4 general categories of meningitis?**

Meningitis can be viral, bacterial, fungal, or aseptic.

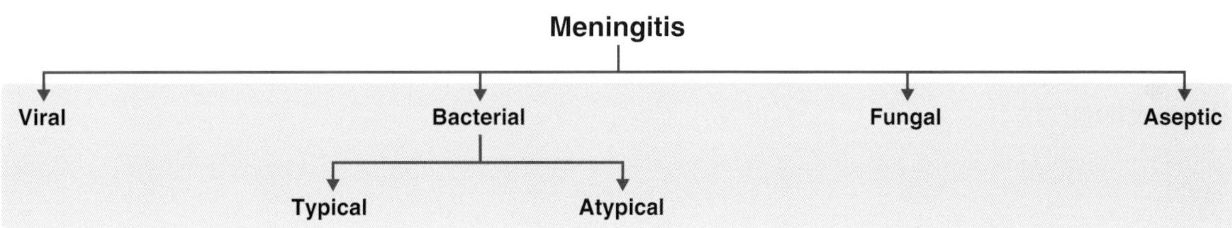


*Historically, viral meningitis has been used synonymously with aseptic meningitis (at a time when viruses were not easily identified in the laboratory). These categories will be considered separate in this chapter.*

**What diagnostic procedure should be performed in patients with suspected meningitis?**

LP should be performed urgently in most patients with suspected meningitis. However, LP can result in cerebral herniation in patients with increased intracranial pressure caused by a mass lesion. In some patients, neuroimaging (eg, computed tomography [CT]) should be performed before LP to evaluate for mass lesions.

**Which patients should undergo neuroimaging before lumbar puncture?**

CT imaging of the head should be performed before LP in patients who are at increased risk for a mass lesion with associated increased intracranial pressure. Such patients include those with immunocompromised status, history of central nervous system disease (eg, mass lesion), new-onset seizure (within 1 week of presentation), papilledema, abnormal level of consciousness, or focal neurologic deficits.[5]

**Should empiric antimicrobial therapy be withheld until a cerebrospinal fluid sample is obtained in patients with suspected meningitis?**

When possible, LP should be performed before antimicrobial therapy is initiated, as this ensures optimal yield of CSF cultures. However, if there is an anticipated delay in performing LP, empiric therapy should be administered first.[6]

**Which of the profiles in Table 30-1 are characteristic of normal cerebrospinal fluid, viral meningitis, typical bacterial meningitis, atypical bacterial meningitis, fungal meningitis, and aseptic meningitis?**

Fluid type A corresponds to normal CSF; type B to typical bacterial meningitis; type C to fungal meningitis (and some types of atypical bacterial meningitis); and type D to viral meningitis, most types of atypical bacterial meningitis, and most types of aseptic meningitis. Fluid types C and D may be characterized by a predominance of neutrophils early in the course of the associated illness. *It is important to note that the numbers provided in Table 30-1 represent general rules of thumb.*[7]

**Table 30-1**

| Fluid type | WBC/µL | Predominant WBC | Glucose (mg/dL) | Protein (mg/dL) |
|---|---|---|---|---|
| A | <5 | Lymphocytes | Normal | <50 |
| B | 500-20,000 | Neutrophils | Low | 100-700 |
| C | 25-500 | Lymphocytes or neutrophils | Low or normal | 50-500 |
| D | 5-1000 | Lymphocytes | Normal | <100 |

**How can it be determined if there is true pleocytosis in the context of a traumatic lumbar puncture?**

After a traumatic LP, peripheral blood contamination of CSF will artificially increase the WBC count. Comparing the ratios of WBCs to red blood cells (RBCs) in both the peripheral blood and CSF can determine if there is true pleocytosis in the context of a traumatic LP. In a purely traumatic tap, the CSF RBC to WBC ratio should be similar to the peripheral RBC to WBC ratio. If the measured CSF WBC count exceeds that predicted by the peripheral ratio, then there were preexisting WBCs in the CSF, independent of the traumatic tap. For example:

| Peripheral RBC (per µL) | Peripheral WBC (per µL) | Peripheral RBC:WBC Ratio | CSF RBC (per µL) | Expected CSF WBC (per µL) |
|---|---|---|---|---|
| 4,000,000 | 10,000 | 400:1 | 20,000 | ≤50 |

If the measured CSF WBC count exceeds 50 cells/µL, then there were preexisting WBCs in the CSF (ie, true pleocytosis).[7]

## VIRAL MENINGITIS

**What is the typical opening pressure of viral meningitis?**

The opening pressure of viral meningitis is typically normal (<18 cm $H_2O$) but can be mildly elevated (up to 35 cm $H_2O$) in some cases.[7]

**What is the characteristic cerebrospinal fluid profile of viral meningitis?**

| Fluid type[7] | WBC (per µL) | WBC Type | Glucose (mg/dL) | Protein (mg/dL) |
|---|---|---|---|---|
| Viral | 5-1000 | Lymphocytes | Normal | <100 |

**Is viral meningitis always associated with a lymphocytic pleocytosis?**

Neutrophils can predominate early in the course of viral meningitis, with a shift to lymphocytes after 12 to 48 hours.[7]

**How is the diagnosis of viral meningitis definitively made?**

Polymerase chain reaction (PCR) of CSF can be used to diagnose specific causes of viral meningitis. PCR is 1000-fold more sensitive than routine viral culture. Definitive diagnosis of viral meningitis reduces unnecessary antibiotic exposure and decreases length of hospital stay.[1]

**What is the treatment for viral meningitis?**

In general, viral meningitis is treated supportively and is usually self-limited. In contrast, viral encephalitis and meningoencephalitis can be life-threatening and antiviral treatment may be life-saving in some cases.[1]

### What are the causes of viral meningitis?

**This group of viruses includes coxsackieviruses A and B, poliovirus, and echovirus and most commonly causes meningitis during the summer and fall seasons in temperate climates.**

Enteroviruses.

**Infection with these viruses may result in recurrent lesions of the oral and genital regions.**

Herpes simplex virus (HSV) types 1 (HSV-1) and 2 (HSV-2).

**A peripheral protein gap can be a clue to infection with this virus.**

Human immunodeficiency virus (HIV).

**Excreted in the urine and feces of rodents.**

Lymphocytic choriomeningitis virus (LCMV).

**Arthropod-borne viruses.**

Arboviruses.

**Parotitis and meningismus in an unvaccinated patient.**

Mumps.

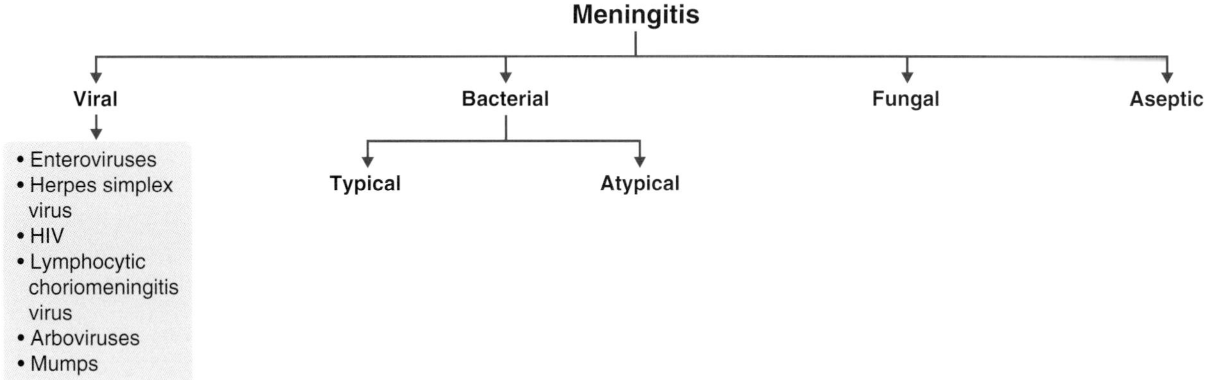


**How common is enterovirus meningitis?**

Enteroviruses are the most common cause of viral meningitis, accounting for most cases across all age groups. Children are most frequently affected. In temperate climates, outbreaks tend to be seasonal, occurring more often in the summer and autumn months. In tropical and subtropical climates, infection rates are high year-round. Most infections are asymptomatic, but a variety of neurologic manifestations can develop, including meningitis, meningoencephalitis, and paralytic poliomyelitis. Meningitis may be associated with mucocutaneous manifestations, such as hand, foot, and mouth disease in patients with coxsackie virus infection. Patients frequently experience moderate to high fever and several days of severe headache. Infection is typically self-limited with good prognosis.[1,8]

**Which type of herpes simplex virus is responsible for most cases of viral meningitis in immunocompetent adults?**

HSV is the second most common cause of viral meningitis. HSV-2 is responsible for most cases of HSV-related viral meningitis in immunocompetent hosts, usually occurring in patients with primary genital herpes infection; it may also occur in the absence of clinical genital herpes. Most cases are self-limited. Nonprimary HSV infection is rarely complicated by meningitis. HSV-2 meningitis can recur; it is the most common etiologic agent of Mollaret's meningitis, a syndrome characterized by recurrent self-limited episodes of meningitis. *HSV encephalitis is caused by HSV-1 in the vast majority of cases (Figure 30-2).*[1,8]

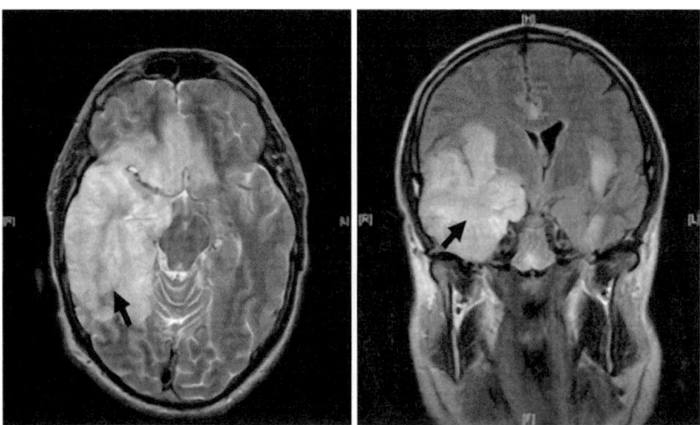

**Figure 30-2.** Axial and coronal T2-weighted magnetic resonance images showing areas of hyperintensity involving the temporal and inferior frontal lobes (arrows), characteristic of herpes simplex encephalitis. (Courtesy of Southampton General Hospital's picture library. Reprinted with permission from BMJ Publishing Group Ltd.)

**When does meningitis usually occur during the course of human immunodeficiency virus infection?**

Meningitis is an early manifestation of HIV infection, occurring in up to one-fifth of patients upon seroconversion. Other features of primary HIV infection may be present, including lymphadenopathy, rash, dermatitis, gastrointestinal disturbances, oral candidiasis, and pharyngitis. Resolution of meningeal symptoms occurs over the course of several weeks. *It is important to consider HIV in patients with self-limited "aseptic" meningitis so as to not miss the diagnosis.*[7]

**What is the treatment for lymphocytic choriomeningitis virus meningitis?**

LCMV meningitis should be considered in any patient with meningitis who has a history of contact with rodent droppings or urine. There is a predilection for the winter months. There is no specific antiviral therapy for LCMV meningitis; the vast majority of patients experience complete recovery.[9]

**What are the arboviruses?**

Viruses that are transmitted via the bite of an arthropod, including mosquitoes, ticks, and flies, are referred to as arboviruses. There are hundreds of such viruses, but only a subset of them cause meningitis, such as West Nile virus, St. Louis encephalitis virus, and California encephalitis viruses (eg, La Crosse virus). Infections generally peak in the summer and early fall. The vast majority of patients are asymptomatic. In symptomatic patients, the most common presentation is a flu-like illness without central nervous system (CNS) involvement after an average incubation period of 3 to 8 days. The most common presentation of CNS involvement is encephalitis, but isolated meningitis can occur. Compared with enteroviruses and herpesviruses, the sensitivity of CSF PCR for arboviruses is significantly lower. Serologies can be complementary. Treatment is supportive.[10]

**What is the prognosis of mumps meningitis?**

Meningitis is the most common neurologic manifestation of infection with mumps virus, occurring in about 15% of patients (with male predominance). It can precede or follow parotid swelling; one-half of cases occur in the absence of parotitis. The vast majority of patients experience complete recovery.[1,9]

*Other viruses that can cause meningitis include Epstein-Barr virus, cytomegalovirus (in immunocompromised patients), varicella-zoster virus, adenovirus, and human herpes virus 6.*[1]

## TYPICAL BACTERIAL MENINGITIS

**What is the opening pressure of typical bacterial meningitis?**

The opening pressure of typical bacterial meningitis is usually elevated (>18 cm $H_2O$).[2]

**What is the characteristic cerebrospinal fluid profile of typical bacterial meningitis?**

| Fluid type[7] | WBC/μL | WBC Type | Glucose (mg/dL) | Protein (mg/dL) |
|---|---|---|---|---|
| Typical bacterial | 500-20,000 | Neutrophils | Low | 100-700 |

**How is the diagnosis of typical bacterial meningitis definitively made?**

The diagnosis of typical bacterial meningitis is made when CSF samples demonstrate the presence of bacteria by Gram stain or culture. In most cases, these tests are associated with detection rates of up to 90%; CSF PCR studies can be adjunctive in some cases. Blood cultures are positive in around one-half of cases.[11]

**What empiric antibiotic regimen is recommended for adult patients with suspected community-acquired bacterial meningitis?**

In adults younger than 50 years of age with community-acquired bacterial meningitis, empiric coverage should include vancomycin (to cover *Streptococcus pneumoniae* with reduced penicillin sensitivity) and a third-generation cephalosporin (to cover *Neisseria meningitidis*); in adults older than 50 years of age, the recommendation is vancomycin, a third-generation cephalosporin, and ampicillin (to cover *Listeria monocytogenes*).[3]

## What are the causes of typical bacterial meningitis?

A common cause of community-acquired pneumonia. — *Streptococcus pneumoniae.*

Associated with Waterhouse-Friderichsen syndrome (adrenal hemorrhage and hypotension). — *Neisseria meningitidis.*

Vaccination has dramatically reduced the incidence of meningitis caused by this organism. — *Haemophilus influenzae.*[6]

The yield of CSF Gram stain for this organism is only about 30%. — *Listeria monocytogenes.*[7]

This gram-positive organism typically causes meningitis in the context of open head trauma or neurosurgery. — *Staphylococcus aureus.*

These organisms are common causes of nosocomial meningitis. — Gram-negative rods.

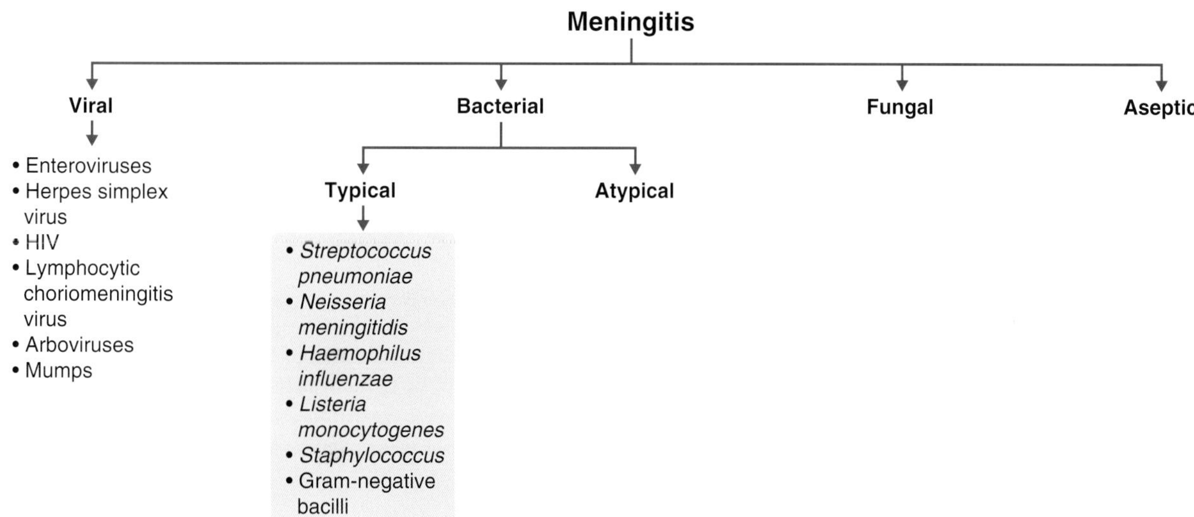


What is the treatment for ***Streptococcus pneumoniae*** meningitis?

*Streptococcus pneumoniae* accounts for more than one-half of bacterial meningitis cases in the industrialized world. Patients younger than 5 years and older than 60 years are at greatest risk. Empiric antimicrobial therapy includes a cephalosporin (eg, ceftriaxone, cefotaxime, cefepime) plus vancomycin. This regimen, which may be subsequently modified based on sensitivity data, should be continued for a total duration of 2 weeks of intravenous therapy. The administration of adjunctive glucocorticoids before or around the same time as antimicrobial therapy improves mortality and morbidity. Despite optimal therapy, up to one-third of patients with *Streptococcus pneumoniae* die; up to one-half of survivors experience chronic neurologic sequelae (eg, hearing loss).[2,11]

**What are the cerebrospinal fluid Gram stain findings in patients with *Neisseria meningitidis* meningitis?**

*Neisseria meningitidis* is a major cause of meningitis worldwide, often occurring in outbreaks. Meningococci are transmitted from person to person via direct contact or droplets. Clinical manifestations of invasive meningococcal disease range from transient bacteremia to a fulminant, life-threatening illness. Meningitis develops in a significant proportion of patients with invasive disease. The majority of these patients develop the characteristic hemorrhagic skin rash (typically petechial, but can be purpuritic or ecchymotic), usually affecting the trunk and lower extremities (Figure 30-3). Gram stain of the CSF demonstrates gram-negative diplococci inside and outside of neutrophils. Empiric antimicrobial therapy includes ceftriaxone or cefotaxime, which can be narrowed to penicillin G in patients with susceptible strains, for a total duration of 7 days in uncomplicated cases. Despite therapy, mortality rate is approximately 10%, and chronic neurologic sequelae develop in about 10% of survivors.[2,12,13]

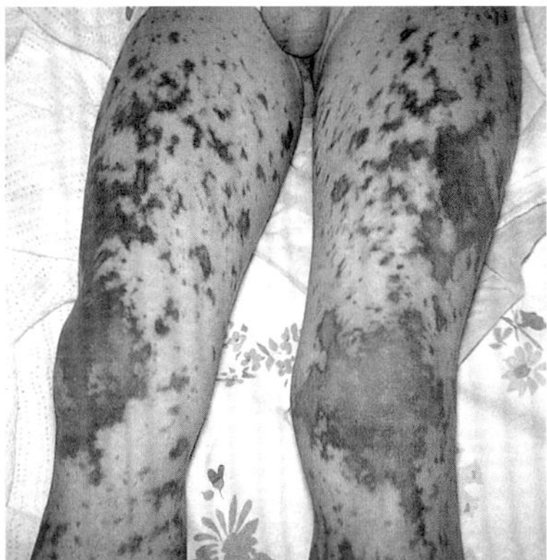

**Figure 30-3.** Fulminant petechial and purpuric rash in a patient with meningococcemia. (From Scheld MW, Whitley RJ, Marra CM. *Infections of the Central Nervous System*. 4th ed. Philadelphia, PA: Lippincott Williams & Wilkens; 2004.)

**How common is *Haemophilus influenzae* meningitis?**

Invasive disease caused by *Haemophilus influenzae* type b (Hib) has nearly been eradicated in regions with widespread use of vaccination. However, strains other than Hib are capable of causing meningitis in these regions, and Hib continues to be a major cause of meningitis worldwide. Antimicrobial therapy of choice is a third-generation cephalosporin (eg, ceftriaxone, cefotaxime) for at least 7 days. Despite therapy, mortality rate is about 7%; chronic neurologic sequelae develop in up to one-third of survivors.[14]

**What is unique about the cerebrospinal fluid profile in *Listeria monocytogenes* meningitis compared with the other typical bacterial organisms?**

*Listeria monocytogenes* is a foodborne pathogen that most often causes meningitis in newborns, immunocompromised patients, and the elderly. Compared with other causes of typical meningitis, it is associated with fewer WBCs, lower protein concentration, and a trend toward a lower percentage of neutrophils and less hypoglycorrhachia. Gram-positive rods on CSF Gram stain is highly suggestive, but yield is low (approximately 30%). Antimicrobial therapy of choice is ampicillin for at least 3 weeks; gentamicin is added in patients with severe disease. Despite therapy, mortality rate is as high as 30%, and there is a high rate of chronic neurologic sequelae in survivors.[2,15]

**What is the treatment for *Staphylococcus aureus* meningitis?**

*Staphylococcus aureus* causes a small but increasing number of cases of acute bacterial meningitis. It occurs as a result of direct inoculation of the CNS from contiguous infection, trauma, or iatrogenic procedures (eg, neurosurgery), or from hematogenous spread of infection originating outside of the CNS. Antimicrobial therapy of choice is nafcillin for susceptible strains, whereas vancomycin is used for methicillin-resistant *Staphylococcus aureus*. Despite therapy, up to one-third of patients die.[2,16]

Which gram-negative bacilli are associated with meningitis?

*Escherichia coli*, *Klebsiella* species, and *Pseudomonas aeruginosa* are among the causes of gram-negative bacillary meningitis. Third-generation cephalosporins are adequate for treating most organisms with the exception of *Pseudomonas aeruginosa*, which should be treated with ceftazidime, cefepime, or meropenem. The recommended duration of therapy is 3 weeks.[2,5]

## ATYPICAL BACTERIAL MENINGITIS

How do the cerebrospinal fluid profiles differ in patients with atypical versus typical bacterial meningitis?

Compared with typical bacterial meningitis, atypical bacterial meningitis is associated with the following CSF profile: WBC count tends to be lower with lymphocytic predominance, protein tends to be lower (but remains elevated), and glucose can be normal or low.[7]

### What are the causes of atypical bacterial meningitis?

Common in the developing world, meningitis related to this organism is challenging to diagnose because of its insidious onset with nonspecific symptoms and the insensitivity of available tests.

*Mycobacterium tuberculosis*.

Gram-negative corkscrew-shaped organisms.

Spirochetes.

An antecedent respiratory illness is typical.

*Mycoplasma pneumoniae*.

A 54-year-old man presents with pneumonia and meningismus 3 weeks after helping in the birthing of sheep.

*Coxiella burnetii* (Q fever).

This organism is most commonly acquired through the ingestion of contaminated raw milk or unpasteurized cheese.

*Brucella* species.

Intracellular organisms carried by arthropods.

*Rickettsia* species.

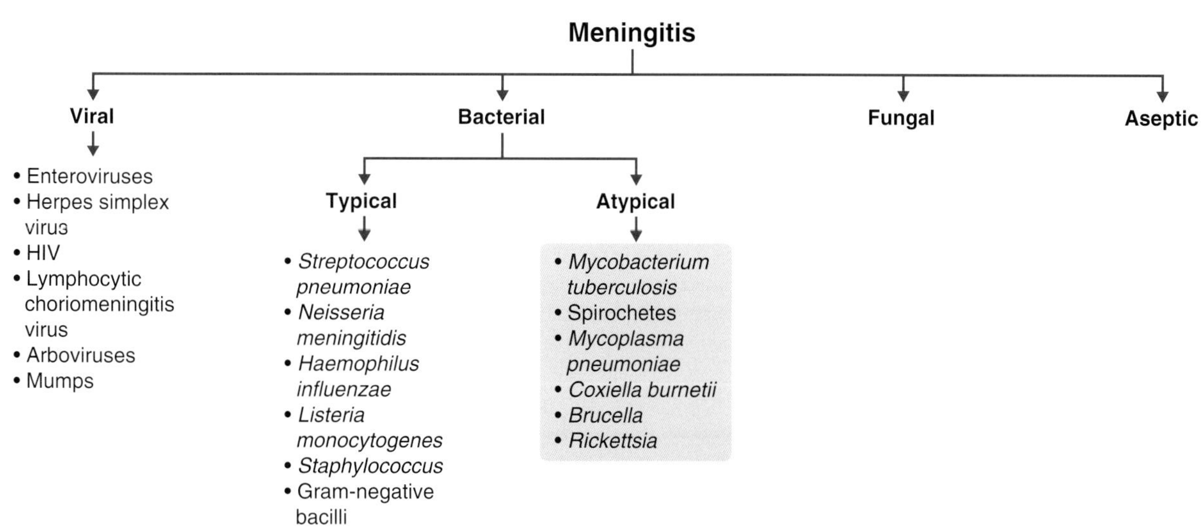

**What is the typical cerebrospinal fluid profile of tuberculous meningitis?**

Tuberculous meningitis is the least common but most severe form of extrapulmonary tuberculosis (TB). HIV infection is an important risk factor in adult patients. The presentation is more insidious than typical bacterial meningitis, occurring over a period of weeks. Patients typically present with headache and subtle mental status changes after a prodrome of low-grade fever, malaise, anorexia, and irritability. The CSF profile resembles fluid type C (see Table 30-1). Early in the course of the illness, there may be a predominance of neutrophils with a gradual shift to lymphocytes over 7 to 10 days. Positive CSF culture confirms the diagnosis, but results take weeks. Ziehl-Neelsen staining for acid-fast bacilli is positive in a minority of cases, although yield may be increased to approximately 60% with large-volume samples or repeat LPs. CSF PCR has a sensitivity of about 80% but a false-positive rate of about 10%.[2,7,17]

**What are the features of meningitis caused by *Borrelia burgdorferi*?**

Lyme meningitis occurs as a result of invasion of the CNS by *Borrelia burgdorferi*, typically occurring within a few months of primary infection. Common symptoms include headache, fatigue, stiff neck, and malaise. Most patients experience antecedent erythema migrans, and many will experience concomitant cranial neuropathy (eg, facial nerve palsy) or peripheral radiculoneuritis. The CSF is abnormal in virtually all patients with Lyme meningitis, resembling fluid type D (see Table 30-1). CSF culture is positive in <5% of cases; serum and CSF antibody testing is helpful in establishing the diagnosis. The antimicrobial treatment of choice is ceftriaxone for several weeks. Other spirochetes capable of causing meningitis include *Treponema pallidum* (ie, syphilis) and *Leptospira* species (ie, leptospirosis).[2,18]

**What is the prognosis of *Mycoplasma pneumoniae* infection of the central nervous system?**

*Mycoplasma pneumoniae* is a common cause of upper and lower respiratory tract infection, particularly in children. CNS involvement occurs in around 7% of patients who are hospitalized for *Mycoplasma pneumoniae* infection. The most common CNS manifestation is encephalitis, but meningitis, transverse myelitis, and polyradiculitis also occur. Most patients experience an antecedent respiratory illness. Serologies and PCR from nasopharyngeal or CSF samples can be helpful in establishing the diagnosis. Macrolide antibiotics are the mainstay of treatment. It is not clear whether adjunctive therapy such as glucocorticoids improves outcomes in patients with CNS disease. Most patients recover, but many experience chronic neurologic sequelae.[19,20]

**What are the features of *Coxiella burnetii* meningitis?**

Infection with *Coxiella burnetii* occurs worldwide and most often develops after exposure to birth fluids of sheep or other mammals, or ingestion of raw milk or fresh goat cheese. The most frequent clinical manifestations include a self-limited flu-like illness, pneumonia, and hepatitis. Meningitis is an uncommon complication but should be considered in patients with exposure history who present with fever, headache, and confusion. CSF is abnormal in most cases, resembling fluid type D (see Table 30-1), except protein may be within the normal range. Serologic testing is the preferred diagnostic method. Doxycycline is the treatment of choice and most patients fully recover.[21,22]

**What are the features of *Brucella* meningitis?**

Brucellosis is the most common zoonosis in the world; it is endemic to certain regions, including the Mediterranean basin, Persian Gulf, India, and parts of Latin America. Neurobrucellosis occurs in about 5% of cases; meningitis is the most frequent manifestation and may have an acute or chronic presentation. Fever and headache are the most frequent presenting complaints, occurring in most patients. CSF is abnormal in virtually all cases, with lymphocytic pleocytosis (mean 250 cells/μL), elevated protein (range 50-500 mg/dL), and normal or low glucose levels. Optimal antimicrobial treatment requires multiple agents, such as the combination of doxycycline, rifampin, and either ceftriaxone or trimethoprim/sulfamethoxazole.[23-25]

What antimicrobial agent is used to treat rickettsial meningitis?

Rickettsial infections occur in endemic regions worldwide. Tick-borne rickettsial infections that are endemic to the Unites States include Rocky Mountain spotted fever (RMSF), other spotted fever group rickettsioses, ehrlichiosis, and anaplasmosis. Most cases occur between April and September. Meningitis can be a manifestation of late-stage RMSF and, when accompanied by the classic petechial rash, can be confused for meningococcemia. Up to one-fifth of patients with ehrlichiosis develop CNS involvement, including meningitis or meningoencephalitis. CNS involvement in anaplasmosis is rare. Doxycycline is the antimicrobial agent of choice for rickettsial infections.[26,27]

## FUNGAL MENINGITIS

What is the typical opening pressure of fungal meningitis?

The opening pressure of fungal meningitis is typically elevated (>18 cm $H_2O$).[2]

What is the characteristic cerebrospinal fluid profile of fungal meningitis?

| Fluid Type[7] | WBC/μL | WBC Type | Glucose (mg/dL) | Protein (mg/dL) |
|---|---|---|---|---|
| Fungal | 25-500 | Lymphocytes or neutrophils | Low or normal | 50-500 |

### What are the causes of fungal meningitis?

A 33-year-old man with acquired immunodeficiency syndrome (AIDS) presents with headache and photophobia and is found to have a markedly elevated opening pressure on LP.

Cryptococcosis.

A 54-year-old woman presents with symptoms and signs of meningitis months after returning from a family reunion in Memphis, Tennessee.

Histoplasmosis or blastomycosis.

A 28-year-old Filipino man presents with fever, headache, and nuchal rigidity 6 weeks after returning home from vacation in Phoenix, Arizona.

Coccidioidomycosis.

Meningitis related to this ubiquitous fungus surprisingly occurs more frequently in immunocompetent hosts than in immunocompromised hosts.

*Aspergillus* species.[28]

Meningitis related to this ubiquitous fungus occurs more frequently in immunocompromised patients, those receiving broad-spectrum antibiotics or parental nutrition, and those who have undergone neurosurgical procedures.

*Candida* species.

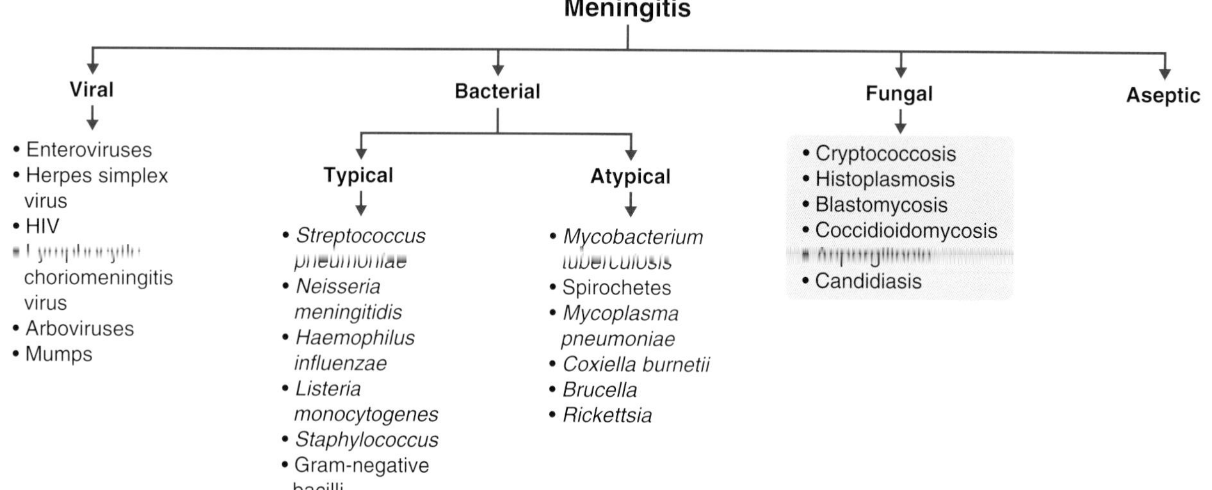


**Which 2 species of *Cryptococcus* cause meningitis?**

*Cryptococcus neoformans* is a ubiquitous fungus that typically affects immunocompromised hosts (eg, patients infected with HIV); *Cryptococcus gattii* is an endemic fungus found in various regions of the world (eg, the Northwestern United States) that often affects immunocompetent hosts. Between the 2, *Cryptococcus neoformans* meningitis is significantly more common.[29]

**How is histoplasmosis of the central nervous system diagnosed?**

Histoplasmosis is one of the most common fungal infections in the world; it is endemic to the Central and Southeastern United States, Latin America, Africa, and parts of Asia. Most infections are asymptomatic or manifest as self-limited pneumonia. Up to one-fifth of patients with disseminated histoplasmosis develop CNS involvement. Diagnosis is challenging and often requires a variety of tests, including CSF culture (considered the gold standard; at least 10 mL of fluid should be sent with prolonged incubation period); blood cultures; and *Histoplasma* antigen and antibody testing of the urine, serum, and CSF. Repeat testing is often required, and more invasive testing (eg, brain biopsy) may be necessary. Mortality and relapse are common.[30]

**How is blastomycosis of the central nervous system treated?**

Blastomycosis has been reported around the world; endemic regions of North America include the Mississippi and Ohio River basins and the areas around the Great Lakes and along the St. Lawrence River. The lungs and skin (Figure 30-4) are common sites of infection; CNS involvement accounts for up to 10% of extrapulmonary disease. The most frequent manifestations include headache, focal neurologic deficits, delirium, vision changes, and seizure. CNS blastomycosis should be treated with a lipid formulation of amphotericin B for 4 to 6 weeks followed by an oral azole for at least 1 year. Despite treatment, mortality rates are high.[31]

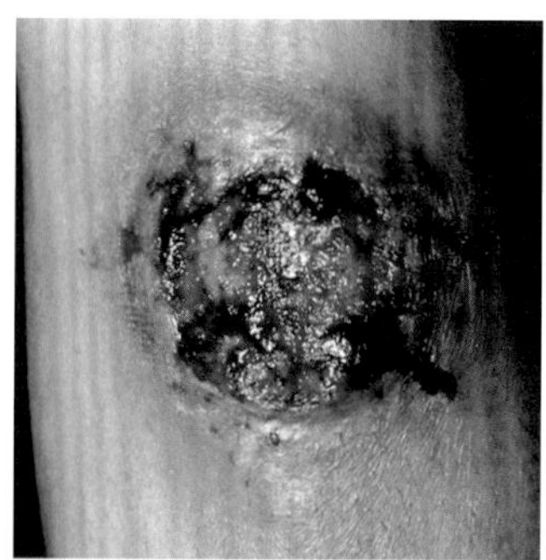

**Figure 30-4.** Cutaneous involvement in a patient with disseminated blastomycosis. The initial lesion is an inflammatory nodule that enlarges and ulcerates, often resembling pyoderma gangrenosum. Lesions evolve to verrucous or crusted plaques with sharply demarcated serpiginous borders. (Reprinted with permission from Goldsmith LA, Katz SI, Gilchrest BA, Paller AS, Leffell DJ, Wolff K. *Fitzpatrick's Dermatology in General Medicine*. 8th ed. New York, NY: McGraw-Hill; 2012:882. Copyright McGraw-Hill Education.)

What are the features of coccidioidal meningitis?

*Coccidioides* species are endemic to desert regions of the Western hemisphere, including parts of Arizona, California, New Mexico, and Texas. Pneumonia is the most common clinical manifestation. One-fifth of patients develop disseminated disease, often months or years later. Dissemination occurs more frequently in some groups, such as Filipino patients. Headache is present in the vast majority of patients with coccidioidal meningitis, often described as bilateral, intense, and throbbing; other manifestations include fever, weight loss, nausea, delirium, and focal neurologic deficits. Without treatment, the vast majority of patients die within 2 years; even with treatment, mortality and relapse rates are high. In contrast, most cases of *Coccidioides* infections involving other organ systems are self-limited.[32-34]

What unique cerebrospinal fluid study can be helpful in the diagnosis of ***Aspergillus*** meningitis?

*Aspergillus* meningitis is an uncommon clinical entity that occurs more frequently in immunocompetent patients. It usually develops as a result of extension from regional infection (eg, orbit, ear, paranasal sinuses), direct inoculation following a procedure (eg, neurosurgery), or hematogenous spread in intravenous drug users. Compared with other causes of fungal meningitis, the pleocytosis tends to be neutrophilic and protein levels are higher. CSF culture is positive in only one-third of cases. However, the CSF galactomannan antigen test is associated with a sensitivity approaching 90%. Prognosis is generally poor.[28]

What are the features of ***Candida*** meningitis?

*Candida* meningitis is uncommon; it occurs more frequently in immunocompromised patients, those receiving broad-spectrum antibiotics or parental nutrition, and those who have undergone neurosurgical procedures. The most common clinical manifestations include fever, headache, delirium, and meningismus. The pleocytosis may be predominantly neutrophilic or lymphocytic. The diagnosis is established with CSF culture; repeat sampling is often required. Treatment requires a prolonged course of combination antifungals (eg, amphotericin B with flucytosine). Despite treatment, mortality rates are high.[35]

## ASEPTIC MENINGITIS

What is the typical opening pressure of aseptic meningitis?

The opening pressure of aseptic meningitis is often normal (<18 cm $H_2O$) but may be mildly elevated in some cases.

What is the characteristic cerebrospinal fluid profile of aseptic meningitis?

| Fluid Type[7] | WBC/μL | WBC Type | Glucose (mg/dL) | Protein (mg/dL) |
|---|---|---|---|---|
| Aseptic | 5-1000 | Lymphocytes or neutrophils | Normal | <100 |

### What are the causes of aseptic meningitis?

A 24-year-old woman with systemic lupus erythematosus (SLE) who had recently been using ibuprofen to treat low back pain presents with headache, confusion, and meningismus.

Drug-induced aseptic meningitis.

A 58-year-old man with a recent diagnosis of gastric adenocarcinoma presents with headache and confusion and is found to have atypical cells on cytologic examination of the CSF.

Malignancy.

A 36-year-old Turkish woman presents with painful oral ulcers, genital ulcers, erythema nodosum, blurry vision, headache, and neck stiffness and is found to have a lymphocytic pleocytosis with elevated CSF protein and normal CSF glucose.

Behçet's disease.

Infection outside of the meninges.

Parameningeal infection.

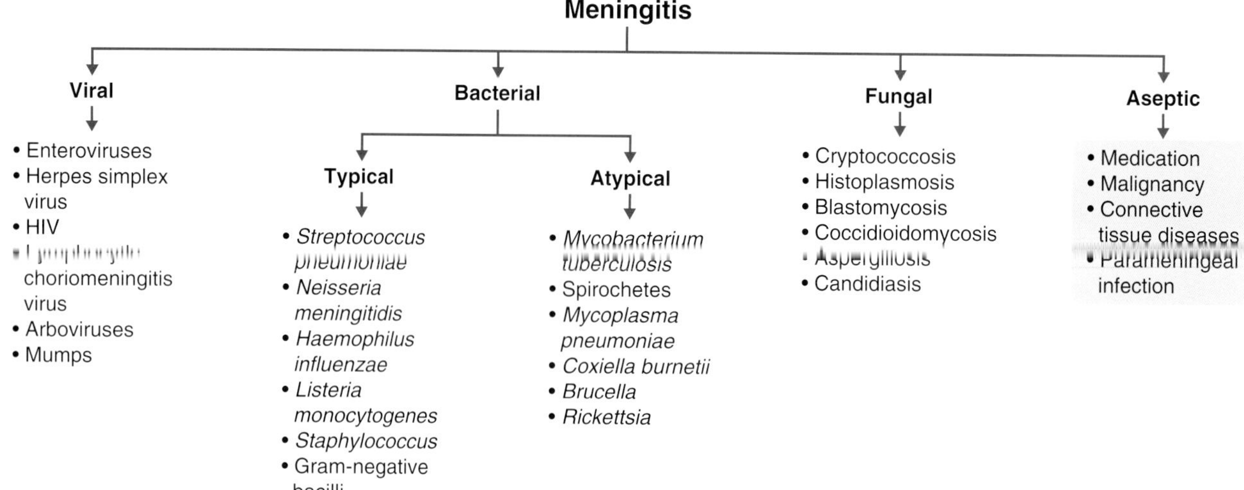


**What are the categories of medications that most frequently cause aseptic meningitis?**

Drug-induced aseptic meningitis is most often caused by nonsteroidal anti-inflammatory drugs, antimicrobials (eg, trimethoprim-sulfamethoxazole), intravenous immunoglobulin, intrathecal agents (eg, methotrexate), and vaccines (eg, measles, mumps, and rubella). Mechanisms include direct irritation of the meninges and immunologic hypersensitivity. There is an association between connective tissue diseases and drug-induced aseptic meningitis, particularly SLE and ibuprofen. The pleocytosis ranges from several hundred to several thousand cells per microliter and is typically neutrophilic but may be lymphocytic or eosinophilic. CSF protein is usually elevated, and CSF glucose is typically normal. Drug-induced aseptic meningitis is a diagnosis of exclusion. If the diagnosis is in doubt, it can be confirmed by a supervised drug re-challenge. Most patients respond fully to withdrawal of the offending agent without long-term sequelae.[36]

**Which malignancies are most frequently associated with aseptic meningitis?**

Metastasis to the leptomeninges is most frequently associated with hematologic malignancies (eg, leukemia and lymphoma), breast cancer, lung cancer, melanoma, and gastrointestinal cancer. CSF analysis is abnormal in the vast majority of cases. Opening pressure is elevated in one-half of patients; pleocytosis, elevated CSF protein, and decreased CSF glucose are typical findings. The identification of cancer cells by cytologic examination is key to making the diagnosis; the sensitivity of cytology is improved by large sampling volumes (>10.5 mL), prompt sampling processing times, and repeat LP. Neuroimaging is also useful in making the diagnosis.[37]

**Which connective tissue diseases are most frequently associated with aseptic meningitis?**

Connective tissue diseases most often associated with aseptic meningitis include SLE, Behçet's disease, rheumatoid arthritis, Sjögren's syndrome, sarcoidosis, ANCA-associated vasculitis, and mixed connective tissue disease. The pleocytosis is most often mild (<500 cells/µL) and lymphocytic. CSF protein is often elevated, and CSF glucose is typically normal.[38,39]

**What types of parameningeal infections can cause aseptic meningitis?**

Aseptic meningitis can be caused by brain abscess, otitis, sinusitis, retropharyngeal abscess, subdural abscess, epidural abscess, and cerebral thrombophlebitis. In the case of brain abscess, it is important to remember that LP carries a risk of brainstem herniation.[7]

## Case Summary

A 34-year-old immunocompromised man presents with acute-onset headache and confusion and is found to have fever, nuchal rigidity, and agitation. An LP showed bloody CSF with normal opening pressure, lymphocytic pleocytosis, normal glucose, and elevated protein. Neuroimaging revealed abnormal signal involving the left medial temporal lobe.

***What is the most likely diagnosis in this patient?***

Herpes simplex meningoencephalitis.

### BONUS QUESTIONS

***Which general types of meningitis would fit the cerebrospinal fluid profile in this case?***

The CSF profile in this case (normal opening pressure, mild lymphocytic pleocytosis, mildly elevated protein, and normal glucose) is consistent with viral meningitis, aseptic meningitis, and most cases of atypical bacterial meningitis.[7]

***What are the causes of bloody cerebrospinal fluid?***

CSF appears cloudy with RBC concentrations between 500 and 6000 cells/µL. The differential diagnosis for grossly bloody CSF includes traumatic LP and true CSF erythrocytosis from intracranial hemorrhage, such as subarachnoid hemorrhage and hemorrhagic meningoencephalitis. Trauma from needle insertion is less likely in this case because the bloody appearance of the fluid did not decrease with serial sampling as would be expected. Subarachnoid hemorrhage is unlikely given the absence of a history of head trauma, and negative imaging.[7]

***What is the most likely cause of bloody cerebrospinal fluid in this case?***

CSF erythrocytosis occurs in approximately 80% of cases of HSV encephalitis and can be an early diagnostic clue. It is thought to be a result of the necrotizing and hemorrhagic nature of the infection.[40]

***What is the significance of the neuroimaging in this case?***

MRI can be helpful in the diagnosis of HSV encephalitis, demonstrating characteristic abnormalities in the vast majority of cases. Typical findings include unilateral or asymmetric bilateral high signal involving the medial temporal lobes, insular cortex, and/or orbital surface of the frontal lobes (see Figure 30-2).[41]

***What evidence suggests the presence of meningoencephalitis (rather than meningitis alone) in this case?***

In this case, HSV encephalitis is suggested by the presence of abnormal cerebral function early in the course of illness, and temporal lobe abnormalities on neuroimaging. Although HSV meningitis is typically a self-limited illness, HSV encephalitis (either as an isolated entity or together with meningitis) is a life-threatening emergency that warrants antiviral therapy.[7]

***How is the diagnosis of herpes simplex virus meningoencephalitis confirmed?***

The detection of HSV DNA in CSF by PCR is highly sensitive and specific for the diagnosis of HSV meningoencephalitis. PCR remains positive at least 5 to 7 days after starting therapy. In up to 10% of cases of HSV encephalitis, the CSF may be completely normal.[41]

***What is the treatment of choice for herpes simplex virus meningoencephalitis?***

HSV meningoencephalitis is a life-threatening illness that should be treated with intravenous acyclovir without delay. Treatment reduces mortality rates from >70% to about 20%. Long-term neurologic sequelae (eg, amnesia) can occur in survivors, particularly when diagnosis and treatment are delayed.[41]

## KEY POINTS

- Meningitis is inflammation of the meninges associated with pleocytosis.
- Symptoms of meningitis include headache, neck stiffness, neck pain, lethargy, confusion (which is usually not prominent in the initial course of the illness), nausea, vomiting, photophobia, and phonophobia.
- Physical findings of meningitis include fever, nuchal rigidity, Kernig's sign, Brudziński's sign, papilledema, and other signs of increased intracranial pressure (eg, sixth nerve palsy). Some physical findings may be specific to underlying organisms (eg, the maculopapular and petechial skin rash of meningococcemia).

- Encephalitis is inflammation of the brain parenchyma, characterized by neurologic dysfunction early in the course of illness.
- Meningoencephalitis is used to describe cases with clinical features of both meningitis and encephalitis.
- Meningitis can be viral, bacterial, fungal, or aseptic.
- The CSF profile (eg, opening pressure, WBC count, protein concentration, and glucose concentration) can be useful in distinguishing between the causes of meningitis.
- CT imaging of the head should be obtained before LP in patients who are at increased risk for the presence of a mass lesion with increased intracranial pressure.

## REFERENCES

1. Logan SA, MacMahon E. Viral meningitis. *BMJ*. 2008;336(7634):36-40.
2. Longo DL, Fauci AS, Kasper DL, Hauser SL, Jameson JL, Loscalzo J, eds. *Harrison's Principles of Internal Medicine*. 18th ed. New York, NY: McGraw-Hill; 2012.
3. Mehndiratta M, Nayak R, Garg H, Kumar M, Pandey S. Appraisal of Kernig's and Brudzinski's sign in meningitis. *Ann Indian Acad Neurol*. 2012;15(4):287-288.
4. Tunkel AR, Glaser CA, Bloch KC, et al. The management of encephalitis: clinical practice guidelines by the Infectious Diseases Society of America. *Clin Infect Dis*. 2008;47(3):303-327.
5. Tunkel AR, Hartman BJ, Kaplan SL, et al. Practice guidelines for the management of bacterial meningitis. *Clin Infect Dis*. 2004;39(9):1267-1284.
6. Brouwer MC, Tunkel AR, van de Beek D. Epidemiology, diagnosis, and antimicrobial treatment of acute bacterial meningitis. *Clin Microbiol Rev*. 2010;23(3):467-492.
7. Walker HK, Hall WD, Hurst JW, eds. *Clinical Methods: The History, Physical, and Laboratory Examinations*. 3rd ed. Boston: Butterworths; 1990.
8. Kupila L, Vuorinen T, Vainionpaa R, Hukkanen V, Marttila RJ, Kotilainen P. Etiology of aseptic meningitis and encephalitis in an adult population. *Neurology*. 2006;66(1):75-80.
9. Meyer HM Jr, Johnson RT, Crawford IP, Dascomb HE, Rogers NG. Central nervous system syndromes of "vital" etiology. A study of 713 cases. *Am J Med*. 1960;29:334-347.
10. Davis LE, Beckham JD, Tyler KL. North American encephalitic arboviruses. *Neurol Clin*. 2008;26(3):727-757, ix.
11. Hoffman O, Weber RJ. Pathophysiology and treatment of bacterial meningitis. *Ther Adv Neurol Disord*. 2009;2(6):1-7.
12. Heckenberg SG, de Gans J, Brouwer MC, et al. Clinical features, outcome, and meningococcal genotype in 258 adults with meningococcal meningitis: a prospective cohort study. *Medicine (Baltimore)*. 2008;87(4):185-192.
13. Manchanda V, Gupta S, Bhalla P. Meningococcal disease: history, epidemiology, pathogenesis, clinical manifestations, diagnosis, antimicrobial susceptibility and prevention. *Indian J Med Microbiol*. 2006;24(1):7-19.
14. Agrawal A, Murphy TF. Haemophilus influenzae infections in the H. influenzae type b conjugate vaccine era. *J Clin Microbiol*. 2011;49(11):3728-3732.
15. Amaya-Villar R, Garcia-Cabrera E, Sulleiro-Igual E, et al. Three-year multicenter surveillance of community-acquired *Listeria monocytogenes* meningitis in adults. *BMC Infect Dis*. 2010;10:324.
16. Aguilar J, Urday-Cornejo V, Donabedian S, Perri M, Tibbetts R, Zervos M. Staphylococcus aureus meningitis: case series and literature review. *Medicine (Baltimore)*. 2010;89(2):117-125.
17. Chin JH. Tuberculous meningitis: diagnostic and therapeutic challenges. *Neurol Clin Pract*. 2014;4(3):199-205.
18. Pachner AR. Early disseminated Lyme disease: Lyme meningitis. *Am J Med*. 1995;98(4A):30S-37S; discussion 7S-43S.
19. Bitnun A, Ford-Jones EL, Petric M, et al. Acute childhood encephalitis and Mycoplasma pneumoniae. *Clin Infect Dis*. 2001;32(12):1674-1684.
20. Koskiniemi M. CNS manifestations associated with Mycoplasma pneumoniae infections: summary of cases at the University of Helsinki and review. *Clin Infect Dis*. 1993;17(suppl 1):S52-S57.
21. Bernit E, Pouget J, Janbon F, et al. Neurological involvement in acute Q fever: a report of 29 cases and review of the literature. *Arch Intern Med*. 2002;162(6):693-700.
22. Kofteridis DP, Mazokopakis EE, Tselentis Y, Gikas A. Neurological complications of acute Q fever infection. *Eur J Epidemiol*. 2004;19(11):1051-1054.
23. Pappas G, Akritidis N, Christou L. Treatment of neurobrucellosis: what is known and what remains to be answered. *Expert Rev Anti Infect Ther*. 2007;5(6):983-990.
24. Pappas G, Papadimitriou P, Akritidis N, Christou L, Tsianos EV. The new global map of human brucellosis. *Lancet Infect Dis*. 2006;6(2):91-99.
25. Yetkin MA, Bulut C, Erdinc FS, Oral B, Tulek N. Evaluation of the clinical presentations in neurobrucellosis. *Int J Infect Dis*. 2006;10(6):446-452.
26. Biggs HM, Behravesh CB, Bradley KK, et al. Diagnosis and management of tickborne rickettsial diseases: Rocky Mountain spotted fever and other spotted fever Group rickettsioses, ehrlichioses, and anaplasmosis–United States. *MMWR Recomm Rep*. 2016;65(2):1-44.
27. Ismail N, Bloch KC, McBride JW. Human ehrlichiosis and anaplasmosis. *Clin Lab Med*. 2010;30(1):261-292.
28. Antinori S, Corbellino M, Meroni L, et al. Aspergillus meningitis: a rare clinical manifestation of central nervous system aspergillosis. Case report and review of 92 cases. *J Infect*. 2013;66(3):218-238.
29. Williamson PR, Jarvis JN, Panackal AA, et al. Cryptococcal meningitis: epidemiology, immunology, diagnosis and therapy. *Nat Rev Neurol*. 2017;13(1):13-24.
30. Hariri OR, Minasian T, Quadri SA, et al. Histoplasmosis with deep CNS involvement: case presentation with discussion and literature review. *J Neurol Surg Rep*. 2015;76(1):e167-e172.

31. Bariola JR, Perry P, Pappas PG, et al. Blastomycosis of the central nervous system: a multicenter review of diagnosis and treatment in the modern era. *Clin Infect Dis*. 2010;50(6):797-804.
32. Crum NF, Lederman ER, Stafford CM, Parrish JS, Wallace MR. Coccidioidomycosis: a descriptive survey of a reemerging disease. Clinical characteristics and current controversies. *Medicine (Baltimore)*. 2004;83(3):149-175.
33. Mathisen G, Shelub A, Truong J, Wigen C. Coccidioidal meningitis: clinical presentation and management in the fluconazole era. *Medicine (Baltimore)*. 2010;89(5):251-284.
34. Vincent T, Galgiani JN, Huppert M, Salkin D. The natural history of coccidioidal meningitis: VA-Armed Forces cooperative studies, 1955-1958. *Clin Infect Dis*. 1993;16(2):247-254.
35. Goldani LZ, Santos RP. Candida tropicalis as an emerging pathogen in Candida meningitis: case report and review. *Braz J Infect Dis*. 2010;14(6):631-633.
36. Jolles S, Sewell WA, Leighton C. Drug-induced aseptic meningitis: diagnosis and management. *Drug Saf*. 2000;22(3):215-226.
37. Le Rhun E, Taillibert S, Chamberlain MC. Carcinomatous meningitis: Leptomeningeal metastases in solid tumors. *Surg Neurol Int*. 2013;4(suppl 4):S265-S288.
38. Jarrin I, Sellier P, Lopes A, et al. Etiologies and management of aseptic meningitis in patients admitted to an internal medicine department. *Medicine (Baltimore)*. 2016;95(2):e2372.
39. Houllis G, Karachalios M, eds. *Meningitis: Causes, Diagnosis and Treatment*. New York: Nova Science Publishers; 2012.
40. Whitley RJ, Soong SJ, Linneman C Jr, Liu C, Pazin G, Alford CA. Herpes simplex encephalitis. Clinical Assessment. *JAMA*. 1982;247(3):317-320.
41. Sabah M, Mulcahy J, Zeman A. Herpes simplex encephalitis. *BMJ*. 2012;344:e3166.

INFECTIOUS DISEASES

Chapter 31

# PNEUMONIA

## Case: A 57-year-old man with shaking chills

A previously healthy 57-year-old man is admitted to the hospital with sudden-onset dyspnea and cough over the course of 2 days. He complains of fever and shaking chills. His cough is productive of brown sputum. He has not had contact with other sick individuals. He has not traveled outside of Oregon during the past 6 years. He does not take any medications and has not had antibiotics recently.

Temperature is 38.8°C, heart rate is 102 beats per minute, and respiratory rate is 32 breaths per minute. The patient is diaphoretic and visibly short of breath. There is an area of dullness to percussion over the left posterior chest with increased tactile fremitus. There are tubular breath sounds, inspiratory rales, and egophony over the same area.

Peripheral white blood cell count is 15.1 K/μL with 82% polymorphonuclear cells and 15% band forms. Sputum Gram stain demonstrates the presence of gram-positive diplococci.

Chest radiographs with frontal (A) and lateral (B) views are shown in Figure 31-1.

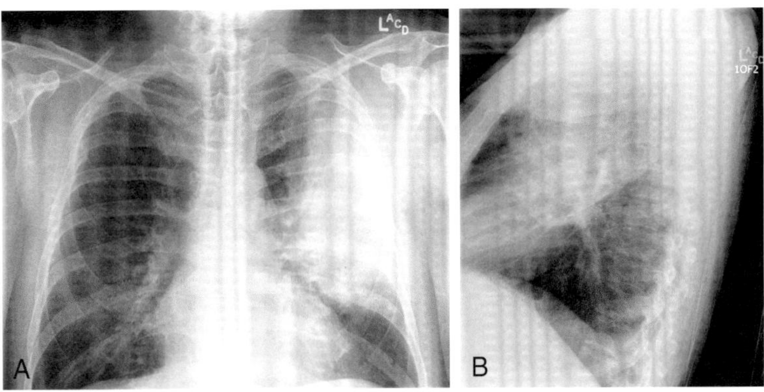


**Figure 31-1.**

***What is the most likely cause of pneumonia in this patient?***

*This chapter reviews the causes of pneumonia in immunocompetent hosts. Immunocompromised hosts are susceptible to a wider spectrum of pathogens, which is outside the scope of this chapter.*

What is pneumonia?

Pneumonia refers to infection of the pulmonary parenchyma with characteristic symptoms, physical findings, and radiographic findings. Acute radiographic findings may be challenging to identify in patients with underlying lung disease.[1,2]

What are the symptoms of pneumonia?

The clinical presentation of pneumonia may vary depending on host factors (eg, age) and the responsible pathogen. Symptoms of pneumonia may include dyspnea, cough, sputum production, pleuritic chest pain, chills, malaise, and confusion.[1,2]

What are the physical findings of pneumonia?

Physical findings of pneumonia may include fever, tachycardia, tachypnea, cachexia, dullness to percussion, increased tactile fremitus, tubular breath sounds, late inspiratory rales, pleural friction rub, egophony, and whispered pectoriloquy.[3]

How does the clinical presentation of pneumonia differ in elderly patients?

Elderly patients with pneumonia may not have cough, sputum production, or peripheral leukocytosis. Up to one-third of these patients are afebrile on presentation.[1]

**What noninfectious conditions can mimic some of the features of pneumonia?**

Up to one-fifth of patients hospitalized for community-acquired pneumonia may have an alternative diagnosis. Noninfectious conditions that can mimic pneumonia include pulmonary edema, lung cancer, pulmonary infarction, cryptogenic organizing pneumonia, eosinophilic pneumonia, acute interstitial pneumonia, sarcoidosis, vasculitis, pulmonary alveolar proteinosis, drug toxicity, and radiation pneumonitis.[1]

**How is pneumonia acquired?**

Most cases of pneumonia occur via microaspiration of upper airway secretions contaminated with microorganisms. Other cases occur via inhalation of airborne organisms or particles, hematogenous spread, or as a result of septic pulmonary emboli (eg, from right-sided endocarditis).[2]

**What tests are available to identify specific microbial pathogens in patients with pneumonia?**

Tests to identify specific microbial pathogens in patients with pneumonia include Gram stain and culture of blood, sputum, and respiratory secretions, antigen testing (eg, legionella and pneumococcal urinary antigens), and polymerase chain reaction (PCR) assays for some pathogens (eg, *Mycoplasma pneumoniae*, viruses). A sputum sample is considered satisfactory when there are >25 polymorphonuclear leukocytes and <10 squamous epithelial cells per lower power field (ie, 100× magnification). Methods of obtaining a respiratory sample include spontaneous expectoration, sputum induction, nasotracheal suctioning, and endotracheal aspiration (in patients who require intubation). Despite the availability and use of these tests, a specific pathogen is not identified in a significant proportion of cases, and empiric treatment is necessary.[1,4]

**What cardiac events are associated with pneumonia?**

Up to one-quarter of hospitalized patients with community-acquired pneumonia experience myocardial infarction, atrial fibrillation, or worsening heart failure. These events are associated with an increase in mortality.[1]

**What are the 2 settings in which pneumonia may be acquired?**

Pneumonia may be acquired within community or hospital settings. The subcategories of pneumonia acquired in the community setting are community-acquired pneumonia (CAP) and endemic pneumonia. The subcategories of pneumonia acquired in the hospital setting are hospital-acquired pneumonia (HAP) and ventilator-associated pneumonia (VAP). Aspiration pneumonia may occur in either setting.

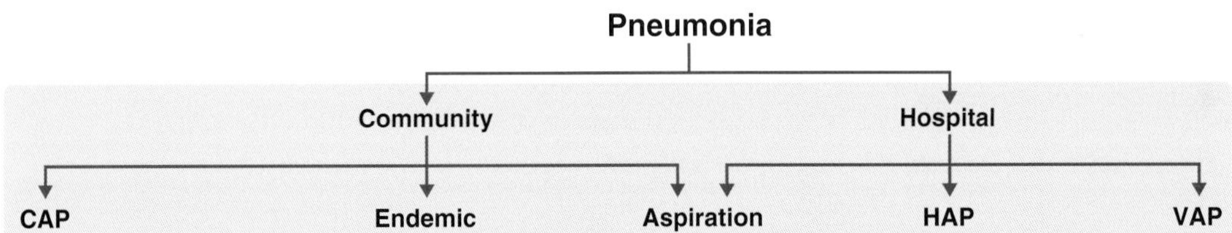


**Why is it important to distinguish between pneumonia acquired in community and hospital settings?**

The typical pathogens and resistance patterns differ between community and hospital settings. These differences inform the choice of empiric treatment before a specific pathogen is identified (or when a pathogen is not identified). Early initiation of antimicrobial treatment improves outcomes in patients with pneumonia. If a specific organism is identified, antimicrobial therapy should be narrowed accordingly.[1]

## COMMUNITY-ACQUIRED PNEUMONIA

**What are the 2 general groups of organisms that cause community-acquired pneumonia?**

CAP can be caused by typical or atypical organisms.

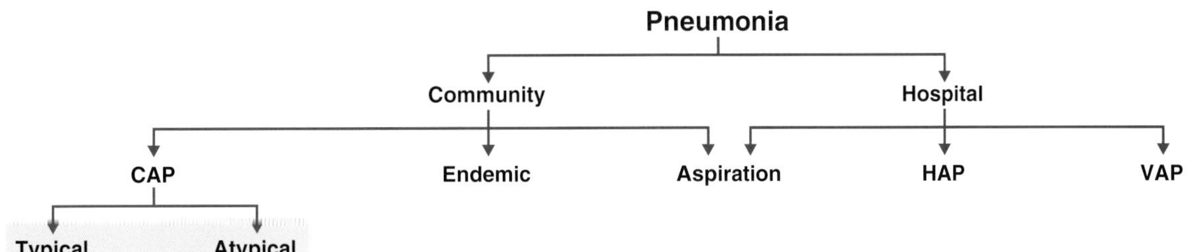

**Why is it important to distinguish between typical and atypical community-acquired pneumonia?**

The usual pathogens differ between typical and atypical CAP, which informs the choice of empiric treatment.

## COMMUNITY-ACQUIRED PNEUMONIA CAUSED BY TYPICAL PATHOGENS

**What clinical features are suggestive of typical community-acquired pneumonia?**

Clinical features that favor typical CAP include acute-onset chills and fever, presentation with septic shock, cough with sputum production, pleuritic chest pain, elevated or depressed peripheral white blood cell count with increased band forms, dense segmental or lobar consolidation on chest radiography, and serum procalcitonin level ≥0.25 μg/L.[1]

**What is the empiric treatment for typical community-acquired pneumonia?**

Outpatients with CAP are generally treated empirically to avoid the cost of diagnostic testing. Most outpatients with CAP without coexisting illness or recent use of antimicrobials may be treated with doxycycline or a macrolide (as long as <25% of pneumococci in the community have high-level macrolide resistance). However, in patients with a clinical syndrome suggestive of a typical organism, empiric treatment with a macrolide may be ineffective and amoxicillin-clavulanate is favored (amoxicillin alone may be ineffective, as there are high rates of β-lactamase production among *Haemophilus influenzae* and *Moraxella catarrhalis* isolates). Alternatives include levofloxacin or moxifloxacin. For hospitalized patients with CAP, a β-lactam (eg, ceftriaxone, cefotaxime, or ceftaroline) plus azithromycin may be used empirically; a quinolone (eg, levofloxacin or moxifloxacin) may be used instead. The recommended duration of treatment is 5 to 7 days.[1]

### What organisms cause typical community-acquired pneumonia?

**Though it is still the most common cause of CAP, the frequency of this pathogen is on the decline (possibly due to vaccination and decreased rates of cigarette smoking).**

*Streptococcus pneumoniae.*[1]

**Present in the nasopharynx of most healthy adults, this organism was so named because when it was discovered in 1892 it was thought to be the cause of influenza.**

*Haemophilus influenzae.*[5]

**A gram-negative, aerobic diplococcus.**

*Moraxella catarrhalis.*

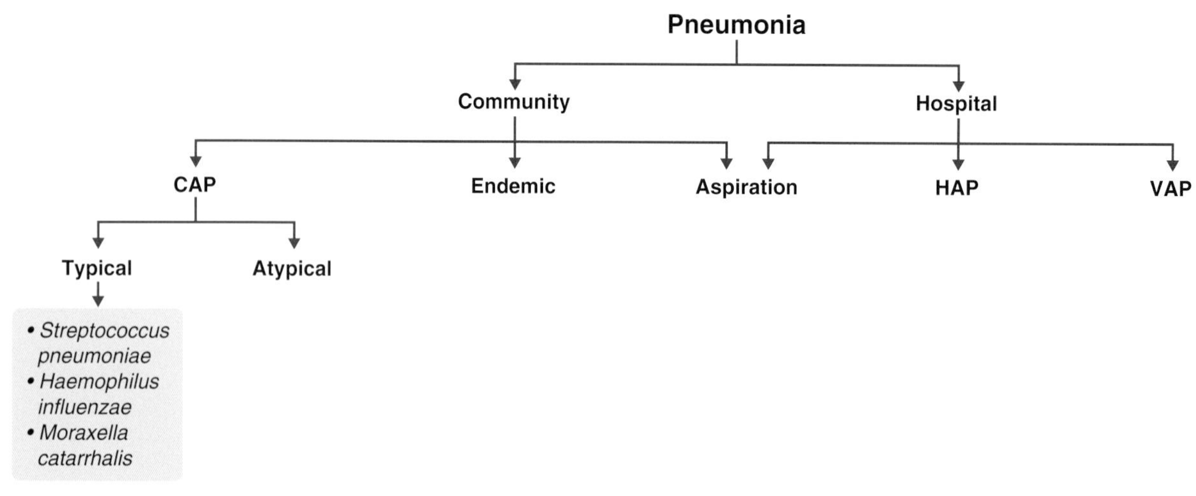

**What tests are available to diagnose *Streptococcus pneumoniae* pneumonia?**

*Streptococcus pneumoniae* is the most common cause of CAP. Risk factors include dementia, seizure disorders, heart failure, cerebrovascular disease, alcoholism, tobacco smoking, chronic obstructive pulmonary disease (COPD), and infection with human immunodeficiency virus. Sputum Gram stain and culture are positive in around 80% of cases (Figure 31-2). Blood culture is positive in up to one-quarter of cases, and urine antigen is positive in most cases; particularly those associated with bacteremia.[1,6]

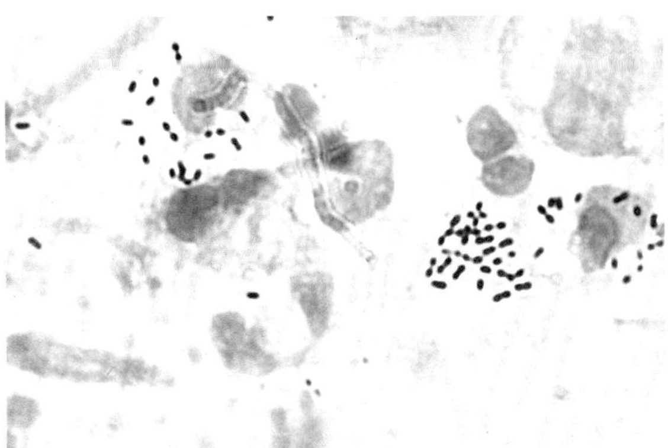

**Figure 31-2.** Gram stain of a smear of purulent sputum demonstrating gram-positive diplococci, characteristic of *Streptococcus pneumoniae*. (From Procop GW, et al. *Koneman's Color Atlas and Textbook of Diagnostic Microbiology*. 7th ed. Philadelphia, PA: Wolters Kluwer; 2017.)

**What are the features of pneumonia caused by *Haemophilus influenzae*?**

*Haemophilus influenzae* is a gram-negative coccobacillus. It is a normal component of the upper respiratory tract, which serves as a reservoir from which infection of the lower respiratory tract may occur, including bronchitis and pneumonia. Most patients with *Haemophilus influenzae* pneumonia present with cough and fever; however, the illness is generally less fulminant compared with pneumococcal pneumonia. Patients with underlying lung disease, particularly COPD, are at increased risk. β-Lactam agents are first-line treatment; some isolates produce β-lactamase and must be treated with a β-lactamase inhibitor.[1,5]

**What are the features of pneumonia caused by *Moraxella catarrhalis*?**

*Moraxella catarrhalis* is a gram-negative diplococcus. Although it is a colonizer of the normal upper respiratory tract, it can cause laryngitis, bronchitis, and pneumonia in adults; particularly the elderly, immunocompromised, and those with COPD. Infections occur more frequently in the winter and spring seasons, a pattern not seen with other causes of typical CAP. Patients often present with cough productive of purulent sputum. High fever, pleuritic chest pain, systemic toxicity, and complications such as empyema and bacteremia are infrequent. Sputum Gram stain, culture, and PCR may be helpful in making the diagnosis; blood cultures are rarely positive. β-Lactamase–producing isolates are widespread.[7]

*Resistant strains of Staphylococcus aureus and Pseudomonas aeruginosa, and other more virulent organisms can cause CAP, but are comparatively less common. The clinical syndrome in patients with pneumonia related to these organisms tends to be more severe. Based on individual risk for drug-resistant pathogens (eg, recent antimicrobial exposure, recent hospitalization, residence in a long-term care facility), empiric coverage of resistant organisms such as Staphylococcus aureus and Pseudomonas aeruginosa should be considered.*[8,9]

## COMMUNITY-ACQUIRED PNEUMONIA CAUSED BY ATYPICAL PATHOGENS

**What clinical features are suggestive of atypical community-acquired pneumonia?**

Clinical features that favor atypical CAP include stable cough lasting >5 days, absence of sputum production, normal or mild peripheral leukocytosis, procalcitonin level ≤0.1 µg/L, and the presence of extrapulmonary manifestations.[1]

**What is the empiric treatment for atypical community-acquired pneumonia?**

Atypical CAP may be treated empirically with a macrolide, doxycycline, or fluoroquinolone.[1]

## What organisms cause atypical community-acquired pneumonia?

**Antibiotics are not helpful.**

Viral pneumonia.

**A 47-year-old woman presents with mild dyspnea and dry cough and is found to have hemolytic anemia.**

*Mycoplasma pneumoniae.*

**After returning from a recent cruise, a 76-year-old man presents with dyspnea, cough, and diarrhea and is found to have a temperature of 39.2°C and heart rate of 68 beats per minute.**

*Legionella* species (Legionnaires' disease).

**Obligate, intracellular bacteria.**

*Chlamydia* species.

**Most cases of infection involving this organism are acute, manifesting as pneumonia or hepatitis. However, chronic infection can manifest months or years later, most often as endocarditis.**

*Coxiella burnetii* (Q fever).[10]

**A 34-year-old man who has recently been hunting and skinning rabbits presents with features of atypical pneumonia.**

*Francisella tularensis* (tularemia).

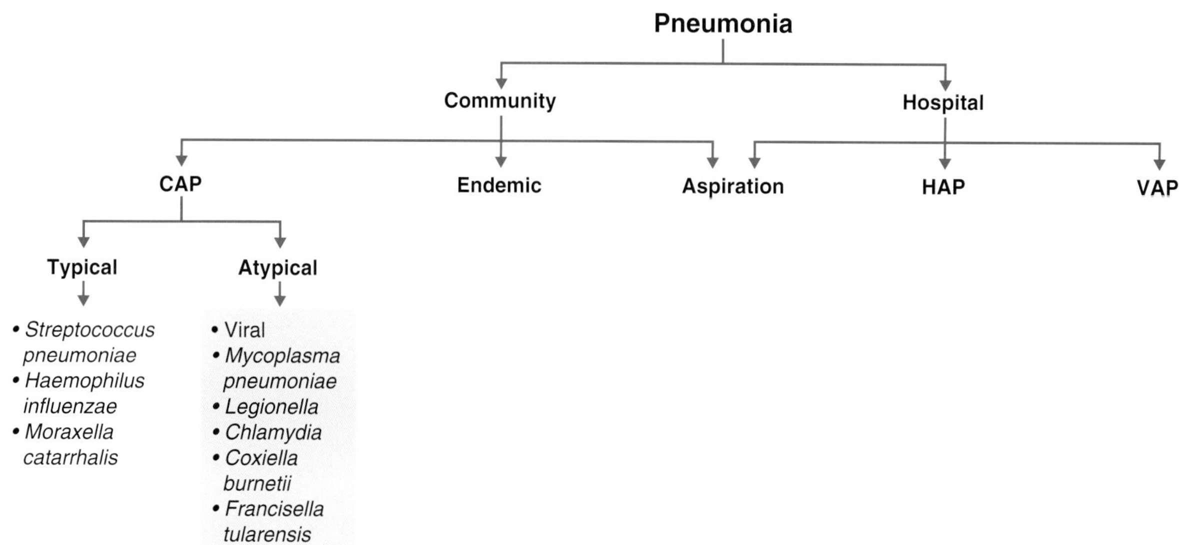


**Which viral pathogens cause pneumonia?**

Influenza virus, respiratory syncytial virus, parainfluenza virus, human metapneumovirus, adenovirus, coronavirus, rhinovirus, and Middle East respiratory syndrome-related coronavirus are among the causes of viral CAP. Analyzing respiratory secretions by PCR is the method of choice in identifying viral pathogens. In some cases the virus is the only source of infection, whereas in others there may be secondary bacterial infection (almost one-fifth of patients with bacterial-proven CAP are coinfected with a virus). A neuraminidase inhibitor (eg, oseltamivir) is the treatment of choice for influenza pneumonia and is more effective when initiated early in the course of illness.[1]

**How common are extrapulmonary manifestations of *Mycoplasma pneumoniae* pneumonia?**

*Mycoplasma pneumoniae* is a common cause of CAP. Extrapulmonary manifestations are present in around one-quarter of cases and can sometimes be more severe and of greater clinical importance than the pneumonia itself. Extrapulmonary manifestations may involve the blood (eg, autoimmune hemolytic anemia), the heart (eg, pericarditis, myocarditis), the skin (eg, Stevens-Johnson syndrome), and the central nervous system (eg, encephalitis, meningitis, optic neuritis).[11]

**How sensitive is the *Legionella* urinary antigen test?**

The *Legionella* urinary antigen test is positive in about 75% of patients with pneumonia caused by *Legionella pneumophilia* serotype 1 (which is responsible for the vast majority of cases). Sputum PCR and culture with selective media can be used to detect other *Legionella* species.[1,12]

**What are the features of *Chlamydia* pneumonia?**

*Chlamydia pneumoniae* is an obligate, intracellular bacterium that causes up to one-fifth of cases of CAP. Clinical manifestations range from a mild, self-limited illness to severe forms of pneumonia, particularly in the elderly and in patients with preexisting cardiopulmonary disease. Serologies and PCR may be useful in diagnosis. *Chlamydia psittaci* should be suspected in patients with recent exposure to birds.[13]

**What are the features of *Coxiella burnetii* pneumonia?**

Q fever is a worldwide zoonotic infection caused by *Coxiella burnetii*. Infection in humans usually occurs via inhalation of bacteria from air contaminated by the excreta of infected animals, particularly birth fluids. Acute infection is symptomatic in one-half of cases, developing after an incubation period of 2 to 3 weeks. It manifests as a nonspecific illness in association with pneumonia or hepatitis. Cough is frequently present but is nonproductive in one-half of patients. Extrapulmonary symptoms are common, including severe headache, myalgias, and arthralgias. Serologies and serum or whole blood PCR assays may be used to establish the diagnosis. Doxycycline is the treatment of choice.[10]

**What is the treatment of choice for pneumonic tularemia?**

Tularemia is a zoonotic infection caused by *Francisella tularensis* and is found predominantly in the Northern Hemisphere. It is most often acquired from arthropod bites or exposure to animal carcasses, such as rabbits and hares. Pneumonia usually develops days to weeks after the start of nonspecific systemic symptoms. Headache and high fever are common early manifestations, followed by a nonproductive cough with or without pleuritic chest pain. Serologies and PCR assays may be used to establish the diagnosis. Unlike most bacterial causes of atypical pneumonia, most strains of *Francisella tularensis* are resistant to macrolide agents. An aminoglycoside agent (eg, streptomycin) is the treatment of choice.[14]

## COMMUNITY-ACQUIRED PNEUMONIA CAUSED BY ENDEMIC PATHOGENS

**What is an endemic pathogen?**

Endemic pathogens are confined to particular geographical locations and usually affect both immunocompetent and immunocompromised hosts.

### What endemic organisms cause community-acquired pneumonia?

**A patient who recently emigrated from Mexico presents with weight loss, night sweats, and hemoptysis and is found to have a right upper lobe cavitary lesion on chest imaging.**

*Mycobacterium tuberculosis* (TB).

**"Valley fever."**

*Coccidioides* species (coccidioidomycosis).

**Urine antigen testing can be useful in the diagnosis of pneumonia related to this pathogen, although there is significant cross-reactivity with other fungi.**

*Histoplasma* species (histoplasmosis).

**Dermatologic findings, including verrucous and ulcerative lesions (see Figure 30-4), are often present in patients with pneumonia caused by this endemic fungus.**

*Blastomyces dermatitidis* (blastomycosis).[15]

**Following a trip to British Columbia, Canada, a previously healthy 48-year-old man presents with chronic cough and is found to have a 2-cm, spiculated, solitary pulmonary nodule on chest imaging concerning for lung cancer.**

*Cryptococcus gattii* (cryptococcosis).

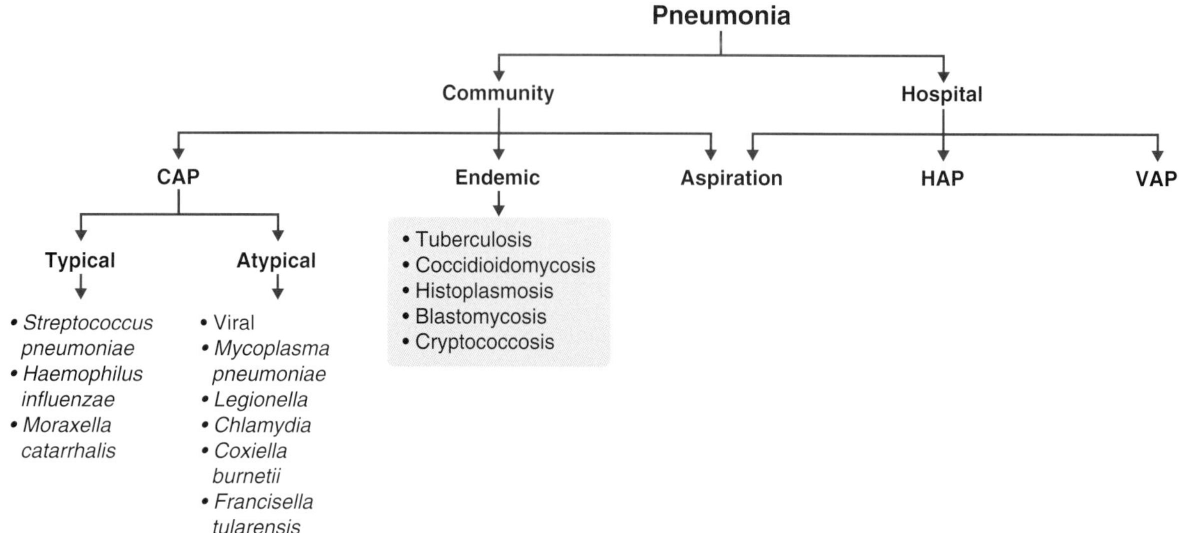


**What is the risk of active pulmonary tuberculosis following initial infection?**

Tuberculosis is common worldwide, particularly in endemic regions. Importantly, TB can also be transmitted from infected hosts in nonendemic areas. A substantial proportion of the world's population has latent TB and is at risk for active disease. The risk of active disease is approximately 5% in the first 18 months after initial infection, and there is a lifetime risk of around 5% thereafter. Pulmonary TB classically presents with chronic cough, sputum production, hemoptysis, fever, night sweats, loss of appetite, and weight loss. Chest imaging (Figure 31-3) and sputum microscopy and culture are the cornerstones of diagnosing active pulmonary TB. PCR assays and histopathology of biopsy samples may be helpful in some cases.[16]

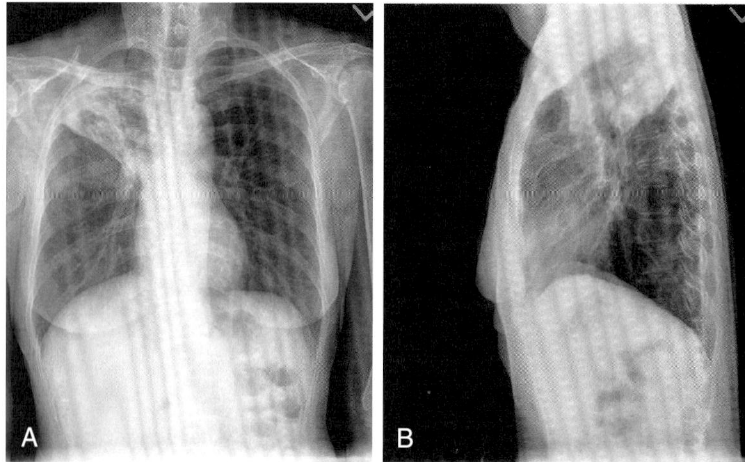


**Figure 31-3.** Chest radiographs (frontal [A] and lateral [B] views) of a 60-year-old Thai woman with fever, hemoptysis, and weight loss demonstrating dense posterior right upper lobe consolidation with cavitation, characteristic of pulmonary TB. Sputum contained numerous *Mycobacterium tuberculosis* organisms. (Courtesy of Cristina Fuss, MD.)

**Where is coccidioidomycosis endemic?**

Coccidioidomycosis is endemic to the Southwestern United States (eg, Arizona), Mexico, and some areas of Central and South America (eg, Argentina). There is some evidence that the endemic borders may be widening with global warming and climate change. Symptomatic cases resemble bronchitis or pneumonia, and most are self-limited over a period of weeks. Features that may help distinguish coccidioidomycosis from typical CAP include exposure history, profound fatigue, cutaneous manifestations (eg, erythema nodosum), and subacute time course. Serology is the most widely used diagnostic test but is not sensitive early in the course of disease.[17]

**What are the features of acute pulmonary histoplasmosis?**

Histoplasmosis is endemic to the Central and Southeastern regions of the United States, Latin America, Africa, and parts of Asia. Infection is common in endemic areas; most are asymptomatic or manifest as pneumonia. Acute pulmonary histoplasmosis is characterized by fever, malaise, headache, weakness, dry cough, and pleuritic chest pain. Chest radiography typically demonstrates patchy areas of consolidation in one or more lobes; a potential distinguishing feature is the presence of hilar and mediastinal lymphadenopathy. The illness is most often self-limited with prompt resolution of symptoms. However, patients with underlying immunocompromised status or those exposed to a large inoculum of the fungus may develop severe pulmonary infection.[18]

**What are the features of pulmonary blastomycosis?**

Blastomycosis has been reported around the world; endemic regions of North America include the Mississippi and Ohio River basins and the areas around the Great Lakes and along the St. Lawrence River. Pneumonia is the most common manifestation of infection. Features include fever, productive cough with or without hemoptysis, myalgias, arthralgias, and pleuritic chest pain. Chest imaging often demonstrates an alveolar or mass-like opacity that can mimic malignancy. Chronic pneumonia develops in a large proportion of untreated patients. Extrapulmonary disease is common and may be an important clue to the diagnosis.[15]

**What are the features of pulmonary cryptococcosis?**

Pulmonary cryptococcosis ranges from asymptomatic disease to severe pneumonia with respiratory failure, depending on the immune status of the host. Manifestations include cough with or without hemoptysis, fever, malaise, pleuritic chest pain, weight loss, dyspnea, and night sweats. The radiographic abnormality is typically focal and often mistaken for lung cancer. The burden of symptoms is lower in immunocompetent hosts, and tends to resolve over a period of weeks to months even without treatment; however, disseminated disease can occur. Immunocompromised hosts experience rapid-onset pulmonary disease with a heavy burden of symptoms; dissemination is common, particularly to the CNS.[19]

## HOSPITAL-ACQUIRED PNEUMONIA

**What is the definition of hospital-acquired pneumonia?**

HAP is defined as the development of pneumonia in a nonintubated patient after 48 hours of hospitalization.[20]

**How common is hospital-acquired pneumonia?**

HAP occurs at a rate of up to 20 cases per 1000 hospital admissions. Those at highest risk include patients who are elderly, immunocompromised, or have underlying lung disease, and those who have undergone recent surgery, or are receiving enteral feeding through a nasogastric tube.[21]

**What organisms should be covered in empiric antibiotic regimens for hospital-acquired pneumonia?**

Any empiric antibiotic regimen for HAP should at least include coverage of enteric gram-negative bacilli, methicillin-sensitive *Staphylococcus aureus*, and *Pseudomonas aeruginosa*. Environmental factors (eg, local antibiogram data) and host factors (eg, drug allergies, severity of illness, risk factors for drug-resistant pathogens) should also guide the choice of empiric therapy. Early empiric treatment is associated with a mortality benefit in patients with HAP and should be initiated as soon as possible after the diagnosis is made. However, there should also be an emphasis on de-escalation based on respiratory and blood culture results when possible, as superfluous treatment increases risk of adverse events (eg, *Clostridium difficile* colitis).[20]

**What is the prognosis of hospital-acquired pneumonia?**

In addition to significant increases in hospital length of stay as well as cost of care, HAP is associated with an overall mortality rate of up to 50%. HAP that develops early in the hospital course (<5 days) has a better prognosis than late-onset HAP (≥5 days).[21,22]

## What organisms cause hospital-acquired pneumonia?

**Enterobacteriaceae.**

Enteric gram-negative bacilli.

**Common causes of community-acquired pneumonia, these organisms tend to cause early-onset hospital-acquired pneumonia.**

*Haemophilus influenzae* and *Streptococcus pneumoniae*.

**A gram-positive organism commonly associated with skin and soft tissue infections and endocarditis.**

*Staphylococcus aureus*.

**These gram-negative organisms often develop resistance to multiple antibiotics.**

*Pseudomonas aeruginosa* and *Acinetobacter baumannii*.

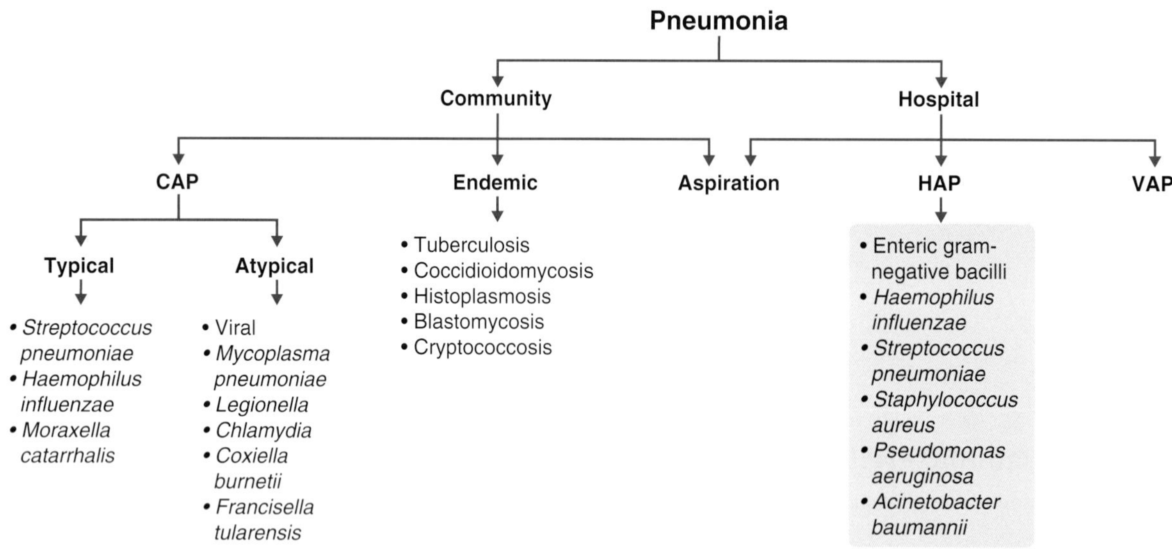


**Which enteric gram-negative bacilli cause hospital-acquired pneumonia?**

Enteric gram-negative bacilli that most frequently cause HAP include *Escherichia coli*, *Klebsiella* species, and *Enterobacter* species. Extended-spectrum β-lactamase activity is becoming increasingly common in these organisms, and there is often fluoroquinolone resistance, necessitating treatment with a carbapenem (eg, meropenem).[22]

**When is hospital-acquired pneumonia more likely to be caused by the pathogens of community-acquired pneumonia (eg, *Haemophilus influenzae* or *Streptococcus pneumoniae*)?**

Cases of early HAP (defined as HAP occurring after <5 days of hospitalization) are more likely to be caused by the usual organisms involved in CAP.[22]

**When should coverage be provided against methicillin-resistant *Staphylococcus aureus* (MRSA) in patients with hospital-acquired pneumonia?**

MRSA is prevalent in the hospital setting and requires specific antibiotic therapy (eg, vancomycin). It is reasonable to provide MRSA coverage in patients with HAP if any of the following risk factors are present: (1) prior intravenous antibiotic use within 90 days, (2) hospitalization in a unit where >20% of *Staphylococcus aureus* isolates are methicillin-resistant, or (3) hospitalization in a unit where prevalence of MRSA is unknown. It is also reasonable to provide MRSA coverage in patients who are known to be carriers of MRSA and those who are severely ill and at high risk for mortality.[20]

**What risk factors are associated with multi-drug-resistant *Pseudomonas aeruginosa*?**

*Pseudomonas aeruginosa* strains are frequently multidrug-resistant. Risk factors include prior use of intravenous antibiotics within 90 days (strongest risk factor) and history of underlying chronic lung disease (eg, COPD, bronchiectasis).[20]

**What is the treatment for *Acinetobacter baumannii*?**

Given the high probability of drug resistance, treatment for *Acinetobacter baumannii* should be driven by susceptibility data. In susceptible strains, a carbapenem or ampicillin-sulbactam is considered first-line therapy. Some strains may only be susceptible to polymyxins (eg, polymyxin B, colistin). In such cases, inhaled colistin may be added to augment therapy.[20]

## VENTILATOR-ASSOCIATED PNEUMONIA

**What is the definition of ventilator-associated pneumonia (VAP)?**

VAP is defined as the development of pneumonia 48 or more hours after endotracheal intubation.[20]

**How common is ventilator-associated pneumonia?**

VAP occurs in up to 40% of intubated patients; it is the most frequent ventilator-associated complication and most frequent ICU-acquired infection. The peak incidence of VAP occurs 5 to 9 days after intubation; cumulative risk is proportional to the duration of intubation.[21]

**What methods are available to aid in the identification of an organism in patients with ventilator-associated pneumonia?**

Noninvasive methods to identify an organism in patients with VAP are preferred and include endotracheal aspiration and blood cultures (positive in about 15% of cases). Invasive methods include bronchoscopy with bronchoalveolar lavage (BAL) and protected specimen brush (PSB).[20]

**What organisms should be covered in empiric antibiotic regimens for ventilator-associated pneumonia?**

As with HAP, any empiric antibiotic regimen for VAP should at least include coverage for enteric gram-negative bacilli, methicillin-sensitive *Staphylococcus aureus*, and *Pseudomonas aeruginosa*. Environmental and host factors should also guide the choice of empiric therapy. Early empiric treatment is associated with mortality benefit in patients with VAP and should be initiated as soon as possible after the diagnosis is made. However, there should also be an emphasis on de-escalation based on respiratory and blood culture results when possible as superfluous treatment increases risk of adverse events.[20]

**When should coverage be provided against MRSA in patients with ventilator-associated pneumonia?**

It is reasonable to provide MRSA coverage in patients with VAP if any of the following are present: (1) any risk factor for multidrug-resistant pathogens, (2) hospitalization in a unit where >10% to 20% of *Staphylococcus aureus* isolates are methicillin-resistant, or (3) hospitalization in a unit where prevalence of MRSA is unknown. It is also reasonable to provide MRSA coverage in patients who are severely ill and at high risk for mortality.[20]

**What are some risk factors for multidrug-resistant pathogens in patients with ventilator-associated pneumonia?**

Risk factors for multidrug-resistant pathogens in patients with VAP include the following: (1) prior intravenous antibiotic use within 90 days, (2) presence of septic shock, (3) acute respiratory distress syndrome (ARDS) before VAP, (4) ≥5 days of hospitalization before VAP, and (5) acute renal replacement therapy before VAP.[20]

**What is the prognosis of ventilator-associated pneumonia?**

VAP is associated with an overall mortality rate of up to 60%.[21]

### What organisms cause ventilator-associated pneumonia?

This group of organisms can develop resistance to most β-lactam antibiotics because of enzymes called extended-spectrum β-lactamases.

Enteric gram-negative bacilli.

The main gram-positive pathogen responsible for VAP.

*Staphylococcus aureus.*

Some authorities recommend the initial use of 2 antibiotic agents to cover this organism.

*Pseudomonas aeruginosa.*[20]

This organism is typically of low virulence outside the hospital but can easily become multidrug-resistant and in some cases is only susceptible to polymyxins.

*Acinetobacter baumannii.*[20]

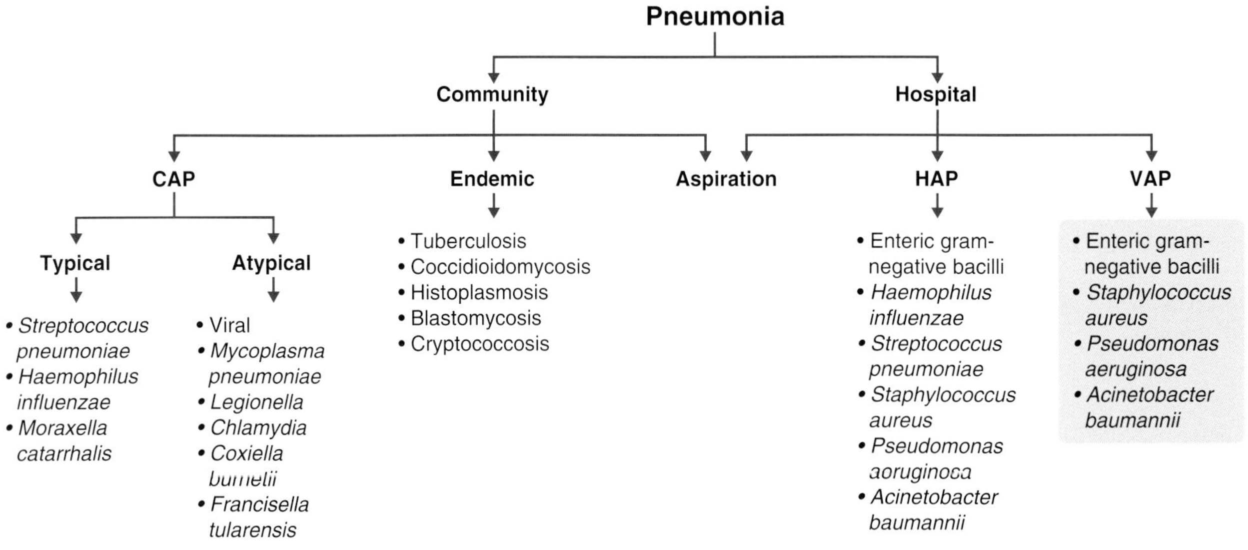


How common is enteric gram-negative bacilli ventilator-associated pneumonia in the United States?

Enteric gram-negative bacilli cause up to 40% of VAP in the United States.[20]

How common is ***Staphylococcus aureus*** ventilator-associated pneumonia in the United States?

*Staphylococcus aureus* causes up to 30% of VAP in the United States.[20]

How common is ***Pseudomonas aeruginosa*** ventilator-associated pneumonia in the United States?

*Pseudomonas aeruginosa* causes up to 20% of VAP in the United States.[20]

How common is ***Acinetobacter baumannii*** ventilator-associated pneumonia in the United States?

*Acinetobacter baumannii* causes up to 10% of VAP in the United States.[20]

## ASPIRATION PNEUMONIA

How is the mechanism of aspiration pneumonia different from the other types of pneumonia?

Most types of pneumonia occur via microaspiration. Organisms such as *Streptococcus pneumoniae* and *Haemophilus influenzae* are relatively virulent, so even a small inoculum can result in pneumonia. In comparison, aspiration pneumonia typically results from the macroaspiration of less virulent pathogens. A large inoculum of organisms is generally required to cause infection.

**What is aspiration pneumonitis?**

Aspiration pneumonitis is characterized by respiratory distress related to the aspiration of toxic material (eg, gastric acid) into the lower airways with an associated inflammatory response, independent of infection. Most patients with aspiration pneumonitis experience rapid recovery with clearing of radiographic abnormalities. However, some patients develop secondary infection and/or acute respiratory distress syndrome.[23]

**What are the risk factors for aspiration pneumonia?**

Healthy patients frequently aspirate during sleep without consequence. For aspiration pneumonia to develop, usually the normal defense mechanisms that protect the lower airways (eg, cough, ciliary action, alveolar macrophages) are impaired, or a large inoculum of organisms is aspirated. Predisposing conditions include chronic neurologic disorders (eg, stroke), esophageal disorders, impaired consciousness, alcoholism, illicit drug abuse, use of acid-suppressive medications, vomiting, instrumentation of the respiratory tract (eg, bronchoscopy), and poor dentition.[4,24]

**Does aspiration pneumonia occur in the community or hospital setting?**

Aspiration pneumonia occurs in both community and hospital settings. The pathogens in these environments differ because hospitalized patients acquire oropharyngeal colonization with nosocomial organisms. Aspiration pneumonia that develops in the community tends to be caused by organisms that are part of the normal oral flora, such as anaerobes and *Streptococcus* species. Aspiration pneumonia that develops in the hospital can additionally include other organisms such as gram-negative bacilli and *Staphylococcus aureus*.[4,25]

**What are the clinical characteristics of aspiration pneumonia?**

The presentation of aspiration pneumonia depends on the organisms involved. Some pathogens (eg, gram-negative bacilli, *Staphylococcus aureus*) cause an acute presentation that is difficult to clinically distinguish from CAP or HAP but should be suspected in patients with predisposing risk factors. When anaerobes are involved, patients experience more indolent symptoms with weeks to months of malaise, low-grade fever, cough, and weight loss. Over time, complications such as necrotizing pneumonia (multiple cavities ≤1 cm in diameter), lung abscess (1 or more cavities >1 cm in diameter that communicate with a bronchus) (Figure 31-4), or empyema may develop. These complications may lead to putrid sputum and hemoptysis. *Nonanaerobes capable of these destructive complications include Staphylococcus aureus, Klebsiella pneumoniae, and Pseudomonas aeruginosa.*[4]

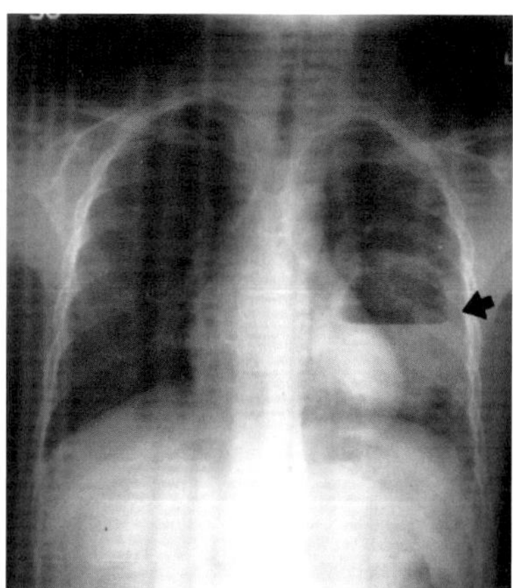

**Figure 31-4.** Chest radiograph showing a large abscess of the left lung with an air-fluid level (arrow). (From Mulholland MW, et al. *Greenfield's Surgery, Scientific Principles and Practice*. 4th ed. Philadelphia, PA: Lippincott Williams & Wilkins; 2005.)

**Which parts of the lungs are typically involved in aspiration pneumonia?**

The right lung is most often involved in aspiration pneumonia because the right mainstem bronchus is wider and straighter than the left. In general, the dependent portions of the lungs are most often involved. In patients who aspirate in the recumbent position, these areas include the posterior segments of the upper lobes and the apical segments of the lower lobes. In patients who aspirate in the upright position, these areas include the basal segments of the lower lobes.[26]

**What methods are available to aid in identifying an organism in patients with aspiration pneumonia?**

Gram stain and culture are the methods of choice for identifying specific organisms involved in aspiration pneumonia. Expectorated sputum is not suitable for anaerobic culture because anaerobes are part of normal oral flora and contaminate samples. Transtracheal aspiration and bronchoscopy with BAL are techniques that bypass the normal flora of the upper respiratory tract and may provide more reliable specimens for anaerobic media. When present, an empyema provides an excellent source for fluid aspiration and identification of a specific organism. Blood cultures are rarely positive in patients with anaerobic pneumonia but may be helpful in cases involving other organisms.[4]

**What is the empiric treatment for aspiration pneumonia?**

Empiric treatment for aspiration pneumonia should take into account the setting in which it occurred. Community-acquired aspiration pneumonia should be treated with agents that cover anaerobes and other constituents of normal oral flora, such as amoxicillin-clavulanate (or ampicillin-sulbactam for patients requiring parenteral therapy). Hospital-acquired aspiration pneumonia may benefit from additional coverage of resistant organisms (eg, *Pseudomonas aeruginosa*) with an agent such as piperacillin-tazobactam; MRSA coverage may be added for patients with risk factors.[4]

## What organisms cause aspiration pneumonia?

**These organisms are part of normal oral flora and cause aspiration pneumonia in the community and hospital settings.**

Anaerobes and *Streptococcus* species.

**These organisms are often responsible for aspiration pneumonia in hospitalized patients.**

Gram-negative bacilli and *Staphylococcus aureus*.

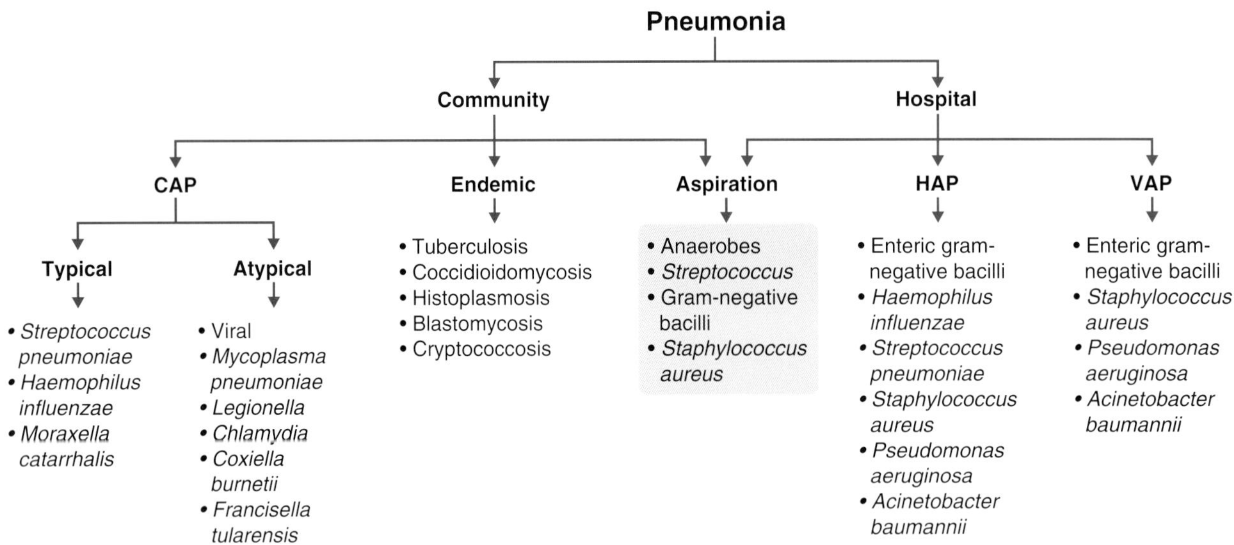


**What are the features of aspiration pneumonia caused by anaerobes?**

Anaerobic organisms are part of normal oral flora and often cause aspiration pneumonia in the community and hospital settings. These pathogens include species of *Peptostreptococcus, Bacteroides, Prevotella, and Fusobacterium*. Aspiration pneumonia caused by anaerobes tends to be insidious in onset and leads to lung abscess and empyema formation, although *Fusobacterium necrophorum* is particularly virulent. Antimicrobial therapy should be prolonged for patients with necrotizing pneumonia, lung abscess, or empyema. In the case of empyema, evacuation of the pleural space is also necessary.[4]

**Which streptococci cause aspiration pneumonia?**

Viridans streptococci are major constituents of normal oral flora and are important causes of aspiration pneumonia in both community and hospital settings. Other streptococci are capable of causing aspiration pneumonia, including *Streptococcus pyogenes*.[4]

**Which gram-negative bacilli cause aspiration pneumonia?**

Hospitalized patients often acquire oropharyngeal colonization with gram-negative bacilli, such as *Klebsiella pneumoniae*, *Enterobacter* species, *Serratia* species, *Pseudomonas aeruginosa*, *Escherichia coli*, and *Proteus* species. Unlike anaerobes, these organisms tend to produce fulminant pneumonia.[4]

**What are the features of *Staphylococcus aureus* pneumonia?**

*Staphylococcus aureus* pneumonia is common in the hospital setting, particularly after aspiration events. Risk factors include advanced age, prolonged hospitalization, underlying lung disease, prior antibiotic therapy, and surgery. The presentation is typically acute, with a tendency toward necrotizing pneumonia, bacteremia, and septic shock. Gram stain and culture of expectorated sputum are sensitive for the presence of *Staphylococcus aureus*. Blood cultures are also helpful in making the diagnosis. Despite treatment, the mortality rate is high.[4,27]

## Case Summary

A previously healthy 57-year-old man presents with acute-onset dyspnea, productive cough, and rigors and is found to have fever, focal findings on lung examination, peripheral leukocytosis, and abnormal findings on chest imaging.

***What is the most likely cause of pneumonia in this patient?***

*Streptococcus pneumoniae.*

### BONUS QUESTIONS

***Why is Streptococcus pneumoniae the most likely organism in this case?***

This case is most suggestive of typical CAP, given the acute-onset of symptoms, productive cough, peripheral leukocytosis with increased band forms, and the presence of lobar consolidation on chest imaging (see Figure 31-1). Typical CAP is most often caused by *Streptococcus pneumoniae*, *Haemophilus influenzae*, and *Moraxella catarrhalis*. The Gram stain in this case demonstrates gram-positive diplococci, which is consistent with *Streptococcus pneumoniae*.

***What is egophony?***

Egophony means "goat sound" (from the Greek "ego"), and refers to the change in timbre of sound as it travels through an area of consolidation. When auscultating the chest, ask the patient to say the word "bee." Egophony is present if the "e" sounds more like "a." *The bleating of a Nubian goat is an excellent example of this sound.*[3]

***What is whispered pectoriloquy?***

Pectoriloquy means "chest speaking." When auscultating the chest, ask the patient to whisper a phrase (such as "66 whiskeys, please"). Normal, aerated lung acts as a filter, making these whispered words garbled and undecipherable. If the words are clearly discernable, then pectoriloquy is present and indicative of underlying nonaerated lung (eg, consolidation, tumor, compressed lung).[3]

***What findings are present on the chest radiograph in this case?***

The chest radiograph in this case (see Figure 31-1) demonstrates a large consolidation with air bronchograms filling much of the left upper lobe. There is no associated pleural effusion.

***Does the patient in this case have risk factors for drug-resistant organisms?***

Factors that increase the likelihood of resistant organisms in CAP include recent antimicrobial exposure, residence in a long-term care facility, tube feeding, prior infection with a drug-resistant organism (within 1 year), recent hospitalization, chronic lung disease, poor functional status, immunocompromised status, and chronic hemodialysis. Based on the information provided, the patient in this case does not appear to be at increased risk for drug-resistant organisms.[8,9]

| | |
|---|---|
| ***How should the patient in this case be treated?*** | Hospitalized patients with CAP without risk factors for drug-resistant pathogens can be treated with an antipneumococcal fluoroquinolone (eg, levofloxacin) or a combination of a β-lactam agent (eg, ceftriaxone) plus a macrolide (eg, azithromycin). Given the signs of systemic toxicity in this case (such as fever, tachycardia, tachypnea, and leukocytosis), it would be reasonable to treat with intravenous antibiotics until there is clinical improvement before transitioning to oral antibiotics.[28] |
| ***What is the prognosis of community-acquired pneumonia requiring hospitalization?*** | The overall 30-day mortality rate in hospitalized patients with CAP is approximately 10%. The 30-day readmission rate is about 20%. Elderly patients may require months to recover, and some never return to their previous state of health.[1] |

## KEY POINTS

- Pneumonia refers to infection of the pulmonary parenchyma with characteristic symptoms, physical findings, and radiographic findings.
- Symptoms of pneumonia include dyspnea, cough, sputum production, pleuritic chest pain, chills, malaise, and confusion.
- Physical findings of pneumonia include fever, tachycardia, tachypnea, cachexia, dullness to percussion, increased tactile fremitus, tubular breath sounds, inspiratory rales, pleural friction rub, egophony, and whispered pectoriloquy.
- Despite a cadre of available diagnostic tests, a specific pathogen may not be identified in many cases of pneumonia. Empiric treatment is often necessary.
- Pneumonia can be acquired in the community or in the hospital.
- The subcategories of pneumonia acquired in the community setting are community-acquired pneumonia and endemic pneumonia.
- Community-acquired pneumonia can be caused by typical or atypical pathogens.
- Typical bacterial pneumonia tends to present acutely with systemic toxicity, whereas atypical pathogens are associated with indolent symptoms and signs.
- The subcategories of pneumonia acquired in the hospital setting are hospital-acquired pneumonia and ventilator-associated pneumonia.
- Hospital-acquired pneumonia is defined as pneumonia occurring after 48 or more hours of hospitalization in nonintubated patients.
- Ventilator-associated pneumonia is defined as pneumonia occurring after 48 or more hours of endotracheal intubation.
- Aspiration pneumonia occurs in both community and hospital settings.
- The common pathogens in each category of pneumonia are distinct and affect the choice of empiric antimicrobials.
- Environmental factors (eg, local antibiogram data) and host factors (eg, drug allergies, severity of illness, presence of risk factors for drug-resistant pathogens) should also be used to guide empiric therapy.

## REFERENCES


1. Musher DM, Thorner AR. Community-acquired pneumonia. *N Engl J Med*. 2014;371(17):1619-1628.
2. Prina E, Ranzani OT, Torres A. Community-acquired pneumonia. *Lancet*. 2015;386(9998):1097-1108.
3. Sapira JD. *The Art & Science of Bedside Diagnosis*. Baltimore, MD: Urban & Schwarzenberg; 1990.
4. Finegold SM. Aspiration pneumonia. *Rev Infect Dis*. 1991;13(suppl 9):S737-S742.
5. King P. Haemophilus influenzae and the lung (Haemophilus and the lung). *Clin Transl Med*. 2012;1(1):10.
6. Longo DL, Fauci AS, Kasper DL, Hauser SL, Jameson JL, Loscalzo J, eds. *Harrison's Principles of Internal Medicine*. 18th ed. New York, NY: McGraw-Hill; 2012.
7. Verduin CM, Hol C, Fleer A, van Dijk H, van Belkum A. *Moraxella catarrhalis*: from emerging to established pathogen. *Clin Microbiol Rev*. 2002;15(1):125-144.
8. Shorr AF, Zilberberg MD, Reichley R, et al. Validation of a clinical score for assessing the risk of resistant pathogens in patients with pneumonia presenting to the emergency department. *Clin Infect Dis*. 2012;54(2):193-198.
9. Webb BJ, Dascomb K, Stenehjem E, et al. Derivation and multicenter validation of the drug resistance in pneumonia clinical prediction score. *Antimicrob Agents Chemother*. 2016;60(5):2652-2663.

10. Anderson A, Bijlmer H, Fournier PE, et al. Diagnosis and management of Q fever–United States, 2013: recommendations from CDC and the Q Fever Working Group. *MMWR Recomm Rep*. 2013;62(RR-03):1-30.
11. Waites KB, Talkington DF. Mycoplasma pneumoniae and its role as a human pathogen. *Clin Microbiol Rev*. 2004;17(4):697-728, table of contents.
12. Yu VL, Plouffe JF, Pastoris MC, et al. Distribution of Legionella species and serogroups isolated by culture in patients with sporadic community-acquired legionellosis: an international collaborative survey. *J Infect Dis*. 2002;186(1):127-128.
13. Blasi F, Tarsia P, Aliberti S. *Chlamydophila pneumoniae*. *Clin Microbiol Infect*. 2009;15(1):29-35.
14. Thomas LD, Schaffner W. Tularemia pneumonia. *Infect Dis Clin North Am*. 2010;24(1):43-55.
15. Saccente M, Woods GL. Clinical and laboratory update on blastomycosis. *Clin Microbiol Rev*. 2010;23(2):367-381.
16. Zumla A, Raviglione M, Hafner R, von Reyn CF. Tuberculosis. *N Engl J Med*. 2013;368(8):745-755.
17. Malo J, Luraschi-Monjagatta C, Wolk DM, Thompson R, Hage CA, Knox KS. Update on the diagnosis of pulmonary coccidioidomycosis. *Ann Am Thorac Soc*. 2014;11(2):243-253.
18. Kauffman CA. Histoplasmosis: a clinical and laboratory update. *Clin Microbiol Rev*. 2007;20(1):115-132.
19. Shirley RM, Baddley JW. Cryptococcal lung disease. *Curr Opin Pulm Med*. 2009;15(3):254-260.
20. Kalil AC, Metersky ML, Klompas M, et al. Management of adults with hospital-acquired and ventilator-associated pneumonia: 2016 Clinical Practice Guidelines by the Infectious Diseases Society of America and the American Thoracic Society. *Clin Infect Dis*. 2016;63(5):e61-e111.
21. Barbier F, Andremont A, Wolff M, Bouadma L. Hospital-acquired pneumonia and ventilator-associated pneumonia: recent advances in epidemiology and management. *Curr Opin Pulm Med*. 2013;19(3):216-228.
22. Kieninger AN, Lipsett PA. Hospital-acquired pneumonia: pathophysiology, diagnosis, and treatment. *Surg Clin North Am*. 2009;89(2):439-461, ix.
23. Mendelson CL. The aspiration of stomach contents into the lungs during obstetric anesthesia. *Am J Obstet Gynecol*. 1946;52:191-205.
24. Taylor JK, Fleming GB, Singanayagam A, Hill AT, Chalmers JD. Risk factors for aspiration in community-acquired pneumonia: analysis of a hospitalized UK cohort. *Am J Med*. 2013;126(11):995-1001.
25. Takayanagi N, Kagiyama N, Ishiguro T, Tokunaga D, Sugita Y. Etiology and outcome of community-acquired lung abscess. *Respiration*. 2010;80(2):98-105.
26. Marik PE. Aspiration pneumonitis and aspiration pneumonia. *N Engl J Med*. 2001;344(9):665-671.
27. Gonzalez C, Rubio M, Romero-Vivas J, Gonzalez M, Picazo JJ. Bacteremic pneumonia due to Staphylococcus aureus: a comparison of disease caused by methicillin-resistant and methicillin-susceptible organisms. *Clin Infect Dis*. 1999;29(5):1171-1177.
28. Mandell LA, Wunderink RG, Anzueto A, et al. Infectious Diseases Society of America/American Thoracic Society consensus guidelines on the management of community-acquired pneumonia in adults. *Clin Infect Dis*. 2007;44(suppl 2):S27-S72.

SECTION 9

# Nephrology

Chapter 32

# ACID-BASE DISORDERS

## Case: An 18-year-old man with polyuria

A previously healthy 18-year-old man presents to the emergency department with progressive nausea, vomiting, and abdominal pain. Several weeks ago he noticed an increase in urinary frequency and volume. Over the past day he has developed abdominal pain and nausea, worsening to the point of intense vomiting. He has experienced weight loss of 10 pounds over the past few weeks.

Heart rate is 134 beats per minute, respiratory rate is 32 breaths per minute, and blood pressure is 94/58 mm Hg. The patient appears acutely ill with deep and rapid breathing. There is a fruity odor on his breath. The abdomen is diffusely tender to palpation.

Serum glucose is 600 mg/dL, sodium ($Na^+$) 126 mEq/L, chloride ($Cl^-$) 82 mEq/L, bicarbonate ($HCO_3^-$) 12 mEq/L, blood urea nitrogen (BUN) 34 mg/dL, and osmolality 305 mOsm/kg (reference range 275-295 mOsm/kg). Arterial blood gas measurement shows a pH of 7.29 and a partial pressure of carbon dioxide ($Paco_2$) of 26 mm Hg.

***What acid-base disturbance(s) is present in this patient?***

**What are the 2 general types of acid produced in the body?**

The body produces volatile acid (ie, $CO_2$) and nonvolatile acid (eg, lactic acid), both of which are created during the metabolism of carbohydrates, proteins, and fats consumed in the diet.[1]

**What is the main extracellular buffer in the body?**

$HCO_3^-$ is the main extracellular buffer. Phosphate and plasma protein also provide extracellular buffering.[2]

**What is the relationship between $CO_2$, water ($H_2O$), $HCO_3^-$, and hydrogen ions ($H^+$)?**

Carbonic anhydrase is an enzyme found inside red blood cells that aids in the interconversion between $CO_2$ and $H_2O$ and $HCO_3^-$ and $H^+$, with carbonic acid ($H_2CO_3$) as an intermediate in the reaction.[3]

$$CO_2 + H_2O \leftrightarrow H_2CO_3 \leftrightarrow HCO_3^- + H^+$$

**What is the relationship between blood pH, serum $HCO_3^-$ and $Paco_2$ in arterial blood?**

The Henderson-Hasselbalch equation describes the relationship between blood pH, $HCO_3^-$, and $Paco_2$.

$$\text{Blood pH} = 6.1 + \log([HCO_3^-]/[0.03 \times Paco_2])$$

*In the above equation, 6.1 is the pKa of the $HCO_3^-$ buffer system, and 0.03 is the solubility coefficient for $CO_2$ in blood.*[3]

**How is acid eliminated from the body?**

Acid is eliminated from the body via metabolic utilization, exhalation of $CO_2$ in the lungs, and excretion of $H^+$ in the kidneys as titratable acid (eg, $H_2PO_4^-$) and $NH_4^+$ (Figure 32-1).[4]

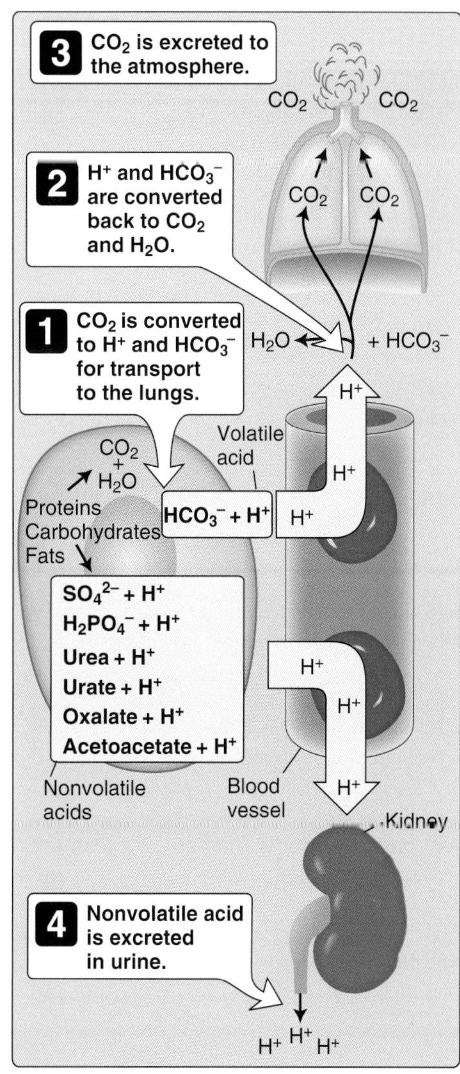


**Figure 32-1.** Volatile and nonvolatile acid elimination. (From Preston RR, Wilson TE. *Lippincott Illustrated Reviews: Physiology.* Philadelphia: Lippincott Williams & Wilkins; 2013.)

**What is normal arterial pH?**

Normal arterial pH is 7.4 ± 0.05. Venous pH is slightly more acidic.[2]

**What arterial pH range is compatible with life?**

An arterial pH between 6.8 and 7.8 is generally compatible with life.[3]

**What is the first diagnostic step in determining the nature of an acid-base disturbance?**

Measurement of the pH of blood (from a blood gas test) is the first diagnostic step in determining the nature of an acid-base disturbance. Acidemia refers to blood pH <7.35; alkalemia refers to blood pH >7.45. *History and physical examination are critical components of the investigation into any acid-base disturbance.*

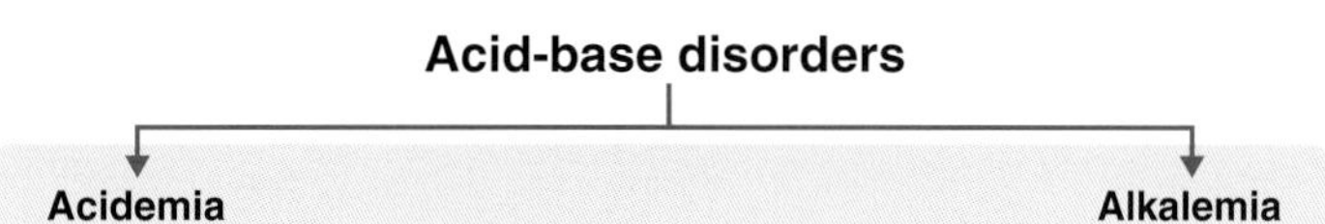

**What is the difference between acidemia/alkalemia and acidosis/alkalosis?**

The suffix -emia refers to the acid-base state of blood (either acidic or alkaline), whereas the suffix -osis refers to system-based disorders that affect the acid-base state of blood. Although there can only be 1 acid-base state of blood at a given time (either acidemia or alkalemia), multiple acid-base disorders can exist simultaneously.

**Once the state of acidemia or alkalemia is determined, what initial laboratory studies are necessary to identify the underlying disorder(s) contributing to the acid-base disturbance?**

Serum $HCO_3^-$ (from the basic metabolic panel or blood gas test) and $Paco_2$ (from the blood gas test) are necessary to identify the underlying disorder(s) involved in an acid-base disturbance.

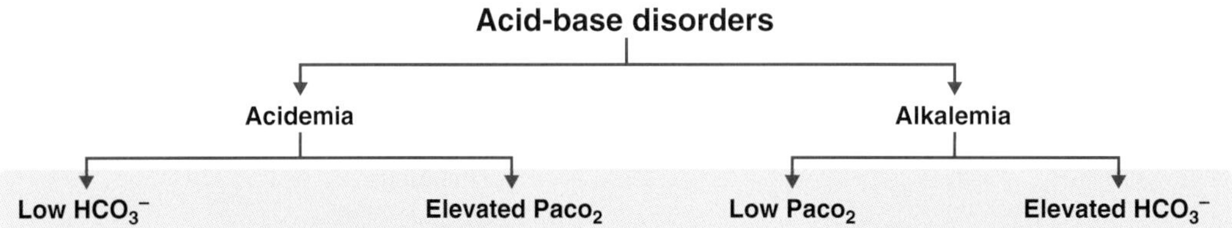


**What is normal serum concentration of $HCO_3^-$?**

Normal serum $HCO_3^-$ is 24 ± 2 mEq/L.[3]

**What is normal $Paco_2$?**

Normal $Paco_2$ is 40 ± 2 mm Hg. It is slightly higher in venous blood.[3]

**What primary acid-base disorder is characterized by the presence of acidemia with low serum $HCO_3^-$?**

Primary metabolic acidosis is characterized by the combination of acidemia and low serum $HCO_3^-$.

**What primary acid-base disorder is characterized by the presence of acidemia with elevated $Paco_2$?**

Primary respiratory acidosis is characterized by the combination of acidemia and elevated $Paco_2$.

**What primary acid-base disorder is characterized by the presence of alkalemia with low $Paco_2$?**

Primary respiratory alkalosis is characterized by the combination of alkalemia and low $Paco_2$.

**What primary acid-base disorder is characterized by the presence of alkalemia with elevated serum $HCO_3^-$?**

Primary metabolic alkalosis is characterized by the combination of alkalemia and elevated serum $HCO_3^-$ (Figure 32-2).

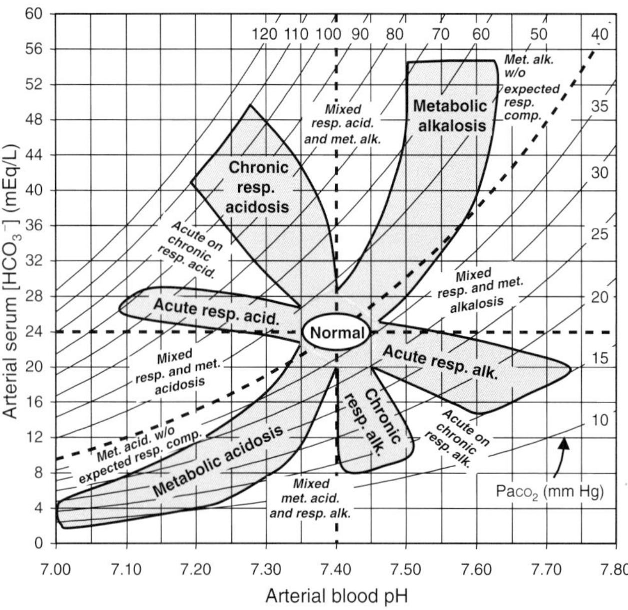


**Figure 32-2.** Acid-base nomogram. Shown are the 95% confidence limits of the normal respiratory and metabolic compensations for primary acid-base disturbances. (From Diepenbrock N. *Quick Reference to Critical Care*. 5th ed. Philadelphia, PA: Wolters Kluwer Health; 2016.)

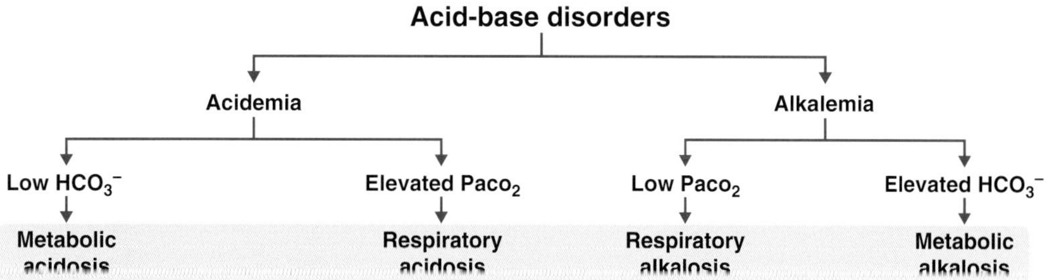


**What systems are responsible for maintaining acid-base homeostasis in the setting of a metabolic disorder?**

The lungs rapidly compensate for acid-base disturbances related to metabolic disorders, with a new steady state $Paco_2$ reached within hours. The kidneys play an integral role in correcting acid-base disturbances by adjusting acid and $HCO_3^-$ elimination, a process that takes several days.[3]

**How is minute ventilation calculated?**

Minute ventilation ($V_E$) is the product of tidal volume ($V_T$) and respiratory rate ($f$) per minute.

$$V_E = V_T \times f$$

**What system is responsible for maintaining acid-base homeostasis in the setting of a persistent respiratory disorder?**

The kidneys compensate for acid-base disturbances related to persistent respiratory disorders. Compensation occurs slowly, with a new steady state serum $HCO_3^-$ reached within 2 to 5 days.[3]

## METABOLIC ACIDOSIS

**What are the 2 general subtypes of metabolic acidosis?**

The subtypes of metabolic acidosis are non-anion gap (non-AG) metabolic acidosis and anion gap (AG) metabolic acidosis.

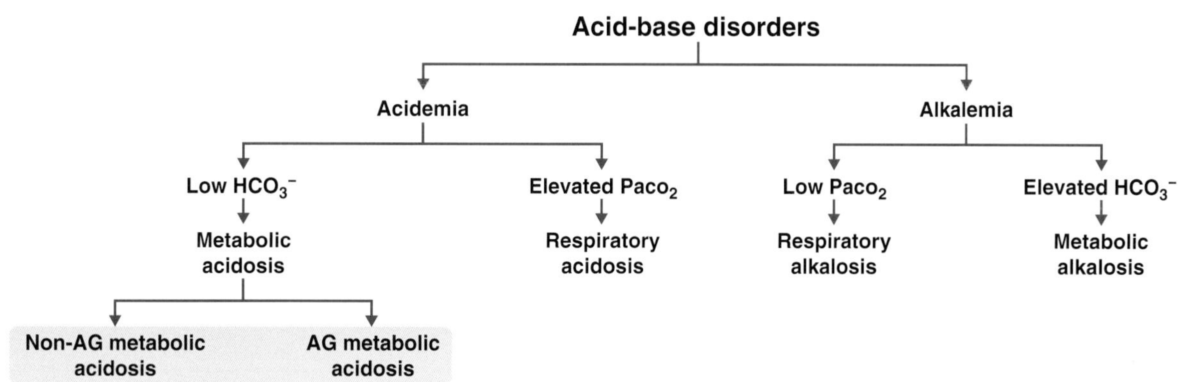


**How is anion gap calculated?**

$AG = [Na^+] - ([Cl^-] + [HCO_3^-])$

**What anion gap value is considered elevated?**

The reference range for AG varies by laboratory. However, in general, AG >12 mEq/L is considered elevated.[4]

**Calculated anion gap should always be corrected for what common condition?**

Calculated AG should always be corrected for hypoalbuminemia, as albumin is a significant unmeasured anion. For every 1 g/dL decrease in serum albumin concentration, 2.5 mEq/L should be added to the calculated AG. Hypophosphatemia may also affect the AG calculation to a smaller degree.[3]

**What conditions are associated with low anion gap?**

Low AG can be observed in conditions associated with high levels of cations, such as paraproteinemia in multiple myeloma, hypercalcemia, hypermagnesemia, and lithium toxicity.[3]

**What alternate term is used to describe non-anion gap (or normal anion gap) metabolic acidosis?**

Non-AG metabolic acidosis is also known as hyperchloremic metabolic acidosis. When $HCO_3^-$ is removed from the blood (eg, through the gastrointestinal [GI] tract), electroneutrality is maintained with a proportional rise in $Cl^-$, which also has a negative charge. Because the sum of serum $HCO_3^-$ and $Cl^-$ is part of the formula for AG, there is no net change in the calculated AG (Figure 32-3).

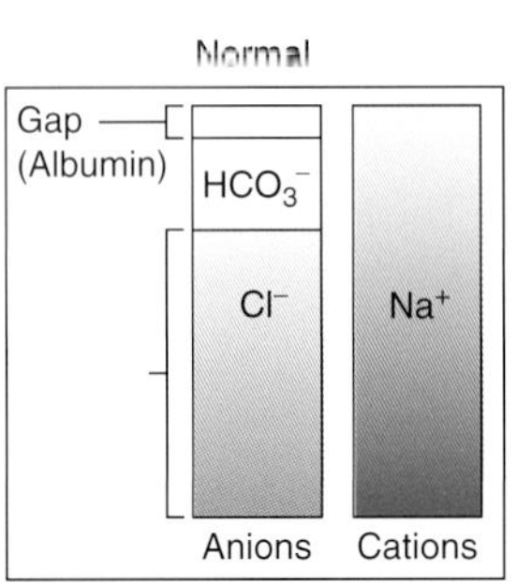


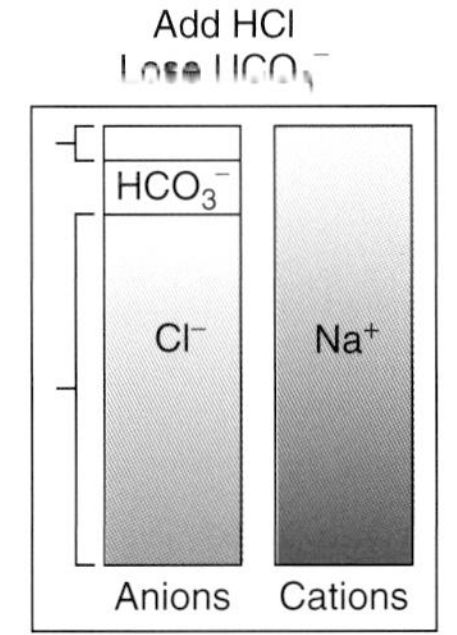


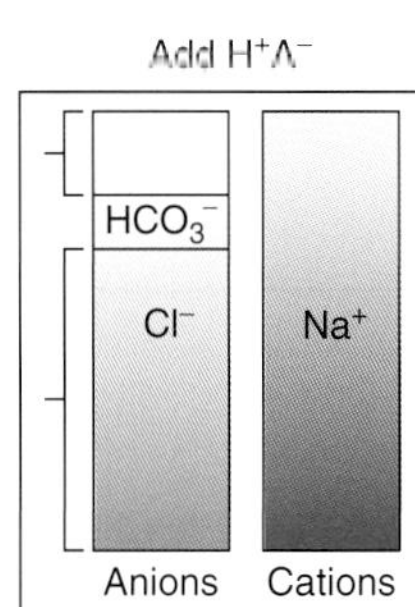


**Figure 32-3.** Balance of anions and cations in the development of metabolic acidosis. The left panel shows the normal state with the sum of $HCO_3^-$ plus unmeasured anions (predominantly albumin) making up the gap. The middle panel shows that a decrease in $HCO_3^-$ accompanied by a corresponding increase in $Cl^-$ results in no change to the anion gap. The right panel shows development of acidosis through the generation or retention of $H^+$ with a different anion (eg, lactate) leading to an increased anion gap. (From Rennke HG, Denker BM. *Renal Pathophysiology: The Essentials*. 4th ed. Philadelphia, PA: Lippincott Williams & Wilkins; 2014.)

**How do the lungs maintain acid-base homeostasis in the setting of metabolic acidosis?**

In the setting of metabolic acidosis, compensatory hyperventilation increases removal of the volatile acid $CO_2$ (see Figure 32-1). When functioning normally, the kidneys also help correct acidemia by excreting acid and reabsorbing $HCO_3^-$.

**When lung function is normal, which formula can be used to predict $Paco_2$ in the setting of metabolic acidosis?**

Winters' formula can be used to calculate the expected $Paco_2$ resulting from respiratory compensation in the setting of metabolic acidosis.[3,5]

Predicted $Paco_2 = (1.5 \times [HCO_3^-]) + 8 \pm 2$

**In the setting of metabolic acidosis, when measured $Paco_2$ is higher than that predicted by the compensation formula, what additional acid-base disorder must be present?**

In the setting of metabolic acidosis, if measured $Paco_2$ is higher than that predicted by the compensation formula, then a concomitant respiratory acidosis is present.

**In the setting of metabolic acidosis, when measured $Paco_2$ is lower than that predicted by the compensation formula, what additional acid-base disorder must be present?**

In the setting of metabolic acidosis, if measured $Paco_2$ is lower than that predicted by the compensation formula, then a concomitant respiratory alkalosis is present.

## NON-ANION GAP METABOLIC ACIDOSIS

### What are the causes of non-anion gap metabolic acidosis?

A 35-year-old American man develops non-AG metabolic acidosis while vacationing in Mexico where he has been sampling local cuisine.

Gastrointestinal loss of $HCO_3^-$ as a result of diarrhea.

An iatrogenic process that can be associated with acute decreases in peripheral white blood cell count, hemoglobin concentration, and platelet count.

Dilution from intravenous fluids.

| | |
|---|---|
| **The non-AG metabolic acidosis related to this organ injury can evolve to AG metabolic acidosis if the insult persists and becomes more severe.** | Mild to moderate acute or chronic kidney disease. |
| **These conditions, of which there are 3 main types, result from impaired renal acid excretion.** | Renal tubular acidosis (RTA). |
| **Used by mountain climbers to prevent and treat altitude sickness.** | Carbonic anhydrase inhibitors. |
| **A surgical procedure that reroutes urine from its natural course out of the body, often used in patients with bladder cancer.** | Ureteral diversion (eg, ileal conduit). |
| **Correction of a respiratory process.** | Post-hypocapnia. |

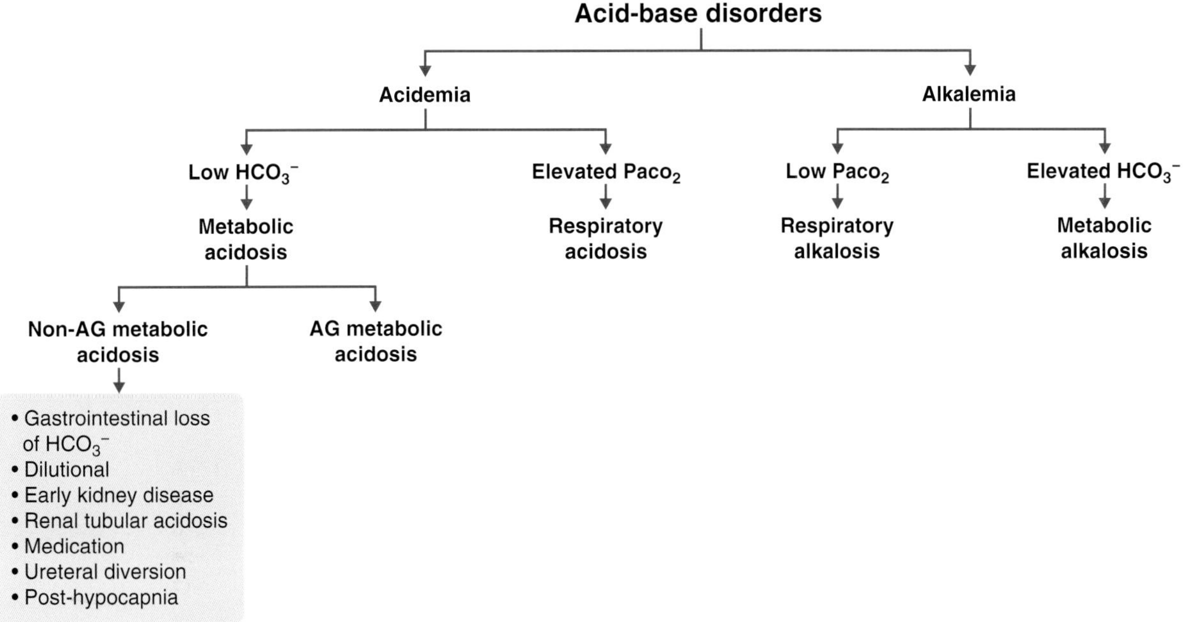


| | |
|---|---|
| **What processes can result in $HCO_3^-$ loss in the gastrointestinal tract?** | GI loss of $HCO_3^-$ can occur as a result of diarrhea, biliary fistula or drain, or pancreatic fistula or drain. |
| **Which type of crystalloid solution can lead to the generation of $HCO_3^-$ in the liver, thereby offsetting the tendency to develop metabolic acidosis related to dilution?** | Ringer's lactate solution contains lactate, which is converted to $HCO_3^-$ in the liver. The generation of $HCO_3^-$ can offset the tendency to develop metabolic acidosis from dilution.[6] |
| **What is the mechanism of non-anion gap metabolic acidosis in early kidney disease?** | The non-AG metabolic acidosis of mild to moderate acute or chronic kidney disease occurs when there is impaired acid excretion as a result of tubular dysfunction, but relatively preserved glomerular filtration rate such that the accumulation of anions that would elevate the AG does not occur.[3,7] |
| **Which types of renal tubular acidosis are associated with non-anion gap metabolic acidosis?** | All 3 types of RTA can result in non-AG metabolic acidosis, including type 1 (distal), type II (proximal), and type IV (hypoaldosteronism).[1] |

**What is the mechanism of the non-anion gap metabolic acidosis produced by acetazolamide?**

Acetazolamide inhibits the action of carbonic anhydrase and therefore retards $HCO_3^-$ reabsorption in the kidney. For mountain climbers, this helps offset the respiratory alkalosis that develops during ascent to high altitude (Figure 32-4).

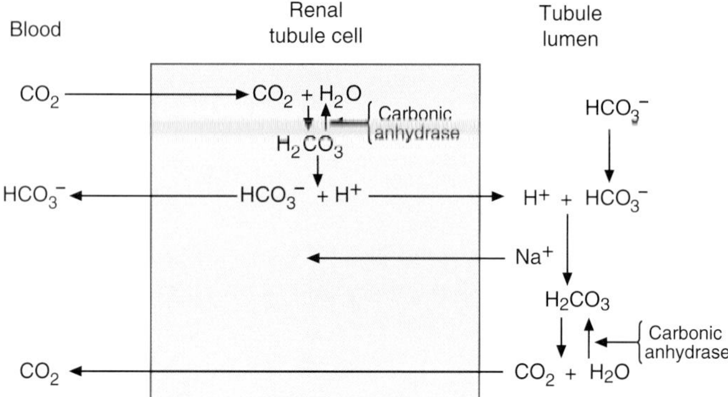


**Figure 32-4.** Renal tubular $HCO_3^-$ reabsorption. (From Alldredge BK, et al. *Applied Therapeutics: The Clinical Use of Drugs*. 10th ed. Philadelphia, PA: Lippincott Williams & Wilkins; 2014.)

**What is the mechanism of non-anion gap metabolic acidosis from ureteral diversion with ileal or colonic conduit?**

Reabsorption of $H^+$ occurs in segments of the bowel that are exposed to urine, such as the conduit in patients with urinary diversion, resulting in a chronic increase in acid load.[8]

**What is the mechanism of non-anion gap metabolic acidosis that follows a period of persistent hyperventilation?**

The kidneys compensate for hypocapnia by increasing $HCO_3^-$ excretion. When $Pa_{CO_2}$ is corrected, transient metabolic acidosis will ensue before the kidneys regenerate the lost $HCO_3^-$.

## ANION GAP METABOLIC ACIDOSIS

**What is the mechanism of increased anion gap in anion gap metabolic acidosis?**

AG metabolic acidosis results from acids that dissociate to produce a hydrogen ion and conjugate base. For example, lactic acid ($C_3H_6O_3$) dissociates into $H^+$ and lactate ($C_3H_5O_3^-$), its conjugate base. The hydrogen ions consume $HCO_3^-$, while the negatively charged conjugate base rises proportionally, maintaining electroneutrality. Consequently, serum $HCO_3^-$ is decreased but $Cl^-$ remains unchanged. The increase in unmeasured anions (ie, the conjugate base) is reflected by an increase in the calculated AG (see Figure 32-3).

**What is the delta anion gap (ΔAG)?**

The ΔAG is the difference between the calculated AG and the upper limit of normal for AG (ie, 12 mEq/L). It should be calculated in patients with AG metabolic acidosis to determine whether the AG metabolic acidosis is pure or mixed with other metabolic disorders (ie, concomitant non-AG metabolic acidosis or concomitant metabolic alkalosis).[12]

**What is the delta anion gap in a patient with serum $Na^+$ of 140 mEq/L, $Cl^-$ of 100 mEq/L, and $HCO_3^-$ of 8 mEq/L?**

$\Delta AG = 32 - 12 = 20$

**How is serum $HCO_3^-$ affected by pure anion gap metabolic acidosis?**

In pure AG metabolic acidosis, the decrease in serum $HCO_3^-$ should be roughly the same as the ΔAG (ie, ratio of ΔAG to $\Delta HCO_3^-$ is roughly 1:1). Some processes result in a ratio very close to 1:1 (eg, diabetic ketoacidosis, early lactic acidosis), whereas other processes result in slightly different ratios (eg, late lactic acidosis results in a ratio of 1.6:1). The serum $HCO_3^-$ can therefore be predicted to a close approximation.[3]

Predicted serum $HCO_3^- = 24 - \Delta AG \pm 5$ mEq/L

**What is the predicted serum $HCO_3^-$ in a patient with pure anion gap metabolic acidosis if the anion gap is 28?**

Predicted serum $HCO_3^-$ = 24 – (28 – 12) ± 5 = 8 ± 5 mEq/L (ie, 3-13 mEq/L)

**How can the predicted serum $HCO_3^-$ be used to determine whether the anion gap metabolic acidosis is pure or mixed with other metabolic disorders?**

Measured serum $HCO_3^-$ should be compared with predicted serum $HCO_3^-$. If measured serum $HCO_3^-$ is within the range of values predicted, then the AG metabolic acidosis is pure. If measured serum $HCO_3^-$ is higher than the upper limit predicted, then there is another process producing excess $HCO_3^-$ (ie, concomitant metabolic alkalosis). If measured serum $HCO_3^-$ is lower than the lower limit predicted, then there is another process reducing $HCO_3^-$ (ie, concomitant non-AG metabolic acidosis).

## What are the causes of anion gap metabolic acidosis?

**A 58-year-old woman with atrial fibrillation presents with acute-onset severe abdominal pain with rigidity, guarding, and rebound tenderness and is found to have AG metabolic acidosis.**

Lactic acidosis from cardioembolic ischemia of the gastrointestinal tract.

**Associated with asterixis.**

Uremia.

**These acids can be detected on urine dipstick.**

Ketoacidosis.

**A 34-year-old man with a history of alcohol dependence presents with blurry vision and AG metabolic acidosis.**

Methanol toxicity.

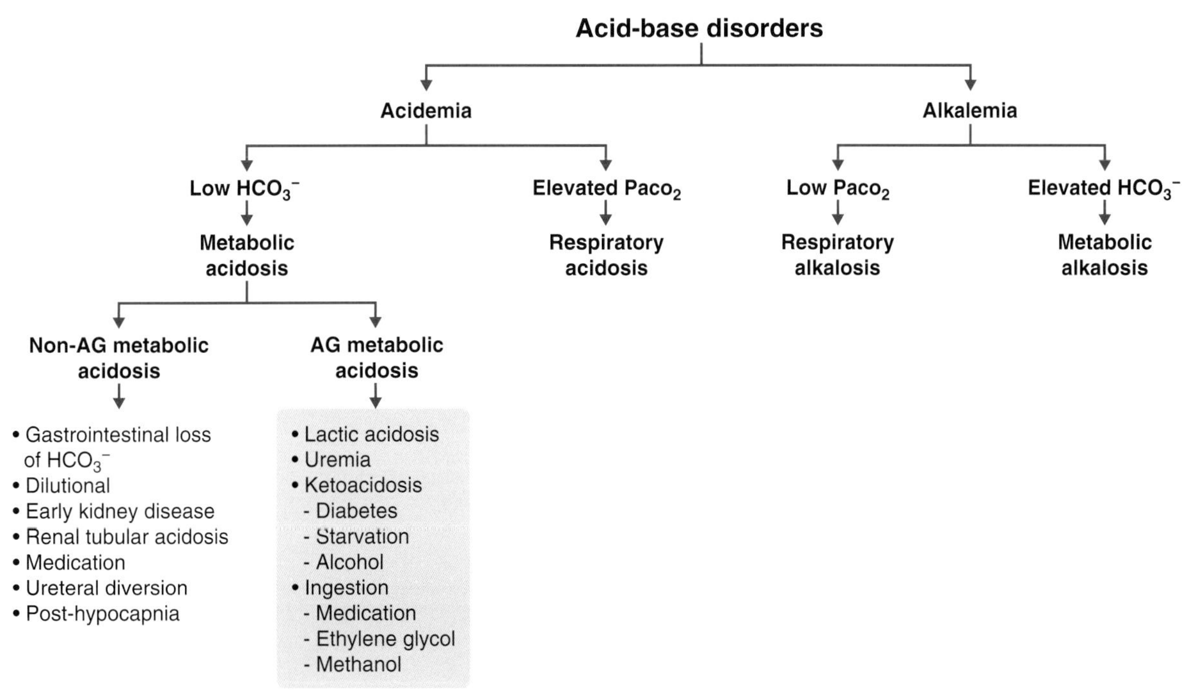


**What are the 2 general types of lactic acidosis?**

The 2 types of lactic acidosis are type A (oxygen delivery to the tissues is impaired) and type B (oxygen delivery to the tissues is not impaired). Common causes of type A lactic acidosis include hypovolemic shock (eg, hemorrhage), cardiogenic shock (eg, myocardial infarction), and distributive shock (eg, sepsis). Common causes of type B lactic acidosis include medications (eg, metformin), toxins (eg, alcohol), and malignancy (eg, lymphoma).

**What is the mechanism of anion gap metabolic acidosis in uremia?**

Mild to moderate acute and chronic kidney disease are associated with non-AG metabolic acidosis when there is impaired acid excretion but relatively preserved glomerular filtration rate. In the setting of uremia or advanced chronic kidney disease, a significant reduction in glomerular filtration leads to the retention of unmeasured anions (eg, phosphate, sulfate, urate), resulting in AG metabolic acidosis.[9]

**Is diabetic ketoacidosis (DKA) more common in patients with type 1 or type 2 diabetes mellitus?**

DKA is more common in patients with type 1 diabetes mellitus. Common precipitants include nonadherence to insulin therapy, infection, and ischemia (eg, myocardial infarction). The cornerstones of management include isotonic fluid resuscitation, insulin administration, and electrolyte replacement as needed.

**What is the significance of ketone bodies during periods of starvation?**

During periods of starvation, the brain switches from a reliance on glucose to ketone bodies as the primary fuel for metabolism. This shift decreases the need for gluconeogenesis, which consumes protein, helping the body to survive for extended periods of time.[10]

**What is the timing of alcoholic ketoacidosis in relation to the consumption of alcohol?**

Alcoholic ketoacidosis typically develops in patients with a recent (hours to days) but not active alcohol binge. Ethanol inhibits lipolysis, so significant generation of ketone bodies occurs only when ethanol levels begin to fall.[11]

**Which medications are associated with anion gap metabolic acidosis?**

Medications associated with AG metabolic acidosis include salicylates (eg, aspirin) and acetaminophen. In addition, numerous medications can cause type B lactic acidosis (eg, isoniazid, linezolid, highly active antiretroviral therapy).[12]

**Which metabolic abnormality can be a clue to the presence of ethanol, ethylene glycol, or methanol toxicity?**

Elevated serum osmolal gap can be a clue to toxic alcohol ingestion. Serum osmolal gap is the difference between measured serum osmolality and calculated serum osmolality (normal is <10 mOsm/kg).

$$\text{Calculated serum osmolality} = (2 \times [Na^+]) + ([\text{glucose}]/18) + ([\text{BUN}]/2.8)$$

*In the above formula, [Na⁺] is measured in mEq/L or mmol/L, and [glucose] and [BUN] are measured in mg/dL.*[3]

**In addition to hemodialysis, what can be used to treat methanol and ethylene glycol poisoning?**

Methanol and ethylene glycol can cause central nervous system depression but are otherwise relatively innocuous. However, toxic metabolites are generated when these parent alcohols are oxidized by alcohol dehydrogenase. Fomepizole or ethanol can be used to inhibit alcohol dehydrogenase, thereby preventing the generation of toxic metabolites.[13]

## RESPIRATORY ACIDOSIS

**What is the basic mechanism of respiratory acidosis?**

Respiratory acidosis is caused by hypoventilation and associated hypercarbia.

**How do the kidneys maintain acid-base homeostasis in the setting of persistent respiratory acidosis?**

The kidneys respond to persistent respiratory acidosis by increasing $HCO_3^-$ reabsorption in the proximal tubule and increasing $H^+$ excretion as titratable acid and $NH_4^+$ (Figure 32-5).

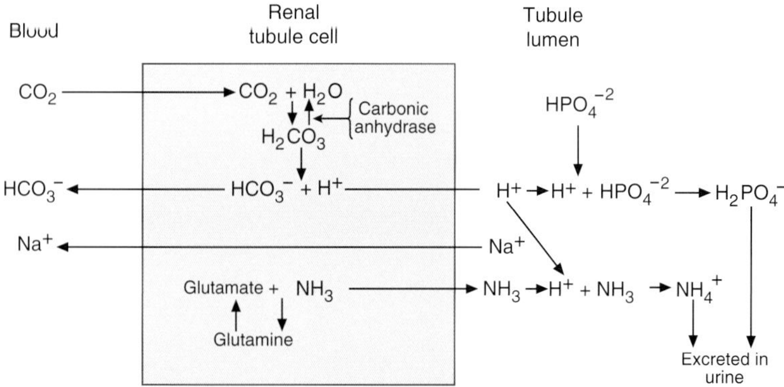


**Figure 32-5.** Renal tubular hydrogen ion (H⁺) excretion. (From Alldredge BK, et al. *Applied Therapeutics: The Clinical Use of Drugs*. 10th ed. Philadelphia, PA: Lippincott Williams & Wilkins; 2014.)

**Which formula can be used to predict serum $HCO_3^-$ in the setting of acute respiratory acidosis?**

In the setting of acute respiratory acidosis, for every 10 mm Hg increase in $Pa_{CO_2}$ above 40 mm Hg, serum $HCO_3^-$ should increase by 1 mEq/L.[3]

**Which formula can be used to predict serum $HCO_3^-$ in the setting of chronic respiratory acidosis?**

In the setting of chronic respiratory acidosis, for every 10 mm Hg increase in $Pa_{CO_2}$ above 40 mm Hg, serum $HCO_3^-$ should increase by 4 to 5 mEq/L.[3]

**In the setting of respiratory acidosis, when measured serum $HCO_3^-$ is higher than that predicted by the compensation formula, what additional acid-base disorder must be present?**

In the setting of respiratory acidosis, if measured serum $HCO_3^-$ is higher than that predicted by the compensation formula, then a concomitant metabolic alkalosis is present.

**In the setting of respiratory acidosis, when measured serum $HCO_3^-$ is lower than that predicted by the compensation formula, what additional acid-base disorder must be present?**

In the setting of respiratory acidosis, if measured serum $HCO_3^-$ is lower than that predicted by the compensation formula, then a concomitant metabolic acidosis is present.

## What are the causes of respiratory acidosis?

**A general decrease in respiratory drive.**

Central nervous system (CNS) depression.

**Difficulty getting air out of the lungs and airways.**

Airway obstruction.

**Excess alveolar ventilation relative to pulmonary capillary perfusion (ie, V/Q >1).**

Increased dead space.

**Diaphragmatic weakness.**

Neuromuscular disease.

**Anatomic abnormalities that can be congenital or acquired.**

Thoracic cage disorders.

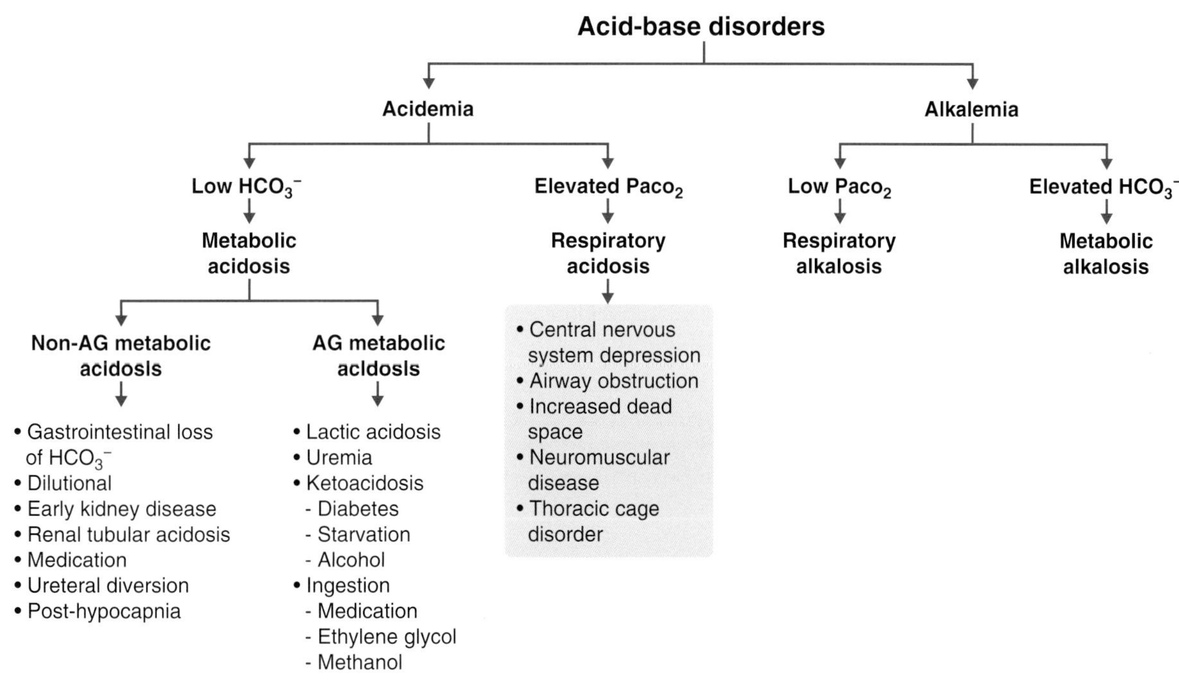


**What are the causes of central nervous system depression?**

Major causes of CNS depression include medications (eg, narcotics, benzodiazepines), stroke, trauma, encephalitis, central sleep apnea, and hypothermia.

What are the causes of airway obstruction?

Major causes of airway obstruction include chronic obstructive pulmonary disease, asthma, obstructive sleep apnea, laryngospasm, tracheomalacia, and foreign body aspiration.

What are the causes of increased dead space?

Major causes of increased dead space include shallow breathing, pulmonary embolism, decreased pulmonary capillary perfusion (eg, from systemic hypotension, pulmonary hypertension, or pulmonary capillaritis), emphysema, and positive pressure ventilation (see chapter 46, Hypoxemia).

Which noninvasive bedside pulmonary function test can be used to gauge severity and progress in a patient with neuromuscular weakness?

Neuromuscular weakness can be evaluated with negative inspiratory force (NIF, or maximal inspiratory pressure [MIP]).

Which thoracic cage disorders can lead to hypoventilation?

Thoracic cage disorders that can lead to hypoventilation include pectus excavatum, kyphoscoliosis, thoracoplasty, fibrothorax, and flail chest.

## RESPIRATORY ALKALOSIS

What is the basic mechanism of respiratory alkalosis?

Respiratory alkalosis is caused by hyperventilation and associated hypocarbia.

How do the kidneys maintain acid-base homeostasis in the setting of persistent respiratory alkalosis?

The kidneys respond to persistent respiratory alkalosis by decreasing $HCO_3^-$ reabsorption in the proximal tubule and decreasing $H^+$ excretion as titratable acid and $NH_4^+$.

Which formula can be used to predict serum $HCO_3^-$ in the setting of acute respiratory alkalosis?

In the setting of acute respiratory alkalosis, for every 10 mm Hg decrease in $Paco_2$ below 40 mm Hg, serum $HCO_3^-$ should decrease by 2 mEq/L.[3]

Which formula can be used to predict serum $HCO_3^-$ in the setting of chronic respiratory alkalosis?

In the setting of chronic respiratory alkalosis, for every 10 mm Hg decrease in $Paco_2$ below 40 mm Hg, serum $HCO_3^-$ should decrease by 4 to 5 mEq/L.[3]

In the setting of respiratory alkalosis, when measured serum $HCO_3^-$ is higher than that predicted by the compensation formula, what additional acid-base disorder must be present?

In the setting of respiratory alkalosis, if measured serum $HCO_3^-$ is higher than that predicted by the compensation formula, then a concomitant metabolic alkalosis is present.

In the setting of respiratory alkalosis, when measured serum $HCO_3^-$ is lower than that predicted by the compensation formula, what additional acid-base disorder must be present?

In the setting of respiratory alkalosis, if measured serum $HCO_3^-$ is lower than that predicted by the compensation formula, then a concomitant metabolic acidosis is present.

### What are the causes of respiratory alkalosis?

An 18-year-old student develops respiratory alkalosis before taking a math final.

Hyperventilation related to anxiety.

Between 37 and 32 BC, a Chinese official warned travelers en route to Afghanistan about "the Little Headache Mountain" and "the Great Headache Mountain," where "men's bodies become feverish, they lose color, and they are attacked with headache and vomiting."

Hypoxemia related to high altitude. The Chinese official was most likely describing acute mountain sickness.[14,15]

Nine months of respiratory alkalosis.

Pregnancy.

**Decreased oxygen delivery to the tissues in a patient with normal cardiac output and normal oxygen hemoglobin saturation.**

Anemia.

**Hyperventilation and respiratory alkalosis can be the first sign of this infectious process associated with end-organ dysfunction and decreased systemic vascular resistance.**

Sepsis.

**Look for spider angiomas on the chest.**

Cirrhosis.

**A 45-year-old man develops respiratory alkalosis after starting treatment for smoking cessation.**

Nicotine therapy.

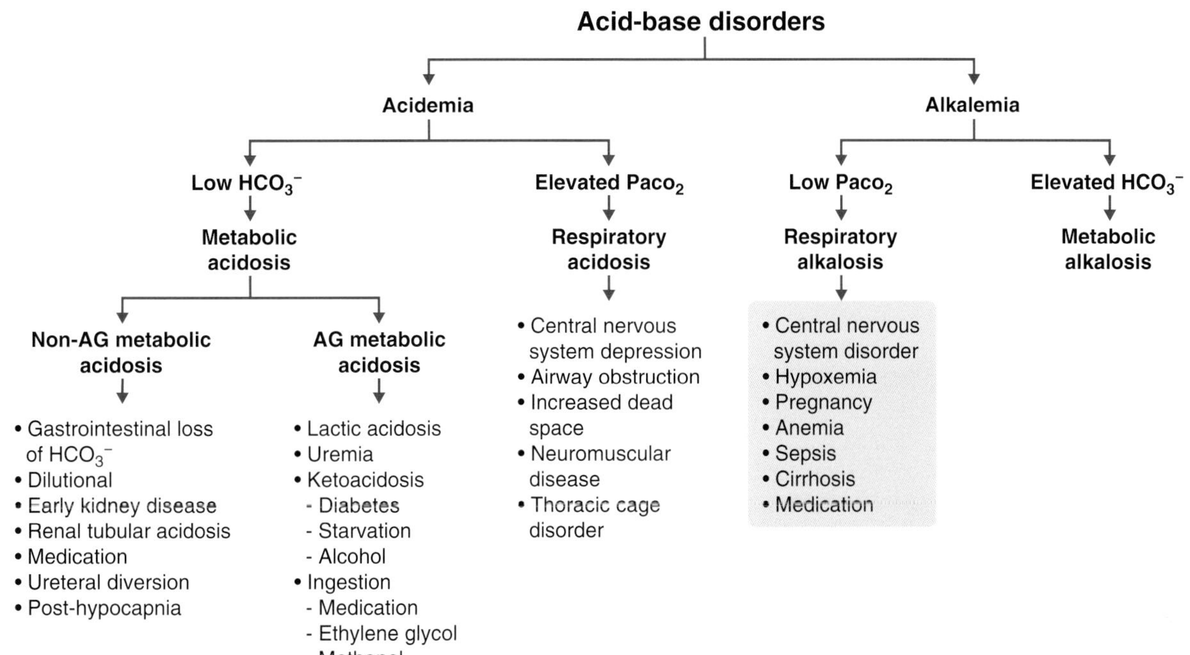


**Which central nervous system disorders are associated with hyperventilation?**

CNS disorders that can cause hyperventilation include anxiety, pain, fever, psychosis, trauma, stroke, infection (eg, meningitis, encephalitis), and space-occupying lesions (eg, tumor).

**Why is hypoxemia associated with respiratory alkalosis?**

Hypoxemia stimulates hyperventilation via the hypoxic ventilatory response. Mechanisms of hypoxemia include reduced inspired oxygen (eg, high altitude), increased dead space ventilation (eg, pulmonary embolism), physiologic shunt (eg, pneumonia), diffusion impairment (eg, interstitial lung disease), and anatomic shunt (eg, atrial septal defect) (see chapter 46, Hypoxemia). *These conditions tend to progress to respiratory acidosis when severe or when there is respiratory muscle fatigue.*[14,16]

**When does respiratory alkalosis develop during the course of pregnancy?**

Minute ventilation begins to increase within the first weeks of pregnancy and is about 50% higher than that in nonpregnant women. However, because of renal compensation, pH during pregnancy is close to normal.[17]

**Which types of anemia can cause respiratory alkalosis?**

Severe anemia from any cause can stimulate hyperventilation as a response to tissue hypoxia.

**While respiratory alkalosis occurs early on, which acid-base disorder eventually predominates in sepsis?**

The predominant acid-base disorder of sepsis is AG metabolic acidosis (ie, lactic acidosis).

**What is the most likely mechanism of respiratory alkalosis in the setting of cirrhosis?**

Progesterone, which is metabolized in the liver and therefore elevated in the serum of patients with cirrhosis, can stimulate hyperventilation via progesterone receptors in the CNS. Estradiol, which is also elevated in the serum of patients with cirrhosis, may potentiate the effects of progesterone by increasing the number of progesterone receptors.[14]

**Which medications are associated with respiratory alkalosis?**

Medications that can cause respiratory alkalosis include salicylates, nicotine, catecholamines, quetiapine, xanthines (eg, theophylline), progesterone, and medroxyprogesterone acetate.[18,19]

## METABOLIC ALKALOSIS

**What 2 pathophysiologic conditions must be present for metabolic alkalosis to occur?**

For metabolic alkalosis to occur, there must be (1) generation of metabolic alkalosis via the addition of new $HCO_3^-$ (either loss of acid or gain of alkali), and (2) impairment in the ability of the kidney to correct the alkalosis (usually a result of decreased effective arterial volume, which augments $HCO_3^-$ reclamation in the kidney).[20]

**How do the lungs maintain acid-base homeostasis in the setting of metabolic alkalosis?**

In the setting of metabolic alkalosis, compensatory hypoventilation decreases removal of the volatile acid $CO_2$. When functioning normally, the kidneys also help correct alkalemia by increasing $HCO_3^-$ excretion and decreasing acid excretion.

**Which formula can be used to predict the $Paco_2$ value in the setting of metabolic alkalosis?**

The following formula can be used to calculate the expected $Paco_2$ resulting from respiratory compensation in the setting of metabolic alkalosis[3]:

$$\text{Predicted } Paco_2 = 0.7 \times ([HCO_3^-] - 24) + 40 \pm 2$$

**In the setting of metabolic alkalosis, when measured $Paco_2$ is higher than that predicted by the compensation formula, what additional acid-base disorder must be present?**

In the setting of metabolic alkalosis, if measured $Paco_2$ is higher than that predicted by the compensation formula, then a concomitant respiratory acidosis is present.

**In the setting of metabolic alkalosis, when measured $Paco_2$ is lower than that predicted by the compensation formula, what additional acid-base disorder must be present?**

In the setting of metabolic alkalosis, if measured $Paco_2$ is lower than that predicted by the compensation formula, then a concomitant respiratory alkalosis is present.

### What are the causes of metabolic alkalosis?

**Metabolic alkalosis on a cruise ship.**

Gastrointestinal loss of $H^+$ related to vomiting from viral gastroenteritis.

**Loss of bicarbonate-free fluid.**

Contraction alkalosis.

**Iatrogenic polyuria.**

Diuretic medications.

**An electrolyte abnormality.**

Hypokalemia

**Hypertension, hypokalemia, metabolic alkalosis, and an adrenal tumor.**

Primary hyperaldosteronism.

**A 42-year-old woman with central obesity, moon facies, and thin skin.**

Cushing's syndrome.

**These 2 inherited conditions mimic the effects of loop and thiazide diuretics, respectively.**

Bartter's and Gitelman's syndromes.

**A 45-year-old man with peptic ulcer disease presents with hypercalcemia and metabolic alkalosis.**

Exogenous alkali.

**Correction of a respiratory process.**

Post-hypercapnia.

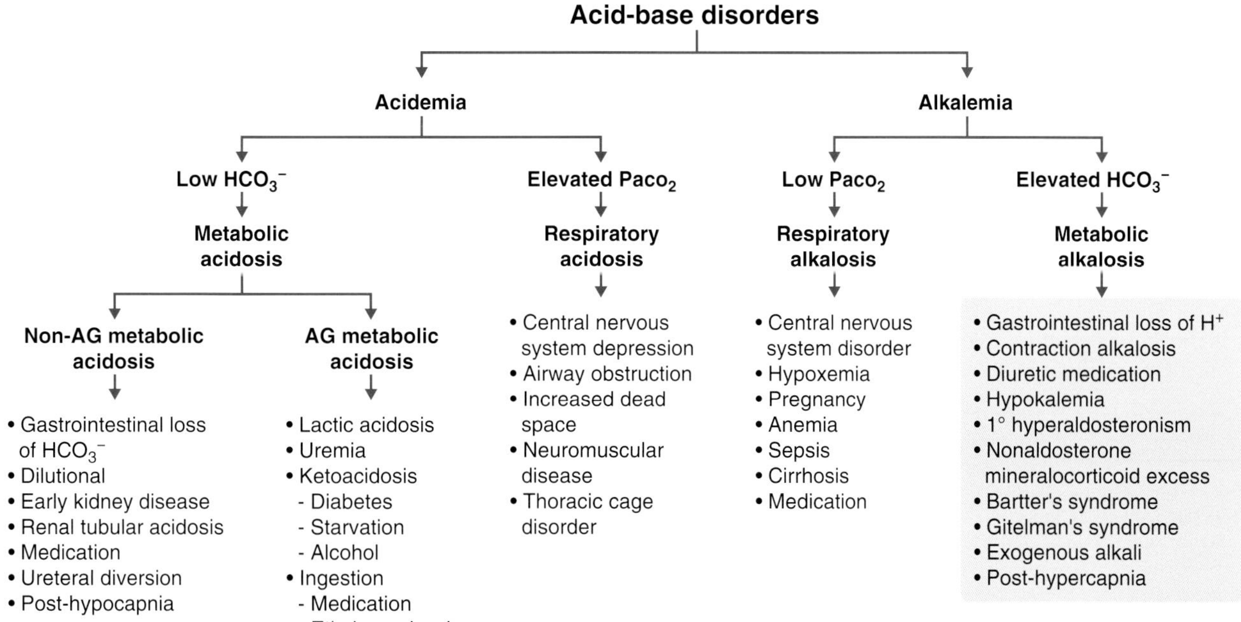


**What are the causes of $H^+$ loss from the gastrointestinal tract?**

Causes of $H^+$ loss from the GI tract include vomiting, nasogastric lavage, and some cases of diarrhea (eg, villous adenoma, laxative abuse).[21]

**What are the main mechanisms by which the metabolic alkalosis of contraction alkalosis is maintained?**

The metabolic alkalosis of contraction alkalosis is maintained as a result of decreased effective arterial blood volume by the following mechanisms: (1) Decrease in glomerular filtration rate reduces the filtered load of $HCO_3^-$, (2) proximal tubule reabsorption of $HCO_3^-$ is enhanced, and (3) decreased $Cl^-$ delivery to the cortical collecting tubule impairs $HCO_3^-$ secretion.[20]

**What is the main mechanism of metabolic alkalosis in loop and thiazide diuretics, and Bartter's and Gitelman's syndromes?**

Loop and thiazide diuretics and Bartter's and Gitelman's syndromes result in elevated renin-angiotensin-aldosterone levels and increased delivery of $Na^+$ and $H_2O$ to the distal nephron, both of which increase urinary $H^+$ secretion, causing metabolic alkalosis. In addition, these conditions often result in contraction alkalosis through the loss of bicarbonate-free fluid, further contributing to metabolic alkalosis.[20]

**What are the mechanisms of metabolic alkalosis related to hypokalemia?**

Hypokalemia can generate and maintain metabolic aklalosis. In the setting of hypokalemia, there is movement of potassium from the intracellular to extracellular fluid compartment, with resultant movement of $H^+$ into the cells to maintain electroneutrality, which increases extracellular pH. In addition, hypokalemia results in decreased $HCO_3^-$ excretion and increased $H^+$ excretion in the kidney.[20]

**What is the mechanism of metabolic alkalosis related to primary hyperaldosteronism?**

Aldosterone acts in the distal nephron to increase $Na^+$ reabsorption in exchange for $H^+$ secretion, augmenting renal acid loss. Coexistent hypertension and hypokalemia can be a clue to the presence of primary hyperaldosteronism. Secondary hyperaldosteronism, with the exception of that generated by diuretics (or Bartter's and Gitelman's), does not generate metabolic alkalosis because increased delivery of $Na^+$ and $H_2O$ to the distal nephron does not occur.[20]

**What are the causes of nonaldosterone mineralocorticoid excess?**

Causes of nonaldosterone mineralocorticoid excess include Cushing's syndrome, Liddle syndrome, and exogenous mineralocorticoids.

**Why are blood products a potential source of exogenous alkali?**

Blood products can be anticoagulated with citrate salts, which are converted in the body to sodium bicarbonate.

**What is the mechanism of metabolic alkalosis that follows a period of persistent hypoventilation?**

The kidneys compensate for hypercapnia by decreasing excretion of $HCO_3^-$. When $Paco_2$ is corrected, transient metabolic alkalosis will ensue before the kidneys excrete the extra $HCO_3^-$.

## Case Summary

A previously healthy 18-year-old man presents with polyuria, nausea, abdominal pain, and vomiting and is found to have multiple metabolic abnormalities.

***What acid-base disturbance(s) is present in this patient?***

Primary anion gap metabolic acidosis with appropriate respiratory compensation and concomitant metabolic alkalosis.

### BONUS QUESTIONS

***What are the steps to determining the primary acid-base disorder in this case? (Recall serum $Na^+$ 126 mEq/L, $Cl^-$ 82 mEq/L, $HCO_3^-$ 12 mEq/L, serum osmolality 305 mOsm/kg, pH 7.29, and $Paco_2$ 26 mm Hg.)***

The blood pH in this case indicates acidemia, which could result from either metabolic or respiratory acidosis. Low serum $HCO_3^-$ indicates that metabolic acidosis is the principal condition.

***What type of metabolic acidosis is present in this case?***

To determine the type of metabolic acidosis (non-AG or AG), the AG must be calculated. In this case, AG = 126 − (82 + 12) = 32 mEq/L, which is elevated (normal is ≤12 mEq/L).

***Is there appropriate respiratory compensation for the metabolic acidosis in this case?***

Using Winters' formula, expected $Paco_2 = (1.5 \times 12) + 8 \pm 2 = 26 \pm 2$ mm Hg. The $Paco_2$ in this case is 26 mm Hg, indicating appropriate compensation. If $Paco_2$ were >28 mm Hg, there would be insufficient respiratory compensation (ie, concomitant respiratory acidosis); if $Paco_2$ were <24 mm Hg, there would be more respiratory compensation than expected (ie, concomitant respiratory alkalosis).

***Is there another metabolic disorder in this case?***

The $\Delta AG = 32 - 12 = 20$ mEq/L. In a pure AG metabolic acidosis, serum $HCO_3^-$ would be expected to decrease by roughly the same amount from 24 to 4 mEq/L. Using the formula (predicted serum $HCO_3^- = 24 - \Delta AG \pm 5$ mEq/L), predicted serum $HCO_3^- = 24 - 20 \pm 5 = 4 \pm 5$ mEq/L. The serum $HCO_3^-$ in this case is >9 mEq/L, indicating concomitant metabolic alkalosis.

***What is the most likely cause of the anion gap metabolic acidosis in this case?***

Given the history of polyuria and the markedly elevated serum glucose level in this case, the most likely cause of AG metabolic acidosis is DKA secondary to a new diagnosis of type 1 diabetes mellitus.

***What is the significance of the deep and rapid breathing described in this case?***

The deep and rapid breathing (Kussmaul's respirations) described in this case is associated with DKA, and reflects the compensatory hyperventilation that occurs in response to metabolic acidosis.

***What is the most likely cause of the concomitant metabolic alkalosis in this case?***

Based on the history in this case, GI loss of $H^+$ from vomiting is the most likely explanation for the concomitant metabolic alkalosis.

***What is the serum osmolal gap in this case?***

Calculated serum osmolality = (126 × 2) + (600/18) + (34/2.8) = 297 mOsm/kg. The measured osmolality in this case is 305 mOsm/kg. The osmolal gap = 305 − 297 = 8 mOsm/kg (normal is <10 mOsm/kg).

***What is the true serum $Na^+$ in this case?***

Measured serum $Na^+$ must be corrected for hyperglycemia. To do this, for every 100 mg/dL increase in glucose above 100 mg/dL, 1.6 to 2.4 mEq/L should be added to the measured $Na^+$. In this case, using a correctional factor of 2.0 mEq/L, the following should be added to the measured $Na^+$: ([600–100]/100) × 2.0 = 10. Corrected serum Na is 126 + 10 = 136 mEq/L.

***What are the main tenets of treating DKA?***

The cornerstones of managing DKA include crystalloid intravenous infusion for rehydration, insulin infusion to decrease the blood glucose level, and electrolyte replacement as needed.

## KEY POINTS

- Normal arterial pH is 7.4 ± 0.05.
- Acidemia is defined by arterial pH <7.35.
- Alkalemia is defined by arterial pH >7.45.
- Acidemia and alkalemia are caused by metabolic and respiratory acid-base disorders.
- History and physical examination are critical components of the investigation of any acid-base disturbance.
- Primary metabolic acidosis is characterized by the combination of acidemia and low serum $HCO_3^-$.
- Primary respiratory acidosis is characterized by the combination of acidemia and elevated $Paco_2$.
- Primary respiratory alkalosis is characterized by the combination of alkalemia and low $Paco_2$.
- Primary metabolic alkalosis is characterized by the combination of alkalemia and elevated serum $HCO_3^-$.
- The subtypes of metabolic acidosis are non-AG metabolic acidosis (AG ≤12 mEq/L) and AG metabolic acidosis (AG >12 mEq/L).
- In cases of AG metabolic acidosis, ΔAG should be calculated to determine whether or not there is a concomitant metabolic disorder.
- The lungs rapidly compensate for metabolic acid-base disorders.
- The kidneys slowly compensate for persistent respiratory acid-base disorders.
- The adequacy of compensation can be determined in any primary acid-base disorder by using disorder-specific formulas.

## REFERENCES


1. Reddy P. Clinical approach to renal tubular acidosis in adult patients. *Int J Clin Pract.* 2011;65(3):350-360.
2. Berne RML, Levy MN. *Physiology*. 4th ed. St. Louis, Missouri: Mosby, Inc.; 1998.
3. Berend K, de Vries AP, Gans RO. Physiological approach to assessment of acid-base disturbances. *N Engl J Med.* 2014;371(15):1434-1445.
4. Costanzo L. *Physiology*. 4th ed. Philadelphia, PA: Lippincott Williams & Wilkins; 2007.
5. Albert MS, Dell RB, Winters RW. Quantitative displacement of acid-base equilibrium in metabolic acidosis. *Ann Intern Med.* 1967;66(2):312-322.
6. Martini WZ, Cortez DS, Dubick MA. Comparisons of normal saline and lactated Ringer's resuscitation on hemodynamics, metabolic responses, and coagulation in pigs after severe hemorrhagic shock. *Scand J Trauma Resusc Emerg Med.* 2013;21:86.
7. Widmer B, Gerhardt RE, Harrington JT, Cohen JJ. Serum electrolyte and acid base composition. The influence of graded degrees of chronic renal failure. *Arch Intern Med.* 1979;139(10):1099-1102.
8. Van der Aa F, Joniau S, Van Den Branden M, Van Poppel H. Metabolic changes after urinary diversion. *Adv Urol.* 2011;2011:764325.
9. Warnock DG. Uremic acidosis. *Kidney Int.* 1988;34(2):278-287.
10. Cahill GF Jr. Starvation in man. *N Engl J Med.* 1970;282(12):668-675.
11. Noor NM, Basavaraju K, Sharpstone D. Alcoholic ketoacidosis: a case report and review of the literature. *Oxf Med Case Reports.* 2016;2016(3):31-33.
12. Pham AQ, Xu LH, Moe OW. Drug-induced metabolic acidosis. *F1000Res.* 2015;4.
13. Jacobsen D, McMartin KE. Antidotes for methanol and ethylene glycol poisoning. *J Toxicol Clin Toxicol.* 1997;35(2):127-143.
14. Lustik SJ, Chhibber AK, Kolano JW, et al. The hyperventilation of cirrhosis: progesterone and estradiol effects. *Hepatology*. 1997;25(1):55-58.
15. Rennie D. The great breathlessness mountains. *JAMA.* 1986;256(1):81-82.
16. Moroz VA, Butrov AV. Mechanisms of compensation of disorders of acid-base status of the blood in patients with chronic anemia. *Ter Arkh.* 1985;57(7):74-79.
17. Huch R. Maternal hyperventilation and the fetus. *J Perinat Med.* 1986;14(1):3-17.
18. Fukuhara Y, Kaneko T, Orita Y. Drug-induced acid-base disorders. *Nihon Rinsho.* 1992;50(9):2231-2236.
19. Palmer BF. Evaluation and treatment of respiratory alkalosis. *Am J Kidney Dis.* 2012;60(5):834-838.
20. Palmer BF, Alpern RJ. Metabolic alkalosis. *J Am Soc Nephrol.* 1997;8(9):1462-1469.
21. Perez GO, Oster JR, Rogers A. Acid-base disturbances in gastrointestinal disease. *Dig Dis Sci.* 1987;32(9):1033-1043.

Chapter 33

# ACUTE KIDNEY INJURY

## Case: A 73-year-old man with blue toes

A 73-year-old man with a history of hypertension, coronary artery disease, type 2 diabetes mellitus, and peripheral artery disease is evaluated in the clinic for skin changes 10 days after undergoing femoropopliteal bypass surgery. The patient had been doing well at home after the procedure until he noticed a new rash over his legs and bluish discoloration of his toes.

Blood pressure is 174/78 mm Hg. There is a lacy erythematous macular rash over the thighs (Figure 33-1) as well as bluish discoloration of the toes bilaterally (Figure 33-2). Dorsalis pedis pulses are palpable.

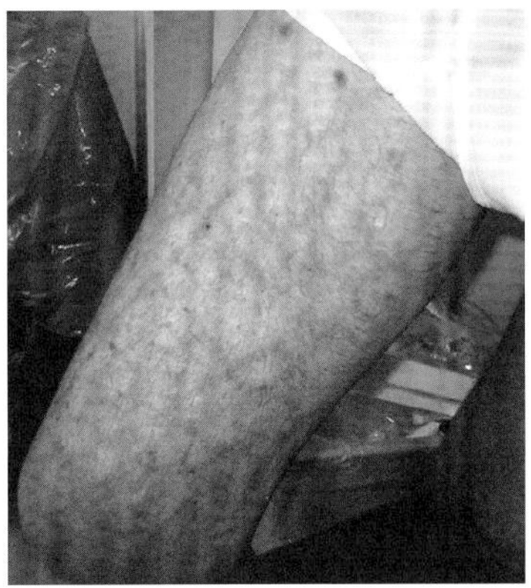

**Figure 33-1.** (Courtesy of Peter D. Sullivan, MD.)

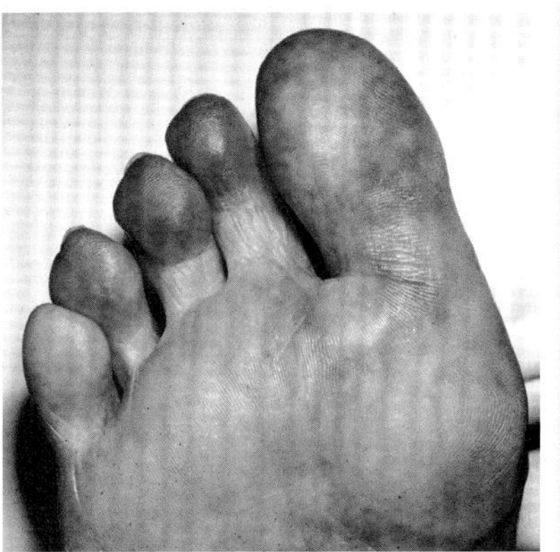

**Figure 33-2.** (Courtesy of Lawrence B. Stack, MD.)

Peripheral white blood cell count is 5.8 K/μL with 14% eosinophils. Blood urea nitrogen (BUN) is 58 mg/dL, and serum creatinine is 4.1 mg/dL. The fractional excretion of sodium ($FE_{Na}$) is 4.8%. Microscopic examination of urine sediment is notable for pyuria, including eosinophils. There are no red blood cells or cellular casts. Renal ultrasound is unremarkable.

***What is the most likely cause of acute kidney injury in this patient?***

**What is acute kidney injury (AKI)?**

AKI is the rapid development (within hours to days) of renal excretory dysfunction, characterized by the accumulation of the products of nitrogen metabolism (ie, urea and creatinine), decreased urine output, or both.[1]

**What is the range of normal for blood urea nitrogen levels?**

BUN is dependent on multiple factors, including protein intake, endogenous protein catabolism, intravascular fluid volume status, hepatic urea synthesis, and kidney function. This is reflected in the wide normal range reported by laboratories (eg, 5-20 mg/dL).[2]

**Is the blood urea nitrogen level a reliable reflection of renal function?**

Elevated BUN can result from high-protein diet, antianabolic medications (eg, glucocorticoids, tetracyclines), catabolic processes (eg, fever, infection), low effective arterial blood volume, and upper gastrointestinal bleeding. Decreased BUN can result from low protein diet, malnutrition, and impaired hepatic function. Given all of these influential factors, serum creatinine concentration is a more reliable predictor of renal function than BUN.[2]

**What is normal serum creatinine concentration?**

Creatinine is produced and released by muscle without significant short-term (day-to-day) variation. Serum creatinine levels are therefore dependent on muscle mass, which is dependent on nutritional status, age, gender, and ethnicity. For the average adult man, the normal range for serum creatinine is 0.6 to 1.2 mg/dL; for the average adult woman, it is approximately 0.5 to 1.1 mg/dL. Normal serum creatinine in individuals with muscle mass above or below average (eg, body builders, elderly, malnourished patients) may be outside of those ranges.[2]

**What is the biochemical laboratory definition of acute kidney injury?**

AKI is defined by any of the following: (1) increase in serum creatinine by ≥0.3 mg/dL within 48 hours, (2) increase in serum creatinine concentration to ≥1.5 times baseline, known or presumed to have occurred within the prior 7 days, or (3) urine volume <0.5 mL/kg per hour for 6 hours.[3]

**What is the expected rise in serum creatinine in a 24-hour period in the average patient with anuric kidney injury?**

In the setting of anuric kidney injury, serum creatinine will increase 1 to 2 mg/dL per day. Higher rates of rise can be seen in patients with extreme catabolic states (2-3 mg/dL per day) or in those with crush injury and rhabdomyolysis (>3 mg/dL per day).[4,5]

**What risk factors are associated with the development of acute kidney injury?**

Risk factors for AKI include preexisting kidney disease (most significant), advanced age, diabetes mellitus, and black race.[6]

**What are the symptoms of acute kidney injury?**

Symptoms are often absent in patients with AKI but, depending on the underlying cause may include decreased urine output, peripheral edema, gross hematuria, dyspnea, and symptoms of uremia if present (eg, nausea).

**What are the physical findings of acute kidney injury?**

Patients with AKI often do not have specific physical findings but, depending on the underlying cause, there may be hypertension, peripheral edema, elevated jugular venous pressure (JVP), inspiratory rales, cutaneous findings associated with specific diagnoses (eg, palpable purpura in patients with small vessel vasculitis), and findings of uremia if present (eg, pericardial friction rub in patients with uremic pericarditis).

**What are the sequelae of severe acute kidney injury?**

Sequelae of severe AKI include electrolyte derangements (eg, hyperkalemia), hypervolemia, metabolic acidosis, and uremia.

**When should renal replacement therapy be considered for patients with acute kidney injury?**

Renal replacement therapy should be considered in patients with anuria (negligible urine output for 6 hours), severe oliguria (urine output <200 mL over 12 hours), severe hyperkalemia (potassium >6.5 mEq/L), severe metabolic acidosis (pH <7.2 with normal or low $Paco_2$), hypervolemia (particularly if pulmonary edema is present), severe azotemia, or clinical sequelae of uremia (eg, pericarditis).[1]

**What is the natural history of acute kidney injury?**

In some patients, AKI leads to new chronic kidney disease (CKD); those with preexisting CKD are at risk for disease progression after an episode of AKI, including the development of end-stage renal disease (ESRD). Renal recovery occurs in many patients with AKI. However, even when renal function initially recovers, patients who experience AKI are at increased risk for later development of CKD.[6]

**What is the definition of chronic kidney disease?**

CKD is defined as the presence of kidney damage (eg, albuminuria) or decreased kidney function (ie, GFR <60 mL/min/1.73 m$^2$) for ≥3 months.[7]

**Which causes of acute kidney injury can lead to chronic kidney disease?**

AKI from any cause can progress to CKD. However, there is a higher rate of progression in patients with acute tubular necrosis (ATN) compared with those without ATN.[6]

**What are the 3 anatomic categories of acute kidney injury?**

AKI can be caused by prerenal, intrarenal (ie, intrinsic), or postrenal processes.

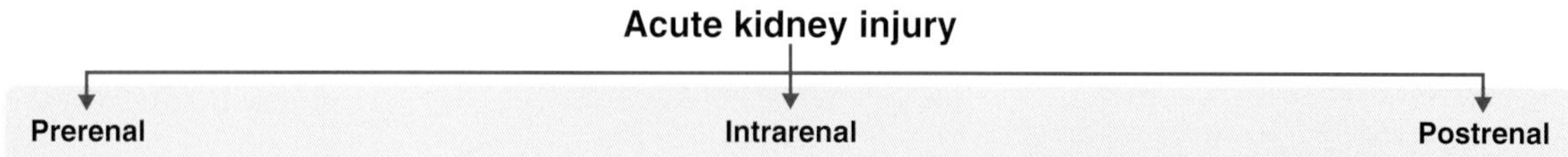


**What structures differentiate the 3 anatomic categories of acute kidney injury?**

Prerenal causes of AKI affect structures up to and including the afferent arteriole (without injuring the renal parenchyma). Intrarenal causes of AKI affect the renal parenchyma (including glomeruli, interstitium, renal tubules, and blood vessels), even if the inciting cause involves a prerenal structure (eg, cardiogenic shock causing ATN). Postrenal causes of AKI include any process that obstructs the flow of urine from the kidneys to the urethra (Figure 33-3).

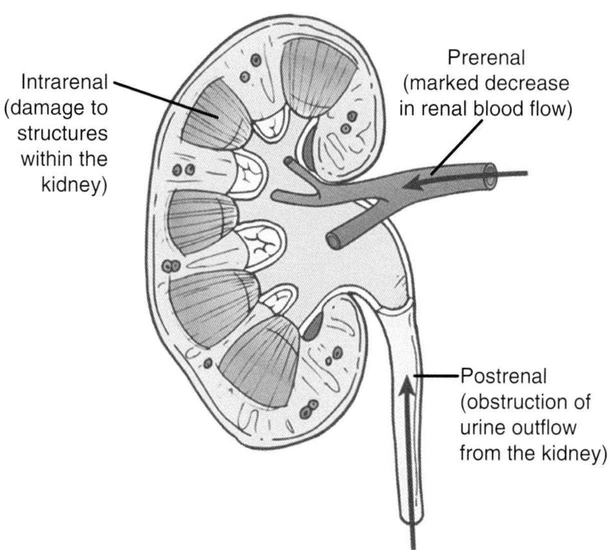


**Figure 33-3.** Acute kidney injury can be related to prerenal, intrarenal, or postrenal processes. (Adapted from Porth CM. *Essentials of Pathophysiology*. 3rd ed. Philadelphia, PA: Lippincott Williams & Wilkins; 2010.)

## PRERENAL ACUTE KIDNEY INJURY

**What is the general mechanism of prerenal acute kidney injury?**

Prerenal AKI generally occurs as a result of decreased renal blood flow.

**What biochemical laboratory data can be suggestive of prerenal acute kidney injury?**

A serum BUN:creatinine ratio >20:1 can occur when there is increased urea reabsorption in the proximal tubule triggered by low effective arterial blood volume. A $FE_{Na}$ of <1% in patients with oliguria is also suggestive of a prerenal etiology. However, $FE_{Na}$ can be influenced by diuretic medications. In patients with recent or active diuretic exposure, the fractional excretion of urea can be used instead (a value <35% is consistent with prerenal AKI).[8–10]

**What are the characteristics of urine sediment in the setting of prerenal acute kidney injury?**

The urine sediment of prerenal AKI is typically bland, but hyaline casts may be present (Figure 33-4).[11]

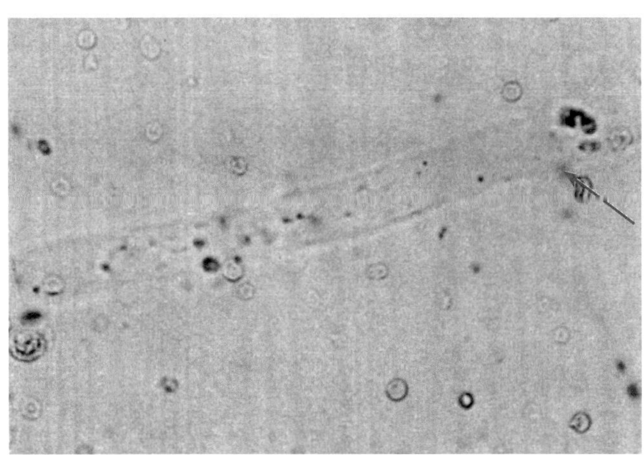

**Figure 33-4.** Hyaline cast (arrow) surrounded by red blood cells. Note the low refractive index of the cast (400×). (From Mundt LA, Shanahan K. *Graff's Textbook of Urinalysis and Body Fluids*. 3rd ed. Philadelphia, PA: Wolters Kluwer; 2016.)

## What are the causes of prerenal acute kidney injury?

**A patient with a recent diagnosis of heart failure is started on dietary restrictions and diuretic therapy and subsequently presents with weight loss of 10 pounds, low JVP, and AKI.**

Hypovolemia.

**A previously healthy 56-year-old woman with a recent back strain develops prerenal AKI after taking escalating doses of over-the-counter analgesic medication.**

Nonsteroidal anti-inflammatory drugs (NSAIDs).

**An increase in total body volume with decreased effective arterial blood volume and an S3 gallop (see Figure 4-3).**

Cardiorenal syndrome.

**A condition characterized by impaired systemic vascular resistance and reduced renal perfusion.**

Distributive shock (eg, sepsis).

**A 63-year-old man with small cell lung cancer develops abdominal pain, confusion, and prerenal AKI.**

Hypercalcemia.

**A decrease in effective arterial blood volume as a result of splanchnic vasodilation.**

Hepatorenal syndrome (HRS).

**A 42-year-old woman with marked hypertension and a bruit over the abdomen.**

Renal artery stenosis (RAS).

**Reduced renal blood flow as a result of compression of the renal veins.**

Abdominal compartment syndrome.

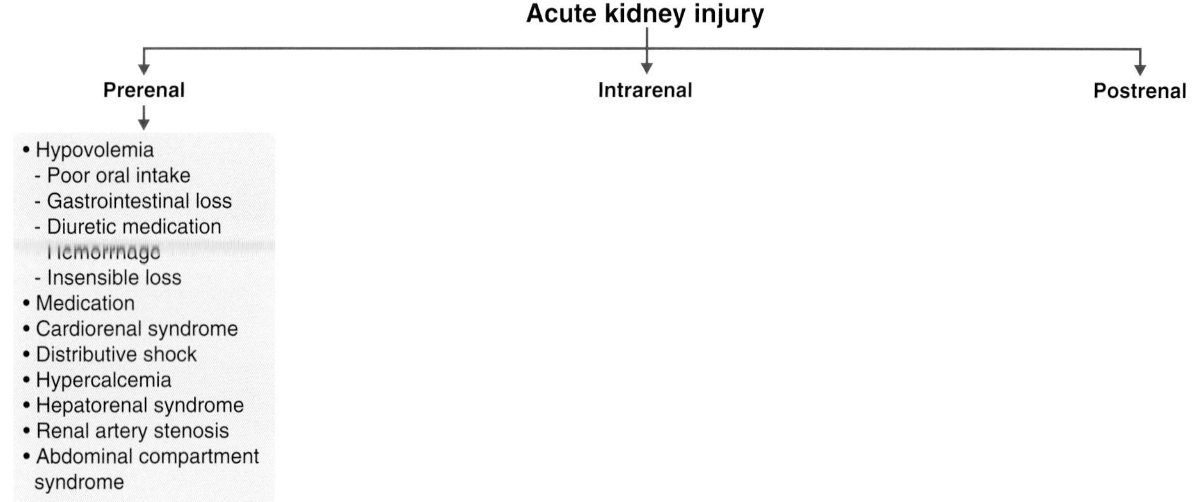


**Which of the following patterns of jugular venous pressure (JVP), cardiac output (CO), and systemic vascular resistance (SVR) are characteristic of hypovolemia, sepsis, and cardiorenal syndrome?**

| | JVP | CO | SVR |
|---|---|---|---|
| A | ↑ | ↓ | ↑ |
| B | ↓ | ↑ | ↓ |
| C | ↓ | ↓ | ↑ |

Hypovolemia is associated with pattern C (low JVP, low CO, and high SVR); sepsis is associated with pattern B (low JVP, high CO, and low SVR); and cardiorenal syndrome is associated with pattern A (high JVP, low CO, and high SVR). Common causes of hypovolemia include poor oral intake, GI loss (eg, diarrhea, vomiting), diuretic use, hemorrhage, and insensible losses.

**What are the mechanisms of prerenal acute kidney injury related to nonsteroidal anti-inflammatory drugs, angiotensin-converting enzyme inhibitors/angiotensin receptor blockers, and calcineurin inhibitors?**

NSAIDs, ACE-I/ARBs, and CIs cause AKI as a result of reduced glomerular filtration pressure via various effects on the afferent and efferent arterioles. NSAIDs impair afferent arteriolar dilation; ACE-I/ARBs impair efferent arteriolar vasoconstriction; and CIs increase afferent arteriolar vasoconstriction.[12]

**What is the mechanism of prerenal acute kidney injury related to hypercalcemia?**

Hypercalcemia causes a reduction in glomerular filtration related to afferent arteriolar constriction. It also causes renal salt wasting, leading to hypovolemia.[4]

**What are the clinical differences between the 2 subtypes of hepatorenal syndrome?**

Type 1 HRS is rapid in onset with a doubling of serum creatinine to a level above 2.5 mg/dL in less than 2 weeks and is commonly associated with multiorgan failure. Type 2 HRS is characterized by a more indolent, stable course and is commonly associated with refractory ascites. Oliguria is more likely to occur in the setting of type 1 HRS.[13]

**What is the mechanism of acute kidney injury in the setting of renal artery stenosis?**

RAS is a chronic process and does not, in and of itself, cause AKI. However, the presence of RAS increases the risk of renal hypoperfusion, leading to AKI. For example, the development of AKI after the initiation of an ACE-I/ARB can be a clue to the diagnosis of RAS.

**At what point does increased abdominal pressure result in oliguria and anuria?**

Oliguria and anuria develop when intra-abdominal pressures reach approximately 15 mm Hg (20 cm $H_2O$) and 30 mm Hg (41 cm $H_2O$), respectively.[14]

## INTRARENAL ACUTE KIDNEY INJURY

**What are the general subcategories of intrarenal acute kidney injury?**

Intrarenal AKI can be caused by vascular disease, glomerulonephritis (GN), ATN, or acute interstitial nephritis (AIN) (Figure 33-5).

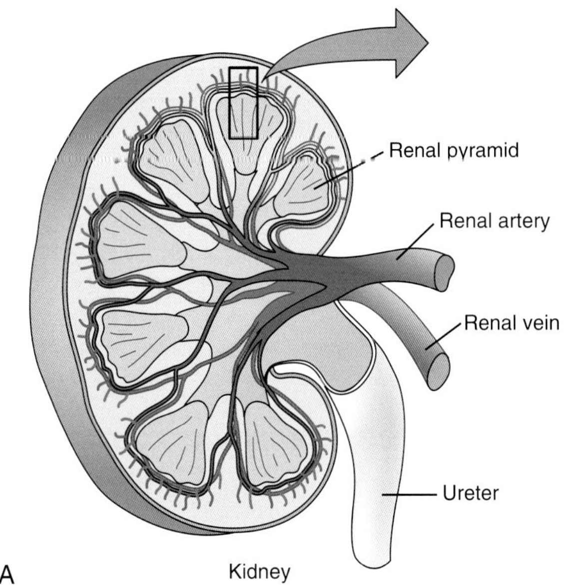


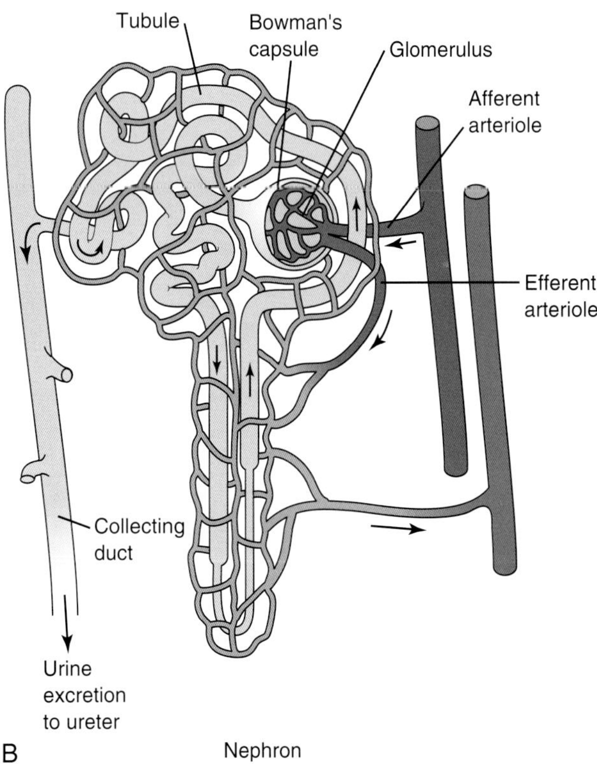


**Figure 33-5.** Cross-section of the kidney (A) and the nephron (B), illustrating the potential structures involved in intrarenal AKI. (From Carter PJ. *Lippincott's Textbook for Nursing Assistants: A Humanistic Approach to Caregiving*. 3rd ed. Philadelphia, PA: Wolters Kluwer Health; 2012.)

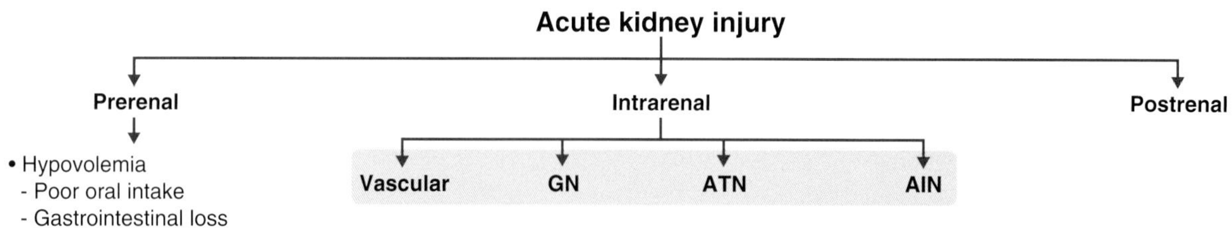


- Hypovolemia
  - Poor oral intake
  - Gastrointestinal loss
  - Diuretic medication
  - Hemorrhage
  - Insensible loss
- Medication
- Cardiorenal syndrome
- Distributive shock
- Hypercalcemia
- Hepatorenal syndrome
- Renal artery stenosis
- Abdominal compartment syndrome

## VASCULAR CAUSES OF INTRARENAL ACUTE KIDNEY INJURY

**What are the names of the arteries between the renal artery and the afferent arteriole?**

Renal artery → segmental artery → interlobar artery → arcuate artery → cortical radiate artery → afferent arteriole.

*Unlike the vascular causes of prerenal AKI that cause low renal blood flow (eg, afferent arteriole constriction), the vascular causes of intrarenal AKI cause renal parenchymal disease.*

### What are the vascular causes of intrarenal acute kidney injury?

**Sudden flank pain and AKI in a patient with atrial fibrillation.**

Renal artery embolism.

**Sudden flank pain and AKI in a patient with atherosclerotic RAS.**

Renal artery thrombosis.

**Inflammation involving the walls of the renal artery.**

Large and medium vessel vasculitis.

**This condition usually follows arterial instrumentation.**

Atheroembolic renal disease.

**Thrombocytopenia, hemolytic anemia, and AKI.**

Thrombotic microangiopathy (TMA).

**A 52-year-old woman with sinus disease, hemoptysis, AKI, and dysmorphic red blood cells (see Figure 34-4) and red blood cell casts on evaluation of urine sediment.**

Small vessel vasculitis related to granulomatosis with polyangiitis (GPA, or Wegener's granulomatosis).

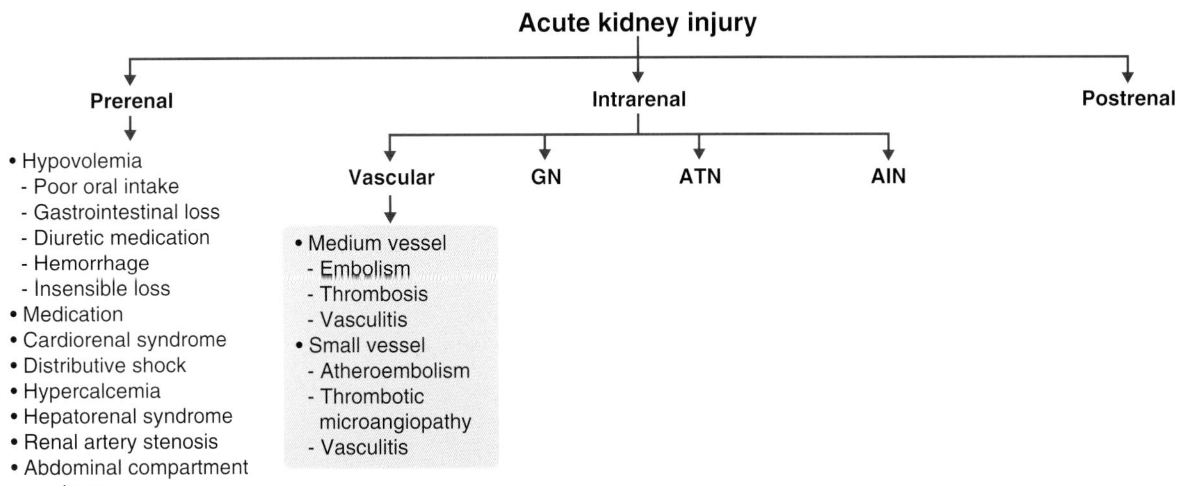


**What are the risk factors for renal artery embolism?**

Risk factors for renal artery embolism include atrial fibrillation, ischemic heart disease, cardiomyopathy, and valvular disease (eg, infective endocarditis).[15]

**What is the most common presenting symptom in patients with renal artery thrombosis?**

Severe flank pain is the most common presenting symptom of renal artery thrombosis. Onset is most often sudden, but can be gradual in some cases, with maximum intensity reached after a few hours. The pain is constant and may radiate to the lower quadrant or chest. Associated gastrointestinal symptoms such as nausea and vomiting are common. AKI develops when the other kidney is diseased at baseline and cannot compensate for the abrupt increase in excretory load.[16]

**Which types of vasculitis can involve the renal artery?**

The renal arteries can be affected by large vessel vasculitis (eg, giant cell arteritis, Takayasu arteritis) and medium vessel vasculitis (eg, polyarteritis nodosa, Kawasaki disease).[17]

**What are the laboratory features of atheroembolic renal disease?**

Atheroembolic renal disease can present with peripheral and urinary eosinophilia and serum hypocomplementemia. Other laboratory abnormalities can indicate additional organ involvement (eg, hepatocellular liver injury suggests hepatic involvement).[18]

**Which causes of thrombotic microangiopathy can present with acute kidney injury?**

In addition to the primary TMA syndromes (eg, thrombotic thrombocytopenic purpura, hemolytic uremic syndrome, drug-induced TMA), other causes of TMA that can present with microangiopathic hemolytic anemia, thrombocytopenia, and AKI include disseminated intravascular coagulation, malignant hypertension, HELLP syndrome, and scleroderma renal crisis.[19]

**Which small vessel vasculitides tend to be associated with intrarenal acute kidney injury?**

The small vessel vasculitides associated with intrarenal AKI include GPA, eosinophilic granulomatosis with polyangiitis (EGPA, or Churg-Strauss syndrome), microscopic polyangiitis, and Henoch-Schönlein purpura. These entities often cause GN.[17]

*Glomerulonephritis is discussed in depth in chapter 34, Glomerular Disease.*

## ACUTE TUBULAR NECROSIS

**What is the mechanism of acute kidney injury in patients with acute tubular necrosis?**

Tubular dysfunction occurs as a result of injury to the tubular epithelial cells, usually ischemic or toxic in nature.[20]

**How common is acute tubular necrosis in hospitalized patients?**

ATN is the most common cause of AKI in the hospital (just under one-half of all cases), and is particularly prevalent in the intensive care unit (more than one-half of all cases).[20]

**What biochemical laboratory data can be suggestive of acute tubular necrosis?**

$FE_{Na}$ >1% to 2% in patients with oliguric AKI is suggestive of ATN. $FE_{Na}$ can be influenced by diuretic medications. In patients with recent or active diuretic exposure, the fractional excretion of urea can be used instead (a value >35%-50% is consistent with ATN).[8,10]

**What are the characteristics of urine sediment in the setting of acute tubular necrosis?**

Examination of urine sediment in the setting of ATN typically reveals the presence of "muddy brown" granular casts (Figure 33-6). ATN is highly likely when at least 6 granular casts are seen.[11]

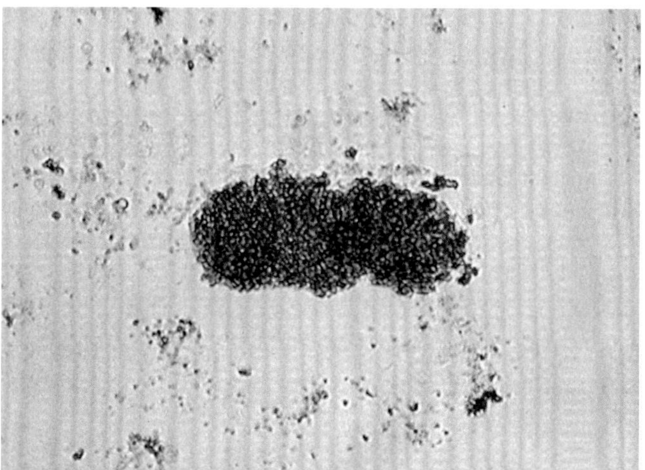

**Figure 33-6.** "Muddy brown" cast (a type of granular cast). (From Mundt LA, Shanahan K. *Graff's Textbook of Urinalysis and Body Fluids*. 3rd ed. Philadelphia, PA: Wolters Kluwer; 2016.)

## What are the causes of acute tubular necrosis?

**A 52-year-old man presents with crushing chest pain, hypotension, elevated JVP, and AKI with muddy brown casts on evaluation of urine sediment.**

Prerenal spectrum resulting in renal ischemia (from cardiogenic shock).

**A 23-year-old immunocompromised man develops ATN after starting treatment for cryptococcal meningitis.**

Amphotericin B.

**A 64-year-old man is hospitalized with diverticulitis and develops AKI 2 days after abdominal cross-sectional imaging is obtained.**

Contrast-induced nephropathy.

**AKI develops after a crush injury.**

Pigment nephropathy.

**Anemia, elevated protein gap, low anion gap, and AKI.**

Protein injury from multiple myeloma.

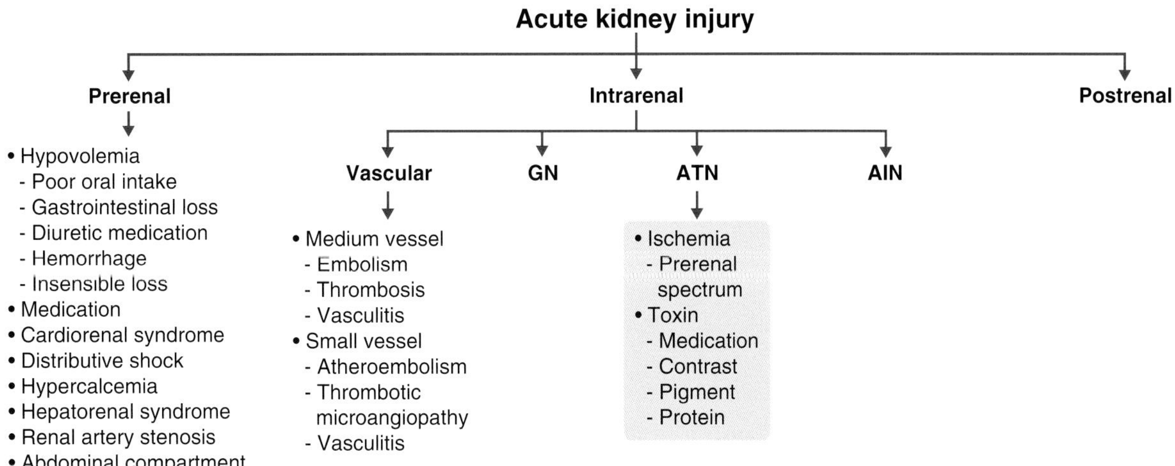


**What laboratory studies can be helpful in recognizing when prerenal acute kidney injury has evolved into acute tubular necrosis?**

In cases of ATN secondary to prerenal AKI, $FE_{Na}$ can be <1%, making this test less useful. The absence or presence of granular casts on evaluation of urine sediment can be helpful. The absence of granular casts is associated with likelihood ratios of 4.5 for prerenal AKI and 0.2 for ATN. The presence of at least 6 granular casts is associated with a likelihood ratio of 10 for ATN and 0.10 for prerenal AKI. A fluid challenge can also be helpful: Renal function recovery after volume repletion is consistent with prerenal AKI but not ATN.[11]

**What is the timing and prognosis of contrast-induced nephropathy?**

Contrast-induced nephropathy typically develops 24 to 48 hours after contrast exposure. Renal recovery occurs in most cases, with function returning to baseline in 7 to 10 days.[21]

**What medications are associated with acute tubular necrosis?**

Medications associated with ATN include NSAIDs, aminoglycosides, vancomycin, polymyxins, pentamidine, amphotericin B, foscarnet, tenofovir, cisplatin, and methotrexate.[21]

**In the setting of pigment nephropathy, what combination of findings on urine dipstick and urine microscopic analysis is classically seen?**

In the setting of pigment nephropathy, urine dipstick will be positive for blood in the absence of red blood cells on microscopic evaluation. The positive dipstick result is caused by the presence of pigment (myoglobin or hemoglobin). This combination of findings can be an important clue to the diagnosis.

**Why are pigment- and contrast-induced nephropathies sometimes associated with $FE_{Na}$ <1%?**

In addition to causing toxicity to the renal tubules, pigment and contrast can induce constriction of the afferent arteriole, resulting in prerenal physiology.[4]

**What has been shown to improve renal recovery in patients with light chain cast nephropathy?**

In patents with light chain cast nephropathy, there is a linear relationship between reduction in serum free light chain concentration (eg, via plasma exchange) and renal recovery.[22]

## ACUTE INTERSTITIAL NEPHRITIS

**What is acute interstitial nephritis?**

AIN is characterized by inflammation and edema within the renal interstitium, often associated with AKI.[23]

**What is the classic clinical triad of acute interstitial nephritis?**

The classic clinical triad of AIN is fever, maculopapular rash, and peripheral eosinophilia. Although each component of the triad occurs commonly, the triad itself is present in a small percentage of patients with AIN overall (about 10%-15%). It may occur more frequently with certain etiologies of AIN (eg, methicillin-induced).[23]

**What are the characteristics of urine sediment in patients with acute interstitial nephritis?**

Examination of urine sediment in the setting of AIN reveals leukocyturia and leukocyte casts in most cases (Figure 33-7). The significance of urine eosinophils is less clear.[23]

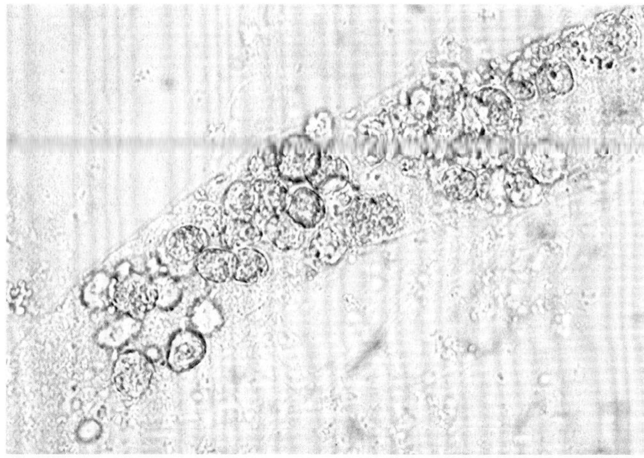

**Figure 33-7.** White blood cell cast (500×). (From Mundt LA, Shanahan K. *Graff's Textbook of Urinalysis and Body Fluids*. 3rd ed. Philadelphia, PA: Wolters Kluwer; 2016.)

**What is the treatment for acute interstitial nephritis?**

The cornerstone of treating AIN is addressing the underlying cause (in most cases, this is the removal of an offending medication). Still, renal function may not fully recover in a significant proportion of patients. Systemic glucocorticoids may be helpful in some cases.[23]

## What are the causes of acute interstitial nephritis?

**Responsible for more than 75% of the cases of AIN.**

Medication.[23]

**Responsible for approximately 15% of cases of AIN; the medications used to treat these illnesses cause AIN more frequently.**

Acute interstitial nephritis associated with infection.[23]

**A 54-year-old black man with hilar lymphadenopathy (see Figure 21-4), hypercalcemia, and AKI.**

Acute interstitial nephritis associated with sarcoidosis.

**A combination of AIN and uveitis.**

Tubulointerstitial nephritis and uveitis (TINU) syndrome.

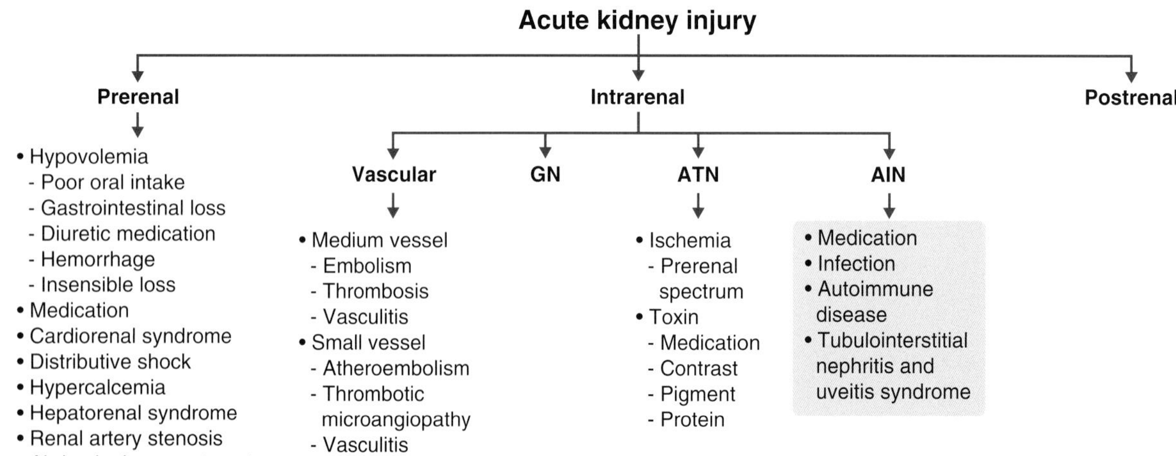

**What medications are associated with acute interstitial nephritis?**

Numerous medications can cause AIN, but the most common agents are NSAIDs and antibiotics (eg, penicillins, cephalosporins, ciprofloxacin, rifampicin, sulfonamides, vancomycin). Other common medications associated with AIN include allopurinol, acyclovir, famotidine, furosemide, omeprazole, and phenytoin.[23]

**When does acute interstitial nephritis usually develop in relation to exposure to a medication?**

The average delay between exposure to a medication and the development of AIN is 7 to 10 days, but it can occur sooner, particularly if there is repeat exposure to an offending drug.[23]

**Which bacterial and viral organisms are associated with acute interstitial nephritis?**

Bacterial organisms associated with AIN include *Brucella, Campylobacter, Escherichia coli, Legionella, Salmonella, Streptococcus, Staphylococcus,* and *Yersinia*; viral organisms include cytomegalovirus, Epstein-Barr virus, hantavirus, and human immunodeficiency virus.[23]

**What autoimmune diseases are associated with acute interstitial nephritis?**

Autoimmune diseases associated with AIN include sarcoidosis, Sjögren's syndrome, and systemic lupus erythematosus.[23]

**What demographic of patients is most commonly affected by tubulointerstitial nephritis and uveitis syndrome?**

TINU syndrome most frequently affects young women. It is characterized by the presence of uveitis, tubulointerstitial nephritis, and constitutional symptoms. Pathogenesis is unknown, but likely involves autoimmunity against elements common to the uveal tract and renal tubulointerstitium. Systemic glucocorticoids are the treatment of choice, and often reverse kidney injury.[24]

## POSTRENAL ACUTE KIDNEY INJURY

**What is the mechanism of postrenal acute kidney injury?**

Postrenal causes of AKI obstruct the flow of urine from the kidneys to the outside world. This obstruction increases pressure within the tubules, resulting in a decrease in glomerular filtration rate.

**What imaging findings are characteristic of postrenal acute kidney injury?**

Hydronephrosis and dilated renal calyces, which can be identified with renal imaging, are characteristic of postrenal AKI.

**What bedside procedure can diagnose and treat some causes of postrenal acute kidney injury?**

Obstruction of the bladder or structures distal to it can often be relieved with placement of a Foley catheter.

**What is the prognosis of postrenal acute kidney injury?**

Renal recovery in patients with postrenal AKI is dependent on the duration and severity of obstruction. In patients with acute obstruction, complete recovery is generally achieved if the obstruction is relieved within 1 week; however, there is little chance for renal recovery if the duration of obstruction exceeds 12 weeks.[25]

### What are the postrenal causes of acute kidney injury?

**A common condition found only in men.**

Benign prostatic hyperplasia (BPH).

**An asymmetric, hard, nodular prostate gland.**

Prostate cancer.

**To cause AKI in patients without preexisting kidney disease, this condition must be bilateral.**

Nephrolithiasis.

**A 28-year-old man who has been taking escalating doses of over-the-counter allergy medication presents with anuria and AKI.**

Neurogenic bladder from anticholinergic medication.

**Patients with this common endocrinopathy are at risk for the development of peripheral neuropathy, gastroparesis, and neurogenic bladder.**

Diabetes mellitus.

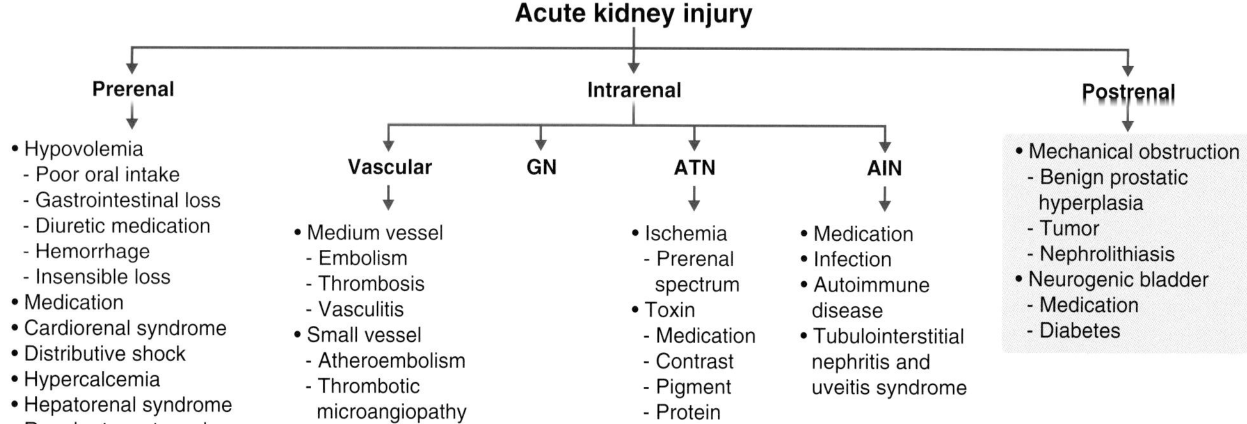


**How common is benign prostatic hyperplasia in men?**

BPH increases in prevalence with age and is found in one-quarter of men who are in the sixth decade of life, one-third of those in the seventh decade of life, and one-half of all men older than 80 years of age.[26]

**What malignancies are associated with renal obstruction?**

Malignancies associated with renal obstruction include prostate cancer, bladder cancer, renal cell carcinoma, transitional cell carcinoma of the collecting system, multiple myeloma, and metastases. Abdominal and pelvic imaging is critical in making the diagnosis.

**Which imaging techniques are most useful in the evaluation of nephrolithiasis?**

Ultrasonography and computed tomography imaging without contrast are the tests of choice in the evaluation of nephrolithiasis. Ultrasonography has the advantage of avoiding radiation exposure when used as the initial imaging technique. Despite the higher sensitivity of computed tomography imaging, there is no evidence that it improves outcomes when used as the initial imaging technique.[27]

**What other causes of mechanical obstruction can lead to postrenal acute kidney injury?**

Other causes of mechanical obstruction include urethral stricture, blood clot (particularly in patients who have recently undergone urinary tract instrumentation), crystal-induced intratubular obstruction (eg, acyclovir, methotrexate, protease inhibitors, ethylene glycol), and retroperitoneal fibrosis.[28]

**What classes of medications are associated with neurogenic bladder?**

Medications associated with neurogenic bladder include anticholinergics, narcotics, sedative hypnotics, antipsychotics, antidepressants, antispasmodics, and calcium channel blockers.[29]

**What is the treatment for bladder dysfunction associated with diabetes mellitus?**

Diabetes mellitus is associated with various types of bladder dysfunction, ranging from detrusor overactivity to poor emptying and bladder outlet obstruction. Treatment options for patients with urinary retention include behavioral modification (eg, voiding at regular intervals), pharmacologic therapy (eg, cholinergic agents), and catheterization to empty the bladder.[30]

**What other causes of neurogenic bladder can lead to postrenal acute kidney injury?**

Other causes of neurogenic bladder include stroke, multiple sclerosis, spinal cord injury, Parkinson's disease, and congenital disorders (eg, spina bifida, cerebral palsy).[29]

## Case Summary

A 73-year-old man with a history of vascular disease presents 10 days after femoropopliteal bypass surgery with new skin changes and is found to have AKI with peripheral and urinary eosinophilia.

***What is the most likely cause of acute kidney injury in this patient?***

Atheroembolic renal disease.

### BONUS QUESTIONS

***What is atheroembolic renal disease?***

Atheroembolic renal disease occurs when atheromatous plaques of the large arteries (eg, aorta) are disrupted and embolize to the small renal arteries and arterioles, causing acute occlusion and ischemia. AKI typically develops in a stepwise fashion in the weeks after plaque disruption.[18]

***What are the epidemiologic risk factors associated with atheroembolic renal disease?***

Risk factors for atheroembolic renal disease include older age (>60 years), male sex, hypertension, diabetes mellitus, vascular disease, cigarette smoking, and white race.[18]

***Which historical clues in this case are suggestive of atheroembolic renal disease?***

The history of vascular disease and recent intravascular procedure in this case are clues to the diagnosis of atheroembolic renal disease.

***Which clinical features in this case are suggestive of atheroembolic renal disease?***

The skin findings (livedo reticularis and blue-colored toes [see Figures 33-1 and 33-2]), as well as the peripheral and urinary eosinophilia in this case are consistent with atheroembolic renal disease.

***What is the utility of the $FE_{Na}$ in this case?***

The $FE_{Na}$ of >1% in this case argues against a prerenal cause of AKI.

***What is the utility of the renal ultrasound in this case?***

The renal ultrasound in this case does not show hydronephrosis or dilated renal calyces, arguing against postrenal AKI.

***Atheroembolism is most commonly precipitated by what procedure?***

Atheroembolism is most commonly associated with coronary angiography.[18]

***What is the treatment and prognosis of atheroembolic renal disease?***

There is no definitive treatment for atheroembolic renal disease other than treatment for underlying risk factors. Prognosis is generally poor: Up to one-half of patients develop dialysis-dependent kidney disease, and mortality is significant at 1 year.[18]

## KEY POINTS

- AKI is the rapid development (within hours to days) of renal excretory dysfunction, characterized by the accumulation of the products of nitrogen metabolism (urea and creatinine), decreased urine output, or both.
- AKI can be caused by prerenal, intrarenal, or postrenal processes.
- Prerenal AKI is caused by decreased renal perfusion without injury to the renal parenchyma.
- Intrarenal AKI is caused by injury to the renal parenchyma, even if the inciting cause involves a prerenal structure.
- Postrenal AKI is caused by obstruction of urine flow anywhere from the kidneys to the urethra.
- Prerenal AKI is associated with elevated serum BUN:creatinine ratio (>20:1) and $FE_{Na}$ of <1%.
- Intrarenal AKI can be caused by vascular disease, GN, ATN, or AIN.
- Vascular causes of intrarenal AKI affect the medium- and small-sized arteries.
- GN is associated with dysmorphic red blood cells and red blood cell casts on evaluation of urine sediment.
- ATN is associated with $FE_{Na}$ >1% to 2% and the presence of granular casts on evaluation of urine sediment.
- AIN is associated with fever, rash, and peripheral and urinary eosinophilia.
- Postrenal AKI is associated with hydronephrosis and dilated renal calyces on imaging.

## REFERENCES


1. Bellomo R, Kellum JA, Ronco C. Acute kidney injury. *Lancet*. 2012;380(9843):756-766.
2. Walker HK, Hall WD, Hurst JW, eds. *Clinical Methods: The History, Physical, and Laboratory Examinations*. 3rd ed. Boston: Butterworths; 1990.
3. KDIGO AKI Work Group. KDIGO clinical practice guidelines for acute kidney injury. *Kidney Int Suppl*. 2012;17:1-138.
4. Abuelo JG, ed. *Renal Failure Diagnosis & Treatment*. Dordrecht, The Netherlands: Kluwer Academic Publishers; 1995.
5. Mosenifar Z, Hoo GWS, eds. *Practical Pulmonary and Critical Care Medicine Disease Management*. New York, NY: Taylor & Francis Group; 2006.
6. Chawla LS, Eggers PW, Star RA, Kimmel PL. Acute kidney injury and chronic kidney disease as interconnected syndromes. *N Engl J Med*. 2014;371(1):58-66.
7. KDIGO. Chapter 1: Definition and classification of CKD. *Kidney Int Suppl*. 2013;3:19.
8. Carvounis CP, Nisar S, Guro-Razuman S. Significance of the fractional excretion of urea in the differential diagnosis of acute renal failure. *Kidney Int*. 2002;62(6):2223-2229.
9. Dossetor JB. Creatininemia versus uremia. The relative significance of blood urea nitrogen and serum creatinine concentrations in azotemia. *Ann Intern Med*. 1966;65(6):1287-1299.
10. Steiner RW. Interpreting the fractional excretion of sodium. *Am J Med*. 1984;77(4):699-702.
11. Perazella MA, Parikh CR. How can urine microscopy influence the differential diagnosis of AKI? *Clin J Am Soc Nephrol*. 2009;4(4):691-693.
12. Macedo E, Mehta RL. Prerenal failure: from old concepts to new paradigms. *Curr Opin Crit Care*. 2009;15(6):467-473.
13. Gines P, Schrier RW. Renal failure in cirrhosis. *N Engl J Med*. 2009;361(13):1279-1290.
14. Richards WO, Scovill W, Shin B, Reed W. Acute renal failure associated with increased intra-abdominal pressure. *Ann Surg*. 1983;197(2):183-187.
15. Kansal S, Feldman M, Cooksey S, Patel S. Renal artery embolism: a case report and review. *J Gen Intern Med*. 2008;23(5):644-647.
16. Goodyear WE, Beard DE. Diagnosis and management of renal-artery thrombosis report of a case. *N Engl J Med*. 1947;237(10):355-358.
17. Jennette JC, Falk RJ. The pathology of vasculitis involving the kidney. *Am J Kidney Dis*. 1994;24(1):130-141.
18. Scolari F, Ravani P. Atheroembolic renal disease. *Lancet*. 2010;375(9726):1650-1660.
19. George JN, Nester CM. Syndromes of thrombotic microangiopathy. *N Engl J Med*. 2014;371(7):654-66.
20. Gill N, Nally JV Jr, Fatica RA. Renal failure secondary to acute tubular necrosis: epidemiology, diagnosis, and management. *Chest*. 2005;128(4):2847-2863.
21. Pazhayattil GS, Shirali AC. Drug-induced impairment of renal function. *Int J Nephrol Renovasc Dis*. 2014;7:457-468.
22. Hutchison CA, Cockwell P, Stringer S, et al. Early reduction of serum-free light chains associates with renal recovery in myeloma kidney. *J Am Soc Nephrol*. 2011;22(6):1129-1136.
23. Praga M, Gonzalez E. Acute interstitial nephritis. *Kidney Int*. 2010;77(11):956-961.
24. Sessa A, Meroni M, Battini G, Vigano G, Brambilla PL, Paties CT. Acute renal failure due to idiopathic tubulo-intestinal nephritis and uveitis: "TINU syndrome". Case report and review of the literature. *J Nephrol*. 2000;13(5):377-380.
25. Better OS, Arieff AI, Massry SG, Kleeman CR, Maxwell MH. Studies on renal function after relief of complete unilateral ureteral obstruction of three months' duration in man. *Am J Med*. 1973;54(2):234-240.
26. McVary KT. BPH: epidemiology and comorbidities. *Am J Manag Care*. 2006;12(5 suppl):S122-S128.
27. Smith-Bindman R, Aubin C, Bailitz J, et al. Ultrasonography versus computed tomography for suspected nephrolithiasis. *N Engl J Med*. 2014;371(12):1100-1110.
28. Yarlagadda SG, Perazella MA. Drug-induced crystal nephropathy: an update. *Expert Opin Drug Saf*. 2008;7(2):147-158.
29. Dorsher PT, McIntosh PM. Neurogenic bladder. *Adv Urol*. 2012;2012:816274.
30. Liu G, Daneshgari F. Diabetic bladder dysfunction. *Chin Med J (Engl)*. 2014;127(7):1357-1364.

Chapter 34

# GLOMERULAR DISEASE

## Case: A 78-year-old man with hematuria

A previously healthy 78-year-old man is admitted to the hospital with hematuria, skin rash, and abdominal pain. The patient reports recovering from an illness 1 to 2 weeks ago that was characterized by cough, sore throat, and runny nose. Several days later he developed abdominal pain. This was followed by the onset of a skin rash involving his legs. After a few days, his urine turned reddish in color. The cough has resolved, and he does not complain of dyspnea.

Blood pressure is 184/93 mm Hg. There is a palpable skin rash on the lower extremities (Figure 34-1).

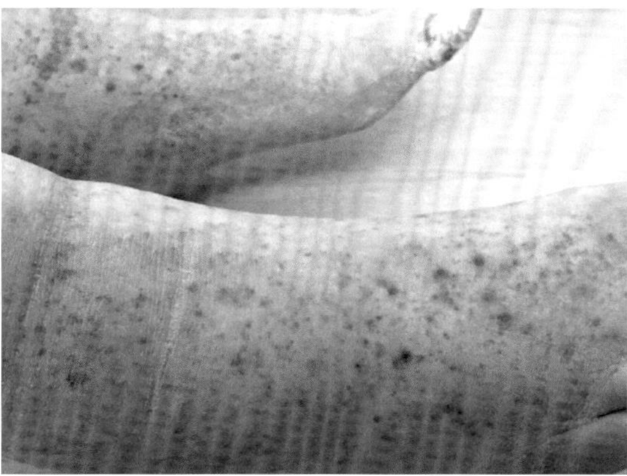

**Figure 34-1.** (Courtesy of Shahana F. Baig-Lewis, MD.)

Peripheral white blood cell count is normal with normal differential. Serum creatinine is 2.9 mg/dL. Urine microscopy identifies 120 red blood cells/hpf. Serum antineutrophil cytoplasmic antibodies (ANCA) and anti–glomerular basement membrane (anti-GBM) antibodies are not identified. Serum complement levels are within normal limits. Urine sediment findings are shown in Figure 34-2A and B.

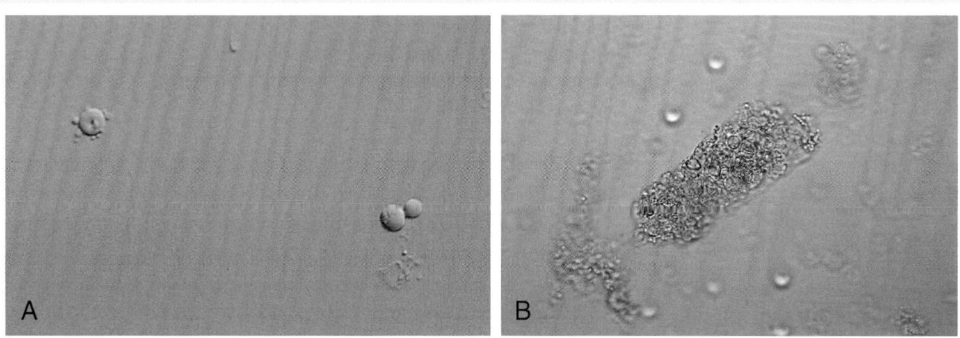


**Figure 34-2.** (From McClatchey KD. *Clinical Laboratory Medicine*. 2nd ed. Philadelphia, PA: Lippincott Williams & Wilkins; 2002.)

***What is the most likely diagnosis in this patient?***

**What is glomerular disease?**

Glomerular disease describes a heterogeneous group of conditions that damage various glomerular structures and produce characteristic clinical, physiologic, biochemical, and histologic manifestations.

**What is the glomerulus?**

The glomerulus is a cluster of capillaries and associated mesangium at the proximal end of the nephron in the kidney. Bowman's capsule surrounds the glomerulus, and together they form the renal corpuscle, the basic filtration unit of the kidney (Figure 34-3).[1]

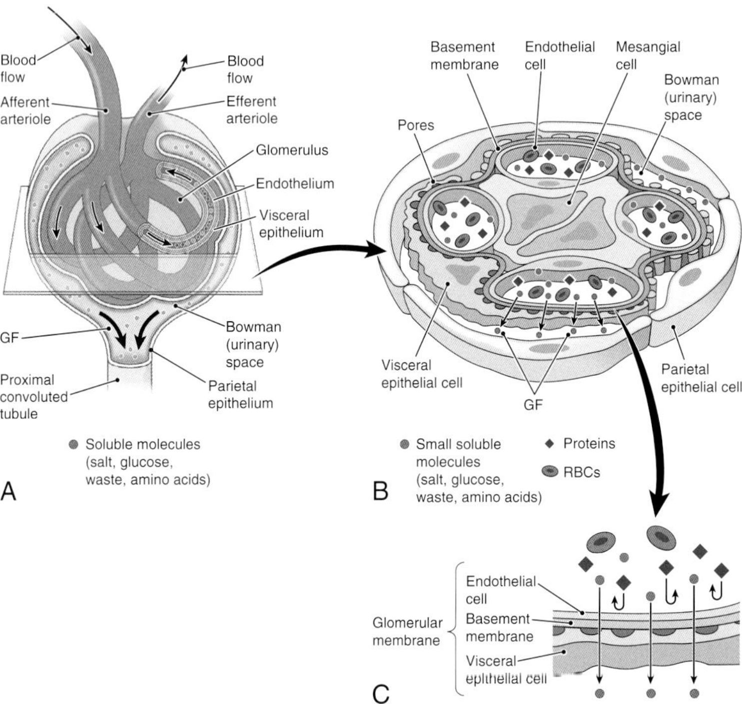


**Figure 34-3.** Anatomy of the glomerulus. A, The relationship of the glomerulus to Bowman's (urinary) space. B, The cellular anatomy of the glomerulus (cross-section). Note the relationships among capillary endothelial cells, basement membrane, and visceral epithelial cells. C, The glomerular membrane is composed of capillary endothelium, basement membrane, and visceral epithelial cells. Small soluble molecules cross the glomerular membrane from blood into Bowman's (urinary) space as glomerular filtrate (GF). In healthy patients, red blood cells and proteins are too large to cross. (McConnell TH. *Nature of Disease: Pathology for the Health Professions*. 2nd ed. Philadelphia, PA: Wolters Kluwer Health; 2013.)

**What are the effects of glomerular injury on the content of urine?**

Glomerular injury results in impaired filtration. Consequently, constituents of blood that are normally excluded from the urinary space (eg, red blood cells [RBCs], white blood cells [WBCs], proteins) pass through the damaged glomerulus and are excreted in urine.[2]

**What are the 2 general clinical syndromes of glomerular disease?**

Glomerular disease generally presents with either nephrotic syndrome or nephritic syndrome. *Some diseases result in both nephrotic and nephritic syndromes, but most are associated with one or the other.*

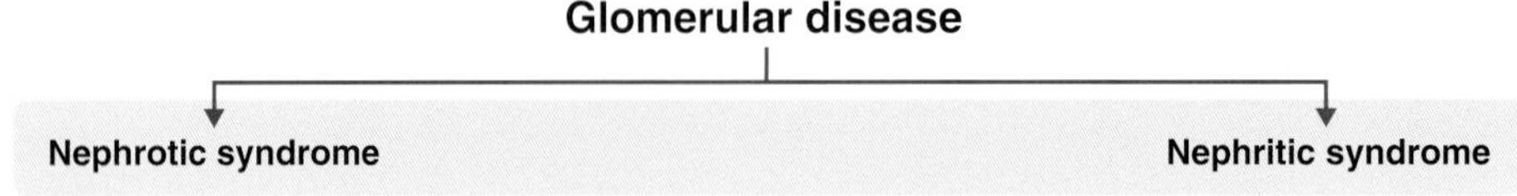


**What are the characteristic urinary findings of nephrotic syndrome?**

Nephrotic syndrome is characterized by proteinuria of at least 3.5 g/d. A minority of patients may also experience microscopic hematuria, but the urine sediment is typically bland. Glomerular diseases that manifest purely as nephrotic syndrome are noninflammatory in nature.[3,4]

**What are the characteristic urinary findings of nephritic syndrome?**

Nephritic syndrome is characterized by active urine sediment consisting of dysmorphic RBCs, RBC casts, and occasionally WBCs and WBC casts. There can be varying degrees of proteinuria that are typically mild to moderate. Glomerular diseases that manifest as nephritic syndrome are inflammatory in nature.[1]

**What name is given to the group of inflammatory glomerular diseases that result in nephritic syndrome?**

Glomerulonephritis (GN) refers to a group of inflammatory glomerular diseases that result in nephritic syndrome.

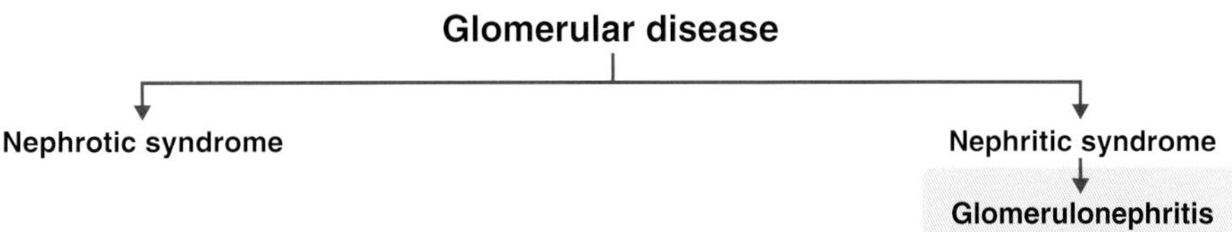


**What is the role of renal biopsy in patients with nephrotic syndrome or glomerulonephritis?**

Renal biopsy includes routine examination of tissue under light, immunofluorescence, and electron microscopy; the patterns of glomerular injury identified by these techniques can often establish a diagnosis. The degree of severity and extent of active versus chronic (irreversible) changes can direct treatment and provide important prognostic information.[2]

## NEPHROTIC SYNDROME

**What is the pathophysiology of nephrotic syndrome?**

Nephrotic syndrome occurs when there is impairment of glomerular charge and size selectivity, which are normally maintained by a combination of the glomerular basement membrane, endothelial cells, and epithelial cells (podocytes) (see Figure 34-3). The resultant increase in glomerular permeability allows large molecules such as albumin to escape into the urine.[4]

**What are the symptoms of nephrotic syndrome?**

Symptoms of nephrotic syndrome may include peripheral edema (often anasarca), fatigue, dyspnea, and foamy urine.

**What are the physical findings of nephrotic syndrome?**

Physical findings of nephrotic syndrome may include hypertension, generalized dependent pitting peripheral edema, ascites, and pleural effusions. Less common findings include abnormalities of the nail (eg, Muehrcke's lines), eruptive xanthomata, and xanthelasma.

**What are the general laboratory features of nephrotic syndrome?**

Nephrotic syndrome is characterized by proteinuria >3.5 g/d, serum albumin <2.5 g/dL, and hyperlipidemia (total cholesterol usually >180 mg/dL). Serum creatinine concentration can be variable in nephrotic syndrome.[3]

**Which validated laboratory calculation can effectively determine the degree of daily proteinuria with a single urine measurement?**

The measurement of protein and creatinine concentrations from a single, untimed (spot) sample of urine can estimate daily proteinuria. The spot protein:creatinine ratio correlates with the protein content of a 24-hour urine collection (in grams per day).[5]

**Why is nephrotic syndrome associated with thromboembolism?**

The mechanism of thrombophilia in nephrotic syndrome is incompletely understood but, in general, is related to an imbalance between prothrombotic and antithrombotic factors. This imbalance occurs as a result of the loss of anticoagulant proteins in the urine, including antithrombin and proteins C and S, and increased production of procoagulant proteins such as fibrinogen. The most common sites of thrombosis in nephrotic syndrome are the renal veins and the veins of the lower extremities.[3]

**Why is nephrotic syndrome associated with infection?**

Patients with nephrotic syndrome develop infections (eg, cellulitis) more frequently than the normal population. Mechanisms include low serum immunoglobulin G (IgG) concentration, reduced complement activity, and diminished T-cell function.[3]

**What pharmacologic agents are available to treat the proteinuria associated with nephrotic syndrome?**

Angiotensin-converting enzyme inhibitors (ACE-I) or angiotensin receptor blockers (ARBs) are effective in decreasing proteinuria in patients with nephrotic syndrome and may slow disease progression.[3]

**What are the 2 general subcategories of nephrotic syndrome?**

Nephrotic syndrome can be primary or secondary.

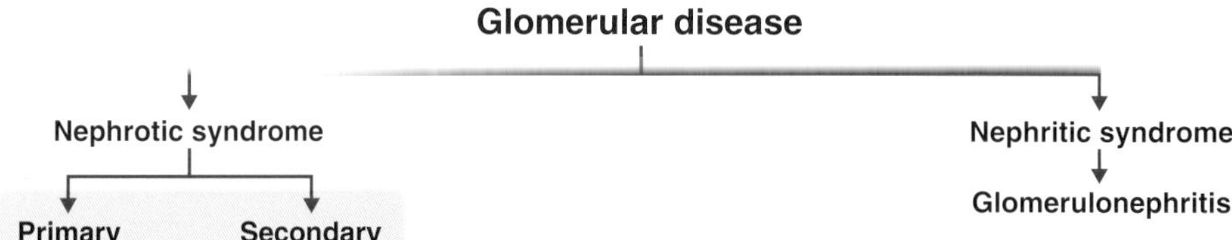


**What are the differences between primary and secondary causes of nephrotic syndrome?**

Primary glomerulonephropathies present with characteristic clinicopathologic patterns but are not related to known or identifiable systemic diseases or exposures (ie, they are idiopathic). Secondary glomerulonephropathies, which are associated with systemic diseases or exposures, tend to present with the clinicopathologic patterns of a particular type of primary glomerulonephropathy. Clues to a secondary cause include multiorgan involvement and other clinical manifestations associated with particular systemic diseases (eg, the malar rash of systemic lupus erythematosus [SLE]).

## PRIMARY CAUSES OF NEPHROTIC SYNDROME

### What are the primary causes of nephrotic syndrome?

**Because of the histologic distribution of this condition, there is a risk of inadvertently missing the involved tissue with biopsy.**

Focal segmental glomerulosclerosis (FSGS).

**This entity is more frequently associated with thromboembolism compared with other causes of nephrotic syndrome.**

Membranous nephropathy.[3]

**This entity is more common in children but is responsible for up to 15% of primary cases of nephrotic syndrome in adults.**

Minimal change disease.[6]

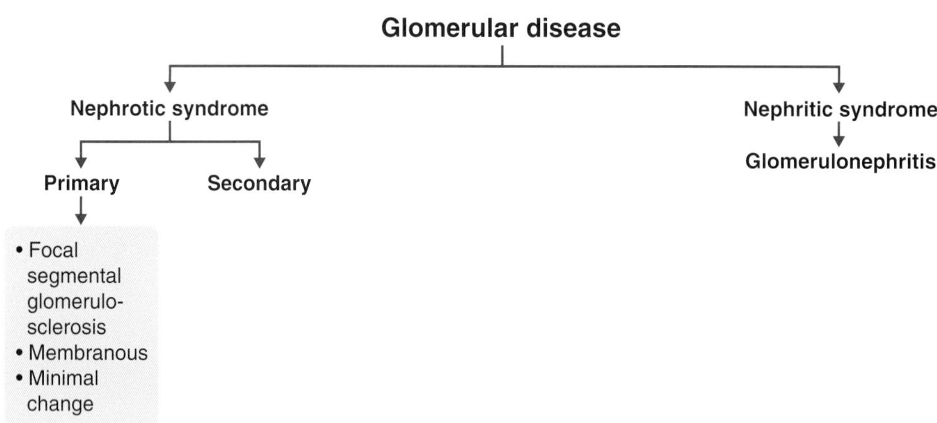


**Which ethnic group is at highest risk for focal segmental glomerulosclerosis?**

FSGS is the most common cause of glomerular disease in black patients (approximately one-half of cases), whereas membranous nephropathy is the most common cause in white patients.[3]

**How frequently is membranous nephropathy related to an underlying condition or exposure?**

Membranous nephropathy is primary (ie, idiopathic) in most cases. The remaining cases are secondary to autoimmune disease (eg, SLE), infection (eg, hepatitis B virus), medication (eg, penicillamine), or malignancy (eg, colon cancer).[7]

**Which pharmacologic agent is considered first-line treatment for minimal change disease in adults?**

Systemic glucocorticoids are used as first-line treatment for minimal change disease in adults, with remission achieved in >80% of cases. However, relapses are common, and these patients require repeated treatments, sometimes becoming dependent on or refractory to steroids.[6,8]

**Which 2 primary glomerular diseases normally associated with nephritic syndrome can present with nephrotic syndrome in a small but significant number of cases?**

Membranoproliferative glomerulonephritis (MPGN) and immunoglobulin A (IgA) nephropathy present with nephrotic syndrome in a small but significant number of cases. *These entities are discussed later in this chapter.*

*Secondary glomerulonephropathies tend to mirror the clinicopathologic patterns of a particular type of primary glomerulonephropathy (eg, SLE can present with a membranous nephropathy pattern) and must be ruled out before a diagnosis of primary (or idiopathic) glomerulonephropathy is given.*

## SECONDARY CAUSES OF NEPHROTIC SYNDROME

### What are the secondary causes of nephrotic syndrome?

**Kimmelstiel-Wilson lesions on histology.**

Diabetes mellitus.

**A 32-year-old woman in her 28th week of pregnancy develops hypertension, peripheral edema, and nephrotic-range proteinuria.**

Preeclampsia.

**A 56-year-old woman with rheumatoid arthritis develops nephrotic syndrome after starting a new therapy.**

Gold or penicillamine therapy.

**A 23-year-old woman with a history of intravenous drug use presents with fever, holosystolic murmur at the apex with radiation to the axilla, positive blood cultures, and nephrotic-range proteinuria.**

Infective endocarditis.

**A 22-year-old man with weight loss, night sweats, generalized lymphadenopathy, and nephrotic syndrome.**

Hodgkin's lymphoma.

**An autoimmune disease capable of causing both nephrotic and nephritic syndromes.**

Systemic lupus erythematosus.

**Diagnosed with Congo red staining and polarized light microscopy.**

Amyloidosis.

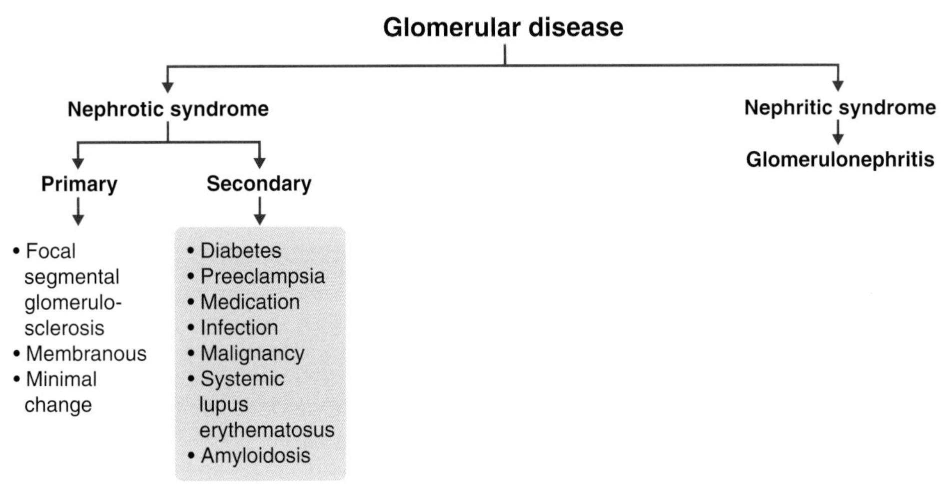

**What clinical features suggest that the development of nephrotic syndrome in a diabetic patient may be related to a condition other than diabetes?**

The suspicion that nephrotic syndrome in diabetic patients may be related to another condition rises when any of the following features are present: nephrotic syndrome with normal renal function, the absence of retinopathy, rapid deterioration of renal function, active urine sediment, gross or microscopic hematuria, and short duration of diabetes.[9]

**What is the prognosis of nephrotic syndrome related to preeclampsia?**

A return to normal renal function without evidence of ongoing proteinuria in the weeks to months after delivery is the rule in most patients with nephrotic syndrome related to preeclampsia. Prognosis for the fetus, on the other hand, is generally poor.[10]

**What medications are associated with nephrotic syndrome?**

Medications most commonly associated with nephrotic syndrome include nonsteroidal anti-inflammatory drugs, lithium, gold, penicillamine, captopril, and tamoxifen.[3,4]

**What infections are associated with nephrotic syndrome?**

Nephrotic syndrome can be associated with bacterial infection (eg, infectious endocarditis, syphilis), viral infection (eg, human immunodeficiency virus, hepatitis B virus, hepatitis C virus), protozoal infection (eg, malaria, toxoplasmosis), and helminthic infection (eg, schistosomiasis, filariasis).[3,4]

**What malignancies are associated with nephrotic syndrome?**

Malignancies most commonly associated with nephrotic syndrome include lymphoma, multiple myeloma, lung cancer, and renal cell carcinoma. The most common histologic patterns of glomerular disease in patients with malignancy-associated nephrotic syndrome are minimal change disease and membranous nephropathy.[11]

**What are the clinical features of membranous lupus nephropathy (MLN)?**

A little more than one-half of all patients with SLE will develop clinically evident kidney disease. Among them, 10% to 15% have MLN. Patients with MLN may not manifest the typical clinical and laboratory findings of SLE. Renal disease does not progress as aggressively as the proliferative forms of lupus nephritis, but a small percentage of patients with MLN will progress to end-stage renal disease. Patients with MLN are at risk for the complications of nephrotic syndrome (eg, thromboembolism).[12]

**What are the renal manifestations of immunoglobulin light chain (AL) amyloidosis?**

Acute or chronic renal insufficiency is present in up to one-half of patients with AL amyloidosis. Proteinuria is common, occurring in most patients at presentation, with half of those cases being in the nephrotic range. Patients with nephrotic syndrome related to AL amyloidosis have a poor prognosis with median survival of 16 months.[13]

**In addition to amyloidosis, what are the other 2 glomerular diseases associated with fibrillar deposits in the mesangium or glomerular basement membrane?**

In addition to amyloidosis, the other main glomerulonephropathies associated with fibrillar deposits in the glomeruli are fibrillary GN (more common) and immunotactoid glomerulopathy (less common). These entities can be distinguished from amyloidosis under the microscope because the fibrils are larger than those seen in amyloidosis and are Congo red–negative. Fibrillary GN and immunotactoid glomerulopathy are idiopathic in most cases but can develop secondary to systemic diseases (eg, multiple myeloma). Nephrotic syndrome is the most common clinical presentation, but many patients also have nephritic syndrome.[14]

## GLOMERULONEPHRITIS

**What are the symptoms of glomerulonephritis?**

Patients with GN may experience hematuria and the symptoms of associated conditions such as acute kidney injury (eg, oliguria, pleuritic chest pain from uremic pericarditis), nephrotic syndrome (eg, peripheral edema), and hypertension (eg, headache).

**What are the physical findings of glomerulonephritis?**

Physical findings of GN may include hypertension, skin findings associated with specific underlying etiologies (eg, palpable purpura in patients with small vessel vasculitis), and findings of uremia if present (eg, pericardial friction rub in patients with uremic pericarditis).

**What are the general laboratory findings of glomerulonephritis?**

General laboratory findings of GN include features of the nephritic syndrome: urine sediment consisting of dysmorphic RBCs, RBC casts, and occasionally WBCs and WBC casts; varying degrees of proteinuria; and varying degrees of acute kidney injury. Other laboratory studies can be indicative of specific underlying causes of GN (eg, serum cryoglobulins in the setting of cryoglobulinemic GN).[1]

**What type of dysmorphic red blood cell is most specific for glomerulonephritis?**

The presence of acanthocytes, ring-shaped RBCs with vesicle-shaped protrusions (commonly described as "Mickey Mouse ears"), is most specific for the presence of GN (Figure 34-4). Acanthocyturia $\geq$5% is associated with a sensitivity of about 50% and specificity of about 98% for GN.[15]

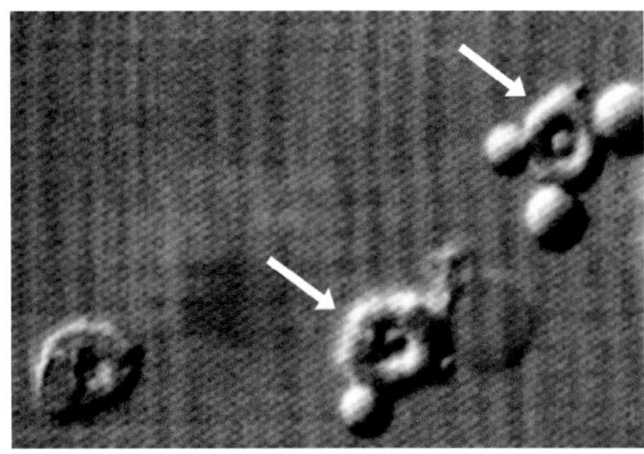

**Figure 34-4.** Dysmorphic red blood cells with vesicle-shaped protrusions (arrows), known as acanthocytes, are specific for glomerulonephritis. (Courtesy of Dr. Mark D. Okusa.)

**What are the subcategories of glomerulonephritis based on serological testing?**

The causes of GN can be separated into the following serologic patterns: positive ANCA, positive anti-GBM antibodies, low complement levels, and other.

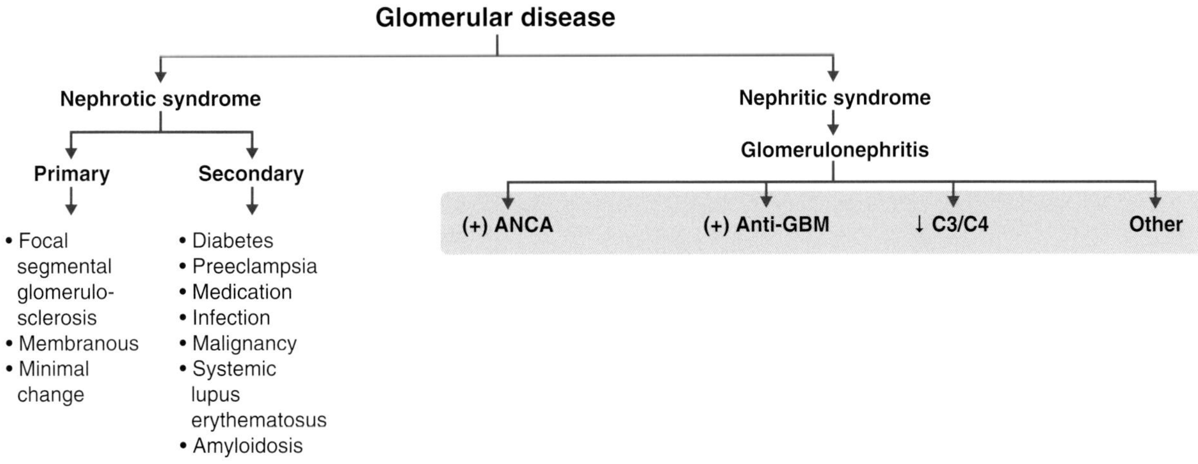


*It is important to recognize that the serologic patterns of GN are not 100% sensitive, and as such, etiologies that belong to these categories can present with a negative serologic workup in some cases. Renal biopsy is the single most definitive investigation into the cause of glomerular disease, including GN.*

## GLOMERULONEPHRITIS ASSOCIATED WITH ANCA

**What does ANCA refer to?**

Antineutrophil cytoplasmic antibodies are a group of autoantibodies directed against proteins found in the cytoplasm of neutrophils, including proteinase 3 (PR3) and myeloperoxidase (MPO).[16]

**In ANCA-positive patients, what are the 2 distinct patterns that may be seen on immunofluorescence microscopy?**

When antibodies to PR3 are present, it results in a cytoplasmic pattern (c-ANCA). Antibodies to MPO are associated with a perinuclear pattern (p-ANCA). Enzyme-linked immunosorbent assays (ELISA) can specifically detect the presence of PR3 and MPO antibodies.[16]

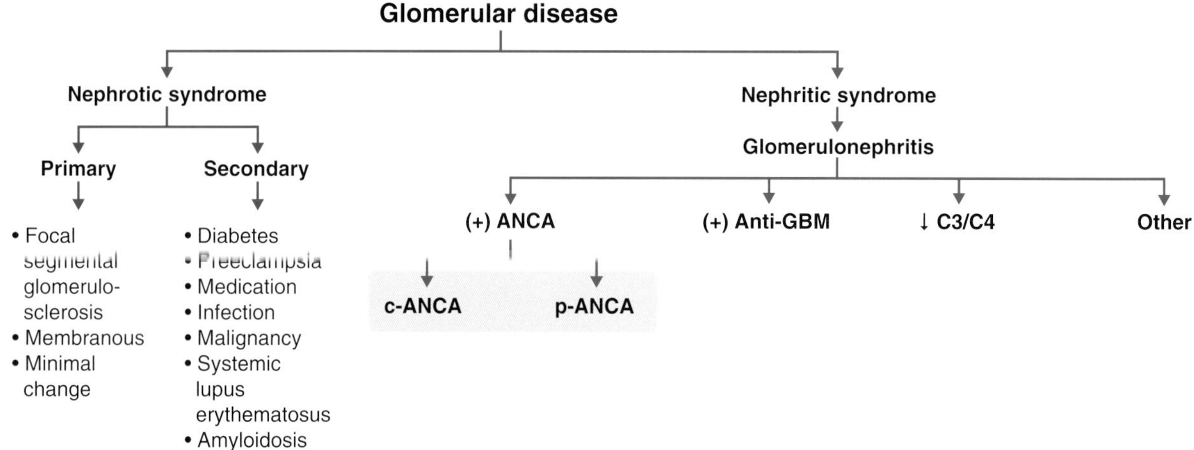


**What characteristic finding on immunofluorescence and electron microscopy distinguishes ANCA-associated glomerulonephritis from other forms of glomerulonephritis?**

The histologic hallmark of ANCA-associated GN is the paucity or lack of glomerular immune deposits (ie, pauci-immune).[16]

## GLOMERULONEPHRITIS ASSOCIATED WITH c-ANCA

### What disease causes glomerulonephritis associated with c-ANCA?

**A 68-year-old woman with a history of sinusitis and saddle-nose deformity (see Figure 50-4) presents with hemoptysis, hematuria, and acute kidney injury and is found to have positive c-ANCA titers.**

Granulomatosis with polyangiitis (GPA, or Wegener's granulomatosis).

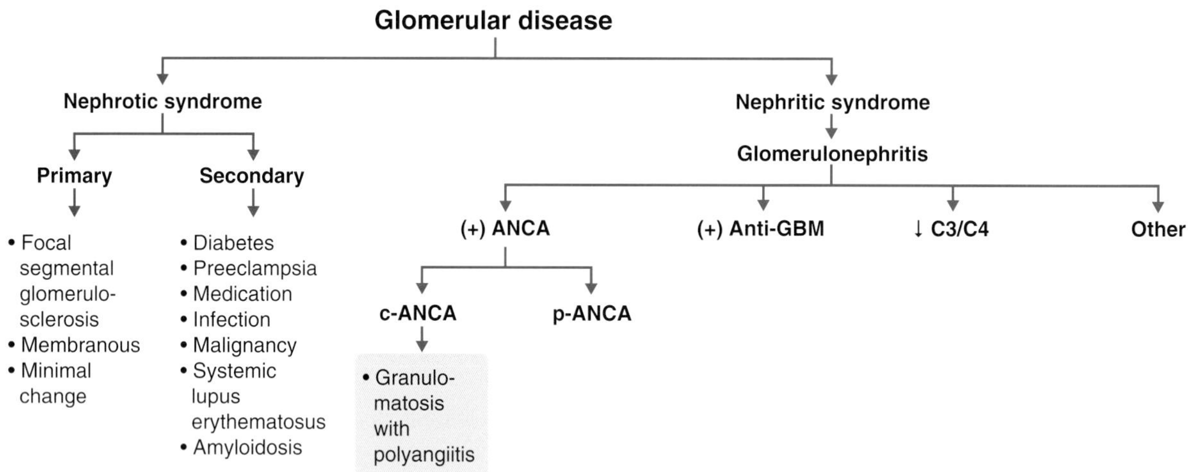


**Are all cases of granulomatosis with polyangiitis associated with ANCA?**

ANCA is positive in up to 90% of cases of systemic GPA. The association is not as strong in patients with limited disease. Among those that are positive, most are c-ANCA. Despite this strong association, the absence of ANCA positivity does not exclude the diagnosis of GPA. Renal biopsy may be necessary to confirm the diagnosis.[17]

**How common is renal involvement in patients with granulomatosis with polyangiitis?**

At the time of presentation, up to one-fifth of patients with GPA will have renal involvement. GN eventually develops in the vast majority of patients within the first 2 years. Treatment consists of an induction phase followed by maintenance therapy. Induction regimens for patients with GN usually consist of glucocorticoids in combination with cyclophosphamide or rituximab, which achieves remission in most patients. Methotrexate or azathioprine is usually used for maintenance therapy.[1,17,18]

## GLOMERULONEPHRITIS ASSOCIATED WITH p-ANCA

### What are the causes of glomerulonephritis associated with p-ANCA?

**The absence of granulomas on histology is a distinguishing feature of this small vessel vasculitis.**

Microscopic polyangiitis (MPA).

**Think of this entity in patients with a history of asthma who present with GN.**

Eosinophilic granulomatosis with polyangiitis (EGPA, or Churg-Strauss syndrome).

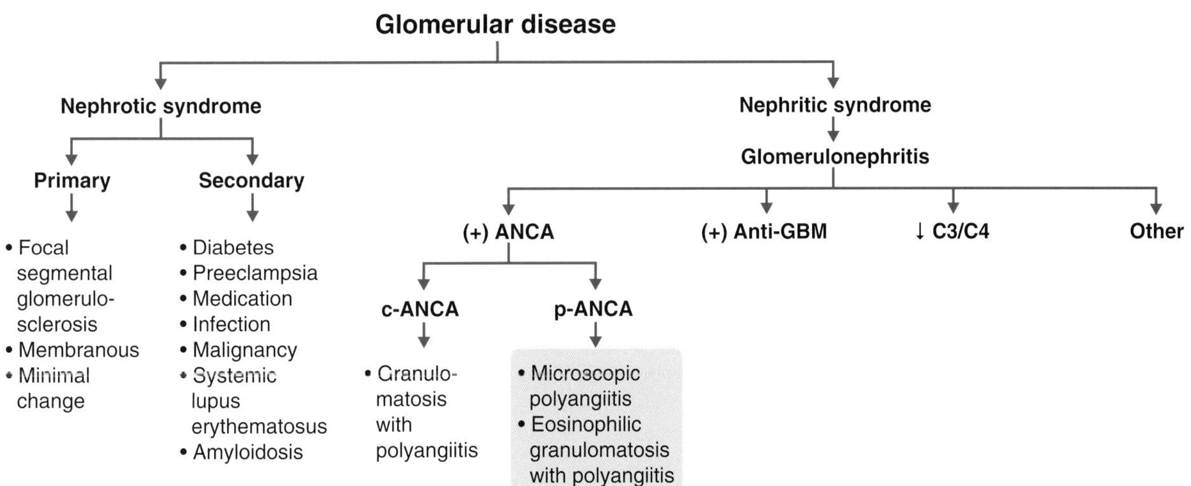


**Are all cases of microscopic polyangiitis associated with ANCA?**

ANCA is positive in up to 75% of patients with MPA. Among those that are positive, most are p-ANCA. Despite this strong association, the absence of ANCA positivity does not exclude the diagnosis of MPA. Renal biopsy may be necessary to confirm the diagnosis.[19]

**How common is renal involvement in patients with microscopic polyangiitis?**

The vast majority of patients with MPA develop renal manifestations (>80%), ranging in severity from asymptomatic proteinuria to rapidly progressive GN. Induction regimens for patients with GN usually consist of glucocorticoids in combination with cyclophosphamide or rituximab, which achieves remission in most patients. Methotrexate or azathioprine is usually used for maintenance therapy.[1,19]

**Are all cases of eosinophilic granulomatosis with polyangiitis associated with ANCA?**

ANCA is positive in approximately one-half of all patients with EGPA but tends to be more common in those with GN. Among those that are positive, most are p-ANCA. The absence of ANCA positivity does not exclude the diagnosis of EGPA. Renal biopsy may be necessary to confirm the diagnosis.[20]

**How common is renal involvement in patients with eosinophilic granulomatosis with polyangiitis?**

Approximately one-quarter of patients with EGPA develop renal manifestations, ranging in severity from asymptomatic urinary abnormalities (eg, microscopic hematuria) to end-stage renal disease. Induction regimens for patients with GN usually consist of glucocorticoids either alone or in combination with cyclophosphamide, which achieves remission in most patients. Azathioprine or methotrexate is usually used for maintenance therapy.[20]

## GLOMERULONEPHRITIS ASSOCIATED WITH ANTI-GBM ANTIBODIES

### What disease causes glomerulonephritis associated with anti-GBM antibodies?

**Aptly named.**

Anti–glomerular basement membrane disease.

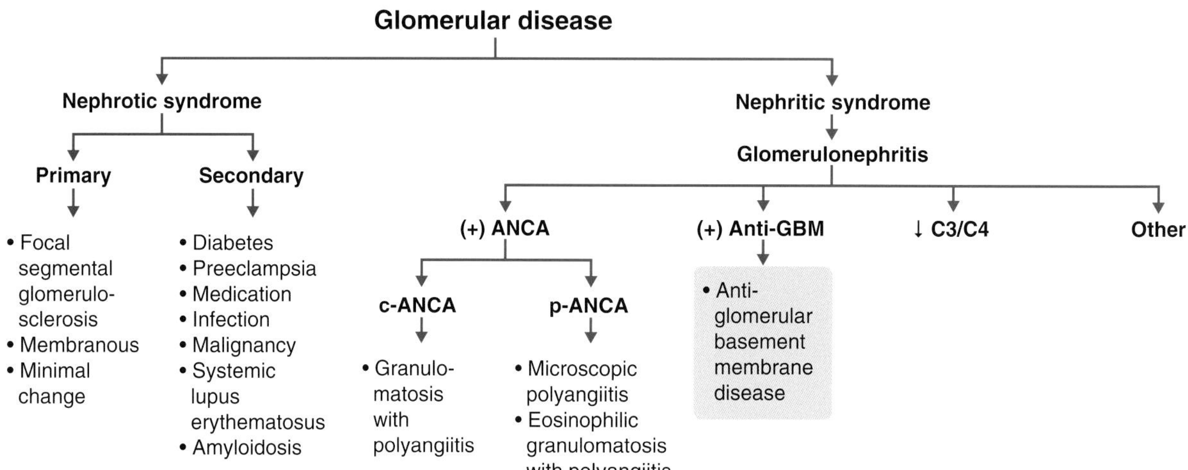


**Are all cases of anti-GBM disease associated with serum anti-GBM antibodies?**

Using conventional methods, serum anti-GBM antibodies are present in up to 90% of patients with anti-GBM disease. Despite this strong association, the absence of anti-GBM antibodies does not exclude the diagnosis of anti-GBM disease. Renal biopsy may be necessary to confirm the diagnosis.[21]

**What is the hallmark of anti-GBM disease on immunofluorescence microscopy?**

Continuous linear deposition of immunoglobulin (usually IgG) along the glomerular basement membrane is the hallmark of anti-GBM disease on immunofluorescence microscopy.[21]

**What syndrome is characterized by the combination of pulmonary hemorrhage and glomerulonephritis related to anti-GBM disease?**

The combination of anti-GBM GN and pulmonary hemorrhage is known as Goodpasture syndrome. It is present in around one-half of patients with anti-GBM disease. In rare cases, pulmonary hemorrhage occurs in the absence of GN.[21]

## GLOMERULONEPHRITIS ASSOCIATED WITH LOW SERUM COMPLEMENT LEVELS

*The pattern of serum hypocomplementemia (ie, the differences in levels of C3 and C4) can be suggestive of particular etiologies.*

### What are the causes of glomerulonephritis associated with low serum complement levels?

**Dark and scant urine following an illness characterized by sore throat, strawberry tongue, and a skin rash that began on the face and progressed to the upper trunk and extremities.**

Post-streptococcal glomerulonephritis (PSGN).

**The most common subtype of this pattern of glomerular injury is characterized by the presence of subendothelial immune deposits on electron microscopy.**

Membranoproliferative glomerulonephritis.

**A 26-year-old woman with renal impairment, active urine sediment, the presence of antinuclear antibodies (ANA), anti–double-stranded deoxyribonucleic acid (anti-dsDNA) antibodies, and low serum complement levels.**

Systemic lupus erythematosus.

**A 25-year-old woman with active intravenous drug use presents with dyspnea and fever and is found to have a decrescendo diastolic murmur over Erb's point, painful nodules on the pulps of her fingers, and hematuria with dysmorphic RBCs.**

Infective endocarditis (IE).

**Chronic hepatitis C infection, palpable purpura, and GN.**

Cryoglobulinemia.

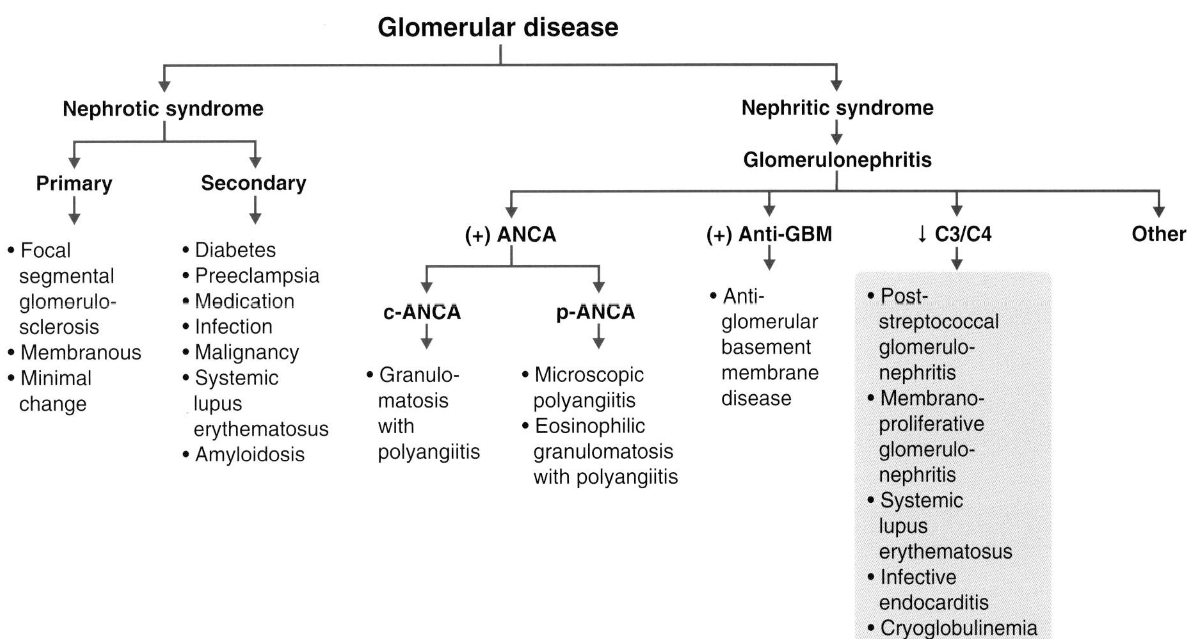


**When does post-streptococcal glomerulonephritis usually develop during the course of streptococcal infection?**

PSGN typically occurs 7 to 10 days after upper respiratory tract infection and 2 to 4 weeks after skin infection. Prognosis is excellent in children, but there is a significant risk of chronic kidney disease or death in adults. *The typical pattern of serum hypocomplementemia in PSGN is low C3 with normal C4 levels (C3 and C4 levels are both reduced in some patients).*[22]

**What are the causes of membranoproliferative glomerulonephritis?**

MPGN can occur as a primary (ie, idiopathic) or secondary glomerular disease, resulting from various conditions such as infection (eg, hepatitis C), autoimmune disease (eg, SLE), and plasma cell dyscrasia (eg, monoclonal gammopathy of unknown significance). *The typical pattern of serum hypocomplementemia in MPGN depends on subtype. Complement-mediated MPGN usually presents with low C3 and normal C4 levels. Immune complex–mediated MPGN usually presents with normal or mildly low C3 and low C4 levels.*[23]

**What is the timing of onset of lupus nephritis during the course of systemic lupus erythematosus?**

Lupus nephritis is more common in younger patients. It can occur at any time during the course of the disease but most commonly presents within 1 year of diagnosis of SLE (it presents within 5 years of diagnosis in the vast majority of cases). *The typical pattern of serum hypocomplementemia in lupus nephritis is reduction in both C3 and C4 levels; however, C4 levels are more often and more profoundly decreased compared with C3.*[24,25]

**What is the differential diagnosis of renal injury in the setting of infective endocarditis?**

The main causes of renal injury related to IE include GN, renal infarction related to septic emboli, acute interstitial nephritis (AIN) related to antibiotic therapy (eg, β-lactams), and acute tubular necrosis (ATN) related to septic physiology or antibiotic therapy (eg, aminoglycosides). GN is typically an early manifestation of IE, occurring at the summit of the illness. Other causes of renal injury related to IE, such as antibiotic-associated AIN, tend to occur later in the course of the illness. *The typical pattern of serum hypocomplementemia in IE-associated GN is low C3 with normal C4 levels (C3 and C4 levels are both reduced in some patients).*[26,27]

**What are the main subtypes of cryoglobulinemia?**

Type I cryoglobulinemia (a monoclonal Ig, usually IgM or IgG) commonly occurs in the setting of hematologic malignancy (eg, Waldenström macroglobulinemia, multiple myeloma). Type II cryoglobulinemia (a mixture of polyclonal Ig with a monoclonal Ig, usually IgM) commonly occurs in the setting of chronic infection (eg, hepatitis C virus, human immunodeficiency virus). Type III cryoglobulinemia (a mixture of polyclonal Ig of all isotypes) commonly occurs in the setting of autoimmune disease (eg, SLE, Sjögren syndrome) but can also occur with chronic infection (eg, hepatitis C virus). *The typical pattern of serum hypocomplementemia in cryoglobulinemia-associated GN is markedly low C4 with normal or mild-to-moderately reduced C3 levels.*[28,29]

## OTHER CAUSES OF GLOMERULONEPHRITIS

### What are the other causes of glomerulonephritis?

**The most common primary glomerular disease worldwide.**

Immunoglobulin A nephropathy.[30]

**Abdominal pain, arthritis, palpable purpura, and GN.**

Henoch-Schönlein purpura (HSP).

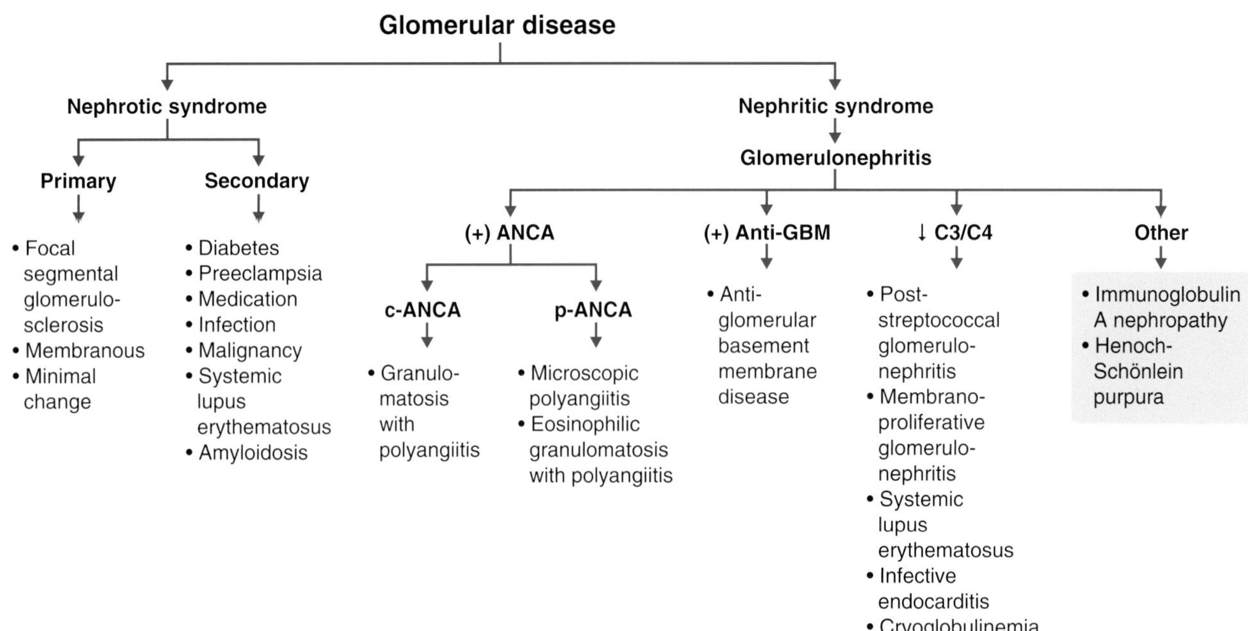

**What are the clinical features of immunoglobulin A nephropathy?**

IgA nephropathy can present at any age but is most common in the second and third decades of life, with a predilection for white and Asian men. The 2 most common presentations of IgA nephropathy are (1) episodes of macroscopic hematuria that often coincide with or occur within 5 days of an upper respiratory tract infection (more common in patients <40 years of age), and (2) asymptomatic patients with abnormal urine sediment and proteinuria (more common in older patients). A minority of patients present with nephrotic syndrome or rapidly progressive GN. Among all patients with IgA nephropathy, up to 40% will eventually progress to end-stage renal disease. Glucocorticoids with or without other immunosuppressive agents may halt disease progression. In patients who progress to end-stage renal disease, kidney transplantation is the treatment of choice. IgA nephropathy recurs in a significant proportion of patients after transplantation.[30]

**How common is glomerulonephritis in patients with Henoch-Schönlein purpura?**

Approximately one-half of patients with HSP develop GN. The histologic features of HSP are identical to that of IgA nephropathy. The 2 conditions are distinguished by the occurrence of extrarenal manifestations in HSP, including palpable purpura, which is universally present.[31]

## Case Summary

A 78-year-old man presents with abdominal pain following a recent upper respiratory tract infection and is found to have hypertension, palpable purpura, acute kidney injury, and hematuria.

***What is the most likely diagnosis in this patient?***

Henoch-Schönlein purpura.

### BONUS QUESTIONS

***What is the significance of the urine sediment in this case?***

The urine sediment in this case shows acanthocytes (a particular type of dysmorphic RBC) (see Figure 34-2A) and an RBC cast (see Figure 34-2B), which indicate glomerular inflammation.

***What is the significance of the recent upper respiratory tract infection in this case?***

Several types of GN can occur in association with infection, including HSP, PSGN, and IgA nephropathy.

***What is the significance of the skin finding in this case?***

The skin rash in this case (see Figure 34-1) is consistent with palpable purpura related to cutaneous small vessel vasculitis. This finding indicates systemic involvement and distinguishes HSP from IgA nephropathy.

***Which procedure would be helpful in confirming the diagnosis of Henoch-Schönlein purpura in this case?***

Skin biopsy with light and immunofluorescence microscopy would reveal leukocytoclastic vasculitis and, more specifically, IgA deposition within the walls of the blood vessels, which is pathognomonic of HSP. Skin biopsy is less invasive than renal biopsy and is generally preferred. However, in cases of severe renal involvement, renal biopsy may have a role in providing prognostic information and guiding therapy. The principal finding of HSP on renal biopsy is globular mesangial IgA deposition on immunofluorescence (also seen with IgA nephropathy).[31]

***What is the treatment for glomerulonephritis associated with Henoch-Schönlein purpura?***

Spontaneous remission of HSP and complete recovery of renal function occur in most cases, but there is a higher risk of progression to chronic kidney disease in adults compared with children. In patients with severe GN, treatment options include glucocorticoids either alone or in combination with plasma exchange or immunosuppressive agents such as azathioprine and intravenous immunoglobulins (IVIG). The efficacy of these modalities is largely unknown. Ultimately, renal transplantation may be necessary for patients who progress to end-stage renal disease.[31]

## KEY POINTS

- Glomerular disease describes a heterogeneous group of entities that damage various glomerular structures and produce characteristic clinical, physiologic, biochemical, and histologic manifestations.
- Glomerular injury results in impaired filtration, allowing constituents of blood into the urinary space that are normally excluded (eg, cells, protein).
- The clinical manifestations of glomerular disease include nephrotic syndrome and nephritic syndrome.
- Nephrotic syndrome describes the constellation of peripheral edema, proteinuria >3.5 g/d, hypoalbuminemia, and hyperlipidemia. Renal excretory function can be variable.
- Important sequelae of nephrotic syndrome include progressive renal failure, thromboembolism, and susceptibility to infection.
- Nephrotic syndrome can be primary (ie, idiopathic) or secondary.
- Nephritic syndrome (ie, glomerulonephritis) describes the constellation of hypertension and active urine sediment (dysmorphic RBCs [acanthocytes in particular], RBC casts, and occasionally WBCs and WBC casts). Renal excretory function and degree of proteinuria can be variable.
- The causes of GN can be separated into the following serologic patterns: positive ANCA, positive anti-GBM antibodies, low complement levels, and other.
- ANCA-associated GN can be associated with c-ANCA or p-ANCA.
- Serologic patterns of GN are not 100% sensitive.
- Renal biopsy is the single most definitive investigation into the cause of glomerular disease.

## REFERENCES


1. Longo DL, Fauci AS, Kasper DL, Hauser SL, Jameson JL, Loscalzo J, eds. *Harrison's Principles of Internal Medicine*. 18th ed. New York, NY: McGraw-Hill; 2012.
2. Madaio MP, Harrington JT. The diagnosis of glomerular diseases: acute glomerulonephritis and the nephrotic syndrome. *Arch Intern Med*. 2001;161(1):25-34.
3. Hull RP, Goldsmith DJ. Nephrotic syndrome in adults. *BMJ*. 2008;336(7654):1185-1189.
4. Orth SR, Ritz E. The nephrotic syndrome. *N Engl J Med*. 1998;338(17):1202-1211.
5. Ginsberg JM, Chang BS, Matarese RA, Garella S. Use of single voided urine samples to estimate quantitative proteinuria. *N Engl J Med*. 1983;309(25):1543-1546.
6. Waldman M, Crew RJ, Valeri A, et al. Adult minimal-change disease: clinical characteristics, treatment, and outcomes. *Clin J Am Soc Nephrol*. 2007;2(3):445-453.
7. Lai WL, Yeh TH, Chen PM, et al. Membranous nephropathy: a review on the pathogenesis, diagnosis, and treatment. *J Formos Med Assoc*. 2015;114(2):102-111.
8. Hogan J, Radhakrishnan J. The treatment of minimal change disease in adults. *J Am Soc Nephrol*. 2013;24(5):702-711.
9. Prakash J. Non-diabetic renal disease (NDRD) in patients with type 2 diabetes mellitus (type 2 DM). *J Assoc Physicians India*. 2013;61(3):194-199.
10. Wei Q, Zhang L, Liu X. Outcome of severe preeclampsia manifested as nephrotic syndrome. *Arch Gynecol Obstet*. 2011;283(2):201-204.
11. Christiansen CF, Onega T, Svaerke C, et al. Risk and prognosis of cancer in patients with nephrotic syndrome. *Am J Med*. 2014;127(9):871-877 e1.
12. Kolasinski SL, Chung JB, Albert DA. What do we know about lupus membranous nephropathy? An analytic review. *Arthritis Rheum*. 2002;47(4):450-455.
13. Korbet SM, Schwartz MM. Multiple myeloma. *J Am Soc Nephrol*. 2006;17(9):2533-2545.
14. Iskandar SS, Falk RJ, Jennette JC. Clinical and pathologic features of fibrillary glomerulonephritis. *Kidney Int*. 1992;42(6):1401-1407.
15. Kohler H, Wandel E, Brunck B. Acanthocyturia–a characteristic marker for glomerular bleeding. *Kidney Int*. 1991;40(1):115-120.
16. Jennette JC, Falk RJ, Andrassy K, et al. Nomenclature of systemic vasculitides. Proposal of an international consensus conference. *Arthritis Rheum*. 1994;37(2):187-192.
17. Kubaisi B, Abu Samra K, Foster CS. Granulomatosis with polyangiitis (Wegener's disease): an updated review of ocular disease manifestations. *Intractable Rare Dis Res*. 2016;5(2):61-69.
18. Almouhawis HA, Leao JC, Fedele S, Porter SR. Wegener's granulomatosis: a review of clinical features and an update in diagnosis and treatment. *J Oral Pathol Med*. 2013;42(7):507-516.
19. Chung SA, Seo P. Microscopic polyangiitis. *Rheum Dis Clin North Am*. 2010;36(3):545-558.
20. Vaglio A, Buzio C, Zwerina J. Eosinophilic granulomatosis with polyangiitis (Churg-Strauss): state of the art. *Allergy*. 2013;68(3):261-273.
21. Troxell ML, Houghton DC. Atypical anti-glomerular basement membrane disease. *Clin Kidney J*. 2016;9(2):211-221.
22. Ferretti JJ, Stevens DL, Fischetti VA, eds. *Streptococcus pyogenes: Basic Biology to Clinical Manifestations*. Oklahoma City, OK; 2016.
23. Sethi S, Fervenza FC. Membranoproliferative glomerulonephritis–a new look at an old entity. *N Engl J Med*. 2012;366(12):1119-1131.

24. Borchers AT, Leibushor N, Naguwa SM, Cheema GS, Shoenfeld Y, Gershwin ME. Lupus nephritis: a critical review. *Autoimmun Rev.* 2012;12(2):174-194.
25. Cameron JS, Vick RM, Ogg CS, Seymour WM, Chantler C, Turner DR. Plasma C3 and C4 concentrations in management of glomerulonephritis. *Br Med J.* 1973;3(5882):668-672.
26. Boils CL, Nasr SH, Walker PD, Couser WG, Larsen CP. Update on endocarditis-associated glomerulonephritis. *Kidney Int.* 2015;87(6):1241-1249.
27. Majumdar A, Chowdhary S, Ferreira MA, et al. Renal pathological findings in infective endocarditis. *Nephrol Dial Transplant.* 2000;15(11):1782-1787.
28. D'Amico G. Renal involvement in hepatitis C infection: cryoglobulinemic glomerulonephritis. *Kidney Int.* 1998;54(2):650-671.
29. Ramos-Casals M, Stone JH, Cid MC, Bosch X. The cryoglobulinaemias. *Lancet.* 2012;379(9813):348-360.
30. Donadio JV, Grande JP. IgA nephropathy. *N Engl J Med.* 2002;347(10):738-748.
31. Roberts PF, Waller TA, Brinker TM, Riffe IZ, Sayre JW, Bratton RL. Henoch-Schonlein purpura: a review article. *South Med J.* 2007;100(8):821-824.

Chapter 35

# HYPERKALEMIA

## Case: A 45-year-old woman with dark urine

A 45-year-old woman with a history of type 1 diabetes mellitus and coronary artery disease is brought to the emergency department after being found down by family. She has a history of poor adherence to prescribed insulin therapy. Other medications include lisinopril and metoprolol succinate.

Heart rate is 124 beats per minute, blood pressure is 140/84 mm Hg, and respiratory rate is 30 breaths per minute. Breathing is deep and labored.

Serum sodium ($Na^+$) is 130 mEq/L; potassium ($K^+$), 6.6 mEq/L; chloride, 94 mEq/L; bicarbonate, 10 mEq/L; blood urea nitrogen, 48 mg/dL; creatinine, 2.1 mg/dL; and glucose, 800 mg/dL. Urine sample is shown in Figure 35-1. No red blood cells are visualized on microscopic urinalysis.

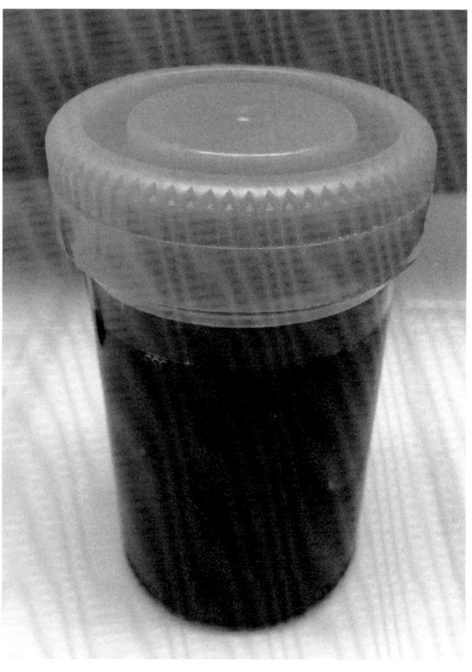

**Figure 35-1.**

***What are the possible causes of hyperkalemia in this patient?***

**What is normal serum $K^+$ concentration?**

The normal range for serum $K^+$ may vary slightly between laboratories but is typically 3.6 to 5 mEq/L.[1]

**What is pseudohyperkalemia?**

Pseudohyperkalemia is the presence of elevated serum $K^+$ in a blood sample due to efflux of $K^+$ from red blood cells during the process of phlebotomy or after the sample has been drawn.

**How is $K^+$ normally distributed within the body?**

Approximately 98% of total body $K^+$ is sequestered within cells (mostly muscle cells), with the remaining 2% in the extracellular fluid compartment.[1]

**Why is it important to maintain normal extracellular K⁺ concentration?**

The ratio of intracellular to extracellular K⁺ is the most important determining factor of the resting membrane potential of neurons and myocytes, which allows for the generation and propagation of action potentials necessary for normal function and stability of the heart and other muscles.[2]

**What processes are responsible for regulating serum K⁺?**

The kidneys maintain total body K⁺ balance by matching excretion with intake, a hormonal process that occurs over a period of hours. The movement of K⁺ between the intracellular and extracellular compartments (ie, transcellular shift) regulates more acute changes in serum K⁺. The gastrointestinal tract normally clears around 10% of K⁺ intake, a contribution that adaptively increases in the setting of renal failure.[2,3]

**What are the symptoms of hyperkalemia?**

Symptoms of hyperkalemia may include muscle weakness, paresthesias, and palpitations.

**What are the electrocardiographic manifestations of hyperkalemia?**

Electrocardiographic manifestations of hyperkalemia include (in order of increasing severity) increased amplitude and peaking of the T wave, prolonged PR interval, decreased amplitude and eventual disappearance of the P wave, prolonged QRS interval, and sine wave pattern (Figure 35-2).[4]

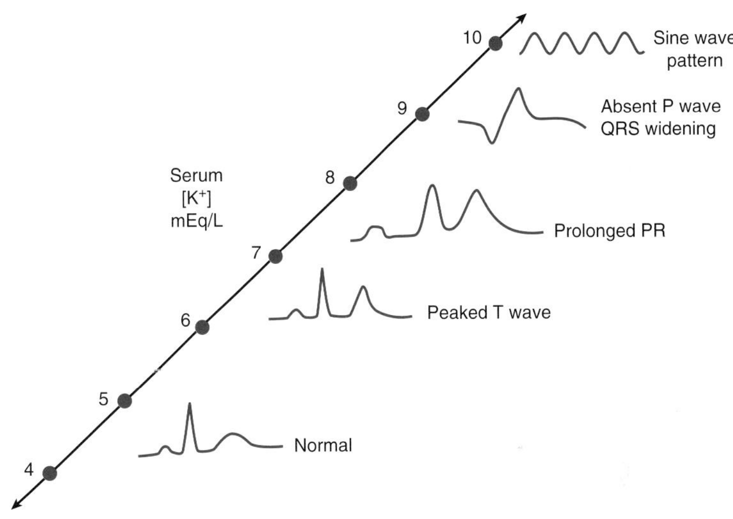


**Figure 35-2.** Electrocardiographic manifestations of hyperkalemia. (Adapted from Marini JJ, Wheeler AP. *Critical Care Medicine: The Essentials*. 4th ed. Philadelphia, PA: Lippincott Williams & Wilkins; 2010.)

**What conduction abnormalities are associated with hyperkalemia?**

Hyperkalemia can result in bundle branch block (right or left), bifascicular block, and atrioventricular block.[5]

**What cardiac dysrhythmias are associated with hyperkalemia?**

Hyperkalemia may be associated with sinus bradycardia, asystole, and idioventricular rhythms (eg, ventricular tachycardia, ventricular fibrillation).[4]

**Which organ is chiefly responsible for maintaining total body K⁺ by matching elimination with intake?**

The kidneys are primarily responsible for maintaining total body K⁺.

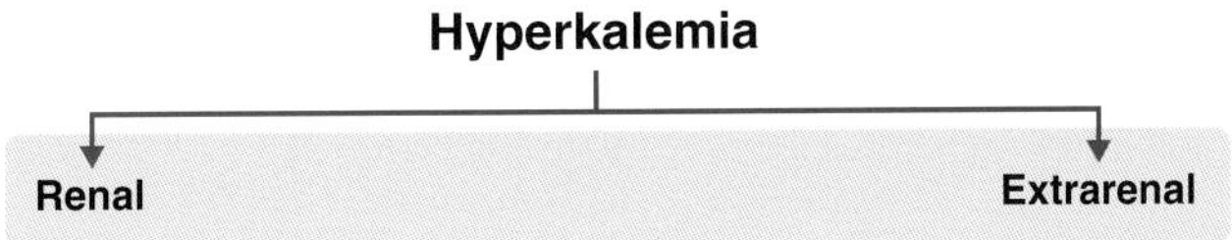


**What are the 2 subcategories of renal-associated hyperkalemia based on renal function?**

Renal-associated hyperkalemia can occur in the setting of decreased renal clearance or normal renal clearance.

Hyperkalemia

- Renal
  - Decreased clearance
  - Normal clearance
- Extrarenal

What is the clinical surrogate for renal function?

Renal clearance can be estimated by calculating the glomerular filtration rate (GFR).

How is glomerular filtration rate estimated?

Several equations are used to predict GFR (most commonly the Modification of Diet in Renal Disease [MDRD] and the Cockcroft-Gault equations), each based primarily on serum creatinine concentration.[6,7]

What is normal serum creatinine concentration?

Creatinine is produced and released by muscle without significant short-term (day-to-day) variation. Serum creatinine levels are therefore dependent on muscle mass, which is dependent on nutritional status, age, gender, and ethnicity. For the average adult man, the normal range for serum creatinine is 0.6 to 1.2 mg/dL; for the average adult woman, it is approximately 0.5 to 1.1 mg/dL. Normal serum creatinine values in individuals with muscle mass above or below average (eg, body builders, elderly, malnourished patients) may be outside of those ranges.[8]

## RENAL CAUSES OF HYPERKALEMIA IN THE SETTING OF DECREASED RENAL CLEARANCE

What is the biochemical definition of acute kidney injury (AKI)?

AKI is defined by any of the following: (1) increase in serum creatinine by ≥0.3 mg/dL within 48 hours, (2) increase in serum creatinine concentration to ≥1.5 times baseline, known or presumed to have occurred within the prior 7 days, or (3) urine volume <0.5 mL/kg per hour for 6 hours.[9]

What is the definition of chronic kidney disease (CKD)?

CKD is defined as the presence of kidney damage (eg, albuminuria) or decreased kidney function (ie, GFR <60 mL/min/1.73 $m^2$) for ≥3 months.[10]

Is severe hyperkalemia more likely to occur with acute kidney injury or chronic kidney disease?

Severe hyperkalemia is more likely to occur in patients with acute rather than chronic kidney injury. Risk increases in parallel with the rate of renal function loss because there is less time for adaptation to occur. In the setting of chronic renal insufficiency, remaining nephrons develop an increased ability to excrete $K^+$, an adaptive mechanism to maintain overall $K^+$ balance. This mechanism is effective until GFR drops below 15 to 20 mL/min. Extrarenal adaptations also occur, including increased cellular uptake and increased gastrointestinal excretion of $K^+$.[3,11]

### What are the causes of hyperkalemia related to decreased renal clearance?

Avocados, spinach, sweet potatoes, oranges, and bananas.

Oral intake (including both dietary and iatrogenic $K^+$ supplementation).

Think of this iatrogenic source of hyperkalemia in hospitalized patients.

Intravenous infusion of $K^+$.

A 56-year-old woman with end-stage renal disease develops a trend of increasing serum $K^+$ after being started on chronic narcotics for pain.

Constipation.

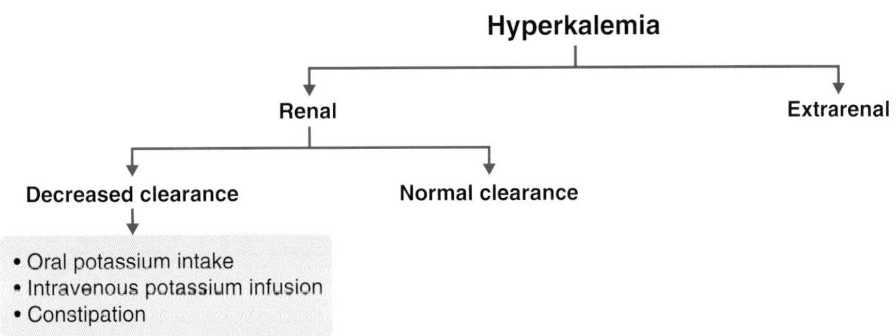


**What natural beverage, readily served at Queen's Park Savannah in Trinidad and Tobago, contains high K⁺ content?**

High concentrations of $K^+$ are found in coconut water. *Dietary $K^+$ restriction is an important part of the long-term management of patients with CKD. Patients should be thoroughly counseled regarding all possible sources of dietary $K^+$.*

**What are the potential sources of intravenous $K^+$?**

Sources of intravenous $K^+$ in the hospital include $K^+$ given to correct hypokalemia (patients with impaired renal function are at particular risk of overcorrection), potassium-containing medication (eg, penicillin G), and blood products.

**What factors increase the risk of hyperkalemia with blood transfusion?**

Risk of hyperkalemia rises with duration of red blood cell storage, irradiation of the blood, and large transfusion volumes (even with fresh products).[12]

**What is the mechanism of hyperkalemia related to constipation?**

Gastrointestinal excretion of $K^+$ increases in patients with CKD, an adaptive mechanism designed to maintain $K^+$ homeostasis. When patients with CKD develop constipation, there is a reduction in overall $K^+$ elimination.[3]

*Exogenous intake of $K^+$, including via oral and intravenous routes, is a rare cause of hyperkalemia in patients with normal renal function.*[13]

## RENAL CAUSES OF HYPERKALEMIA IN THE SETTING OF NORMAL RENAL CLEARANCE

### What are the renal causes of hyperkalemia in the setting of normal renal clearance?

**A 56-year-old man develops hyperkalemia after starting treatment for hypertension.**

Angiotensin-converting enzyme inhibitor (ACE-I).

**Also known as renal tubular acidosis type IV.**

Hypoaldosteronism.

**Normal renal function, hyperkalemia, metabolic acidosis, and elevated serum aldosterone level.**

Pseudohypoaldosteronism.

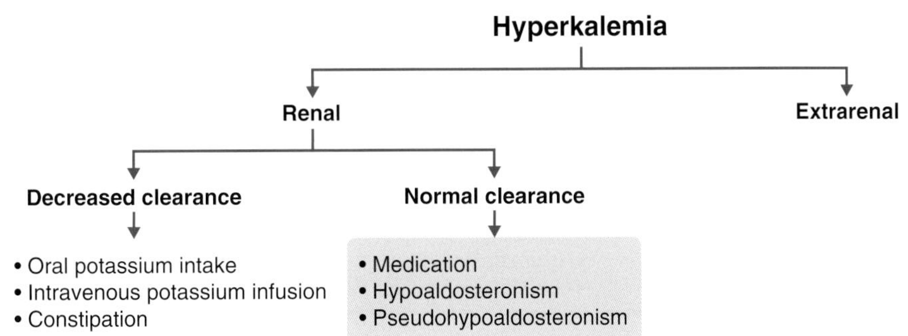

**What are the mechanisms of medication-induced hyperkalemia related to the kidney?**

Mechanisms of medication-induced hyperkalemia related to the kidney include impaired aldosterone secretion (eg, ACE-I, nonsteroidal anti-inflammatory drugs) and impaired action of aldosterone (eg, aldosterone antagonists, potassium-sparing diuretics) (Figure 35-3).[14]

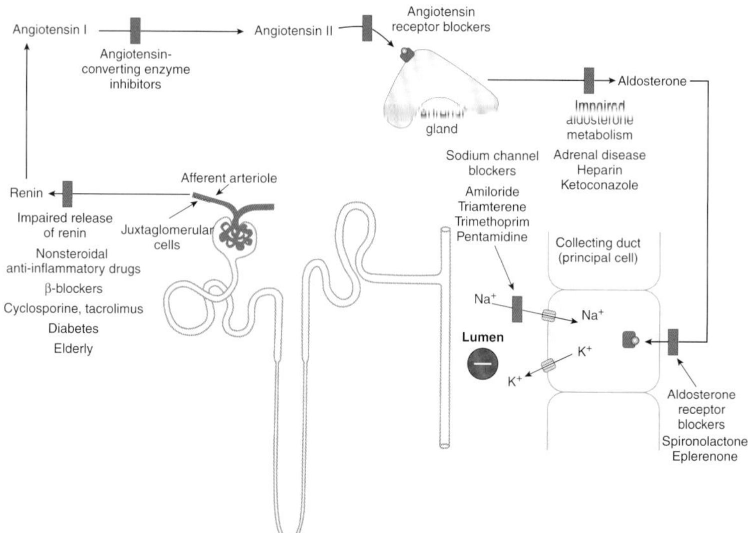


**Figure 35-3.** The renin-angiotensin-aldosterone system and regulation of renal $K^+$ excretion. Aldosterone binds to a cytosolic receptor in the principal cell and stimulates $Na^+$ reabsorption across the luminal membrane. As $Na^+$ is reabsorbed, the electronegativity of the lumen increases thereby providing a more favorable driving force for $K^+$ secretion. Disease states or drugs that interfere at any point along this process can impair renal $K^+$ secretion and lead to hyperkalemia. (From Schrier RW. *Diseases of the Kidney and Urinary Tract*. 8th ed. Philadelphia, PA: Lippincott Williams & Wilkins; 2007.)

**What are the causes of hypoaldosteronism?**

Causes of hypoaldosteronism include medications (eg, ACE-I), hyporeninemia, and primary adrenal insufficiency.

**What is pseudohypoaldosteronism?**

Pseudohypoaldosteronism describes a group of disorders characterized by renal tubular unresponsiveness to aldosterone. It results in hyperkalemia, metabolic acidosis, and increased serum aldosterone concentration.

*Although these causes of hyperkalemia can occur in patients with normal renal function, incidence and severity are generally amplified when superimposed on renal dysfunction.*

## EXTRARENAL CAUSES OF HYPERKALEMIA

**What is the principal mechanism of hyperkalemia unrelated to the kidney?**

Hyperkalemia unrelated to the kidney occurs as a result of transcellular shift.

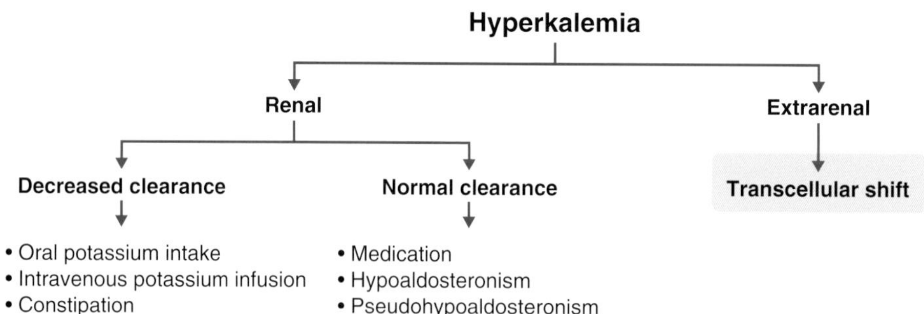

**How is the concentration gradient of $K^+$ between the intracellular and extracellular fluid compartments maintained?**

The concentration gradient of $K^+$ between the intracellular and extracellular fluid compartments is maintained by the $Na^+$-$K^+$-adenosine triphosphatase (ie, $Na^+/K^+$-ATPase or $Na^+/K^+$ pump), which uses energy to move $K^+$ against its concentration gradient from the extracellular to the intracellular compartment (Figure 35-4).[2]

**What are the chief factors that affect transcellular shifts of $K^+$?**

Under normal conditions, insulin and catecholamines are the primary drivers of transcellular shifts of $K^+$. Acid-base derangements and plasma tonicity also affect transcellular shifts of $K^+$.[2]

**What is the effect of insulin on the $Na^+/K^+$ pump?**

Insulin increases the activity of the $Na^+/K^+$ pump, thereby accelerating the movement of $K^+$ into the intracellular compartment. *Insulin is often used in the treatment of hyperkalemia.*[2]

**What are the effects of catecholamines on the $Na^+/K^+$ pump?**

β-Adrenergic receptors activate the $Na^+/K^+$ pump, whereas α-adrenergic receptors impair cellular entry of $K^+$. *$\beta_2$-Agonists are often used in the treatment of hyperkalemia.*[2]

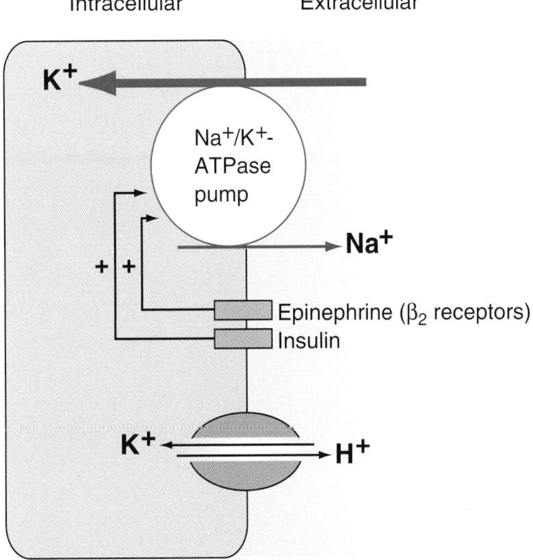


**Figure 35-4.** Mechanisms regulating transcellular shifts in potassium. (From Porth CM. *Essentials of Pathophysiology: Concepts of Altered Health States*. 4th ed. Philadelphia, PA: Wolters Kluwer; 2015.)

## What are the causes of hyperkalemia related to transcellular shift?

**Hyperkalemia on induction of anesthesia.**

Succinylcholine.

**This condition can be identified with an arterial blood gas test.**

Acidemia.

**A metabolic abnormality common to hyperglycemia, mannitol, ethylene glycol, ethanol, and methanol toxicity.**

Serum hyperosmolality.

**A cause of pseudohematuria, often associated with crush injuries.**

Rhabdomyolysis.

**A 43-year-old woman develops hyperkalemia shortly after starting treatment for lymphoma.**

Tumor lysis syndrome.

**A result of pancreatic endocrine dysfunction.**

Insulin deficiency.

**Episodes of transient weakness or paralysis beginning in infancy.**

Hyperkalemic periodic paralysis.

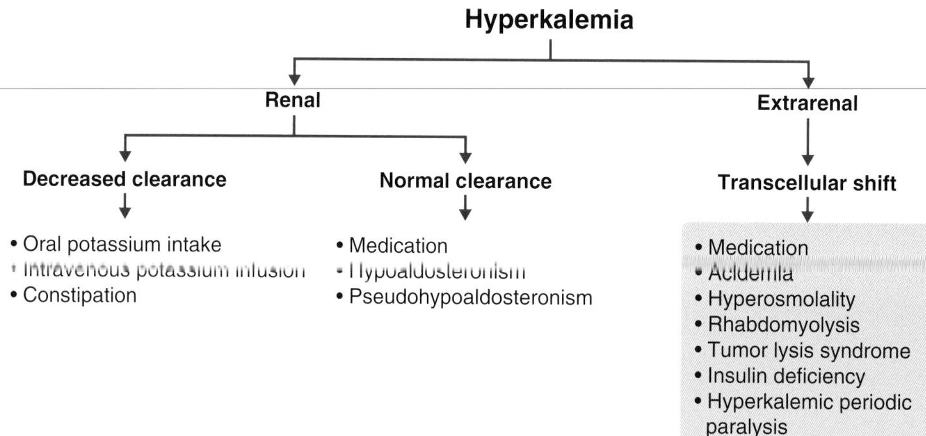


**Which medications promote movement of $K^+$ to the extracellular compartment?**

Medications that lead to $K^+$ movement out of cells include β-blockers, digoxin, and succinylcholine.

**What is the mechanism of acidemia-associated transcellular shift of $K^+$?**

The increase in extracellular $K^+$ related to acidemia results from the interplay between various ion channels. For example, lower extracellular pH decreases the rate of $Na^+$-$H^+$ exchange, which lowers intracellular $Na^+$, reducing the activity of the $Na^+/K^+$ pump and leading to higher extracellular $K^+$.[2]

**What is the mechanism of hyperkalemia associated with hyperosmolality?**

In the setting of hyperosmolality, $K^+$ moves with water from the intracellular to the extracellular compartment through the process of solvent drag. As water moves out of cells, intracellular $K^+$ increases, producing a higher concentration gradient that favors the efflux of $K^+$.[2]

**What are the classic urinalysis findings in the setting of rhabdomyolysis?**

Rhabdomyolysis is associated with positive blood on urine dipstick (a result of myoglobinuria) in the absence of red blood cells on microscopic evaluation. This combination of findings can be an important clue to the diagnosis.

**What is the classic laboratory pattern associated with tumor lysis syndrome?**

Tumor lysis syndrome describes a characteristic pattern of metabolic disturbances, including hyperkalemia, hyperphosphatemia, hyperuricemia, and hypocalcemia, which develop as a result of the release of intracellular content into the bloodstream when there is massive tumor cell lysis, either spontaneously or as a result of therapy. The clinical consequences can be severe, including renal failure, cardiac dysrhythmias, seizure, and death. In patients at risk for tumor lysis syndrome, preventative strategies include intravenous hydration and the use of hypouricemic agents (eg, allopurinol, rasburicase).[15]

**What are some scenarios in which there may be a deficiency of insulin that leads to hyperkalemia?**

Insulin deficiency can occur in the setting of diabetes mellitus (both types 1 and 2), fasting (particularly in dialysis patients), and treatment with somatostatin or somatostatin-agonists (particularly in dialysis patients).[16,17]

**What are the precipitants of weakness in patients with hyperkalemic periodic paralysis?**

Precipitants of weakness in patients with hyperkalemic periodic paralysis include cold exposure, rest after exercise (often aborted by resuming exercise), hunger, low-carbohydrate meals, and potassium-rich meals.[18,19]

*Although these causes of hyperkalemia can occur in patients with normal renal function, incidence and severity are generally amplified when superimposed on renal dysfunction.*

## Case Summary

A 45-year-old woman with a history of type 1 diabetes mellitus and coronary artery disease is brought to the hospital after being found down and is discovered to have multiple metabolic derangements, including hyperkalemia.

| | |
|---|---|
| ***What are the possible causes of hyperkalemia in this patient?*** | Rhabdomyolysis, acute kidney injury, medication (ACE-I and β-blocker), insulin deficiency, and hyperosmolality. |

BONUS QUESTIONS

| | |
|---|---|
| ***What is the significance of the urine sample in this case?*** | Rhabdomyolysis and associated myoglobinuria can result in red-brown–, tea-, or cola-colored urine (see Figure 35-1). The absence of RBCs on microscopic analysis of the urine indicates that the color is not related to the presence of blood. *It is not possible to differentiate hemoglobinuria and myoglobinuria based on the appearance of urine alone.* |
| ***What is the cause of low serum bicarbonate in this case?*** | The low serum bicarbonate in this case is the result of anion gap metabolic acidosis, likely caused by diabetic ketoacidosis. |
| ***What are the most likely causes of acute kidney injury in this case?*** | Diabetic ketoacidosis results in osmotic diuresis, which can lead to prerenal AKI. Rhabdomyolysis can also cause AKI via afferent arteriole vasoconstriction and direct tubular toxicity. |
| ***What is the calculated serum osmolality in this case? (Recall serum $Na^+$ is 130 mEq/L, BUN 48 mg/dL, and glucose 800 mg/dL.)*** | In this case, serum osmolality = $(130 \times 2) + (48/2.8) + (800/18) = 322$ mOsm/kg. This is elevated (reference range 275-295 mOsm/kg) and could be contributing to the hyperkalemia. |
| ***What medication can be given to stabilize the myocytes in the setting of hyperkalemia?*** | An intravenous infusion of calcium chloride (10%) or calcium gluconate (10%) can be used to stabilize myocytes in the setting of hyperkalemia. Calcium gluconate is less irritating to the veins at the injection site.[13] |
| ***What medications can be used to temporarily shift $K^+$ into the intracellular compartment?*** | $\beta_2$-Agonists (eg, albuterol), insulin (along with an ampule of dextrose in patients with normal serum glucose concentration), and sodium bicarbonate are often used to temporarily shift $K^+$ into the intracellular compartment (see Figure 35-4).[13] |
| ***What medications can be used to increase elimination of $K^+$ from the body?*** | Ion-exchange resins (eg, sodium polystyrene) can be used to increase gastrointestinal excretion of $K^+$, and loop diuretics (eg, furosemide) can be used to increase renal excretion of $K^+$.[13] |
| ***In addition to pharmacologic therapy, what therapeutic intervention may be necessary in cases of severe hyperkalemia?*** | In severe cases of hyperkalemia, renal replacement therapy (RRT) may ultimately be necessary to remove $K^+$ from the body. Hemodialysis is more effective than continuous forms of RRT.[13] |

## KEY POINTS

- Potassium homeostasis is regulated by the balance between exogenous intake, excretion in urine and stool, and transcellular shift.
- Transcellular shift of $K^+$ occurs rapidly and is primarily driven by insulin and catecholamines.
- Maintenance of normal serum $K^+$ levels is important for a variety of reasons, including stability of the heart and other muscles.
- Hyperkalemia is generally defined as serum $K^+$ >5 mEq/L.
- Clinical manifestations of hyperkalemia include weakness, paresthesias, palpitations, electrocardiographic changes, and dysrhythmia.
- The kidney is the principal organ responsible for regulating total body $K^+$.
- Hyperkalemia can be caused by renal or extrarenal processes.
- Renal causes of hyperkalemia can be separated according to renal function.

- In patients with impaired renal function, the risk of hyperkalemia is generally higher with AKI, as adaptive mechanisms occur in the setting of CKD to maintain $K^+$ homeostasis.
- Extrarenal causes of hyperkalemia are primarily related to transcellular shift.
- The etiologies of hyperkalemia in the setting of normal renal function also occur in the setting of renal dysfunction, generally with more severe results.
- Management of hyperkalemia depends on its severity and rate of development.
- Intravenous calcium can be used to stabilize the myocytes in hyperkalemic patients.
- Pharmacologic agents can be used to promote influx of $K^+$ into cells (eg, albuterol) and increase $K^+$ excretion in urine (eg, furosemide) and stool (eg, sodium polystyrene).
- Renal replacement therapy may ultimately be necessary to treat hyperkalemia, particularly in severe cases.

## REFERENCES


1. Aronson PS, Giebisch G. Effects of pH on potassium: new explanations for old observations. *J Am Soc Nephrol.* 2011;22(11):1981-1989.
2. Palmer BF. Regulation of potassium homeostasis. *Clin J Am Soc Nephrol.* 2015;10(6):1050-1060.
3. Hayes CP Jr, McLeod ME, Robinson RR. An extrarenal mechanism for the maintenance of potassium balance in severe chronic renal failure. *Trans Assoc Am Physicians.* 1967;80:207-216.
4. Mattu A, Brady WJ, Robinson DA. Electrocardiographic manifestations of hyperkalemia. *Am J Emerg Med.* 2000;18(6):721-729.
5. Bashour T, Hsu I, Gorfinkel HJ, Wickramesekaran R, Rios JC. Atrioventricular and intraventricular conduction in hyperkalemia. *Am J Cardiol.* 1975;35(2):199-203.
6. Cockcroft DW, Gault MH. Prediction of creatinine clearance from serum creatinine. *Nephron.* 1976;16(1):31-41.
7. Levey AS, Bosch JP, Lewis JB, Greene T, Rogers N, Roth D. A more accurate method to estimate glomerular filtration rate from serum creatinine: a new prediction equation. Modification of Diet in Renal Disease Study Group. *Ann Intern Med.* 1999;130(6):461-470.
8. Walker HK, Hall WD, Hurst JW, eds. *Clinical Methods: The History, Physical, and Laboratory Examinations.* 3rd ed. Boston: Butterworths; 1990.
9. KDIGO AKI Work Group. KDIGO clinical practice guidelines for acute kidney injury. *Kidney Int Suppl.* 2012;17:1-138.
10. KDIGO. Chapter 1: Definition and classification of CKD. *Kidney Int Suppl.* 2013;3:19.
11. Schultze RG, Taggart DD, Shapiro H, Pennell JP, Caglar S, Bricker NS. On the adaptation in potassium excretion associated with nephron reduction in the dog. *J Clin Invest.* 1971;50(5):1061-1068.
12. Vraets A, Lin Y, Callum JL. Transfusion-associated hyperkalemia. *Transfus Med Rev.* 2011;25(3):184-196.
13. Lehnhardt A, Kemper MJ. Pathogenesis, diagnosis and management of hyperkalemia. *Pediatr Nephrol.* 2011;26(3):377-384.
14. Ben Salem C, Badreddine A, Fathallah N, Slim R, Hmouda H. Drug-induced hyperkalemia. *Drug Saf.* 2014;37(9):677-692.
15. Howard SC, Jones DP, Pui CH. The tumor lysis syndrome. *N Engl J Med.* 2011;364(19):1844-1854.
16. Adabala M, Jhaveri KD, Gitman M. Severe hyperkalaemia resulting from octreotide use in a haemodialysis patient. *Nephrol Dial Transplant.* 2010;25(10):3439-3442.
17. Allon M, Takeshian A, Shanklin N. Effect of insulin-plus-glucose infusion with or without epinephrine on fasting hyperkalemia. *Kidney Int.* 1993;43(1):212-217.
18. Fontaine B, Lapie P, Plassart E, et al. Periodic paralysis and voltage-gated ion channels. *Kidney Int.* 1996;49(1):9-18.
19. Miller TM, Dias da Silva MR, Miller HA, et al. Correlating phenotype and genotype in the periodic paralyses. *Neurology.* 2004;63(9):1647-1655.

Chapter 36

# HYPERNATREMIA

## Case: A 28-year-old woman with polyuria

A 28-year-old woman with no known medical conditions is brought to the emergency department after developing confusion. The patient was camping in eastern Oregon before symptoms began. During the trip, friends noticed that she was unusually thirsty and had been making frequent trips to urinate. She acknowledged at that time that she had noticed these symptoms for several months but had not sought medical evaluation. On the third day, after the water supply started to diminish, the patient reported to friends that she was feeling unwell. She was taken to the emergency room when she began saying things that did not make sense.

Heart rate is 75 beats per minute, and blood pressure is 123/84 mm Hg. The patient is somnolent and not oriented. Mucous membranes and axillae are moist. Jugular venous pressure is estimated to be 6 cm $H_2O$. There is no peripheral edema.

Serum sodium ($Na^+$) is 158 mEq/L, blood urea nitrogen (BUN) is 12 mg/dL, creatinine is 0.7 mg/dL, and osmolality is 326 mOsm/kg (reference range 275 to 295 mOsm/kg). Urine $Na^+$ is 70 mEq/L and osmolality is 152 mOsm/kg.

***What is the most likely cause of hypernatremia in this patient?***

**What is hypernatremia?**

Hypernatremia is defined as an elevated serum $Na^+$ concentration that occurs when there is a deficit of water relative to $Na^+$ in the extracellular fluid compartment.[1]

**What is normal serum $Na^+$ concentration?**

Normal serum $Na^+$ is 135 to 142 mEq/L.[2]

**How is $Na^+$ normally distributed within the body?**

Most $Na^+$ resides in extracellular fluid, and its distribution between extracellular and intracellular fluid is regulated by the $Na^+/K^+$-adenosine triphosphatase (ie, $Na^+/K^+$-ATPase or $Na^+/K^+$ pump).[3]

**How is water homeostasis regulated?**

The central nervous system and the kidneys work in concert to maintain water homeostasis, which ultimately controls serum $Na^+$ concentration. Osmoreceptors located in the hypothalamus detect extracellular tonicity and respond by adjusting thirst and the secretion of vasopressin (ie, arginine vasopressin [AVP], or antidiuretic hormone [ADH]). Vasopressin acts in the kidney to increase the reabsorption of free water; it can concentrate urine to a maximum of 1200 mOsm/kg. In the absence of vasopressin, urine osmolality can drop to a minimum of 50 mOsm/kg. In the setting of hypernatremia, thirst and vasopressin secretion should be stimulated. A significant decrease in blood volume also stimulates vasopressin secretion (Figure 36-1).[2]

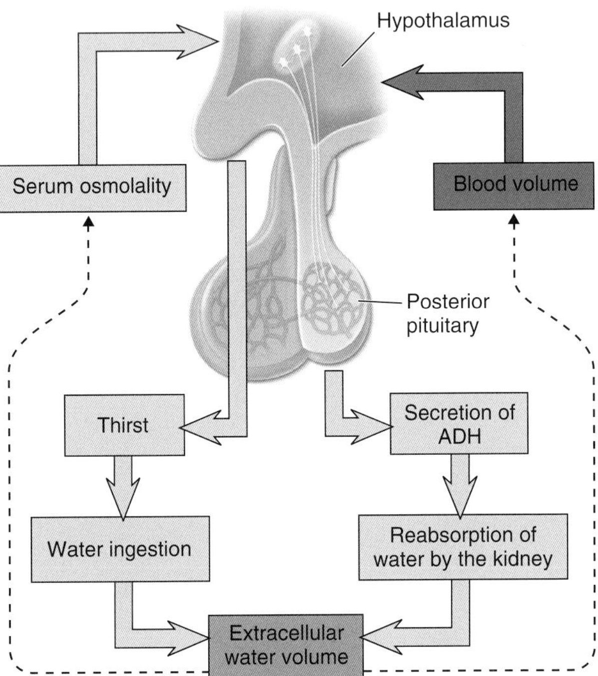


**Figure 36-1.** When osmoreceptors in the hypothalamus sense an increase in solute concentration, or when baroreceptors in the hypothalamus sense a decrease in blood volume, there is an increase in the sensation of thirst and the secretion of vasopressin (ADH) from the posterior pituitary, which leads to water reabsorption in the distal tubules of the kidneys. Homeostasis is maintained by a negative feedback loop. (Modified from Porth CM. *Essentials of Pathophysiology: Concepts of Altered Health States*. Philadelphia, PA: Lippincott Williams & Wilkins; 2003, with permission.)

**What are the effects of serum $Na^+$ concentration on cell volume?**

Sodium is an effective solute and therefore contributes to overall serum tonicity. Water moves freely between fluid compartments in response to differences in tonicity. Accordingly, the presence of hypernatremia, which is always associated with hypertonicity, causes a shift of water out of cells, resulting in cellular contraction. Conversely, hypotonic hyponatremia causes a shift of water into cells, resulting in cellular swelling (Figure 36-2).[3]

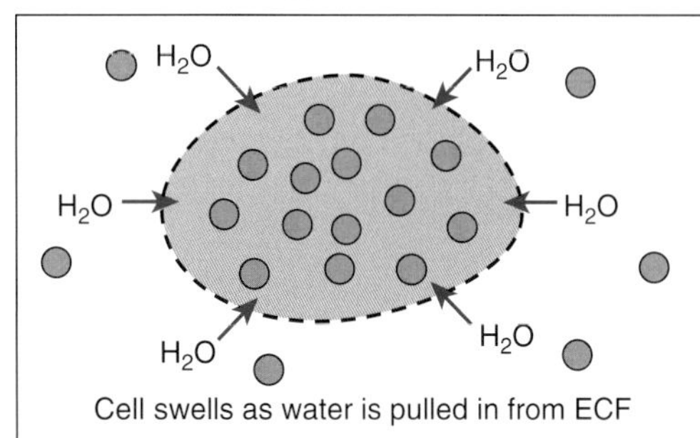


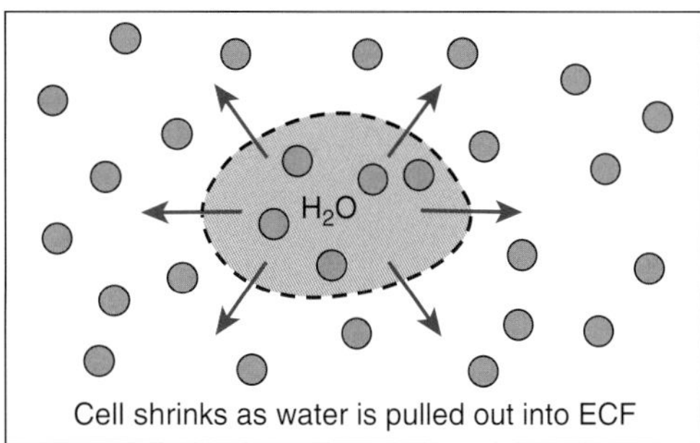


**Figure 36-2.** The effects of hypernatremia and hyponatremia on cell volume and extracellular fluid (ECF). (From Smeltzer SC, Hinkle JL, Bare BG, Cheever KH. *Brunner and Suddarth's Textbook of Medical-Surgical Nursing*. 12th ed. Philadelphia, PA: Wolters Kluwer; 2010.)

**What are the effects of serum $Na^+$ concentration on brain tissue?**

In most tissues of the body, the $Na^+$ concentrations of serum and interstitial fluid are virtually identical due to free movement of $Na^+$ through the capillary membrane. In contrast, capillaries in the brain are impermeable to $Na^+$. The result is that an abnormal serum $Na^+$ concentration will cause water to move into or out of brain tissue, with subsequent swelling or contraction, respectively. Only minimal changes in the volume of brain tissue are compatible with life.[2]

**What adaptive mechanisms occur in the setting of chronic hypernatremia?**

In the setting of chronic hypernatremia, defined by at least 24 to 48 hours' duration, osmotically active intracellular molecules (osmolytes) (eg, glutamate, taurine, myo-inositol) are increased within cells, including brain cells. This helps decrease the gradient of tonicity between extracellular and intracellular fluid, which in turn, decreases movement of water out of cells. This adaptation is particularly important in brain tissue.[2]

**What are the clinical differences between acute and chronic hypernatremia?**

Given the adaptation that occurs in response to chronic hypernatremia, patients are often asymptomatic. In contrast, patients with acute hypernatremia (developed over a period of hours) are almost always symptomatic, and changes in brain volume can be life-threatening. The physiologic adaptation that occurs in chronic hypernatremia limits the rate with which hypernatremia can be corrected (Figure 36-3). In cases where duration is unknown, chronicity should be assumed.[2]

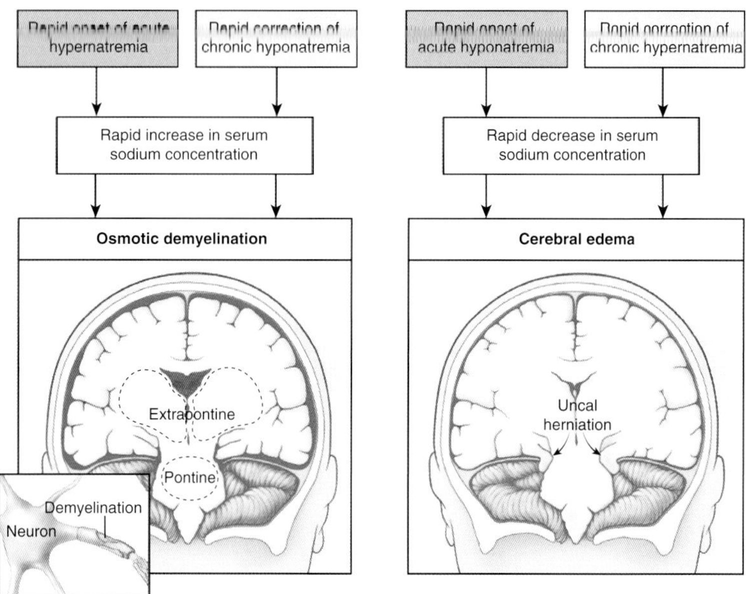


**Figure 36-3.** Rapid onset or rapid correction of either hyponatremia or hypernatremia can cause brain damage. A rapid increase in the level of serum sodium, either from acute hypernatremia or from rapid correction of chronic hyponatremia, can cause osmotic demyelination (which can involve pontine and extrapontine regions of the brain). Cerebral edema is a complication of rapid decreases in serum sodium concentration, which can lead to brain herniation in severe cases. (Adapted with permission from Sterns RH. Disorders of plasma sodium–causes, consequences, and correction. *N Engl J Med.* 2015;372(1):55-65.)

**What are the clinical manifestations of acute hypernatremia?**

Clinical manifestations of acute hypernatremia may include thirst (with some exceptions), muscle weakness, decreased consciousness, delirium, convulsions, coma, and brain shrinkage, which can lead to osmotic demyelination, and vascular rupture with intracranial hemorrhage.[2]

**What is the first step in establishing the cause of hypernatremia?**

Determining extracellular fluid volume status is the first step in establishing the cause of hypernatremia.

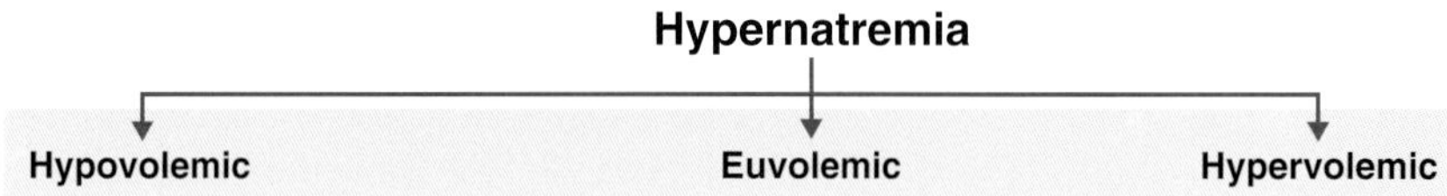


**What physical findings are associated with hypovolemia?**

Hypovolemia may be associated with decreased skin turgor, dry mucous membranes and axillae, increased capillary refill time, sunken eyes, and low jugular venous pressure.

**What physical findings are associated with hypervolemia?**

Hypervolemia may be associated with elevated jugular venous pressure, ascites, rales on lung auscultation (due to pulmonary edema), dullness to percussion of the lung bases (due to pleural effusions), and peripheral edema.

## HYPOVOLEMIC HYPERNATREMIA

*Hypovolemic hypernatremia can be thought of as extracellular loss of hypotonic fluid (water > salt).*

**What are the 2 subcategories of hypovolemic hypernatremia?**

Hypovolemic hypernatremia can be caused by renal or extrarenal processes.

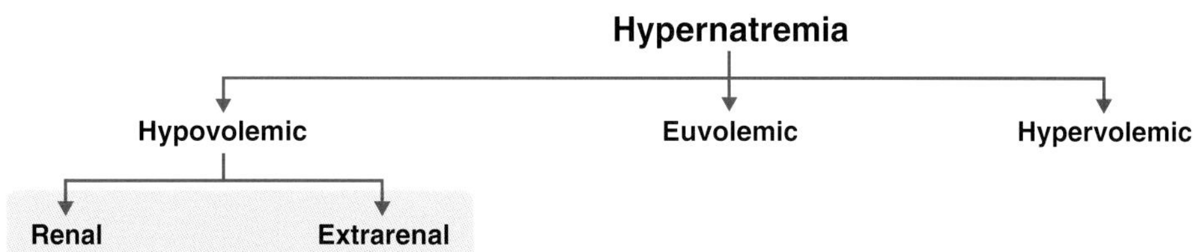


**What laboratory test can be helpful in distinguishing renal from extrarenal causes of hypovolemic hypernatremia?**

Spot urine $Na^+$ concentration can be suggestive of whether the source of volume depletion is renal ($U_{Na}$ > 20 mEq/L) or extrarenal ($U_{Na}$ < 20 mEq/L, especially <10 mEq/L).[4]

### What are the renal causes of hypovolemic hypernatremia?

**Iatrogenic loss of hypotonic fluid (relative to serum).**

Diuretic medication, particularly loop diuretics.

**Water follows the solute load.**

Osmotic diuresis.

**Opening the floodgates.**

Postobstructive diuresis.

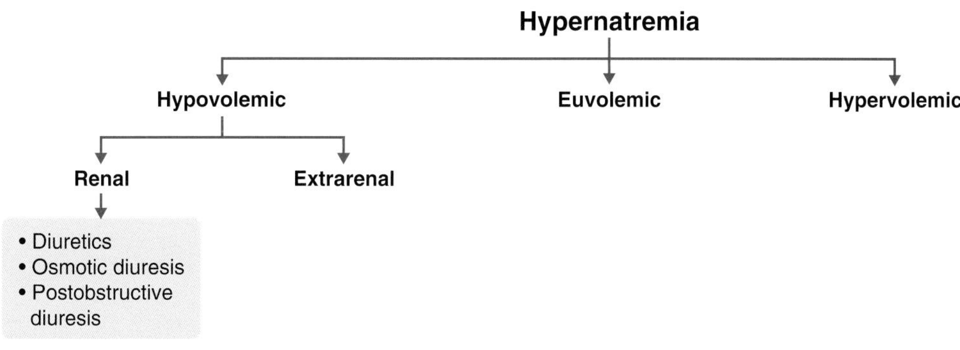

**What is the mechanism of hypernatremia related to loop diuretics?**

Loop diuretics decrease the reabsorption of $Na^+$ and chloride in the thick ascending limb of the loop of Henle (within the renal medulla), which ultimately impairs the ability of the kidneys to make concentrated urine (Figure 36-4). If the osmolality of excreted urine is lower than that of serum, then hypernatremia will eventually occur. *Patients with diuretic-induced hypernatremia may be euvolemic or hypervolemic.*[5]

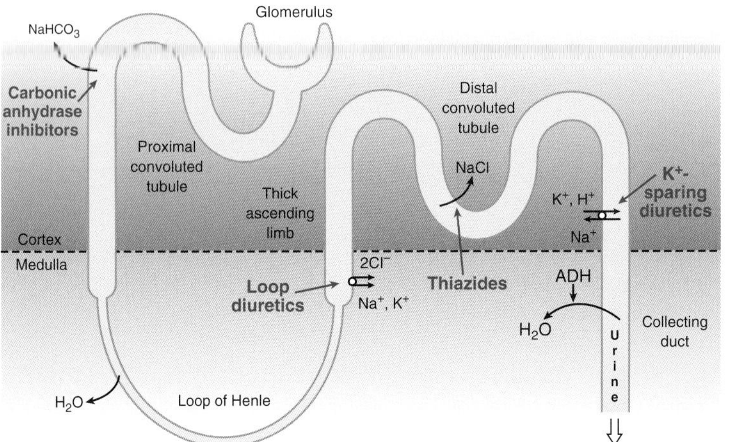


**Figure 36-4.** Diuretic drugs are secreted into the proximal convoluted tubule and act at the sites shown. Approximately 70% of filtered sodium is reabsorbed in the proximal convoluted tubule; 25%, in the thick ascending limb of the loop of Henle; 5%, in the distal convoluted tubule; and 1% to 2%, in the cortical collecting tubule (mediated by the action of aldosterone). Vasopressin (ADH) increases the permeability of the distal nephron for water. (Adapted with permission from Lilly LS. *Pathophysiology of Heart Disease: A Collaborative Project of Medical Students and Faculty*. 6th ed. Philadelphia, PA: Wolters Kluwer Health; 2016.)

**Does hyperglycemia cause hyponatremia or hypernatremia?**

Hyperosmolality caused by either effective solutes (eg, glucose) or ineffective solutes (eg, urea) can lead to the excretion of hypotonic urine through osmotic diuresis. *Under certain circumstances, ineffective solutes can become effective urine solutes.* In the case of osmotic diuresis caused by an effective solute, such as glucose, the increased tonicity of extracellular fluid will trigger movement of water from the intracellular to the extracellular fluid compartment, resulting in dilutional hyponatremia. However, if free water intake does not keep up with urinary water loss, then hypernatremia will eventually ensue.

**What is postobstructive diuresis?**

Postobstructive diuresis refers to a state of polyuria that occurs after relief of urinary tract obstruction, such as from bladder outlet obstruction or bilateral ureteral obstruction. Patients are at risk for dehydration, electrolyte disturbances (eg, hypernatremia), and death.[6]

## What are the extrarenal causes of hypovolemic hypernatremia?

**A patient develops hypernatremia after treatment for small bowel obstruction is initiated.**

Loss of hypotonic fluid (relative to serum) related to nasogastric tube drainage.

**Marathon runners and burn victims.**

Cutaneous (integumentary) loss of hypotonic fluid (relative to serum).

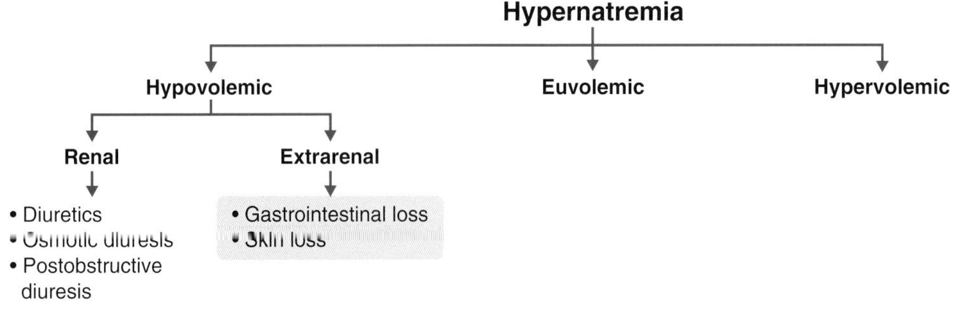

**What are some causes of hypotonic fluid loss from the gastrointestinal (GI) tract?**

Loss of hypotonic fluid (relative to serum) from the GI tract can occur as a result of diarrhea, vomiting, or tube drainage.

**What is the concentration of $Na^+$ in sweat?**

The average concentration of $Na^+$ in sweat is approximately 40 mEq/L, but there is variation according to the site of the body and the rate of sweat production. Sweat $Na^+$ concentration rises with increased rates of sweat production but is always lower than serum $Na^+$ concentration.[7]

## EUVOLEMIC HYPERNATREMIA

*Euvolemic hypernatremia can be thought of as extracellular deficiency of pure water.*

### What are the causes of euvolemic hypernatremia?

**Hypernatremia develops despite minimal loss of free water in the kidneys, GI tract, or skin.**

Low free water intake.

**Hypernatremia and polyuria.**

Diabetes insipidus (DI).

**Transient hypernatremia (resolving within minutes).**

Intracellular water shift.

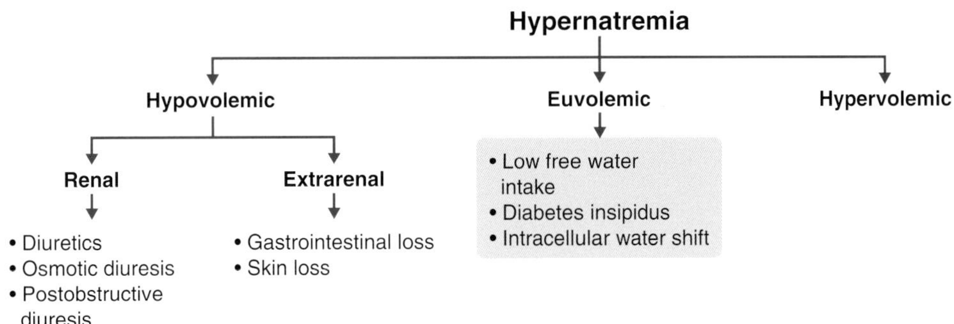


**What are the risk factors for hypernatremia due to low free water intake?**

Risk factors for hypernatremia from low free water intake include older age, delirium, and intubation.[1]

**What are the 2 general types of diabetes insipidus?**

DI can be central (ie, deficient vasopressin secretion) or nephrogenic (ie, vasopressin resistance). In the setting of hypernatremia, low urine osmolality (<300 mOsm/kg) is suggestive of DI. Unlike nephrogenic DI, central DI is responsive to treatment with desmopressin.[8]

**What are the causes of intracellular water shift?**

An increase in intracellular osmolality, which is accompanied by the movement of water from the extracellular to the intracellular fluid compartment, can be caused by intensive exercise and seizure from electroconvulsive therapy.[9,10]

## HYPERVOLEMIC HYPERNATREMIA

*Hypervolemic hypernatremia can be thought of as extracellular gain of hypertonic fluid (salt > water).*

### What are the causes of hypervolemic hypernatremia?

**Look for concurrent hypertension.**

Mineralocorticoid excess.

**A castaway should never drink seawater.**

Exogenous $Na^+$ intake.

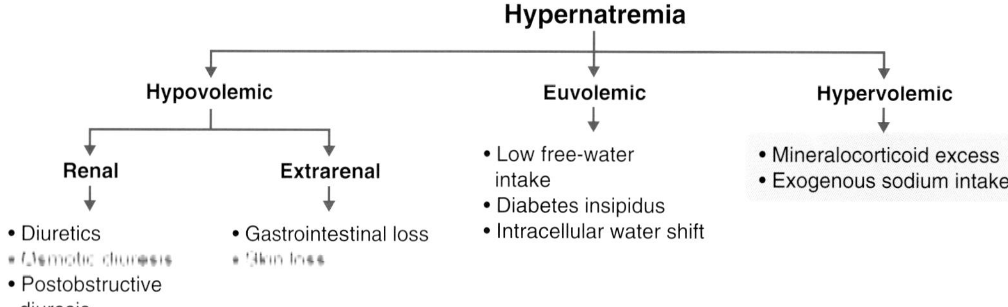


**What are the causes of primary hyperaldosteronism?**

Primary hyperaldosteronism (ie, Conn's syndrome) refers to a group of disorders in which production of aldosterone is excessively high relative to serum $Na^+$ concentration. Manifestations may include hypertension, mild hypernatremia, and hypokalemia. Causes of primary hyperaldosteronism include adrenal hyperplasia, adrenal adenoma, adrenocortical carcinoma, and familial hyperaldosteronism.[11]

**What are the sources of exogenous $Na^+$ intake?**

Sources of exogenous $Na^+$ intake include hypertonic sodium bicarbonate infusion, hypertonic sodium chloride infusion, hypertonic tube feeds, ingestion of sodium chloride, ingestion of seawater, emetics rich in sodium chloride, hypertonic saline enemas, hypertonic dialysis, and intrauterine injection of hypertonic saline.[1]

## Case Summary

A 28-year-old woman with chronic thirst and polyuria presents with acute confusion and somnolence, and is found to have hypernatremia.

***What is the most likely cause of hypernatremia in this patient?***

Diabetes insipidus.

### BONUS QUESTIONS

***Which general category of hypernatremia applies to this case?***

This case can be described as euvolemic hypernatremia.

***What features in this case are suggestive of euvolemic volume status?***

The normal jugular venous pressure and absence of peripheral edema in this case effectively rule out hypervolemia. Euvolemia and hypovolemia can be difficult to differentiate clinically. However, the presence of moist mucous membranes and axillae, low BUN, and high urine $Na^+$ concentration suggest that extracellular fluid volume is not low.[12]

***What is diabetes insipidus?***

DI is a syndrome characterized by the production of excessive volumes (>50 mL/kg body weight per 24 hours) of dilute urine (osmolality < 300 mOsm/kg). Symptoms include thirst, polyuria, enuresis, and nocturia. Dehydration does not usually occur unless fluid intake is impaired.[13]

***What is central diabetes insipidus?***

Central DI is characterized by insufficient secretion of vasopressin in the central nervous system, which leads to hypotonic polyuria and hypernatremia. It can be inherited or acquired. Common associations in adults include head trauma, neurosurgery, autoimmune destruction of the neurohypophysis, infiltrative disorders (eg, sarcoidosis), malignancy, and ischemia. A significant proportion of cases are idiopathic.[8]

***What is nephrogenic diabetes insipidus?***

Nephrogenic DI is characterized by renal resistance to vasopressin, which leads to hypotonic polyuria and hypernatremia. It can be inherited or acquired. Common associations in adults include medications (eg, lithium), hypercalcemia, hypokalemia, and infiltrative disorders (eg, amyloidosis).[8]

***Does the patient in this case have central or nephrogenic diabetes insipidus?***

Based on the information given, it is not clear whether the patient in this case has central DI or nephrogenic DI. Testing would be needed to first confirm the diagnosis of DI; once confirmed, additional tests can delineate between central and nephrogenic forms.

***How can the diagnosis of diabetes insipidus be confirmed in this case?***

The water deprivation test can be used to confirm the diagnosis of DI. The patient is restricted from water and monitored closely for changes in laboratory parameters (eg, serum and urine osmolality) until 1 of 2 endpoints is reached. If urine osmolality does not rise appropriately (>300 mOsm/kg) before serum osmolality (or serum $Na^+$ concentration) rises above the upper limit of normal (295 mOsm/kg), then a diagnosis of complete DI is made. If urine osmolality does rise to >300 mOsm/kg, then complete DI is not present, and other causes of polyuria should be considered, including partial DI and primary polydipsia (a higher threshold of urine osmolality can be used to rule out partial DI, eg, 600 mOsm/kg). Assays have recently been developed to diagnose DI, including measurement of serum copeptin, which may obviate the need for water deprivation testing.[8,13,14]

***What laboratory test can be used to differentiate central from nephrogenic diabetes insipidus?***

Following the water deprivation test, when serum osmolality is sufficiently high and urine osmolality is inappropriately low, the patient should be given desmopressin, a synthetic vasopressin analogue. In patients with central DI, a full response to desmopressin would be expected (urine volume will decline while urine osmolality rises). In patients with nephrogenic DI, because of resistance to desmopressin, there would be no appreciable changes to urine volume and osmolality.[13]

***Is the hypernatremia in this case acute or chronic?***

Given that the patient in this case is symptomatic, acute hypernatremia is most likely. The recent history of water deprivation during the camping trip is also indicative of an acute process.

***What is the significance of the history of polyuria and increased thirst in this case?***

Given the history of polyuria and increased thirst, it is likely that the patient in this case has had DI for at least several months. With an intact thirst mechanism, most patients with DI are able to achieve relatively normal serum $Na^+$ concentrations, assuming there is adequate access to water. In this case, a lack of adequate water access led to an abrupt rise in serum $Na^+$.

***What is the management of hypernatremia?***

For symptomatic acute hypernatremia (<24-48 hours), rapid treatment is imperative. This can be achieved by infusing a hypotonic fluid (eg, 5% dextrose in water) with the aim of immediately restoring normal serum $Na^+$ concentration. Chronic hypernatremia should be corrected more cautiously to prevent events such as cerebral edema and seizure. Correction of serum $Na^+$ at a rate of <0.5 mEq/L per hour (<12 mEq/d) is recommended in cases of chronic hypernatremia.[2]

## KEY POINTS

- Water homeostasis, which controls serum $Na^+$ concentration, is regulated by thirst and the hormonal interplay between the central nervous system and the kidneys.
- Maintenance of normal serum $Na^+$ concentration is important for preserving cell volume.
- Hypernatremia is generally defined as serum $Na^+$ >142 mEq/L.
- Clinical manifestations of hypernatremia depend on its duration and severity.
- Acute hypernatremia is often symptomatic with manifestations that include thirst, muscle weakness, decreased consciousness, delirium, convulsions, coma, and brain shrinkage, which can lead to osmotic demyelination, and vascular rupture with intracranial hemorrhage.
- Chronic hypernatremia is often asymptomatic.
- Hypernatremia can be associated with extracellular hypovolemia, euvolemia, or hypervolemia.
- Hypovolemic hypernatremia results from extracellular loss of hypotonic fluid (water > salt).

## KEY POINTS—CONT'D

- Hypovolemic hypernatremia can be caused by renal or extrarenal processes.
- Euvolemic hypernatremia results from extracellular deficiency of pure water.
- Hypervolemic hypernatremia results from extracellular gain of hypertonic fluid (salt > water).
- Acute symptomatic hypernatremia should be corrected rapidly with infusion of hypotonic fluid and serial monitoring of serum $Na^+$ concentration.
- Chronic hypernatremia should be corrected judiciously to prevent cerebral edema and seizures.

## REFERENCES


1. Adrogue HJ, Madias NE. Hypernatremia. *N Engl J Med*. 2000;342(20):1493-1499.
2. Sterns RH. Disorders of plasma sodium–causes, consequences, and correction. *N Engl J Med*. 2015;372(1):55-65.
3. Spital A, Sterns RD. The paradox of sodium's volume of distribution. Why an extracellular solute appears to distribute over total body water. *Arch Intern Med*. 1989;149(6):1255-1257.
4. Liamis G, Filippatos TD, Elisaf MS. Evaluation and treatment of hypernatremia: a practical guide for physicians. *Postgrad Med*. 2016;128(3):299-306.
5. Szatalowicz VL, Miller PD, Lacher JW, Gordon JA, Schrier RW. Comparative effect of diuretics on renal water excretion in hyponatraemic oedematous disorders. *Clin Sci (Lond)*. 1982;62(2):235-238.
6. Halbgewachs C, Domes T. Postobstructive diuresis: pay close attention to urinary retention. *Can Fam Physician*. 2015;61(2):137-142.
7. Schwartz IL, Thaysen JH. Excretion of sodium and potassium in human sweat. *J Clin Invest*. 1956;35(1):114-120.
8. Fenske W, Allolio B. Clinical review: current state and future perspectives in the diagnosis of diabetes insipidus: a clinical review. *J Clin Endocrinol Metab*. 2012;97(10):3426-3437.
9. Felig P, Johnson C, Levitt M, Cunningham J, Keefe F, Boglioli B. Hypernatremia induced by maximal exercise. *JAMA*. 1982;248(10):1209-1211.
10. Welt LG, Orloff J, Kydd DM, Oltman JE. An example of cellular hyperosmolarity. *J Clin Invest*. 1950;29(7):935-939.
11. Funder JW, Carey RM, Mantero F, et al. The management of primary aldosteronism: case detection, diagnosis, and treatment: an Endocrine Society Clinical Practice Guideline. *J Clin Endocrinol Metab*. 2016;101(5):1889-1916.
12. Ellison DH, Berl T. Clinical practice. The syndrome of inappropriate antidiuresis. *N Engl J Med*. 2007;356(20):2064-2072.
13. Kalra S, Zargar AH, Jain SM, et al. Diabetes insipidus: the other diabetes. *Indian J Endocrinol Metab*. 2016;20(1):9-21.
14. Timper K, Fenske W, Kuhn F, et al. Diagnostic accuracy of copeptin in the differential diagnosis of the polyuria-polydipsia syndrome: a Prospective Multicenter Study. *J Clin Endocrinol Metab*. 2015;100(6):2268-2274.

Chapter 37

# HYPOKALEMIA

## Case: A 43-year-old woman with dry mouth

A 43-year-old woman presents to the clinic with several weeks of generalized weakness, muscle aches, and episodes of muscle cramps that have been increasing in frequency. Before these symptoms began, she reports a long-standing history of dry eyes, dry mouth with difficulty swallowing, and vaginal dryness. Recent medical history is notable for spontaneous passage of a kidney stone. She denies diarrhea. She does not take any medications.

Blood pressure is 118/82 mm Hg, and respiratory rate is 22 breaths per minute. There is bilateral conjunctival erythema. A small strip of filter paper is placed inside the lower eyelids, and the patient is asked to close her eyes. After 5 minutes, there is 2.8 mm of moisture on the paper strip from the right eye and 3.1 mm of moisture on the paper strip from the left eye (normal wetting is ≥5 mm).

Serum sodium ($Na^+$) is 138 mEq/L; potassium ($K^+$), 1.8 mEq/L; chloride ($Cl^-$), 116 mEq/L; bicarbonate ($HCO_3^-$), 12 mEq/L; blood urea nitrogen, 21 mg/dL; creatinine, 1.1 mg/dL; and glucose, 102 mg/dL. Serum pH is 7.30. Urine sodium is 30 mEq/L, potassium is 40 mEq/L, and chloride is 38 mEq/L. Urine pH is 6.80.

Electrocardiogram is shown in Figure 37-1.

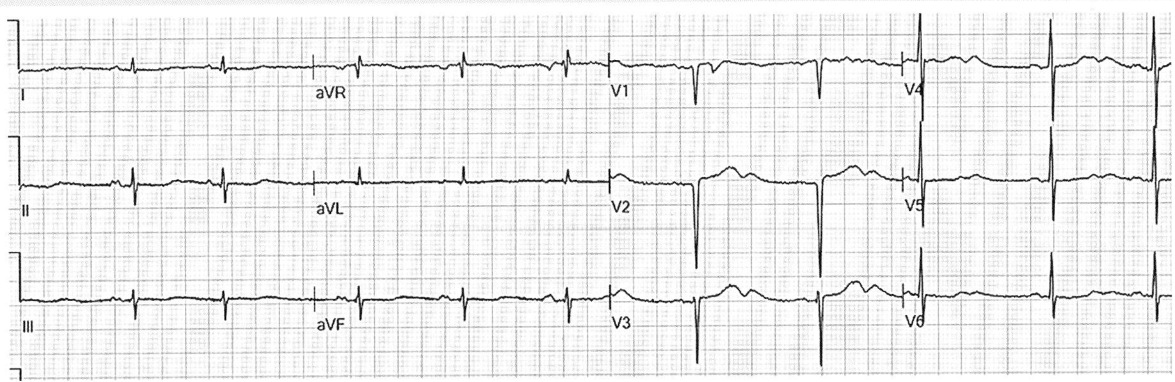


**Figure 37-1.** (Courtesy of Ignatius Zarraga, MD.)

***What is the most likely cause of hypokalemia in this patient?***

**What is normal serum $K^+$ concentration?**

The normal range for serum $K^+$ may vary slightly between laboratories, but is typically 3.6 to 5 mEq/L.[1]

**How common is hypokalemia?**

Hypokalemia is one of the most common electrolyte abnormalities, affecting around one-fifth of hospitalized patients.[2]

**How is $K^+$ normally distributed within the body?**

Approximately 98% of total body $K^+$ is sequestered within cells (mostly muscle cells), with the remaining 2% in the extracellular fluid compartment.[1]

**Why is it important to maintain a normal extracellular $K^+$ concentration?**

The ratio of intracellular to extracellular $K^+$ is the most important determining factor of the resting membrane potential of neurons and myocytes, which allows for the generation and propagation of action potentials necessary for normal function and stability of the heart and other muscles.[3]

**What systems are responsible for regulating serum K⁺ concentration?**

The kidneys maintain total body $K^+$ balance by matching excretion with intake, a hormonal process that occurs over a period of hours. The movement of $K^+$ between the intracellular and extracellular compartments (ie, transcellular shift) regulates more acute changes in serum $K^+$ concentration. The gastrointestinal (GI) tract normally clears around 10% of $K^+$ intake.[3]

**What are the symptoms of hypokalemia?**

Symptoms of hypokalemia may include malaise, muscle weakness, myalgias, cramping, and constipation.[4]

**What are the electrocardiographic manifestations of hypokalemia?**

Electrocardiographic manifestations of hypokalemia include (in order of increasing severity) decreased amplitude and broadening of the T wave, depression of the ST segment, increase in P-wave amplitude and duration, increase in QRS duration, the emergence of the U wave (most commonly seen in precordial leads $V_2$ and $V_3$), and fusion of the T and U waves (Figure 37-2).[2]

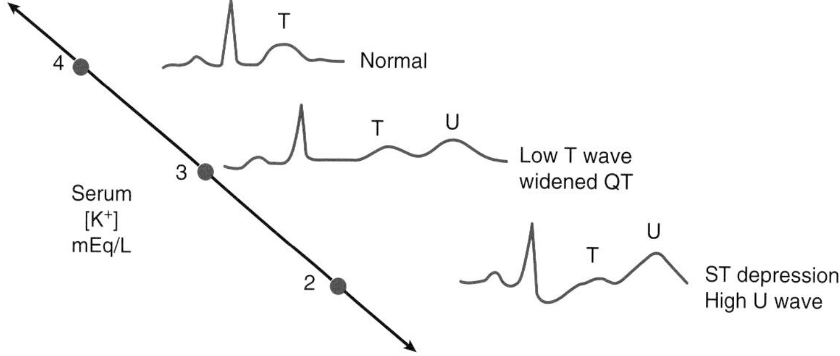


**Figure 37-2.** ECG manifestations of hypokalemia. (From Marino PL. *Marino's The ICU Book*. 4th ed. Philadelphia, PA: Wolters Kluwer Health/Lippincott Williams & Wilkins; 2014.)

**Which cardiac dysrhythmias are associated with hypokalemia?**

Hypokalemia can result in tachyarrhythmia (including ventricular tachycardia and ventricular fibrillation) and atrioventricular block.[2]

**What are the 3 general mechanisms of hypokalemia?**

Hypokalemia can be caused by low intake, excess loss, or transcellular shift of $K^+$.

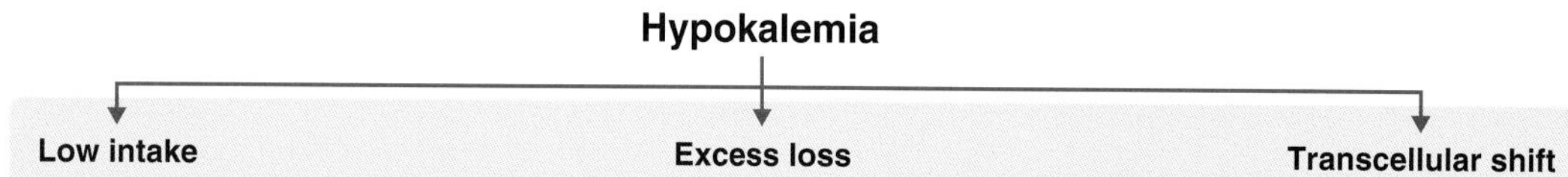


## HYPOKALEMIA RELATED TO LOW ORAL INTAKE OF POTASSIUM

**When K⁺ intake is zero, what happens to total body K⁺?**

Despite the presence of compensatory mechanisms to maintain total body $K^+$, when intake is zero, obligatory $K^+$ losses in urine and stool still occur, resulting in the net loss of $K^+$ over time.[5]

### What are the causes of hypokalemia related to poor intake?

**A 48-year-old man with a history of chronic heavy alcohol consumption presents with weakness and is found to have hypophosphatemia and hypokalemia.**

Poor oral intake.

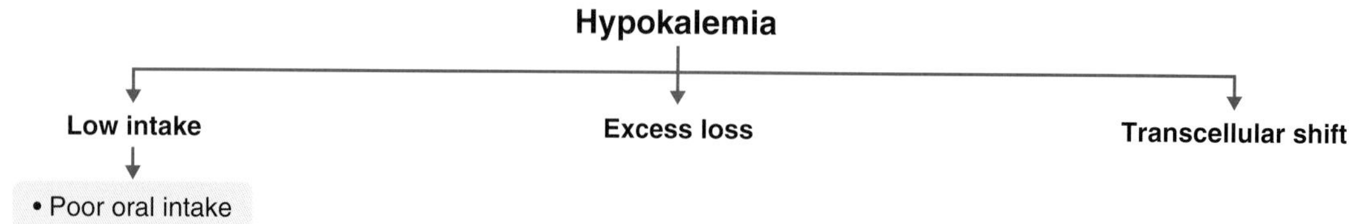

**What is the average daily oral $K^+$ intake in the industrialized world?**

The average oral $K^+$ intake in the industrialized world is approximately 75 mEq/d for men and 55 mEq/d for women.[5]

**Under normal circumstances, what proportion of dietary $K^+$ is absorbed in the gastrointestinal tract?**

Approximately 85% to 90% of dietary $K^+$ is absorbed in the GI tract, the vast majority of which occurs in the small intestine.[5]

**What compensatory mechanism preserves $K^+$ homeostasis when oral intake is low?**

When oral intake of $K^+$ is low, there is a compensatory reduction in renal and GI excretion of $K^+$. When dietary $K^+$ intake is zero, obligatory renal losses decrease to approximately 5 to 10 mEq/d.[5]

## HYPOKALEMIA RELATED TO EXCESS LOSS OF POTASSIUM

**What is the main source of $K^+$ loss from the body?**

The kidneys are the main source of $K^+$ excretion (Figure 37-3).

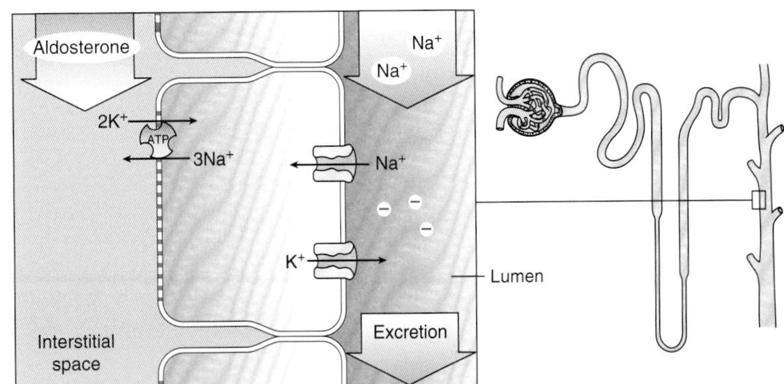


Figure 37-3. $K^+$ excretion depends on 2 factors. First, the hormone aldosterone must be present. Aldosterone increases the activity of the basolateral $Na^+/K^+$- ATPase, which generates the gradient for $Na^+$ movement from the tubule into the cell. Second, there must be adequate distal delivery of $Na^+$ to supply the epithelial $Na^+$ channel. Intracellular movement of $Na^+$ generates a negative charge within the tubular lumen, which is the driving force for $K^+$ excretion via apical channels. (From Danziger J, Zeidel M, Parker MJ, Schwartzstein RM. *Renal Physiology: A Clinical Approach*. Philadelphia, PA: Lippincott Williams & Wilkins; 2012.)

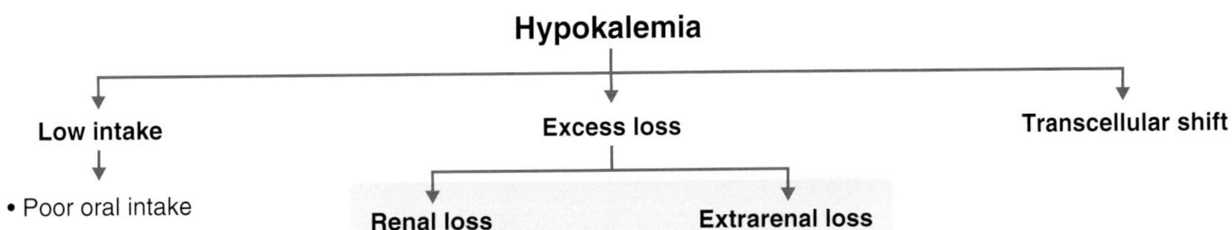


## HYPOKALEMIA RELATED TO RENAL LOSS OF POTASSIUM

### What are the causes of hypokalemia related to renal loss of potassium?

**Iatrogenic.**

Medication.

**Another electrolyte is to blame.**

Hypomagnesemia.

**Polyuria in a patient with hyperglycemia.**

Osmotic diuresis.

**Hypertension and hypokalemia.**

Mineralocorticoid excess.

**Increased intraluminal negative charge promotes $K^+$ excretion in the kidney.**

Nonreabsorbable anions.

**A cause of non-anion gap metabolic acidosis.**

Renal tubular acidosis (RTA).

This genetic condition mimics the mechanism of thiazide diuretics. — Gitelman's syndrome.

This genetic condition mimics the mechanism of loop diuretics. — Bartter's syndrome.

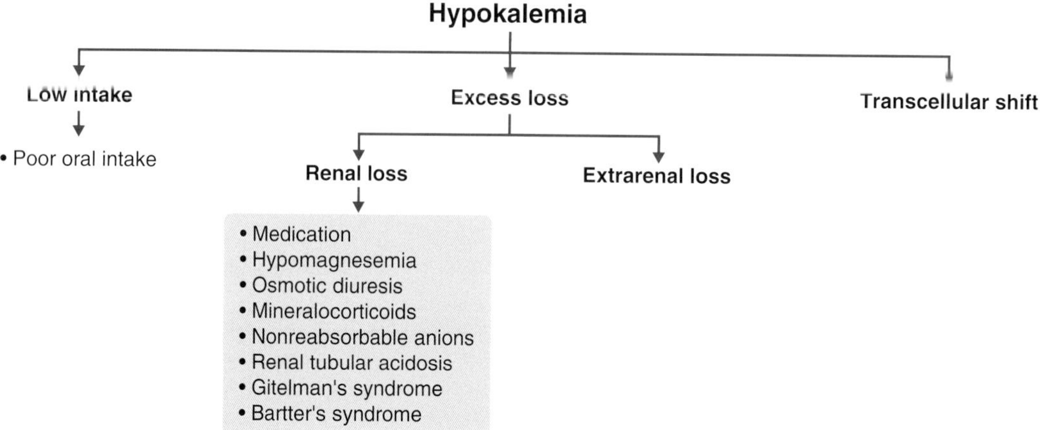


**Which medications are associated with renal $K^+$ loss?**

Medications commonly associated with hypokalemia include loop diuretics, thiazide diuretics, antimicrobials (eg, amphotericin B), mineralocorticoids (eg, fludrocortisone), and glucocorticoids (eg, prednisone).[4]

**Why is it important to evaluate for hypomagnesemia in patients with hypokalemia?**

Coexistent hypomagnesemia can impair $K^+$ repletion. It must be corrected for $K^+$ supplementation to be completely effective.[6]

**What is the mechanism of hypokalemia in patients with osmotic diuresis?**

Osmotic diuresis results in increased $Na^+$ and water delivery to the distal tubule, which promotes $Na^+$ and $K^+$ exchange (see Figure 37-3).

**What are the causes of aldosterone-independent syndromes of mineralocorticoid excess?**

Aldosterone-independent causes of mineralocorticoid excess include Cushing's syndrome, congenital adrenal hyperplasia, apparent mineralocorticoid excess, licorice ingestion, glucocorticoid resistance, exogenous mineralocorticoids, Liddle syndrome, and Geller syndrome.

**What are some examples of nonreabsorbable anions?**

Examples of nonreabsorbable anions include bicarbonate in patients with vomiting, β-hydroxybutyrate in diabetic ketoacidosis, and penicillin antibiotics. These anions increase the intraluminal negative charge of the distal nephron, promoting $K^+$ excretion.[7]

**Which types of renal tubular acidosis are associated with hypokalemia?**

Non-anion gap metabolic acidosis is a consequence of all types of RTA. Types 1 and 2 in particular are associated with hypokalemia. RTA type 4 (ie, hypoaldosteronism) is associated with hyperkalemia.[8]

**Which syndrome is more common, Bartter's or Gitelman's?**

Gitelman's syndrome is significantly more prevalent in the general population (1 in 40,000) compared with Bartter's syndrome (1 in 1,000,000).[9]

## HYPOKALEMIA RELATED TO EXTRARENAL LOSS OF POTASSIUM

### What are the causes of hypokalemia related to extrarenal loss of potassium?

The most common extrarenal source of $K^+$ loss from the body. — Gastrointestinal losses (eg, diarrhea, vomiting, tube drainage).

Hypokalemia in marathon runners. — Excessive perspiration.

Iatrogenic losses. — Dialysis and plasmapheresis.

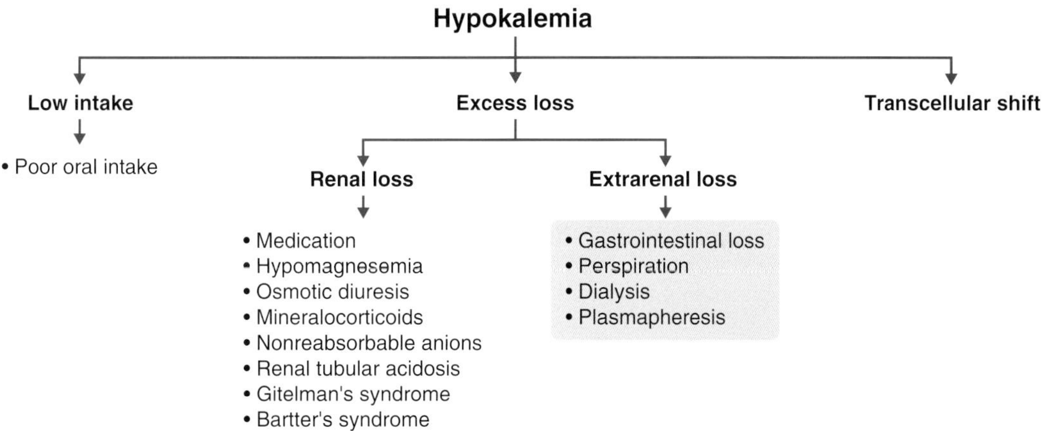


**What is average fecal $K^+$ excretion per day?**

In the industrialized world, normal fecal $K^+$ excretion averages 9 mEq/d. Excretion >16 to 22 mEq/d is excessive and may cause hypokalemia, particularly if it occurs over a prolonged period of time.[5]

**What is the concentration of $K^+$ in sweat?**

The average concentration of $K^+$ in sweat is approximately 9 mEq/L. Individuals who exercise in hot climates are capable of secreting >12 L of sweat per day.[10]

**How common is hypokalemia in peritoneal dialysis patients?**

Hypokalemia affects up to one-third of patients on peritoneal dialysis. It tends to occur more often in older patients and those with diabetes mellitus.[11]

**What is the mechanism of hypokalemia related to plasmapheresis?**

Hypokalemia associated with plasmapheresis occurs as a result of dilution when plasma is removed and replaced with a potassium-free solution (eg, albumin).

## HYPOKALEMIA RELATED TO TRANSCELLULAR SHIFT OF POTASSIUM

**How is the concentration gradient of $K^+$ between the intracellular and extracellular fluid compartments maintained?**

The concentration gradient of $K^+$ between the intracellular and extracellular fluid compartments is maintained by the $Na^+/K^+$-adenosine triphosphatase (ie, $Na^+/K^+$-ATPase or $Na^+/K^+$ pump), which uses energy to move $K^+$ against its concentration gradient from the extracellular to the intracellular compartment (see Figure 35-4).[3]

**What are the chief factors that affect transcellular shifts of $K^+$?**

Under normal conditions, insulin and catecholamines are the primary drivers of transcellular shifts of $K^+$. Acid-base derangements and plasma tonicity also affect transcellular shifts of $K^+$ (see Figure 35-4).[3]

### What are the causes of hypokalemia related to transcellular shift?

**The acid-base state of blood associated with Bartter's and Gitelman's syndromes.**

Alkalemia.

**Stress, exercise, and medications.**

Adrenergic excess.

**This hormone is often used as treatment for hyperkalemia.**

Insulin.

**Often induced therapeutically in some cases of cardiac arrest.**

Hypothermia.

**A familial disease resulting in transient episodes of weakness and paralysis with a male to female predominance of 3:1.**

Hypokalemic periodic paralysis.[12]

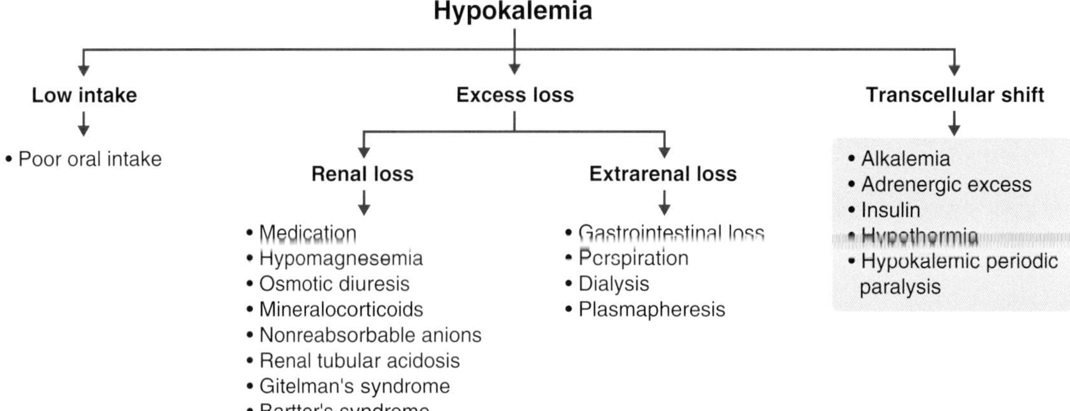


**In addition to being a cause of hypokalemia itself, alkalemia is associated with what other causes of hypokalemia?**

Alkalemia is associated with mineralocorticoid excess, Gitelman's syndrome, Bartter's syndrome, and excess GI loss (eg, vomiting) and can contribute to the hypokalemia generated by those conditions. Hypokalemia can be an important factor in the maintenance of alkalemia by impairing $HCO_3^-$ excretion and augmenting $H^+$ excretion in the kidney.[13]

**What are the effects of catecholamines on the $Na^+/K^+$ pump?**

β-Adrenergic receptors activate the $Na^+/K^+$ pump, whereas α-adrenergic receptors impair cellular entry of $K^+$ (see Figure 35-4).[3]

**What is the effect of insulin on the $Na^+/K^+$ pump?**

Insulin increases the activity of the $Na^+/K^+$ pump, thereby accelerating the movement of $K^+$ into the intracellular compartment (see Figure 35-4).[3]

**What syndrome can result in insulin-mediated cellular influx of $K^+$ after nutrition is given to a patient following a period of prolonged malnutrition?**

Refeeding syndrome is associated with insulin-mediated cellular influx of $K^+$.

**What dangerous electrolyte disturbance can occur in hypothermic patients who are supplemented with $K^+$ and subsequently rewarmed?**

Hyperkalemia can occur in patients with hypothermia during rewarming, as there is rapid efflux of $K^+$ from the intracellular to the extracellular compartment.[14]

**How common is hypokalemic periodic paralysis?**

The prevalence of hypokalemic periodic paralysis in the industrialized world is approximately 1 in 100,000 persons. It is transmitted in an autosomal dominant pattern and usually presents within the second decade of life. Factors that may trigger episodes of paralysis include emotion, stress, cold exposure, and alcohol ingestion. Attacks occur more often at night and are characterized by flaccid paralysis of all four limbs. The associated hypokalemia may be profound, with serum $K^+$ levels as low as 1 mEq/L.[12]

## Case Summary

A 43-year-old woman with a history of kidney stones presents with subacute weakness and myalgias, chronic dry eyes, dry mouth, and vaginal dryness, and is found to have severe hypokalemia and other metabolic derangements.

***What is the most likely cause of hypokalemia in this patient?***

Renal tubular acidosis type 1 (distal).

### BONUS QUESTIONS

***What is renal tubular acidosis?***

RTA describes a group of conditions in which there is impaired capacity for urinary acidification despite relatively preserved glomerular filtration, resulting in net acid retention, non-anion gap metabolic acidosis, and various electrolyte disturbances. The 3 major forms include RTA type 1 (distal), RTA type 2 (proximal), and RTA type 4 (ie, hypoaldosteronism). The 2 forms of distal RTA (types 1 and 4) occur as a result of impaired $H^+$ excretion, whereas RTA type 2 occurs as a result of impaired bicarbonate reabsorption.[8]

***What is the significance of the urine pH in this case?***

In the setting of acidemia, renal acidification of urine (measured by urine pH) can be used as a marker of renal compensatory capacity. In general, appropriate compensation results in urine pH <5.3. If the urine pH is >5.5 (as in this case) it suggests impaired renal acidification of urine, consistent with RTA. Urine pH >5.5 is typical of RTA type 1 but is a less reliable finding in other types of RTA.[8,15]

***What is the significance of the positive urine anion gap (UAG) in this case?***

$UAG = (Na^+_{urine} + K^+_{urine}) - Cl^-_{urine}$. Ammonium ($NH_4^+$) is the major unmeasured cation in urine. In the setting of acidemia and normal renal function, there is a compensatory increase in acid elimination by the kidney via $NH_4^+$ excretion, which is reflected by a negative UAG. A negative UAG therefore indicates a source of acidemia with intact renal $NH_4^+$ excretion (eg, diarrhea). If the UAG is positive, as in this case, then urine $NH_4^+$ is low, indicating impairment in $NH_4^+$ excretion (eg, distal RTA). The UAG is typically negative in the setting of RTA type 2 because distal acidification is intact. The UAG can be helpful in differentiating proximal and distal RTAs.[8]

***Which additional laboratory finding in this case is suggestive of renal tubular acidosis type 1 as opposed to type 4?***

The presence of hypokalemia in this case is suggestive of RTA type 1. RTA type 4, on the other hand, is associated with hyperkalemia.[8]

***What finding is present on the electrocardiogram in this case?***

The electrocardiogram in this case (see Figure 37-1) demonstrates prominent U waves (particularly in the precordial leads V2 and V3), a characteristic electrocardiographic feature of hypokalemia.

***What is the mechanism of hypokalemia in patients with renal tubular acidosis type 1?***

The chronic metabolic acidosis of RTA type 1 increases the flow rate and delivery of $Na^+$ and water to the distal nephron through a variety of mechanisms. This leads to volume depletion, which stimulates renin and aldosterone secretion. Increased $Na^+$ delivery and elevated aldosterone levels are potent stimulants of $K^+$ secretion in the distal nephron, leading to hypokalemia.[1]

***How much $K^+$ should be given to correct hypokalemia?***

In patients with normal renal function, 10 mEq of $K^+$ would be expected to raise the serum $K^+$ concentration by approximately 0.1 mEq/L.

***What is the significance of the history of kidney stones in this case?***

RTA type 1 is associated with hypercalciuria, hypocitraturia, and alkaline urine. Such an environment promotes the formation of calcium phosphate stones.[16]

***What is the pathophysiology of renal tubular acidosis type 1?***

RTA type 1 is caused by inherited or acquired defects of the $\alpha$-intercalated cells of the collecting duct (eg, impaired activity of the luminal $H^+$-ATPase) that retard $H^+$ excretion.[8]

| | |
|---|---|
| ***What is the treatment for renal tubular acidosis type 1?*** | Because urinary acid excretion is impaired in patients with RTA type 1, exogenous alkali therapy is necessary to balance daily acid production. Sodium bicarbonate or sodium citrate is typically used. Citrate salts have the added benefit of correcting hypocitraturia, which can prevent the formation of kidney stones. Correction of the underlying metabolic acidosis usually corrects the associated hypokalemia. However, some patients may require chronic $K^+$ supplementation.[17] |
| ***What is the significance of the dry mucous membranes and minimal tear production in this case?*** | In this case, the history of dry eyes, dry mouth, vaginal dryness, and minimal tear production on Schirmer's test are indicative of Sjögren's syndrome, which can be associated with RTA type 1.[8] |

## KEY POINTS

- Potassium homeostasis is regulated by the interplay between exogenous intake, excretion in urine and stool, and transcellular shifts.
- Maintenance of normal serum $K^+$ concentration is important for the stability of heart and muscle cells.
- Hypokalemia is generally defined as serum $K^+$ <3.6 mEq/L.
- Clinical manifestations of hypokalemia include malaise, muscle weakness, myalgias, cramps, constipation, electrocardiographic changes (eg, U waves), and dysrhythmia.
- Hypokalemia can be caused by low intake, excess loss, or transcellular shift of $K^+$.
- Excess $K^+$ loss can be renal or extrarenal in nature.
- Transcellular shift of $K^+$ occurs rapidly and is primarily driven by insulin and catecholamines.
- In patients with normal renal function, 10 mEq of $K^+$ would be expected to raise the serum $K^+$ concentration by approximately 0.1 mEq/L.

## REFERENCES


1. Aronson PS, Giebisch G. Effects of pH on potassium: new explanations for old observations. *J Am Soc Nephrol*. 2011;22(11):1981-1989.
2. El-Sherif N, Turitto G. Electrolyte disorders and arrhythmogenesis. *Cardiol J*. 2011;18(3):233-245.
3. Palmer BF. Regulation of potassium homeostasis. *Clin J Am Soc Nephrol*. 2015;10(6):1050-1060.
4. Veltri KT, Mason C. Medication-induced hypokalemia. *P T*. 2015;40(3):185-190.
5. Agarwal R, Afzalpurkar R, Fordtran JS. Pathophysiology of potassium absorption and secretion by the human intestine. *Gastroenterology*. 1994;107(2):548-571.
6. Whang R, Whang DD, Ryan MP. Refractory potassium repletion. A consequence of magnesium deficiency. *Arch Intern Med*. 1992;152(1):40-45.
7. Mohr JA, Clark RM, Waack TC, Whang R. Nafcillin-associated hypokalemia. *JAMA*. 1979;242(6):544.
8. Reddy P. Clinical approach to renal tubular acidosis in adult patients. *Int J Clin Pract*. 2011;65(3):350-360.
9. Ji W, Foo JN, O'Roak BJ, et al. Rare independent mutations in renal salt handling genes contribute to blood pressure variation. *Nat Genet*. 2008;40(5):592-599.
10. Knochel JP, Dotin LN, Hamburger RJ. Pathophysiology of intense physical conditioning in a hot climate. I. Mechanisms of potassium depletion. *J Clin Invest*. 1972;51(2):242-255.
11. Kim HW, Chang JH, Park SY, et al. Factors associated with hypokalemia in continuous ambulatory peritoneal dialysis patients. *Electrolyte Blood Press*. 2007;5(2):102-110.
12. Fontaine B, Lapie P, Plassart E, et al. Periodic paralysis and voltage-gated ion channels. *Kidney Int*. 1996;49(1):9-18.
13. Palmer BF. Evaluation and treatment of respiratory alkalosis. *Am J Kidney Dis*. 2012;60(5):834-838.
14. Zydlewski AW, Hasbargen JA. Hypothermia-induced hypokalemia. *Mil Med*. 1998;163(10):719-721.
15. Yaxley J, Pirrone C. Review of the diagnostic evaluation of renal tubular acidosis. *Ochsner J*. 2016;16(4):525-530.
16. Pereira PC, Miranda DM, Oliveira EA, Silva AC. Molecular pathophysiology of renal tubular acidosis. *Curr Genomics*. 2009;10(1):51-59.
17. Batlle D, Haque SK. Genetic causes and mechanisms of distal renal tubular acidosis. *Nephrol Dial Transplant*. 2012;27(10):3691-3704.

Chapter 38

# HYPONATREMIA

## Case: A 68-year-old man with hemoptysis

A previously healthy 68-year-old man presents to the clinic after coughing up streaks of blood over the past week. He has experienced mild nausea and malaise over the same period of time. His wife has insisted he maintain his normal food and fluid intake. He smokes 1.5 packs of cigarettes per day, a nearly lifelong habit.

Heart rate is 80 beats per minute, blood pressure is 123/81 mm Hg, and respiratory rate is 22 breaths per minute. Mucous membranes and axillae are moist. Jugular venous pressure is estimated to be 6 cm $H_2O$. There is no peripheral edema.

Serum sodium ($Na^+$) is 120 mEq/L; blood urea nitrogen (BUN), 13 mg/dL; serum creatinine, 0.8 mg/dL; serum osmolality, 264 mOsm/kg; urine $Na^+$, 60 mEq/L; and urine osmolality, 620 mOsm/kg.

Contrast-enhanced computed tomography imaging of the chest with coronal (Figure 38-1A) and axial (Figure 38-1B) views reveals a right hilar mass measuring 9.5 × 7.5 cm with encasement of the right main bronchus and bronchus intermedius; there are associated enlarged right paratracheal, subcarinal, and supraclavicular lymph nodes.

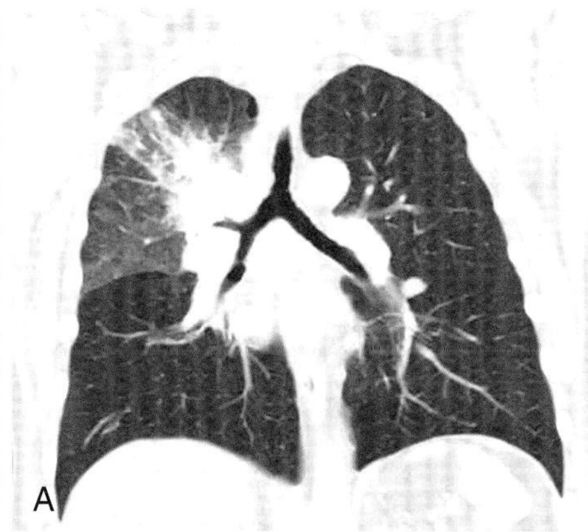

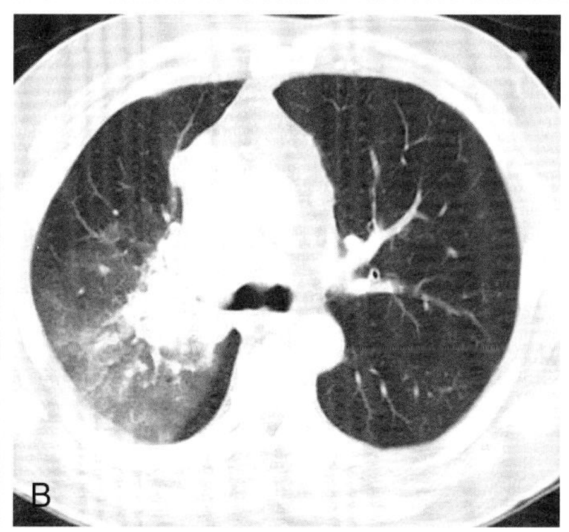


**Figure 38-1.**

***What is the most likely cause of hyponatremia in this patient?***

**What is hyponatremia?**

Hyponatremia is defined as low serum $Na^+$ concentration that occurs when there is an excess of water relative to $Na^+$ in the extracellular fluid compartment.[1]

**What is normal serum $Na^+$ concentration?**

Normal serum $Na^+$ is 135 to 142 mEq/L.[2]

**How is the severity of hyponatremia defined?**

Severity of hyponatremia is variably defined, but the following thresholds provide a rule of thumb: serum $Na^+$ 130 to 135 mEq/L is mild, serum $Na^+$ 125 to 129 mEq/L is moderate, and serum $Na^+$ <125 mEq/L is severe.[1]

**How common is hyponatremia?**

Hyponatremia is one of the most common electrolyte abnormalities in hospitalized patients, with at least mild hyponatremia occurring in up to one-fifth of patients.[1]

**How is $Na^+$ normally distributed within the body?**

Most $Na^+$ resides in extracellular fluid, and its distribution between extracellular and intracellular fluid is regulated by the $Na^+/K^+$-adenosine triphosphatase (ie, $Na^+/K^+$-ATPase or $Na^+/K^+$ pump).[3]

**How is water homeostasis regulated?**

The central nervous system and the kidneys work in concert to maintain water homeostasis, which ultimately controls serum $Na^+$ concentration. Osmoreceptors located in the hypothalamus detect extracellular tonicity and respond by adjusting thirst and the secretion of vasopressin (ie, arginine vasopressin [AVP], or antidiuretic hormone [ADH]). Vasopressin acts in the kidney to increase the reabsorption of free water; it can concentrate the urine to a maximum of 1200 mOsm/kg. In the absence of vasopressin, urine osmolality can drop to a minimum of 50 mOsm/kg. In the setting of hyponatremia, thirst and vasopressin secretion should be inhibited. A significant decrease in blood volume also stimulates vasopressin secretion (see Figure 36-1).[2]

**What are the effects of serum $Na^+$ concentration on cell volume?**

Sodium is an effective solute and therefore contributes to overall serum tonicity. Water moves freely between fluid compartments in response to differences in tonicity. Accordingly, the presence of hypernatremia, which is always associated with hypertonicity, will result in a shift of water out of cells, causing cellular contraction. Conversely, hypotonic hyponatremia will result in a shift of water into cells, causing cellular swelling (see Figure 36-2).[3]

**What are the effects of serum $Na^+$ concentration on brain tissue?**

In most tissues of the body, the $Na^+$ concentrations of serum and interstitial fluid are virtually identical due to free movement of $Na^+$ through the capillary membrane. In contrast, capillaries in the brain are impermeable to $Na^+$. The result is that an abnormal serum $Na^+$ concentration will cause water to move into or out of brain tissue, with subsequent swelling or contraction, respectively. Only minimal changes in the volume of brain tissue are compatible with life.[2]

**What adaptive mechanisms occur in the setting of chronic hyponatremia?**

In the setting of chronic hypotonic hyponatremia, defined by at least 24 to 48 hours' duration, osmotically active intracellular molecules (osmolytes) (eg, glutamate, taurine, myo-inositol) are leaked out of the cell. This helps decrease the difference in tonicity between extracellular and intracellular fluid, which in turn, decreases movement of water into cells. This adaptation is particularly important in brain tissue (Figure 38-2).[1,2]

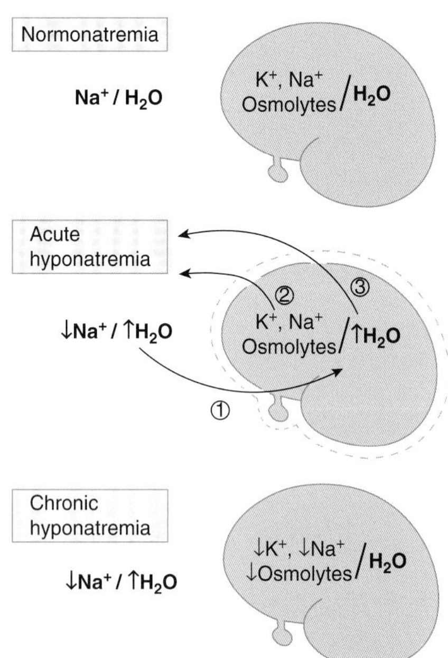


**Figure 38-2.** Schematic diagram of brain volume adaptation to hyponatremia. Under normal conditions brain tonicity and extracellular fluid tonicity are in equilibrium (top). Following the induction of extracellular fluid hypotonicity, water moves into the brain, producing brain edema (dotted line, middle, #1). However, in response to the induced swelling, the brain rapidly loses intracellular solutes (middle, #2). As water losses accompany the losses of brain solute, the expanded brain volume then decreases back toward normal (middle, #3). If hypotonicity is sustained, brain volume eventually normalizes completely, and the brain becomes fully adapted to hyponatremia (bottom). (From Schrier RW. *Diseases of the Kidney and Urinary Tract*. 8th ed. Philadelphia, PA: Lippincott Williams & Wilkins; 2007.)

**After correction of hypotonicity, how long does it take for the recovery of lost intracellular osmolytes to occur?**

After chronic hypotonicity is corrected, the recovery of lost intracellular electrolytes can take a week or longer.[2]

**What are the clinical differences between acute and chronic hyponatremia?**

Given the adaptation that occurs in response to chronic hyponatremia, patients are often asymptomatic. In contrast, patients with acute hyponatremia (developed over a period of hours) are almost always symptomatic, and changes in brain volume can be life-threatening. The physiologic adaptation that occurs in chronic hyponatremia limits the rate with which hyponatremia can be corrected (see Figure 36-3). In cases where duration is unknown, chronic hyponatremia should be assumed.[2]

**What are the clinical manifestations of acute hyponatremia?**

Clinical manifestations of acute hyponatremia may include nausea, malaise, lethargy, headache, delirium, obtundation, seizure, and coma.[2]

**What is the first step in establishing the cause of hyponatremia?**

Determining serum tonicity is the first step in establishing the cause of hyponatremia.

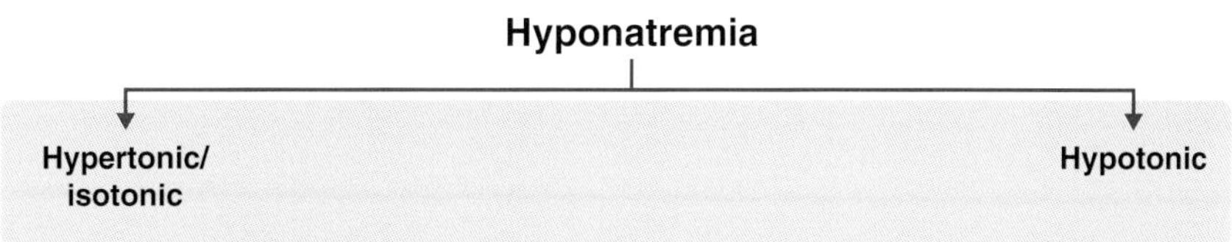


**What are the laboratory definitions of hypertonicity, isotonicity, and hypotonicity?**

Hypertonicity is present when the effective serum osmolality is >295 mOsm/kg, hypotonicity is present when the effective serum osmolality is <275 mOsm/kg, and isotonicity is present when the effective serum osmolality is 275 to 295 mOsm/kg.[4]

**What is the difference between serum osmolality and serum tonicity?**

Serum osmolality takes into account all solutes, including those that are effective (ie, solutes that do not freely move between the intracellular and extracellular fluid compartments) and those that are ineffective (ie, solutes that move freely). In contrast, serum tonicity (also called effective osmolality) takes into account only effective solutes.

**What is the clinical difference between effective and ineffective solutes?**

Ineffective solutes contribute to serum osmolality, but move freely between intracellular and extracellular fluid compartments to maintain an even concentration gradient and, therefore, do not generate an osmotic gradient. Without an osmotic gradient, movement of water between extracellular and intracellular fluid compartments does not occur. Effective solutes, in contrast, do not move freely, giving rise to osmotic gradients that trigger movement of water.

**What are the main contributors to serum osmolality?**

The main contributors to serum osmolality include serum $Na^+$, glucose, and BUN.

$$\text{Calculated serum osmolality (mOsm/kg)} = (2 \times [Na^+]) + ([\text{glucose}]/18) + ([\text{BUN}]/2.8)$$

*In the above formula, [Na⁺] is measured in mEq/L or mmol/L, and [glucose] and [BUN] are measured in mg/dL.*[5]

**Are $Na^+$, glucose, and urea effective or ineffective solutes?**

Sodium and glucose are effective solutes, whereas urea is an ineffective solute.

**How could the formula for serum osmolality be modified to better reflect serum tonicity?**

To better reflect serum tonicity, the contribution of urea should be subtracted from the formula for serum osmolality because it is an ineffective solute.[1]

## HYPERTONIC AND ISOTONIC HYPONATREMIA

### What are the causes of hypertonic or isotonic hyponatremia?

**A common cause of hypertonic hyponatremia that is not associated with a serum osmolal gap.**

Hyperglycemia.

**This agent may be used to acutely reduce intracranial pressure.**

Hypertonic mannitol.

**Laboratory artifact.**

Pseudohyponatremia.

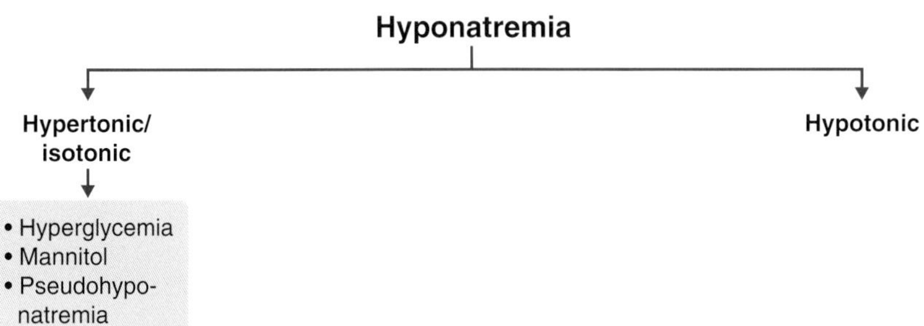


**What is the expected decrease in serum $Na^+$ concentration caused by hyperglycemia?**

For each 100 mg/dL increase in serum glucose concentration above 100 mg/dL, the serum $Na^+$ decreases by 1.6 to 2.4 mEq/L. Using a correctional factor of 2.0 mEq/L, the following formula can be used to determine the value that should be added to the measured serum $Na^+$ concentration[1]:

([measured glucose–100]/100) × 2.0

**What are the effects on cell volume of hyperosmolar hyponatremia related to either hyperglycemia or hypertonic mannitol?**

The hyperosmolality associated with hyperglycemia and hypertonic mannitol results in cellular contraction. Because glucose and mannitol are effective solutes, the resultant high serum tonicity acts to draw water out of cells and into the extracellular fluid compartment. This dilutes the serum $Na^+$ concentration, resulting in hyponatremia.

**Are there any circumstances in which hyperosmolar hyponatremia may be associated with cellular swelling?**

Serum hyperosmolality related to ineffective solutes (eg, urea, alcohol) does not trigger the movement of water into the extracellular fluid compartment. If there is coexistent hyponatremia, it must be driven by an unrelated process, which could include those associated with serum hypotonicity. If overall serum tonicity is lower than intracellular tonicity, water will move into the intracellular fluid compartment, causing cellular swelling.

**What clinical conditions are associated with pseudohyponatremia?**

Pseudohyponatremia is associated with hyperlipidemia and paraproteinemia.[1]

## HYPOTONIC HYPONATREMIA

**What is the first step in establishing the cause of hypotonic hyponatremia?**

Determining extracellular fluid volume status is the first step in establishing the cause of hypotonic hyponatremia.

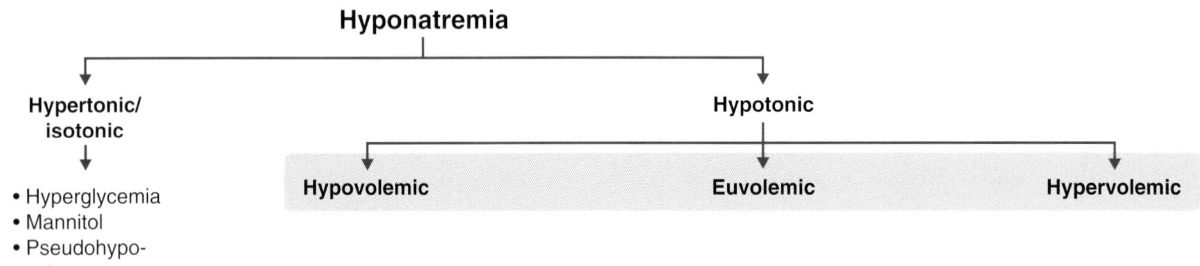

**What physical findings are associated with hypovolemia?**

Hypovolemia may be associated with decreased skin turgor, dry mucous membranes and axillae, increased capillary refill time, sunken eyes, and low jugular venous pressure.

**What physical findings are associated with hypervolemia?**

Hypervolemia may be associated with elevated jugular venous pressure, ascites, rales on lung auscultation (due to pulmonary edema), dullness to percussion of the lung bases (due to pleural effusions), and peripheral edema.

**What laboratory test can be helpful in distinguishing hypovolemic patients from euvolemic patients?**

In patients who are not hypervolemic, spot urine $Na^+$ concentration can be helpful in distinguishing between hypovolemia ($U_{Na}$ < 30 mEq/L) and euvolemia ($U_{Na}$ > 30 mEq/L). *Cases of hypovolemia due to renal $Na^+$ wasting (eg, primary adrenal insufficiency, diuretic use) can be associated with relatively higher $U_{Na}$, possibly exceeding 30 mEq/L.*[6]

## HYPOVOLEMIC HYPONATREMIA

*Hypovolemic hyponatremia can be thought of as extracellular loss of hypertonic fluid (salt > water).*

**What is the status of vasopressin levels in patients with hypovolemic hyponatremia?**

Decreased effective arterial blood volume (reduced by at least 10%-20%) with inadequate circulation results in baroreceptor-mediated release of vasopressin, which acts to maintain intravascular volume at the expense of serum tonicity (see Figure 36-1).[2]

**What are the 2 subcategories of hypovolemic hyponatremia?**

Hypovolemic hyponatremia can be caused by renal or extrarenal processes.

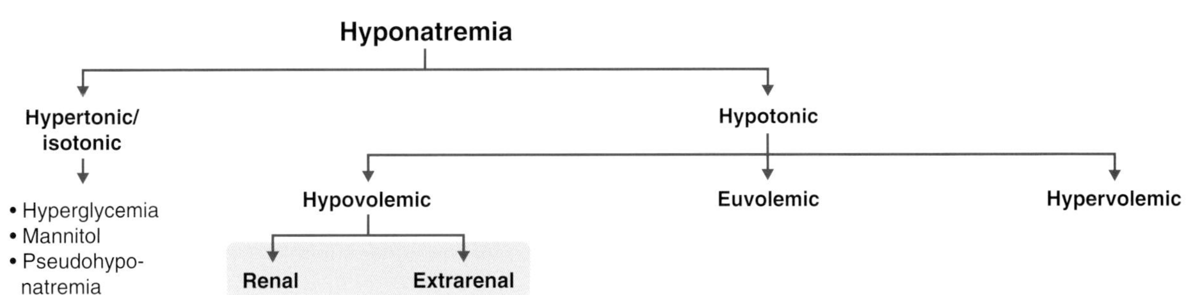


**Which laboratory test can be helpful in distinguishing renal from extrarenal causes of hypovolemic hyponatremia?**

Spot urine $Na^+$ concentration can be suggestive of whether the source of volume depletion is renal ($U_{Na}$ > 20 mEq/L) or extrarenal ($U_{Na}$ < 20 mEq/L, especially <10 mEq/L).[7,8]

## RENAL CAUSES OF HYPOVOLEMIC HYPONATREMIA

### What are the renal causes of hypovolemic hyponatremia?

**Iatrogenic loss of hypertonic fluid (relative to serum).**

Diuretic medication, particularly thiazide diuretics.

**Hyponatremia, hyperkalemia, and hypotension.**

Primary adrenal insufficiency.

**A 34-year-old woman with a subarachnoid hemorrhage related to a motor vehicle accident develops hypovolemic hyponatremia.**

Cerebral salt wasting.

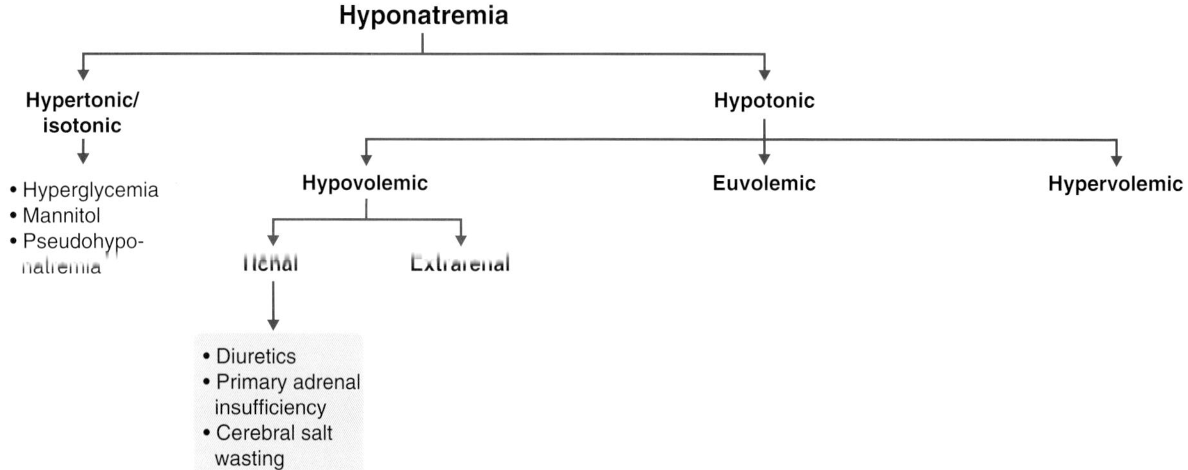


**What is the mechanism of hyponatremia related to thiazide diuretics?**

Thiazide diuretics decrease the reabsorption of $Na^+$ and chloride in the distal convoluted tubule (within the renal cortex), which ultimately impairs the ability of the kidneys to make dilute urine (see Figure 36-4). If the osmolality of the excreted urine exceeds that of serum, then hyponatremia will eventually occur. In addition, intravascular hypovolemia related to diuresis stimulates the secretion of vasopressin, which may contribute to the development of hyponatremia. *Patients with diuretic-induced hyponatremia may be euvolemic or hypervolemic.*[9]

**What is the treatment for hyponatremia related to adrenal insufficiency?**

Hyponatremia related to adrenal insufficiency should be treated with cortisol to decrease vasopressin release and intravenous fluids to improve the effective arterial blood volume.[10]

**What is cerebral salt wasting?**

Cerebral salt wasting occurs in the setting of central nervous system disease, particularly subarachnoid hemorrhage. It is characterized by hypovolemic hyponatremia, which develops as a result of renal $Na^+$ wasting. The pathogenesis is poorly understood. The timing of cerebral salt wasting can be variable, with some cases occurring within days of head injury and others occurring up to 2 months later. It may be confused with the syndrome of inappropriate antidiuretic hormone secretion (SIADH), but distinguishing between the two is important as treatment differs. For example, unlike SIADH, cerebral salt wasting should not be treated with water restriction. Volume repletion with isotonic saline is the treatment of choice.[11]

## EXTRARENAL CAUSES OF HYPOVOLEMIC HYPONATREMIA

### What are the extrarenal causes of hypovolemic hyponatremia?

**You cannot lose what you do not have.**

Poor oral intake.

**True isotonic fluid loss, resulting in decreased effective arterial blood volume.**

Gastrointestinal losses.

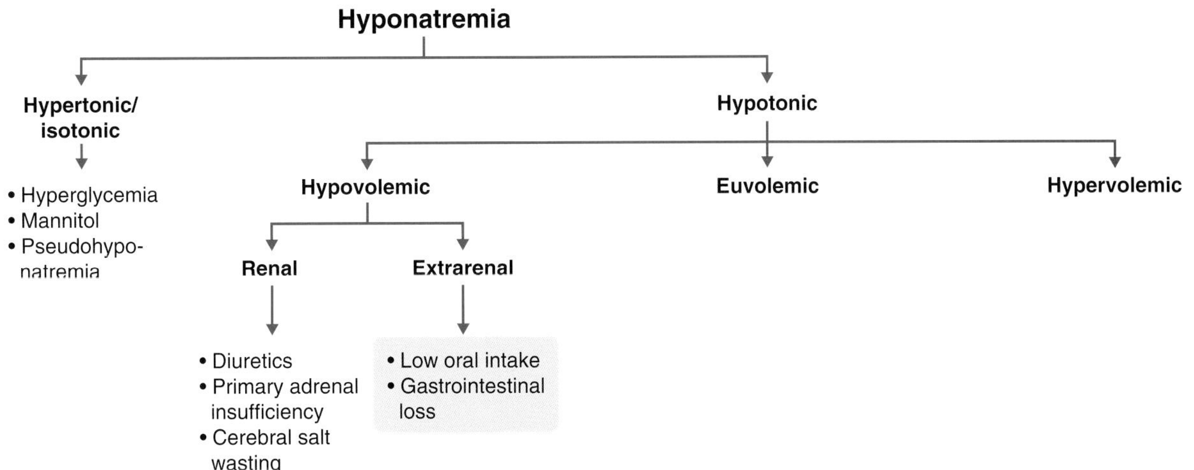


**Which groups of adults are at increased risk for low oral intake?**

Adult patients at risk for low oral intake include the elderly, alcoholics, the economically disadvantaged, and patients with eating disorders. Volume repletion with isotonic saline is the treatment of choice. Patients may be at risk for refeeding syndrome when oral intake resumes or increases.

**What are some causes of isotonic or hypertonic fluid loss from the gastrointestinal (GI) tract?**

Loss of isotonic or hypertonic fluid (relative to serum) from the GI tract can occur as a result of diarrhea, vomiting, or tube drainage. Volume repletion with isotonic saline is the treatment of choice.

## EUVOLEMIC HYPONATREMIA

*Euvolemic hyponatremia can be thought of as extracellular gain of pure water.*

**What is the status of vasopressin levels in patients with euvolemic hyponatremia?**

In euvolemic patients with hyponatremia, vasopressin is either present (vasopressin-dependent) or suppressed (vasopressin-independent), depending on the underlying cause.

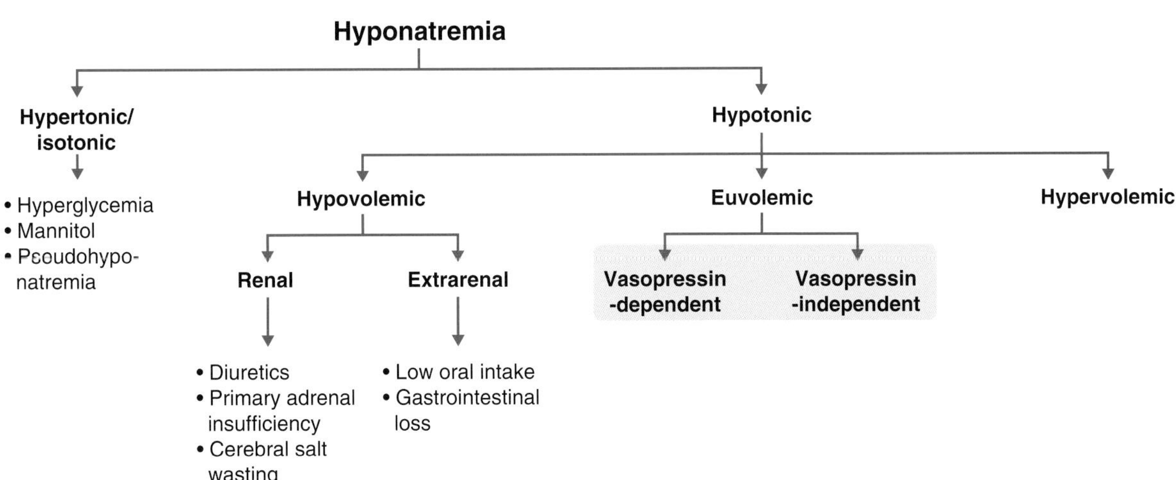


**Which laboratory test can be helpful in establishing whether euvolemic hyponatremia is related to a vasopressin-dependent or vasopressin-independent process?**

Urine osmolality can be suggestive of whether euvolemic hyponatremia is vasopressin-mediated or not. In the setting of hyponatremia, urine osmolality >100 mOsm/kg is consistent with a vasopressin-dependent process. In general, urine osmolality greater than serum osmolality nearly always indicates the presence of vasopressin.[1]

## VASOPRESSIN-DEPENDENT CAUSES OF EUVOLEMIC HYPONATREMIA

### What are the vasopressin-dependent causes of euvolemic hyponatremia?

**A 22-year-old woman with epilepsy is started on a new antiepileptic medication and is subsequently found to have a serum Na⁺ concentration of 122 mEq/L. She is euvolemic with a urine osmolality of 560 mOsm/kg.**

Syndrome of inappropriate antidiuretic hormone secretion.

**Endocrinopathies.**

Hypothyroidism and secondary adrenal insufficiency.

**In patients with this condition, thirst and vasopressin secretion may be stimulated at a serum Na⁺ concentration >132 mEq/L, and inhibited at values <132 mEq/L.**

Reset osmostat.

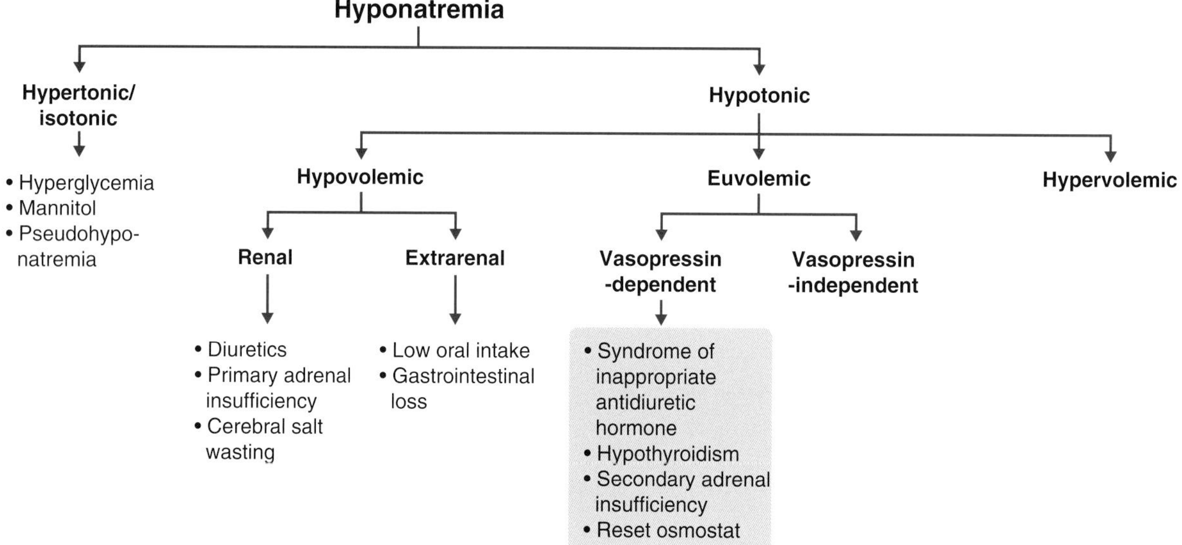


**What are the causes of syndrome of inappropriate antidiuretic hormone secretion?**

Causes of SIADH include medication (eg, antipsychotics), lung disease (eg, pneumonia), malignancy (eg, small cell lung cancer), central nervous system disease (eg, brain tumor), pain, nausea, and stress.[1]

**Under what conditions is hypothyroidism associated with hyponatremia?**

Although it is rare, hyponatremia can develop in patients with severe hypothyroidism (particularly myxedema coma). As a result of its effects on cardiac output and systemic vascular resistance, severe hypothyroidism causes a decrease in renal perfusion and an increase in baroreceptor-mediated vasopressin secretion, leading to impaired renal free water excretion (see Figure 36-1). The association between hypothyroidism of lesser severity and hyponatremia is not as clear.[12]

**Why does secondary adrenal insufficiency cause euvolemic hyponatremia rather than hypovolemic hyponatremia (as seen in primary adrenal insufficiency)?**

The hypocortisolism characteristic of both primary and secondary adrenal insufficiency leads to a loss of hypothalamic inhibition, with an associated increase in corticotropin-releasing hormone from the hypothalamus, which is a vasopressin secretagogue. The increased vasopressin levels impair renal free water excretion, leading to hyponatremia. In primary adrenal insufficiency, direct involvement of the adrenal cortex may lead to an additional deficiency of mineralocorticoids. Hypoaldosteronism results in renal Na⁺ and water wasting, leading to hypovolemia and baroreceptor-mediated stimulation of vasopressin (ie, hypovolemic hyponatremia). In secondary adrenal insufficiency, mineralocorticoid activity remains intact because it is not dependent on adrenocorticotropic hormone and is instead under the control of the renin-angiotensin system. While isolated hypocortisolism may lead to hyponatremia, sufficient levels of aldosterone in these patients prevent renal Na⁺ and water wasting, thereby maintaining euvolemia (ie, euvolemic hyponatremia).[4,13]

What are the characteristics of reset osmostat?

Reset osmostat describes a serum osmotic threshold (the level at which thirst and vasopressin secretion are stimulated and inhibited) that is lower than normal. The resultant hyponatremia is typically chronic, mild to moderate, and asymptomatic. Reset osmostat is technically a subtype of SIADH, but treatment is usually not necessary since thirst and vasopressin secretion are inhibited once the lower osmotic threshold is reached, which halts any further reduction in serum $Na^+$.[4,8]

## VASOPRESSIN-INDEPENDENT CAUSES OF EUVOLEMIC HYPONATREMIA

### What are the vasopressin-independent causes of euvolemic hyponatremia?

Commonly associated with psychiatric disorders.

Primary polydipsia.

Low solute intake.

Beer potomania (ie, "tea and toast" potomania).

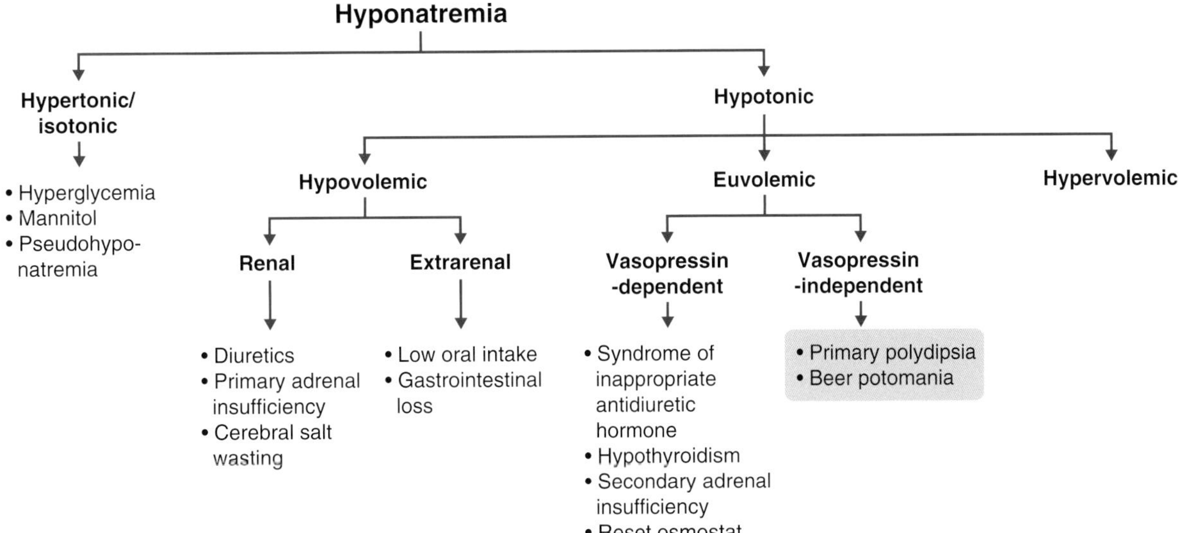


What is primary polydipsia?

Hyponatremia caused by primary polydipsia occurs most often in patients with psychiatric disorders, particularly schizophrenia. It develops when water ingestion overwhelms renal excretory capacity. The capacity of the kidney to excrete free water is dependent on solute excretion and urinary diluting capability. A typical Western diet results in solute excretion of around 800 mOsm/d. The maximum urinary dilution capability of healthy kidneys is 50 mOsm/L. Therefore, the maximum volume of free water that can be excreted in a day is around 16 liters (800 mOsm/day / 50 mOsm/L = 16 L per day). If water ingestion exceeds this threshold (as in primary polydipsia), then the resultant free water excess will cause hyponatremia. Primary polydipsia is treated with free water restriction. Associated mental health disorders should also be addressed.[4,14]

What is the mechanism of hyponatremia related to beer potomania?

Low solute intake can occur in a variety of settings, most often affecting patients who drink large volumes of beer with little food intake and those on low protein diets. Low solute excretion limits the volume of urinary free water that can be removed from the body. For example, in a patient with 250 mOsm of obligatory solute excretion per day, assuming maximal urinary dilution of 50 mOsm/L, the maximum daily volume of urinary free water excretion is 5 liters (250 mOsm/d / 50 mOsm/L = 5 L per day). If the daily ingestion of free water exceeds 5 liters (14 cans of beer), then hyponatremia will develop. These patients must be monitored carefully as an increased solute load will result in brisk diuresis and dangerously rapid correction of hyponatremia.[14]

## HYPERVOLEMIC HYPONATREMIA

*Hypervolemic hyponatremia can be thought of as extracellular gain of hypotonic fluid (water > salt).*

**What is the status of vasopressin levels in patients with hypervolemic hyponatremia?**

Despite the presence of total body hypervolemia, the conditions that lead to hypervolemic hyponatremia are associated with a decrease in effective arterial blood volume, resulting in baroreceptor-mediated release of vasopressin, which acts to maintain intravascular volume at the expense of serum tonicity.

**What are the 2 subcategories of hypervolemic hyponatremia?**

Hypervolemic hyponatremia can be caused by renal or extrarenal processes.

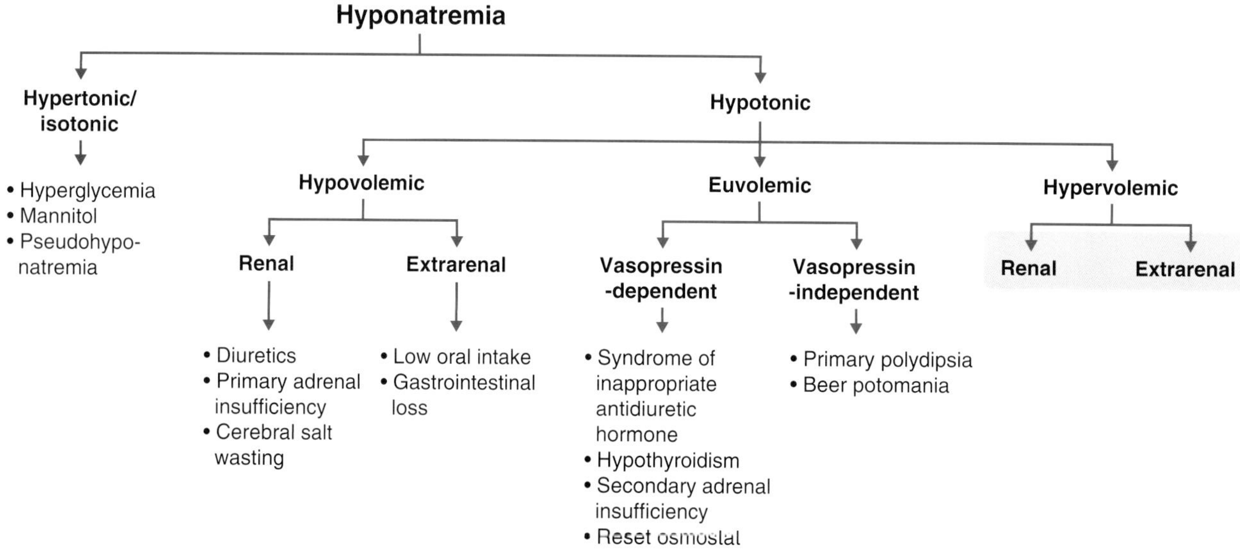


## RENAL CAUSES OF HYPERVOLEMIC HYPONATREMIA

### What are the renal causes of hypervolemic hyponatremia?

**Asterixis and a pericardial friction rub.**

Renal failure.

**Associated with anasarca and foamy urine.**

Nephrotic syndrome.

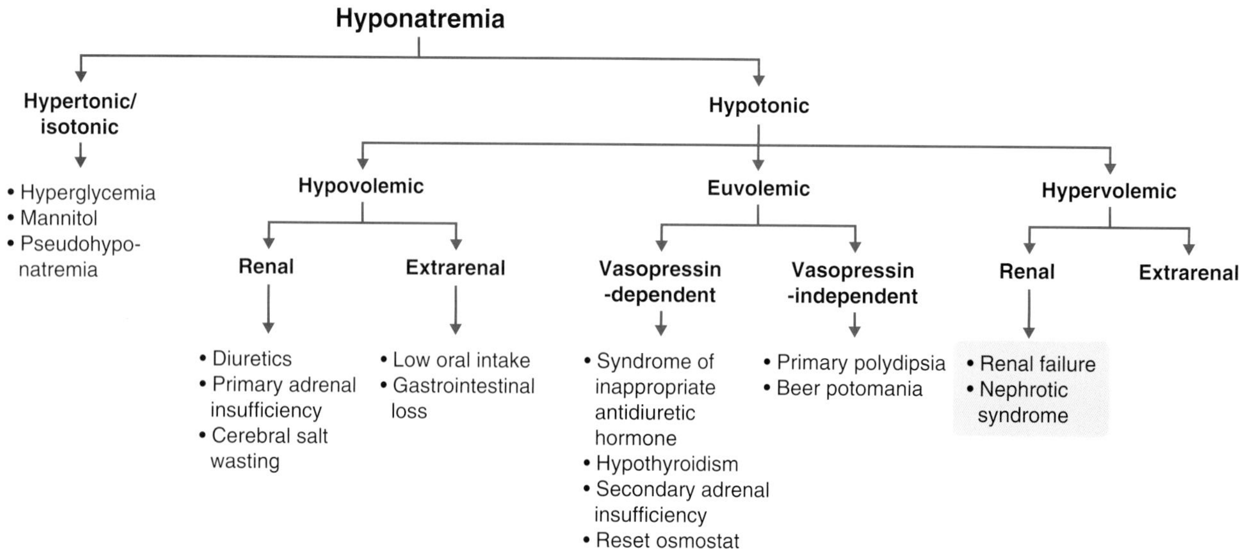

**What is the mechanism of hyponatremia related to renal failure?**

In advanced renal failure, the capacity of the kidneys to dilute urine becomes impaired, such that minimum urine osmolality may be as high as 200 to 250 mOsm/kg. This chronic impairment in free water excretion eventually leads to free water retention and hyponatremia.[15]

**What are the characteristic urinary findings of nephrotic syndrome?**

Nephrotic syndrome is characterized by proteinuria of at least 3.5 g/d. A minority of patients may also experience microscopic hematuria, but the urine sediment is typically bland. Hyponatremia is not common early in the course of nephrotic syndrome. However, when serum albumin concentration falls below 2 g/dL, intravascular volume depletion may stimulate vasopressin secretion, followed by the development of hyponatremia.[4,16]

## EXTRARENAL CAUSES OF HYPERVOLEMIC HYPONATREMIA

### What are the extrarenal causes of hypervolemic hyponatremia?

**Poor forward blood flow to the kidneys.**

Heart failure.

**A middle-aged man with a history of alcohol abuse is found to have hypervolemic hyponatremia associated with spider angiomas, flank fullness, and asterixis.**

Cirrhosis.

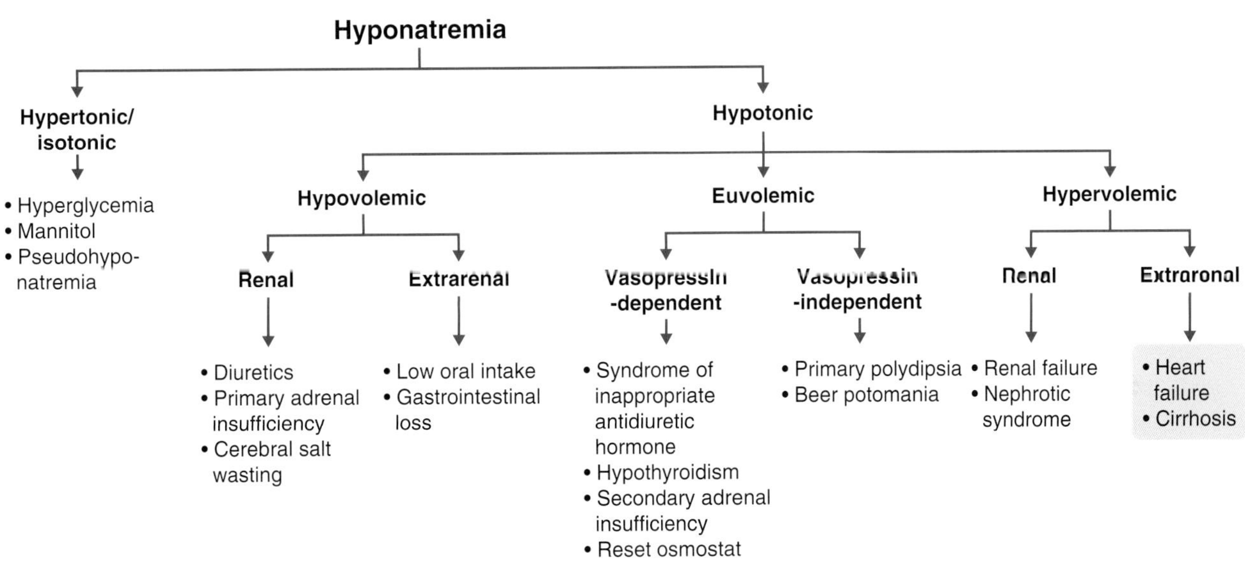


**Is diuresis effective in the treatment for hyponatremia associated with heart failure?**

Diuretics often improve hyponatremia associated with heart failure by optimizing preload, which improves cardiac output and effective arterial blood volume, thereby inhibiting baroreceptor-mediated vasopressin release. However, diuretic therapy, particularly thiazide agents, may worsen hyponatremia in some patients.[17]

**Is diuresis effective in the treatment for hyponatremia associated with cirrhosis?**

Hyponatremia is common in patients with cirrhosis, but only rarely occurs in the absence of ascites. It develops when vasodilation of the splanchnic circulation results in baroreceptor-mediated vasopressin secretion. Diuretics, including loop and thiazide agents, often exacerbate the hyponatremia associated with cirrhosis because these medications contribute to intravascular hypovolemia, stimulating the secretion of vasopressin.[18]

## Case Summary

A 68-year-old man with an extensive smoking history presents with nausea, malaise, and hemoptysis and is found to have hyponatremia, elevated urine osmolality, and a lung mass on chest imaging.

***What is the most likely cause of hyponatremia in this patient?***

Syndrome of inappropriate antidiuretic hormone secretion.

### BONUS QUESTIONS

***Which general categories of hyponatremia apply to this case?***

This case can be described as hypotonic, euvolemic, vasopressin-dependent hyponatremia. Categorizing hyponatremia in this way significantly narrows the differential diagnosis.

***What features in this case are suggestive of euvolemic volume status?***

The normal jugular venous pressure and absence of peripheral edema in this case effectively rule out hypervolemia. Euvolemia and hypovolemia can be difficult to differentiate clinically. However, there is no history of poor oral intake or excess fluid loss to suggest hypovolemia. Moreover, the presence of moist mucous membranes and axillae, low BUN, and urine $Na^+$ concentration >30 mEq/L suggest that extracellular fluid volume is not low.[1]

***What information in this case indicates that the hyponatremia is vasopressin-dependent?***

In the setting of hyponatremia, urine osmolality >100 mOsm/kg is indicative of a vasopressin-mediated process.[1]

***What is the most likely underlying cause of syndrome of inappropriate antidiuretic hormone secretion in this case?***

Lung disease is a common cause of SIADH; in this case, given the smoking history, lung mass (see Figure 38-1), and evidence of SIADH, the most likely diagnosis is lung cancer. Small cell lung cancer in particular is most often associated with SIADH.[1]

***Is the hyponatremia in this case most likely acute or chronic?***

In this case, chronic hyponatremia is suggested by the lack of symptoms. In cases where the duration of hyponatremia is unknown, chronicity should be presumed, which has implications on management strategies.

***What is the definitive management of syndrome of inappropriate antidiuretic hormone secretion?***

Elimination of the underlying cause is the definitive therapy for SIADH; most cases related to malignancy resolve with effective antineoplastic therapy.[1]

***In addition to addressing the underlying cause, what other management strategies should be considered in this case?***

Given that the hyponatremia in this case is most likely chronic, care must be taken not to treat too aggressively. In cases of chronic hyponatremia, a rate of correction of no more than 0.5 to 1 mEq/L per hour is reasonable (with a maximum of 8 mEq/L per 24-hour period); close monitoring of the serum $Na^+$ concentration is prudent. Fluid restriction is key to treating chronic hyponatremia related to SIADH. Other options include the use of salt tablets, hypertonic saline infusion, furosemide, urea, and vasopressin antagonists.[1,2]

***Why is it dangerous to correct chronic hyponatremia too quickly?***

Within 24 to 48 hours of the onset of hypotonic hyponatremia, brain tissue begins to adapt to increases in water content and associated cerebral edema. One such adaptation is the leakage of osmolytes from brain cells, which acts to reduce the tonicity gradient between the extracellular and intracellular environments, mitigating the influx of water (see Figure 38-2). Once this compensatory mechanism has occurred, rapid correction of the serum $Na^+$ concentration will result in an abrupt difference in tonicity between extracellular and intracellular fluid, favoring the movement of water out of the cells, which can lead to osmotic demyelination, a devastating complication.[2]

***What are the clinical manifestations of osmotic demyelination?***

Osmotic demyelination is a biphasic syndrome, with initial manifestations typically occurring days after overcorrection of hyponatremia (there may be a lag of up to a week in some cases). Neurologic symptoms may improve initially, but this is followed by the gradual onset of new and variable neurologic manifestations, including seizures, behavioral abnormalities, and movement disorders. In severe cases, when there is involvement of the pons, patients develop a "locked-in" syndrome with quadriparesis and the inability to speak or swallow. Patients may recover from osmotic demyelination, sometimes completely, but many others develop permanent disability or die.[2,19]

***What is the management of symptomatic acute hyponatremia?***

For symptomatic and severe acute hyponatremia (<24-48 hours), rapid treatment is imperative. This can be achieved by infusing 3% saline intravenously with a goal rate of correction of 1 to 2 mEq/L per hour (with a maximum of 8-10 mEq/L per 24-hour period); close monitoring of the serum $Na^+$ concentration is prudent. Once the neurologic symptoms have abated (usually after the initial increase in serum $Na^+$ of 4-6 mEq/L), the rate can generally be slowed.[1,2]

## KEY POINTS

- Water homeostasis, which controls serum $Na^+$ concentration, is regulated by thirst and the hormonal interplay between the central nervous system and the kidneys.
- Maintenance of normal serum $Na^+$ concentration is important for preserving cell volume.
- Hyponatremia is generally defined as serum $Na^+$ <135 mEq/L.
- Clinical manifestations of hyponatremia depend on its duration and severity.
- Acute hyponatremia is defined by duration <24 to 48 hours.
- Acute hyponatremia is often symptomatic with manifestations that include nausea, malaise, lethargy, headache, delirium, obtundation, seizure, and coma.
- Chronic hyponatremia is often asymptomatic.
- Hyponatremia can be associated with serum hypertonicity, isotonicity, or hypotonicity.
- Hypotonic hyponatremia can be associated with extracellular hypovolemia, euvolemia, or hypervolemia.
- Hypovolemic hyponatremia results from extracellular loss of hypertonic fluid (salt > water).
- Hypovolemic hyponatremia can be caused by renal or extrarenal processes.
- Euvolemic hyponatremia results from extracellular gain of pure water.
- Euvolemic hyponatremia can be caused by vasopressin-dependent or vasopressin-independent processes.
- Hypervolemic hyponatremia results from extracellular gain of hypotonic fluid (water > salt).
- Hypervolemic hyponatremia can be caused by renal or extrarenal processes.
- Acute symptomatic hyponatremia should be corrected rapidly with infusion of hypertonic saline and serial monitoring of the serum $Na^+$ concentration.
- Management of chronic hyponatremia depends on the underlying cause but can include fluid restriction, salt tablets, hypertonic saline infusion, furosemide, urea, and vasopressin antagonists. The rate of serum $Na^+$ correction should be carefully considered to prevent the development of osmotic demyelination.

## REFERENCES

1. Ellison DH, Berl T. Clinical practice. The syndrome of inappropriate antidiuresis. *N Engl J Med*. 2007;356(20):2064-2072.
2. Sterns RH. Disorders of plasma sodium–causes, consequences, and correction. *N Engl J Med*. 2015;372(1):55-65.
3. Spital A, Sterns RD. The paradox of sodium's volume of distribution. Why an extracellular solute appears to distribute over total body water. *Arch Intern Med*. 1989;149(6):1255-1257.
4. Verbalis JG, Goldsmith SR, Greenberg A, et al. Diagnosis, evaluation, and treatment of hyponatremia: expert panel recommendations. *Am J Med*. 2013;126(10 suppl 1):S1-S42.

5. Berend K, de Vries AP, Gans RO. Physiological approach to assessment of acid-base disturbances. *N Engl J Med*. 2014;371(15):1434-1445.
6. Chung HM, Kluge R, Schrier RW, Anderson RJ. Clinical assessment of extracellular fluid volume in hyponatremia. *Am J Med*. 1987;83(5):905-908.
7. Schrier RW. Body water homeostasis: clinical disorders of urinary dilution and concentration. *J Am Soc Nephrol*. 2006;17(7):1820-1832.
8. Longo DL, Fauci AS, Kasper DL, Hauser SL, Jameson JL, Loscalzo J, eds. *Harrison's Principles of Internal Medicine*. 18th ed. New York, NY: McGraw-Hill; 2012.
9. Ashraf N, Locksley R, Arieff AI. Thiazide-induced hyponatremia associated with death or neurologic damage in outpatients. *Am J Med*. 1981;70(6):1163-1168.
10. Ahmed AB, George BC, Gonzalez-Auvert C, Dingman JF. Increased plasma arginine vasopressin in clinical adrenocortical insufficiency and [illegible]
11. Leonard J, Garrett RE, Salottolo K, et al. Cerebral salt wasting after traumatic brain injury: a review of the literature. *Scand J Trauma Resusc Emerg Med*. 2015;23:98.
12. Pantalone KM, Hatipoglu BA. Hyponatremia and the thyroid: causality or association? *J Clin Med*. 2014;4(1):32-36.
13. van der Hoek J, Hoorn EJ, de Jong GM, Janssens EN, de Herder WW. Severe hyponatremia with high urine sodium and osmolality. *Clin Chem*. 2009;55(11):1905-1908.
14. Sanghvi SR, Kellerman PS, Nanovic L. Beer potomania: an unusual cause of hyponatremia at high risk of complications from rapid correction. *Am J Kidney Dis*. 2007;50(4):673-680.
15. Tannen RL, Regal EM, Dunn MJ, Schrier RW. Vasopressin-resistant hyposthenuria in advanced chronic renal disease. *N Engl J Med*. 1969;280(21):1135-1141.
16. Hull RP, Goldsmith DJ. Nephrotic syndrome in adults. *BMJ*. 2008;336(7654):1185-1189.
17. Verbrugge FH, Steels P, Grieten L, Nijst P, Tang WH, Mullens W. Hyponatremia in acute decompensated heart failure: depletion versus dilution. *J Am Coll Cardiol*. 2015;65(5):480-492.
18. Sherlock S, Senewiratne B, Scott A, Walker JG. Complications of diuretic therapy in hepatic cirrhosis. *Lancet*. 1966;1(7446):1049-1052.
19. King JD, Rosner MH. Osmotic demyelination syndrome. *Am J Med Sci*. 2010;339(6):561-567.

Chapter 39

# SECONDARY HYPERTENSION

## Case: A 24-year-old man with discordant peripheral pulses

A 24-year-old man presents to the clinic for evaluation of hypertension. He has no known medical conditions and does not regularly see a physician. His blood pressure was measured at the local grocery store, and he was told it was elevated. He does not take any medications, including over-the-counter agents or supplements. Review of systems is notable for headache and exertional shortness of breath over the past few months.

Blood pressure is 182/98 mm Hg in the right upper extremity, 178/94 mm Hg in the left upper extremity, 103/72 mm Hg in the right lower extremity, and 98/64 mm Hg in the left lower extremity. Jugular venous pressure is 8 cm $H_2O$. The carotid pulses are bounding. The radial pulses are strong, but the dorsalis pedis pulses are weakly palpable. There is an extra heart sound heard just before S1 with the bell of the stethoscope over the apex. No murmurs are present.

Electrocardiogram is notable for left ventricular hypertrophy. A close-up of the chest radiograph is shown in Figure 39-1.

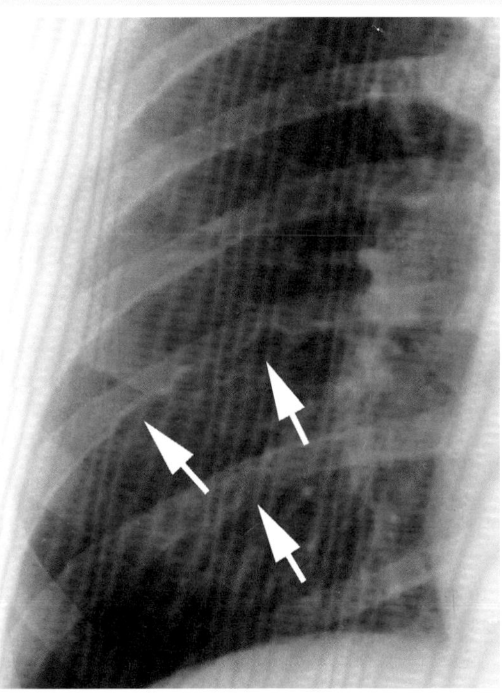

**Figure 39-1.** (From Daffner RH, Hartman MS. *Clinical Radiology: The Essentials.* 4th ed. Philadelphia, PA: Lippincott Williams & Wilkins; 2014.)

***What is the most likely cause of hypertension in this patient?***

**What is essential hypertension?**

Essential hypertension is characterized by a chronic abnormal elevation in systolic or diastolic arterial blood pressure (BP) without a clear underlying etiology. There are likely multiple underlying factors involved in the development of essential hypertension, including genetic and environmental elements (eg, diet).[1]

**What is secondary hypertension?**

Secondary hypertension is defined as abnormal elevation in systolic arterial BP resulting from an identifiable, and often correctable, underlying cause. Primary and secondary hypertension can coexist in the same patient, so some degree of hypertension may persist despite appropriate treatment of secondary causes.[2]

**How common is secondary hypertension?**

In the industrialized world, secondary hypertension affects approximately 5% to 10% of the general hypertensive population.[2]

**What clinical characteristics are suggestive of secondary hypertension?**

Any of the following clinical characteristics are suggestive of secondary hypertension: onset of hypertension at a young age (ie, <30-40 years), few risk factors for essential hypertension (eg, family history, obesity), resistant hypertension (BP >140/90 mm Hg) despite several antihypertensive drugs, episodes of severe hypertension (>180/100 mm Hg), abrupt increase in systolic BP in a previously stable patient, labile hypertension, and evidence of target organ damage (eg, left ventricular hypertrophy).[1,2]

**What is the clinical significance of hypertension?**

Hypertension is a key risk factor for stroke, myocardial infarction, heart failure, and kidney failure.[1]

**How is blood pressure regulated?**

Moment-to-moment regulation of blood pressure is controlled by the neurally mediated baroreceptors found in the carotid sinus and aortic arch. Long-term regulation of blood pressure is controlled by the hormone-based renin-angiotensin-aldosterone system, and atrial and brain natriuretic peptides (see Figure 22-2).[3]

**The causes of secondary hypertension can be separated into which general categories?**

The causes of secondary hypertension can be separated into the following categories: vascular, endocrinologic, toxic, and other.

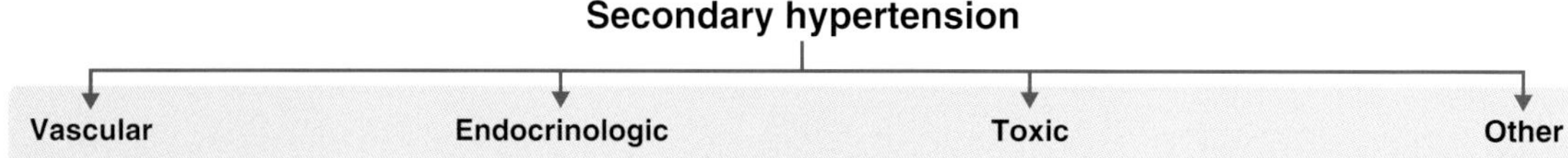


## VASCULAR CAUSES OF SECONDARY HYPERTENSION

### What are the vascular causes of secondary hypertension?

**A 35-year-old woman with new-onset hypertension and an abdominal bruit on examination.**

Renal artery stenosis.

**Rib notching on chest radiography.**

Coarctation of aorta.

**A 43-year-old man with testicular pain, hypertension, and chronic hepatitis B infection.**

Polyarteritis nodosa.

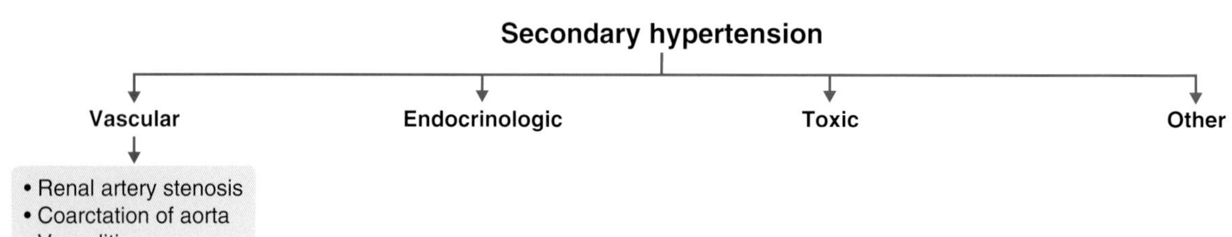

**What are the most common causes of renal artery stenosis in younger and older populations?**

Renal artery stenosis may be responsible for up to 20% of cases of resistant hypertension. Fibromuscular dysplasia is the most common cause in children and young adults, whereas atherosclerosis is the most common cause in older adults. Clues to the diagnosis include an abdominal bruit (particularly when diastolic) and acute renal function deterioration after starting an angiotensin-converting enzyme inhibitor or angiotensin receptor blocker. Conventional renal angiography (Figure 39-2) is the diagnostic gold standard, but other less invasive imaging studies are available for initial testing, including duplex ultrasonography.[2]

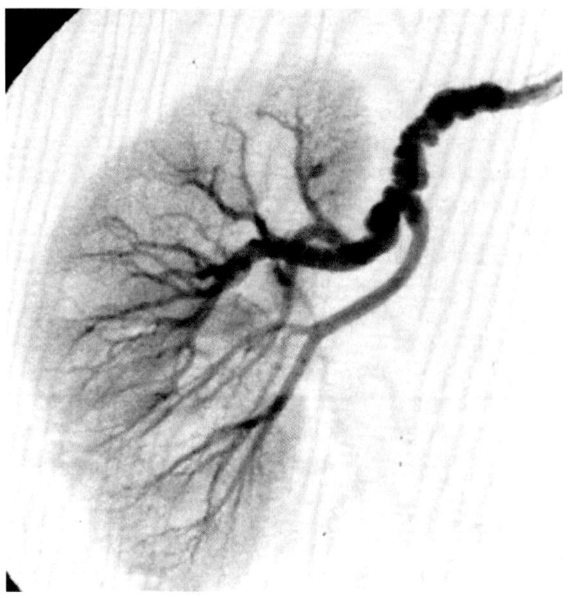

**Figure 39-2.** Typical arteriographic "string of beads" appearance of fibromuscular dysplasia. (From Schrier RW. *Diseases of the Kidney and Urinary Tract*. 8th ed. Philadelphia, PA: Lippincott Williams & Wilkins; 2007.)

**What blood pressure finding can be a clue to the diagnosis of coarctation of the aorta?**

Coarctation of the aorta can be associated with discordant blood pressure readings between upper and lower extremities.

**Which types of large and medium vessel vasculitis are associated with secondary hypertension?**

Secondary hypertension can occur in patients with medium vessel vasculitides, including polyarteritis nodosa and Kawasaki disease, and large vessel vasculitides, including giant cell arteritis and Takayasu arteritis.[4]

## ENDOCRINOLOGIC CAUSES OF SECONDARY HYPERTENSION

### What are the endocrinologic causes of secondary hypertension?

**Weight gain, cold intolerance, and constipation.**

Hypothyroidism.

**Hypertension, hypokalemia, and metabolic alkalosis.**

Mineralocorticoid excess.

**Anxiety, heat intolerance, weight loss, and tremor.**

Hyperthyroidism.

**Treatment for this condition often includes intravenous fluids, calcitonin, and bisphosphonates.**

Hypercalcemia.

**Central obesity, thin skin, ecchymosis, and osteoporosis.**

Cushing's syndrome.

**Arthralgias, macroglossia, jaw enlargement, and headache.**

Acromegaly.

**Flushing, palpitations, headache, chest pain, and perspiration.**

Pheochromocytoma.

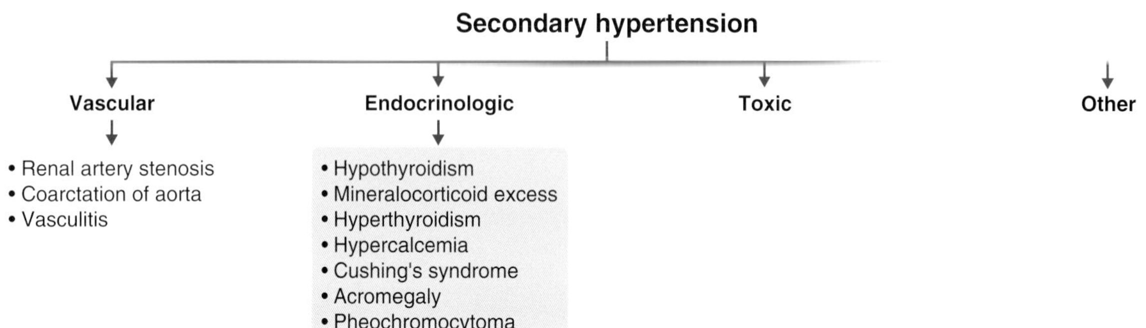


**How common is hypertension in patients with hypothyroidism?**

Hypertension is present in around one-fifth of patients with hypothyroidism. Serum thyroid stimulating hormone (TSH) and free thyroxine ($T_4$) are the initial tests of choice. Hypertension usually resolves with thyroid hormone replacement therapy.[5]

**What pattern of electrolyte and metabolic abnormalities is classically associated with primary hyperaldosteronism?**

Primary hyperaldosteronism (ie, Conn's syndrome) may be present in up to 10% of hypertensive patients. The most common causes are bilateral idiopathic hyperplasia of the adrenal glands and unilateral aldosterone-secreting adrenal adenoma. Primary hyperaldosteronism is classically associated with mild hypernatremia, hypokalemia, and metabolic alkalosis, but this pattern of metabolic abnormalities is not always present. The initial test of choice is plasma aldosterone (ng/dL) to plasma renin activity (ng/mL/hr) ratio (a ratio >30 is suggestive of the diagnosis).[5]

**What is characteristic about the hypertension associated with hyperthyroidism?**

Hyperthyroidism is often associated with an isolated elevation in systolic blood pressure (generating a wide pulse pressure). Serum TSH and $T_4$ are the initial tests of choice. β-Blockers may be useful in treating hypertension until there is definitive management of the underlying hyperthyroidism.[5,6]

**What is the mechanism of hypertension related to hypercalcemia?**

The main mechanism of hypertension in the setting of hypercalcemia is direct calcium-mediated increase in systemic vascular resistance (including renal vascular resistance). The hypertension usually resolves with management of hypercalcemia. Thiazide agents should be avoided in hypercalcemic patients.[7]

**How common is hypertension in patients with Cushing's syndrome?**

Hypertension is present in around one-fifth of patients with iatrogenic Cushing's syndrome; there is a dramatic increase in occurrence among patients with endogenous Cushing's syndrome (hypertension is present in as many as 95% of patients with ectopic ACTH secretion). In patients with a clinical syndrome compatible with Cushing's syndrome (see Figure 8-3), the urine free cortisol test, which measures the quantity of free cortisol secreted in the urine in a 24-hour period, is the most reliable confirmatory test.[8]

**How common is hypertension in patients with acromegaly?**

Hypertension occurs in around one-third of patients with acromegaly. Most cases of acromegaly are caused by pituitary tumors that secrete growth hormone; other sources of growth hormone secretion include small cell lung cancer and pancreatic cancer. In patients with a compatible clinical syndrome (see Figure 41-4), serum insulin-like growth factor (IGF-1) is the initial test of choice. Hypertension typically improves with management of acromegaly.[5,9,10]

**How common is hypertension in patients with pheochromocytoma?**

Hypertension is the most common sign of pheochromocytoma, occurring in the vast majority of patients (about 95%). Elevated blood pressure may be sustained or paroxysmal (acute-on-chronic elevations are also common). Initial test options include urinary and plasma fractionated metanephrines and catecholamines. α-Blockers (eg, prazosin) are the treatment of choice for hypertension in patients with pheochromocytoma. β-Blockers may be added, but only after α-blockade has been instituted in order to avoid hypertensive crisis caused by unopposed α-receptor mediated vasoconstriction.[11]

## TOXIC CAUSES OF SECONDARY HYPERTENSION

### What are the toxic causes of secondary hypertension?

**Cyclooxygenase inhibitors.**

Nonsteroidal anti-inflammatory drugs (NSAIDs).

**Iatrogenic Cushing's syndrome.**

Corticosteroids.

**Used to treat the symptoms of menopause.**

Estrogens.

**Stimulant medications.**

Sympathomimetics.

**A beverage.**

Alcohol.

**Illicit sympathomimetics.**

Cocaine and amphetamines.

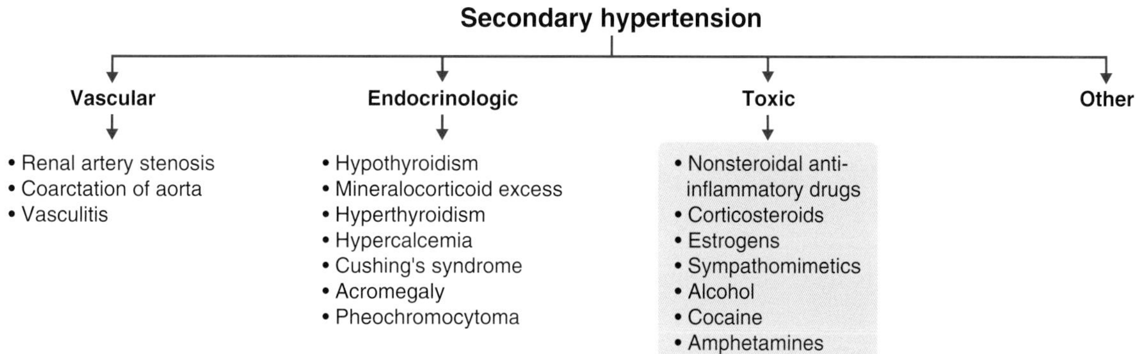


**What is the average increase in blood pressure related to the use of nonsteroidal anti-inflammatory drugs?**

NSAIDs are associated with a relatively modest increase in mean blood pressure of 5 mm Hg, but the increase can be more pronounced in patients with a history of hypertension controlled with antihypertensive medications.[12]

**What is the mechanism of glucocorticoid-induced hypertension?**

Glucocorticoid activity at the mineralocorticoid receptor causes sodium and fluid retention, leading to hypertension. However, synthetic glucocorticoids have less mineralocorticoid activity than cortisol, so hypertension is more prevalent in patients with endogenous Cushing's syndrome. When the use of corticosteroid medication is unavoidable, hypertension is often responsive to dietary restrictions (eg, salt, fluid), and diuretic agents.[12]

**What are the risk factors for hypertension related to exogenous estrogen?**

Hypertension is more common in women taking oral contraceptives by a factor of 2 to 3. Risk factors include a history of gestational hypertension, family history of hypertension, cigarette use, black race, obesity, and diabetes mellitus. If the medication cannot be stopped, hypertension is generally responsive to low-dose diuretic agents.[12]

**What are some sympathomimetic agents?**

Common examples of sympathomimetic agents include methylphenidate, ephedrine, pseudoephedrine, oxymetazoline, and phenylpropanolamine. Some of these agents can be found in over-the-counter nasal sprays, oral decongestants, and appetite suppressants. When these agents cannot be stopped, antihypertensive therapy may be necessary. β-Blockers should be avoided because unopposed α-adrenergic vasoconstriction can lead to hypertensive crisis.[12]

**How much alcohol consumption is associated with increases in blood pressure?**

For most patients, moderate alcohol intake (1 drink per day for women and 1-2 drinks per day for men) has limited effect on blood pressure. Chronic consumption of alcohol that exceeds this threshold is associated with hypertension, the severity of which follows a dose-dependent relationship. In some cases, complete abstinence from alcohol is required to control blood pressure. *It is important to note that hypertension frequently develops in the setting of alcohol withdrawal, usually 2 to 3 days after the last drink.*[5,12-14]

**What is the mechanism of hypertension related to cocaine?**

Tachycardia and hypertension are common manifestations of cocaine intoxication. Cocaine blocks norepinephrine reuptake in the synaptic cleft, resulting in its accumulation and subsequent activation of the sympathetic nervous system. β-Blockers should be avoided in patients with acute cocaine toxicity because unopposed α-adrenergic vasoconstriction can lead to hypertensive crisis and exacerbate myocardial ischemia. Nitroglycerin, calcium channel blockers, and benzodiazepines are safe and effective alternative agents.[12]

**What complication involving the pulmonary vasculature can develop in patients who abuse cocaine or amphetamines?**

Acute amphetamine intoxication has a presentation similar to that of cocaine toxicity. Tachycardia and hypertension are common findings. Cocaine and amphetamines can affect the pulmonary vasculature, leading to the development of chronic pulmonary arterial hypertension.[12,15]

## OTHER CAUSES OF SECONDARY HYPERTENSION

### What are the other causes of secondary hypertension?

**Hematuria and hypertension.**

Renal parenchymal disease related to glomerulonephritis.

**A large neck circumference can be a clue to the presence of this condition.**

Obstructive sleep apnea (OSA).

**Discordance between blood pressure recordings in the office and those taken by the patient at home.**

White-coat hypertension.

**Only women are at risk.**

Pregnancy-associated hypertension (including gestational hypertension and preeclampsia).

**This group of disorders is often associated with labile blood pressures, including supine hypertension and orthostatic hypotension.**

Neurologic disorders.

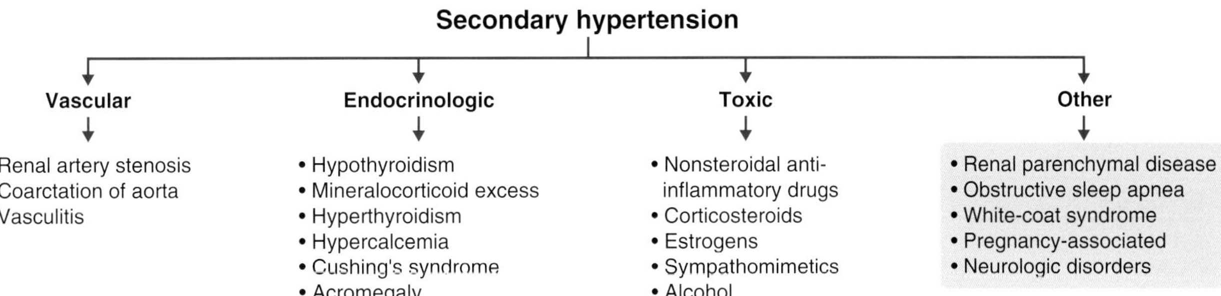


**What types of renal parenchymal disease are associated with hypertension?**

Renal parenchymal diseases associated with hypertension include chronic kidney disease (hypertension is present in the majority of these patients), acute glomerulonephritis, and scleroderma renal crisis.[16]

**How common is hypertension in patients with obstructive sleep apnea?**

Hypertension is present in most patients with OSA. Among those without hypertension, there is a 3-fold increase in the risk of developing it. Continuous positive airway pressure (CPAP) is the most effective therapy for OSA and has been shown to improve associated hypertension.[5]

**What diagnostic tool can be useful in assessing for white-coat hypertension?**

24-hour ambulatory blood pressure monitoring can be helpful in determining whether hypertension is situational or not.

**What is the first-line agent for pregnancy-induced hypertension?**

Methyldopa is first-line for pregnancy-associated hypertension. Teratogenicity must be considered before starting any medication in pregnant women.[5]

**What neurologic disorders are associated with secondary hypertension?**

Neurologic disorders associated with hypertension include increased intracranial pressure (Cushing's response), quadriplegia, dysautonomia, and Guillain–Barré syndrome.[5]

## Case Summary

A 24-year-old man with no known medical conditions presents for evaluation of hypertension, and is found to have isolated hypertension of the upper extremities, bounding carotid pulses, discordant peripheral pulses, the presence of an extra heart sound, and an abnormal chest radiograph.

***What is the most likely cause of hypertension in this patient?***

Coarctation of the aorta.

### BONUS QUESTIONS

***What is coarctation of the aorta?***

Coarctation of the aorta is a narrowing of the aorta, usually congenital in origin. Coarctation is commonly classified based on the location of the narrowing relative to structures of the aortic arch such as the ductus arteriosus (preductal, juxtaductal, or postductal) or the left subclavian artery (proximal or distal).[17]

***What is the significance of the extra heart sound in this case?***

The extra sound in this case is most likely an S4 gallop associated with left ventricular hypertrophy, a common sequela of long-standing coarctation of the aorta. The S4 is a low-frequency late diastolic sound that is best appreciated over the apex of the heart with the bell of the stethoscope (see Figure 4-4).[18]

***Why is coarctation of the aorta associated with asymmetric peripheral pulses?***

The pattern of asymmetry of the peripheral pulses in coarctation of the aorta is dependent on the location of narrowing. Distal to the narrowed portion of the aorta, blood flow is compromised, whereas blood flow proximal to this narrowed area is intensified.

***Where is the general location of the coarctation in this case?***

The coarctation in this case must be distal to all of the great vessels of the aortic arch, as there are strong pulses and hypertension in the upper extremities. If the coarctation were proximal to the left subclavian artery, then blood flow to the left upper extremity would be compromised.

***What is the abnormal finding on the chest radiograph in this case?***

The chest radiograph in this case shows "notching" of the ribs (see Figure 39-1, arrows). This finding represents erosions of the bone caused by increased pressure and blood flow through dilated intercostal arteries that have developed to supply collateral flow to the postcoarctation segment of the aorta. Rib notching is typically bilateral and affects the inferior border of the posterior third to ninth ribs.[19]

***What is the most frequent congenital cardiac condition associated with coarctation of the aorta?***

Patients with coarctation of the aorta commonly have coexistent bicuspid aortic valve (up to 85% of cases).[20]

***What is the natural history of coarctation of the aorta?***

Coarctation of the aorta is associated with a wide range of outcomes, depending on its severity. Without correction, the mean life expectancy in patients with coarctation of the aorta is 35 years (90% of patients die before the age of 50 years). It is associated with coronary artery disease, stroke, aortic dissection, and congestive heart failure.[20]

***What is the medical treatment for coarctation of the aorta?***

Medical management of coarctation of the aorta focuses on treatment for hypertension. First-line agents include β-blockers, angiotensin-converting enzyme inhibitors, and angiotensin receptor blockers.[20]

## KEY POINTS

- Hypertension is a key risk factor for stroke, myocardial infarction, heart failure, and kidney failure.
- Secondary hypertension is the abnormal elevation in systolic arterial BP resulting from an identifiable, and often correctable, underlying cause.
- Secondary hypertension affects 5% to 10% of the general hypertensive population.
- Clinical features suggestive of secondary hypertension include the following: young age at onset, few risk factors for essential hypertension, resistant hypertension, episodes of severe hypertension, abrupt increase in BP in a previously stable patient, labile hypertension, and evidence of target organ damage.
- The causes of secondary hypertension can be separated into the following categories: vascular, endocrinologic, toxic, and other.
- History and physical examination are instrumental in identifying the cause of secondary hypertension.

## REFERENCES

1. Sukor N. Secondary hypertension: a condition not to be missed. *Postgrad Med J.* 2011;87(1032):706-713.
2. Rimoldi SF, Scherrer U, Messerli FH. Secondary arterial hypertension: when, who, and how to screen? *Eur Heart J.* 2014;35(19):1245-1254.
3. Berne RML, Levy MN. *Physiology*. 4th ed. St. Louis, Missouri: Mosby, Inc.; 1998.
4. Jennette JC, Falk RJ. The pathology of vasculitis involving the kidney. *Am J Kidney Dis.* 1994;24(1):130-141.
5. Chiong JR, Aronow WS, Khan IA, et al. Secondary hypertension: current diagnosis and treatment. *Int J Cardiol.* 2008;124(1):6-21.
6. Prisant LM, Gujral JS, Mulloy AL. Hyperthyroidism: a secondary cause of isolated systolic hypertension. *J Clin Hypertens (Greenwich).* 2006;8(8):596-599.
7. Eiam-Ong S, Eiam-Ong S, Punsin P, Sitprija V, Chaiyabutr N. Acute hypercalcemia-induced hypertension: the roles of calcium channel and alpha-1 adrenergic receptor. *J Med Assoc Thai.* 2004;87(4):410-418.
8. Magiakou MA, Smyrnaki P, Chrousos GP. Hypertension in Cushing's syndrome. *Best Pract Res Clin Endocrinol Metab.* 2006;20(3):467-482.
9. Bondanelli M, Ambrosio MR, degli Uberti EC. Pathogenesis and prevalence of hypertension in acromegaly. *Pituitary.* 2001;4(4):239-249.
10. Colao A, Ferone D, Marzullo P, Lombardi G. Systemic complications of acromegaly: epidemiology, pathogenesis, and management. *Endocr Rev.* 2004;25(1):102-152.
11. Zuber SM, Kantorovich V, Pacak K. Hypertension in pheochromocytoma: characteristics and treatment. *Endocrinol Metab Clin North Am.* 2011;40(2):295-311, vii.
12. Gyamlani G, Geraci SA. Secondary hypertension due to drugs and toxins. *South Med J.* 2007;100(7):692-699; quiz 700, 8.
13. Husain K, Ansari RA, Ferder L. Alcohol-induced hypertension: mechanism and prevention. *World J Cardiol.* 2014;6(5):245-252.

14. Kaplan NM. Alcohol and hypertension. *Lancet*. 1995;345(8965):1588-1589.
15. Montani D, Seferian A, Savale L, Simonneau G, Humbert M. Drug-induced pulmonary arterial hypertension: a recent outbreak. *Eur Respir Rev*. 2013;22(129):244-250.
16. Whaley-Connell AT, Sowers JR, Stevens LA, et al. CKD in the United States: Kidney Early Evaluation Program (KEEP) and National Health and Nutrition Examination Survey (NHANES) 1999-2004. *Am J Kidney Dis*. 2008;51(4 suppl 2):S13-S20.
17. Nance JW, Ringel RE, Fishman EK. Coarctation of the aorta in adolescents and adults: a review of clinical features and CT imaging. *J Cardiovasc Comput Tomogr*. 2016;10(1):1-12.
18. Tavel ME. *Clinical Phonocardiography and External Pulse Recording*. 2nd ed. Chicago, Illinois: Year Book Medical Publishers, Inc.; 1967.
19. Gooding CA, Glickman MG, Suydam MJ. Fate of rib notching after correction of aortic coarctation. *Am J Roentgenol Radium Ther Nucl Med*. 1969;106(1):21-23.
20. Jurcut R, Daraban AM, Lorber A, et al. Coarctation of the aorta in adults: what is the best treatment? Case report and literature review. *J Med Life*. 2011;4(2):189-195.

# SECTION 10

# Neurology

## Chapter 40

## HEADACHE

### Case: A 50-year-old man with tinnitus

A previously healthy 50-year-old man is evaluated in the clinic for 6 months of fatigue, headache, and intermittent fever. He was previously evaluated for these symptoms and was thought to have infectious mononucleosis or viral labyrinthitis. However, his symptoms are progressing, and he is seeking another opinion. The headache is diffuse and constant and has become more intense over time. Recently, the patient has developed ringing in the ears. He estimates weight loss of 15 pounds since the symptoms began. The patient lives with his wife in Portland, Oregon. Over the past few years, he has visited Morocco, British Columbia, Texas, and California. He has no pets.

Temperature is 37.5°C. The patient is alert and oriented. The sinuses are nontender. Fundoscopic examination reveals bilateral papilledema. There are no focal neurologic abnormalities on examination. Computed tomography (CT) imaging of the brain is unremarkable.

Human immunodeficiency virus (HIV) antibodies are not detected in the serum. Lumbar puncture reveals the following cerebrospinal fluid (CSF) profile:

| Appearance | Pressure (cm $H_2O$) | WBC/μL | Glucose (mg/dL) | Total protein (mg/dL) |
|---|---|---|---|---|
| Clear | 42 | 84 (72% lymphocytes) | 17 | 210 |

Magnetic resonance imaging (MRI) of the brain with axial (Figure 40-1A) and sagittal (Figure 40-1B) views reveals a ring-enhancing 1 × 1.2 cm right cerebellar mass (arrows) and diffuse leptomeningeal nodularity.

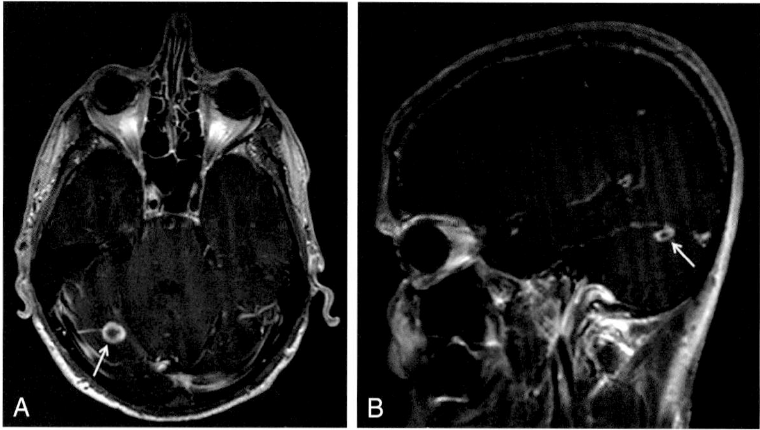


**Figure 40-1.**

***What is the most likely cause of headache in this patient?***

**How common is headache in the general population?**

Headache is one of the most common presenting complaints in the primary care clinic, affecting the vast majority of men and women at some point during life.[1,2]

**What are the 2 general categories of headache disorders?**

Headache disorders can be primary or secondary.

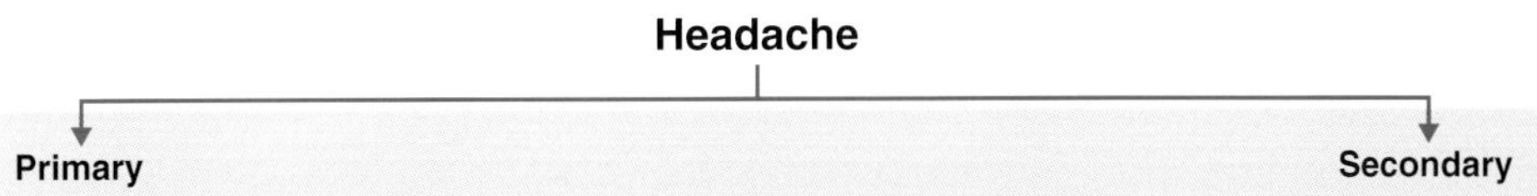


**Are primary or secondary headaches more common?**

Primary disorders account for most cases of headache, particularly in the primary care clinic. However, the frequency of secondary headache increases in certain populations (eg, immunocompromised patients, patients with a history of malignancy).[1,2]

**What are the clinical clues to the presence of a secondary headache disorder?**

Secondary headache disorders are suggested by the presence of any of the following features: sudden- or new-onset headache at an older age (>40 years), change in the quality of chronic headache, systemic symptoms or illness (eg, fever, history of malignancy, nausea or vomiting, neck stiffness, immunocompromised status, use of anticoagulant medications), neurologic symptoms or signs (eg, confusion, focal neurologic deficits, seizure, papilledema), headaches that wake patients from sleep, and headaches that are worsened with Valsalva maneuvers.[3]



## PRIMARY HEADACHE DISORDERS

### What are the primary headache disorders?

**Bilateral, mild in intensity, "tightening" or "pressing" in quality, often associated with stress, and lasting for minutes to days.**

Tension headache.[2]

**A 23-year-old woman with an 8-month history of recurring unilateral pulsatile headache lasting anywhere from a few hours to a few days, associated with nausea, and typically preceded by visual disturbance.**

Migraine headache.

**This primary headache disorder is more common in men and is characterized by unilateral retro-orbital pain associated with lacrimation, conjunctival erythema, and nasal drainage.**

Cluster headache.[2]

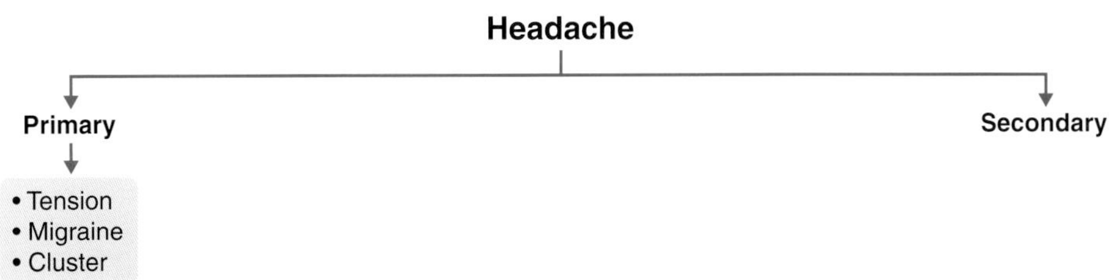


**What are the pharmacologic treatment options for tension headaches?**

Acetaminophen or nonsteroidal anti-inflammatory drugs (NSAIDs) are generally effective for tension headaches.[2]

**What are the characteristics of migraine headaches?**

Migraine headaches are typically unilateral, pulsatile, moderate to severe in intensity, aggravated by routine physical activity, and often associated with nausea, photophobia, or phonophobia. Migraines may be preceded by aura, which is a reversible focal neurologic symptom that develops over 5 to 20 minutes and lasts for <60 minutes.[2]

**How often are migraines associated with aura?**

Aura occurs in up to one-fifth of patients with migraine (ie, "classic" migraine) and is most commonly visual in nature. The headache tends to be similar in quality to migraine without aura (ie, "common" migraine) but may lack some features. Aura can occur without an associated headache in some cases.[2]

**What are the pharmacologic treatment options for migraine headaches?**

Abortive and preventive medications are the 2 main approaches to treating migraines. First-line abortive therapies for mild to moderate migraines include NSAIDs or caffeine-containing combination analgesics, whereas triptans and ergotamines are first-line for moderate to severe migraines. There are multiple options for preventive therapies, including antiepileptic drugs (eg, topiramate), β-blockers, calcium channel blockers, and some antidepressants (eg, tricyclics). The choice of therapy should be guided by patient-specific factors.[4,5]

**Cluster headaches are part of what group of primary headache disorders?**

Cluster headaches are considered one of the trigeminal autonomic cephalalgias (TACs), a group of primary headache disorders characterized by the presence of unilateral pain in the distribution of the trigeminal nerve associated with ipsilateral cranial autonomic features (eg, ptosis, conjunctival injection, lacrimation, nasal congestion, rhinorrhea).[6]

**What other conditions belong to the trigeminal autonomic cephalalgias?**

The TACs include cluster headaches, paroxysmal hemicranias, hemicranias continua, short-lasting unilateral neuralgiform headache attacks with conjunctival injection and tearing (SUNCT), and short-lasting unilateral neuralgiform headache attacks with cranial autonomic features (SUNA).[6]

**How common are cluster headaches?**

Cluster headaches, which occur predominantly in men, are the most common of the TACs but are rare overall (affecting approximately 0.1% of the general population).[6]

**What are the pharmacologic treatment options for cluster headaches?**

Like migraine headaches, there are abortive and preventive approaches to managing cluster headaches. For acute termination of a cluster headache, nonoral routes of administration are required. Subcutaneously administered sumatriptan is a first-line option. Oxygen inhalation via a nonrebreather facemask (10-15 L/min for 15-20 minutes) is also considered to be first-line abortive therapy. For prevention, verapamil is considered the drug of choice, but there are other options (eg, topiramate, sodium valproate, melatonin, lithium).[6]

## SECONDARY HEADACHE DISORDERS

**What are the 2 anatomic subcategories of secondary headache disorders?**

Secondary headache disorders can be caused by intracranial or extracranial processes.

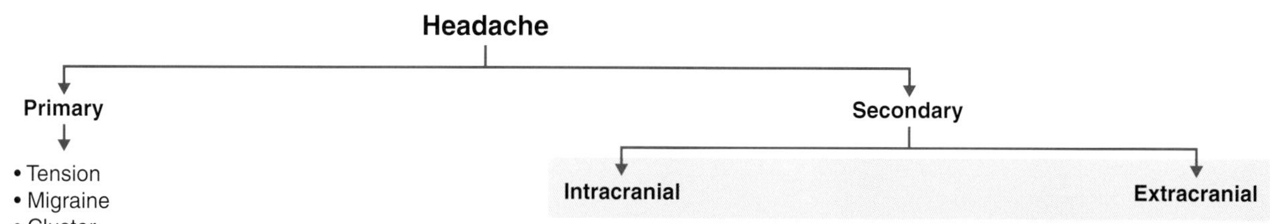


**The intracranial causes of secondary headache can be separated into which general subcategories?**

The intracranial causes of secondary headache can be separated into the following subcategories: vascular, infectious, tumor, cerebrospinal fluid, and other.

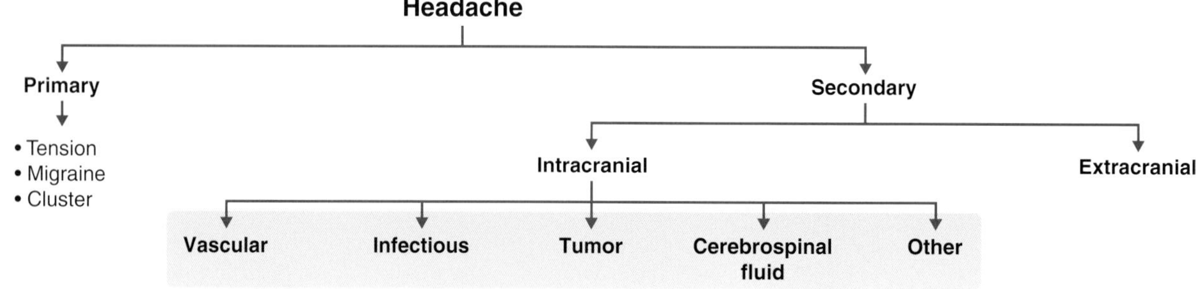

## INTRACRANIAL VASCULAR CAUSES OF HEADACHE

### What are the intracranial vascular causes of headache?

Arteriovenous nicking, flame-shaped hemorrhages, cotton wool spots, and papilledema may be present on fundoscopic examination.

Severe systemic hypertension.

A 72-year-old man with vascular disease presents with acute-onset vertigo, ataxia, and homonymous hemianopsia.

Posterior circulation stroke.

A 24-year-old woman with homozygous factor V Leiden presents with sudden-onset headache after recently starting estrogen-based contraception.

Cerebral venous thrombosis.

This acute vascular event is a common cause of stroke in young patients and may occur within the anterior or posterior circulations.

Arterial dissection.

Nosebleeds, hemoptysis, and cutaneous telangiectasias (Figure 40-2).

Arteriovenous malformation (AVM) related to hereditary hemorrhagic telangiectasia.

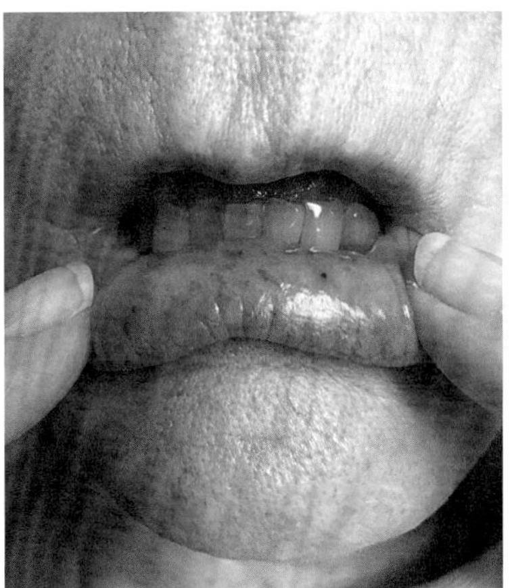

**Figure 40-2.** Multiple telangiectasias involving the mucosa of the lower lip in a patient with hereditary hemorrhagic telangiectasia.

Headache in a patient with polycystic kidney disease.

Cerebral aneurysm.

"Thunderclap" headache in a patient with polycystic kidney disease.

Subarachnoid hemorrhage from ruptured cerebral aneurysm.

Treatment for this vascular condition generally includes immunosuppressive medications.

Vasculitis, including primary angiitis of the central nervous system (PACNS), systemic vasculitis (eg, Behçet's disease), and vasculitis associated with systemic disease (eg, systemic lupus erythematosus).

A mimic of primary angiitis of the central nervous system; this entity usually presents with "thunderclap" headache (which is unusual in primary angiitis of the central nervous system).

Reversible cerebral vasoconstriction syndrome (RCVS).[7]

This vascular condition is most common in Asian populations, with a bimodal age distribution of children around 5 years of age and adults 40 to 50 years of age.

Moyamoya disease.[8]

NEUROLOGY

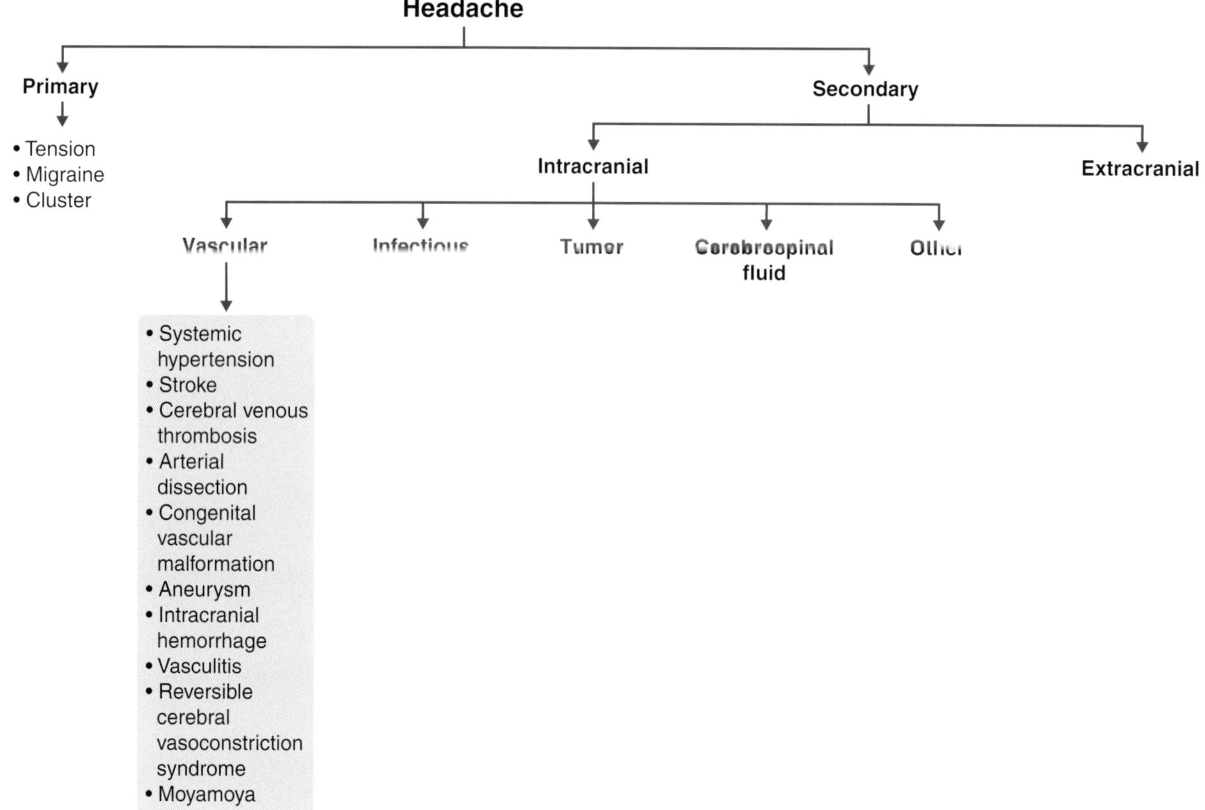


**Under what conditions can systemic hypertension cause headache?**

Headache can occur in association with acute systemic hypertension, where an abrupt rise in blood pressure within the range of autoregulation results in increased transmural pressure in the larger cerebral arteries, which are sensitive to pain; hypertensive encephalopathy, where an abrupt rise in blood pressure outside the range of autoregulation results in extravasation of plasma and erythrocytes into brain tissue; and chronic systemic hypertension.[9]

**What are the characteristics of headache associated with chronic systemic hypertension?**

The headache of chronic systemic hypertension is typically bilateral and located in the back of the head. It tends to be nocturnal, present on waking in the morning, and improved on rising. This pattern occurs because at night, when blood pressure generally tends to be lower, patients with chronic systemic hypertension experience a state of relative hypotension, which triggers compensatory cerebral vasodilation via autoregulation, leading to increased cerebral blood flow and headache. On rising, the erect position increases blood pressure, reversing vasodilation and improving the headache.[9,10]

**How often is headache associated with stroke?**

Headache occurs in around one-third of patients with stroke (it also occurs in some patients with transient ischemic attack), and usually localizes to the affected hemisphere. It occurs more commonly in patients with posterior circulation stroke where it often localizes to the occipital region.[11]

**How common is headache in patients with cerebral venous thrombosis?**

Headache occurs in most patients with cerebral venous thrombosis and is often the initial symptom. Associated manifestations are frequent and include papilledema, focal neurologic deficits, seizure, drowsiness, and confusion. Common causes include infection (eg, otitis media), pregnancy, oral contraceptive use, underlying malignancy, connective tissue disease (eg, Behçet's disease), and thrombophilia (eg, antithrombin III deficiency). CT imaging of the brain is often unrevealing. MRI of the brain combined with magnetic resonance venography is the diagnostic method of choice. Treatment options include anticoagulation, thrombolysis, and surgery.[11]

**Which 2 major intracranial vessels are most commonly involved in arterial dissection?**

The carotid and vertebral arteries are the intracranial vessels most often associated with arterial dissection. Carotid artery dissection is relatively more common.[11]

**What are the 4 general types of congenital cerebral vascular malformation?**

The 4 types of congenital cerebral vascular malformation are developmental venous anomaly, capillary telangiectasia, cavernous malformation, and arteriovenous malformation.

**What are the characteristics of the headache associated with nonruptured cerebral aneurysms?**

The headache associated with nonruptured cerebral aneurysms can be acute or chronic. When acute, it is sudden in onset and severe in intensity, comparable to that of subarachnoid hemorrhage. Other clinical manifestations include facial pain, vision loss, seizure, and cranial neuropathy.[12]

**What are the general types of intracranial hemorrhage?**

There are 5 main types of intracranial hemorrhage: epidural, subdural, subarachnoid, intraparenchymal, and intraventricular. Headache can occur with any of these entities.

**What diagnostic studies are helpful in the diagnosis of primary angiitis of the central nervous system?**

CSF evaluation and neuroimaging are helpful in the workup of PACN. The CSF profile is abnormal in most patients and characterized by modest lymphocytic pleocytosis, elevated protein, and the occasional presence of oligoclonal bands. Brain biopsy is ultimately required to make the diagnosis in most cases (it also has the advantage of ruling out mimics such as infection or malignancy).[7]



**What is the prognosis of reversible cerebral vasoconstriction syndrome?**

RCVS occurs most often in women with a mean age of onset of 42 years. It is caused by transient dysregulation of cerebral vascular tone. Underlying triggers include recent pregnancy, exposure to vasoactive substances (eg, cocaine), and sexual intercourse. The headache is sudden-onset and severe (ie, thunderclap) and is frequently associated with nausea, vomiting, photophobia, confusion, and blurred vision. Most patients with RCVS recover without disability, but stroke with long-term deficits and death have been reported.[13]

**What are the characteristics of the headache associated with moyamoya disease?**

The headache of moyamoya disease is similar to migraine in quality but generally does not respond to pharmacologic therapy. Neuroimaging is required to make the diagnosis (see Figure 42-3). Headache subsides in some patients within a year of surgical treatment, but it is persistent in others.[8]

## INTRACRANIAL INFECTIOUS CAUSES OF HEADACHE

### What are the intracranial infectious causes of headache?

**A 19-year-old military recruit presents with headache, neck stiffness, and photophobia.**

Meningitis.

**Similar to meningitis, but this condition is associated with neurocognitive dysfunction early in the course of illness and can be associated with a normal CSF profile.**

Encephalitis.

**This condition typically requires surgical drainage and a long duration of intravenous antibiotics.**

Brain abscess.

**A 24-year-old woman with active intravenous drug use is admitted with aortic valve endocarditis and develops new headache and focal neurologic deficits.**

Cerebral septic emboli.

**Common in patients with acquired immunodeficiency syndrome (AIDS) as a result of reactivation of previously acquired infection, often through exposure to feline feces**

Cerebral toxoplasmosis.

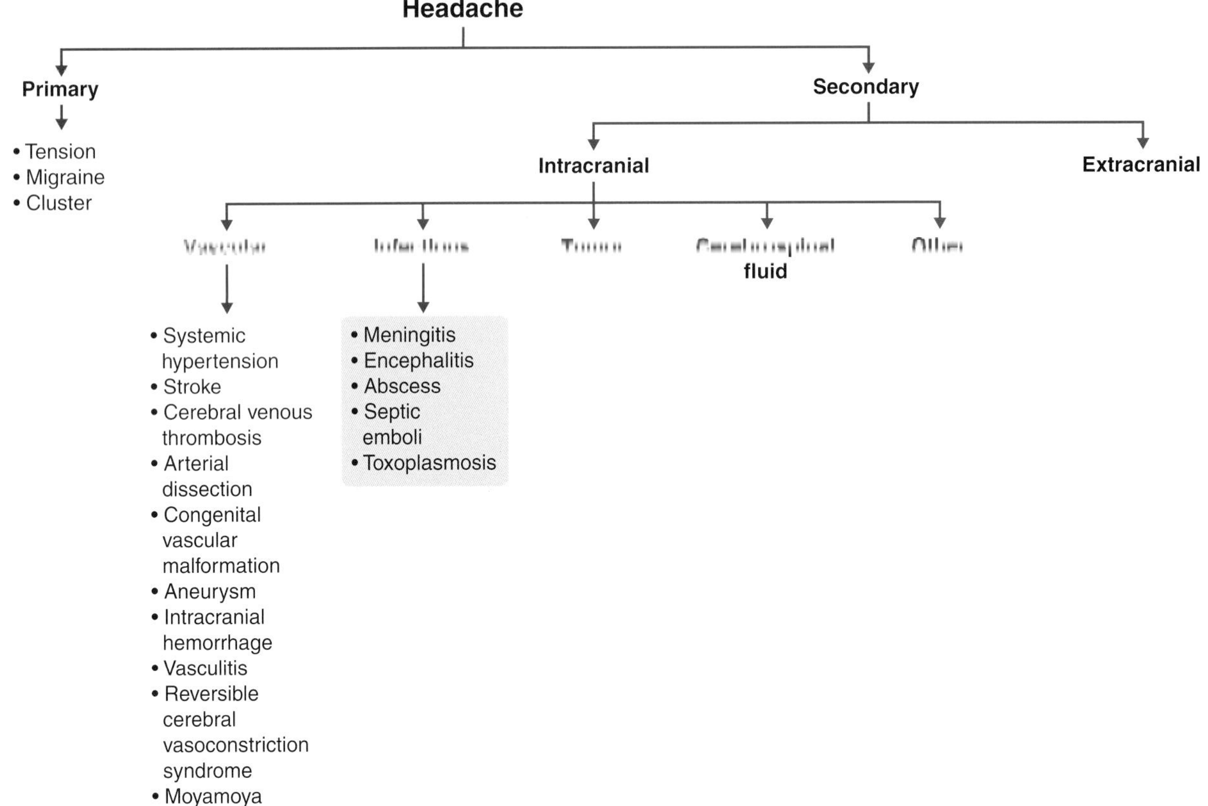


**Which of the following cerebrospinal fluid profiles are characteristic of these conditions: normal, viral meningitis, typical bacterial meningitis, atypical bacterial meningitis, fungal meningitis, and aseptic meningitis?**

| Fluid type | WBC/ μL | WBC type | Glucose (mg/dL) | Protein (mg/dL) |
|---|---|---|---|---|
| A | <5 | Lymphocytes | 40-80 | <50 |
| B | 500-20,000 | Neutrophils | <40 | 100-700 |
| C | 25-500 | Lymphocytes or neutrophils | <40 | 50-500 |
| D | 5-1000 | Lymphocytes | 40-80 | <100 |

Fluid type A corresponds to normal CSF; type B to typical bacterial meningitis; type C to fungal meningitis (and some types of atypical bacterial meningitis, eg, tuberculosis); and type D to viral meningitis, most types of atypical bacterial meningitis, and most types of aseptic meningitis. Fluid types C and D may be characterized by a predominance of neutrophils early in the course of illness.[14]

**What finding may be present on electroencephalography (EEG) in patients with herpes simplex encephalitis?**

In most patients with herpes simplex encephalitis, EEG reveals a temporal focus demonstrating periodic lateralizing epileptiform discharges (ie, lateralized periodic discharges).[15]

**What are the 3 general mechanisms of brain abscess development?**

Brain abscess can occur as a result of direct extension from extracranial infection (eg, dental abscess), hematogenous spread, or direct inoculation following head injury or neurosurgery. Neuroimaging is required to make the diagnosis.

**Is the risk of cerebral septic emboli limited to left-sided infective endocarditis?**

Paradoxical systemic septic emboli, including cerebral emboli, can occur in patients with right-sided endocarditis and coexistent right-to-left shunt. In patients with patent foramen ovale or other intracardiac shunt, transient right-to-left shunting can occur when right-sided pressures are abruptly increased (eg, during Valsalva).[16]

**In patients with human immunodeficiency virus (HIV) infection, what peripheral CD4 cell count is associated with a significant increase in risk of cerebral toxoplasmosis?**

A CD4 cell count <200/μL is associated with a significantly increased risk of cerebral toxoplasmosis and should trigger initiation of specific prophylactic medication (eg, trimethoprim-sulfamethoxazole).[17]

## HEADACHE RELATED TO INTRACRANIAL TUMOR

**How common are intracranial tumors?**

In the industrialized world, the incidence of intracranial tumor is approximately 12 per 100,000 persons.[18]

**How common is headache in patients with intracranial tumors?**

Headache occurs in about one-half of patients with intracranial tumors. Other manifestations include nausea, vomiting, seizure, focal neurologic deficits, and neurocognitive dysfunction.[18]

**What are the characteristics of the headache associated with intracranial tumors?**

The headache associated with intracranial tumors is usually bifrontal but worse on the side of the tumor, similar to tension headache in quality, worse with bending over, associated with nausea or vomiting, and can be more noticeable in the morning.[18,19]

**What is the study of choice to evaluate for the presence of an intracranial tumor?**

MRI of the brain is the study of choice to evaluate for intracranial tumor. CT imaging can miss lesions of the posterior fossa or nonenhancing tumors (eg, low-grade gliomas).[18]

**What are the 2 general types of intracranial tumors?**

Intracranial tumors can be metastatic or primary.

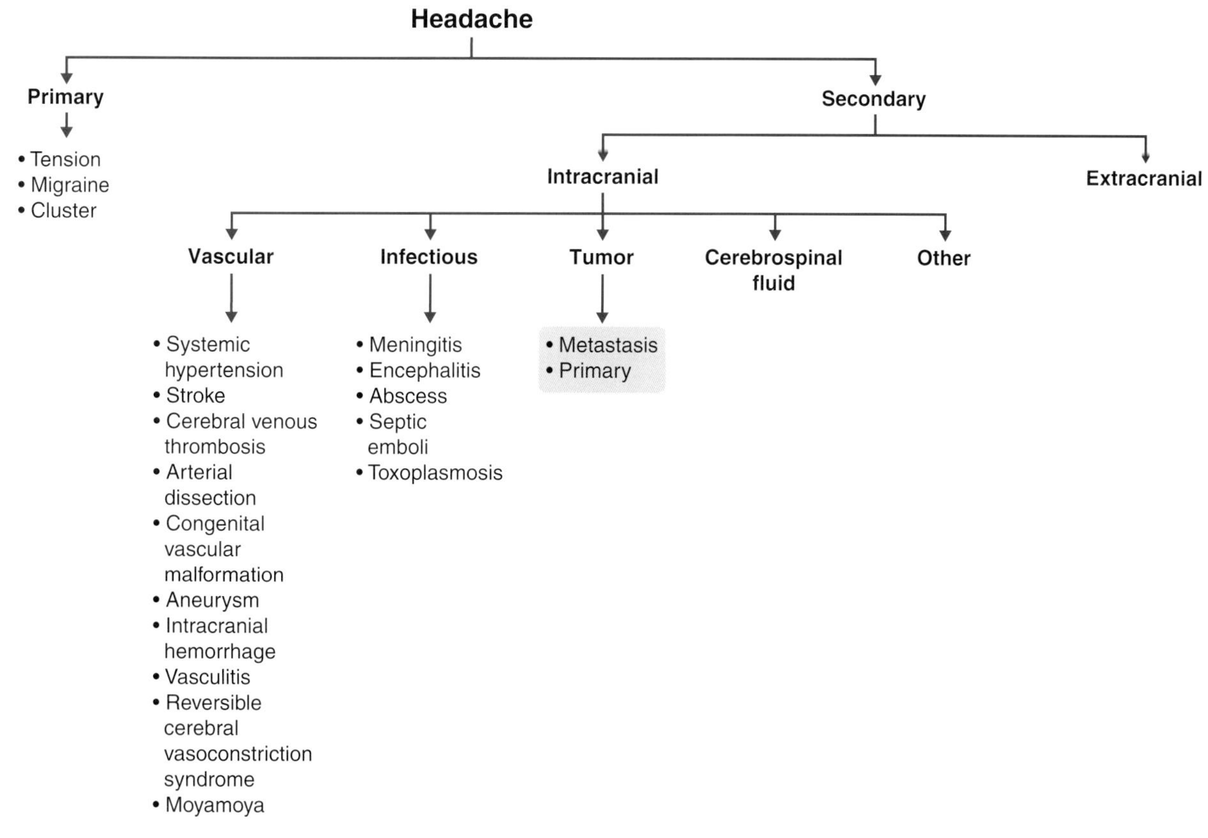

**How common are metastatic brain tumors?**

Brain metastases are the most common type of intracranial metastases and are increasing in frequency (likely due to increasing survival rates), occurring in close to one-half of adult cancer patients according to autopsy reports.[20]

**Which types of cancers are most commonly associated with brain metastases?**

Lung cancer accounts for more than one-half of all cases of brain metastases. Breast cancer, melanoma, renal cell carcinoma, and colorectal cancer make up most of the other cases.[20]

**What is the prognosis of patients with intracranial metastases?**

The prognosis associated with the presence of intracranial metastasis varies according to patient and tumor characteristics but, overall, is quite poor. Virtually all cases are associated with fatal outcomes.[21]

**What is the most common type of primary intracranial tumor in adults?**

Gliomas are the most common type of primary intracranial tumor, accounting for more than one-half of all cases. Glioblastoma multiforme is the most frequent subtype.[22]

**What is the prognosis of glioblastoma multiforme?**

The prognosis of glioblastoma multiforme is poor, with a median survival on the order of months and few survivors at 5 years after diagnosis.[22]

## HEADACHE RELATED TO CEREBROSPINAL FLUID

### What are the causes of headache related to cerebrospinal fluid?

**A 23-year-old obese woman with chronic daily headache is found to have papilledema (Figure 40-3), normal blood pressure, normal neuroimaging, and an opening pressure of 48 cm $H_2O$ on lumbar puncture with an otherwise normal CSF profile.**

Pseudotumor cerebri (ie, idiopathic intracranial hypertension).

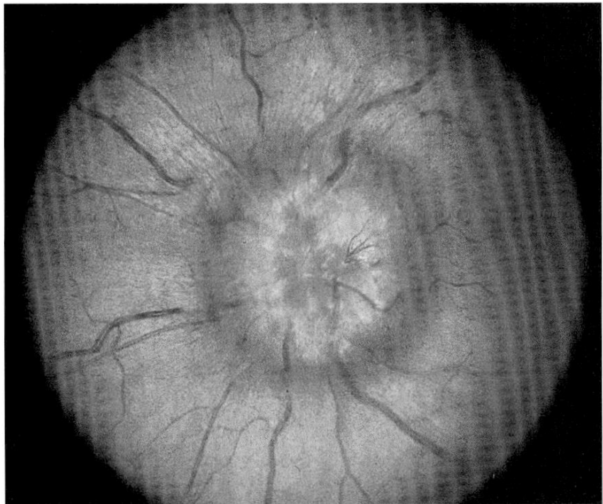

**Figure 40-3.** Chronic papilledema secondary to increased intracranial pressure. There is optic disc edema with indistinct disc margins and obscured blood vessels. (From Rubin R, Strayer DS. *Rubin's Pathology: Clinicopathologic Foundations of Medicine*. 5th ed. Philadelphia, PA: Lippincott Williams & Wilkins; 2008.)

**Accumulation of CSF related to a disturbance in formation, flow, or absorption.**

Hydrocephalus.[23]

**May be associated with clear drainage from the nose or ear.**

Spontaneous cerebrospinal fluid leak.

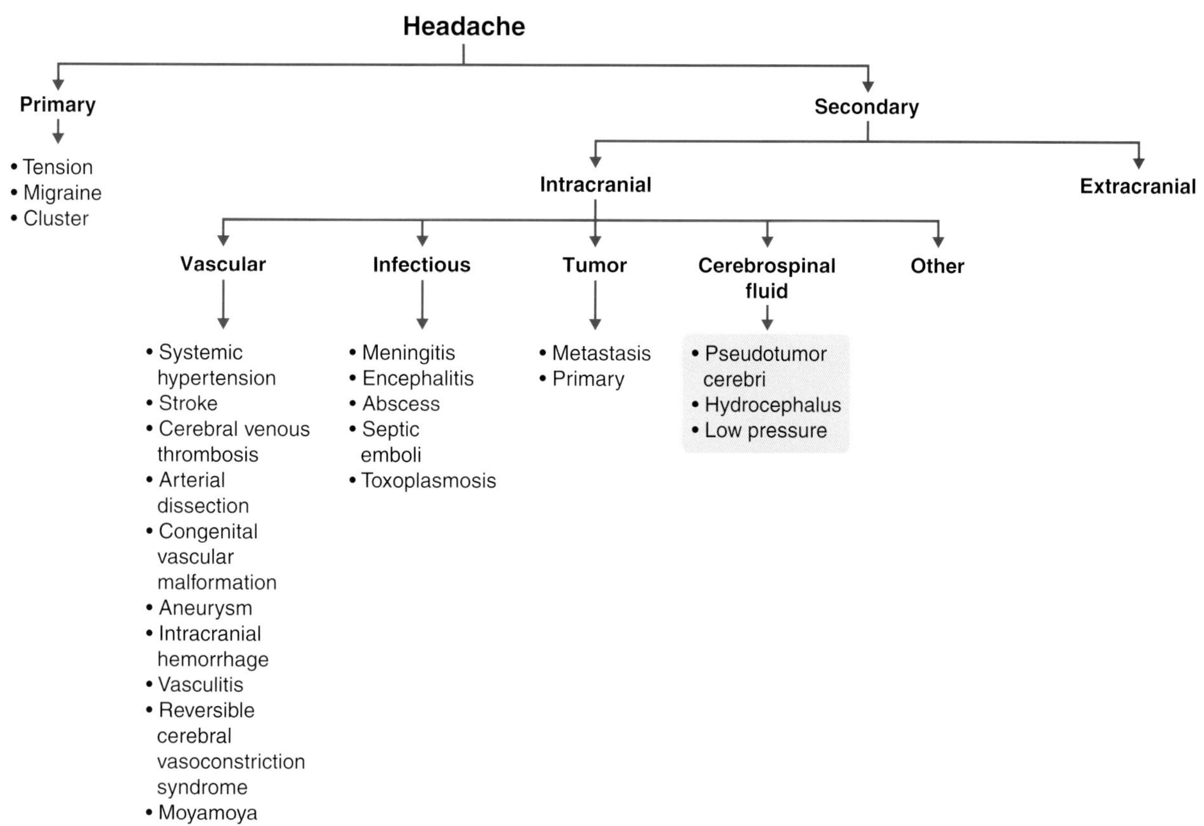




**What is the most severe sequela of pseudotumor cerebri?**

Headache is present in most patients with pseudotumor cerebri. Associated symptoms include blurred vision and visual loss. Permanent vision loss occurs in a significant number of patients. Systemic hypertension is a major risk factor for the development of vision loss in these patients.[24]

**What are the causes of acquired hydrocephalus?**

Acquired hydrocephalus can occur as a result of tumors and cysts (eg, colloid cyst), inflammation (eg, meningitis), and absorption blockages (eg, intracranial hemorrhage, normal pressure hydrocephalus).[23]

**What quality is highly characteristic of the headache associated with low cerebrospinal fluid pressure?**

The headache related to CSF leak is typically positional, worse in the upright position and improved with recumbence. *Lumbar puncture is a more common cause of low CSF pressure than spontaneous CSF leak.*

## OTHER INTRACRANIAL CAUSES OF HEADACHE

### What are the other intracranial causes of headache?

**Recurrent episodes of sudden-onset, brief, unilateral, and stabbing pain in the distribution of 1 or more branches of the fifth cranial nerve.**

Trigeminal neuralgia.

**A college football player complains of chronic daily headache after sustaining a concussion during a game 6 months ago.**

Post-traumatic headache.

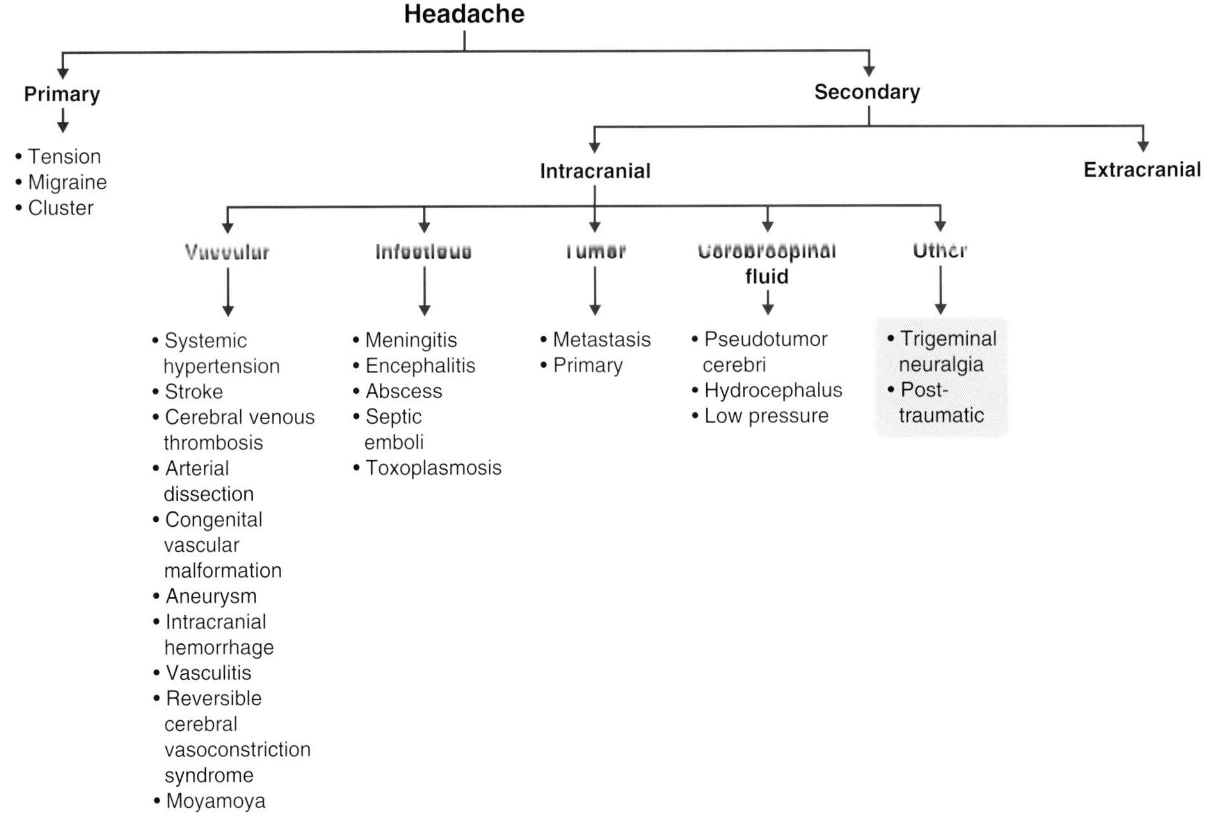


**What is first-line pharmacologic treatment for trigeminal neuralgia?**

Trigeminal neuralgia is a clinical diagnosis, based on characteristic paroxysms of pain in the distribution of one or more branches of the fifth cranial nerve. Carbamazepine is considered first-line pharmacologic treatment. Oxcarbazepine may be an effective alternative agent.[25]

**How common is post-traumatic headache after traumatic brain injury (TBI)?**

At 1 year after TBI, almost one-half of patients experience post-traumatic headache. Women and patients with a baseline headache disorder pre-TBI are more likely to experience post-traumatic headache. Incidence appears to be unrelated to the severity of TBI.[26]

## EXTRACRANIAL CAUSES OF HEADACHE

### What are the extracranial causes of headache?

**A 66-year-old man with coronary artery disease complains of headache after starting a medication for chronic stable angina.**

Nitrates.

**Associated with anxiety, sweats, tactile hallucinations, agitation, and tremor.**

Alcohol withdrawal.

**Extracranial infections.**

Sinusitis and dental abscess.

**Headache may be accompanied by clicking or grating sounds with chewing.**

Temporomandibular joint disorder (TMJ).

**Neck pain often occurs in association with headache caused by this condition.**

Cervical spine disease (ie, cervicogenic headache).

**A marathon runner presents shortly after a race with acute headache, confusion, and vomiting.**

Hypotonic hyponatremia.

**A painful red eye associated with headache, nausea, and vomiting.**

Primary angle-closure glaucoma.

| | |
|---|---|
| **A 32-year-old man presents with sudden-onset neck pain and headache after visiting a chiropractor for a neck strain and is found to have ipsilateral ptosis and miosis.** | Extracranial carotid artery dissection. |
| **A 78-year-old woman complains of headache, scalp tenderness, and jaw discomfort with meals and is found to have an erythrocyte sedimentation rate of 80 mm/h.** | Giant cell (or temporal) arteritis. |

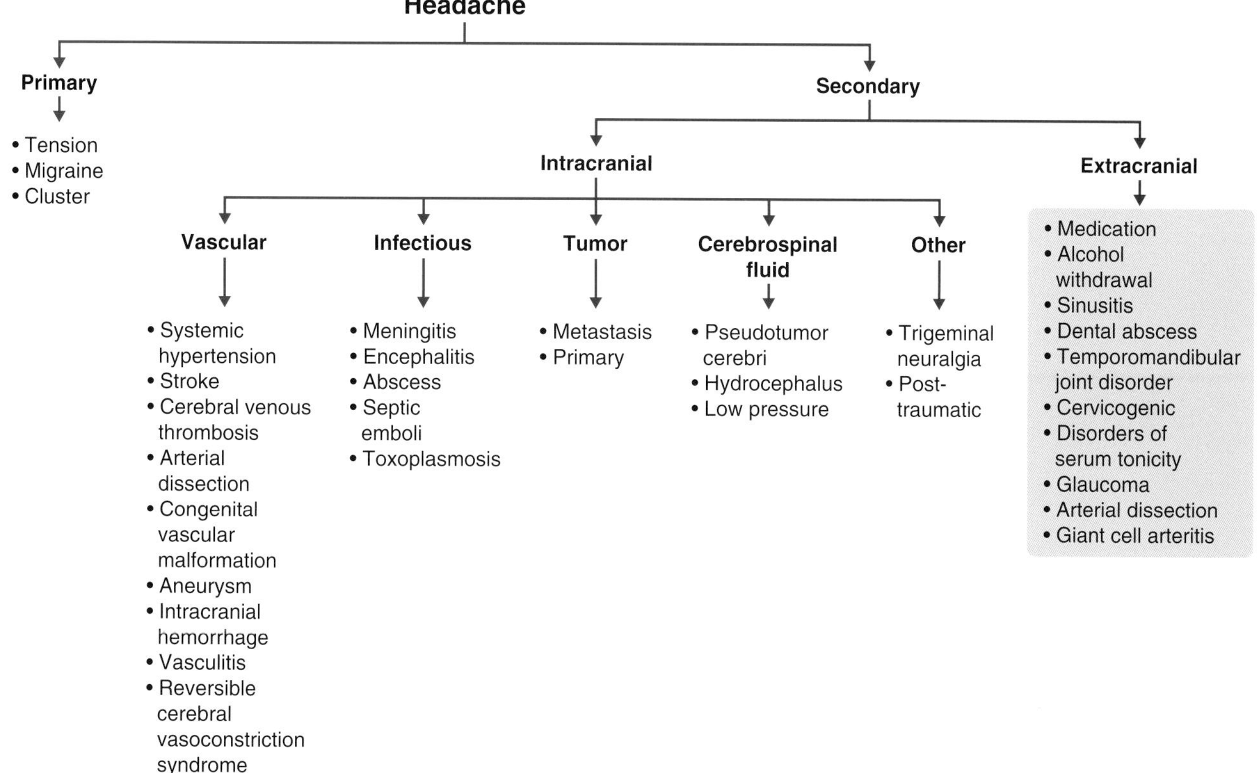


| | |
|---|---|
| **What are the various ways in which medication can cause or contribute to headache?** | Headache can occur as a side effect of appropriate medication use (eg, nitrates), as a result of medication overuse (eg, ibuprofen), or from medication withdrawal (eg, estrogens). |
| **When does headache typically occur during the course of alcohol withdrawal?** | Minor withdrawal symptoms, including headache, typically occur within 8 hours of cessation of chronic alcohol consumption.[27] |
| **What are the characteristics of the headache caused by sinusitis?** | Headache associated with sinusitis is typically periorbital with radiation to the ears, has a quality of pressure or dullness, is worse in the morning but improves over the course of the day, and is associated with nasal congestion.[28] |
| **What serious complication must be considered in a patient with a dental abscess, headache, and a focal neurologic deficit?** | Any patient with a dental abscess who develops headache and a focal neurologic deficit should be evaluated with neuroimaging for a brain abscess as a result of contiguous spread of infection. |
| **What are the characteristics of headache associated with temporomandibular joint disorder?** | Headache occurs in most patients with TMJ and is often the only manifestation. It is most commonly bilateral and can be located in the temporal, periorbital, or frontal regions. It is often precipitated by jaw movements, excessive talking, chewing gum, eating tough-textured food, and stress.[29] |
| **What are the characteristics of cervicogenic headache?** | Cervicogenic headache is 4 times more likely to occur in women. It is typically unilateral, starting at the back of the head before migrating to the front. It can be aggravated by certain neck positions.[30] |

NEUROLOGY

**What is the mechanism of headache in patients with serum hypotonicity?**

Serum hypotonicity leads to a shift of fluid from the extracellular the intracellular fluid compartment, with resultant cerebral edema and associated headache. A similar mechanism occurs when chronic hypertonicity is corrected too quickly.

**What is the treatment for acute primary angle-closure glaucoma?**

Acute primary angle-closure glaucoma is a medical emergency that requires prompt recognition and treatment to avoid blindness. Patients typically present with a painful red eye with blurred vision, headache, and nausea and vomiting. Topical and systemic pharmacologic agents (eg, topical timolol maleate and systemic acetazolamide) should be started immediately to lower intraocular pressure, followed by iridotomy. When recognized and treated promptly, most patients with acute primary angle-closure glaucoma recover without permanent vision damage.[31]

**What is the typical location of the headache related to vertebral artery dissection?**

Vertebral artery dissection classically results in pain over the occipital region. When there is cerebral ischemia, headache may be accompanied by neurologic deficits in a posterior distribution pattern (eg, vision loss, nystagmus, cerebellar signs). The diagnosis is made with CT or magnetic resonance angiography.[11]

**How common is headache in patients with giant cell arteritis?**

Giant cell arteritis typically affects patients older than 50 years. Headache is present in more than 90% of cases. It tends to be localized and progressive in nature, and may be accompanied by vision changes, systemic symptoms (eg, fever, weight loss, myalgias), and superficial temporal artery swelling and tenderness (see Figure 50-2). Elevation of the erythrocyte sedimentation rate (>50 mm/h) is characteristic. When giant cell arteritis is suspected, patients should immediately be started on high dose glucocorticoids (eg, 1 mg/kg of prednisone) followed by urgent biopsy of the temporal artery.[11]

## Case Summary

A previously healthy 50-year-old man with recent travel to British Columbia presents with chronic fatigue, fever, headache, and tinnitus and is found to have an abnormal CSF profile with a ring-enhancing brain lesion on neuroimaging.

***What is the most likely cause of headache in this patient?***

Fungal meningitis.

### BONUS QUESTIONS

***What features of this case are suggestive of a secondary headache disorder?***

Features of this case concerning for a secondary headache disorder include onset after 40 years of age, the presence of systemic symptoms and signs (fever and weight loss), and the presence of neurologic deficits (tinnitus, papilledema).

***What features of this case are characteristic of fungal meningitis?***

In this case, fungal meningitis is suggested by the indolent nature of the symptoms as well as the presence of the typical CSF profile of fungal meningitis (some atypical bacterial infections, such as *Coxiella*, can present with a similar CSF profile; see chapter 30, Meningitis).

***Which organism is the most likely cause of fungal meningitis in this case?***

*Cryptococcus gattii* is the organism most likely to be involved in this case because it is endemic to British Columbia, Canada (where the patient had recently traveled) and can infect immunocompetent hosts. The markedly elevated opening pressure on lumbar puncture is also characteristic of cryptococcal meningitis.

***What cerebrospinal fluid studies can confirm the diagnosis of cryptococcal meningitis?***

CSF samples should be sent for India ink preparation, culture, and assays for cryptococcal antigen (including the recently developed lateral flow assay). However, these studies are not 100% sensitive, particularly in cases involving *Cryptococcus gattii*. Repeat large-volume CSF samples can improve sensitivity.[32]

***What is the most likely cause of the ring-enhancing lesion on brain imaging in this case?***

The brain lesion demonstrated by the neuroimaging in this case (see Figure 40-1, arrows) is most likely a cryptococcoma.

| | |
|---|---|
| *What findings on MRI of the brain may be present in patients with cryptococcal meningitis?* | In addition to crytpococcomas, brain MRI in patients with cryptococcal meningitis may demonstrate dilated Virchow-Robin spaces, pseudocysts, cortical and lacunar infarcts, and hydrocephalus.[32] |
| *How is Cryptococcus acquired?* | *Cryptococcus* is acquired via inhalation, where it can then disseminate. Sometimes dissemination occurs after a latent period, during which the fungus is contained within the lymph nodes of the lungs.[32] |
| *Which 2 species of Cryptococcus cause meningitis, and which demographic groups are affected by each?* | *Cryptococcus neoformans* is a ubiquitous fungus that typically infects immunocompromised hosts (eg, HIV-positive patients); *Cryptococcus gattii* is an endemic fungus found in various regions of the world (eg, British Columbia, Canada) that can infect immunocompromised and immunocompetent hosts. |
| *What is the natural history of cryptococcal meningitis?* | Without treatment, cryptococcal meningitis progresses and patients develop confusion, seizure, impaired consciousness, and eventually coma and death.[32] |
| *What is the treatment for cryptococcal meningitis?* | Cryptococcal meningitis is treated with antifungal therapy in 3 phases which include induction (2-6 weeks), consolidation (8 weeks), and maintenance (≥1 year). The induction phase typically consists of the combination of liposomal amphotericin B plus flucytosine. Consolidation and maintenance therapies consist of varying doses of fluconazole monotherapy. The recommended induction phase for immunocompetent patients (including those with *Cryptococcus gattii* infection) is longer (4-6 weeks). The presence of cerebral cryptococcomas may require prolonged therapy.[32] |
| *What is the prognosis of cryptococcal meningitis in HIV-positive patients?* | Outcomes are not appreciably different between HIV-positive patients infected with *Cryptococcus gattii* and those infected with *Cryptococcus neoformans*. In the industrialized world, the 10-week mortality in HIV-infected patients is as high as 25% despite treatment. Factors associated with poor outcomes include delirium at the time of presentation, older age, lower weight, and higher fungal burden (assessed via CSF colony-forming unit count).[32] |
| *What is the prognosis of cryptococcal meningitis in HIV-negative patients?* | In the industrialized world, cryptococcal meningitis in HIV-negative patients is associated with a 90-day mortality rate of approximately 30%. Factors associated with poor outcomes include delirium at the time of presentation, the absence of headache, higher fungal burden, and lower CSF white blood cell count.[32] |
| *What therapeutic option exists for patients with cryptococcal meningitis who have elevated intracranial pressure?* | Cryptococcal meningitis with high CSF opening pressure is associated with a greater burden of symptoms (eg, headache, nausea, delirium). Therapeutic lumbar punctures can be used to control high CSF pressure in these patients, improving symptoms and other outcomes, including mortality. One approach is to reduce the opening pressure by 50% (when extremely elevated) or to a normal pressure of <20 cm $H_2O$.[33,34] |

## KEY POINTS

- There is a high lifetime prevalence of headache in the general population, and it is one of the most common presenting complaints in the primary care setting.
- Headache disorders can be primary or secondary.
- The most common primary headache disorders include tension headache, migraine headache, and cluster headache.
- In general, primary headache disorders are more common than secondary disorders, but the risk of a secondary disorder increases in certain populations (eg, immunocompromised patients).
- Clues to the presence of secondary headache include sudden or new-onset headache at an older age (>40 years), change in the quality of chronic headache, systemic symptoms or illness (eg, fever), neurologic symptoms or signs (eg, seizure), headaches that wake patients from sleep, and headaches that are worsened with Valsalva.
- Secondary headache disorders can be caused by intracranial or extracranial processes.
- Intracranial causes of secondary headache can be separated into the following subcategories: vascular, infectious, tumor, cerebrospinal fluid, and other.

## REFERENCES


1. Bigal ME, Bordini CA, Speciali JG. Etiology and distribution of headaches in two Brazilian primary care units. *Headache*. 2000;40(3):241-247.
2. Hale N, Paauw DS. Diagnosis and treatment of headache in the ambulatory care setting: a review of classic presentations and new considerations in diagnosis and management. *Med Clin North Am*. 2014;98(3):505-527.
3. Venkatesan A. Case 13: a man with progressive headache and confusion. *MedGenMed*. 2006;8(3):19.
4. Estemalik E, Tepper S. Preventive treatment in migraine and the new US guidelines. *Neuropsychiatr Dis Treat*. 2013;9:709-720.
5. Gilmore B, Michael M. Treatment of acute migraine headache. *Am Fam Physician*. 2011;83(3):271-280.
6. Newman LC. Trigeminal autonomic cephalalgias. *Continuum (Minneap Minn)*. 2015;21(4 Headache):1041-1057.
7. Hajj-Ali RA, Calabrese LH. Primary angiitis of the central nervous system. *Autoimmun Rev*. 2013;12(4):463-466.
8. Scott RM, Smith ER. Moyamoya disease and moyamoya syndrome. *N Engl J Med*. 2009;360(12):1226-1237.
9. Spierings EL. Acute and chronic hypertensive headache and hypertensive encephalopathy. *Cephalalgia*. 2002;22(4):313-316.
10. Moser M, Wish H, Friedman AP. Headache and hypertension. *JAMA*. 1962;180:301-306.
11. Dodick D. Headache as a symptom of ominous disease. What are the warning signals? *Postgrad Med*. 1997;101(5):46-50, 5-6, 62-4.
12. Raps EC, Rogers JD, Galetta SL, et al. The clinical spectrum of unruptured intracranial aneurysms. *Arch Neurol*. 1993;50(3):265-268.
13. Sattar A, Manousakis G, Jensen MB. Systematic review of reversible cerebral vasoconstriction syndrome. *Expert Rev Cardiovasc Ther*. 2010;8(10):1417-1421.
14. Walker HK, Hall WD, Hurst JW, eds. *Clinical Methods: The History, Physical, and Laboratory Examinations*. 3rd ed. Boston: Butterworths; 1990.
15. Tunkel AR, Glaser CA, Bloch KC, et al. The management of encephalitis: clinical practice guidelines by the Infectious Diseases Society of America. *Clin Infect Dis*. 2008;47(3):303-327.
16. Pittenger B, Young JW, Mansoor AM. Subretinal abscess. *BMJ Case Rep*. 2017;2017.
17. Belanger F, Derouin F, Grangeot-Keros L, Meyer L. Incidence and risk factors of toxoplasmosis in a cohort of human immunodeficiency virus-infected patients: 1988-1995. HEMOCO and SEROCO Study Groups. *Clin Infect Dis*. 1999;28(3):575-581.
18. DeAngelis LM. Brain tumors. *N Engl J Med*. 2001;344(2):114-123.
19. Forsyth PA, Posner JB. Headaches in patients with brain tumors: a study of 111 patients. *Neurology*. 1993;43(9):1678-1683.
20. Rivkin M, Kanoff RB. Metastatic brain tumors: current therapeutic options and historical perspective. *J Am Osteopath Assoc*. 2013;113(5):418-423.
21. Owonikoko TK, Arbiser J, Zelnak A, et al. Current approaches to the treatment of metastatic brain tumours. *Nat Rev Clin Oncol*. 2014;11(4):203-222.
22. Ohgaki H. Epidemiology of brain tumors. *Methods Mol Biol*. 2009;472:323-342.
23. Pople IK. Hydrocephalus and shunts: what the neurologist should know. J Neurol Neurosurg Psychiatry. 2002;73(suppl 1):i17-i22.
24. Corbett JJ, Savino PJ, Thompson HS, et al. Visual loss in pseudotumor cerebri. Follow-up of 57 patients from five to 41 years and a profile of 14 patients with permanent severe visual loss. *Arch Neurol*. 1982;39(8):461-474.
25. Zakrzewska JM, Linskey ME. Trigeminal neuralgia. *BMJ Clin Evid*. 2014;2014.
26. Hoffman JM, Lucas S, Dikmen S, et al. Natural history of headache after traumatic brain injury. *J Neurotrauma*. 2011;28(9):1719-1725.
27. Schuckit MA. Recognition and management of withdrawal delirium (delirium tremens). *N Engl J Med*. 2014;371(22):2109-2113.
28. Tarabichi M. Characteristics of sinus-related pain. *Otolaryngol Head Neck Surg*. 2000;122(6):842-847.
29. Lupoli TA, Lockey RF. Temporomandibular dysfunction: an often overlooked cause of chronic headaches. *Ann Allergy Asthma Immunol*. 2007;99(4):314-318.
30. Page P. Cervicogenic headaches: an evidence-led approach to clinical management. *Int J Sports Phys Ther*. 2011;6(3):254-266.
31. Weinreb RN, Aung T, Medeiros FA. The pathophysiology and treatment of glaucoma: a review. *JAMA*. 2014;311(18):1901-1911.
32. Williamson PR, Jarvis JN, Panackal AA, et al. Cryptococcal meningitis: epidemiology, immunology, diagnosis and therapy. *Nat Rev Neurol*. 2017;13(1):13-24.
33. Graybill JR, Sobel J, Saag M, et al. Diagnosis and management of increased intracranial pressure in patients with AIDS and cryptococcal meningitis. The NIAID Mycoses Study Group and AIDS Cooperative Treatment Groups. *Clin Infect Dis*. 2000;30(1):47-54.
34. Perfect JR, Dismukes WE, Dromer F, et al. Clinical practice guidelines for the management of cryptococcal disease: 2010 update by the Infectious Diseases Society of America. *Clin Infect Dis*. 2010;50(3):291-322.

Chapter 41

# POLYNEUROPATHY

## Case: A 42-year-old woman with a painful tongue

A 42-year-old woman with a history of hypertension, obesity, and gastric bypass surgery complicated by chronic diarrhea is evaluated in the clinic for a painful tongue and numbness of the lower extremities. The tongue has been swollen, red, and painful over the past few weeks. She also describes progressively worsening numbness and "pins and needles" sensations in the hands and feet over the same period of time. She describes difficulty with balance and walking. The patient underwent gastric bypass surgery at 38 years of age. She stopped taking all medications 8 months ago because of financial reasons. She does not drink alcohol.

There is erythema and scaling of the oral commissures, and the tongue is beefy and red (Figure 41-1). There are sharply marginated patches of scaly erythema around the anogenital region. There is symmetric weakness of the hip and knee flexors. Patellar tendon reflexes are brisk, however Achilles tendon reflexes are absent. Stimulation of the plantar aspect of the foot results in dorsiflexion of the hallux (ie, positive Babinski sign). There are symmetric distal deficits in light touch, vibratory sensation, and proprioception in all 4 extremities, and there are less severe deficits in pain and temperature sensations. Romberg test is positive. There is frank ataxia on gait examination.

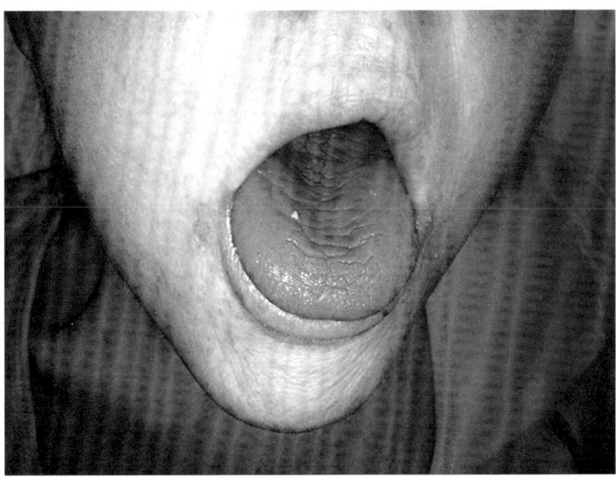

**Figure 41-1.** (Courtesy of OHSU Chief Residents, 2012-2013.)

***What is the most likely cause of polyneuropathy in this patient?***

**What is neuropathy?**

Neuropathy describes injury to any part of the central or peripheral nervous systems (Figure 41-2).

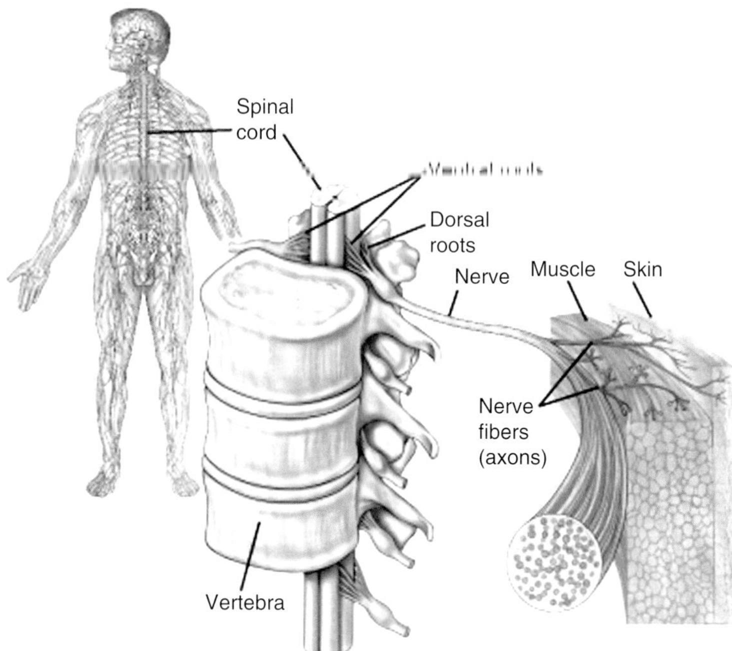


**Figure 41-2.** The central and peripheral nervous systems.

**What is peripheral neuropathy?**

The peripheral nervous system is composed of the cranial nerves (excluding the optic nerve), the spinal nerve roots (ventral and dorsal), the dorsal root ganglia, the peripheral nerve trunks and associated terminal branches, and the peripheral autonomic nervous system. Peripheral neuropathy refers to injury or dysfunction in any part of the peripheral nervous system, encompassing conditions such as radiculopathy, plexopathy, mononeuropathy, and polyneuropathy. The somatic (ie, motor, sensory) and autonomic nervous systems may be involved. Clinical manifestations may include pain, impaired sensation and strength, and autonomic symptoms (eg, abnormal sweating). *The term peripheral neuropathy is often incorrectly used as a synonym for polyneuropathy.*[1–3]

**What is radiculopathy?**

Radiculopathy is a type of peripheral neuropathy in which injury occurs at the level of the nerve root, where the nerve exits the spinal cord. Clinical manifestations involve the corresponding dermatome and myotome. Sensory symptoms (eg, numbness, tingling, pain) often start in the back or neck and radiate to an extremity in a dermatomal distribution.[4]

**What is plexopathy?**

Plexopathy is a type of peripheral neuropathy involving groups of nerves called plexuses, usually related to trauma or entrapment (ie, compression), resulting in symptoms and signs in the distribution of the plexus. For example, brachial plexopathy results in disturbances in strength, sensation, and reflexes along the C5-T1 distribution.[5]

**What is mononeuropathy?**

Mononeuropathy is a type of peripheral neuropathy involving a single peripheral nerve, usually related to trauma or entrapment. Clinical manifestations are typically acute to subacute in onset and correlate with an individual nerve distribution. Carpal tunnel syndrome is an example of mononeuropathy.[4]

**What is mononeuritis multiplex?**

Mononeuritis multiplex (ie, multiple mononeuropathy or mononeuropathy multiplex) is a type of peripheral neuropathy that involves at least 2 noncontiguous peripheral nerves. It is commonly associated with vasculitis, where inflammation and thrombosis of the vasa nervorum results in ischemic injury to the nerve. Other causes of mononeuritis multiplex include diabetes, leprosy, sarcoidosis, and hereditary neuropathy with liability to pressure palsy.[3,6]

**What is polyneuropathy?**

Polyneuropathy is a type of peripheral neuropathy that is generalized, affecting many peripheral nerves. Clinical manifestations typically occur in symmetric nerve distributions, usually in a length-dependent fashion (ie, disturbances begin at the terminal ends of the longest nerves), and with an early predominance of sensory symptoms (weakness is a late finding). *Although mononeuritis multiplex is technically a form of polyneuropathy and can mimic a generalized condition (particularly when it is advanced), it is considered separate by convention.*[4]

NEUROLOGY

**What are the 2 main pathophysiologic and electrophysiologic patterns of nerve injury in patients with polyneuropathy?**

Neuropathy can be associated with axonal or demyelinating patterns of injury (Figure 41-3). Axonal neuropathy involves degeneration and loss of axons. Demyelinating neuropathy involves degeneration of the myelin surrounding axons. Causes of neuropathy can be associated with patterns of axonal or demyelinating injury, which can guide the differential diagnosis.[1]

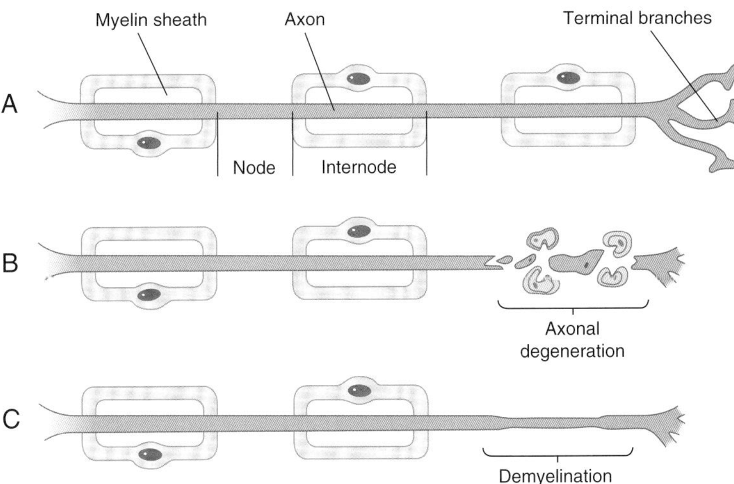


**Figure 41-3.** Axonal degeneration and demyelinating disease of peripheral nerve fibers. A, The normal axon surrounded by myelin, which provides an insulating sheath that allows for rapid saltatory conduction of action potentials. B, Axonal degeneration ("dying-back" phenomenon). C, Demyelination, with loss of the myelin sheath. (From Krishnan AV, Pussell BA, Kiernan MC. Neuromuscular disease in the dialysis patient: an update for the nephrologist. *Semin Dial*. 2009;22:267-278.)

**What are the symptoms of polyneuropathy?**

Symptoms of polyneuropathy may include, in varying combinations, numbness or loss of sensation (hypoesthesia), "pins and needles" or tingling sensations (paresthesia), pain or burning (dysesthesia), early satiety or other autonomic disturbances, and weakness (typically a late finding).[4]

**What parts of the neurologic examination are important in the evaluation of patients with suspected polyneuropathy?**

Physical examination is essential in patients with polyneuropathy. The cranial nerve examination is important for identifying proximal involvement. Motor examination should assess for strength, muscle bulk, tone, and the presence of fasciculations. Reflexes should be evaluated. Sensory examination should separately evaluate the large fibers (ie, vibration and joint position) and small fibers (ie, pain [assessed by pinprick testing] and temperature). The pattern of motor and sensory involvement should be noted (ie, symmetric or asymmetric, distal or proximal, focal or nonfocal). Other useful tests include the Romberg test and evaluation of gait.[3,7]

**What are the physical findings of polyneuropathy?**

Physical findings of polyneuropathy depend on the predominant type of nerve fibers involved (ie, motor or sensory), but may include, in varying combinations, hypoesthesia, hyperesthesia, allodynia, sensory ataxia, hyporeflexia, generalized weakness, and autonomic disturbances (eg, orthostatic hypotension).[8]

**Why is it helpful to determine the size of fibers involved in patients with polyneuropathy?**

Different causes of polyneuropathy often affect nerve fibers in specific patterns. Physical testing can identify the fibers involved, thus narrowing the differential diagnosis. Large fiber neuropathies manifest with combinations of disturbances in strength, vibratory sense, and proprioception; whereas small fiber neuropathies manifest with combinations of disturbances in pain and temperature sensations, and autonomic function. Reflexes are generally diminished or absent in patients with large fiber neuropathies, but remain intact in patients with small fiber neuropathies.[3]

**In addition to polyneuropathy, what other lower motor neuron conditions should be considered in patients who present with pure motor disturbance?**

Although some types of polyneuropathies predominantly involve motor fibers, a pure motor disorder (ie, weakness without sensory or autonomic disturbances) should prompt consideration of motor neuron diseases (eg, amyotrophic lateral sclerosis), neuromuscular junction disorders (eg, myasthenia gravis), and myopathies (eg, polymyositis).

**What is the role of electrodiagnostic testing in the workup of polyneuropathy?**

Electrodiagnostic studies (ie, nerve conduction study [NCS] and electromyography [EMG]) are useful for identifying disorders involving large myelinated fibers but not small fibers. The combination of NCS and EMG can localize the lesion, determine the pattern of injury (ie, axonal or demyelinating), determine the fiber type involved (ie, motor, sensory, or both), and provide a sense of severity and time course of the disease (ie, acute or chronic).[9,10]

**What studies are available to test for autonomic dysfunction?**

Autonomic function can be assessed via the following methods: (1) measuring the heart rate response to respiration, Valsalva maneuver, or tilting (ie, tilt table testing); (2) measuring the blood pressure response to hand grip, Valsalva maneuver, or tilting; and (3) measuring the sympathetic skin response (ie, sudomotor testing).[10]

**What supplementary studies can be helpful in select patients with polyneuropathy?**

Genetic studies, cerebrospinal fluid (CSF) examination, skin biopsy, and nerve biopsy can each play a role in the evaluation of polyneuropathy in select patients.

**How common is polyneuropathy?**

Polyneuropathy affects about 4% of the general population in the industrialized world, and is more common in patients older than 75 years.[4]

**What are the 4 general categories of polyneuropathy?**

Polyneuropathy can be metabolic, toxic, inflammatory, or hereditary.

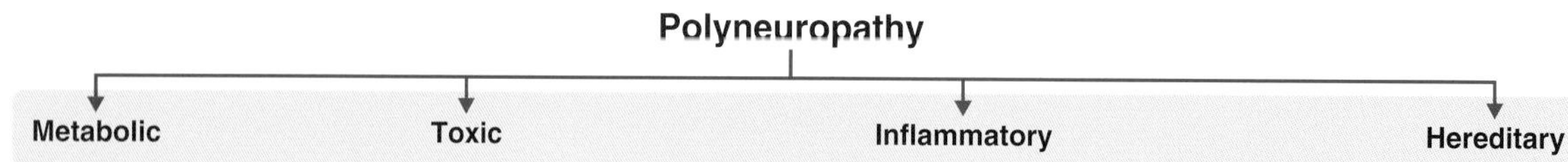


**How often is a diagnosis made in patients presenting with polyneuropathy?**

The combination of history, physical examination, laboratory testing (eg, serum protein electrophoresis [SPEP]), and ancillary testing (eg, electrodiagnostic tests) reveals a diagnosis in up to 80% of cases of polyneuropathy. A diagnosis is not made in the remainder of cases despite a thorough workup. Idiopathic polyneuropathy typically progresses slowly and does not often result in severe physical disability.[10]

## METABOLIC CAUSES OF POLYNEUROPATHY

**What pathophysiologic or electrophysiologic pattern of nerve injury is most commonly associated with metabolic causes of polyneuropathy?**

Metabolic causes of polyneuropathy are most commonly associated with axonal injury, but demyelinating injury can predominate in some conditions.[2]

## What are the metabolic causes of polyneuropathy?

**The single most common cause of polyneuropathy in the industrialized world.**

Diabetes mellitus.

**Weight gain, bradycardia, and Queen Anne's sign (thinning of the lateral third of the eyebrows).**

Hypothyroidism.

**In patients with this condition, progressive polyneuropathy is an indication to initiate dialysis, which is often successful in halting further neuropathic progression.**

Chronic kidney disease (CKD).[11]

**A patient with celiac sprue presents with paresthesias of the feet.**

Nutritional deficiency.

**Spider angiomas, palmar erythema, and caput medusae.**

Chronic liver disease.

**Frontal bossing, protruding jaw (Figure 41-4), and hyperglycemia.**

Acromegaly.

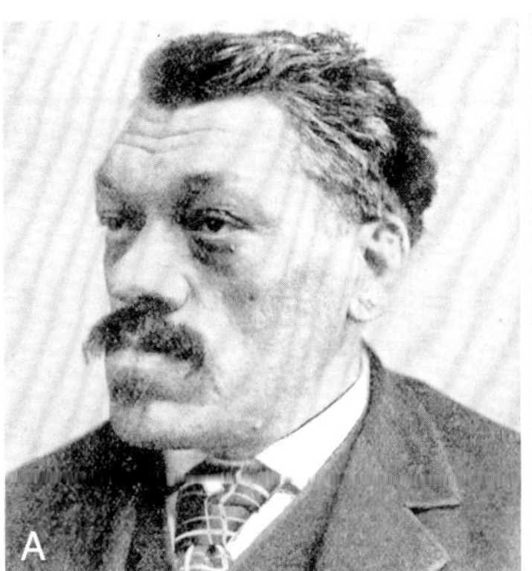


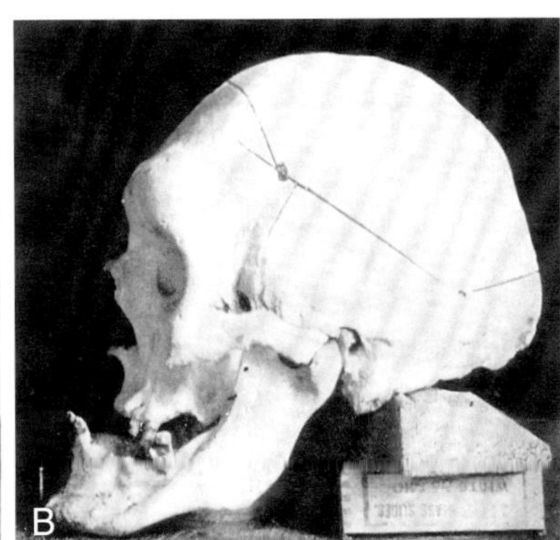


**Figure 41-4.** A, Typical coarse facial features of acromegaly. The nose, eyelids, and ears are enlarged and thickened. The supraorbital ridges are prominent. The lower lip is thick and projecting. The bones of the lower jaw are enlarged, leading to prognathism. B, Skull of a patient with acromegaly, demonstrating prognathism and prominent supraorbital ridges. (From Osborne OT. Acromegaly. In: Buck AH, ed. *A Reference Handbook of the Medical Sciences*. Vol 1. New York: William Wood and Co.; 1900.)

**Polyneuropathy**

- **Metabolic**
  - Diabetes mellitus
  - Hypothyroidism
  - Chronic kidney disease
  - Nutritional deficiency
  - Chronic liver disease
  - Acromegaly
- **Toxic**
- **Inflammatory**
- **Hereditary**

**Which screening tests can be performed in the clinic to evaluate for polyneuropathy in patients with diabetes?**

Diabetes mellitus accounts for up to one-half of cases of polyneuropathy in the industrialized world. In diabetic patients, impairment in vibratory perception using a 128-Hz tuning fork is associated with a positive likelihood ratio of polyneuropathy of up to 35; impairment in pressure sensation with a 5.07 monofilament is associated with a positive likelihood ratio of up to 15. *Prediabetes (eg, impaired glucose tolerance) can also cause polyneuropathy.*[4]

**What are the clinical characteristics of polyneuropathy related to hypothyroidism?**

Polyneuropathy related to hypothyroidism is common, although typically mild. Electrodiagnostic testing most often reveals a sensory neuropathy. Paresthesia is the most commonly reported symptom.[12]

**How common is polyneuropathy in patients with chronic kidney disease?**

Polyneuropathy is present in the majority of patients with CKD who are dialysis-dependent. The high prevalence in this population is likely a reflection of the coexistence of diabetes and CKD. Patients with the combination of CKD and diabetes tend to have more severe polyneuropathy than those with CKD alone.[11]

**Which nutritional deficiencies are associated with polyneuropathy?**

Polyneuropathy can be caused by deficiencies of vitamin B12 (cobalamin), vitamin B1 (thiamine), vitamin B6 (pyridoxine), vitamin E, and copper.[13]

**Acquired copper deficiency can develop in association with exposure to high levels of which other micronutrient?**

High zinc exposure (eg, related to nutritional supplementation or exposure to some denture pastes) is associated with copper deficiency.[10]

**What are the clinical characteristics of polyneuropathy related to chronic liver disease?**

Most patients with polyneuropathy related to chronic liver disease are asymptomatic. Sensory neuropathy is the most commonly identified type, the pattern of nerve injury is usually axonal, and the severity of polyneuropathy is independent of the cause of chronic liver disease.[14]

**Which type of peripheral neuropathy is most common in patients with acromegaly?**

Polyneuropathy is an uncommon complication of acromegaly. More typically, these patients develop mononeuropathies (eg, carpal tunnel syndrome) related to entrapment by bone and soft tissue hypertrophy.[15]

## TOXIC CAUSES OF POLYNEUROPATHY

**What pathophysiologic or electrophysiologic pattern of nerve injury is most commonly associated with toxic causes of polyneuropathy?**

Toxic causes of polyneuropathy are most commonly associated with axonal injury, but demyelinating injury can predominate in some conditions.[3]

### What are the toxic causes of polyneuropathy?

**The second most common cause of polyneuropathy in the industrialized world, usually occurring after decades of daily exposure.**

Alcohol.[4]

**Iatrogenic.**

Medication.

**A patient develops polyneuropathy after spending the past several weeks in an intensive care unit with acute respiratory distress syndrome.**

Critical illness polyneuropathy.

**A 56-year-old man who works in a factory producing batteries for vehicles presents with bilateral lower extremity paresthesias and is found to have microcytic anemia and basophilic stippling of the erythrocytes on peripheral blood smear (Figure 41-5).**

Lead toxicity.

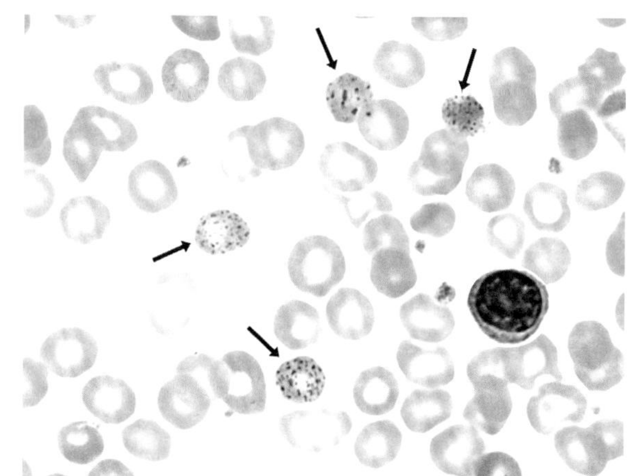

**Figure 41-5.** Microcytic red blood cells with coarse basophilic stippling (arrows) in a patient with lead poisoning. (From: Pereira I, George TI, Arber DA. *Atlas of Peripheral Blood: The Primary Diagnostic Tool*. Philadelphia, PA: Wolters Kluwer Health; 2012.)

**A 21-year-old college student presents with polyneuropathy after starting a job as a technician in a biochemistry laboratory where he uses gel electrophoresis to study proteins.**

Acrylamide toxicity.

**A 54-year-old farmer presents with a motor-predominant polyneuropathy 2 weeks after experiencing an episode of excessive eye tearing, excessive sweating, diarrhea, and vomiting.**

Organophosphate poisoning.

**This vitamin is unique in that it can be associated with polyneuropathy when it is either deficient or present in excess.**

Vitamin B6.

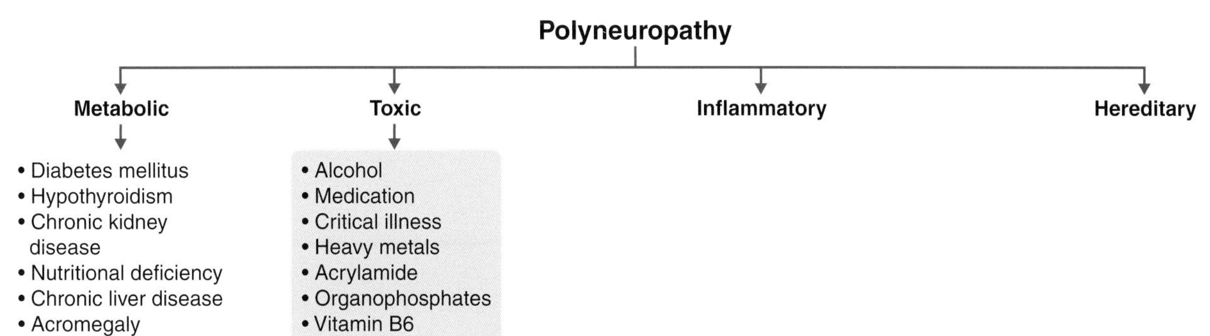


**Which metabolic causes of polyneuropathy are often present in alcoholic patients?**

Long-term excessive alcohol use can cause polyneuropathy via direct neurotoxicity. These patients often additionally suffer from nutritional deficiencies and chronic liver disease, both of which may contribute to the polyneuropathy of alcoholism.[10]

**What medications are associated with polyneuropathy?**

Numerous medications are associated with polyneuropathy, including chemotherapeutic agents (eg, vincristine, paclitaxel), antibiotics (eg, metronidazole, nitrofurantoin, isoniazid, dapsone), antiretroviral agents (eg, zalcitabine, didanosine), cardiac medications (eg, amiodarone), colchicine, phenytoin, cimetidine, lithium, and disulfiram.[3]

**What risk factors are associated with critical illness polyneuropathy?**

Risk factors for critical illness polyneuropathy include sepsis, systemic inflammatory response syndrome, and multiple organ failure.[16]

**Which heavy metals are associated with polyneuropathy?**

Exposure to lead, thallium, arsenic, or mercury can result in polyneuropathy.[17]

**What is the prognosis of polyneuropathy related to acrylamide toxicity?**

Nearly complete reversal of polyneuropathy occurs when exposure to acrylamide is removed.[17]

**What is the prognosis of polyneuropathy related to organophosphate toxicity?**

Mild cases of polyneuropathy related to organophosphate toxicity are associated with good recovery; in cases where myelopathy is also present, recovery is generally poor.[17]

**What dose of vitamin B6 is associated with polyneuropathy?**

The polyneuropathy related to vitamin B6 toxicity usually occurs when doses are greater than 2 g/d, but it has also been reported when lower doses are consumed over long periods of time.[17]

**What additional occupational toxins can lead to polyneuropathy?**

Polyneuropathy can occur as a result of exposure to allyl chloride, carbon disulfide, dimethylaminopropionitrile, ethylene oxide, and hexacarbons (eg, *n*-hexane).[17]

## INFLAMMATORY CAUSES OF POLYNEUROPATHY

**What pathophysiologic or electrophysiologic pattern of nerve injury is most commonly associated with inflammatory causes of polyneuropathy?**

Inflammatory causes of polyneuropathy are most commonly associated with demyelinating injury, but axonal injury can predominate in some conditions.[3]

**What are the typical cerebrospinal fluid findings in patients with polyneuropathy related to inflammatory conditions?**

Inflammatory causes of polyneuropathy are often associated with elevated CSF protein concentration with or without pleocytosis.[7]

**What are the 2 subcategories of inflammatory polyneuropathy?**

Inflammatory polyneuropathy can be infectious or noninfectious.

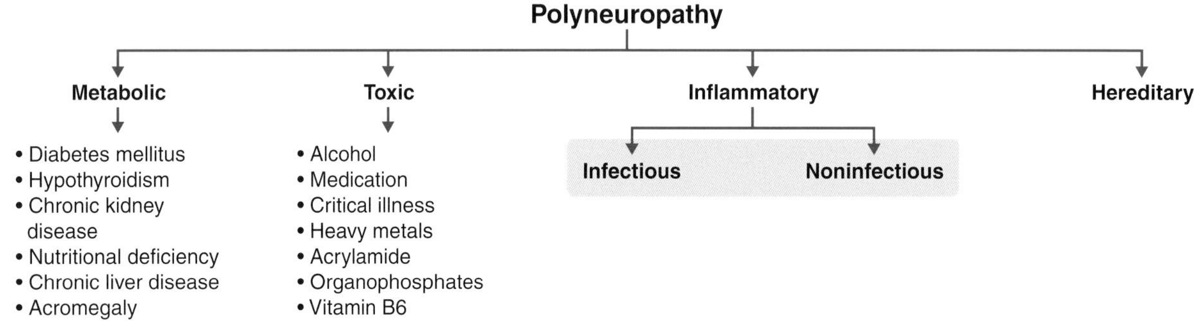


## INFECTIOUS CAUSES OF INFLAMMATORY POLYNEUROPATHY

### What are the infectious causes of inflammatory polyneuropathy?

**Polyneuropathy can be associated with this chronic viral infection or its treatment.**

Human immunodeficiency virus (HIV).

**A patient visits a clinic in Boston for evaluation of symmetric, distal paresthesias. He recalls a target-shaped rash on his leg approximately 8 months prior.**

Lyme disease.

**Development of cranial and upper extremity neuropathy 4 weeks after an upper respiratory tract infection characterized by ulcerative oropharyngeal mucosa and the presence of a pseudomembrane.**

Diphtheria.

**One of the most common causes of peripheral neuropathy worldwide, this infection most typically presents with mononeuropathy or mononeuritis multiplex, particularly of the upper extremities; patients may also have hypopigmented skin lesions with hypoesthesia.**

Leprosy.[18]

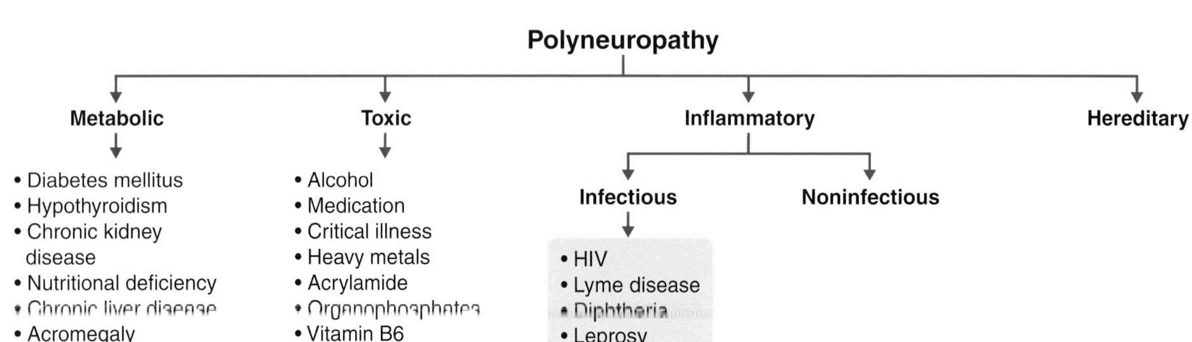

**How common is polyneuropathy in patients with HIV infection?**

Polyneuropathy is estimated to affect up to one-third of patients with HIV. It commonly develops within months of HIV transmission. Most patients complain of symmetric distal numbness, burning pain, and paresthesias. Examination reveals decreased or absent Achilles tendon reflexes, and deficits in vibratory and temperature sensations in a stocking-glove distribution.[19]

**What is the prognosis of polyneuropathy associated with Lyme disease?**

Most cases of polyneuropathy associated with Lyme disease resolve or improve after treatment of the underlying infection.[20]

**How common is polyneuropathy in patients with diphtheria?**

Polyneuropathy develops in the majority of patients with severe respiratory infection from diphtheria and in a minority but significant proportion of patients with asymptomatic infection. The first indication of neuropathy related to diphtheria is paralysis of the soft palate and posterior pharyngeal wall; the descendent nature of the polyneuropathy can help distinguish it from Guillain-Barré syndrome (GBS).[21]

**Are anesthetic skin lesions universally present in patients with neuropathy related to leprosy?**

Classic leprosy neuropathy presents with anesthetic skin lesions, but pure neuritic leprosy presents with neuropathy in the absence of cutanous manifestations. Nerve biopsy is the gold standard for diagnosis in such cases.[18]



## NONINFECTIOUS CAUSES OF INFLAMMATORY POLYNEUROPATHY

### What are the noninfectious causes of inflammatory polyneuropathy?

**Two weeks after a diarrheal illness, a 36-year-old woman presents with ascending paralysis and is found to have elevated CSF protein concentration without pleocytosis (ie, albuminocytologic dissociation).**

Guillain-Barré syndrome.

**A heterogeneous group of disorders that result in the deposition of misassembled fibril proteins that alter the structure and function of normal tissues, most commonly within the kidneys, liver, and heart.**

Acquired amyloidosis.[22]

**Diagnosed using SPEP, and sometimes associated with a low serum anion gap.**

Paraproteinemia.

**A 63-year-old man with an extensive smoking history presents with idiopathic polyneuropathy and is found to have positive serum anti-Hu antibodies.**

Paraneoplastic syndrome.

**Malar rash, pancytopenia, and polyarticular inflammatory arthritis.**

Systemic lupus erythematosus (SLE).

**A patient with palpable purpura, hematuria with dysmorphic erythrocytes (see Figure 34-4), and foot drop.**

Vasculitis (eg, cryoglobulinemia).

**A 44-year-old woman presents with progressive symmetric polyneuropathy and hyporeflexia over the course of 10 weeks and is found to have slowed nerve conduction on electrodiagnostic testing and albuminocytologic dissociation on evaluation of CSF.**

Chronic inflammatory demyelinating polyneuropathy (CIDP).

**A granulomatous condition.**

Sarcoidosis.

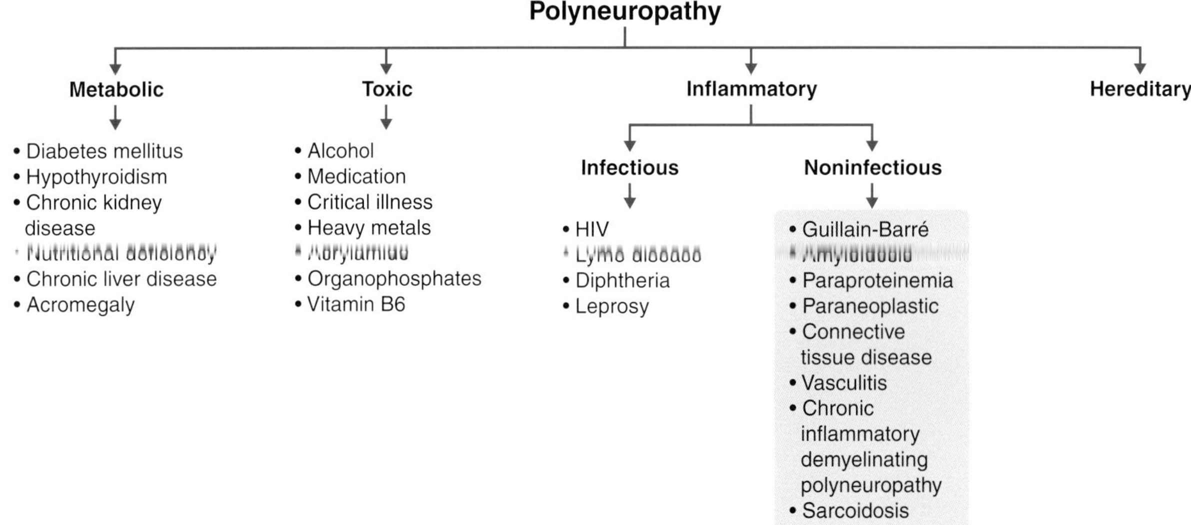


**What is the treatment for Guillain-Barré syndrome?**

Treatment with plasma exchange or intravenous immunoglobulin (IVIG) hastens recovery in patients with Guillain-Barré syndrome, particularly when initiated within 2 weeks of disease onset. Despite treatment, mortality is around 5% and long-term severe disability occurs in approximately 20% of patients.[23]

**What are the characteristics of polyneuropathy related to acquired amyloidosis?**

Peripheral neuropathy most commonly occurs in the setting of immunoglobulin light chain (AL) amyloidosis. It is a length-dependent sensorimotor polyneuropathy, but involves the autonomic nervous system in most cases, causing patients to present with symptoms such as nausea, vomiting, early satiety, bloating, constipation, diarrhea, postural light-headedness, and erectile dysfunction. Peripheral neuropathy is rare in inflammatory (AA) amyloidosis.[22]

**What conditions are associated with paraproteinemic polyneuropathy?**

Paraproteinemic polyneuropathy can occur with monoclonal gammopathy of unknown significance (most common), multiple myeloma, AL amyloidosis, POEMS syndrome (**P**olyneuropathy, **O**rganomegaly, **E**ndocrinopathy, **M**onoclonal gammopathy, and **S**kin changes), Waldenström macroglobulinemia, cryoglobulinemia (types I and II), and lymphoproliferative disorders (eg, chronic lymphocytic leukemia).[24]

**When does paraneoplastic polyneuropathy usually occur during the course of malignancy?**

In patients with paraneoplastic polyneuropathy, the polyneuropathy often precedes the diagnosis of the underlying malignancy, which can sometimes be discovered with investigative imaging studies, including whole body positron emission tomography (PET).[25]

**Which connective tissue diseases are associated with polyneuropathy?**

Polyneuropathy can occur in patients with SLE, rheumatoid arthritis, and Sjögren's syndrome.[26]

**What types of peripheral neuropathy occur in patients with vasculitis?**

Patients with vasculitis most frequently develop polyneuropathies and mononeuropathies, including mononeuritis multiplex.[6]

**What treatments are associated with improved outcomes in patients with chronic inflammatory demyelinating polyneuropathy?**

Systemic glucocorticoids, IVIG, and plasma exchange are associated with improved outcomes in patients with CIDP. Treatment choice depends on variables related to the host and features of the disease (eg, patients with pure motor CIDP should not be treated with glucocorticoids, as there is risk of deterioration with this modality). Sometimes switching or combining modalities may be necessary.[27]

**How common is peripheral neuropathy in patients with sarcoidosis?**

Sarcoidosis involves the nervous system in approximately 5% of cases. Cranial neuropathy (especially involving the facial nerve) is the most common manifestation, affecting up to one-half of patients. Other peripheral neuropathies, including mononeuritis multiplex, radiculopathy, and polyneuroapthy, are less common. In some cases, an acute GBS-like polyneuropathy can occur. However, the CSF profile shows elevated protein and pleocytosis, distinguishing it from GBS, which typically presents with albuminocytologic dissociation.[28]

## HEREDITARY CAUSES OF POLYNEUROPATHY

**What pathophysiologic or electrophysiologic pattern of nerve injury is most commonly associated with hereditary causes of polyneuropathy?**

Hereditary causes of polyneuropathy are most commonly associated with demyelinating injury, but axonal injury can predominate in some conditions.[3]

### What are the hereditary causes of polyneuropathy?

**The most common hereditary cause of polyneuropathy, ultimately diagnosed in one-fifth of patients presenting to neuromuscular clinics with chronic peripheral neuropathy.**

Charcot-Marie-Tooth (also known as hereditary motor and sensory neuropathy) type 1.[29,30]

**A 39-year-old Portuguese man presents with numbness in the feet, early satiety, and light-headedness on standing and is subsequently diagnosed with a fat pad biopsy.**

Familial amyloidosis.

**A 25-year-old woman presents with recurrent episodes of bilateral lower extremity weakness and numbness that usually occur after periods of prolonged sitting and last for weeks at a time.**

Hereditary neuropathy with liability to pressure palsy (HNPP).

**Intermittent acute attacks of diffuse abdominal pain, paresthesias, and red urine (see Figure 42-4).**

Acute porphyria.

**A group of hereditary disorders, most of which present at birth with a variety of sensory and autonomic abnormalities.**

Hereditary sensory and autonomic neuropathies (HSAN). *Some of the HSANs are misnomers, as motor neuropathy occurs with a high frequency in many of these disorders.*[31]

**Disorders of maternal lineage.**

Mitochondrial disorders.

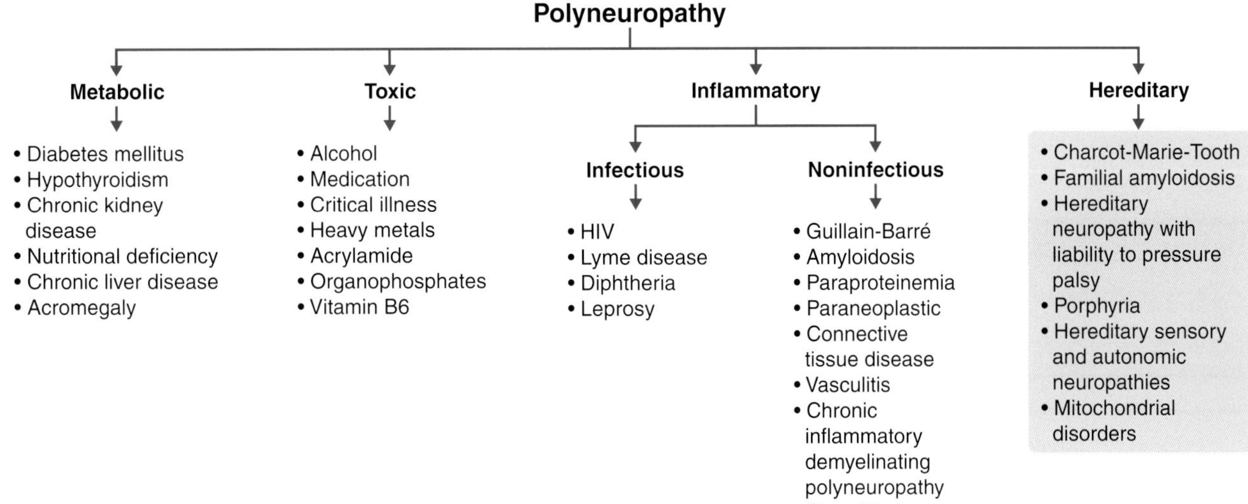


NEUROLOGY

**What foot deformities are common in patients with Charcot-Marie-Tooth disease?**

Pes cavus (high arched feet) and hammertoes (the proximal interphalangeal joint of the toe is bent upward) are common in patients with Charcot-Marie-Tooth disease (Figure 41-6).[30]

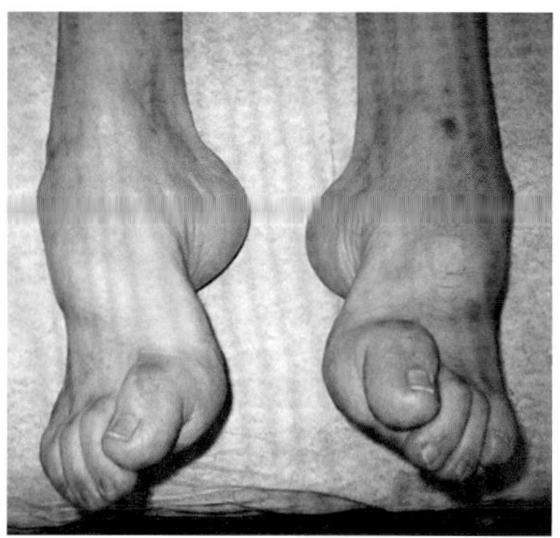

**Figure 41-6.** Pes cavus with hammertoes in a patient with Charcot-Marie-Tooth disease. (From Louis ED, Mayer SA, Rowland LP. *Merritt's Neurology*. 13th ed. Philadelphia, PA: Wolters Kluwer; 2016.)

**What patterns of peripheral neuropathy are characteristic of familial amyloidosis?**

Patients with familial amyloidosis can develop mononeuropathy, sensorimotor polyneuropathy, autonomic neuropathy, or a combination of the 3. The most common and earliest site of involvement is the median nerve at the wrist, which presents like carpal tunnel syndrome.[22]

**What is the prognosis of hereditary neuropathy with liability to pressure palsy?**

Patient with HNPP usually recover completely from acute neuropathies, but it can sometimes take several months. Chronic (usually mild) symptoms may persist, and the phenotype of patients with residual symptoms can resemble that of CMT. Life expectancy is normal.[29]

**What are the characteristics of the peripheral neuropathy associated with porphyria?**

In patients with porphyria, motor and autonomic disturbances predominate, with an axonal pattern of nerve injury. Motor neuropathy can be asymmetric, affecting proximal (including facial) and distal muscles. Attacks can be precipitated by hormonal factors, medications, nutritional status, and alcohol consumption.[32]

**Which of the hereditary sensory and autonomic neuropathies can present in adulthood?**

HSAN type 1 often presents in early adulthood (median age of 20 years with a range of 15-55 years) with sensory symptoms, followed by weakness, ulcers, pain, and balance difficulties.[31]

**How common is peripheral neuropathy in patients with mitochondrial disorders?**

Peripheral neuropathy is present in almost one-half of patients with mitochondrial disorders and can be the predominant feature, often presenting in adulthood (eg, mitochondrial neurogastrointestinal encephalopathy).[33]

**What are some general hereditary disorders associated with polyneuropathy?**

Spinocerebellar ataxia, Tangier disease, abetalipoproteinemia, Chediak-Higashi syndrome, and lysosomal storage diseases can be associated with polyneuropathy.

*Some hereditary disorders associated with peripheral neuropathy that manifest predominantly in infancy or childhood (eg, giant axonal neuropathy) have been omitted to limit the scope of this chapter.*

## Case Summary

A 42-year-old woman with a history of gastric bypass surgery presents with skin changes, glossitis, and evidence of myeloneuropathy.

***What is the most likely cause of polyneuropathy in this patient?***

Vitamin B12 deficiency.

## BONUS QUESTIONS

***Why is the patient in this case at risk for vitamin B12 deficiency?***

Bariatric surgery can lead to malabsorption of micronutrients such as vitamin B12, folate, iron, zinc, and copper. The patient in this case stopped taking supplemental micronutrients, which is usually necessary for patients after bariatric surgery, putting her at increased risk for deficiencies.

***What is the significance of the skin findings in this case?***

The scaling and erythema of the oral commissures described in this case is suggestive of angular cheilitis, which is associated with a number of nutritional deficiencies, including vitamin B12. The scaly erythematous rash around the anogenital area probably represents acquired acrodermatitis enteropathica related to zinc deficiency.

***What is the significance of the positive Romberg test in this case?***

The Romberg test evaluates for deficits in proprioception (large fibers). The patient is asked to stand with the feet together. To maintain balance in this position, at least 2 of the following senses are necessary: normal vision, normal vestibular function, and normal proprioception. In a patient with a disturbance in proprioception, balance can be maintained by normal vestibular function and vision. However, when the eyes are closed, a loss of balance occurs as the patient becomes solely reliant on the vestibular system, which is not enough to maintain balance.

***What is the significance of the combination of brisk patellar tendon reflexes and absent Achilles tendon reflexes in this case?***

The brisk patellar tendon reflexes, proximal muscle weakness, positive Babinski sign, and impairment in vibratory/proprioceptive sense greater than the impairment in pain/temperature sense are suggestive of spinal cord (corticospinal tract and dorsal column) involvement. The absent Achilles tendon reflexes indicate peripheral nerve involvement. The combination of both spinal cord and peripheral nerve involvement is known as myeloneuropathy. Patients with vitamin B12 deficiency often present with myeloneuropathy, which can be a clue to the diagnosis.[13,34]

***What would be the expected electrodiagnostic pattern of nerve injury in this case?***

The polyneuropathy of vitamin B12 deficiency is axonal in most cases.[34]

***How common is peripheral neuropathy in patients with vitamin B12 deficiency?***

Peripheral neuropathy is seen in one-quarter of patients with vitamin B12 deficiency.[34]

***What are the major dietary sources of vitamin B12?***

Foods rich in vitamin B12 include animal proteins, such as meats and eggs.[34]

***What is the recommended daily intake of vitamin B12?***

The recommended daily allowance of vitamin B12 is 2.4 μg for men and nonpregnant women, 2.6 μg for pregnant women, 2.8 μg for lactating women, and 1.5 to 2 μg for children up to 18 years of age.[34]

***In the industrialized world, how much vitamin B12 is found in the average diet?***

The average non-vegetarian diet in the industrialized world contains around 5 to 8 μg of vitamin B12 per day; a vegetarian diet contains ≤0.5 μg of vitamin B12 per day, putting these individuals at risk for deficiency.[34]

***What is the basic physiology of vitamin B12 absorption?***

The low pH of the stomach allows for the release of vitamin B12 from its coenzyme form via the actions of pepsin. Vitamin B12 then binds to haptocorrin (R-protein), and the complex travels to the second part of the duodenum, where pancreatic proteases free vitamin B12. It then binds intrinsic factor (IF), and the complex is absorbed in the ileum.[34]

***What is the most common cause of vitamin B12 deficiency in the industrialized world?***

The most common cause of vitamin B12 in the industrialized world is pernicious anemia, where immune-mediated atrophy of the gastric parietal cells results in impaired secretion of IF and hydrochloric acid, which are both integral to vitamin B12 absorption.[34]

***What abnormalities can be revealed on a complete blood count in the setting of vitamin B12 deficiency?***

Vitamin B12 deficiency is associated with macrocytosis, with or without anemia.

***What biochemical laboratory tests are useful in the diagnosis of vitamin B12 deficiency?***

No single biochemical laboratory test should be considered diagnostic of vitamin B12 deficiency in the absence of a compatible clinical syndrome or other corroborating biochemical tests. Serum vitamin B12 concentration is useful, particularly in patients with compatible hematologic or neurologic manifestations, where it is below normal in virtually all cases. However, a number of conditions (eg, multiple myeloma) can influence serum concentrations of vitamin B12, leading to falsely low or high values. In patients with borderline vitamin B12 levels (between 200 and 300 pg/mL) or when clinical suspicion remains high despite vitamin B12 levels at the lower end of normal (<350 pg/mL), testing serum concentrations of methylmalonic acid and homocysteine may be useful; both metabolites are elevated in vitamin B12 deficiency (normal levels suggest the absence of vitamin B12 deficiency). A number of variables (eg, renal insufficiency, age) can falsely elevate the serum concentrations of methylmalonic acid and homocysteine. A reduction in serum concentration of these metabolites after vitamin B12 supplementation can provide confirmation of true vitamin B12 deficiency.[8,34,35]

***What is the management of vitamin B12 deficiency?***

Vitamin B12 should be adminstered to patients with B12 deficiency. The preferred route of administration depends on the severity of deficiency and patient-specific factors (eg, patients with altered gastrointestinal absorption of vitamin B12 may not benefit from oral supplementation). An effective vitamin B12 replacement regimen includes 1 mg/d of vitamin B12 given intramuscularly for 1 week, followed by 1 mg/wk for 4 weeks, and finally 1 mg/mo for life. After vitamin B12 stores have been augmented by parenteral therapy, oral daily vitamin B12 supplementation (1-2 mg daily) can be effective in some patients. In this case, zinc and other micronutrient supplementation should also be provided.[34]

***When do the clinical manifestations of vitamin B12 deficiency begin to reverse after therapy is initiated?***

In patients with vitamin B12 deficiency, evidence of clinical improvement occurs within hours of initiation of effective vitamin B12 therapy. Megaloblastosis reverses in 24 hours; normal hematopoiesis is established within 48 hours; and anemia begins to improve within a week (normalization requires around 8 weeks).[34]

## KEY POINTS

- Peripheral neuropathy describes injury to any part of the peripheral nervous system, including the somatic (motor, sensory) and autonomic nervous systems.
- Polyneuropathy is a type of generalized peripheral neuropathy that is distinct from radiculopathy, plexopathy, mononeuropathy, and mononeuritis multiplex.
- Symptoms of polyneuropathy include varying combinations of numbness, paresthesias, pain, autonomic disturbances, and weakness.
- Physical findings of polyneuropathy include varying combinations of hypoesthesia, hyperesthesia, allodynia, sensory ataxia, hyporeflexia, and autonomic disturbances (eg, orthostatic hypotension).
- In patients with polyneuropathy, physical examination can identify the pattern of nerve fibers involved, narrowing the differential diagnosis.
- Electrodiagnostic studies can be helpful in patients with peripheral neuropathy to localize the lesion, determine the pattern of nerve injury (ie, axonal or demyelinating), determine the fiber type involved (ie, motor, sensory, or both), and give a sense of the time course and severity of the disease.
- Tests are available to evaluate the autonomic nervous system (eg, tilt table testing).
- Additional studies that can be helpful in select patients with polyneuropathy include genetic studies, CSF examination, skin biopsy, and nerve biopsy.
- Polyneuropathy can be metabolic, toxic, inflammatory, or hereditary.
- Inflammatory polyneuropathy can be infectious or noninfectious.
- In general, metabolic and toxic causes of polyneuropathy result in axonal neuropathy (with exceptions), whereas inflammatory and hereditary causes of polyneuropathy result in demyelinating neuropathy (with exceptions).
- The combination of history, physical examination, blood tests, and ancillary tests (eg, electrodiagnostic studies) establishes an underlying diagnosis in most cases of polyneuropathy.

## REFERENCES


1. Callaghan BC, Price RS, Chen KS, Feldman EL. The importance of rare subtypes in diagnosis and treatment of peripheral neuropathy: a review. *JAMA Neurol.* 2015;72(12):1510-1518.
2. Hughes RA. Peripheral neuropathy. *BMJ.* 2002;324(7335):466-469.
3. Poncelet AN. An algorithm for the evaluation of peripheral neuropathy. *Am Fam Physician.* 1998;57(4):755-764.
4. Callaghan BC, Price RS, Feldman EL. Distal symmetric polyneuropathy: a review. *JAMA.* 2015;314(20):2172-2181.
5. Bowen BC, Seidenwurm DJ. Expert panel on neurologic I. Plexopathy. *AJNR Am J Neuroradiol.* 2008;29(2):400-402.
6. Finsterer J. Systemic and non-systemic vasculitis affecting the peripheral nerves. *Acta Neurol Belg.* 2009;109(2):100-113.
7. Misra UK, Kalita J, Nair PP. Diagnostic approach to peripheral neuropathy. *Ann Indian Acad Neurol.* 2008;11(2):89-97.
8. Ropper AH, Samuels MA, Klein JP, eds. *Adam and Victor's Principles of Neurology.* 10th ed. China: McGraw-Hill Education; 2014.
9. Feinberg J. EMG: myths and facts. *HSS J.* 2006;2(1):19-21.
10. Watson JC, Dyck PJ. Peripheral neuropathy: a practical approach to diagnosis and symptom management. *Mayo Clin Proc.* 2015;90(7):940-951.
11. Krishnan AV, Kiernan MC. Neurological complications of chronic kidney disease. *Nat Rev Neurol.* 2009;5(10):542-551.
12. Beghi E, Delodovici ML, Bogliun G, et al. Hypothyroidism and polyneuropathy. *J Neurol Neurosurg Psychiatry.* 1989;52(12):1420-1423.
13. Hammond N, Wang Y, Dimachkie MM, Barohn RJ. Nutritional neuropathies. *Neurol Clin.* 2013;31(2):477-489.
14. Chaudhry V, Corse AM, O'Brian R, Cornblath DR, Klein AS, Thuluvath PJ. Autonomic and peripheral (sensorimotor) neuropathy in chronic liver disease: a clinical and electrophysiologic study. *Hepatology.* 1999;29(6):1698-1703.
15. Stewart BM. The hypertrophic neuropathy of acromegaly; a rare neuropathy associated with acromegaly. *Arch Neurol.* 1966;14(1):107-110.
16. Hermans G, De Jonghe B, Bruyninckx F, Van den Berghe G. Clinical review: critical illness polyneuropathy and myopathy. *Crit Care.* 2008;12(6):238.
17. Staff NP, Windebank AJ. Peripheral neuropathy due to vitamin deficiency, toxins, and medications. *Continuum (Minneap Minn).* 2014;20(5 Peripheral Nervous System Disorders):1293-1306.
18. Nascimento OJ. Leprosy neuropathy: clinical presentations. *Arq Neuropsiquiatr.* 2013;71(9B):661-666.
19. Kaku M, Simpson DM. HIV neuropathy. *Curr Opin HIV AIDS.* 2014;9(6):521-526.
20. Logigian EL, Steere AC. Clinical and electrophysiologic findings in chronic neuropathy of Lyme disease. *Neurology.* 1992;42(2):303-311.
21. Manikyamba D, Satyavani A, Deepa P. Diphtheritic polyneuropathy in the wake of resurgence of diphtheria. *J Pediatr Neurosci.* 2015;10(4):331-334.
22. Shin SC, Robinson-Papp J. Amyloid neuropathies. *Mt Sinai J Med.* 2012;79(6):733-748.
23. Yuki N, Hartung HP. Guillain-Barre syndrome. *N Engl J Med.* 2012;366(24):2294-2304.
24. Zivkovic SA, Lacomis D, Lentzsch S. Paraproteinemic neuropathy. *Leuk Lymphoma.* 2009;50(9):1422-1433.
25. Koike H, Sobue G. Paraneoplastic neuropathy. *Handb Clin Neurol.* 2013;115:713-726.
26. Bougea A, Anagnostou E, Konstantinos G, George P, Triantafyllou N, Kararizou E. A systematic review of peripheral and central nervous system involvement of rheumatoid arthritis, systemic lupus erythematosus, primary Sjogren's syndrome, and associated immunological profiles. *Int J Chronic Dis.* 2015;2015:910352.
27. Vallat JM, Sommer C, Magy L. Chronic inflammatory demyelinating polyradiculoneuropathy: diagnostic and therapeutic challenges for a treatable condition. *Lancet Neurol.* 2010;9(4):402-412.
28. Hoyle JC, Jablonski C, Newton HB. Neurosarcoidosis: clinical review of a disorder with challenging inpatient presentations and diagnostic considerations. *Neurohospitalist.* 2014;4(2):94-101.
29. Adam MP, Ardinger HH, Pagon RA, et al, eds. *GeneReviews(R).* Seattle, WA; 1993.
30. Hoyle JC, Isfort MC, Roggenbuck J, Arnold WD. The genetics of Charcot-Marie-Tooth disease: current trends and future implications for diagnosis and management. *Appl Clin Genet.* 2015;8:235-243.
31. Fridman V, Oaklander AL, David WS, et al. Natural history and biomarkers in hereditary sensory neuropathy type 1. *Muscle Nerve.* 2015;51(4):489-495.
32. Tracy JA, Dyck PJ. Porphyria and its neurologic manifestations. *Handb Clin Neurol.* 2014;120:839-849.
33. Menezes MP, Ouvrier RA. Peripheral neuropathy associated with mitochondrial disease in children. *Dev Med Child Neurol.* 2012;54(5):407-414.
34. Briani C, Dalla Torre C, Citton V, et al. Cobalamin deficiency: clinical picture and radiological findings. *Nutrients.* 2013;5(11):4521-4539.
35. Matchar DB, McCrory DC, Millington DS, Feussner JR. Performance of the serum cobalamin assay for diagnosis of cobalamin deficiency. *Am J Med Sci.* 1994;308(5):276-283.

Chapter 42

# SEIZURE

## Case: A 68-year-old man with pronator drift

A previously healthy 68-year-old man is admitted to the hospital after his wife witnessed an unusual event. The two were eating breakfast when the patient suddenly extended his left arm and leg and flexed his right arm and leg; moments later the patient turned his head and eyes toward the left. This was followed by rhythmic flexion and extension of his arms and legs for 2 minutes, during which time he was unresponsive. The patient was confused for 15 minutes afterward, and does not recall much of the event. He has not been feeling well for a few months, and endorses malaise, drenching night sweats, and an unintentional weight loss of 18 pounds. The patient underwent a tooth extraction procedure 6 months ago. He has no prior history of seizures.

Temperature is 37.7°C. The patient appears cachectic. There is a 3/6 holosystolic murmur best heard over the apex with radiation to the axilla. Cranial nerves are intact. There is pronator drift of the left upper extremity. Reflexes and sensation are intact.

Magnetic resonance imaging (MRI) of the brain with axial (Figure 42-1A and C), coronal (Figure 42-B), and sagittal (Figure 42-1D) views demonstrates multiple ring-enhancing cystic lesions involving the bilateral frontal and temporal lobes, the largest of which is 2.2 × 2.1 cm.

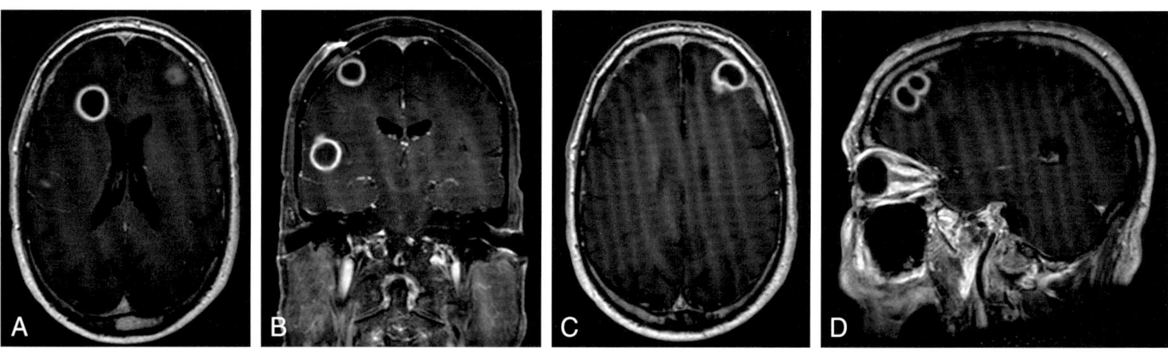


**Figure 42-1.**

***What is the most likely cause of seizure in this patient?***

What is a seizure?

A seizure is defined as abnormal excessive or synchronous neuronal activity in the brain resulting in transient symptoms and signs.[1]

What conditions are commonly confused with seizure?

Migraine headache, syncope, transient ischemic attack, psychogenic seizure, Ménière's disease, and movement disorders can be confused with seizure.[2]

What are the symptoms and signs of a seizure?

The clinical manifestations of seizures vary by type and contributing factors but can involve disturbances in sensory, motor, and autonomic function, consciousness, emotional state, memory, cognition, and behavior. These features can occur in isolation or in combination. Common manifestations include myoclonic jerking, alteration of awareness, tonic or clonic activity (or both), atonic activity, automatisms, tongue biting, incontinence, and postictal confusion.[2,3]

What is myoclonus?

Myoclonus describes sudden-onset, brief (<100 ms), and involuntary isolated or repetitive contraction of a muscle or groups of muscles.[4]

**What is tonic activity?**

Tonic activity describes an increase in muscle contraction that is sustained and can last from a few seconds to several minutes.[4]

**What is clonic activity?**

Clonic activity describes myoclonus that is regular, repetitive (at a rate of 2-3 contractions per second), and sustained for prolonged periods of time, involving the same muscle groups.[4]

**What is tonic-clonic activity?**

Tonic-clonic activity describes the paired sequence of tonic movement followed by clonic movement.[4]

**What is atonic activity?**

Atonic activity describes sudden loss of or decreased muscle tone involving the head, trunk, jaw, or limb musculature without preceding myoclonic or tonic activity, lasting ≥1 to 2 seconds.[4]

**What is dystonic activity?**

Dystonic activity describes simultaneous sustained contraction of agonist and antagonist muscles, resulting in athetoid or twisting movements, which may produce abnormal postures.[4]

**What are automatisms?**

Automatisms are coordinated, repetitive, motor activity (eg, lip smacking) that can resemble voluntary movement but occur when cognition is impaired. Afterward, the patient is usually amnestic.[4]

**What is an aura?**

Aura describes an ictal symptom (eg, visual disturbance) that occurs without a change in awareness and may precede an observable seizure. When it occurs in isolation, an aura is considered to be a focal sensory seizure.[4]

**What is status epilepticus?**

Status epilepticus is reached when the duration of a typical seizure is longer than expected (usually >5 minutes), or when seizures recur in succession without interval return to baseline consciousness.[4,5]

**What is a postictal state?**

A postictal state describes the period immediately following a seizure characterized by changes in behavior, motor function, and neuropsychological performance, lasting until baseline status returns, which may take anywhere from seconds to days.[6]

**What is the role of physical examination in the evaluation of a patient with a suspected seizure disorder?**

Physical examination can identify neurologic deficits and findings indicative of systemic disease (eg, lymphadenopathy), which can be suggestive of an underlying cause of the seizure.[2]

**What is the role of electroencephalography (EEG) in the evaluation of a patient with a possible seizure disorder?**

EEG can confirm the presence of abnormal electrical activity, determine the location of the seizure focus, and provide information about the type of seizure disorder.[2]

**How sensitive is electroencephalography in epileptic patients?**

The initial EEG is normal in around one-half of patients with epilepsy. If suspicion remains, the EEG should be repeated after the patient has been deprived of sleep (which lowers the seizure threshold). In a small proportion of epileptic patients, electroencephalographic abnormalities cannot be detected despite multiple EEGs.[2]

**What supplementary studies can be useful in some patients with suspected seizure?**

Blood tests (eg, basic metabolic panel, serologies), cerebrospinal fluid evaluation, and neuroimaging (eg, brain MRI) can be useful in select patients with a suspected seizure disorder.[2]

**When is emergency neuroimaging recommended after a first seizure?**

Emergency neuroimaging should be performed after a first seizure in patients on therapeutic anticoagulation, and in those with new focal neurologic deficits, persistent delirium, fever, recent trauma, persistent headache, a history of malignancy, and risk factors for acquired immunodeficiency syndrome.[2]

**What is the pharmacologic treatment of choice for an active seizure?**

Most seizures resolve spontaneously within a few minutes. Immediately identifiable and reversible etiologies (eg, hypoglycemia) should be treated. If the seizure is prolonged or status epilepticus has been reached, and no reversible cause is apparent, then first-line treatment is a short-acting benzodiazepine administered intravenously.[5]

**What are the 2 general categories of seizures?**

Seizures can be unprovoked or provoked.

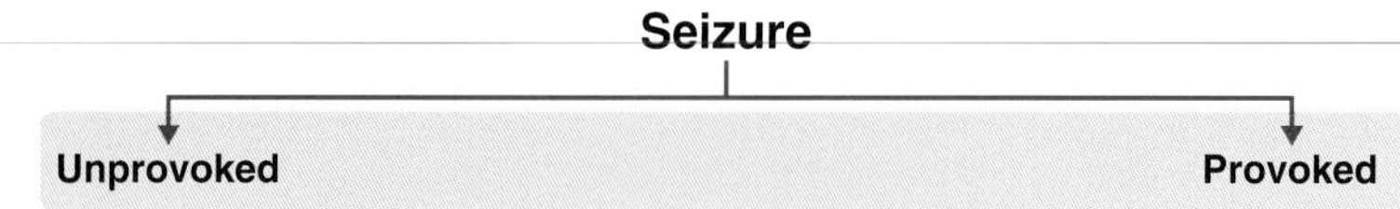


**What is an unprovoked seizure?**

An unprovoked seizure occurs in the absence of a temporary or reversible associated condition.[1]

**What is a provoked seizure?**

A provoked seizure occurs in close temporal relationship with an acquired precipitating condition; these seizures are also referred to as "acute symptomatic seizures."[1,7,8]

*For the purposes of the framework in this chapter, seizures associated with acquired conditions are categorized as provoked. However, conditions that result in residual brain alteration (eg, head trauma, stroke) or those that are irreversible (eg, brain tumor) can also lead to a long-term predisposition for "unprovoked" seizures outside of the acute period (ie, "remote symptomatic seizures").*[3,7,8]

**After a single unprovoked seizure, what is the risk of a second seizure?**

Following a single unprovoked seizure, the risk for a second seizure over the next 2 to 8 years is approximately 40% to 50%.[1]

**After 2 unprovoked seizures, what is the risk of a third seizure?**

Following 2 unprovoked seizures, the risk for a third seizure over the next 4 years is approximately 60% to 90%.[1]

**What is epilepsy?**

Epilepsy is a disorder of the brain characterized by recurrent unprovoked seizures (at least 2 seizures occurring >24 hours apart), or 1 unprovoked seizure with a high probability for a second seizure (≥60% over the next 10 years). The likelihood of a second seizure is based on risk factors such as permanent structural disease of the brain. Patients with epilepsy syndromes (eg, juvenile myoclonic epilepsy) experience seizures along with other characteristic clinical, genetic, and electroencephalographic features.[1]

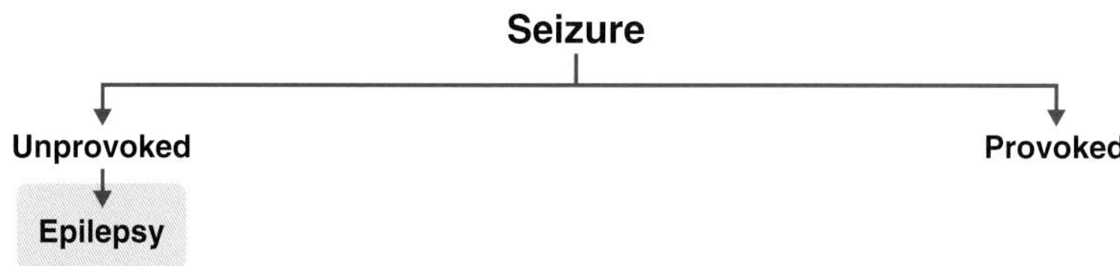


*The seizure threshold is generally lower in epileptics, and as such, these patients are at higher risk for provoked seizures compared with nonepileptic patients under similar seizure-precipitating conditions.*

**How common is epilepsy?**

Epilepsy is a common neurologic condition worldwide; approximately 3% of the general population in the industrialized world will have epilepsy at some point during life.[2]

**Is epilepsy a lifelong disorder?**

Epilepsy can be a lifelong disorder. However, it is considered to be resolved when patients with age-related epilepsy syndromes are outside of the age range or when patients are seizure-free for at least 10 years without antiepileptic medications for the most recent 5 years.[1]

**What are the causes of epilepsy?**

In most cases, epilepsy is either genetic (ie, due to a known mutation) or "idiopathic" (these cases are most likely due to undiscovered genetic conditions). Residual brain alteration from acute conditions, such as head trauma, stroke, brain tumors, and intracranial infection, can lead to a long-term predisposition for seizures and epilepsy.[3,9,10]

**What are the triggers for seizure activity in epileptic patients?**

Stimuli such as flashing lights, intense exercise, loud music, and strong emotions can trigger seizures in epileptic patients. Additionally, the seizure threshold in epileptic patients can be lowered by various factors, including lack of sleep, fever, hormonal changes, hyperventilation, stress, and certain medications (eg, bupropion).[11]

**What are the nonpharmacologic long-term treatment options for patients with epilepsy?**

Lifestyle modification (eg, avoiding sleep deprivation, abstaining from alcohol) and behavioral techniques (eg, biofeedback) can effectively reduce the seizure burden for some patients with epilepsy.[12]

**How effective are antiepileptic drugs in the long-term treatment of epilepsy?**

Overall long-term remission is achieved with antiepileptic drugs in most patients with epilepsy. A combination of agents is commonly required, as monotherapy is effective in less than one-half of patients. The choice between the various antiepileptic drugs must take into account patient and drug-related factors.[13]

**What are the 2 main subtypes of seizures in patients with epilepsy?**

Patients with epilepsy can experience focal (ie, "partial") or generalized seizures.

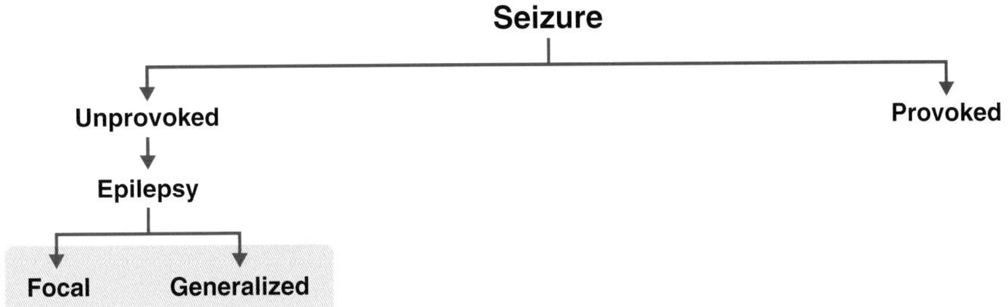




**What general regions of the brain are affected by focal and generalized seizures?**

Focal seizures involve a portion of the brain at onset and are limited to 1 hemisphere; consciousness may or may not be impaired. Generalized seizures involve both cerebral hemispheres simultaneously with resultant loss of consciousness. Focal seizures may become secondarily generalized (ie, focal seizure evolving to a bilateral, convulsive seizure) (Figure 42-2).[9,10,14]

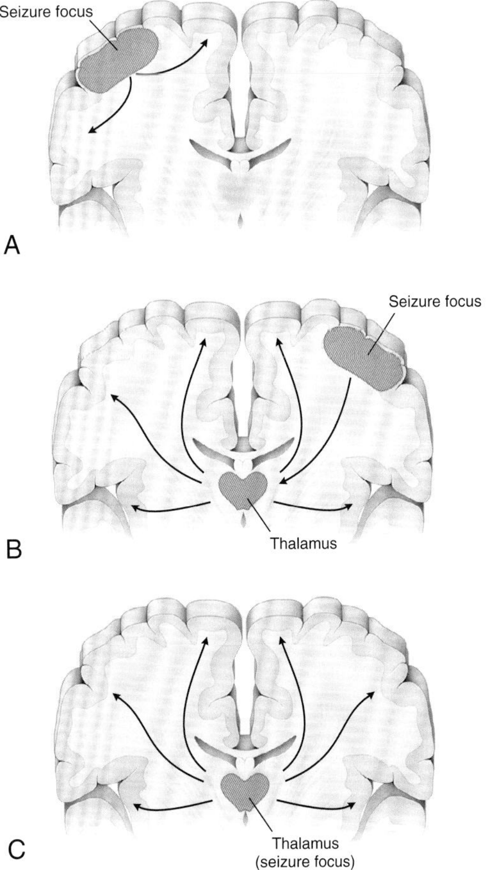


**Figure 42-2.** Pathways of seizure propagation. A, Focal seizure. B, Focal seizure with secondary generalization. C, Primary generalized seizure. (Adapted from Golan DE, et al. *Principles of Pharmacology: The Pathophysiologic Basis of Drug Therapy*. 3rd ed. Philadelphia, PA: Lippincott Williams & Wilkins; 2011.)

**Why is it important to distinguish between focal and generalized seizures?**

Distinguishing between focal and generalized seizures is needed to direct strategies for therapy. Some antiepileptic agents specifically treat focal seizure disorders but are ineffective for generalized seizure disorders (and may even lower the seizure threshold in these patients). Other agents treat generalized seizure disorders but are ineffective for focal seizure disorders. Furthermore, there are surgical treatment options for some types of focal, but not generalized, seizure disorders.[15]

## FOCAL SEIZURES

### What are the 2 main subtypes of focal seizures?

**A fully alert 18-year-old man experiences sudden stiffening of the right arm that persists for 1 minute.**

Simple focal seizure (ie, focal seizure without impairment of consciousness).

**During a lecture, a 43-year-old algebra teacher suddenly appears to stare into space and then begins to rhythmically pick at thin air for 45 seconds; the students are unable to get her attention, and she is confused for several minutes after the event.**

Complex focal seizure (ie, focal seizure with impairment of consciousness).

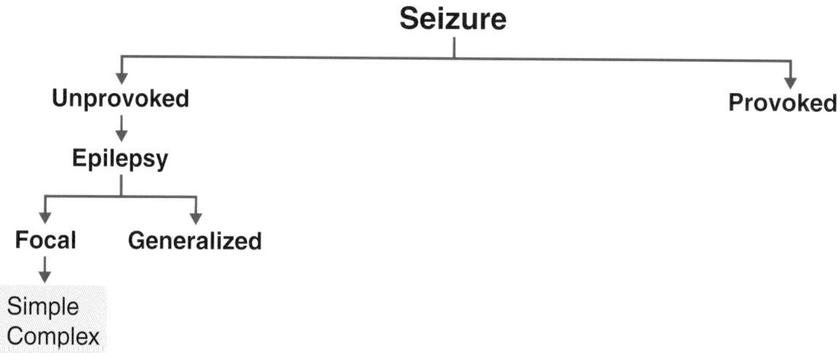


**What is the principle difference between simple and complex focal seizures?**

Consciousness is impaired in complex focal seizures but preserved in simple focal seizures.

**Why is it important to distinguish between simple focal and complex focal seizures?**

The distinction between simple focal and complex focal seizures is needed to accurately assess seizure risk and patient safety. Patients with complex focal seizure disorders may be subject to activity restrictions, including driving and the use of machinery.[12]

**What are the clinical manifestations of focal-onset seizures?**

Depending on the region of the brain that is affected, focal-onset seizures can present with a variety of manifestations including motor (eg, focal limb movement), somatosensory (eg, paresthesia), special sensory (eg, visual, auditory, olfactory, gustatory, vertiginous), autonomic (eg, sweating), and psychic (eg, fear). For example, seizures originating from the temporal lobe often present with lip smacking or other oral and alimentary automatisms, whereas those originating from the occipital lobe present with visual symptoms. Manifestations may spread to adjacent areas of the body when the motor cortex is involved (ie, Jacksonian march).[12,16]

**What is Todd's paralysis?**

Temporary postictal weakness in the region of the body affected by a focal motor seizure is referred to as Todd's paralysis.[12]

**How effective is pharmacologic monotherapy for patients with a focal seizure disorder?**

Pharmacologic monotherapy is effective in around one-third of patients with a focal seizure disorder. Combination therapy is often necessary.[13]

Which antiepileptic drugs are effective as initial monotherapy in adult patients with focal seizure disorders?

Initial monotherapy options with established efficacy for adult patients with focal seizure disorders include carbamazepine, levetiracetam, phenytoin, and zonisamide. Options that are probably or possibly efficacious include valproic acid, gabapentin, lamotrigine, oxcarbazepine, phenobarbital, topiramate, and vigabatrin. Lacosamide is an effective and well-tolerated adjuvant agent in patients with focal seizure disorders.[13,17]

Which antiepileptic drugs are effective as initial monotherapy in elderly patients with focal seizure disorders?

Initial monotherapy options with established efficacy for elderly patients with focal seizure disorders include gabapentin and lamotrigine.[17]

## GENERALIZED SEIZURES

### What are the main subtypes of generalized seizures?

A 16-year-old boy is evaluated for recurrent episodes of staring lasting up to 10 seconds, during which time he is unresponsive. After the episodes he is alert and oriented. The events are reproduced when the patient is asked to hyperventilate.

Absence seizure (ie, petit mal seizure).

A 33-year-old woman with early morning episodes of sudden-onset, brief, and involuntary dysrhythmic contractions of the proximal limbs.

Myoclonic seizure.

A 54-year-old man is evaluated after his wife complains of recurrent episodes of sudden-onset flexion of the waist for around 15 seconds during sleep.

Tonic seizure.

Rhythmic contractions of the shoulder muscles at a rate of 2 to 3 per second followed by confusion.

Clonic seizure.

A 46-year-old woman is evaluated for an episode of sudden loss of postural tone resulting in a fall and is found to have an abnormal EEG.

Atonic seizure.

A 28-year-old man is observed suddenly stiffening, then jerking the extremities for nearly 2 minutes; he is confused after the event.

Tonic-clonic seizure (ie, grand mal seizure).

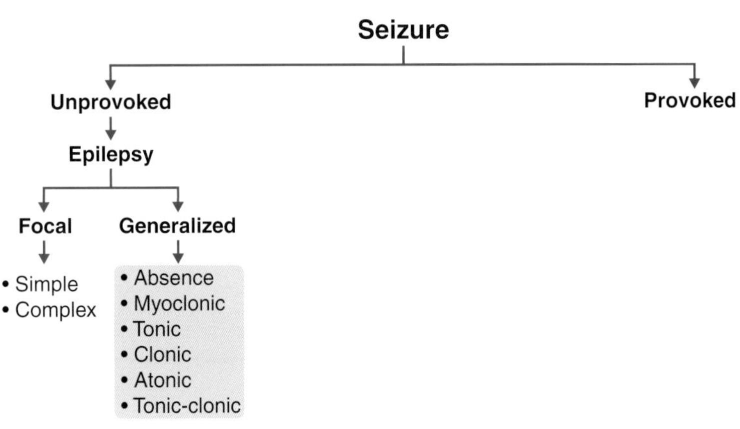

**Which antiepileptic drugs are effective as initial monotherapy in patients with absence seizures?**

Initial monotherapy options with established efficacy for patients with absence seizures include ethosuximide and valproic acid. Lamotrigine is an option with possible efficacy.[17]

**Which antiepileptic drugs may precipitate or aggravate myoclonic seizures in susceptible patients?**

Myoclonic seizures can be precipitated or aggravated by carbamazepine, gabapentin, oxcarbazepine, phenytoin, tiagabine, and vigabatrin.[17]

**What is the typical duration of tonic seizures?**

Tonic seizures typically last for 15 to 20 seconds.[17]

**What is the difference between myoclonic and clonic seizures?**

Clonic seizures are characterized by sustained and rhythmic myoclonus and are usually associated with a postictal state.[4]

**What is the typical duration of atonic seizures?**

Atonic seizures typically last for several seconds and rarely longer than 1 minute.[12]

**Which antiepileptic drugs are typically used as initial monotherapy in adults with generalized tonic-clonic seizure disorders?**

Initial monotherapy options with possible efficacy for adult patients with generalized tonic-clonic seizure disorders include carbamazepine, lamotrigine, oxcarbazepine, phenobarbital, phenytoin, topiramate, levetiracetam, and valproic acid.[17]

## PROVOKED SEIZURES

**How common are provoked seizures?**

Provoked seizures account for almost one-half of all first seizures.[8]

**The causes of provoked seizures can be separated into which general subcategories?**

The causes of provoked seizures can be separated into the following subcategories: vascular, toxic, structural, infectious, and metabolic.

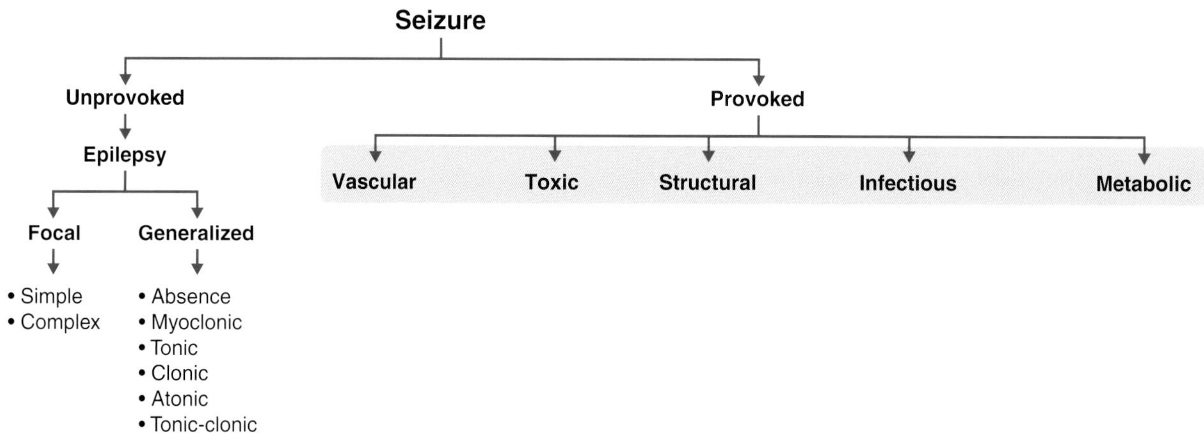


**Are provoked seizures usually generalized or focal?**

Provoked seizures related to nonstructural conditions typically present as generalized seizures (eg, hypoglycemia is usually associated with generalized tonic-clonic seizures). However, provoked seizures related to structural conditions (eg, cerebral aneurysm) typically present as focal seizures.

## VASCULAR CAUSES OF SEIZURE

### What are the vascular causes of seizure?

**A 68-year-old man with a history of coronary artery disease and peripheral vascular disease develops sudden-onset hemiparesis.**

Stroke.

| | |
|---|---|
| **Associated with posterior reversible encephalopathy syndrome (PRES).** | Hypertension. |
| **A 34-year-old woman presents in status epilepticus immediately after complaining of the most severe headache of her life.** | Subarachnoid hemorrhage. |
| **A young woman on combination oral contraceptive pills presents with worsening headache over the course of a week and is found to have papilledema on fundoscopic examination.** | Cerebral venous thrombosis (CVT). |
| **Congenital in nature.** | Cerebral vascular malformation, including developmental venous anomaly, capillary telangiectasia, cavernous malformation (CM), and arteriovenous malformation (AVM). |
| **A common source of atraumatic subarachnoid hemorrhage.** | Cerebral aneurysm. |
| **An immune-mediated condition that can be limited to the central nervous system (CNS) or involve it as part of a systemic condition (eg, Behçet's disease).** | Vasculitis. |
| **Most cases are reversible as the name implies but some result in long-term disability.** | Reversible cerebral vasoconstriction syndrome (RCVS). |
| **"Puff of smoke" (Figure 42-3).** | Moyamoya disease. |

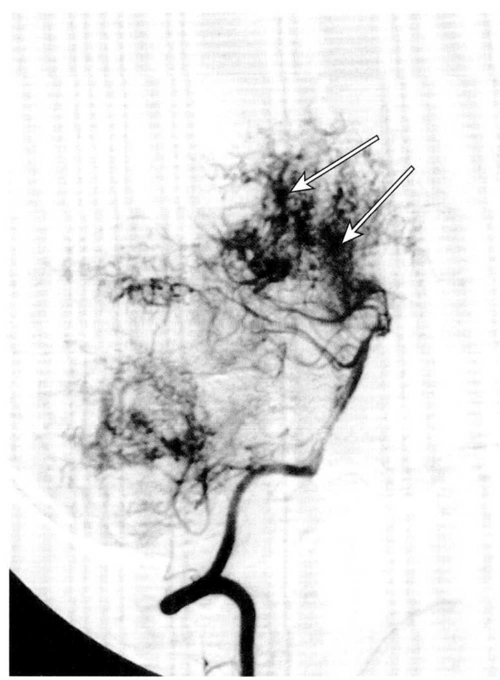

**Figure 42-3.** An extensive collateral network of blood vessels (arrows) gives rise to the typical "puff of smoke" appearance of moyamoya disease during cerebral angiography. (From Von Schulthess GK. *Molecular Anatomic Imaging: PET/CT, PET/MR, and SPECT/CT.* 3rd ed. Philadelphia, PA: Wolters Kluwer; 2016.)

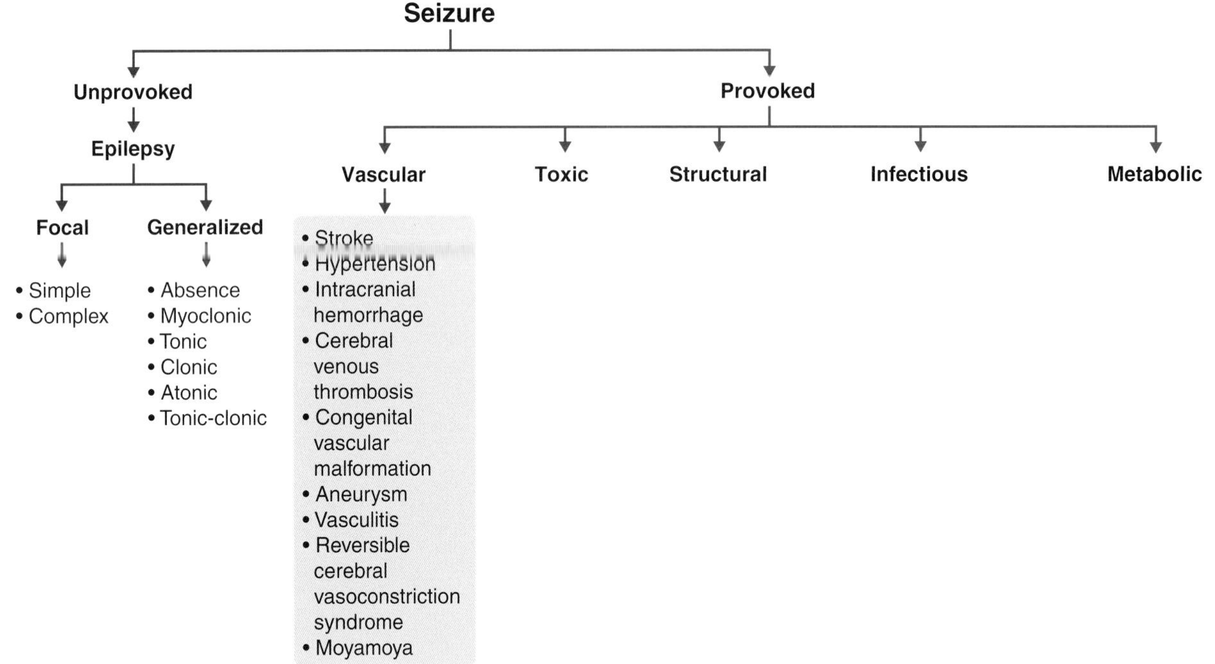


**What are the characteristics of seizures related to acute stroke?**

Seizures occur in up to 7% of patients with acute stroke, typically within the first 48 hours after the event. Focal seizures are most common and usually originate within the ischemic penumbra.[8]

**How often are seizures associated with posterior reversible encephalopathy syndrome?**

Seizures occur in most patients with PRES, and are often the presenting manifestation. Generalized tonic-clonic seizures are typical. Most patients do not progress to epilepsy.[8]

**What is the risk of seizure after intracranial hemorrhage?**

The risk of seizure is increased in patients with intracranial hemorrhage; it occurs in around 15% of patients with subarachnoid hemorrhage and around 5% of patients with intracerebral hemorrhage. The risk of developing epilepsy is substantial: compared to the general population, epilepsy is 34 times more likely to develop in patients with subarachnoid hemorrhage.[8]

**What is the risk of experiencing a seizure after cerebral venous thrombosis?**

Seizures occur on presentation in nearly one-half of patients with CVT, while a smaller proportion of patients will go on to experience a seizure within 2 weeks of the event.[8]

**What are the characteristics of seizures related to cavernous malformation?**

Seizures are part of the initial presentation in most patients with CM. Seizures are more likely to occur when the malformation is located in the frontal or temporal lobes. Focal seizures are the predominant type, but secondary generalized seizures also occur.[18]

**How often are seizures associated with unruptured cerebral aneurysms?**

Seizures are an uncommon occurrence in patients with unruptured cerebral aneurysms (around 5% of patients); aneurysms of the middle cerebral artery are most commonly associated with seizures.[19]

**What are the clinical manifestations of primary angiitis of the central nervous system (PACNS)?**

Headache is the most common manifestation of PACNS; others include delirium, transient ischemic attack, stroke, seizure, behavioral change, focal neurologic deficit, ataxia, visual disturbance, cranial neuropathy, myelopathy, and radiculopathy.[20]

**How often are seizures associated with reversible cerebral vasoconstriction syndrome?**

Seizures occur in a minority of patients with RCVS. Recurrent headache is the most common symptom and is often described as "thunderclap" in onset and intensity.[20]

What chronic vascular changes are associated with moyamoya disease?

Progressive bilateral stenosis of the intracranial portion of the internal carotid arteries and proximal branches can occur in patients with moyamoya disease.[21]

## TOXIC CAUSES OF SEIZURE

### What are the toxic causes of seizure?

Seizures related to this substance occur more commonly as a result of withdrawal than intoxication.

Alcohol.

Iatrogenic.

Medication (including intoxication and withdrawal).

These substances are ingested, snorted, inhaled, and injected.

Recreational drugs.

A 29-year-old man is found with seizure-like activity inside his garage with his car running.

Carbon monoxide poisoning.

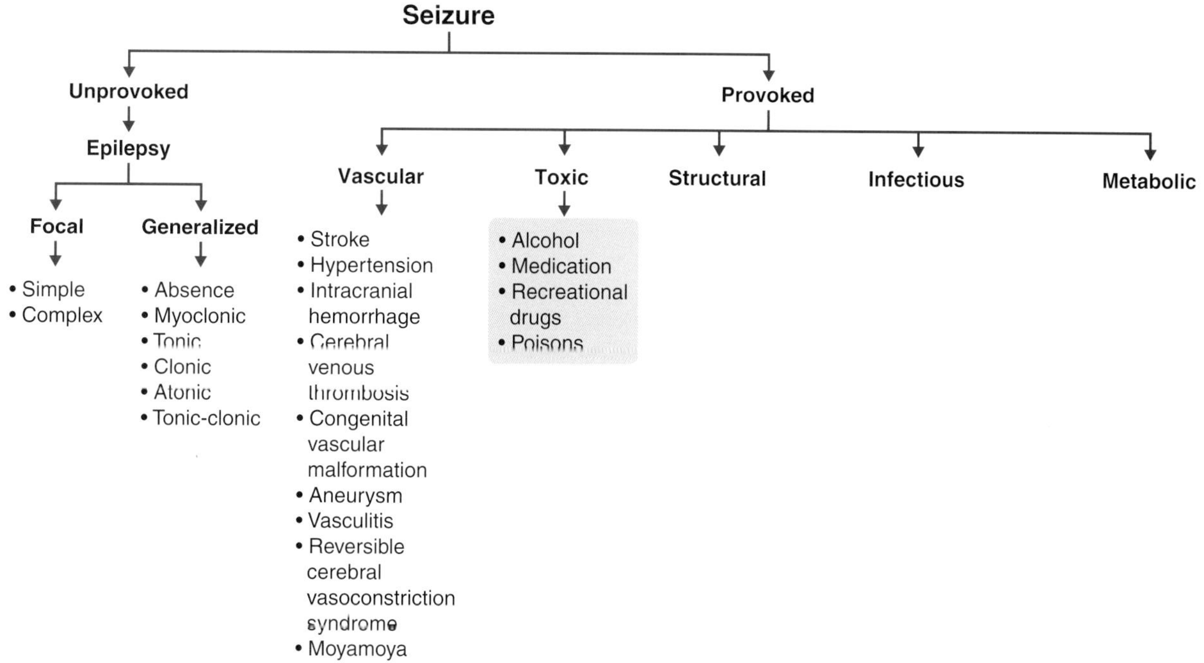


What are the characteristics of seizures related to alcohol withdrawal?

Alcohol withdrawal seizures are common, constituting around one-third of total hospital admissions related to seizures. Onset is typically 6 to 48 hours after cessation of alcohol and the seizure type is usually generalized.[8]

Intoxication with which medications are associated with the highest risk for seizure?

The tricyclic antidepressants, such as maprotiline, clomipramine, and amoxapine, are associated with a high rate of seizures when therapeutic levels are exceeded (seizure occurs up to one-fifth of patients who overdose). Other medications associated with seizures include theophylline, isoniazid, cyclosporine, chlorpromazine, clozapine, bupropion, meperidine, and flumazenil.[8]

Seizures can occur as a result of withdrawal from what commonly prescribed medications?

Withdrawal from barbiturates, benzodiazepines, and other sedatives (eg, zolpidem) can result in seizures.[8]

**Seizures can occur with intoxication from which recreational drugs?**

Intoxication with cocaine, amphetamines, and hallucinogens can result in seizures.[8]

**What treatment should be given as soon as possible to patients with carbon monoxide poisoning?**

In patients with carbon monoxide poisoning, oxygen should be given at a concentration of 100% via either a nonrebreather mask or hyperbaric chamber.

## STRUCTURAL CAUSES OF SEIZURE

### What are the structural causes of seizure?

**A 64-year-old man with a history of non–small cell lung cancer, thought to be in remission, presents with a focal complex seizure characterized by lip smacking.**

Metastatic brain tumor.

**A 76-year-old woman experiences a focal complex seizure 8 hours after being admitted to the hospital following a ground-level fall and is found to have normal neuroimaging.**

Traumatic brain injury (TBI).

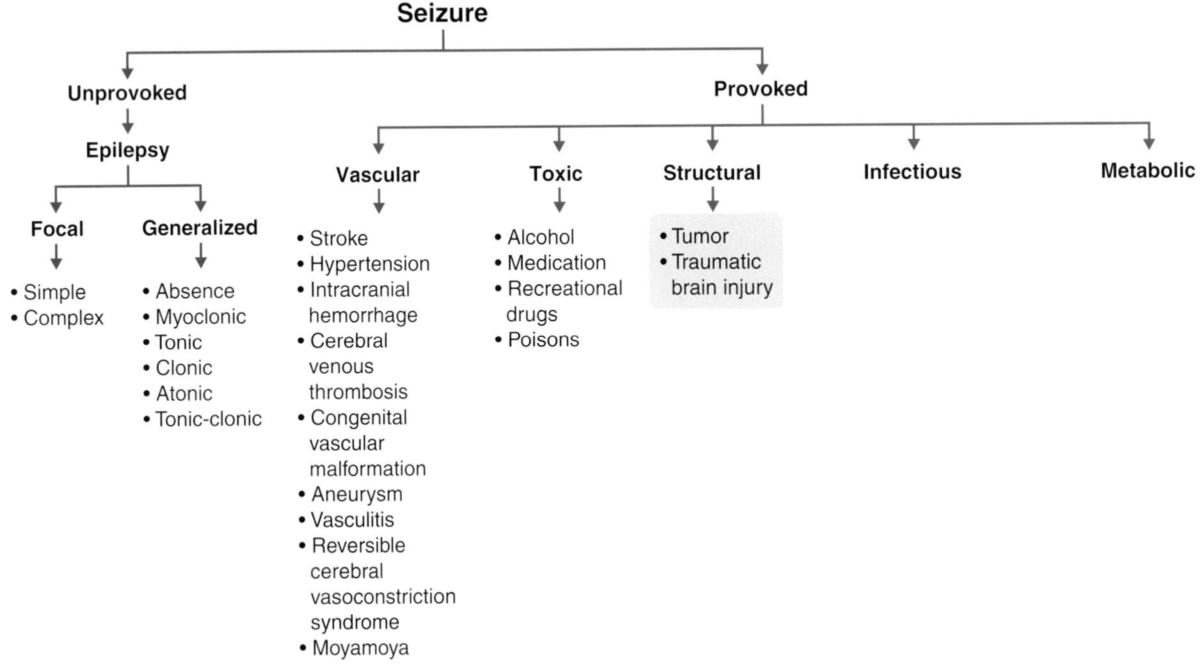


**How often is seizure the presenting clinical sign of a brain tumor?**

Seizures are the presenting manifestation of brain tumors in up to one-half of patients and are more common with low-grade tumors.[22]

**Which inherited condition that results in the development of brain tumors should be suspected in a patient with seizures and multiple hypopigmented macules?**

Tuberous sclerosis complex should be suspected in a patient with a seizure disorder who is found to have hypopigmented macules (ie, ash leaf spots) on physical examination.

**What is the risk of developing epilepsy after traumatic brain injury?**

The risk of developing epilepsy (ie, future seizures outside of the acute setting) after TBI increases with severity of injury and is higher in patients who experience acute seizure. Epilepsy is approximately 15 times more common in adult patients with severe TBI compared with the general population. Most develop epilepsy within the first year after the event, but it may occur many years later.[8]

## INFECTIOUS CAUSES OF SEIZURE

### What are the infectious causes of seizure?

| | |
|---|---|
| **A 20-year-old college student presents with headache, photophobia, neck stiffness, and a generalized seizure.** | Meningitis. |
| **A 55-year-old woman with a history of kidney transplant presents with confusion and headache and is found to have periodic lateralized epileptiform discharges (ie, lateralized periodic discharges) on EEG.** | Herpes simplex or human herpesvirus 6 encephalitis. |
| **A 48-year-old man with an untreated dental abscess presents with a complex focal seizure.** | Brain abscess. |
| **Parasites.** | Toxoplasmosis and neurocysticercosis. |
| **A viral-mediated demyelinating condition of the central nervous system found in immunocompromised patients.** | Progressive multifocal leukoencephalopathy (PML). |



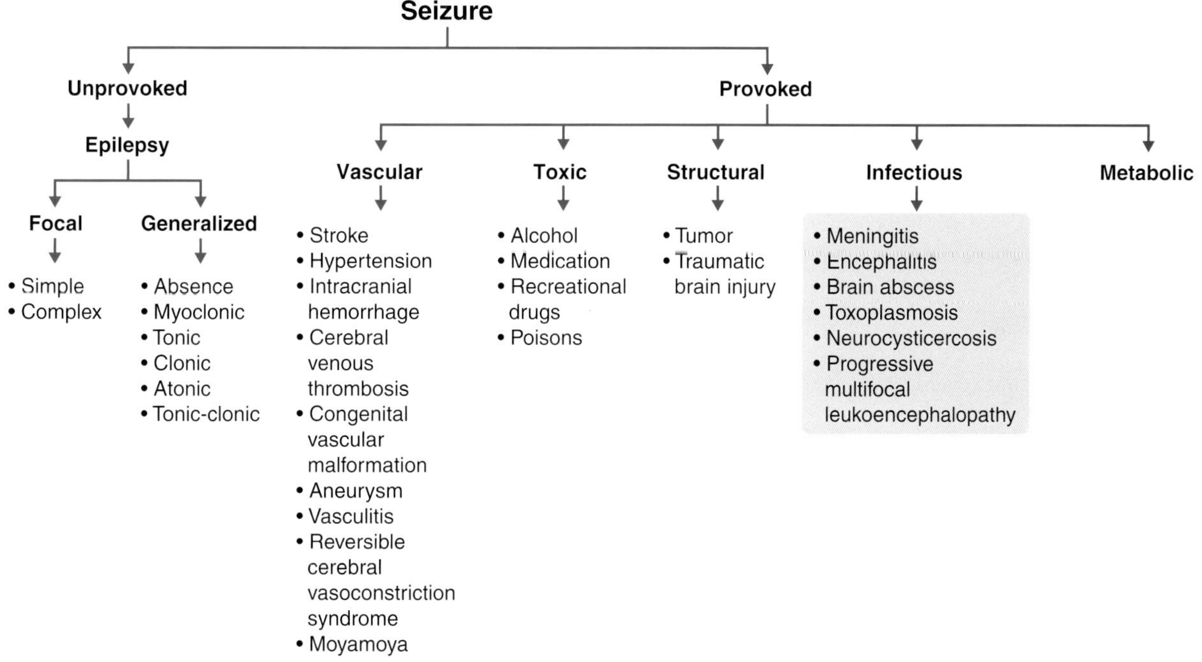


| | |
|---|---|
| **How often do seizures occur in patients with bacterial meningitis?** | Seizures occur in around one-fifth of patients with community-acquired bacterial meningitis; when seizures do occur, there is a significantly increased risk of mortality.[23] |
| **How often do seizures occur in patients with herpes simplex encephalitis?** | Seizures are part of the presenting manifestations in about one-half of patients with herpes simplex encephalitis, probably as a result of involvement of the frontotemporal cortex, which is highly epileptogenic.[24] |
| **How often do seizures occur in patients with brain abscess?** | Seizures are the presenting manifestation in around one-quarter of patients with brain abscess. Epilepsy subsequently develops in a significant proportion of patients.[25,26] |

**What is the risk of seizure related to toxoplasmosis?**

It is estimated that one-third of the world's population is infected with toxoplasmosis. There is an associated 1.5- to 4-fold risk of seizure in these patients.[27]

**What is the risk of epilepsy in patients with neurocysticercosis who have persistent abnormalities on neuroimaging (eg, cysts and calcified cysts)?**

Epilepsy develops in just over one-half of patients with neurocysticercosis who have persistent abnormalities on neuroimaging. Neurocysticercosis is the most common cause of epilepsy in the developing world, responsible for around one-third of all seizures.[8]

**What are the characteristics of seizures related to progressive multifocal leukoencephalopathy?**

Seizures occur in around one-fifth of patients with PML. The most frequent seizure types include simple focal, complex focal, and simple focal with secondary generalization. Seizures are generally responsive to antiepileptic drugs and do not affect survival.[28]

## METABOLIC CAUSES OF SEIZURE

### What are the metabolic causes of seizure?

**This condition should be ruled out in the immediate evaluation of anyone with impaired consciousness.**

Hypoglycemia.

**Hypertonicity and polyuria in a diabetic patient.**

Hyperglycemia.

**Seizure in a marathon runner who rehydrates with water.**

Hyponatremia.

**Seizure in a patient with diabetes insipidus.**

Hypernatremia.

**These electrolyte disturbances are associated with Chvostek's sign.**

Hypocalcemia and hypomagnesemia.

**Tissue death.**

Cerebral hypoxia with anoxic brain injury.

**Asterixis on examination.**

Uremia.

**Delirium, jaundice, and coagulopathy.**

Liver failure.

**A 28-year-old woman who is 32 weeks pregnant presents with hypertension, proteinuria, and a generalized tonic-clonic seizure.**

Eclampsia.

**Acute episodes of abdominal pain, polyneuropathy, and urine that turns red over time (Figure 42-4).**

Acute porphyria.

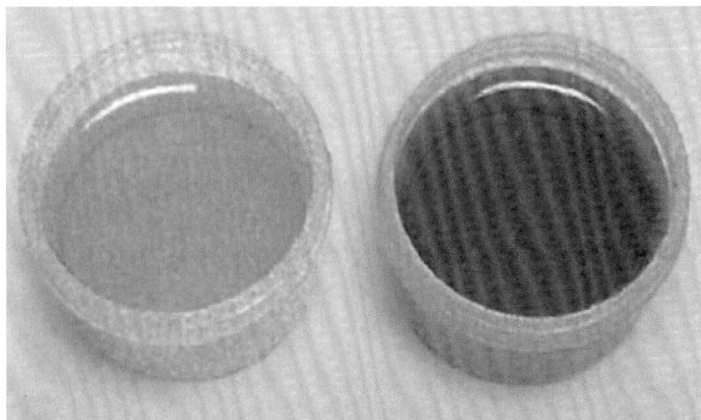

**Figure 42-4.** Urine from a patient with porphyria cutanea tarda (right) and from a patient with normal porphyrin excretion (left). From Champe PC, Harvey RA, Ferrier DR. *Biochemistry*. 4th ed. Philadelphia, PA: Wolters Kluwer Health/Lippincott Williams & Wilkins, 2000, with permission.

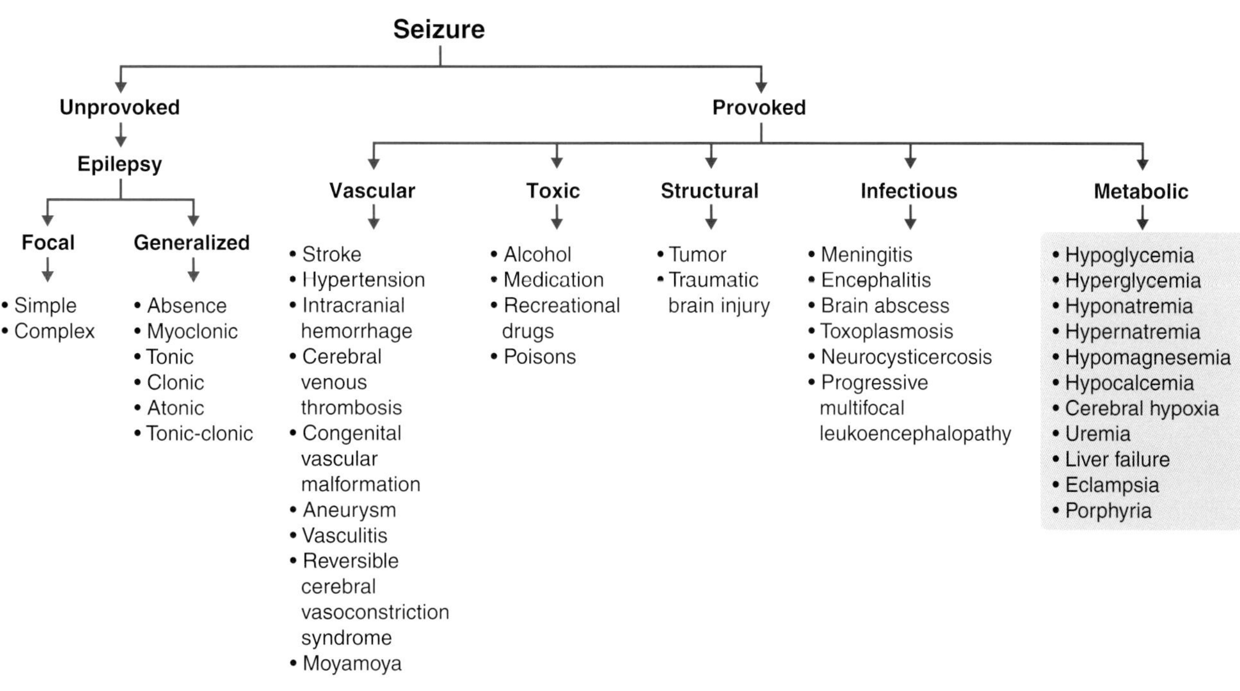




**What is the most common type of seizure related to hypoglycemia?**

Patients with hypoglycemia most often experience generalized tonic-clonic seizures.[29]

**Are seizures more common in patients with diabetic ketoacidosis or nonketotic hyperosmolar state?**

Seizures tend to occur in patients with nonketotic hyperosmolar state but are rare in patients with diabetic ketoacidosis, likely related to the anticonvulsant effect of ketosis. Focal motor seizure is the most common type.[29]

**What treatment should be immediately administered to patients with seizures related to hyponatremia?**

Intravenous hypertonic saline (3%) should be given immediately to patients with seizures related to hyponatremia.[30]

**Under what circumstance do seizures occur most often in patients with hypernatremia?**

Seizures related to hypernatremia most commonly occur when chronic hypernatremia is corrected too quickly.[30]

**What degree of hypomagnesemia is generally required to cause seizures?**

Seizures generally occur in association with severe hypomagnesemia (<1 mEq/L) and are usually generalized tonic-clonic.[30]

**How often do seizures occur in patients with symptomatic hypoparathyroidism?**

Seizures occur in around one-half of patients with symptomatic hypoparathyroidism.[30]

**What conditions can lead to cerebral hypoxia?**

Cerebral hypoxia can occur with any of the following conditions: impaired arterial oxygen content (eg, anemia, hypoxemia), impaired oxygen delivery (eg, low cardiac output), impaired binding of oxygen to hemoglobin (eg, methemoglobinemia), and impaired uptake or use of oxygen by the tissues (eg, carbon monoxide poisoning, sepsis, cyanide poisoning).

**What is dialysis disequilibrium syndrome (DDS)?**

DDS may occur when rapid removal of urea during hemodialysis results in an osmotic gradient, leading to cerebral edema. Manifestations include nausea, headache, vomiting, tremor, and seizure.[31]

**What type of liver disease is associated with seizures?**

Seizures can occur in patients with acute (ie, fulminant) liver failure, probably related to the cerebral edema that can develop with this condition, but are an unusual manifestation of chronic liver disease.[32]

**When do seizures usually occur in patients with eclampsia?**

Seizures associated with eclampsia occur prepartum in around one-half of patients and postpartum in the other half. A small proportion of patients experience seizures during childbirth.[8]

**Which antiepileptic drugs can potentially worsen an acute attack of porphyria?**

Antiepileptic drugs that can worsen an acute attack of porphyria include phenytoin, phenobarbital, clonazepam, and valproic acid.[33]

## Case Summary

A 68-year-old man presents with a first-time seizure after several months of malaise, night sweats, and weight loss and is found to have a low-grade fever, heart murmur, focal neurologic deficit, and multiple ring-enhancing lesions on neuroimaging.

***What is the most likely cause of seizure in this patient?***

Brain abscess.

### BONUS QUESTIONS

***What type of seizure is described in this case?***

The patient in this case experienced a focal seizure with secondary generalization (ie, focal seizure evolving to a bilateral, convulsive seizure).

***What region of the brain is likely to have been the epileptic focus in this case?***

The "fencing" posturing described in this case (extending the arm and leg on one side while flexing the contralateral limbs) is reflective of a focus in the supplementary motor area of the frontal lobe; contralateral gaze deviation is also classically seen with frontal lobe foci (it can also be seen with temporal lobe foci). The most likely culprit lesion in this case is in the right frontal lobe (see Figure 42-1). Localizing seizure foci based only on clinical history and examination can be challenging, and EEG is usually necessary. Localizing the origin of focal seizures is important when surgical treatment options are being explored.

***What features of this case suggest a provoked seizure?***

In this case, features suggestive of a provoked seizure include older age of onset, systemic symptoms and signs (eg, night sweats, weight loss), and the focal neurologic finding (ie, pronator drift).

***What are the mechanisms through which brain abscesses occur?***

Brain abscesses form via contiguous spread through disrupted barriers surrounding the brain in around one-half of cases; hematogenous spread is the mechanism in one-quarter of cases; and the mechanism is unknown in the remaining quarter of cases.[25]

***What are some examples of regional infection that can lead to brain abscess via contiguous spread?***

Brain abscess is a potential complication of otitis media, mastoiditis, sinusitis, and dental abscess.[25]

***What is the most likely mechanism of brain abscess in this case?***

Multiple bilateral foci on neuroimaging in this case are suggestive of hematogenous spread. The presence of a holosystolic murmur and preceding dental work suggest subacute bacterial endocarditis.

***What specimens for culture can be collected in patients with brain abscess to identify the culprit organism(s)?***

The causative organism of a brain abscess can be identified via blood and cerebrospinal fluid cultures in around one-quarter of cases. Caution should be exercised before performing lumbar puncture in these patients given the risk of brain herniation. Regional infections, if present, should be cultured. Ultimately, neurosurgical stereotactic aspiration may be necessary to obtain positive cultures. Almost any brain abscess >1 cm in diameter is amenable to this technique. Gram stain and aerobic and anaerobic cultures should be obtained. Other specific studies (eg, acid-fast smear) should be obtained depending on patient-specific factors.[25]

***How are brain abscesses managed?***

A combination of neurosurgical drainage and intravenous antibiotics is typically used to treat brain abscesses. The course of intravenous antibiotics is often long (about 6-8 weeks). Serial imaging studies should be performed to monitor clinical response and guide the duration of therapy.[25]

***What dangerous complications are associated with brain abscess?***

In patients with brain abscess, ventriculitis can occur from abscess rupture into the ventricular system and is associated with a high mortality rate. Other dangerous complications include status epilepticus, hydrocephalus, and brain herniation.[25]

***What is the prognosis of patients with brain abscess?***

Overall, good outcomes with no or minimal long-term sequelae are observed in most patients treated for brain abscess. However, epilepsy develops in a significant proportion of patients.[25,26]

## KEY POINTS

- A seizure is defined as abnormal excessive or synchronous neuronal activity resulting in transient symptoms and signs, including sensory, motor, and autonomic manifestations.
- Status epilepticus is reached when the duration of a typical seizure is longer than expected (usually >5 minutes), or when seizures recur in succession without interval return to baseline consciousness.
- A postictal state is the transient period after a seizure characterized by changes in behavior, motor function, and neuropsychological performance.
- Seizures can be focal or generalized.
- Focal seizures involve a portion of the brain at onset and are limited to 1 hemisphere. Generalized seizures involve both cerebral hemispheres simultaneously with loss of consciousness.
- Focal seizures can be simple (without impaired awareness) or complex (with impaired awareness).
- Focal seizures can become secondarily generalized (ie, focal seizure evolving to a bilateral, convulsive seizure).
- Seizures can be unprovoked or provoked.
- An unprovoked seizure is one that occurs in the absence of a temporary or reversible precipitant.
- Epilepsy is a disorder of the brain characterized by recurrent unprovoked seizures.
- Long-term remission is achieved with antiepileptic drugs in most patients with epilepsy.
- The causes of provoked seizures can be separated into the following subcategories: vascular, toxic, structural, infectious, and metabolic.
- Causes of provoked seizures that result in residual brain alteration (eg, stroke) or those that are not temporary (eg, brain tumor) can lead to a long-term predisposition for seizures and epilepsy.
- Treatment for provoked seizures should focus on reversing the underlying cause if possible. Antiepileptic medications may be necessary at least temporarily.
- Most acute seizures resolve spontaneously within a few minutes. If a seizure is prolonged or status epilepticus is reached, then first-line pharmacologic therapy is an intravenously-administered short-acting benzodiazepine (unless there is an immediately reversible provoking condition such as hypoglycemia).



## REFERENCES


1. Fisher RS, Acevedo C, Arzimanoglou A, et al. ILAE official report: a practical clinical definition of epilepsy. *Epilepsia*. 2014;55(4):475-482.
2. Browne TR, Holmes GL. Epilepsy. *N Engl J Med*. 2001;344(15):1145-1151.
3. Fisher RS, van Emde Boas W, Blume W, et al. Epileptic seizures and epilepsy: definitions proposed by the International League Against Epilepsy (ILAE) and the International Bureau for Epilepsy (IBE). *Epilepsia*. 2005;46(4):470-472.
4. Blume WT, Luders HO, Mizrahi E, Tassinari C, van Emde Boas W, Engel J Jr. Glossary of descriptive terminology for ictal semiology: report of the ILAE task force on classification and terminology. *Epilepsia*. 2001;42(9):1212-1218.
5. Brophy GM, Bell R, Claassen J, et al. Guidelines for the evaluation and management of status epilepticus. *Neurocrit Care*. 2012;17(1):3-23.
6. Remi J, Noachtar S. Clinical features of the postictal state: correlation with seizure variables. *Epilepsy Behav*. 2010;19(2):114-117.
7. Beghi E, Carpio A, Forsgren L, et al. Recommendation for a definition of acute symptomatic seizure. *Epilepsia*. 2010;51(4):671-675.
8. Beleza P. Acute symptomatic seizures: a clinically oriented review. *Neurologist*. 2012;18(3):109-119.
9. Berg AT, Berkovic SF, Brodie MJ, et al. Revised terminology and concepts for organization of seizures and epilepsies: report of the ILAE Commission on Classification and Terminology, 2005-2009. *Epilepsia*. 2010;51(4):676-685.
10. Sander JW, Hart YM, Johnson AL, Shorvon SD. National General Practice Study of Epilepsy: newly diagnosed epileptic seizures in a general population. *Lancet*. 1990;336(8726):1267-1271.
11. Nakken KO, Solaas MH, Kjeldsen MJ, Friis ML, Pellock JM, Corey LA. Which seizure-precipitating factors do patients with epilepsy most frequently report? *Epilepsy Behav*. 2005;6(1):85-89.
12. Bromfield EB, Cavazos JE, Sirven JI, eds. *An Introduction to Epilepsy [Internet]*. West Hartford, CT: American Epilepsy Society; 2006.
13. Becerra JL, Ojeda J, Corredera E, Ruiz Gimenez J. Review of therapeutic options for adjuvant treatment of focal seizures in epilepsy: focus on lacosamide. *CNS Drugs*. 2011;25(suppl 1):3-16.
14. Chang BS, Lowenstein DH. Epilepsy. *N Engl J Med*. 2003;349(13):1257-1266.
15. Luders HO, Turnbull J, Kaffashi F. Are the dichotomies generalized versus focal epilepsies and idiopathic versus symptomatic epilepsies still valid in modern epileptology? *Epilepsia*. 2009;50(6):1336-1343.
16. Ahmed SN, Spencer SS. An approach to the evaluation of a patient for seizures and epilepsy. *WMJ*. 2004;103(1):49-55.
17. Glauser T, Ben-Menachem E, Bourgeois B, et al. Updated ILAE evidence review of antiepileptic drug efficacy and effectiveness as initial monotherapy for epileptic seizures and syndromes. *Epilepsia*. 2013;54(3):551-563.
18. Cosgrove GR. Occult vascular malformations and seizures. *Neurosurg Clin N Am*. 1999;10(3):527-535.
19. Kamali AW, Cockerell OC, Butlar P. Aneurysms and epilepsy: an increasingly recognised cause. *Seizure*. 2004;13(1):40-44.

20. Hajj-Ali RA, Calabrese LH. Primary angiitis of the central nervous system. *Autoimmun Rev*. 2013;12(4):463-466.
21. Scott RM, Smith ER. Moyamoya disease and moyamoya syndrome. *N Engl J Med*. 2009;360(12):1226-1237.
22. van Breemen MS, Wilms EB, Vecht CJ. Epilepsy in patients with brain tumours: epidemiology, mechanisms, and management. *Lancet Neurol*. 2007;6(5):421-430.
23. Zoons E, Weisfelt M, de Gans J, et al. Seizures in adults with bacterial meningitis. *Neurology*. 2008;70(22 Pt 2):2109-2115.
24. Misra UK, Tan CT, Kalita J. Viral encephalitis and epilepsy. *Epilepsia*. 2008;49(suppl 6):13-18.
25. Brouwer MC, Tunkel AR, McKhann GM 2nd, van de Beek D. Brain abscess. *N Engl J Med*. 2014;371(5):447-456.
26. Muzumdar D, Jhawar S, Goel A. Brain abscess: an overview. *Int J Surg*. 2011;9(2):136-144.
27. Ngoungou EB, Bhalla D, Nzoghe A, Darde ML, Preux PM. Toxoplasmosis and epilepsy–systematic review and meta analysis. *PLoS Negl Trop Dis*. 2015;9(2):e0003525.
28. Lima MA, Drislane FW, Koralnik IJ. Seizures and their outcome in progressive multifocal leukoencephalopathy. *Neurology*. 2006;66(2):262-264.
29. Verrotti A, Scaparrotta A, Olivieri C, Chiarelli F. Seizures and type 1 diabetes mellitus: current state of knowledge. *Eur J Endocrinol*. 2012;167(6):749-758.
30. Castilla-Guerra L, del Carmen Fernandez-Moreno M, Lopez-Chozas JM, Fernandez-Bolanos R. Electrolytes disturbances and seizures. *Epilepsia*. 2006;47(12):1990-1998.
31. Patel N, Dalal P, Panesar M. Dialysis disequilibrium syndrome: a narrative review. *Semin Dial*. 2008;21(5):493-498.
32. Lewis M, Howdle PD. The neurology of liver failure. *QJM*. 2003;96(9):623-633.
33. Tracy JA, Dyck PJ. Porphyria and its neurologic manifestations. *Handb Clin Neurol*. 2014;120:839-849.

# Chapter 43

# STROKE

## Case: A 48-year-old woman with flank pain

A previously healthy 48-year-old woman is admitted to the hospital with acute-onset severe right-sided flank pain with radiation to the back and associated nausea. The patient recently flew home to the United States after vacationing in England. She has had left leg swelling and pain since returning home. The patient takes combination oral contraceptive pills but no other medications. She is not a smoker.

There is erythema and pitting edema of the left lower extremity. The abdomen is soft, and there is no tenderness to palpation. Right-sided costovertebral angle tenderness is present. Urinalysis demonstrates hematuria without dysmorphic red blood cells.

Doppler ultrasound of the left lower extremity demonstrates thrombosis of the deep femoral vein. Computed tomography (CT) imaging with intravenous contrast of the abdomen (Figure 43-1) shows a lack of enhancement of the right kidney (arrow). Shortly after completing the imaging study, the patient suddenly becomes unintelligible. On examination, the head and eyes are deviated toward the left and there is a right-sided facial droop. There is full strength of the left upper and lower extremities but no movement on the right. The patient responds to painful stimuli on the left but not the right. The biceps, patellar, and Achilles reflexes are brisk on the right. Urgent CT imaging of the brain shows loss of gray-white matter differentiation in the territory of the left middle cerebral artery. CT imaging of the brain 24 hours later is shown in Figure 43-2.

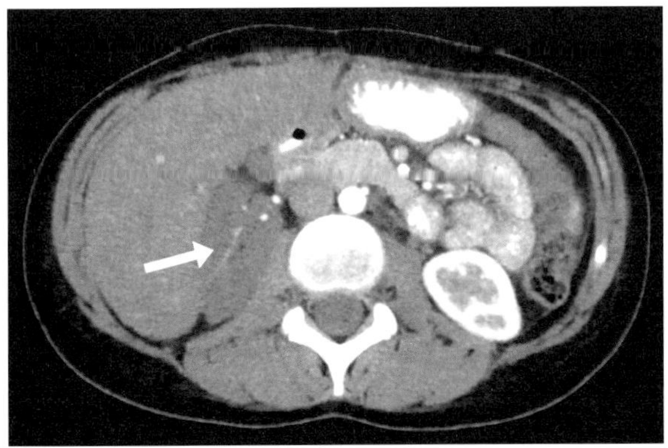

**Figure 43-1.**

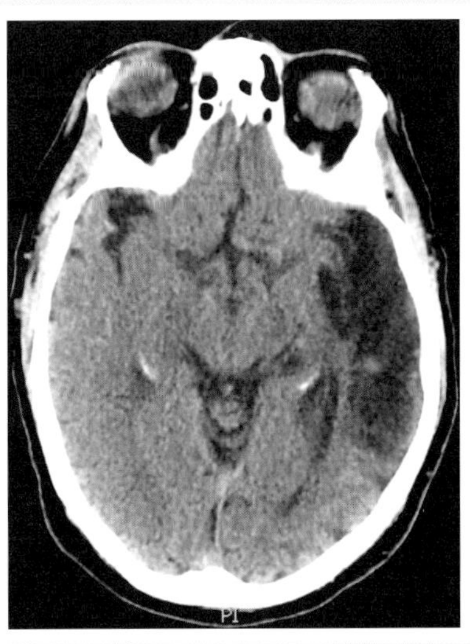


**Figure 43-2.**

***What is the most likely cause of stroke in this patient?***

**What is a stroke?**

A stroke (ie, cerebrovascular accident) occurs when there is acute infarction of brain tissue, spinal cord, or retina, resulting in neurologic deficits. The nature and severity of neurologic deficits can vary according to the distribution and size of the stroke. There are well-described ischemic stroke syndromes according to the distribution of infarction. Hemorrhagic stroke tends to be more variable in presentation because the area of injury often crosses multiple vascular territories.[1]

**What is a transient ischemic attack (TIA)?**

A TIA is defined as transient neurologic dysfunction caused by focal ischemia of brain tissue, spinal cord, or retina without acute infarction.[2]

**What is the risk of stroke in patients with transient ischemic attack?**

The risk of stroke after TIA depends on underlying risk factors, but it occurs in up to 10% of patients at 2 days and 15% at 90 days.[3]

**How common is stroke?**

In the United States, it is estimated that a stroke occurs every 40 seconds. Prevalence increases with age and is approximately 15% in adults older than 80 years. Stroke is the second leading cause of death worldwide.[3]

**What are the risk factors for stroke?**

Chronic hypertension, defined by a systolic blood pressure ≥140 mm Hg or a diastolic blood pressure ≥90 mm Hg. It is the strongest risk factor for stroke and is present in most stroke patients. Other risk factors include diabetes mellitus, cardiac dysrhythmias (eg, atrial fibrillation), dyslipidemia, smoking, physical inactivity, poor nutrition, family history and genetics, and chronic kidney disease.[2]

**What conditions are commonly confused with stroke or transient ischemic attack?**

Migraine, postictal paresis (ie, Todd's paralysis), hypoglycemia, subdural hematoma, mass lesions (eg, brain tumor), and conversion disorder can be confused with stroke or TIA.

**What is the prognosis of stroke?**

The prognosis of stroke depends largely on the type of stroke and the size and territory of infarction. Overall, the 30-day mortality rate of stroke in the industrialized world is approximately 10%; 1-year mortality is around 20%; and 5-year mortality is around 40%. Factors that increase the likelihood of a poor outcome include older age, comorbid ischemic heart disease or diabetes mellitus, and larger size of infarction.[3]

**What are the 2 general types of stroke?**

Strokes can be hemorrhagic or ischemic (Figure 43-3).

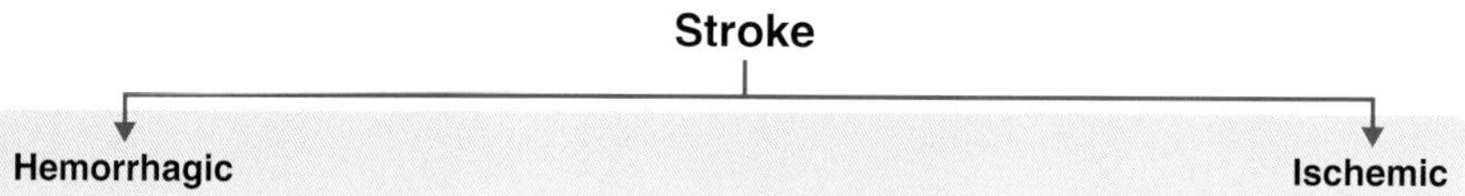


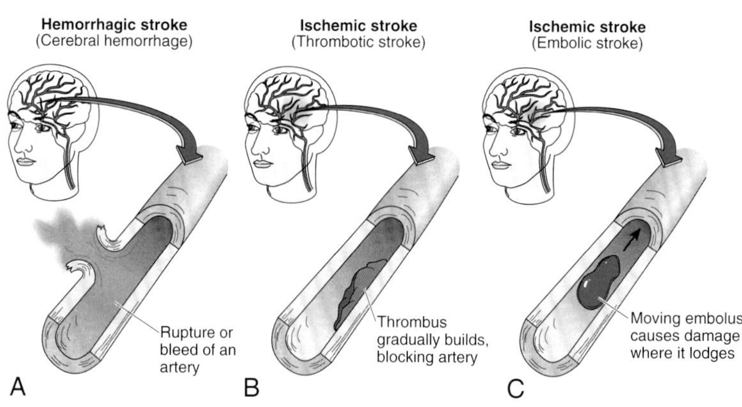


**Figure 43-3.** Mechanisms of hemorrhagic and ischemic stroke. (Adapted with permission from Walton T. *Medical Conditions and Massage Therapy: A Decision Tree Approach*. Philadelphia, PA: Wolters Kluwer Health; 2010.)

**Why is it important to differentiate between hemorrhagic and ischemic stroke?**

Underlying causes and general treatment considerations vary between hemorrhagic and ischemic stroke.

**What are the mechanisms of tissue injury in hemorrhagic and ischemic stroke?**

Hemorrhagic stroke causes injury due to mechanical compression of brain tissue and local toxicity from blood breakdown products; ischemic stroke causes injury due to insufficient oxygen and nutrient delivery to brain tissue. *Hemorrhagic stroke can generally be thought of as a consequence of the presence of blood, and ischemic stroke, a consequence of the absence of blood.*

**What are the relative rates of hemorrhagic and ischemic stroke?**

In the industrialized world, around 80% of strokes are ischemic and the remaining 20% are hemorrhagic.[3,4]

**Is hemorrhagic or ischemic stroke associated with higher morbidity and mortality?**

Hemorrhagic stroke is associated with higher morbidity and mortality in the acute poststroke period compared with ischemic stroke, with a 30-day mortality rate approaching 50% (5 times greater than ischemic stroke). Long-term functional status among survivors is similar between the two.[3,5]

**How can the type of stroke (ie, hemorrhagic or ischemic) be established?**

Neuroimaging is necessary to determine whether a stroke is hemorrhagic or ischemic, as symptoms and signs alone cannot distinguish between the two. CT imaging or magnetic resonance imaging (MRI) should be performed. Noncontrast CT imaging is highly sensitive for acute intracranial hemorrhage and is more widely available, faster, less susceptible to motion artifact, and less expensive compared with MRI. Lumbar puncture with evaluation of cerebrospinal fluid (CSF) for the presence of blood or xanthochromia can be suggestive of subarachnoid hemorrhage (SAH), a subtype of hemorrhagic stroke.[4]

**Is CT imaging adequate for the evaluation of ischemic stroke?**

MRI is associated with a significantly higher sensitivity for ischemic stroke compared with CT imaging, particularly for lesions in the posterior fossa and within the first hours after the event.[4]



## HEMORRHAGIC STROKE

**Hemorrhagic strokes occur within which 2 anatomic spaces of the brain?**

Hemorrhagic stroke can occur within the brain parenchyma (ie, intracerebral) or subarachnoid space (ie, between the arachnoid and pia mater) (Figure 43-4).

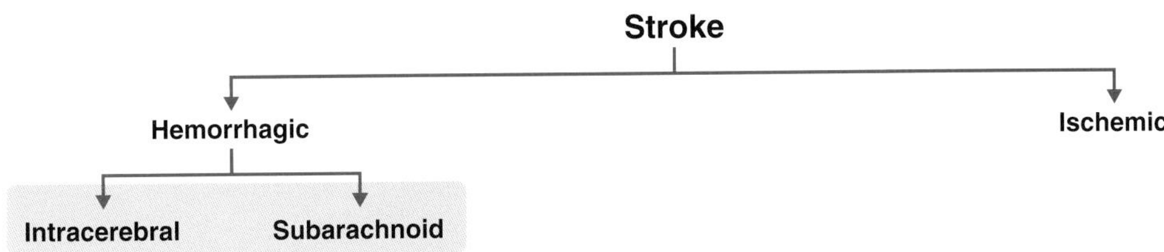


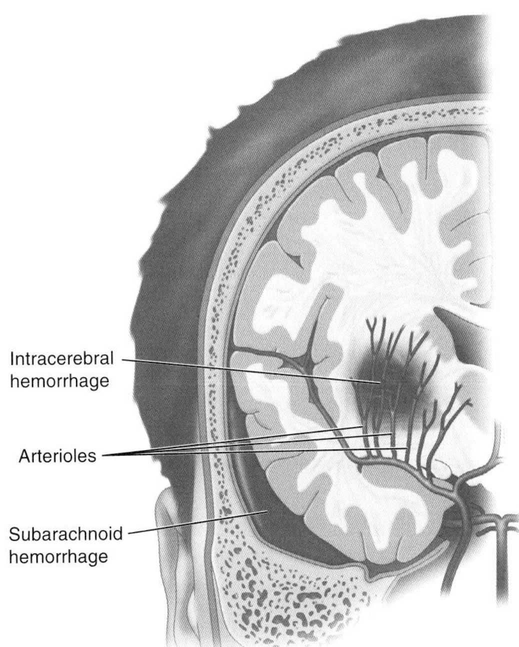


**Figure 43-4.** Hemorrhagic stroke can occur within the brain (intracerebral hemorrhage) or on the surface (subarachnoid hemorrhage). (From Werner R. *A Massage Therapist's Guide to Pathology,* 6th ed. Philadelphia, PA: Wolters Kluwer; 2016.)

**Why is it important to differentiate between strokes caused by intracerebral hemorrhage and subarachnoid hemorrhage?**

The underlying causes and general treatment considerations vary between strokes caused by intracerebral hemorrhage and SAH.

**What are the relative rates of intracerebral hemorrhage and subarachnoid hemorrhage?**

Intracerebral hemorrhage is more common than SAH, accounting for 10% to 15% of all strokes. SAH accounts for around 5% of all strokes.[5]

## HEMORRHAGIC STROKE CAUSED BY INTRACEREBRAL HEMORRHAGE

**What risk factors are associated with intracerebral hemorrhage?**

Risk factors for intracerebral hemorrhage include hypertension, older age, race (eg, blacks, Asians), high levels of alcohol consumption, and lower levels of low density lipoprotein and triglycerides.[6,7]

**What are the findings of intracerebral hemorrhage on CT imaging?**

Intracerebral hemorrhage typically appears as a round or oval hyperattenuating lesion on noncontrast CT imaging (Figure 43-5). Early on, the mass measures 40 to 60 Hounsfield units (HU) and can be heterogeneous in appearance. Over time as the clot organizes, it becomes more homogenous and hyperdense, measuring 60 to 80 HU within hours to days and 80 to 100 HU over the course of a few days.[5]

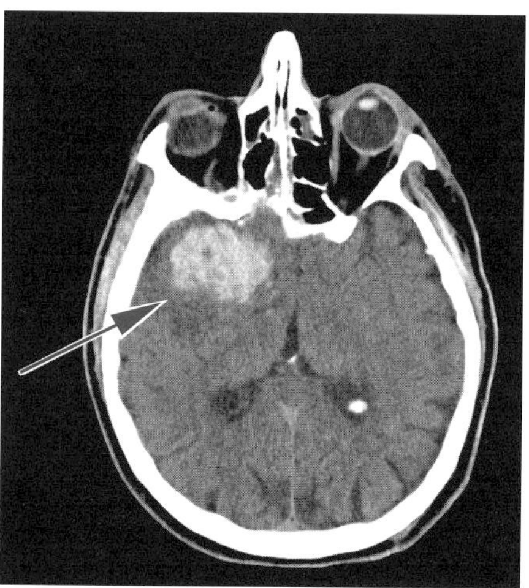

Figure 43-5. Noncontrast CT imaging showing hyperdensity (arrow) in the area of the right temporal lobe corresponding to the presence of intracerebral hemorrhage. (From Garcia MJ. *Noninvasive Cardiovascular Imaging: A Multimodality Approach*. Philadelphia, PA: Lippincott Williams & Wilkins; 2010.)

**What general medical treatment should be considered for acute spontaneous intracerebral hemorrhage?**

In patients with acute spontaneous intracerebral hemorrhage, underlying bleeding diatheses should be identified and addressed (eg, reversal of elevated international normalized ratio); systolic blood pressure (SBP) should be lowered if elevated (for patients with SBP 150 to 220 mm Hg, it is safe to acutely decrease it to 140 mm Hg); blood sugar should be managed to avoid hyperglycemia or hypoglycemia; and seizures should be treated with antiepileptic medications. In patients with elevated intracranial pressure, additional measures including intubation and sedation, elevation of the head of the bed, hypertonic fluid administration, and hemicraniectomy may be necessary.[8]

**What is the short-term mortality of intracerebral hemorrhage?**

The 30-day mortality of intracerebral hemorrhage is nearly 50%.[5]

### What are the causes of intracerebral hemorrhage?

**An S4 gallop on auscultation of the heart and evidence of left ventricular hypertrophy on electrocardiography.**

Hypertension (HTN).

**A disease of older patients resulting from protein deposition within cerebral blood vessels.**

Cerebral amyloid angiopathy (CAA).

| | |
|---|---|
| A 65-year-old woman suffers a ground-level fall, hitting her head on the pavement, and subsequently develops confusion and focal neurologic deficits. | Trauma. |
| A 29-year-old man is admitted with gingival bleeding, epistaxis, and confusion after a recent upper respiratory tract infection and is found to have a petechial rash on the lower extremities. | Immune thrombocytopenic purpura. |
| Congenital lesions. | Cerebral vascular malformation (CVM). |
| A 38-year-old woman with a recent diagnosis of melanoma presents with focal neurologic deficits. | Metastatic brain tumor. |
| Intracerebral hemorrhage related to this acquired vascular lesion almost always occurs in association with SAH. | Cerebral aneurysm. |
| A nonarterial vascular source of intracerebral hemorrhage. | Cerebral venous thrombosis (CVT). |
| This vascular condition predominates in Asians. | Moyamoya disease. |
| A patient's neurologic status suddenly deteriorates 10 days after an ischemic stroke. | Hemorrhagic transformation of an ischemic stroke. |

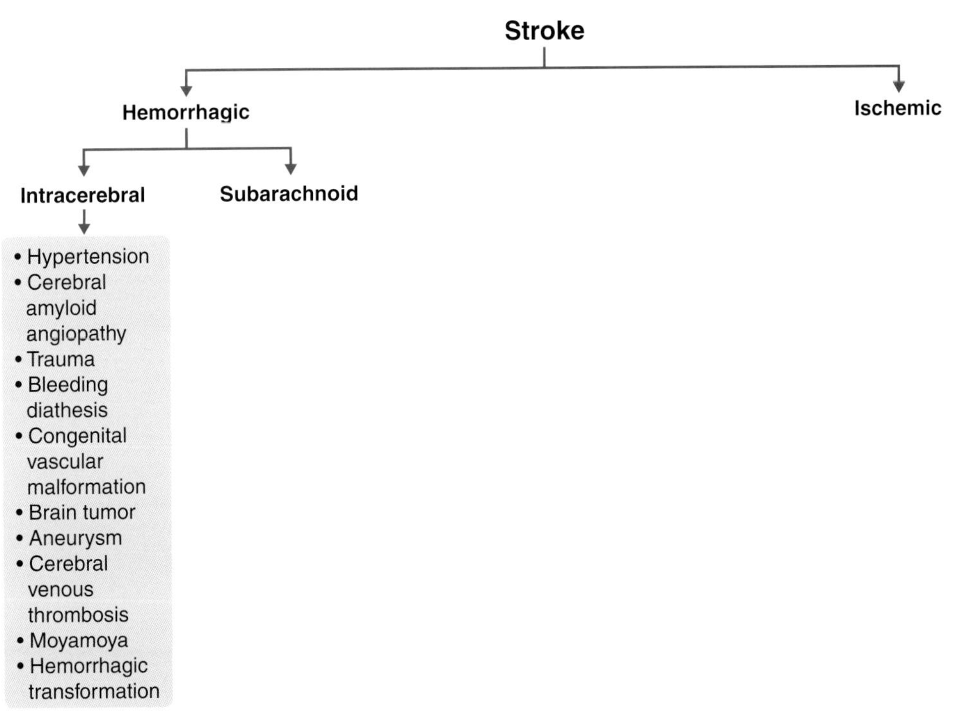

**What are the most common locations of intracerebral hemorrhage related to hypertension?**

Intracerebral hemorrhage related to HTN tends to occur within deep brain structures. The putamen and internal capsule account for most cases; other common sites include the thalamus and pons.[5]

**Which cerebral vessels are involved in cerebral amyloid angiopathy?**

Amyloid deposition occurs in the small- and medium-sized vessels of the leptomeninges and cortex, while there is relative sparing of the vessels of the basal ganglia, white matter, and posterior fossa. Intracerebral hemorrhage related to CAA tends to be lobar.[5]

**What is the frequency of intracerebral hemorrhage in patients with traumatic brain injury?**

Approximately one-half of patients with traumatic brain injury will develop some type of intracranial hemorrhage. Among those patients, intracerebral hemorrhage occurs in one-half. The risk of mortality increases by a factor of 3 when the size of the intracerebral hemorrhage increases from small to large.[9]

**Why is it important to determine whether a bleeding diathesis is present in patients with intracerebral hemorrhage?**

Identifying a bleeding diathesis in patients with intracerebral hemorrhage represents an opportunity for targeted treatment; diatheses should be corrected when possible.

**Which types of cerebral vascular malformation are associated with increased risk of intracerebral hemorrhage?**

Arteriovenous malformation (AVM) and cavernous malformation (CM) are associated with intracerebral hemorrhage.[5]

**What imaging findings are suggestive of intracerebral hemorrhage associated with underlying tumor?**

Intracerebral hemorrhage associated with underlying tumors tend to be more heterogeneous in appearance, slower to degrade over time, associated with thick or nodular enhancement, and associated with a greater degree of surrounding vasogenic edema. Because tumors may be obscured by the hemorrhage, delayed repeat imaging should be considered in patients without an identified alternative cause.[5]

**How often do ruptured cerebral aneurysms result in intracerebral hemorrhage?**

Up to one-third of ruptured aneurysms result in intracerebral hemorrhage; SAH is also present in the vast majority of these cases.[5]

**How common is intracerebral hemorrhage in the setting of cerebral venous thrombosis?**

Almost half of patients with CVT have an associated intracerebral hemorrhage. The presence of a hyperattenuating cortical or deep vein adjacent to the hematoma on CT imaging is highly suggestive of CVT. Most cases of CVT occur in women.[5]

**What unique imaging finding is characteristic of moyamoya disease?**

Moyamoya disease is characterized by progressive bilateral stenosis of the intracranial portion of the internal carotid arteries and proximal branches, resulting in extensive collateral circulation. This network of collateral arteries resembles a "puff of smoke" on angiography (see Figure 42-3).[10]

**When does spontaneous hemorrhagic transformation occur during the course of an ischemic stroke?**

Spontaneous hemorrhagic transformation typically occurs in the second week after ischemic stroke. Early transformation is usually related to thrombolytic therapy or mechanical clot removal.[5]

## HEMORRHAGIC STROKE CAUSED BY SUBARACHNOID HEMORRHAGE

**What are the risk factors for subarachnoid hemorrhage?**

Positive family history of SAH, hypertension, hyperlipidemia, and active smoking are the 4 strongest risk factors for SAH.[11]

**What "warning" symptom may occur in patients with subarachnoid hemorrhage?**

Before the major bleeding event, some patients with SAH experience a sentinel headache, which is described as sudden in onset and unusually severe. The sentinel headache typically occurs within 2 weeks before SAH, with a peak incidence within 1 day.[12]

**What are the findings of subarachnoid hemorrhage on CT imaging?**

SAH typically appears as high attenuation material conforming to the subarachnoid space on noncontrast CT imaging (Figure 43-6). It can be focal or diffuse and present within the sulci, fissures, or basal cisterns. Noncontrast CT imaging is approximately 98% sensitive for SAH within 12 hours, but this decreases to around 93% 24 hours after the event due to the decreased density of blood over time. A sentinel bleed (a relatively small bleed that precedes the major event) can be missed on imaging.[5]

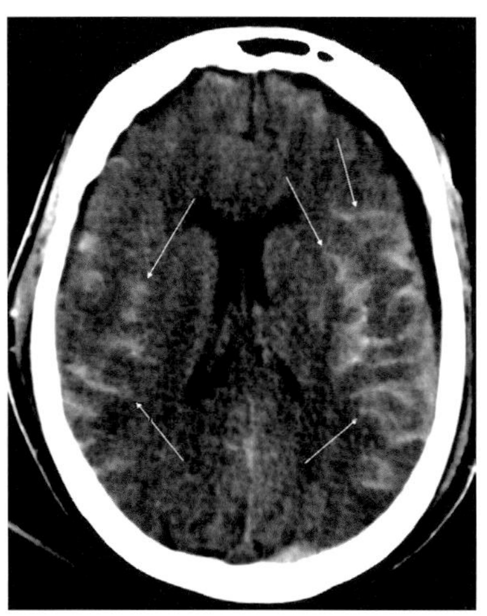

**Figure 43-6.** Noncontrast CT imaging showing diffuse subarachnoid hemorrhage (arrows). When it is visualized within the cortical sulci, fissures, and cisterns, hemorrhage is confirmed to be located within the subarachnoid space. (From Pope TL Jr, Harris JH Jr. *Harris & Harris' The Radiology of Emergency Medicine*. 5th ed. Philadelphia, PA: Lippincott Williams & Wilkins; 2013.)



**Which procedure should be performed when suspicion of subarachnoid hemorrhage remains strong despite negative CT imaging of the head?**

Lumbar puncture with CSF analysis should be performed in patients suspected of SAH when neuroimaging is negative. Typical findings of SAH include elevated opening pressure and CSF erythrocytosis or xanthochromia, depending on how long the blood has been in the subarachnoid space.

**How can true cerebrospinal fluid erythrocytosis be distinguished from trauma related to needle insertion?**

When CSF erythrocytosis occurs as a result of trauma, the bloody appearance of the fluid (as well as the CSF red blood cell count) should lessen over time as fluid is collected. The first and last vials provide the most obvious comparison.

**What general medical treatment should be considered for acute spontaneous subarachnoid hemorrhage?**

In patients with acute spontaneous SAH, underlying bleeding diatheses should be identified and addressed, elevated SBP should be lowered carefully (eg, without overly-rapid reduction to a target <160 mm Hg), and oral nimodipine should be administered. In patients with hydrocephalus, extraventricular drain placement should be considered. Additional measures may be necessary in patients with elevated intracranial pressure.[13]

**What is the short-term mortality of subarachnoid hemorrhage?**

The 30-day mortality of SAH is approximately 40%.[5]

## What are the causes of subarachnoid hemorrhage?

**Usually identifiable from the history, this is the most common overall cause of SAH.**

Craniospinal trauma.[5]

**The leading cause of nontraumatic SAH, accounting for the vast majority of cases.**

Ruptured cerebral aneurysm.[5]

**A predictable pattern of bleeding on neuroimaging, centered immediately anterior to the midbrain, with a negative angiographic study.**

Perimesencephalic nonaneurysmal subarachnoid hemorrhage (PM-NASAH).[5]

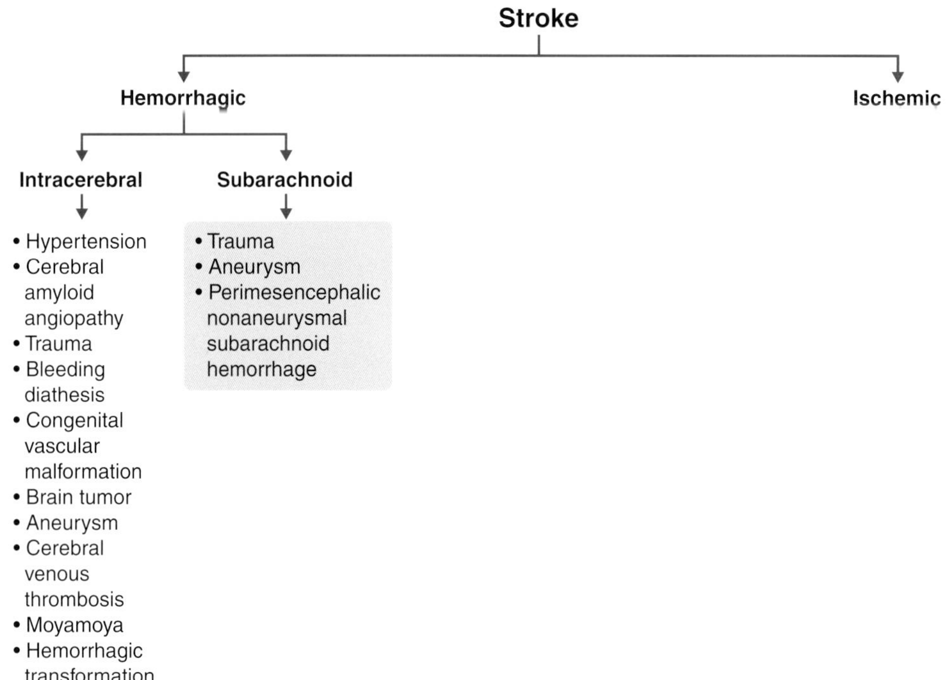


**What is the management of minor traumatic subarachnoid hemorrhage?**

Most cases of traumatic SAH are mild and do not require specific treatment. Serial imaging should be obtained to document stability.[5,14]

**What are the general characteristics of cerebral aneurysms?**

Asymptomatic cerebral aneurysms exist in around 2% of adults. Most are located in the anterior circulation and tend to occur at the branch points of cerebral vessels. Risk of rupture is about 0.7% annually but increases with size, particularly when aneurysms are >7 mm in diameter in the anterior circulation or >5 mm in the posterior circulation.[5]

**What studies are available to evaluate for the presence of a cerebral aneurysm?**

Conventional angiography is considered the gold standard for detection of cerebral aneurysms. CT angiography (CTA) and magnetic resonance angiography (MRA) are noninvasive options but are less sensitive, particularly when the aneurysms are small (<3 mm). In the case of a negative initial study, repeat studies are often required, and conventional angiography is the preferred modality.[13]

**What is the prognosis of perimesencephalic nonaneurysmal subarachnoid hemorrhage?**

Most cases of PM-NASAH are not associated with a cerebral aneurysm and the underlying cause remains elusive. The presentation of PM-NASAH is similar to other types of SAH. However, it is associated with excellent prognosis.[5]

**What are the rare causes of subarachnoid hemorrhage?**

Rare causes of SAH include vascular malformations (both cerebral and spinal), intracranial arterial dissection, brain tumors, sickle cell anemia, vasculitis, coagulopathy, and pituitary apoplexy.[5]

## ISCHEMIC STROKE

**Which 2 main arteries supply the brain?**

The internal carotid arteries (ICAs) give rise to the anterior circulation, and the vertebral arteries give rise to the posterior circulation. The circle of Willis is an anastomosis between the 2 major systems, allowing for redundant flow when parts of either system become compromised (Figure 43-7).[15]

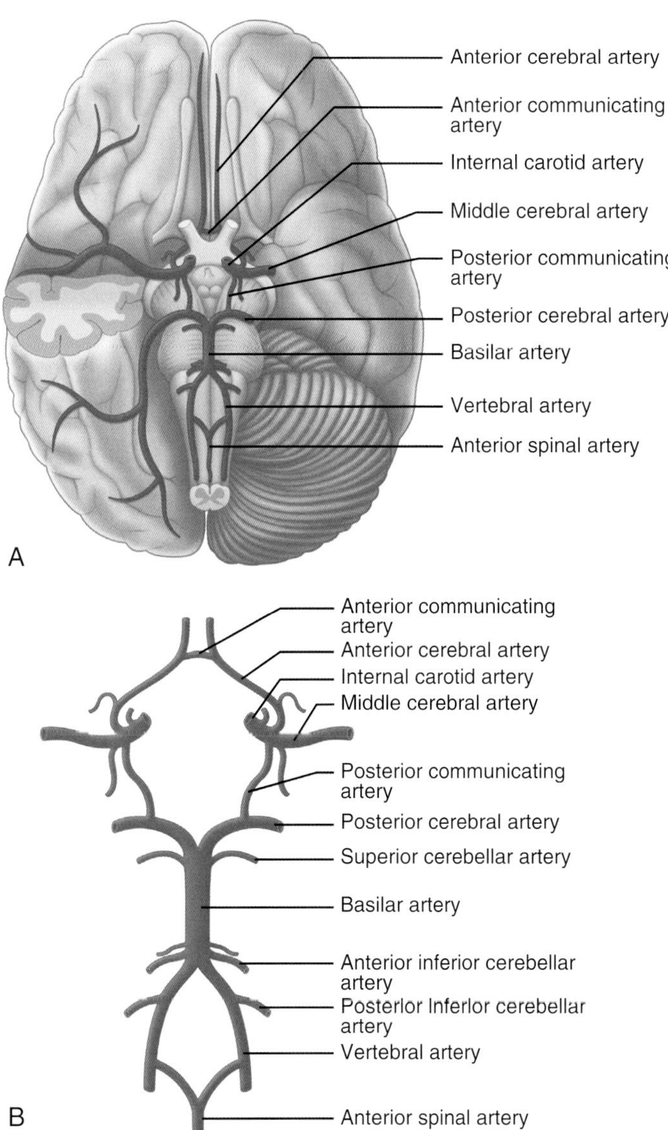


**Figure 43-7.** A, The circle of Willis seen from below the brain. B, The arteries of the circle of Willis. (Adapted from Morton PG, Fontaine DK. *Critical Care Nursing: A Holistic Approach,* 10th ed. Philadelphia, PA: Wolters Kluwer Health; 2013.)

**Which major vessels constitute the anterior and posterior circulations?**

The vessels of the anterior circulation include the ICA, middle cerebral artery (MCA), and anterior cerebral artery (ACA). The vessels of the posterior circulation include the vertebral artery, basilar artery, and posterior cerebral artery (PCA).[15]

**What areas of the brain are supplied by the anterior and posterior systems?**

The anterior circulation supplies the majority of the cerebral hemispheres, with the exceptions of the occipital and medial temporal lobes, which are fed from the posterior circulation. The posterior circulation supplies the brainstem, cerebellum, and posterior portions of the cerebral hemispheres (ie, occipital and medial temporal lobes).[15,16]

**What are the 3 subcategories of ischemic stroke?**

Ischemic stroke can occur as a result of in situ occlusion, embolism, or watershed infarction.

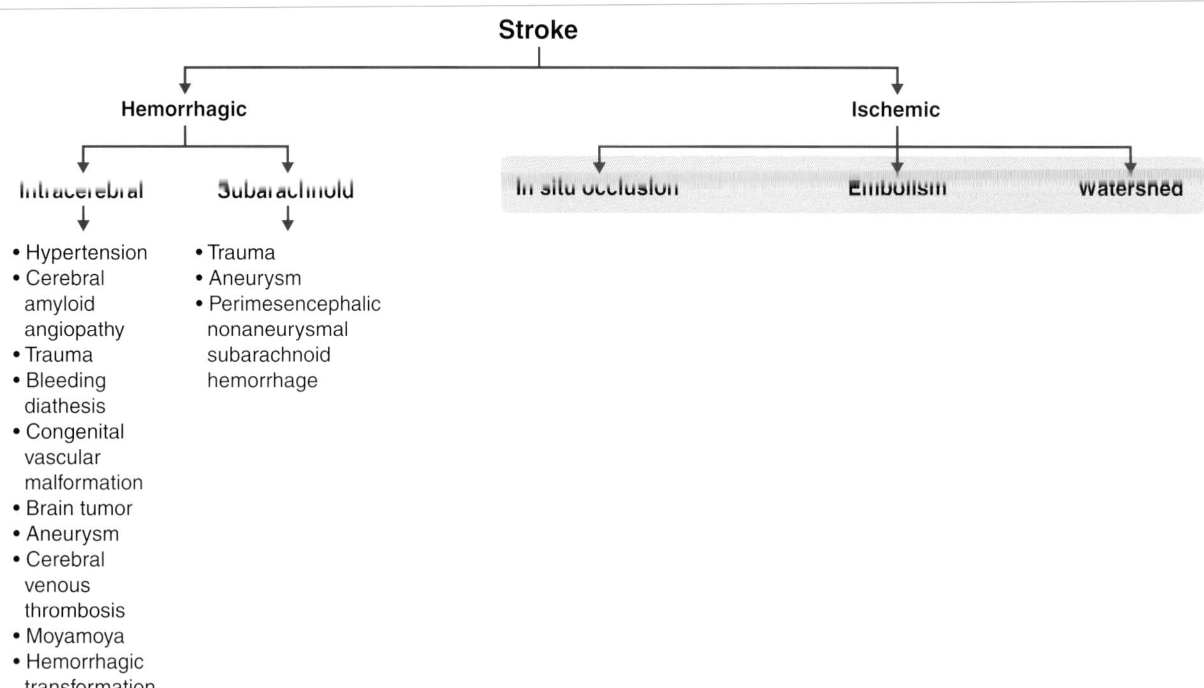


**What are the mechanisms of in situ occlusive, embolic, and watershed strokes?**

In all types of ischemic stroke, brain infarction occurs as a result of decreased cerebral perfusion, with associated decreased delivery of oxygen and nutrients. In situ occlusive stroke can involve large or small arteries. Large artery involvement occurs as a result of thrombosis, whereas small artery involvement occurs as a result of other mechanisms (eg, lipohyalinosis). Embolic stroke occurs when debris travels from a remote source and lodges within a cerebral artery. If the source is a cerebral vessel, then the stroke is both thrombotic and embolic. Watershed stroke occurs when a systemic process results in cerebral hypoperfusion that affects the most vulnerable regions of the brain, which are typically the zones between neighboring vascular territories.

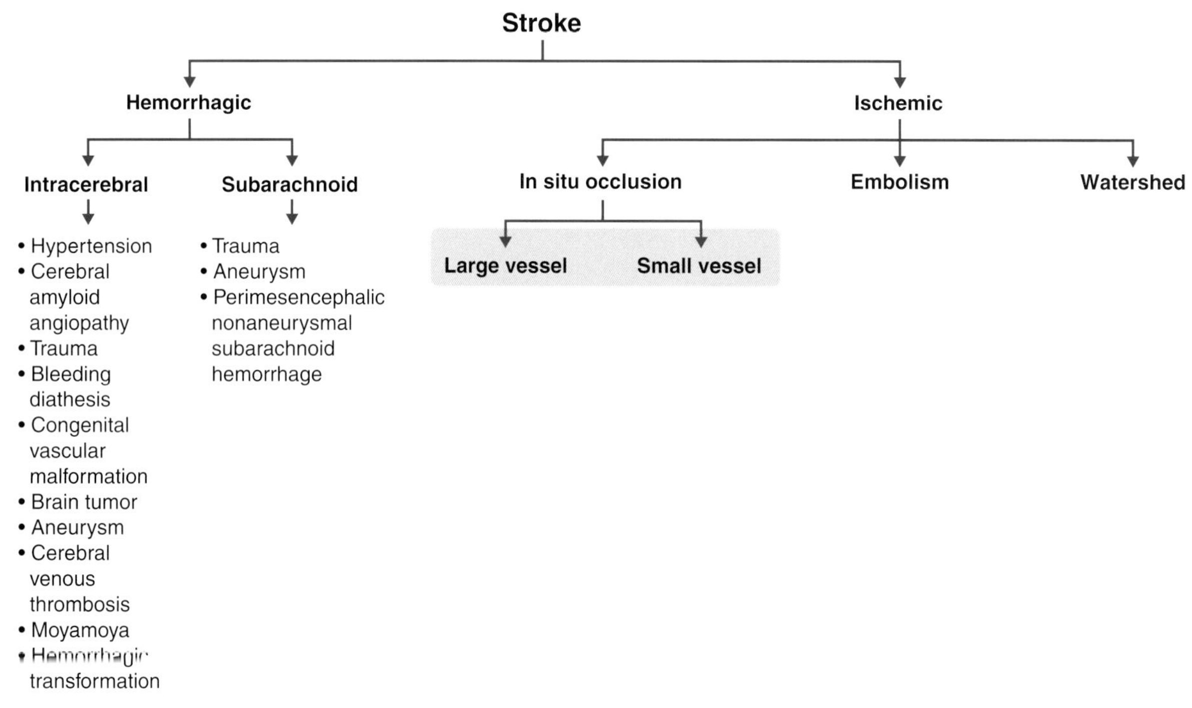

**Why is it important to differentiate between the mechanisms of ischemic stroke?**

Underlying causes and general treatment considerations differ between in situ occlusive, embolic, and watershed strokes.

**In addition to addressing the underlying cause, what general medical treatment should be considered for ischemic stroke related to acute occlusion?**

In patients with ischemic stroke related to acute occlusion, blood pressure should be lowered when it is severely elevated (SBP >220 mm Hg or diastolic blood pressure >120 mm Hg) with a goal of around 15% reduction during the first 24 hours (BP should be <185/110 mm Hg in patients who are to receive thrombolytics). It is reasonable to try to achieve blood glucose levels in a range of 140 to 180 mg/dL. Intravenous recombinant tissue plasminogen activator (tPA) should be administered to select patients within a limited window of time from onset of ischemic stroke (or from when patient was last seen to be normal if time of onset is unknown). A window of 3 to 4.5 hours is used, depending on patient-specific factors. Mechanical thrombectomy may be beneficial in select patients with large vessel occlusions (eg, terminal ICA, proximal ACA, proximal MCA). Oral administration of aspirin within 24 to 48 hours after stroke (but not within 24 hours of fibrinolytic therapy if it is given) is recommended. Additional measures may be necessary in patients with elevated intracranial pressure, and hemicraniectomy may be beneficial in patients with malignant cerebral edema.[17,18]

## ISCHEMIC STROKE CAUSED BY ACUTE IN SITU OCCLUSION OF A LARGE VESSEL

**Which cerebral arteries are classified as large vessels?**

Large cerebral arteries include the ICA, vertebral artery, basilar artery, and the circle of Willis and its proximal branches (eg, MCA).

**What is the tempo of stroke caused by large vessel thrombosis?**

Compared with strokes caused by embolism and small vessel in situ occlusion, large vessel thrombotic strokes are typically associated with a slowly evolving or "stuttering" onset.[15]

**What are the most common mechanisms of infarction involving the internal carotid arteries?**

All 3 of the major mechanisms of ischemic stroke, including acute in situ occlusion (from acute thrombosis), embolism, and watershed, can occur in relation to ICA disease. The most common mechanism is acute thrombosis.[16]

**What clinical syndromes are associated with acute internal carotid artery occlusion?**

Unlike the more distal large arteries, the clinical syndromes of ICA occlusion are variable and dependent on the constitution of the circle of Willis. When there is a competent circle of Willis (which provides redundant blood flow), no area of the brain is entirely dependent on a single ICA, and therefore occlusion may be asymptomatic. However, if the circle of Willis does not provide blood flow to the ipsilateral side, the consequence of ICA occlusion is massive hemispheric infarction, with resultant sensorimotor deficits of the contralateral face, arm, and leg (ie, hemiparesis and hemihypesthesia), aphasia when the dominant hemisphere is involved, and contralateral neglect when the nondominant hemisphere is involved. When there is chronic occlusion of the contralateral ICA, then acute occlusion may result in bihemispheric infarction, with resultant coma and quadriparesis.[15,16]

**What clinical syndrome is associated with acute occlusion of the stem of the middle cerebral artery?**

Acute occlusion of the MCA stem results in sensorimotor deficits of the contralateral face, arm, and, to a lesser degree, leg; homonymous hemianopsia; deviation of the head toward the side of the lesion, ipsilateral gaze preference; global aphasia when the dominant hemisphere is involved; and contralateral neglect (including anosognosia in severe cases) when the nondominant hemisphere is involved.[15,16]

| | |
|---|---|
| **What clinical syndrome is associated with acute occlusion of the superior division of the middle cerebral artery?** | Acute occlusion of the superior division of the MCA results in dense sensorimotor deficits of the contralateral face, arm, and, to a lesser degree, leg; ipsilateral deviation of the head, ipsilateral gaze preference; and global aphasia (that later improves to Broca's aphasia) when the dominant hemisphere is involved.[15,16] |
| **What clinical syndrome is associated with acute occlusion of the inferior division of the middle cerebral artery?** | Acute occlusion of the inferior division of the MCA results in superior quadrantanopsia; Wernicke's aphasia when the dominant hemisphere is involved; and contralateral neglect when the nondominant hemisphere is involved.[15,16] |
| **What clinical syndrome is associated with acute occlusion of the anterior cerebral artery distal to the anterior communicating artery?** | Acute occlusion of the ACA distal to the anterior communicating artery results in motor deficits involving the contralateral foot, leg, and, to a lesser degree, upper extremity, with sparing of the hand and face. *Acute occlusion of the ACA proximal to the anterior communicating artery is usually well tolerated as a result of collateral blood flow.*[15,16] |
| **What clinical syndromes are associated with acute occlusion of the large arteries of the posterior circulation?** | Acute occlusion of the large arteries of the posterior circulation results in complex and variable presentations owing to the potential involvement of multiple structures (eg, brainstem, cerebellum, visual cortex), and individual differences in vascular anatomy. Manifestations may include sensorimotor deficits of the ipsilateral face and contralateral extremities, loss of vision of one or both homonymous visual fields, ataxia, vertigo, diplopia or oculomotor deficits (eg, skew deviation), dysphagia, and dysarthria. Non-neurological manifestations may include cardiac dysrhythmias and respiratory dysfunction owing to medullary involvement.[15,16,19] |

## What are the underlying causes of acute large artery thrombosis?

| | |
|---|---|
| **The most common cause of acute large vessel thrombosis; risk factors include hypertension, diabetes mellitus, smoking, and advancing age.** | Atherosclerosis.[20] |
| **A 38-year-old woman with Ehlers-Danlos syndrome presents with sudden-onset neck and head pain followed by visual deficits and vertigo.** | Vertebral artery dissection. |
| **A young woman presents with neurologic deficits after an episode of migraine with aura and is found to have associated infarction on neuroimaging.** | Pathologic cerebral vasoconstriction (ie, vasospasm). |
| **The primary cause of renal artery stenosis in young and middle-aged women.** | Fibromuscular dysplasia. |
| **Treatment for this vascular condition usually includes immunosuppressive therapy.** | Vasculitis. |
| **Also associated with hemorrhagic stroke, this condition is described by bilateral stenosis of the internal carotid arteries and proximal branches.** | Moyamoya disease. |
| **A 58-year-old man presents with stroke and is found to have a hematocrit of 60%.** | Polycythemia vera. |

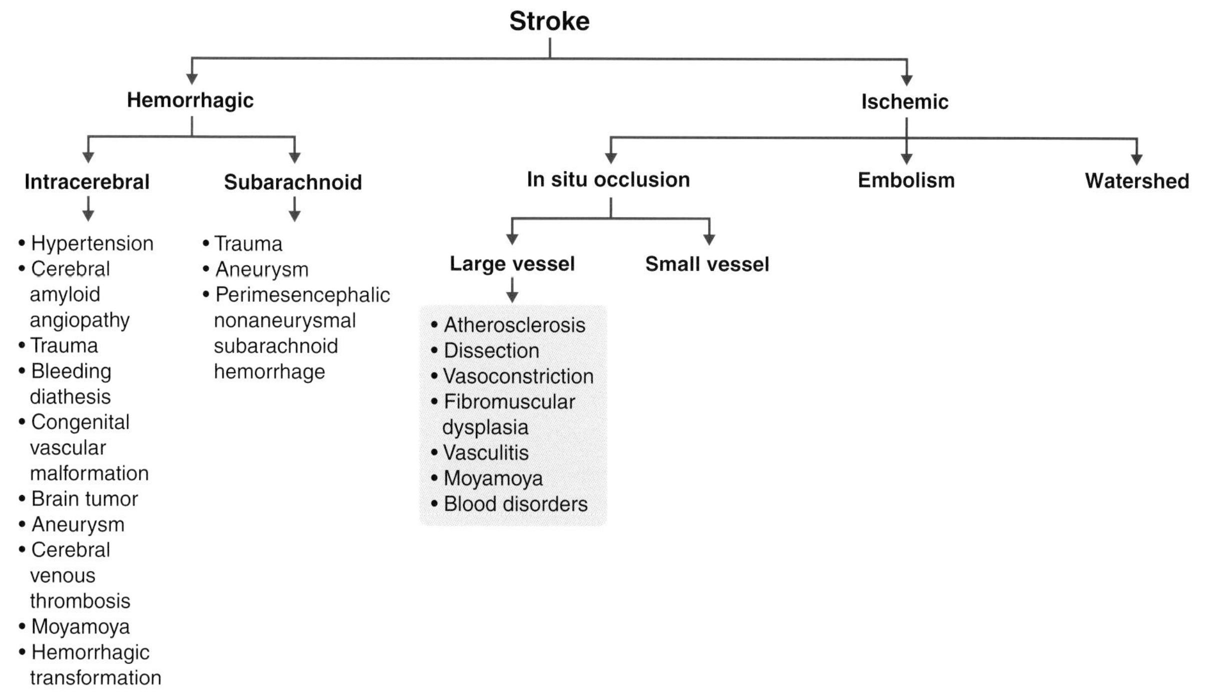




**What noninvasive studies are available for the evaluation of cerebral artery atherosclerosis?**

Noninvasive imaging options to evaluate for cerebral artery atherosclerosis include transcranial Doppler ultrasonography, CTA, and MRA. CTA is associated with a sensitivity of approximately 97% and specificity of approximately 99.5% for the detection of lesions with >50% stenosis (compared with conventional angiography).[20]

**How often is ischemic stroke caused by arterial dissection?**

Cervical artery dissection (ie, carotid or vertebral artery dissection) causes around 20% of ischemic strokes in young and middle-aged patients. Carotid dissection is more common than vertebral dissection.[21,22]

**What are the causes of pathologic cerebral vasoconstriction?**

Causes of pathologic cerebral vasoconstriction include migraine headache, recreational drug use (eg, cocaine), massive subarachnoid hemorrhage, eclampsia, and reversible cerebral vasoconstriction syndrome.[15]

**Which arteries are most commonly affected by fibromuscular dysplasia?**

The renal arteries are most commonly involved in patients with fibromuscular dysplasia (80%) (see Figure 39-2), followed by the extracranial carotid arteries (75%), vertebral arteries (35%), mesenteric arteries (25%), and the intracranial carotid arteries (20%).[23]

**Primary angiitis of the central nervous system (PACNS) affects cerebral arteries of what size?**

PACNS predominantly affects the medium- and small-sized arteries. Radiographic findings involving the large-sized arteries should raise suspicion for an alternative diagnosis.[24]

**What are the demographic differences among adult patients with moyamoya disease who present with hemorrhagic and ischemic strokes?**

In the United States, adults with moyamoya disease overwhelmingly present with ischemic stroke (approximately 80%). In Asian countries, there is a higher rate of hemorrhagic stroke in adults with moyamoya disease.[10]

**Which blood disorders are associated with thrombotic stroke?**

Thrombotic stroke can be related to the following blood disorders: sickle cell anemia, polycythemia vera, thrombocytosis, disseminated intravascular coagulation, protein C or S deficiency, antithrombin III deficiency, antiphospholipid antibody syndrome, heparin-induced thrombocytopenia, and hyperhomocysteinemia. Blood disorders account for up to 5% of all strokes.[19]

## ISCHEMIC STROKE CAUSED BY ACUTE IN SITU OCCLUSION OF A SMALL VESSEL

**Which cerebral arteries are classified as small vessels?**

Small cerebral arteries include the penetrating arteries that come off the vertebral artery, basilar artery, MCA, and the circle of Willis, feeding subcortical structures such as the basal ganglia (eg, putamen, caudate, globus pallidus, thalamus), subcortical white matter (eg, internal capsule, corona radiata), and pons.[15]

**What is the tempo of a stroke related to small vessel occlusion?**

Small vessel strokes tend to develop more quickly than large vessel strokes, but not as suddenly as embolic strokes.[11]

**What is a lacunar infarction?**

A lacunar infarction occurs as a result of the occlusion of a small artery (50-200 μm in diameter). When macrophages remove the involved tissue, a small cavity, or *lacune*, is left behind. These range from 3 to 15 mm in diameter.[15]

**What are the risk factors for lacunar infarction?**

The strongest risk factor for lacunar infarction is chronic hypertension, which is present in the vast majority of patients. Other risk factors include diabetes mellitus and hyperlipidemia.[15]

**How common are lacunar infarctions?**

In the industrialized world, lacunar strokes account for around one-quarter of all ischemic strokes.[25]

**In what locations of the brain do lacunar infarctions most often occur?**

In descending order of frequency, lacunes occur in the putamen, caudate, thalamus, pons, internal capsule, and deep in the central hemispheral white matter (Figure 43-8).[15]

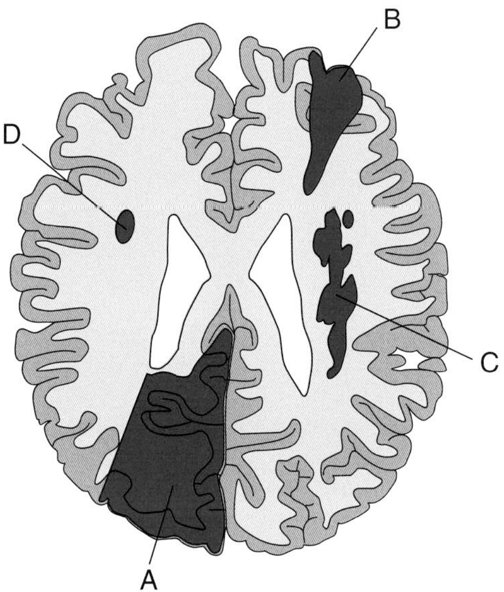


**Figure 43-8.** Topographic patterns of cerebral infarction. A, Territorial infarction (from posterior cerebral artery occlusion). B, Watershed border-zone infarction (between the territories of the anterior cerebral artery and the middle cerebral artery). C, Internal border-zone infarction (deep middle cerebral artery territory). D, Lacunar infarction (lenticulostriate-penetrating artery occlusion). (Adapted from Marshall R, Mayer S. *On Call Neurology*. 3rd ed. Philadelphia, PA: Saunders; 2007.)

**What clinical syndromes are associated with lacunar infarctions?**

The quality and severity of deficits associated with lacunar infarctions are dependent on location. The most common syndromes include, in descending order of frequency, pure motor hemiparesis (eg, when the posterior limb of the internal capsule is involved), pure hemisensory stroke (eg, when the thalamus is involved), ataxic hemiparesis (eg, when the pons, midbrain, internal capsule, or parietal white matter is involved), and clumsy hand dysarthria syndrome (eg, when the midpons is involved). Multiple lacunes deep in both hemispheres can result in gait disorders and dementia. In virtually all forms of lacunar infarction, there is an absence of cortical deficits (eg, seizure, aphasia, amnesia, agnosia, apraxia, dysgraphia, alexia), which can be a clue to the diagnosis.[15,26]

**How are lacunar infarctions diagnosed?**

Unlike occlusions of large arteries, involvement of the smaller arteries cannot be visualized on angiography. Diagnosis is based on the clinical syndrome and the presence of characteristic noncortical infarctions on head imaging, which are more likely to be found on MRI than CT.[15]

**What general medical treatment should be considered for acute lacunar infarction?**

There is some evidence that administering intravenous thrombolytics in select patients with acute lacunar infarction may be beneficial, using the same eligibility criteria as in patients with large vessel ischemic stroke. However, more data is needed in this subgroup of ischemic stroke. Aspirin should be given within 24 to 48 hours after stroke (but not within 24 hours of fibrinolytic therapy if it is given).[25]

**What is the prognosis of lacunar infarction?**

In general, short-term recovery is more favorable in patients with lacunar infarction compared with other causes of ischemic stroke, sometimes with complete recovery even after a severe event. However, many patients experience some degree of long-term sequelae.[15]



## What are the underlying causes of acute small vessel in situ occlusion?

**This abnormal vascular process occurs within the small arteries and is associated with chronic hypertension and diabetes mellitus.**

Lipohyalinosis.

**This vasculopathy is the leading cause of large vessel thrombotic stroke.**

Atherosclerosis.

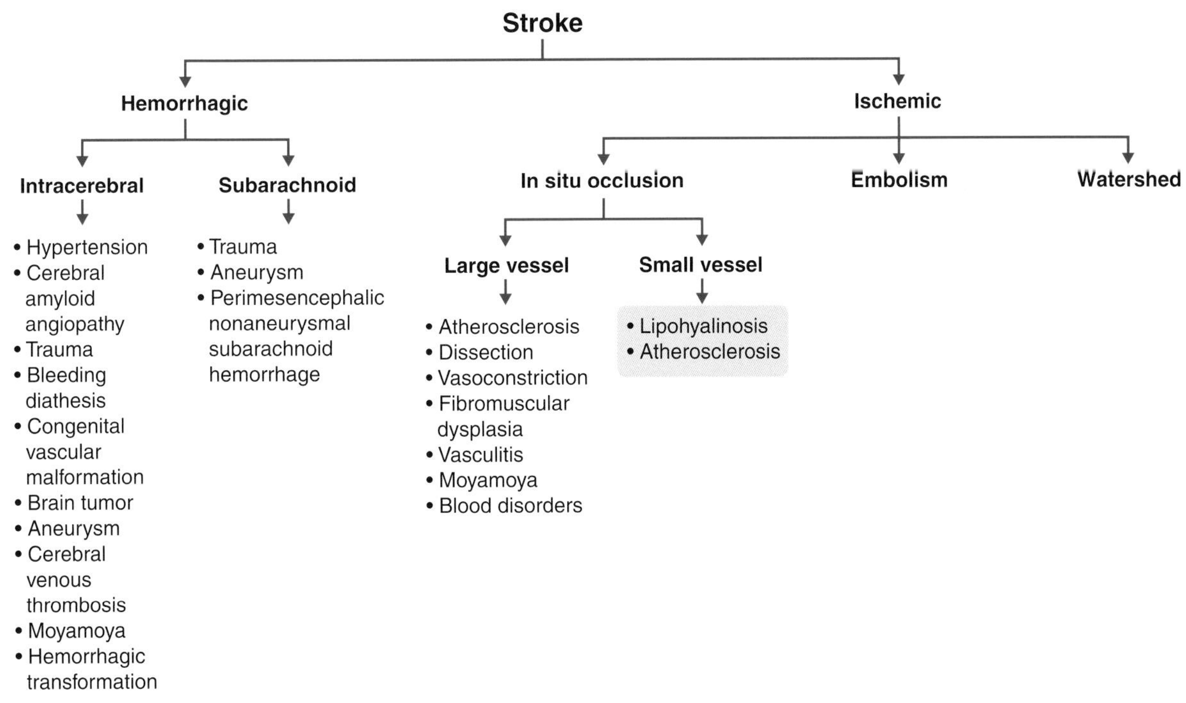


**What is the mechanism of small vessel occlusion related to lipohyalinosis?**

Lipohyalinosis, which is a vascular lesion characterized pathologically by the presence of fibrinoid material and lipid deposition within the arterial wall with associated medial hypertrophy, leads to encroachment on the arterial lumen with eventual obliteration.[27]

**What is the mechanism of small vessel occlusion related to atherosclerosis?**

The origins of the small arteries can become blocked by atheromata found within the parent arteries, resulting in occlusion.[27]

## EMBOLIC STROKE

**What is the tempo of stroke related to embolism?**

Embolic strokes tend to occur suddenly with maximal deficits at onset. Some patients with chronic significant cerebral atherosclerotic disease develop robust collateral circulation, mitigating the effects of an acute embolic event.[15,28]

**What pattern of infarction can be a clue to the presence of an embolic source of ischemic stroke?**

In contrast to thrombotic strokes, which typically present in a single vascular territory, embolic strokes can involve multiple cerebral vascular territories, as well as noncerebral vascular territories (eg, kidney).

### What are the general mechanisms of embolic stroke?

**A large proportion of cardiac output goes to the brain.**

Cardioembolism.

**A gift from one artery to another.**

Artery-to-artery embolism.

**Venous thromboembolism.**

Paradoxical embolism.

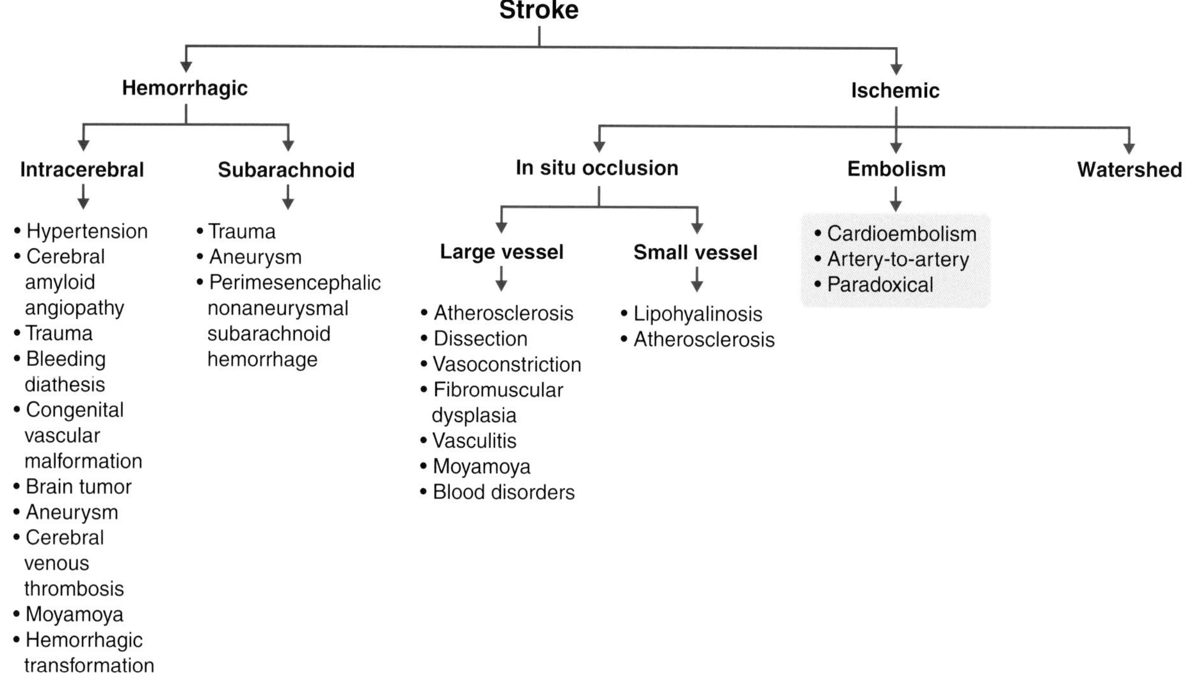


**How common is cardioembolic stroke?**

Cardioembolic stroke is the most common underlying cause of embolic stroke and accounts for one-quarter of all strokes in the general population of the industrialized world.[19]

**What are the major risk factors for cardioembolic stroke?**

Risk factors for cardioembolic stroke include atrial fibrillation, mitral valve stenosis, prosthetic cardiac valve, recent myocardial infarction, left ventricular or atrial thrombus, infectious and non-infectious endocarditis, dilated cardiomyopathy, and intracardiac tumors (eg, atrial myxoma).[19]

**What are the most common sites of atherosclerotic lesions that give rise to artery-to-artery embolic stroke?**

The aortic arch is a common source of atheroembolic stroke. In the anterior circulation, the most common sites include the carotid artery (most commonly at the carotid artery bifurcation and siphon) and the M1 segment of the MCA. In the posterior circulation, the most common sites include the first and fourth segments of the vertebral artery and the first segment of the basilar artery.[29]

**What features of atherosclerotic disease confer increased risk for embolic stroke?**

For atherosclerotic disease of the aorta, the size of the plaques correlates with risk of ischemic stroke (plaques >4 mm in thickness confer highest risk). Transesophageal echocardiography allows for the detection and measurement of aortic arch disease. For the cerebral arteries, the size of the plaque also correlates with risk of ischemic stroke (there is increased risk with lesions causing >50% stenosis and an even greater risk with >70% stenosis). Noninvasive imaging modalities used to assess the burden of cerebral atherosclerotic disease include transcranial Doppler ultrasonography, MRA, and CTA. Conventional angiography may be necessary in some patients.[28,29]

**What is the cornerstone of medical therapy for patients at risk for artery-to-artery embolism?**

Antiplatelet therapy (either mono or dual depending on clinical factors) is the cornerstone of medical therapy used to prevent ischemic stroke in patients at risk for artery-to-artery embolism.[28]

**What clinical syndromes are associated with emboli from the internal carotid arteries?**

The clinical manifestations of ICA-related emboli are variable owing to individual disparity in collateral flow that develops as a result of long-standing ICA disease, ranging from asymptomatic to devastating hemispheric infarction.[16]

**What clinical scenario is described by the expression "spectacular shrinking deficit"?**

"Spectacular shrinking deficit" is an expression used to describe the clinical manifestations of a migrating embolus originating from the ICA. The initial embolus lodges in the stem of the MCA, resulting in a major hemispheric deficit, but the deficit improves as the embolus moves to one of the smaller branches of the MCA.[16]

**What coexistent conditions must be present for paradoxical embolism to occur?**

Paradoxical embolism, which occurs when embolic material from the venous circulation transfers to the arterial circulation, requires both venous emboli and a right-to-left shunt (eg, patent foramen ovale [PFO], atrial septal defect, or ventricular septal defect). Right-to-left shunting can occur in patients with left-to-right intracardiac shunt when right-sided pressures are transiently increased (eg, during Valsalva).[30]

**What is the prevalence of patent foramen ovale in the general population?**

PFO occurs in one-quarter of the general population. It is present in one-half of patients with cryptogenic stroke.[31]

## WATERSHED STROKE

**How common is watershed infarction?**

Based on autopsy studies, watershed infarctions account for approximately 10% of all strokes. This may be an underestimation because watershed infarction is rarely fatal.[32]

**Where are the watershed areas of the brain?**

The cortical (external) watershed zones include the anterior region within the frontal and parietal parasagittal cortex (MCA/ACA territory) and the posterior region within the parieto-temporo-occipital cortex (MCA/PCA). The incidences of anterior and posterior watershed infarctions are similar. The subcortical (internal) watershed zones include the corona radiata (deep/superficial perforators of the MCA) and the centrum semiovale (superficial perforators of the ACA/MCA) (see Figure 43-8).[16,32]

**What are the 2 main clinical manifestations of cortical watershed infarction?**

Anterior watershed ischemia (MCA/ACA territory) results in a (proximal greater than distal) sensorimotor deficit of the upper extremity with possible involvement of the lower extremity and sparing of the face and hand (described as "man-in-the-barrel" syndrome when the infarction is bilateral). Posterior watershed ischemia (MCA/PCA territory) results in visual agnosias, various degrees of visual field deficits (eg, hemianopsia, quadrantanopia, cortical blindness), transcortical aphasia or contralateral neglect (depending on involvement of the dominant or nondominant hemisphere), and, when the infarction is bilateral, the Balint syndrome (ie, simultagnosia, optic ataxia, and oculomotor apraxia). Rarely, both syndromes may occur together. Other features of watershed infarction include syncope at onset and focal limb shaking.[15,16]

**What are the clinical manifestations of subcortical watershed infarction?**

Confluent subcortical watershed infarction may result in contralateral sensorimotor deficits of the arm, leg, and face, and focal cognitive and behavioral dysfunction (with poor recovery), whereas partial subcortical watershed infarction may result in brachiofacial sensorimotor deficits and focal cognitive and behavioral dysfunction (with good recovery).[33]

## What are the causes of watershed stroke?

**A 65-year-old man with elevated jugular venous pressure, an S3 gallop, pulsus alternans, and cold extremities.**

Cardiogenic shock.

**Global cerebral hypoperfusion with or without systemic hypotension.**

Diffuse atherosclerosis of the cerebral arteries.

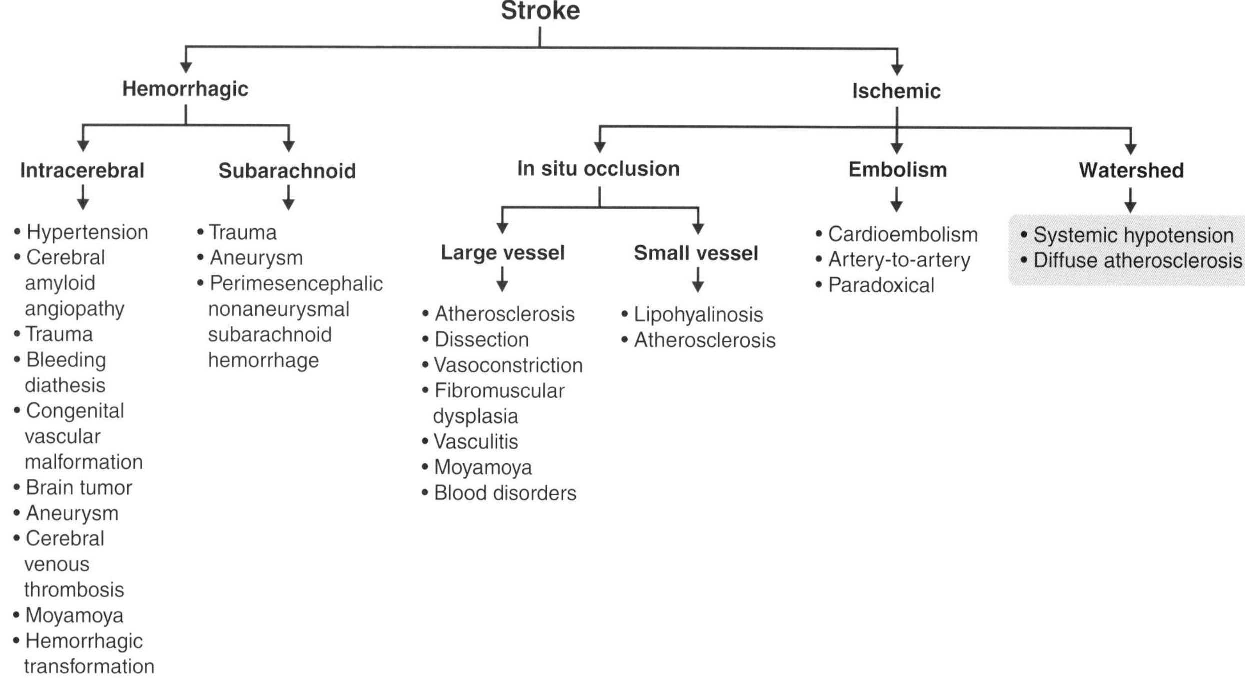


**Is systemic hypotension more likely to result in cortical or subcortical watershed stroke?**

Systemic hypotension is associated with both types of watershed infarctions but most often results in subcortical watershed stroke.[32]

**Which cerebral artery is most commonly associated with watershed stroke as a result of atherosclerotic disease?**

The ICA, being the most proximal cerebral artery, is most likely to cause watershed stroke when there is severe atherosclerotic disease. The condition can be unilateral or bilateral.[16,32]

*It should be recognized that cerebral hypoxia caused by entities such as hypoxemia and carbon monoxide poisoning (although not traditionally considered to be causes of stroke) could result in brain tissue infarction.*

## Case Summary

A 48-year-old woman on combined oral contraceptive pill presents with sudden-onset right flank pain followed by the development of focal neurologic deficits and is found to have lower extremity deep vein thrombosis, a lack of contrast enhancement of the right kidney on imaging, and evidence of an ischemic stroke involving the distribution of the left middle cerebral artery.

***What is the most likely cause of stroke in this patient?***

Paradoxical embolism.

## BONUS QUESTIONS

| | |
|---|---|
| ***What is the most likely explanation for the flank pain, hematuria, and lack of contrast enhancement of the right kidney in this case?*** | The constellation of flank pain, hematuria, and lack of right kidney enhancement on imaging in this case (see Figure 43-1) is most likely explained by an embolic event to the right renal artery with resultant acute obstruction and ischemic injury. |
| ***Which features of this case make embolic stroke likely?*** | The neurologic deficits in this case occurred suddenly and were maximal at onset, characteristic of the tempo of embolic stroke. Involvement of multiple tissue beds in the body is also suggestive of embolic phenomena. |
| ***What is the most likely source of paradoxical embolism in this case?*** | The deep vein thrombosis of the left leg is the likely source of emboli in this case. In order for paradoxical embolism to occur, there must also be a coexistent right-to-left shunt; a patent foramen ovale is statistically most likely, present in one-quarter of the general population.[31] |
| ***What acute medical treatment should be considered for the patient in this case?*** | Given that the onset of the stroke is within 3 hours and there are no contraindications (eg, active internal bleeding), the patient in this case should be treated with an intravenous fibrinolytic agent (eg, tPA). Aspirin should be given within 24 to 48 hours of stroke (but not within 24 hours of intravenous thrombolytic administration). |
| ***What is the role of mechanical thrombectomy in patients with ischemic stroke?*** | In the setting of proximal large artery occlusion of the anterior circulation, such as in this case, mechanical thrombectomy is beneficial in patients who do and do not receive intravenous thrombolytics, and should be pursued unless there are contraindications. Proximal large artery occlusions of the posterior circulation may also benefit from mechanical thrombectomy.[17] |
| ***What study should be performed in this case to investigate the paradoxical nature of the stroke?*** | A transthoracic echocardiogram with agitated saline contrast should be performed to evaluate for intracardiac shunt. |
| ***If a patent foramen ovale is discovered on echocardiography in this case, what treatment strategies should be used for secondary prevention of stroke?*** | Antiplatelet or systemic anticoagulants are recommended for patients with cryptogenic stroke who are found to have a patent foramen ovale. In some cases, such as when there are recurrent paradoxical emboli despite appropriate medical therapy, it may be reasonable to consider mechanical closure of the PFO.[34] |

## KEY POINTS

- Stroke occurs when there is acute infarction of brain tissue resulting in neurologic deficits.
- Chronic hypertension is the most significant risk factor for stroke. Others include diabetes mellitus, atrial fibrillation, dyslipidemia, smoking, and family history.
- Strokes can be hemorrhagic (20%) or ischemic (80%).
- Hemorrhagic stroke causes injury due to mechanical compression of brain tissue and local toxicity from blood breakdown products; ischemic stroke causes injury due to insufficient oxygen and nutrient delivery to brain tissue.
- Neuroimaging is necessary to distinguish between hemorrhagic and ischemic stroke.
- Hemorrhagic stroke is associated with higher 30-day mortality compared with ischemic stroke, but long-term functional status among survivors is similar between the two.
- Hemorrhagic stroke can occur as a result of intracerebral hemorrhage or SAH, each with different underlying causes and treatments.
- Ischemic stroke can occur as a result of acute in situ occlusion (including large vessel and small vessel), embolism, or watershed infarction, each with different underlying causes and treatments.
- There are well-described large vessel and small vessel ischemic stroke syndromes depending on the distribution of infarction.
- Involvement of noncontiguous vascular territories is suggestive of embolic stroke.

## KEY POINTS—CONT'D

- Embolic stroke can occur as a result of cardioembolism (most common), artery-to-artery embolism, or paradoxical embolism.
- Eligible patients with acute ischemic stroke related to thrombosis or embolism may benefit from intravenous tPA if given within a certain time from confirmed or estimated stroke onset.
- Mechanical thrombectomy may be beneficial in select patients with proximal large artery occlusion.
- Watershed stroke occurs when a systemic process results in global cerebral hypoperfusion that affects the vulnerable regions of the brain located between neighboring vascular territories, and is best managed by addressing the underlying systemic process.

## REFERENCES


1. Prabhakaran S, Ruff I, Bernstein RA. Acute stroke intervention: a systematic review. *JAMA*. 2015;313(14):1451-1462.
2. Kernan WN, Ovbiagele B, Black HR, et al. Guidelines for the prevention of stroke in patients with stroke and transient ischemic attack: a guideline for healthcare professionals from the American Heart Association/American Stroke Association. *Stroke*. 2014;45(7):2160-2236.
3. Benjamin EJ, Blaha MJ, Chiuve SE, et al. Heart disease and stroke statistics-2017 update: a report from the American Heart Association. *Circulation*. 2017; 135(10):e146-e603.
4. van der Worp HB, van Gijn J. Clinical practice. Acute ischemic stroke. *N Engl J Med*. 2007;357(6):572-579.
5. Smith SD, Eskey CJ. Hemorrhagic stroke. *Radiol Clin North Am*. 2011;49(1):27-45.
6. Ariesen MJ, Claus SP, Rinkel GJ, Algra A. Risk factors for intracerebral hemorrhage in the general population: a systematic review. *Stroke*. 2003;34(8):2060-2065.
7. Sturgeon JD, Folsom AR, Longstreth WT Jr, Shahar E, Rosamond WD, Cushman M. Risk factors for intracerebral hemorrhage in a pooled prospective study. *Stroke*. 2007;38(10):2718-2725.
8. Hemphill JC III, Greenberg SM, Anderson CS, et al. Guidelines for the management of spontaneous intracerebral hemorrhage: a guideline for healthcare professionals from the American Heart Association/American Stroke Association. *Stroke*. 2015;46(7):2032-2060.
9. Perel P, Roberts I, Bouamra O, Woodford M, Mooney J, Lecky F. Intracranial bleeding in patients with traumatic brain injury: a prognostic study. *BMC Emerg Med*. 2009;9:15.
10. Scott RM, Smith ER. Moyamoya disease and moyamoya syndrome. *N Engl J Med*. 2009;360(12):1226-1237.
11. Vlak MH, Rinkel GJ, Greebe P, Greving JP, Algra A. Lifetime risks for aneurysmal subarachnoid haemorrhage: multivariable risk stratification. *J Neurol Neurosurg Psychiatry*. 2013;84(6):619-623.
12. Polmear A. Sentinel headaches in aneurysmal subarachnoid haemorrhage: what is the true incidence? A systematic review. *Cephalalgia*. 2003;23(10):935-941.
13. Connolly ES Jr, Rabinstein AA, Carhuapoma JR, et al. Guidelines for the management of aneurysmal subarachnoid hemorrhage: a guideline for healthcare professionals from the American Heart Association/American Stroke Association. *Stroke*. 2012;43(6):1711-1737.
14. Armin SS, Colohan AR, Zhang JH. Traumatic subarachnoid hemorrhage: our current understanding and its evolution over the past half century. *Neurol Res*. 2006;28(4):445-452.
15. Ropper AH, Samuels MA, Klein JP, eds. *Adam and Victor's Principles of Neurology*. 10th ed. China: McGraw-Hill Education; 2014.
16. Gavrilescu T, Kase CS. Clinical stroke syndromes: clinical-anatomical correlations. *Cerebrovasc Brain Metab Rev*. 1995;7(3):218-239.
17. Goyal M, Menon BK, van Zwam WH, et al. Endovascular thrombectomy after large-vessel ischaemic stroke: a meta-analysis of individual patient data from five randomised trials. *Lancet*. 2016;387(10029):1723-1731.
18. Jauch EC, Saver JL, Adams HP Jr, et al. Guidelines for the early management of patients with acute ischemic stroke: a guideline for healthcare professionals from the American Heart Association/American Stroke Association. *Stroke*. 2013;44(3):870-947.
19. Flemming KD, Brown RD Jr, Petty GW, Huston J III, Kallmes DF, Piepgras DG. Evaluation and management of transient ischemic attack and minor cerebral infarction. *Mayo Clin Proc*. 2004;79(8):1071-1086.
20. Banerjee C, Chimowitz MI. Stroke caused by atherosclerosis of the major intracranial arteries. *Circ Res*. 2017;120(3):502-513.
21. Dodick D. Headache as a symptom of ominous disease. What are the warning signals? *Postgrad Med*. 1997;101(5):46-50, 5-6, 62-4.
22. Griffiths D, Sturm J. Epidemiology and etiology of young stroke. *Stroke Res Treat*. 2011;2011:209370.
23. Varennes L, Tahon F, Kastler A, et al. Fibromuscular dysplasia: what the radiologist should know: a pictorial review. *Insights Imaging*. 2015;6(3):295-307.
24. Berlit P. Diagnosis and treatment of cerebral vasculitis. *Ther Adv Neurol Disord*. 2010;3(1):29-42.
25. Behrouz R, Malek AR, Torbey MT. Small vessel cerebrovascular disease: the past, present, and future. *Stroke Res Treat*. 2012;2012:839151.
26. Arboix A, Marti-Vilalta JL, Garcia JH. Clinical study of 227 patients with lacunar infarcts. *Stroke*. 1990;21(6):842-847.
27. Caplan LR. Lacunar infarction and small vessel disease: pathology and pathophysiology. *J Stroke*. 2015;17(1):2-6.
28. Holmstedt CA, Turan TN, Chimowitz MI. Atherosclerotic intracranial arterial stenosis: risk factors, diagnosis, and treatment. *Lancet Neurol*. 2013;12(11):1106-1114.
29. Mohr JP, Albers GW, Amarenco P, et al. American Heart Association Prevention Conference. IV. Prevention and rehabilitation of stroke. Etiology of stroke. *Stroke*. 1997;28(7):1501-1506.
30. Pittenger B, Young JW, Mansoor AM. Subretinal abscess. *BMJ Case Rep*. 2017;2017.
31. Saver JL. Clinical practice. Cryptogenic stroke. *N Engl J Med*. 2016;374(21):2065-2074.

32. Momjian-Mayor I, Baron JC. The pathophysiology of watershed infarction in internal carotid artery disease: review of cerebral perfusion studies. *Stroke*. 2005;36(3):567-577.
33. Bladin CF, Chambers BR. Clinical features, pathogenesis, and computed tomographic characteristics of internal watershed infarction. *Stroke*. 1993;24(12):1925-1932.
34. Nayor M, Maron BA. Contemporary approach to paradoxical embolism. *Circulation*. 2014;129(18):1892-1897.

Chapter 44

# WEAKNESS

## Case: A 52-year-old man with a "waddling" gait

A previously healthy 52-year-old man presents to the clinic complaining of weakness. Several weeks ago he developed soreness and heaviness of the legs, which forced him to stop his daily exercise routine. The symptoms progressed, and he soon began having difficulty rising from a seated position. He additionally describes recent voice changes and swallowing difficulties. The symptoms do not change over the course of the day. He does not describe any ocular symptoms.

Vital signs are unremarkable. The patient has a "waddling" gait. Cranial nerves are intact. Mild atrophy of the proximal muscles is present. Strength of the deltoids and hip flexors are graded 3/5; handgrip strength is 5/5; and toe raises are performed without difficulty. Sensation is intact. Reflexes are normal and symmetric. There is discoloration around the eyes (Figure 44-1). There are violaceous and scaly papules over the dorsum of the metacarpophalangeal and interphalangeal joints (Figure 44-2).

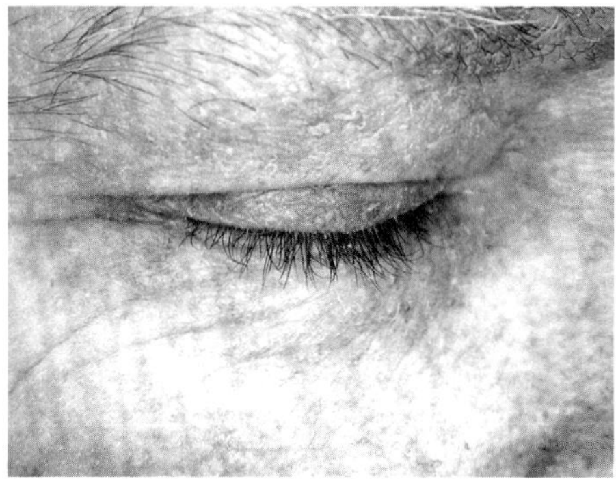

**Figure 44-1.** (From Schalock PC, Hsu JTS, Arndt KA. *Lippincott's Primary Care Dermatology*. Philadelphia, PA: Wolters Kluwer Health; 2011.)

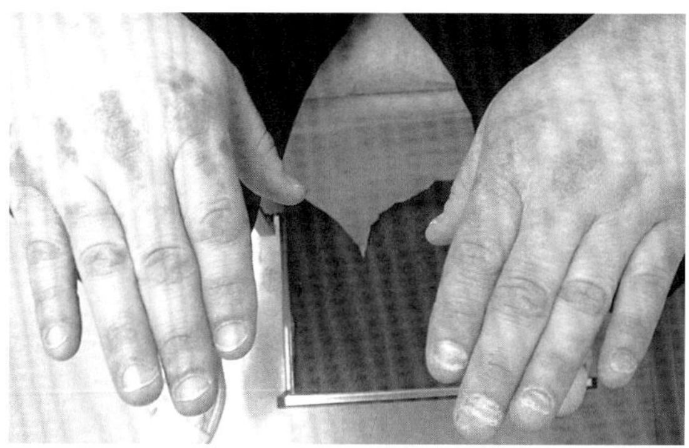

**Figure 44-2.** (Courtesy of Peter D. Sullivan, MD.)

***What is the most likely cause of weakness in this patient?***

What is muscle weakness?

Weakness is a reduction in the power that can be generated by muscle.[1]

**What is a motor unit?**

A motor unit consists of a nerve cell, the axon from that nerve cell, and the muscle fibers innervated by the terminal branches of that axon (Figure 44-3).[2]

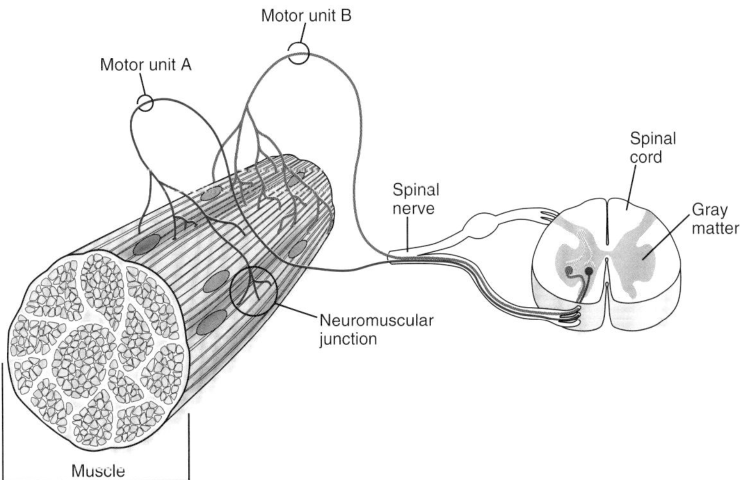


**Figure 44-3.** A motor unit is made up of a motor neuron cell body (which resides in the gray matter of the spinal cord) along with its axon (which exits the spinal cord) and the muscle fibers innervated by the terminal branches of the axon. (From Ives JC, *Motor Behavior: Connecting Mind and Body for Optimal Performance*, 2nd ed. Philadelphia, PA: Wolters Kluwer; 2018.)



**What is fatigability?**

Fatigability describes a gradual reduction in power with repetitive use of a muscle. It can be a feature of neuromuscular disease, such as myasthenia gravis. Fatigability should not be confused with fatigue such as that experienced by patients with systemic conditions (eg, anemia), in which true weakness is not present.[2]

**What is asthenia?**

Asthenia, often confused with weakness, is characterized by feelings of weariness, exhaustion, and disinclination to engage in and sustain physical activity, in the absence of true muscle weakness. Similar terms include fatigue, lassitude, and lethargy.[2]

**What is bradykinesia?**

Bradykinesia, sometimes misinterpreted as weakness, is an abnormal increase in the time required to initiate and complete movement.[1]

**What is muscle bulk?**

Bulk refers to overall muscle mass. Atrophy, which can be symmetric or asymmetric, occurs with certain causes of muscle weakness, particularly lower motor neuron (LMN) processes.

**What is muscle tone?**

Tone refers to the involuntary resistance of muscle to passive stretch. Spasticity is a type of velocity-dependent (ie, more obvious with fast movements) hypertonicity that predominantly affects the antigravity muscles (ie, upper limb flexors and lower limb extensors), and is seen with upper motor neuron (UMN) disorders. Rigidity is a type of velocity-independent hypertonicity that affects flexors and extensors equally, and is seen with extrapyramidal disorders such as Parkinson's disease. Flaccidity describes a decrease in tone, and is seen with LMN disorders (it can also be seen in the acute phase of UMN disorders [eg, spinal shock]).[1]

**What is muscle fibrillation?**

Fibrillation refers to involuntary contraction of individual muscle fibers as a result of denervation. It is too fine to be visualized with the naked eye but can be observed on electromyography.[2]

**What is muscle fasciculation?**

Fasciculation refers to involuntary contraction of 1 or more motor units resulting in a visible twitch of a muscle fascicle. It can occur as a result of increased neuromuscular irritability associated with lower motor neuron disease.[2]

**What is clonus?**

Clonus refers to sustained and rhythmic involuntary muscular contractions that occur with a frequency of 5 to 7 Hz in response to a stretch reflex. It is a manifestation of the hyperreflexic state of spasticity and may be an indication of upper motor neuron disease.[2]

**What is paralysis?**

Paralysis refers to the complete loss of voluntary movement related to interruption of the motor pathway anywhere from the cerebral cortex to the muscle fiber.[2]

**What is the meaning of the term "plegia"?**

The term plegia denotes severe weakness or paralysis. Monoplegia refers to paralysis of 1 limb; hemiplegia refers to paralysis of 1 side of the body (involving the arm, the leg, and sometimes the face); paraplegia refers to paralysis of both legs; and quadriplegia refers to paralysis of all 4 extremities.[2]

**What is the meaning of the term "paresis"?**

The term paresis denotes partial loss of motor function.[2]

**What scale can be used to grade muscle strength?**

The following 0-5 scale is commonly used for grading muscle weakness[2]:

0—Complete paralysis
1—Minimal contraction
2—Active movement when gravity is eliminated
3—Full movement against gravity but cannot provide resistance against manual muscle opposition
4—Active movement against gravity and resistance but overcome by manual muscle opposition
5—Normal strength

**How can true involuntary muscle weakness be distinguished from voluntary weakness during resistance testing?**

True weakness gives way smoothly to resistance. In voluntary release, the patient may successfully resist for a few moments before suddenly letting go (ie, "giveaway" weakness). In other cases, the patient may attempt to mimic the gradual release of true weakness, but this produces a series of small phases akin to a "cogwheel" (not to be confused with true cogwheeling in basal ganglia disorders). In some circumstances, voluntary release does not rule out the presence of true weakness (eg, concurrent pain may lead to voluntary release in those with true weakness).[3]

**What are the 4 anatomic categories of weakness?**

Weakness can be caused by disorders of the UMN, LMN, neuromuscular junction (NMJ), or muscle (Figure 44-4).

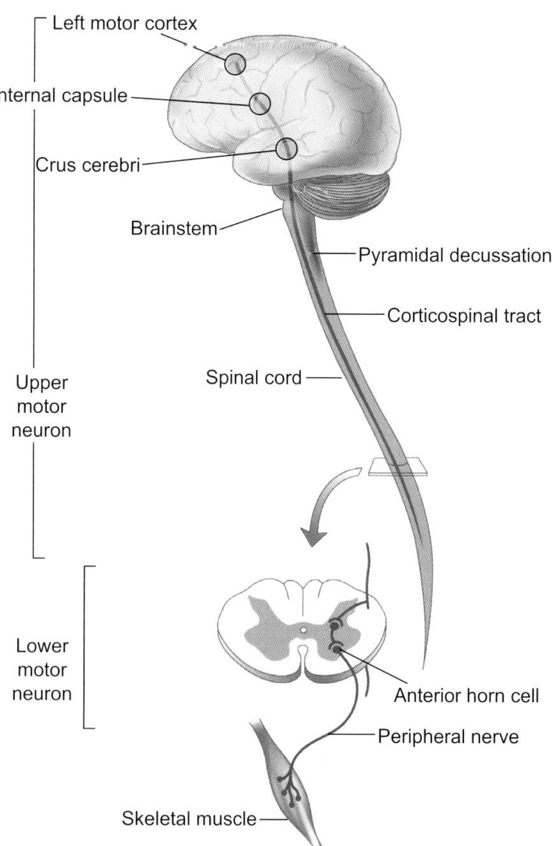


**Figure 44-4.** Relationship between the upper motor neuron, lower motor neuron, neuromuscular junction, and muscle. (Adapted From Drislane FW, Acosta J, Caplan L, Chang B, Tarulli A. *Blueprints Neurology*, 4rd ed. Philadelphia, PA: Wolters Kluwer Health; 2013.)

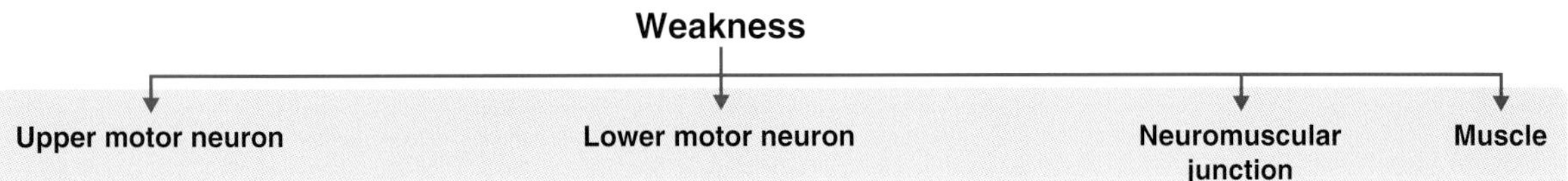


**What are the general characteristics of the 4 categories of weakness?**

UMN lesions are proximal to the anterior horn cell and are characterized by increased tone (spasticity), hyperreflexia, and minimal atrophy; proximal muscles are typically affected more than distal muscles. LMN lesions involve the structures distal to and including the anterior horn cell and are characterized by flaccid tone, diminished reflexes, fasciculations, and atrophy; distal muscles are typically affected more than proximal muscles. NMJ disorders present with variable distributions of weakness (classically proximal > distal). Myopathic weakness tends to be symmetric and most pronounced in the proximal muscles.[1]

**What are the effects of upper motor neuron lesions, lower motor neuron lesions, and myopathies on muscle bulk, fasciculations, tone, tendon reflexes, and Babinski reflex?**

| Sign | UMN | LMN | Myopathy |
|---|---|---|---|
| Atrophy | None/minimal | Severe | Mild |
| Fasciculations | None | Common** | None |
| Tone | Increased (spastic)* | Decreased | Normal/decreased |
| Reflexes | Increased* | Decreased | Normal/decreased |
| Babinski | Present | Absent | Absent |

**Reflexes and tone may be decreased in UMN lesions in the period immediately following the injury (eg, spinal shock).*
***Fasciculations are most often seen in LMN disorders involving the anterior horn cell and/or nerve root.*[1]

**What finding on physical examination is suggestive of a disorder of the neuromuscular junction?**

The presence of fatigable weakness is suggestive of disorders that affect the NMJ, particularly postsynaptic disorders (eg, myasthenia gravis).

## WEAKNESS RELATED TO UPPER MOTOR NEURON LESIONS

**What is an upper motor neuron?**

UMNs are neurons originating in the motor cortex that synapse with LMNs of the brainstem (brainstem nuclei) and spinal cord (anterior horn cells), which in turn innervate effector organs (eg, muscle) (see Figure 44-4).

**Upper motor neuron lesions occur within which 2 general anatomic structures?**

UMN lesions can involve the brain or spinal cord (see Figure 44-4).

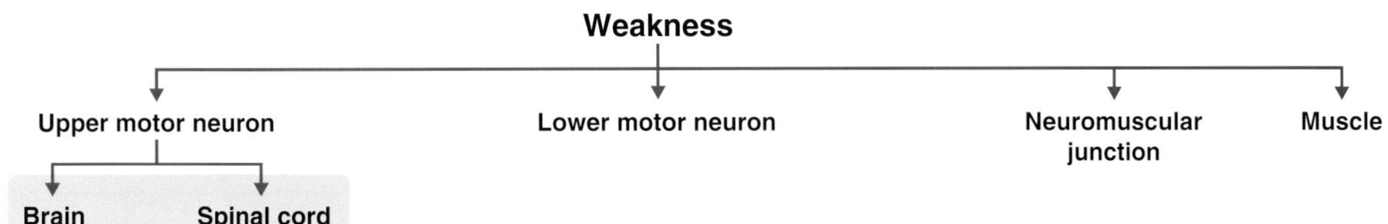

**What direct connections between the brain and spinal cord control voluntary movement?**

The cell bodies of the UMNs (gray matter) reside mainly in the motor cortex. The axons from these neurons (white matter) form the corticobulbar and corticospinal tracts, which travel through the subcortical white matter and internal capsule to the brainstem. The corticobulbar tracts innervate the LMNs of the brainstem, whereas the corticospinal tracts continue on to innervate the LMNs of the spinal cord (Figure 44-5). The indirect pathways between the brain and spinal cord include the rubrospinal, reticulospinal, vestibulospinal, and tectospinal (extrapyramidal) tracts.[1,2]

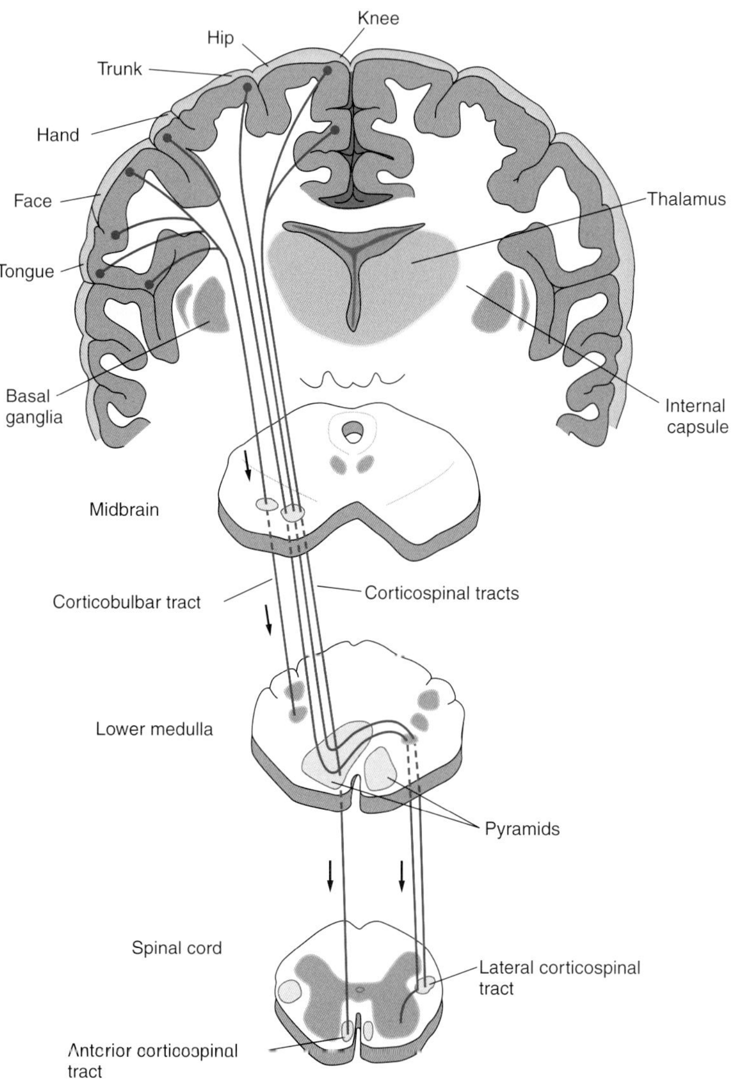


**Figure 44-5.** Motor pathways: corticospinal and corticobulbar tracts. (From Hogan-Quigley B, Palm ML, *Bickley LS. Bates' Nursing Guide to Physical Examination and History Taking,* 2nd ed. Philadelphia, PA: Wolters Kluwer; 2017.)

**In which general regions of the brain do upper motor neuron lesions occur?**

Within the brain, UMN lesions can occur in the cerebral cortex, subcortical white matter, internal capsule, and brainstem.[1]

**What are the general characteristics of the weakness caused by upper motor neuron lesions?**

UMN lesions always affect a group of muscles (never an individual muscle), with proximal > distal involvement, disproportionately affecting the upper limb extensors (causing pronator drift) and lower limb flexors. Facial movements that are bilateral (eg, eyes, jaw) are spared or affected to a small degree because of bilateral innervation (Broadbent's law). Deficits in fine motor movement (eg, finger tapping) may also be observed.[2]

What are the characteristics of the facial weakness caused by lesions of the corticobulbar tracts?

Lesions of the corticobulbar tracts usually involve the contralateral muscles of the lower face and tongue while there is sparing of the muscles that habitually produce bilateral movement, including extraocular, upper facial (eg, forehead), pharyngeal, and jaw muscles. This occurs as a result of the bilateral innervation of those muscles.[1,2]

Restricted weakness (eg, hand and arm or foot and leg) can result from upper motor neuron lesions involving which general regions of the brain?

Because of the somatotopic organization of the corticospinal system, a discrete lesion of the cortex or subcortex could result in limited zones of weakness (see Figure 44-5).[7]

Hemiparesis can result from upper motor neuron lesions involving which general regions of the brain or spinal cord?

Hemiparesis, the most frequent form of paralysis, can occur as a result of lesions of the corticospinal tracts above the midcervical spinal cord.[1,2]

What additional neurologic manifestations often occur along with hemiparesis in patients with lesions of the cerebral cortex?

Lesions of the cerebral cortex often result in disorders of language and visual-spatial integration (eg, neglect), and can cause cortical sensory disturbances (eg, agraphesthesia), apraxia, and seizure. The presence of any of these findings in addition to hemiparesis is suggestive of a lesion within the cerebral cortex.[1]

Pure motor hemiparesis of the face, arm, and leg can result from upper motor neuron lesions involving which regions of the brain?

Because the descending motor fibers from the cortex converge and collect within the posterior limb of the internal capsule, cerebral peduncle, and upper pons, even small lesions in these regions can result in pure motor hemiparesis, where the face, arm, hand, leg, and foot are affected to a similar degree.[1]

Ipsilateral cranial nerve signs with contralateral hemiparesis can result from upper motor neuron lesions involving which region of the brain?

Lesions of the brainstem can result in ipsilateral cranial nerve signs with contralateral hemiparesis.[1]

Hemiparesis in the absence of cranial nerve signs or facial weakness is suggestive of upper motor neuron lesions involving which region of the spinal cord?

Lesions of the high cervical spinal cord can result in ipsilateral hemiparesis in the absence of cranial nerve signs or facial weakness.[1]

Paraparesis can result from upper motor neuron lesions involving which region of the spinal cord?

Lesions at or below the thoracic spinal cord that involve both corticospinal tracts can result in paraparesis.[1]

Quadriparesis can result from upper motor neuron lesions involving which region of the spinal cord?

Like hemiparesis, quadriparesis can occur as a result of lesions of the corticospinal tracts above the midcervical spinal cord; however, in the case of quadriparesis, both corticospinal tracts must be involved.

## WEAKNESS RELATED TO UPPER MOTOR NEURON LESIONS OF THE BRAIN

### What are the causes of weakness related to the brain?

Risk factors for this condition include hypertension, smoking, hyperlipidemia, and atrial fibrillation.

Stroke.

A 67-year-old man with non–small cell lung cancer presents with insidious-onset weakness of the left arm with increased muscle tone and tendon reflexes.

Metastatic brain tumor.

Fever, papilledema, and focal neurologic deficits in a patient with recent otitis media.

Brain abscess.

A young woman with optic neuritis.

Multiple sclerosis (MS).

An acute demyelinating condition that typically follows a viral infection.

Acute disseminated encephalomyelitis (ADEM).

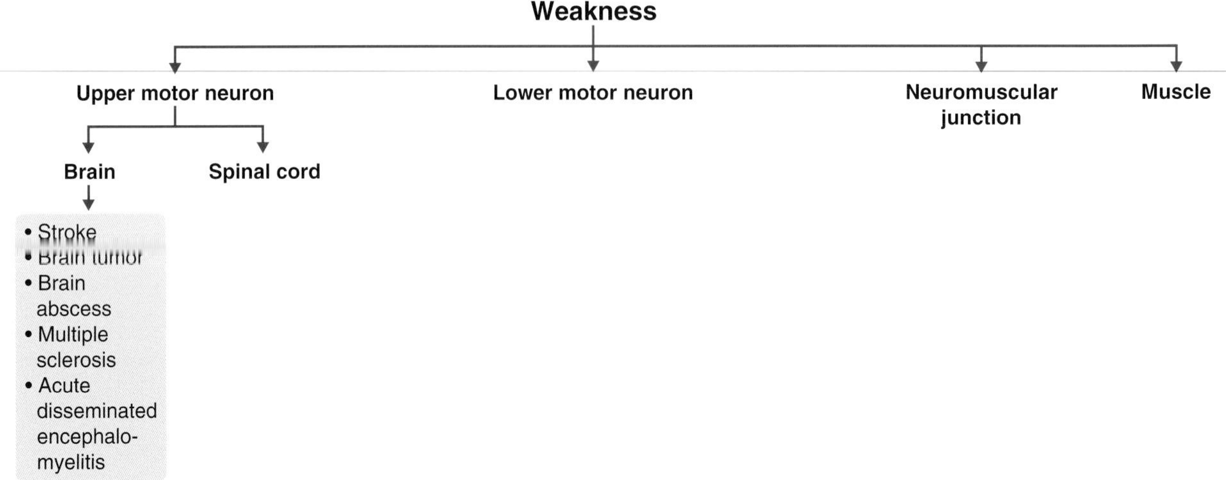


**Which side of the body would be affected by a stroke involving the right cerebral cortex, cerebral white matter, or internal capsule?**

Lesions involving the right cerebral cortex, cerebral white matter (ie, corona radiata), or internal capsule result in hemiparesis of the contralateral (left) side.

**What proportion of metastatic brain tumors involve the cerebral hemispheres (where the motor cortex is located) compared with the posterior fossa (where the brainstem is located)?**

Metastatic lesions predominate in the cerebral hemispheres (80%) compared with the posterior fossa (20%), reflecting the relative size and blood flow of those regions; brain metastases typically involve the gray-white junction.[2]

**What are the 3 general mechanisms of brain abscess development?**

Brain abscesses occur as a result of direct extension from extracranial infection (eg, sinusitis), hematogenous spread, or direct inoculation following head injury or neurosurgery.

**What are the manifestations of brainstem involvement in patients with multiple sclerosis?**

Diplopia is the most common manifestation of brainstem involvement in MS; others include facial sensory symptoms, unstable gait, vertigo, oscillopsia, facial weakness, nausea or vomiting, trigeminal neuralgia, dysarthria, hypoacusia, dysgeusia, somnolence, and dysphagia.[4]

**How is the evaluation of cerebrospinal fluid (CSF) helpful in distinguishing multiple sclerosis from acute disseminated encephalomyelitis?**

Although CSF is abnormal in most patients with ADEM (characterized by moderate pleocytosis and elevated protein), the presence of oligoclonal bands occurs in only a minority and is more suggestive of MS.[5]

## WEAKNESS RELATED TO UPPER MOTOR NEURON LESIONS OF THE SPINAL CORD

**What are the origins and routes of the corticospinal tracts within the spinal cord?**

The axons of the UMNs descend through the brainstem; at the cervicomedullary junction, most axons (70%-90%) decussate (cross) into the contralateral corticospinal tract of the lateral spinal cord while a smaller proportion remain ipsilateral in the anterior spinal cord. The axons continue on to innervate the LMNs of the spinal cord (see Figure 44-5).[1]

**How are the corticospinal tracts organized?**

The corticospinal tracts are organized somatotopically. The axons that control upper extremity movement are positioned medially, whereas those controlling lower extremity movement are positioned laterally (see Figure 44-5). Central cord syndrome, for example, results in loss of motor function predominantly in the upper extremities with relative sparing of the lower extremities.[2]

**Which arteries supply the spinal cord?**

The anterior spinal artery supplies the ventral two-thirds of the spinal cord, whereas the posterior spinal arteries supply the dorsal one-third.[2]

**What would be the expected result of complete spinal cord transection?**

Spinal cord transection results in interruption of all ascending and descending tracts below the level of the lesion, leading to bilateral complete loss of sensation, motor, and autonomic function. Spinal shock may result from acute cord transection, which is characterized by a temporary state of flaccid paralysis, loss of sensation below the level of the lesion, atonic paralysis of the bladder and bowel, gastric atony, and diminished reflexes.[2]

**Cessation of respiration would result from complete transection of what level of the spinal cord?**

Transection of the spinal cord above C3 results in complete cessation of respiration and is commonly fatal.[2]

**What are the characteristics of anterior cord syndrome?**

Anterior cord syndrome refers to damage to the ventral two-thirds of the spinal cord (supplied by the anterior spinal artery), which contains the corticospinal tracts (resulting in motor deficits below the level of the lesion) and spinothalamic tracts (resulting in loss of pain and temperature sensation below the level of the lesion). There is preservation of fine touch, vibration, and proprioception (carried by the dorsal columns).[2]

**What are the characteristics of posterior cord syndrome?**

Posterior cord syndrome is characterized by damage to the dorsal columns (fine touch, vibration, and proprioception), resulting in manifestations such as gait (sensory) ataxia and paresthesias. There is preservation of motor function, pain, and temperature (carried by the corticospinal and spinothalamic tracts). Posterior cord syndrome related to vascular disease is much less common than anterior cord syndrome.[2]

**What is Brown-Séquard syndrome?**

Brown-Séquard syndrome occurs as a result of damage to a single lateral side of the spinal cord. Involved structures include the unilateral corticospinal tract, dorsal column, and spinothalamic tract. Clinical sequelae include ipsilateral weakness, ipsilateral loss of proprioception and vibration, and contralateral loss of pain and temperature.[2]

**Is spinal cord disease associated with upper motor neuron involvement only?**

Most spinal cord diseases (ie, myelopathies) produce UMN lesions via involvement of the corticospinal tracts; however, LMN signs may be present at the level of the spinal cord lesion when there is local involvement of the anterior horn cell.[2]

NEUROLOGY

## What are the causes of weakness related to the spinal cord?

**Mass effect.**

Spinal cord compression (eg, from disc herniation).

**A 44-year-old man becomes quadriplegic after falling off a horse.**

Trauma.

**Fever and paraparesis.**

Infection (eg, epidural abscess).

**Damage to the anterior spinal artery, which supplies the area of the spinal cord housing the corticospinal tracts.**

Vascular disease (eg, vasculitis).

**A 34-year-old woman with anorexia nervosa slowly develops angular cheilitis, paresthesias, spastic paraparesis, brisk reflexes, and a positive Romberg sign.**

Vitamin $B_{12}$ deficiency.

**A 28-year-old woman develops pain with left eye movement and acute-onset paraparesis associated with a white matter lesion of the cervical spine on magnetic resonance imaging (MRI), followed by resolution of symptoms over the next few weeks.**

Multiple sclerosis.

**Development of myelopathy following immunization.**

Acute disseminated encephalomyelitis.

| | |
|---|---|
| **This entity, which is on a continuum with inflammatory disorders such as multiple sclerosis and acute disseminated encephalomyelitis, can be idiopathic or secondary to other conditions (usually autoimmune diseases).** | Transverse myelitis. |
| **A noninfectious granulomatous disease.** | Sarcoidosis. |
| **A neoplastic process without evidence of spinal cord compression or direct cord involvement.** | Paraneoplastic syndrome. |
| **Palmar erythema, spider angiomas, and caput medusae.** | Hepatic myelopathy. |
| **These myelopathies run in families.** | Hereditary myelopathy (eg, hereditary spastic paraparesis). |
| **Myelopathy on vacation in Hawaii.** | Surfer's myelopathy. |
| **Scuba divers are at risk.** | Caisson's disease (ie, decompression sickness). |

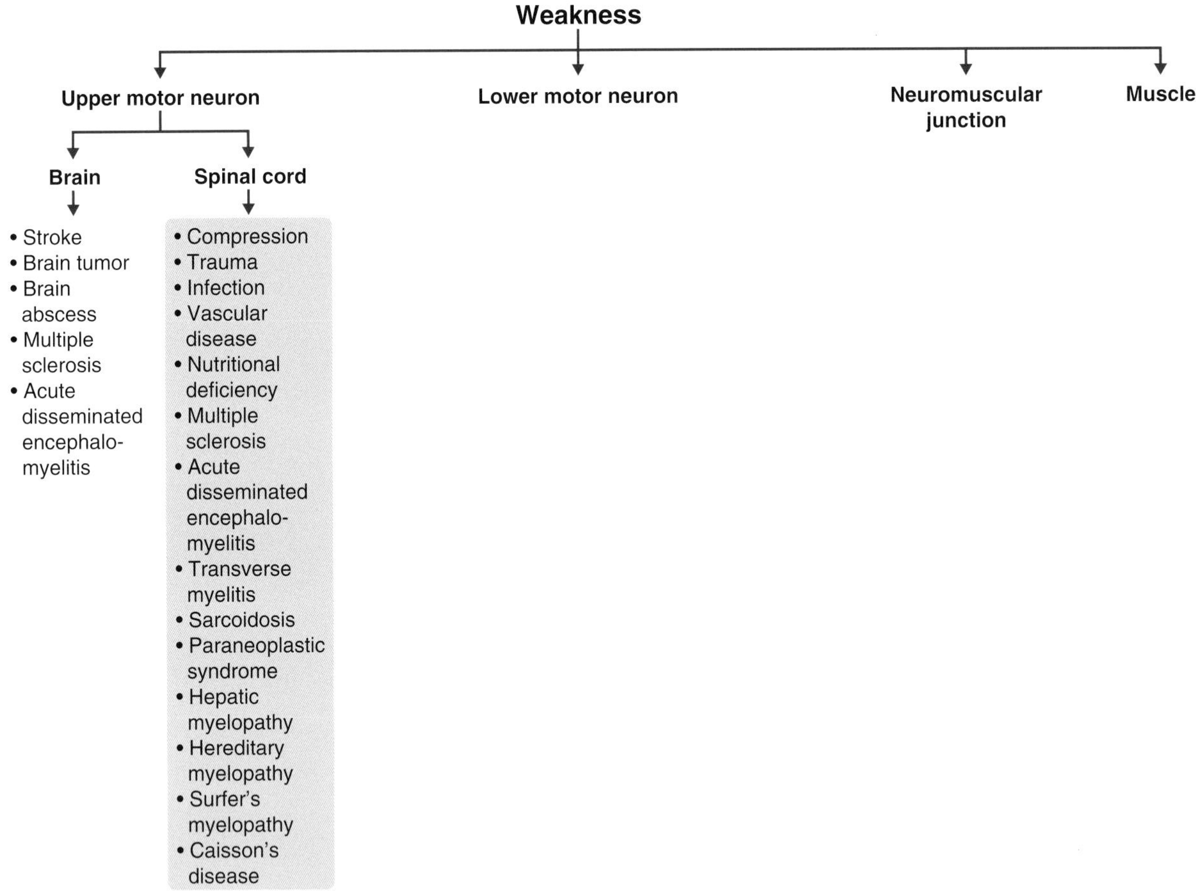


| | |
|---|---|
| **What are the compressive causes of myelopathy?** | Compressive causes of myelopathy include degenerative disease (eg, osteoarthritis), spondylolisthesis, spinal stenosis, disc herniation, tumor (benign or malignant), syringomyelia, epidural abscess, and hematoma. |
| **What are the traumatic causes of myelopathy?** | Motor vehicle accidents account for about one-half of all traumatic causes of myelopathy; other causes include falls, inflicted injuries (eg, gunshots), sports-related injuries, radiation treatment, and electrical injury.[6] |

**What are the infectious causes of myelopathy?**

Infectious causes of myelopathy include epidural abscess, acute viral myelitis, human immunodeficiency virus (HIV), tuberculosis, syphilis, fungi (eg, *Blastomyces dermatitidis*), and parasites (eg, *Schistosoma mansoni*).[7]

**What are the vascular causes of myelopathy?**

Vascular causes of myelopathy include thrombi, emboli, vasculitis, hematoma, and vascular malformation (eg, dural arteriovenous fistula).[2]

**Which nutritional deficiencies can result in myelopathy?**

Deficiencies of vitamin $B_{12}$ or copper can result in myelopathy, often presenting as myeloneuropathy (the combination of spinal cord and peripheral nerve involvement).[2]

**What are the patterns of spinal cord involvement in multiple sclerosis?**

The vast majority of patients with MS develop spinal cord lesions, which can be helpful in making the diagnosis when identified with MRI. Most lesions are focal, usually involving the cervical cord although diffuse abnormalities occur in a minority of cases.[8]

**What is the prognosis of acute disseminated encephalomyelitis?**

ADEM is a rare inflammatory demyelinating condition of the central nervous system that can be triggered by viral infections and vaccinations. Immunosuppressive medications with or without plasma exchange is the mainstay of treatment. Most children with ADEM improve, with many achieving complete recovery. The prognosis of adults with ADEM is less favorable; permanent disability, recurrence, and death occur at higher rates in adults.[9]

**What is the prognosis of transverse myelitis?**

Transverse myelitis is an acquired inflammatory disorder of the spinal cord that results in acute or subacute motor, sensory, and/or autonomic deficits below the level of the lesion. It is most often triggered by infection or vaccination, but can be associated with an underlying systemic disease (eg, systemic lupus erythematosus) or a demyelinating disease such as MS. Immunosuppressive medications with or without plasma exchange is the mainstay of treatment. The prognosis of transverse myelitis is highly variable. When associated with MS, patients may have complete or substantial recovery. When idiopathic or associated with other diseases, residual neurologic deficits are common. Most recovery occurs within the first 3 months after the initial event.[10]

**What is the typical cerebrospinal fluid profile in patients with sarcoid myelopathy?**

The granulomatous inflammation of sarcoidosis can involve the spinal cord. There is usually evidence of systemic sarcoidosis in affected patients (the presence of hilar lymphadenopathy can be a clue). MRI of the spine can be suggestive of the diagnosis. CSF evaluation often reveals mononuclear pleocytosis with elevated protein and normal glucose. Ultimately, biopsy may be necessary to confirm the diagnosis. Sarcoid myelopathy is often responsive to treatment with glucocorticoids.[2]

**Which laboratory test can be helpful in diagnosing paraneoplastic syndromes of the central nervous system?**

A paraneoplastic syndrome is suggested by the detection of paraneoplastic antibodies in serum or CSF.

**What is the most common presentation of hepatic myelopathy?**

Hepatic myelopathy is rare, usually occurring in patients with chronic liver disease and associated portosystemic shunt. The most common deficit is progressive spastic paraparesis. Prognosis may be improved with early recognition and treatment with liver transplantation.[11]

**What hereditary conditions are associated with myelopathy predominantly involving upper motor neurons?**

Hereditary myelopathies predominantly involving UMNs include hereditary spastic paraplegias (HSP), adrenoleukodystrophy, and Friedreich's ataxia.[12]

**What is the timing of onset of surfer's myelopathy?**

Surfer's myelopathy describes a nontraumatic myelopathy that develops when prolonged prone positioning is followed by vigorous activity and assumption of the upright position. It is characterized by the onset of upper lumbar or thoracic pain, progressive paraparesis or paraplegia, and urinary retention, usually within an hour of surfing. It tends to affect novice surfers. Prognosis is variable; some experience full recovery and others are left with permanent paralysis.[2]

**What is the mechanism of Caisson's disease?**

Caisson's disease occurs when patients ascend too rapidly after exposure to high pressures under water. Under these conditions, nitrogen bubbles form and become trapped in spinal vessels, resulting in ischemia. The thoracic spine is most frequently affected. Immediate recompression in a hyperbaric chamber is the treatment of choice. Some patients recover whereas others are left with permanent disability.[2]

## WEAKNESS RELATED TO LOWER MOTOR NEURON LESIONS

**What is a lower motor neuron?**

LMNs are motor neurons that reside in the brainstem and spinal cord and are controlled by UMNs.

**Lower motor neuron lesions occur within which 3 general anatomic structures?**

LMN lesions can involve the anterior horn cell, nerve root or plexus, or peripheral nerve.

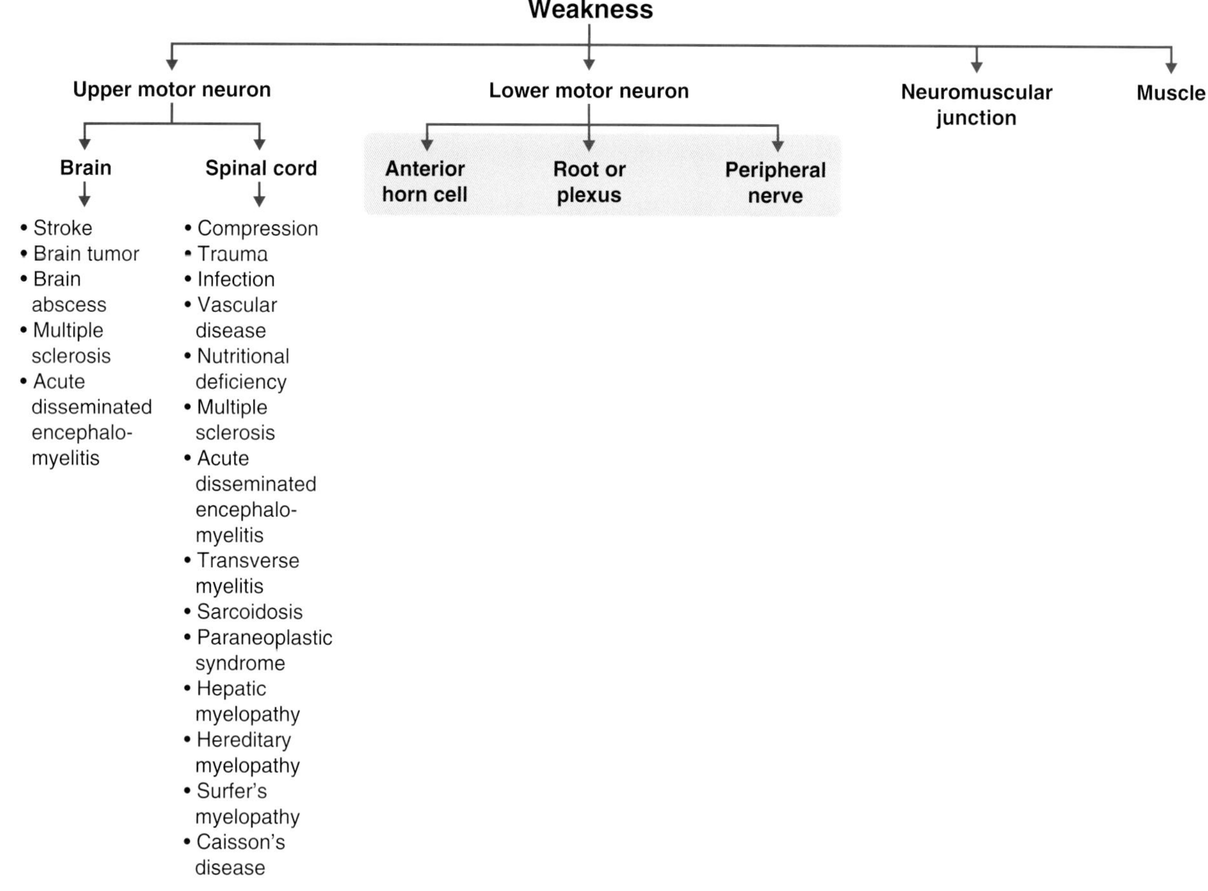

**What are the relationships between the anterior horn cells, spinal nerve roots, nerve plexuses, and peripheral nerves?**

Motor nerve fibers originating from the anterior horn cells of the spinal cord form the ventral nerve roots; neighboring roots join together to form plexuses that give rise to peripheral nerves (Figure 44-6).[2]

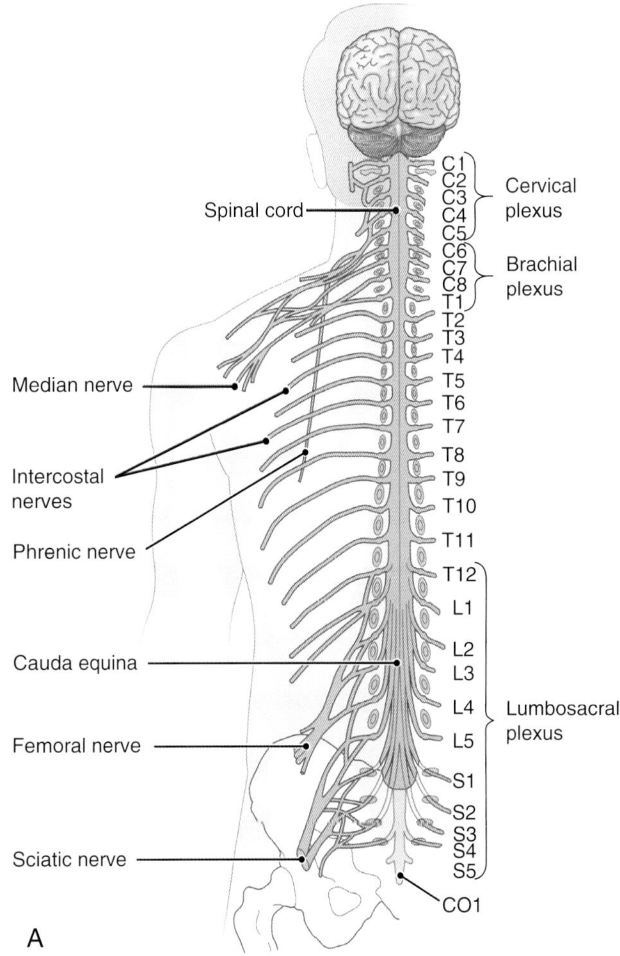


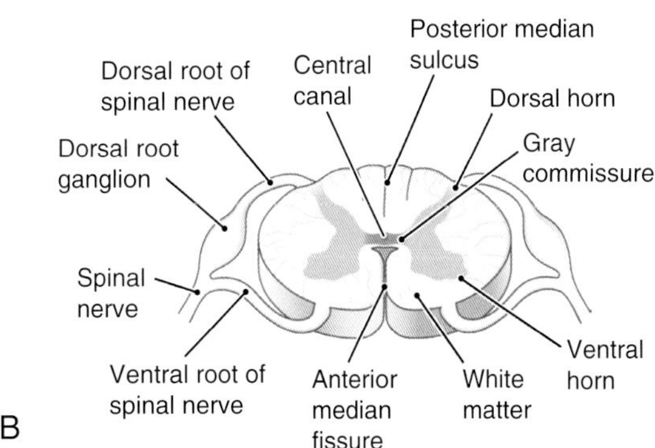


**Figure 44-6.** Spinal cord and spinal nerves. A, Posterior view showing nerve plexuses and some peripheral nerves. B, Cross-section of the spinal cord showing the organization of the gray and white matter. The roots of the spinal nerves are also shown. (From Cohen BJ, Hull KL. *Memmler's The Human Body in Health and Disease.* 13th ed. Philadelphia, PA: Wolters Kluwer Health; 2015.)

## WEAKNESS RELATED TO LOWER MOTOR NEURON LESIONS OF THE ANTERIOR HORN CELL

### What are the causes of weakness related to the anterior horn cell?

**Lou Gehrig's disease.**

Amyotrophic lateral sclerosis (ALS).

**Related to amyotrophic lateral sclerosis; this disease affects lower motor neurons only.**

Progressive muscular atrophy (PMA).

NEUROLOGY

| | |
|---|---|
| **An upper and lower motor neuron disorder of the cranial nerves.** | Progressive bulbar palsy (PBP). |
| **Related to amyotrophic lateral sclerosis; this motor neuron disease predominantly affects the upper extremities.** | Flail arm syndrome (FAS). |
| **Related to amyotrophic lateral sclerosis; this motor neuron disease predominantly affects the lower extremities.** | Flail leg syndrome (FLS). |
| **A mosquito-borne virus.** | West Nile Virus. |
| **Vaccination has almost eradicated this virus from parts of the world.** | Poliomyelitis. |
| **Muscular atrophy is a prominent feature of this disease that predominantly occurs in children.** | Spinal muscular atrophy (SMA). |

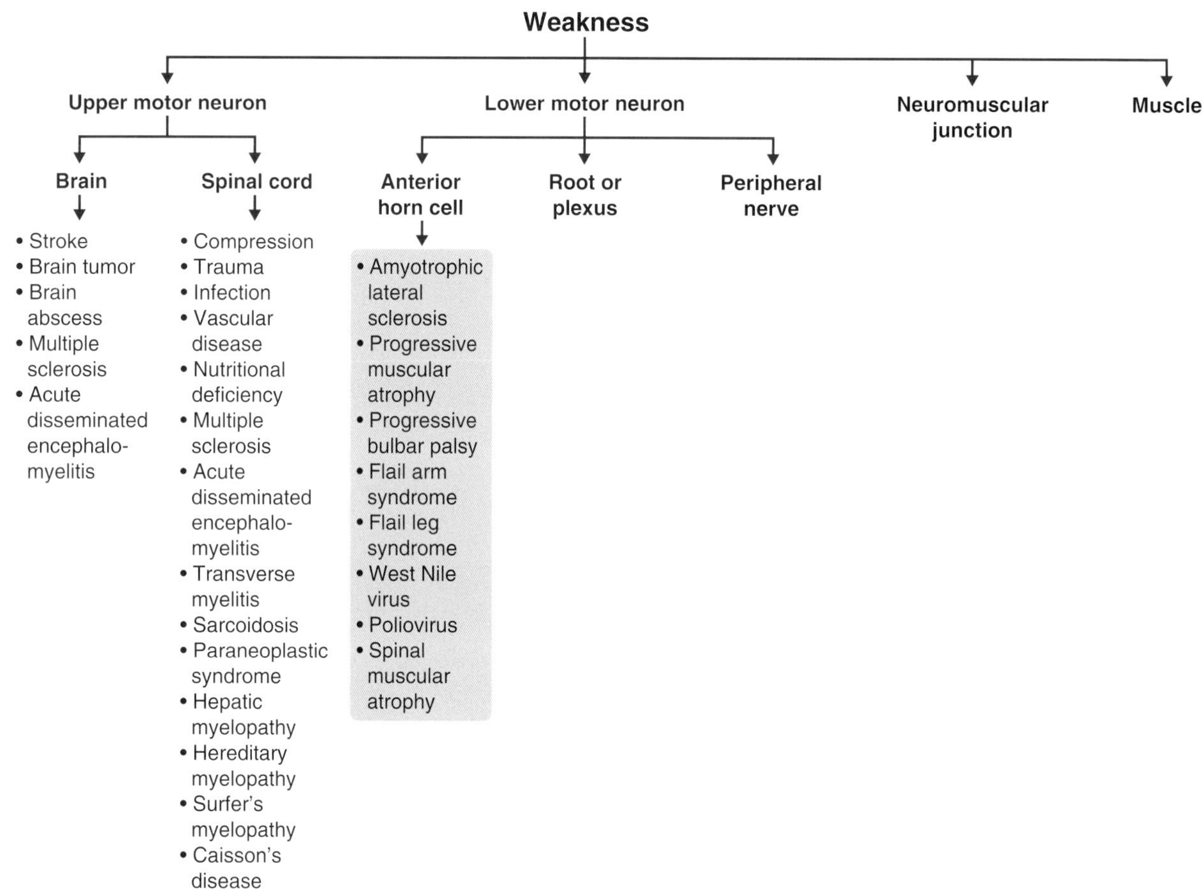


| | |
|---|---|
| **Does amyotrophic lateral sclerosis exclusively involve the anterior horn cell?** | ALS is a progressive neurodegenerative disorder that results in gradually worsening muscle weakness and eventual death. Degeneration involves the anterior horn cells as well as the corticobulbar and corticospinal tracts resulting in the characteristic combination of both lower and upper motor neuron signs. The disease is familial in around 10% of cases. Men are disproportionately affected by a ratio of 2:1. Onset is above 45 years of age in most cases. *Primary lateral sclerosis is a condition closely related to ALS that only affects UMNs.*[2] |

**What is the prognosis of progressive muscular atrophy?**

PMA is more common in men by a ratio of 4:1. The clinical course tends to progress more slowly compared with ALS. The 5-year survival rate is approximately 70% in patients whose onset is before 50 years of age, and is around 40% in those diagnosed after 50 years of age.[2]

**What is the prognosis of progressive bulbar palsy?**

PBP is a disorder that first involves the upper and lower motor neurons of the brainstem, resulting in weakness of the cranial muscles (eg, jaw, face, tongue, pharynx, larynx). The prognosis of PBP is poor; most patients die within 2 to 3 years of onset when weakness spreads to the respiratory muscles.[2]

**What are some of the clinical differences between flail arm syndrome and amyotrophic lateral sclerosis?**

Compared with ALS, FAS demonstrates an even stronger predominance in men, has a predilection for the proximal muscles of the upper extremities without significant weakness of the legs or bulbar sites, has less UMN involvement, and is associated with better prognosis.[13]

**What are the clinical characteristics of flail leg syndrome?**

In patients with FLS, weakness and atrophy begin in the distal lower extremities and there is slow progression and subtle or late UMN involvement. Like FAS, FLS is associated with better prognosis compared with ALS.[14]

**What are the characteristics of the weakness associated with West Nile virus infection?**

West Nile virus infection results in acute asymmetric flaccid paralysis, absent deep tendon reflexes, and preserved sensation. Although the major site of involvement is the anterior horn cell, other sites can be involved, including the adjacent white matter, dorsal root ganglia, and peripheral nerves.[15]

**How is poliovirus spread in humans?**

Poliovirus is mainly spread human-to-human, usually through the fecal-oral route. The vast majority of infections are either asymptomatic or associated with an influenza-like illness, whereas a small proportion involves the central nervous system, most typically causing acute, asymmetric, and flaccid weakness predominantly involving the lower extremities.[16]

**What other viral infections cause weakness related to involvement of anterior horn cells?**

Viruses that can involve anterior horn cells include non-polio enteroviruses (eg, enteroviruses D68 and 71), Japanese encephalitis virus, and HTLV-I.[16]

**What are the characteristics of adult-onset spinal muscular atrophy?**

Adult-onset (type 4) SMA is an autosomal recessive disease that typically presents after 30 years of age, causing proximal limb and diaphragmatic weakness. It is slowly progressive and patients eventually become wheelchair bound but have normal life expectancy.[2]

## WEAKNESS RELATED TO LOWER MOTOR NEURON LESIONS OF THE ROOT OR PLEXUS

**What is a myotome?**

A myotome refers to the group of muscles innervated by a single spinal nerve root. Myotomes are helpful in localizing lesions of the neuromuscular system.

**What are the characteristic manifestations of injury to the nerve root?**

Nerve root injury (ie, radiculopathy) usually results in weakness, pain, sensory loss, and diminished reflexes in the sensorimotor distribution of the involved nerve root (ie, the associated myotomes and dermatomes). If more than 1 root is involved, the term polyradiculopathy is used.[2]

**Why is weakness caused by radiculopathy usually only mild in severity?**

Many muscles, particularly the larger ones, receive innervation from multiple nerve roots, which preserves strength in the setting of radiculopathy.[2]

**What are the characteristic manifestations of injury to the nerve plexus?**

Nerve plexus injury, also called plexopathy, results in motor, sensory, and reflex loss involving 1 extremity, but the patterns of deficits are often variable and complex.[2]

**What are the 2 main plexopathies?**

Brachial and lumbosacral plexopathies are the 2 main types. *Lumbar and sacral plexuses are sometimes considered separate.*

NEUROLOGY

## What are the causes of weakness related to the nerve root or plexus?

| | |
|---|---|
| **A 76-year-old man complains of weakness and numbness of his legs when he stands or walks for prolonged periods of time; the symptoms resolve after he sits down.** | Lumbar spinal stenosis. |
| **An endocrinopathy commonly associated with polyneuropathy.** | Diabetes mellitus. |
| **A 47-year-old man with right arm weakness after a motorcycle accident.** | Brachial plexopathy related to avulsion or stretch injury. |
| **A 28-year-old woman presents with bilateral facial droop and right leg pain and weakness after a camping trip in Massachusetts.** | Lyme disease. |
| **Misplacement of an epidural injection could result in this chronic inflammatory process.** | Arachnoiditis. |
| **A patient with hilar adenopathy develops lower back pain, numbness of the perineum, bladder and bowel incontinence, and decreased anal sphincter tone.** | Sarcoidosis, complicated by cauda equina syndrome. |
| **A patient is awoken in the middle of the night with sudden-onset severe "shooting" pain that radiates from the right shoulder to the arm, which is followed a few days later by weakness of the right arm, and is found to have a "winged" scapula.** | Neuralgic amyotrophy (ie, Parsonage-Turner syndrome). |

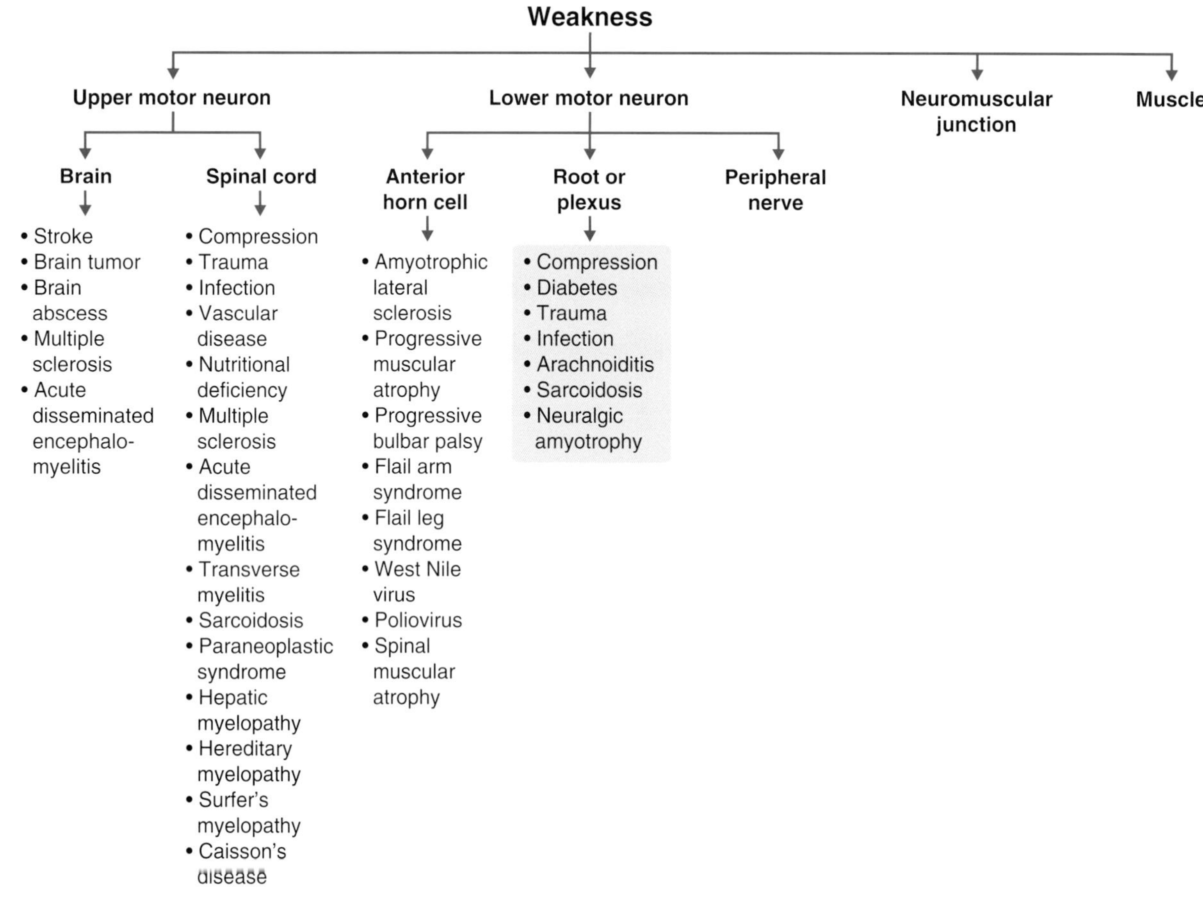

**What are the compressive causes of neuropathy involving the nerve root or plexus?**

Compressive causes of neuropathy involving the nerve root or plexus include degenerative disease (eg, osteoarthritis), spondylolisthesis, spinal stenosis, disc herniation, benign or malignant tumor, syringomyelia, epidural abscess, hematoma, and thoracic outlet obstruction.

**What physical examination maneuver is highly specific for compressive cervical radiculopathy?**

Spurling test is specific for compressive cervical radiculopathy. The patient's head is extended and rotated toward the side of the pain, then downward pressure is applied on the top of the head. The test is positive if symptoms in the arm are reproduced in a radicular distribution.[17]

**What are the characteristics of diabetic lumbosacral radiculoplexus neuropathy?**

Diabetic patients can develop a variety of disorders of the peripheral nervous system. Diabetic lumbosacral radiculoplexus neuropathy (ie, diabetic amyotrophy) refers to a distinct neuropathy that involves the lumbosacral radiculoplexus. Affected patients tend to be older with relatively well-controlled or undiagnosed diabetes. Pain starts in the low back or hip and spreads unilaterally to the thigh and knee. It is described as deep and aching and tends to be worse at night. Later, weakness and atrophy develop in the pelvic girdle and thigh muscles. The pain generally begins to subside spontaneously after several days. Motor recovery virtually always occurs, but usually requires months to years.[2]

**What are the iatrogenic causes of traumatic root or plexus injury?**

Iatrogenesis accounts for up to 10% of brachial plexopathies. Root or plexus injury can occur during surgery (from direct injury or surgical positioning), attempted reduction of shoulder dislocations, anesthetic regional blocks, and radiation therapy.[18]

**What are the infectious causes of root or plexus pathology?**

Infectious causes of root or plexus pathology include *Mycobacterium tuberculosis* (ie, Pott's disease), varicella-zoster virus, cytomegalovirus, syphilis, Lyme disease, schistosomiasis, and strongyloides.[1]

**What imaging finding is associated with arachnoiditis?**

In patients with arachnoiditis, inflammation and subsequent proliferation of connective tissue results in thickening of the arachnoid membrane and eventual obliteration of the subarachnoid space, which is evident on imaging of the spine.[2]

**What are the characteristics of sarcoid radiculopathy?**

Sarcoidosis of the peripheral nervous system most commonly involves the cranial nerves (eg, facial nerve palsy). Polyradiculopathy, which is less common, primarily involves the thoracic and lumbar roots and may improve with systemic glucocorticoid therapy. Laminectomy may be considered for refractory cases.[19]

**What is neuralgic amyotrophy?**

Neuralgic amyotrophy (ie, Parsonage-Turner syndrome) is an acquired clinical syndrome characterized by episodes of neuropathic pain and patchy paresis of the upper extremities. It most often involves the upper part of the brachial plexus, resulting in weakness of the infraspinatus and serratus anterior muscles (leading to a winged scapula). The pathophysiology of this condition is incompletely understood but is thought to be immune-mediated. Most patients recover over the course of a few years, but some will experience chronic pain and motor dysfunction. A rare familial form exists, known as hereditary neuralgic amyotrophy. Patients with inherited neuralgic amyotrophy tend to be younger, experience more frequent recurrent attacks, and are more likely to develop nerve involvement outside the brachial plexus.[20]

## WEAKNESS RELATED TO LOWER MOTOR NEURON LESIONS OF THE PERIPHERAL NERVE

### What are the causes of weakness related to the peripheral nerve?

**A single peripheral nerve is affected.**

Mononeuropathy.

**At least 2 noncontiguous individual nerves are affected.**

Mononeuritis multiplex.

**Usually characterized by a generalized neuropathy affecting many peripheral nerves in a symmetric, length-dependent fashion.**

Polyneuropathy.

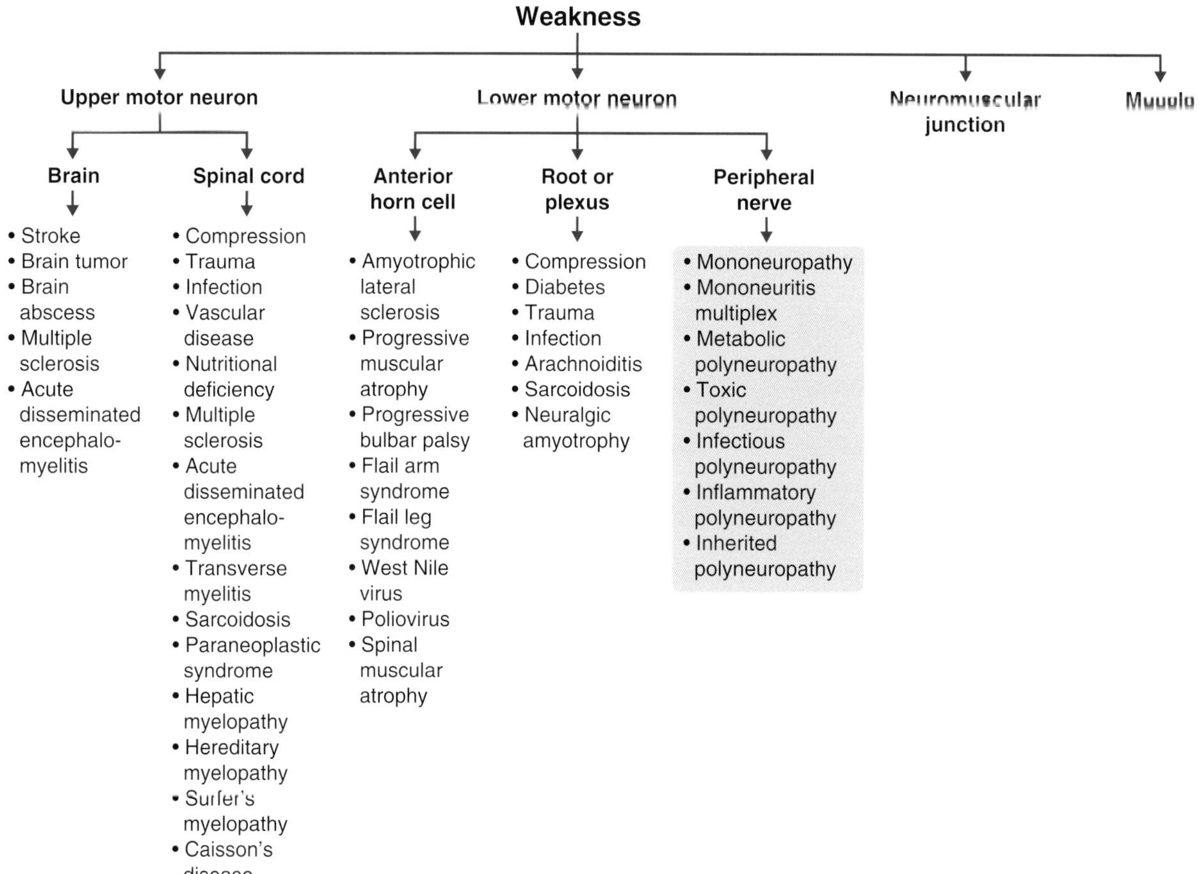


**What physical findings are present in the setting of mononeuropathy involving the median nerve?**

Mononeuropathy involving the median nerve (ie, carpal tunnel syndrome) is characterized by the presence of neuropathic symptoms and signs along the distribution of the median nerve (ie, involving the thumb, index, middle finger, and the radial side of the ring finger). Tinel's test (tapping the volar surface of the wrist) or Phalen's test (flexion of the wrist for >60 seconds) may be positive for pain or paresthesias in the distribution of the median nerve. Atrophy of the thenar eminence and weakness and atrophy of the abductor pollicis brevis and opponens pollicis become evident in advanced cases.[21]

**What are the causes of mononeuritis multiplex?**

Mononeuritis multiplex describes the presence of neuropathy involving 2 or more noncontiguous individual nerves. More than one-half of all cases are caused by involvement of the vasa nervorum by a systemic vasculitis such as polyarteritis nodosa. Other causes include diabetes mellitus, Lyme disease, sarcoidosis, HIV infection, and leprosy.[2]

*For a detailed discussion of polyneuropathy, see chapter 41, Polyneuropathy.*

## WEAKNESS RELATED TO DISORDERS OF THE NEUROMUSCULAR JUNCTION

**What is the neuromuscular junction?**

The NMJ is the interface between a single nerve fiber and its corresponding muscle fiber; it is the junction where electrical activity of the nerve is translated into muscle contraction (Figure 44-7).[2]

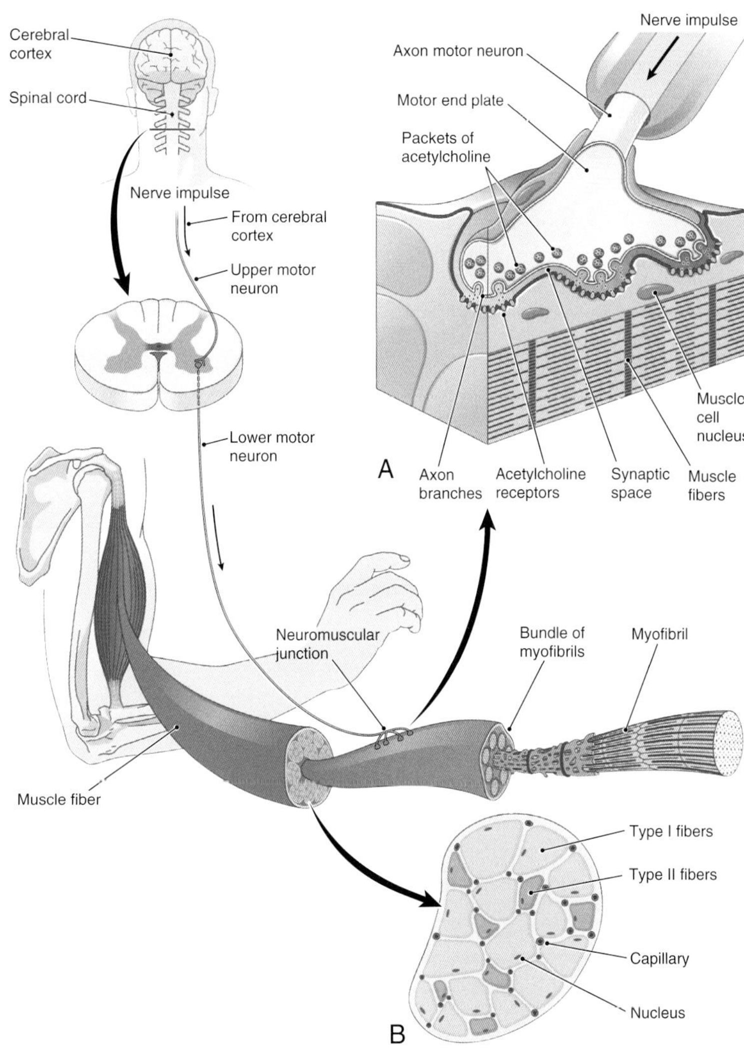


**Figure 44-7.** Relationship between the upper motor neuron, lower motor neuron, neuromuscular junction, and muscle. A, Detail of the neuromuscular junction. B, Detail of skeletal muscle. (Adapted from McConnell TH. *The Nature of Disease Pathology for the Health Professions*, 2nd ed. Philadelphia, PA: Wolters Kluwer Health, 2017.)

**Which molecule is primarily involved in the communication between nerve and muscle?**

Acetylcholine (ACh) is the primary neurotransmitter of the NMJ.[2]

**What triggers the release of acetylcholine from the nerve terminal to the synaptic cleft?**

The arrival of an axonal action potential triggers several steps that ultimately result in the release of ACh into the synaptic cleft via an exocytotic process.[2]

**How does acetylcholine stimulate muscle action?**

After ACh is released into the synaptic cleft, it binds to receptors on the postsynaptic membrane, which triggers depolarization, entry of calcium ions, and generation of an action potential in the muscle membrane, leading to contraction of the muscle.[2]

**What enzyme is involved in hydrolyzing bound acetylcholine?**

ACh is hydrolyzed by acetylcholinesterase. This serves to terminate the action potential, allowing for sequential muscle activation.[2]

## What are the causes of weakness related to the neuromuscular junction?

A young woman presents with weakness that worsens toward the end of the day and is found to have a mediastinal mass.

Myasthenia gravis associated with thymoma.

A 74-year-old man with small cell lung cancer presents with fluctuating weakness.

Lambert-Eaton syndrome.

Bacteria, ticks, snakes, lizards, spiders, scorpions, plants, and insecticides.

Toxins.

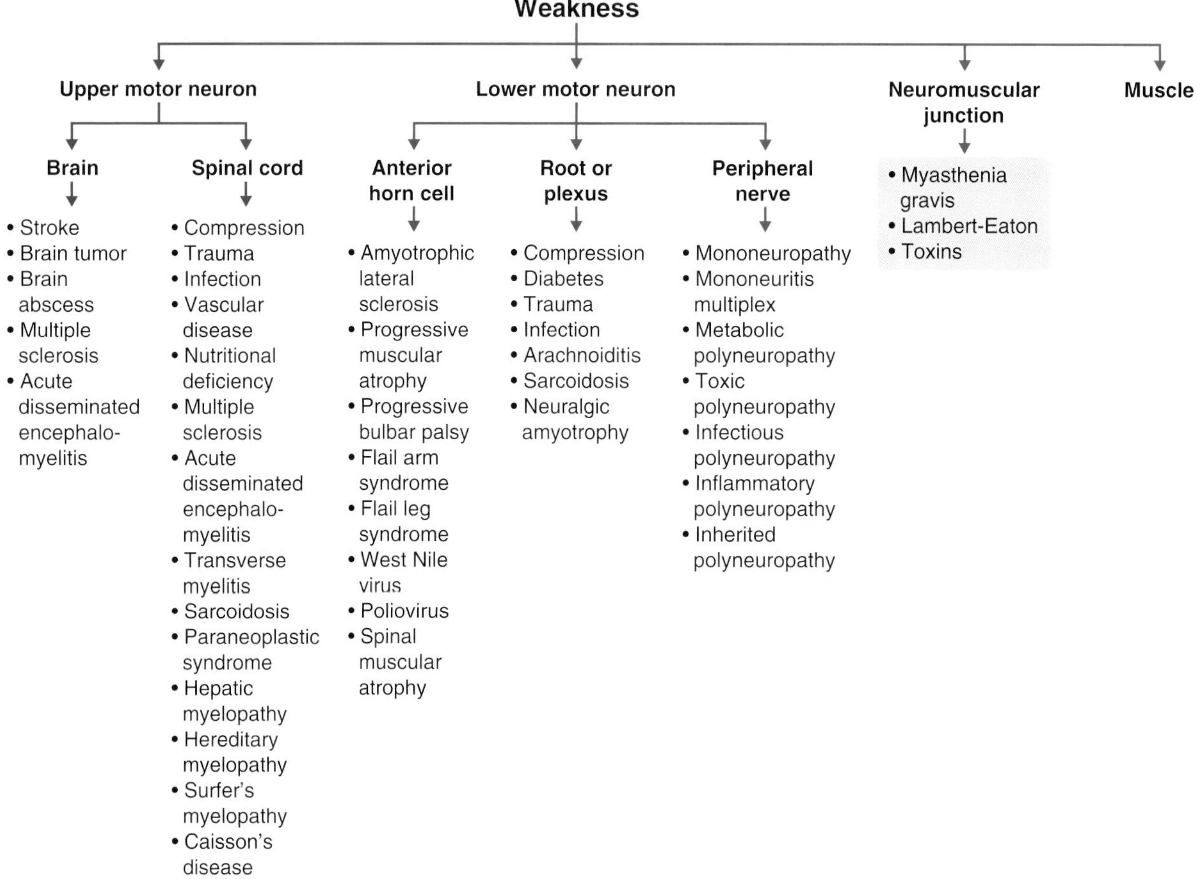


What physical finding is characteristic of myasthenia gravis?

Myasthenia gravis is the most common disorder of the NMJ. It is an autoimmune condition in which ACh receptors are blocked or destroyed, resulting in impaired neuromuscular transmission. The hallmark clinical manifestation of myasthenia gravis is weakness that presents or worsens with repetitive activity (ie, fatigability). The muscles of the eyes, face, jaw, throat, and neck are often the first to be affected, resulting in manifestations such as diplopia, ptosis, dysphagia, difficulty chewing, and dysarthria. Although the course can be variable, disease activity typically begins intermittently and becomes more persistent over time. Pharmacologic management includes anticholinesterases and immunosuppressants (eg, glucocorticoids). Other therapeutic modalities include plasma exchange and thymectomy.[2]

What physical finding is characteristic of Lambert-Eaton syndrome?

Lambert-Eaton syndrome is a disorder of the NMJ that is strongly associated with small cell lung cancer. It is caused by the presence of autoantibodies that result in the functional loss of voltage-gated calcium channels on the presynaptic motor nerve terminal. Muscles of the trunk, shoulder girdle, pelvic girdle, and lower extremities are disproportionately affected. Weakness that improves with repetition (the opposite of myasthenia gravis) is characteristic of Lambert-Eaton syndrome.[2]

What are the typical clinical manifestations of botulism? — Within 12 to 36 hours of exposure to botulinum toxin (usually by ingestion), patients experience nausea, vomiting, and anorexia. The initial neurologic manifestations include blurred vision and diplopia related to ptosis, strabismus, and extraocular muscle palsies. This is followed quickly by other bulbar manifestations including voice changes, dysarthria, and dysphagia. Progressive weakness of the face, neck, trunk, and extremities are usually the last manifestations.[2]

Which ticks are most commonly responsible for dysfunction of the neuromuscular junction? — Ticks that cause NMJ dysfunction vary by region. For example, in Canada and the northwestern United States, the most common offender is the wood tick *Dermacentor andersoni*, whereas in the southeastern United States, it is the dog tick *Dermacentor variabilis*.[2]

Which spider is most commonly associated with dysfunction of the neuromuscular junction? — Venom from the black widow spider (*Latrodectus*) can cause NMJ dysfunction.[2]

Which insecticides are most commonly associated with dysfunction of the neuromuscular junction? — Exposure to organophosphates and carbamates can result in NMJ dysfunction.[22]



## WEAKNESS RELATED TO MYOPATHY

What is a muscle fiber? — Muscle fibers are multinucleated cells that vary in length and diameter. Each muscle fiber receives innervation from a terminal branch of an axon originating from an anterior horn cell in the spinal cord or the motor nuclei of a cranial nerve in the brainstem. A single muscle is composed of thousands of fibers (see Figure 44-7).[2]

What are the most common symptoms and signs of myopathy? — Symptoms of myopathy may include weakness (most frequent), pain, spasm, cramping, twitching, myotonia, and a change in muscle size (usually atrophy).[2]

Which electrolyte is particularly important in regulating muscle contraction? — The regulation of muscle contraction is principally dependent on calcium.[2]

What are the 2 main contractile proteins in muscle? — Actin and myosin are the main contractile proteins in muscle.[2]

What is the source of chemical energy for muscle contraction? — Adenosine triphosphate (ATP) provides the chemical energy for muscle contraction.[2]

What enzyme, found in high concentrations within muscle cells, can be an important serologic marker of myopathy? — Creatine kinase (CK) can be found in high concentrations in the serum of patients with myopathy.[2]

### What are the myopathic causes of weakness?

A 47-year-old woman presents with lower extremity discomfort and weakness a few weeks after starting a medication for hypercholesterolemia. — Statin-induced myopathy.

The elevation of aspartate aminotransferase and alanine aminotransferase in a ratio >2:1 may be a clue to the underlying diagnosis. — Alcohol-induced myopathy.

An electrolyte disturbance associated with primary hyperaldosteronism (ie, Conn's syndrome). — Hypokalemia.

Prolonged immobility. — Deconditioning.

A 50-year-old woman with central obesity, abdominal striae, and progressive proximal muscle weakness. — Cushing's syndrome.

**A condition often associated with the intensive care unit.**

Critical illness myopathy.

**Following a tropical storm in Thailand, a young woman develops cola-colored urine and weakness after being removed from her damaged home.**

Rhabdomyolysis.

**A patient develops strabismus, diplopia, and dysarthria after consuming undercooked pork.**

Trichinosis.

**An immune-mediated condition.**

Inflammatory myopathy.

**A progressive hereditary degenerative muscle disease.**

Muscular dystrophy.

**Disorders of the breakdown, use, and storage of the sources of energy for muscle contraction.**

Metabolic myopathy.

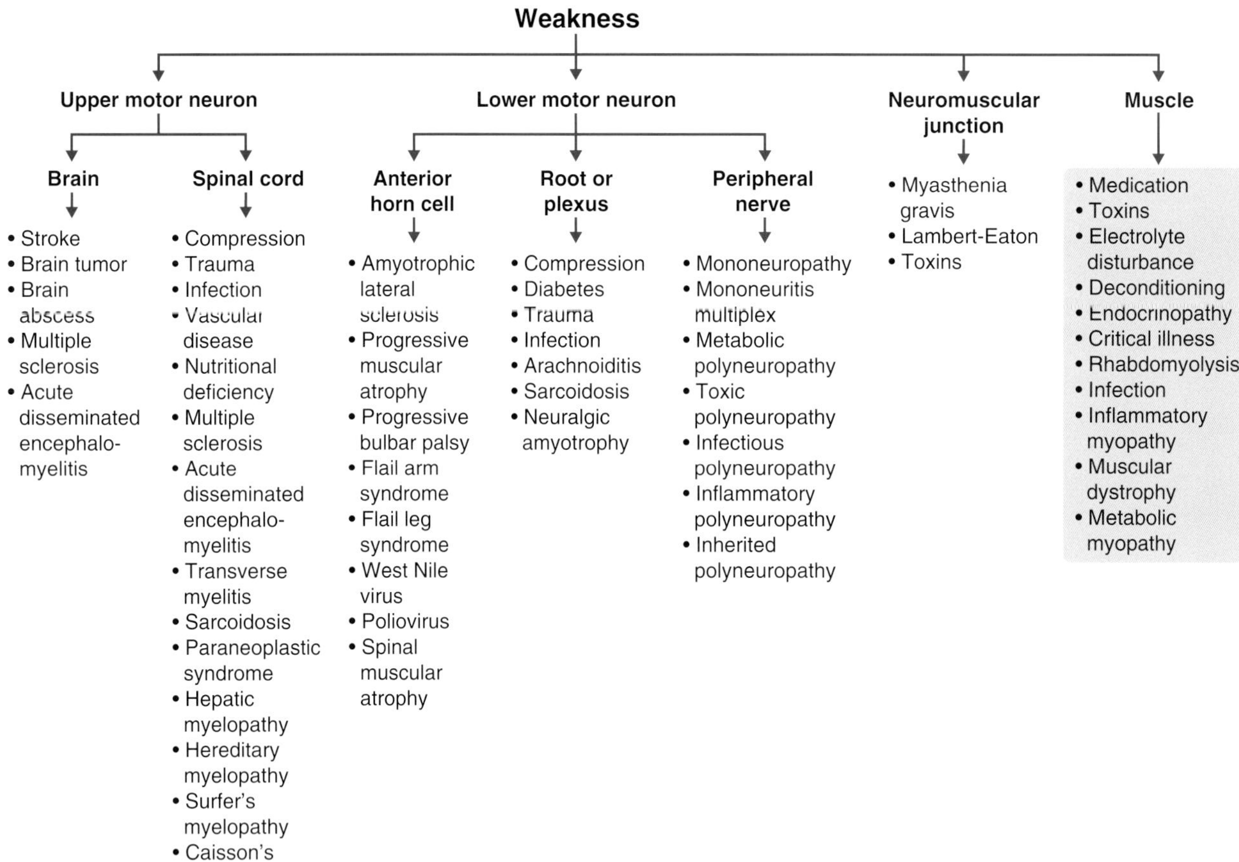


**What are the clinical hallmarks of medication-induced myopathy?**

Medication-induced myopathy typically occurs in patients without preexisting muscular symptoms. It is suggested by a delay in the development of symptoms after exposure to a causative agent and the complete or partial improvement of symptoms after withdrawal of the agent. The absence of an alternative cause of myopathy is additionally supportive. The prognosis of medication-induced myopathy is variable, mirroring the wide-ranging mechanisms and degrees of severity of the condition. However, most cases completely or at least partially resolve after discontinuation of the offending agent.[2]

**What toxins are associated with myopathy?**

Toxins associated with myopathy include alcohol, cocaine, amphetamines, heroin, mushroom poisoning (eg, *Amanita phalloides*), and exogenous or endogenous glucocorticoids.[2]

**Which electrolyte disturbances are associated with myopathy?**

Numerous electrolyte disturbances are associated with myopathy, including hyper/hyponatremia, hyper/hypokalemia, hypophosphatemia, hypocalcemia, and hypomagnesemia.[23]

**What is the timing of onset of deconditioning during the course of inactivity?**

Deconditioning occurs within days to weeks following a sudden decrease in activity. It appears to be primarily mediated through a downregulation of protein synthesis resulting in loss of muscle mass.[24]

**Which endocrinopathies can cause myopathy?**

Endocrinopathies associated with myopathy include hypothyroidism, hyperthyroidism, Cushing's syndrome, acromegaly, and others that are associated with electrolyte disturbances (eg, primary hyperaldosteronism).[2]

**How can critical illness polyneuropathy be distinguished from critical illness myopathy?**

Electromyography can be used to localize a lesion and distinguish neuropathy from myopathy. In some cases, both conditions may be present. Most cases of critical illness myopathy develop in association with the administration of high doses of glucocorticoids, but it can occur in patients with sepsis and shock who are not exposed to steroids.[2]

**What is rhabdomyolysis?**

Rhabdomyolysis occurs when there is rapid skeletal muscle breakdown (eg, from a crush injury), manifesting with painful and sometimes weak muscles, elevated serum CK, myoglobinuria, and acute kidney injury.[2]

**What are the infectious causes of myopathy?**

Infectious causes of myopathy include parasites (eg, trichinosis, toxoplasmosis), viruses (eg, HIV, HTLV-I, influenza), bacteria (eg, *Staphylococcus aureus*), and rarely, fungi.[25]

**What are the inflammatory myopathies?**

The main 3 inflammatory myopathies are dermatomyositis (DM), polymyositis (PM), and inclusion body myositis (IBM). Others include eosinophilic myositis, vasculitis, immune-mediated necrotizing myopathy, granulomatous myositis (eg, sarcoidosis), myositis related to graft-versus-host disease, and myositis related to connective tissue disease (eg, systemic lupus erythematosus).

**How can a handshake provide a clue to the diagnosis of myotonic dystrophy?**

Myotonic dystrophy, which is the most common adult muscular dystrophy, is associated with prolonged failure of relaxation after muscle contraction, called myotonia. This delayed relaxation can be appreciated on shaking hands with an affected individual.[2]

**Which energy substrates are necessary for the sustenance of normal muscular activity?**

During early exercise, glucose is the main source of energy; when glycogen stores become depleted, the principle source of energy comes from the oxidation of fatty acids.[2]

## Case Summary

A 52-year-old man presents with progressive proximal muscle weakness and is found to have abnormal skin findings.

***What is the most likely cause of weakness in this patient?***

Dermatomyositis.

NEUROLOGY

## BONUS QUESTIONS

***What is the primary phenotypic difference between dermatomyositis and polymyositis?***

DM is characterized by involvement of the skin (ie, dermatitis).[2]

***What is the significance of the skin findings in this case?***

The discoloration around the patient's eyes in this case (see Figure 44-1) is known as a "heliotrope" rash (ie, lilac-colored change in the skin over the eyelids and around the eyes, sometimes with edema). The [illegible] papules over the dorsal joints of the hands (see Figure 44-2) are known as Gottron's papules. Other skin findings characteristic of DM include an erythematous rash over the neck and chest, known as the "V" sign (when present over the shoulders and upper arms, it is known as the "shawl" sign), cutaneous calcifications, and erythroderma.[2]

***What is the timing of onset of dermatitis relative to myositis in patients with dermatomyositis?***

The skin findings of DM typically precede the muscle findings.[2]

***What systemic conditions are associated with dermatomyositis and polymyositis?***

DM and PM are often associated with connective tissue diseases (eg, rheumatoid arthritis), malignancy, and other autoimmune conditions (eg, myasthenia gravis). Antisynthetase syndrome occurs in some patients with DM or PM and is characterized by a constellation of clinical manifestations, including fever, interstitial lung disease, inflammatory myopathy, polyarticular inflammatory arthritis, Raynaud's phenomenon, and mechanic's hands (see Figure 47-4).[2,26]

***Which malignancies are most often linked to dermatomyositis and polymyositis?***

Underlying malignancies most often associated with DM and PM in men are those of the lung and colon; in women, breast and ovarian malignancies are most common.[2]

***What are the epidemiologic differences between the 3 main inflammatory myopathies (dermatomyositis, polymyositis, and inclusion body myositis)?***

DM equally affects adults and children with a propensity for females in adulthood but an equal propensity for the sexes in childhood; most patients with PM are adults (30-60 years of age), and there is a propensity for women; IBM occurs most commonly in patients over 50 years of age, and there is a 3:1 predominance of males:females.[2]

***What laboratory tests can be helpful in the diagnosis of the inflammatory myopathies, including dermatomyositis?***

Serum levels of muscle enzymes, such as CK and aldolase, are often elevated in patients with inflammatory myopathy. Various antibodies may also be present in patients with PM or DM, particularly in the setting of an underlying connective tissue disease (eg, anti-histidyl-tRNA synthetase [anti-Jo-1] in patients with antisynthetase syndrome).[2]

***What supplementary tests can be helpful in the diagnosis of the inflammatory myopathies?***

EMG, MRI, and biopsy of the muscle are often helpful in establishing the diagnosis of inflammatory myopathy.[2]

***What is the treatment of choice for patients with acute inflammatory myopathy?***

Systemic glucocorticoids are considered first-line treatment for acute PM and DM. IBM does not consistently respond to treatment with glucocorticoids.[2]

***What is the prognosis of inflammatory myopathy?***

PM and DM are typically responsive to glucocorticoids and prognosis is generally favorable, except in cases associated with underlying malignancy or connective tissue disease. IBM typically progresses over many years, sometimes quite slowly, but most patients become disabled over time.[2]

## KEY POINTS

- Weakness is defined as a reduction in power generated by muscle.
- Fatigue and asthenia are often confused with weakness, but sometimes these conditions coexist.
- Weakness can be caused by disorders of the upper motor neuron, lower motor neuron, neuromuscular junction, or muscle.
- UMN lesions occur proximal to the anterior horn cell and predominantly involve the extensors and abductors of the upper limbs and the flexors of the lower limbs, and affect proximal > distal muscles.
- UMN weakness is associated with the following physical findings: little to no atrophy, absence of fasciculations, increased tone (spasticity), hyperreflexia, and positive Babinski reflex.
- UMN lesions can involve the brain or spinal cord.
- LMN lesions involve the structures distal to and including the anterior horn cell and affect distal > proximal muscles.
- LMN weakness is associated with the following physical findings: severe atrophy, fasciculations, diminished tone, diminished reflexes, and absent Babinski reflex.
- LMN lesions can involve the anterior horn cell, nerve root or plexus, or peripheral nerve.
- NMJ disorders present with variable distributions of weakness.
- The prototypic cause of NMJ disease is myasthenia gravis, which is characterized by fatigable weakness.
- Myopathic weakness tends to be symmetric and affect proximal > distal muscles.
- Myopathic weakness is associated with the following physical findings: mild atrophy, absence of fasciculations, normal or diminished tone, normal or diminished reflexes, and absent Babinski reflex.



## REFERENCES


1. Longo DL, Fauci AS, Kasper DL, Hauser SL, Jameson JL, Loscalzo J, eds. *Harrison's Principles of Internal Medicine*. 18th ed. New York, NY: McGraw-Hill; 2012.
2. Ropper AH, Samuels MA, Klein JP, eds. *Adam and Victor's Principles of Neurology*. 10th ed. China: McGraw-Hill Education; 2014.
3. Sapira JD. *The Art & Science of Bedside Diagnosis*. Baltimore, Maryland, USA: Urban and Schwarzenberg; 1990.
4. Habek M. Evaluation of brainstem involvement in multiple sclerosis. *Expert Rev Neurother*. 2013;13(3):299-311.
5. Alexander M, Murthy JM. Acute disseminated encephalomyelitis: treatment guidelines. *Ann Indian Acad Neurol*. 2011;14(suppl 1): S60-S64.
6. Devivo MJ. Epidemiology of traumatic spinal cord injury: trends and future implications. *Spinal Cord*. 2012;50(5):365-372.
7. Berger JR, Sabet A. Infectious myelopathies. *Semin Neurol*. 2002;22(2):133-142.
8. Bot JC, Barkhof F, Polman CH, et al. Spinal cord abnormalities in recently diagnosed MS patients: added value of spinal MRI examination. *Neurology*. 2004;62(2):226-233.
9. Ketelslegers IA, Visser IE, Neuteboom RF, Boon M, Catsman-Berrevoets CE, Hintzen RQ. Disease course and outcome of acute disseminated encephalomyelitis is more severe in adults than in children. *Mult Scler*. 2011;17(4):441-448.
10. Frohman EM, Wingerchuk DM. Clinical practice. Transverse myelitis. *N Engl J Med*. 2010;363(6):564-572.
11. Nardone R, Buratti T, Oliviero A, Lochmann A, Tezzon F. Corticospinal involvement in patients with a portosystemic shunt due to liver cirrhosis: a MEP study. *J Neurol*. 2006;253(1):81-85.
12. Ginsberg L. Disorders of the spinal cord and roots. *Pract Neurol*. 2011;11(4):259-267.
13. Yang H, Liu M, Li X, Cui B, Fang J, Cui L. Neurophysiological differences between flail arm syndrome and amyotrophic lateral sclerosis. *PLoS One*. 2015;10(6):e0127601.
14. Wijesekera LC, Mathers S, Talman P, et al. Natural history and clinical features of the flail arm and flail leg ALS variants. *Neurology*. 2009;72(12):1087-1094.
15. Leis AA, Stokic DS. Neuromuscular manifestations of west nile virus infection. *Front Neurol*. 2012;3:37.
16. Howard RS. Poliomyelitis and the postpolio syndrome. *BMJ*. 2005;330(7503):1314-1318.
17. Caridi JM, Pumberger M, Hughes AP. Cervical radiculopathy: a review. *HSS J*. 2011;7(3):265-272.
18. Wilbourn AJ. Iatrogenic nerve injuries. *Neurol Clin*. 1998;16(1):55-82.
19. Koffman B, Junck L, Elias SB, Feit HW, Levine SR. Polyradiculopathy in sarcoidosis. *Muscle Nerve*. 1999;22(5):608-613.
20. van Alfen N, van Engelen BG. The clinical spectrum of neuralgic amyotrophy in 246 cases. *Brain*. 2006;129(Pt 2):438-450.
21. Ibrahim I, Khan WS, Goddard N, Smitham P. Carpal tunnel syndrome: a review of the recent literature. *Open Orthop J*. 2012;6:69-76.
22. Jokanovic M. Medical treatment of acute poisoning with organophosphorus and carbamate pesticides. *Toxicol Lett*. 2009;190(2): 107-115.

23. Yu J. Endocrine disorders and the neurologic manifestations. *Ann Pediatr Endocrinol Metab*. 2014;19(4):184-190.
24. Berry MJ, Morris PE. Early exercise rehabilitation of muscle weakness in acute respiratory failure patients. *Exerc Sport Sci Rev*. 2013;41(4):208-215.
25. Crum-Cianflone NF. Bacterial, fungal, parasitic, and viral myositis. *Clin Microbiol Rev*. 2008;21(3):473-494.
26. Katzap E, Barilla-LaBarca ML, Marder G. Antisynthetase syndrome. *Curr Rheumatol Rep*. 2011;13(3):175-181.

SECTION 11

# Pulmonology

## Chapter 45

# HEMOPTYSIS

### Case: A 29-year-old woman with a diastolic murmur

A 29-year-old woman who emigrated from Mexico at 10 years of age presents to the emergency department with sudden-onset severe abdominal pain. Three days prior, the patient experienced transient hemiparesthesias and dysarthria. Cross-sectional imaging of the abdomen (Figure 45-1) and chest (Figure 45-2) are shown.

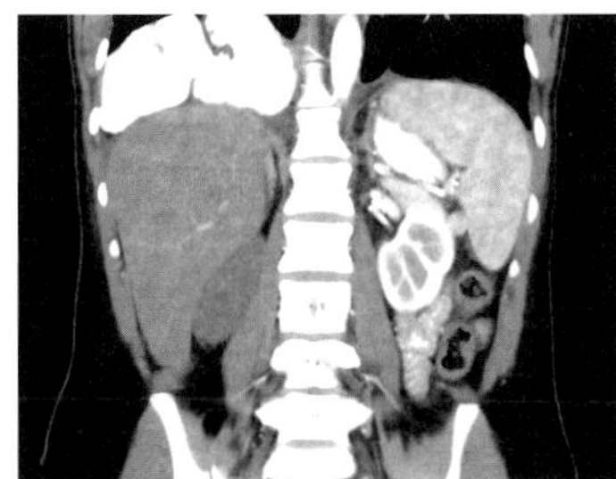

**Figure 45-1.**

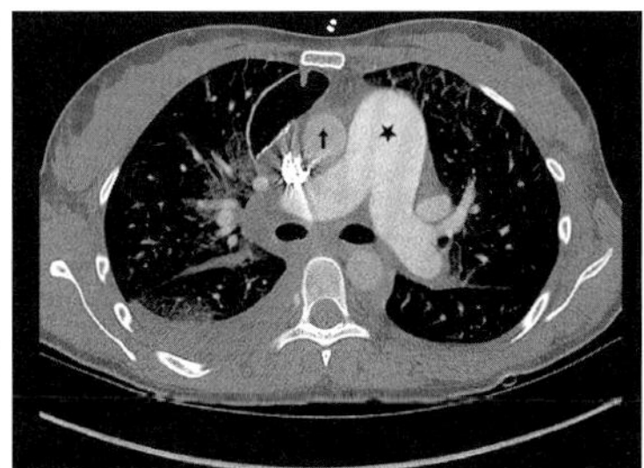

**Figure 45-2.**

The patient is taken for emergency right renal artery embolectomy. After the procedure, she develops acute-onset dyspnea, hypoxemia, and hemoptysis. The sputum is bright red in color with a volume of one-half cup over the course of an hour.

Cardiac auscultation reveals a regular rhythm with a pronounced S1, an extra sound just after S2 best heard with the diaphragm of the stethoscope over the apex, and a rumbling diastolic murmur with presystolic accentuation best heard with the bell of the stethoscope over the apex. Phonocardiograms of the heart sounds are shown in Figure 45-3. *For audio of the heart sounds in this case, see the associated reference.*[1]

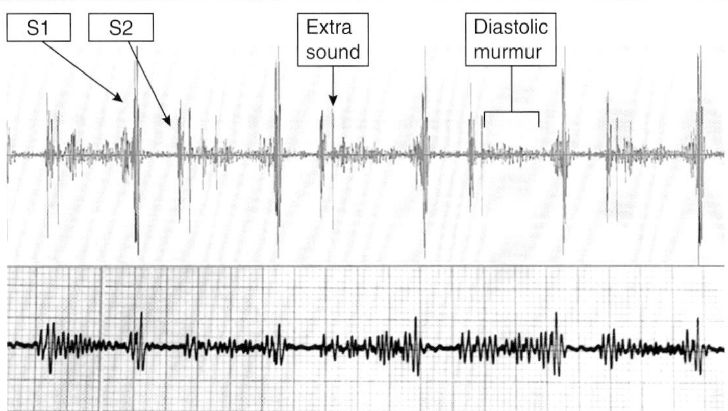


**Figure 45-3.** Phonocardiogram from a contemporary electronic stethoscope (top). Phonocardiogram from a mid-20th century antique phonocardiograph (bottom). (Reprinted with permission from Oehler AC, Sullivan PD, Mansoor AM. Mitral stenosis. *BMJ Case Rep*. 2017;2017.)

***What is the most likely cause of hemoptysis in this patient?***

**What is hemoptysis?**

Hemoptysis is the expectoration of blood produced within the lower respiratory tract, anywhere from the trachea to the alveoli.[2]

**What conditions can mimic hemoptysis and should always be considered in a patient who expectorates blood?**

Hematemesis, expectorated blood from a source originating in the upper gastrointestinal tract, and bleeding from the upper respiratory tract are often confused for hemoptysis. Epistaxis with drainage down the throat into the lungs is common, underscoring the importance of nasal examination in patients with suspected hemoptysis.

**What historical features can help distinguish hemoptysis from hematemesis?**

The following features are suggestive of hematemesis: nausea and vomiting; preexisting gastric or hepatic disease; and brown, black, or coffee ground appearance of the expectorated material. The following are suggestive of hemoptysis: absence of nausea and vomiting, preexisting lung disease associated with hemoptysis (eg, bronchiectasis), and frothy, bright red, liquid, or clotted appearance of the expectorated material.[3]

**Which arteries supply blood to the lungs?**

The pulmonary arteries supply 99% of blood to the lungs, while the bronchial arteries supply the remaining 1%. The pulmonary arteries are involved in gas exchange, while the bronchial arteries supply circulation to the airways, lung parenchyma, and pulmonary arteries (Figure 45-4). Capillary anastomoses between the 2 systems exist.[4]

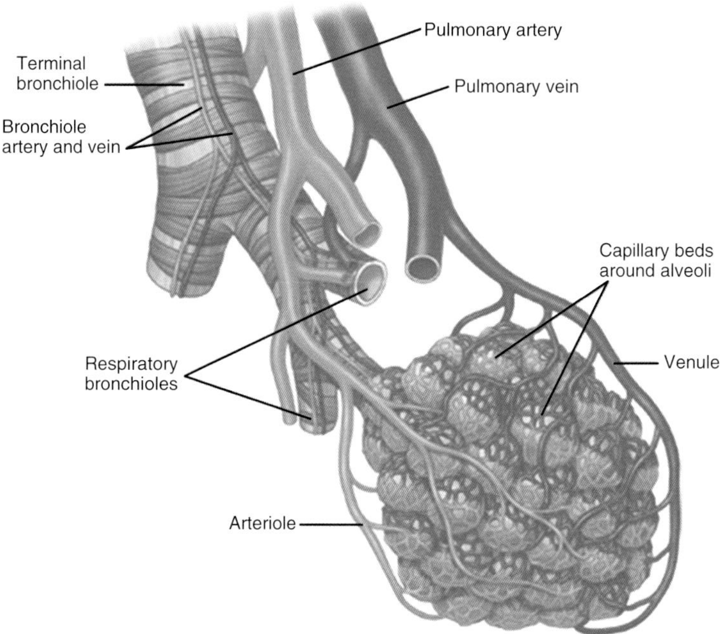


**Figure 45-4.** Blood supply of the lungs. The bronchial circulation contributes to the pulmonary microvasculature by supplying blood to the bronchovascular bundles, pulmonary interstitium, and the vasa vasorum of the pulmonary arteries and veins. (From Saremi F. *Perfusion Imaging in Clinical Practice: A Multimodality Approach to Tissue Perfusion Analysis*. Philadelphia, PA: Wolters Kluwer; 2015.)

**Which arterial system is involved in hemoptysis?**

Both the pulmonary arteries and the bronchial arteries may be involved in hemopytsis, but the higher-pressure bronchial arteries are the most common source of massive hemoptysis (around 90% of cases) compared with the lower-pressure pulmonary arteries (around 5% of cases); pulmonary and bronchial capillaries and veins cause the remaining cases.[4]

**How is the severity of hemoptysis defined?**

The severity of hemoptysis is usually graded as massive or submassive. No universal criteria have been established, but volume thresholds between 100 and 1000 mL over a 24-hour period have been suggested to define massive hemoptysis. A reasonable threshold to use is 300 mL/d. *Quantification of hemoptysis is not always possible or practical, underscoring the importance of clinical judgment.*[4]

**Why is it important to determine the quantity of hemoptysis?**

Massive hemoptysis is a life-threatening condition with a significant mortality rate when it is not promptly managed. The first step is to maintain a safe airway and then identify the source of bleeding with chest imaging and/or bronchoscopy. The patient should be positioned such that the side of bleeding is gravity-dependent (ie, bleeding side down) until definitive management occurs (usually arterial endovascular embolization or surgery).[4]

**What is the role of conventional chest radiography in patients with hemoptysis?**

Chest radiography is important in the initial workup of hemoptysis because it is widely available, inexpensive, and prompt. The sensitivity of conventional radiography for localizing the source of bleeding is approximately 50%.[4]

**What is the role of computed tomography (CT) imaging in patients with hemoptysis?**

In patients with hemoptysis, CT imaging with intravenous contrast is more sensitive than conventional radiography for localizing the source of bleeding. It also has the advantage of providing a more detailed evaluation of lung anatomy and may be able to diagnose the underlying etiology (eg, bronchiectasis).[4]

**What is the role of bronchoscopy in patients with hemoptysis?**

In patients with hemoptysis, bronchoscopy is complementary to chest imaging in detecting the site and underlying cause of bleeding. Advantages of bronchoscopy include the ability to localize endobronchial lesions, although massive bleeding may obscure a bleeding site. Sampling for culture and histopathology are additional advantages. Sometimes bleeding can be controlled with bronchoscopic techniques (eg, cold saline, balloon inflation, or laser coagulation).[4]

**Which 2 systems are involved in most cases of hemoptysis?**

Most cases of hemoptysis involve the cardiovascular or pulmonary systems.

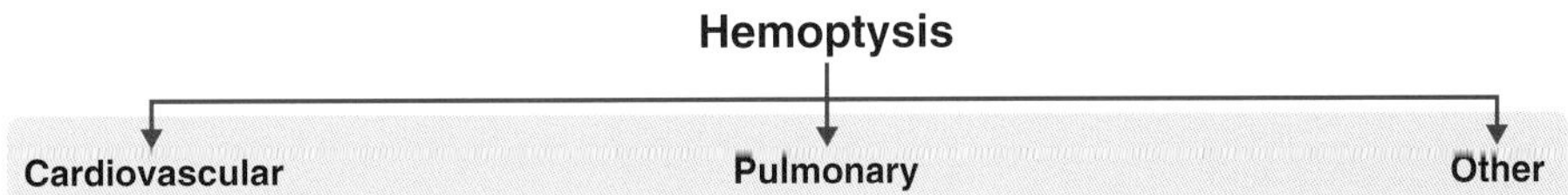


## CARDIOVASCULAR CAUSES OF HEMOPTYSIS

### What are the cardiovascular causes of hemoptysis?

**Acute pulmonary arterial hypertension.**

Pulmonary embolism (PE) and infarction (Figure 45-5).

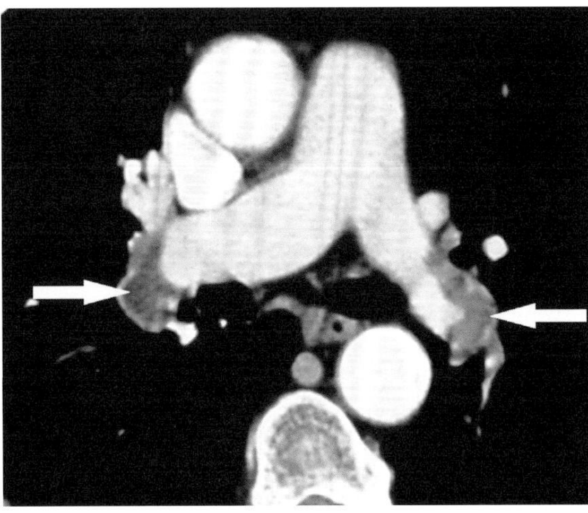

**Figure 45-5.** Contrast-enhanced CT showing bilateral filling defects in the pulmonary arteries (arrows) in a patient with pulmonary embolism. (From Brant WE, Helms CA. *Fundamentals of Diagnostic Radiology*. 4th ed. Philadelphia, PA: Lippincott Williams & Wilkins; 2012.)

**Elevated left atrial pressure leading to rupture of the alveolar capillaries.**

Heart failure.

PULMONOLOGY

**This group of inflammatory conditions often presents with protean manifestations, reflecting the wide range of potential organ system involvement.**

Vasculitis.

**Associated with a murmur on auscultation of the heart.**

Valvular disease.

**A 32-year-old woman with cutaneous telangiectasias and episodes of hemoptysis and epistaxis.**

Arteriovenous malformation (AVM)

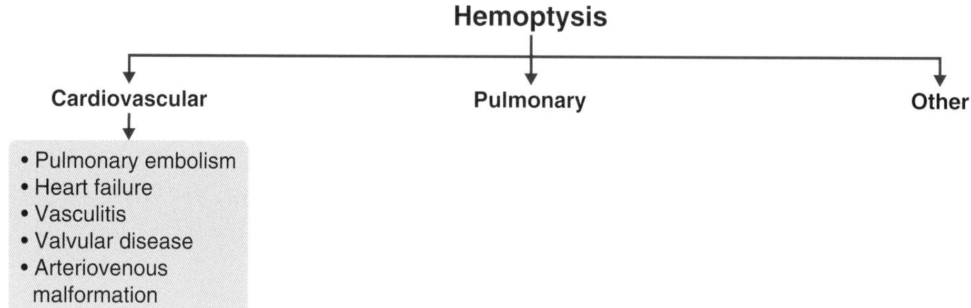


**How common is hemoptysis in patients with pulmonary embolism?**

Hemoptysis is more likely in patients with PE who have an associated pulmonary infarction, but occurs in a minority of patients overall. More common manifestations of PE include dyspnea, pleuritic chest pain, tachypnea, tachycardia, and syncope.[5]

**What are the characteristics of hemoptysis associated with congestive heart failure?**

Hemoptysis caused by congestive heart failure is nonmassive and often described as "pink, frothy" sputum.

**Which vasculitides are associated with hemoptysis?**

Hemoptysis is generally associated with the antineutrophil cytoplasmic antibody–associated small vessel systemic vasculitides, including granulomatosis with polyangiitis (GPA, or Wegener's granulomatosis), microscopic polyangiitis, and eosinophilic granulomatosis with polyangiitis (EGPA, or Churg-Strauss syndrome). Pulmonary capillaritis can also be associated with antiglomerular basement membrane disease (ie, Goodpasture syndrome) and underlying rheumatologic diseases (eg, systemic lupus erythematosus).

**Which valvular lesions are associated with hemoptysis?**

Any valvular lesion that results in left-sided heart failure can lead to hemoptysis via pulmonary venous hypertension. However, 3 lesions can cause hemoptysis via other mechanisms and deserve special attention: tricuspid valve endocarditis, which can result in septic pulmonary emboli; mitral stenosis, which can result in sudden elevation of left atrial pressure; and mitral regurgitation with flail posterior leaflet, which can result in asymmetric right upper lobe pulmonary edema and a focal increase in pulmonary capillary pressure.

**What underlying genetic condition commonly causes pulmonary arteriovenous malformations?**

Hereditary hemorrhagic telangiectasia (HHT, or Osler-Weber-Rendu syndrome) is an autosomal dominant condition characterized by the development of vascular malformations in various organs of the body. Patients most often present with cutaneous telangiectasias (see Figure 40-2) and frequent epistaxis. Some patients develop pulmonary AVMs that are at risk for spontaneous rupture, which can result in massive hemoptysis or hemothorax.

## PULMONARY CAUSES OF HEMOPTYSIS

**The pulmonary causes of hemoptysis can be separated into which 2 anatomic subcategories?**

Pulmonary causes of hemoptysis can involve the airways or parenchyma.

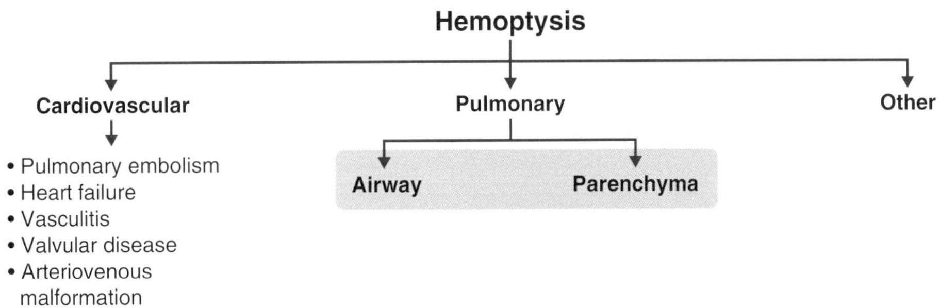


## What are the causes of hemoptysis related to the airways?

**Most commonly caused by a viral or bacterial infection.**

Acute bronchitis.

**Dilation and thickening of the airways on chest imaging (see Figure 20-3).**

Bronchiectasis.

**A 66-year-old man with a history of chronic obstructive pulmonary disease (COPD) and active cigarette use presents with subacute weight loss, night sweats, and hemoptysis.**

Malignancy (eg, bronchogenic carcinoma).

**A 24-year-old man emerges from a bar fight with missing teeth and a new cough.**

Foreign body aspiration.

**A patient develops hemoptysis 2 hours after bronchoscopy with endobronchial biopsy.**

Iatrogenic.

**Communication between blood vessel and airway.**

Bronchovascular fistula.

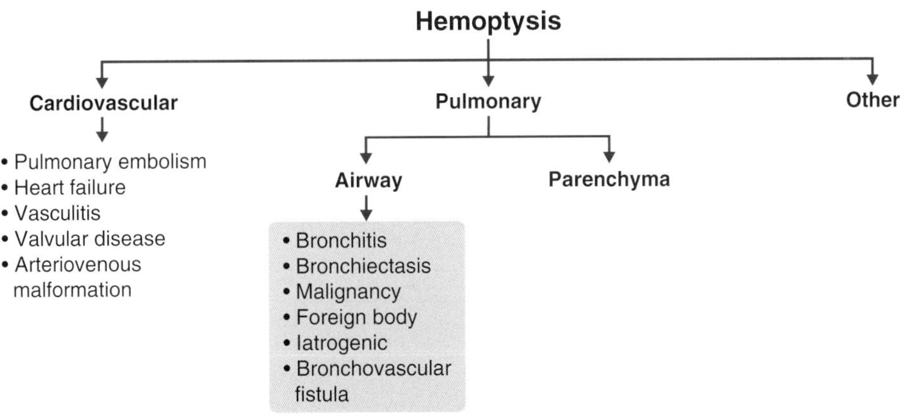


**How often is bronchitis the cause of hemoptysis?**

Acute bronchitis accounts for up to one-half of cases of hemoptysis in the industrialized world. In addition to infection, inhalation of various gases, fumes, or dusts (ie, inhalation injury) can cause acute bronchitis.[6,7]

**What are the mechanisms of hemoptysis in the setting of bronchiectasis?**

Hemoptysis results from denudation and proliferative neovascularization of the airway mucosa that occurs in patients with bronchiectasis. Airway dilation, which brings the bronchial arteries closer to the mucosal surface, is a contributing factor.[2]

**How often is hemoptysis part of the initial presentation in patients with primary lung cancer?**

Only around 10% of patients with primary lung cancer present with hemoptysis. It is more likely to occur in cancers arising centrally, such as squamous cell carcinoma and small cell lung cancer. Massive hemoptysis can occur in these patients when there is erosion into the hilar blood vessels. Endobronchial tumors, such as carcinoid, can also cause hemoptysis.[2]

**How can the presence of an aspirated foreign body be confirmed?**

Depending on the foreign body, conventional chest radiography can confirm aspiration in most cases. CT is more sensitive for small objects. Bronchoscopy can be both diagnostic and therapeutic.[8]

**What are the iatrogenic causes of hemoptysis?**

Hemoptysis can be caused by bronchoscopy with endobronchial or transbronchial biopsy, vascular injury related to catheters, percutaneous lung biopsy, airway stents, and bone marrow transplantation (BMT).

**What is the nature and timing of hemoptysis in patients who have undergone bone marrow transplantation?**

Some patients present with sudden-onset massive hemoptysis within 100 days of BMT as a result of diffuse alveolar hemorrhage. The pathogenesis of this complication has not been completely elucidated.[2]

**What are the characteristics of hemoptysis related to a bronchovascular fistula?**

Massive hemoptysis is typical of bronchovascular fistulae, sometimes preceded by a sentinel bleed. Bronchovascular fistulae usually occur as a result of invasive infection (eg, aspergillosis) or pulmonary procedures (eg, lung resection, lung transplantation).[9]

## What are the causes of hemoptysis related to the pulmonary parenchyma?

**Infection of the alveoli.**

Pneumonia.

**A 56-year-old man with a history of heavy alcohol abuse presents with low-grade fever and malaise, and chest imaging reveals parenchymal consolidation with an air-fluid level (see Figure 31-4).**

Lung abscess.

**The leading cause of hemoptysis worldwide.**

Pulmonary tuberculosis (TB).[6]

**A 33-year-old woman with a history of heart transplantation for familial dilated cardiomyopathy presents with fever, weight loss, and hemoptysis and is found to have a crescentic cavitation on chest imaging.**

Pulmonary aspergillosis.

**A 63-year-old man presents with fever, cough, and hemoptysis 8 weeks after eating freshwater crabs.**

Pulmonary paragonimiasis.

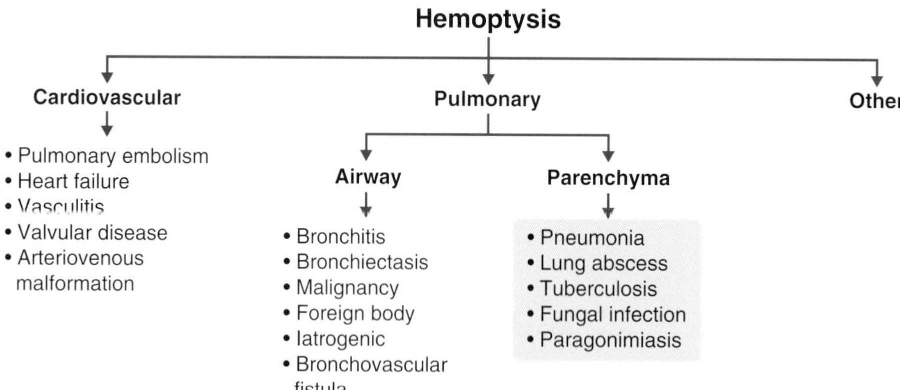


**Hemoptysis most commonly occurs in association with pneumonia caused by which organisms?**

Organisms that cause necrotizing pneumonia are more likely to result in hemoptysis, including *Staphylococcus aureus* and gram-negative rods (eg, *Klebsiella pneumoniae, Pseudomonas aeruginosa*). Distortion of lung architecture that might occur as a result of severe pneumonia can predispose patients to hemoptysis during subsequent infections.[2]

**What organisms are commonly associated with lung abscess?**

Lung abscesses are usually polymicrobial. Anaerobic organisms of the oral cavity are commonly involved, including gram-negatives (eg, *Bacteroides* species) and gram-positives (eg, *Peptostreptococcus* species). Aerobic organisms (eg, *Staphylococcus aureus*) are less commonly involved.[10]

**How common is hemoptysis in patients with active pulmonary tuberculosis?**

Hemoptysis develops in around one-quarter of patients with active pulmonary TB. Most patients present with blood-streaked sputum. However, massive hemoptysis can occur when cavitations erode into surrounding vascular structures such as the bronchial arteries.[2]

**Which populations are at highest risk of acquiring fungal infection of the lungs?**

Immunocompromised patients and those with chronically diseased lungs (eg, COPD) are at highest risk for acquiring pulmonary fungal infections. As with pulmonary TB, massive hempoptysis can occur when cavitations erode into surrounding vascular structures.[6]

**Where is *Paragonimus westermani* endemic?**

*Paragonimus westermani* is a lung fluke endemic to Southeast Asia and China. It typically presents with fever, cough, and hemoptysis, and is frequently mistaken for pulmonary TB. Cases in the United States have been reported in patients who have ingested crayfish or small crabs.[2]

## OTHER CAUSES OF HEMOPTYSIS

### What are the other causes of hemoptysis?

**"Hemoptysis in a woman is removed by eruption of the menses."—Hippocrates.**

Catamenial hemoptysis.[11]

**More common in children, this condition should be considered when there are recurrent episodes of diffuse alveolar hemorrhage without an identifiable cause.**

Idiopathic pulmonary hemosiderosis.

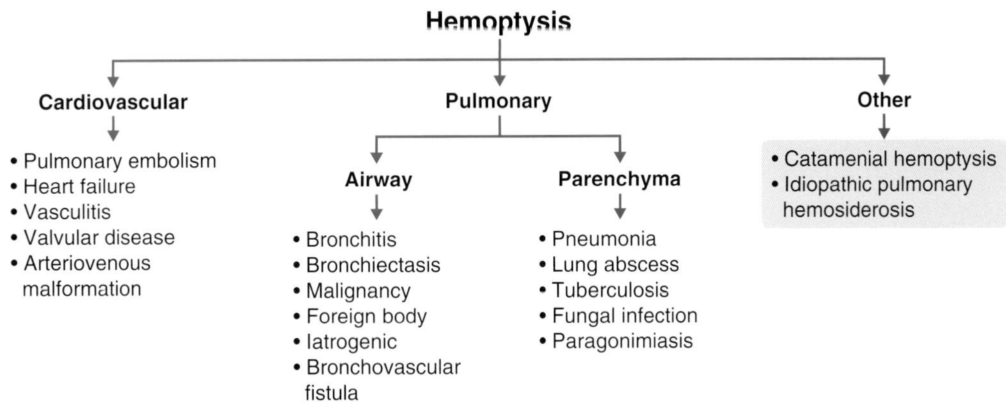


**What is the pathogenesis of catamenial hemoptysis?**

Catamenial hemoptysis results from the presence of ectopic endometrial tissue within the lower respiratory tract, including the parenchyma and airways, possibly as a result of entry through small defects in the diaphragm. Hormonal suppression of endometrial proliferation may be effective in some cases. Surgery can be offered in refractory cases, but there is risk of recurrence.[12]

**What is the long-term effect of idiopathic pulmonary hemosiderosis on the lungs?**

Idiopathic pulmonary hemosiderosis is a rare condition of unknown etiology, characterized by recurrent episodes of diffuse alveolar hemorrhage. Bleeding can be severe and life-threatening. The accumulation of iron in the alveoli over time can lead to pulmonary fibrosis. Glucocorticoids have been shown to reduce the development of pulmonary fibrosis, as well as overall morbidity and mortality. There may also be a role for other immunosuppressive medications.[13]

## Case Summary

A 29-year-old woman from Mexico develops acute-onset hemoptysis after undergoing a thrombectomy procedure and is found to have an abnormal cardiac examination, including an extra heart sound and a rumbling diastolic murmur.[1]

***What is the most likely cause of hemoptysis in this patient?***

Mitral valve stenosis.

### BONUS QUESTIONS

***What is the significance of the embolic events in this case?***

Embolic phenomena occur in patients with mitral stenosis and can be part of the initial presentation. Emboli are usually, but not always, related to concomitant atrial fibrillation.[1]

***What is the most likely source of the extra heart sound in this case?***

Extra heart sounds that occur near S2 include split S2, S3 gallop, opening snap, pericardial knock, and tumor plop. The extra sound in this case (see Figure 45-3) is most likely the opening snap of mitral stenosis, based on location, pitch, the associated diastolic murmur, and clinical history. *For audio of the heart sounds in this case, see the associated reference.*[1,14]

***What 4 main auscultatory findings are found in patients with significant mitral stenosis?***

The main auscultatory findings of mitral stenosis include the following: (1) pronounced S1, (2) early diastolic opening snap, (3) rumbling diastolic murmur at the apex best heard with the bell of the stethoscope, and (4) presystolic accentuation of the murmur. An irregularly irregular heart rhythm will be present in patients with atrial fibrillation.[1]

***What cardiac event causes presystolic accentuation of the murmur of mitral stenosis?***

At the end of diastole, left atrial contraction against a stenotic mitral valve increases turbulent blood flow, augmenting the intensity of the associated murmur. This finding is absent in patients with atrial fibrillation because there is no coordinated atrial contraction.

***What long-term sequela of mitral stenosis is present on CT imaging in this case?***

CT imaging of the chest in this case (see Figure 45-2) demonstrates that the pulmonary trunk (star) is significantly larger than the adjacent ascending aorta (arrow), a clue to the presence of pulmonary hypertension. The ratio of the diameter of the main pulmonary artery to that of the ascending aorta is normally <1 in adults.[15]

***What are the causes of hemoptysis in patients with mitral stenosis?***

The hemoptysis of mitral stenosis occurs via 2 primary mechanisms: (1) pulmonary edema related to pulmonary venous hypertension, resulting in pink, frothy sputum and (2) rupture of the thin-walled bronchial veins (ie, pulmonary apoplexy) from sudden increases in left atrial pressure, resulting in massive but typically self-limited hemoptysis.[16,17]

***What likely triggered hemoptysis in this case?***

In this case, it is likely that hemodynamic changes related to renal artery embolism or the embolectomy procedure resulted in a sudden increase in left atrial pressure. Unlike aortic stenosis, mitral stenosis is associated with minimal functional reserve, and decompensation occurs easily in the setting of tachycardia or high flow.[16]

***What is the most common cause of mitral stenosis worldwide?***

Rheumatic heart disease is the most common cause of mitral stenosis worldwide.[16]

***What is the prognosis of severe mitral stenosis?***

Without treatment, the prognosis of severe mitral stenosis is poor. Morbidity and mortality are significantly improved with treatment, including percutaneous balloon valvuloplasty, surgical valvotomy, or mitral valve replacement.[16]

## KEY POINTS

- Hemoptysis is the expectoration of blood produced in the lower respiratory tract.
- Hematemesis, bleeding from the upper airway, and nasal bleeding can be confused with hemoptysis and should be ruled out.
- The severity of hemoptysis is graded as massive or submassive; 300 mL/d is a reasonable threshold to distinguish the two.
- Massive hemoptysis is life-threatening and requires prompt management, including maintaining the airway and placing the bleeding lung in a dependent position.
- Conventional radiography, CT imaging, and bronchoscopy play complementary roles in the evaluation of hemoptysis.
- The causes of hemoptysis can be separated into the following categories: cardiovascular, pulmonary, and other.
- Pulmonary causes of hemoptysis can involve the airways or parenchyma.
- The most common causes of hemoptysis include acute bronchitis, pneumonia, lung abscess, lung cancer, tuberculosis, heart failure, and bronchiectasis.

## REFERENCES


1. Oehler AC, Sullivan PD, Mansoor AM. Mitral stenosis. *BMJ Case Rep*. 2017;2017.
2. Longo DL, Fauci AS, Kasper DL, Hauser SL, Jameson JL, Loscalzo J, eds. *Harrison's Principles of Internal Medicine*. 18th ed. New York, NY: McGraw-Hill; 2012.
3. Bidwell JL, Pachner RW. Hemoptysis: diagnosis and management. *Am Fam Physician*. 2005;72(7):1253-1260.
4. Larici AR, Franchi P, Occhipinti M, et al. Diagnosis and management of hemoptysis. *Diagn Interv Radiol*. 2014;20(4):299-309.
5. Kostadima E, Zakynthinos E. Pulmonary embolism: pathophysiology, diagnosis, treatment. *Hellenic J Cardiol*. 2007;48(2):94-107.
6. Kapur S, Louie BE. Hemoptysis and thoracic fungal infections. *Surg Clin North Am*. 2010;90(5):985-1001.
7. Reisz G, Stevens D, Boutwell C, Nair V. The causes of hemoptysis revisited. A review of the etiologies of hemoptysis between 1986 and 1995. *Mo Med*. 1997;94(10):633-635.
8. Qureshi A, Behzadi A. Foreign-body aspiration in an adult. *Can J Surg*. 2008;51(3):E69-E70.
9. Sellke FW, del Nido PJ, Swanson SJ, eds. *Sabiston & Spencer Surgery of the Chest*. 9th ed. Philadelphia, PA: Elsevier, Inc.; 2015.
10. Kuhajda I, Zarogoulidis K, Tsirgogianni K, et al. Lung abscess-etiology, diagnostic and treatment options. *Ann Transl Med*. 2015;3(13):183.
11. Eastman TJ. Periodical hemoptysis. *Boston Med Surg J*. 1910(162):320-322.
12. Augoulea A, Lambrinoudaki I, Christodoulakos G. Thoracic endometriosis syndrome. *Respiration*. 2008;75(1):113-119.
13. Ioachimescu OC, Sieber S, Kotch A. Idiopathic pulmonary haemosiderosis revisited. *Eur Respir J*. 2004;24(1):162-170.
14. Marriott HJL. *Bedside Cardiac Diagnosis*. Philadelphia, Pennsylvania: Lippincott Company; 1993.
15. Pena E, Dennie C, Veinot J, Muniz SH. Pulmonary hypertension: how the radiologist can help. *Radiographics*. 2012;32(1):9-32.
16. Chandrashekhar Y, Westaby S, Narula J. Mitral stenosis. *Lancet*. 2009;374(9697):1271-1283.
17. Scarlat A, Bodner G, Liron M. Massive haemoptysis as the presenting symptom in mitral stenosis. *Thorax*. 1986;41(5):413-414.

# Chapter 46

# HYPOXEMIA

## Case: A 51-year-old man with positional dyspnea

A 51-year-old man with a history of chronic hepatitis C infection complicated by cirrhosis presents to the emergency department with shortness of breath. He has been followed by a hepatologist for management of hepatic encephalopathy, ascites, and esophageal varices, which have been stable for several years. The patient has a history of shortness of breath that typically resolves following large volume paracentesis, which he has occasionally required. However, over the past few months the patient has noticed progressive dyspnea despite control of the ascites. Breathing seems to improve when he lies on his back.

Heart rate is 100 beats per minute, and respiratory rate is 24 breaths per minute. Hemoglobin oxygen saturation by pulse oximetry ($Spo_2$) is 85% on room air with the patient in the upright position; it improves to 96% in the supine position. There are multiple spider angiomas on the anterior chest. Jugular venous pressure is 7 cm $H_2O$. The lungs are clear to auscultation. An image of the patient's hand is shown in Figure 46-1.

Arterial blood gas on room air shows that pH is 7.48, partial pressure of carbon dioxide ($Paco_2$) is 32 mm Hg, and partial pressure of oxygen is 56 mm Hg. An image from a transthoracic echocardiogram with agitated saline contrast shows the presence of microbubbles in the right-sided cardiac chambers (Figure 46-2A). An image from the same study is captured 8 cardiac cycles after initial opacification of the right-sided cardiac chambers (Figure 46-2B).

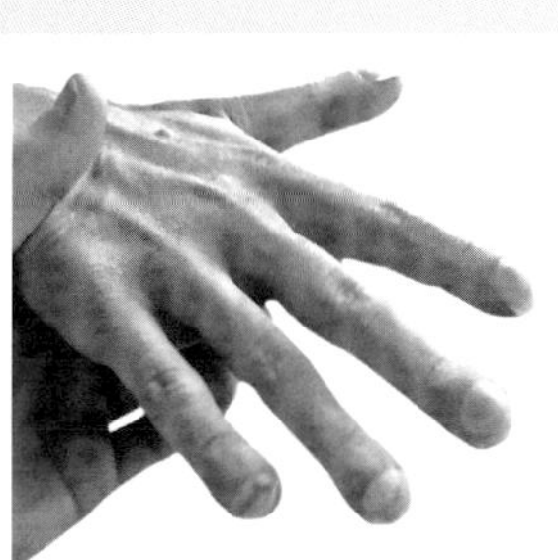

**Figure 46-1.**

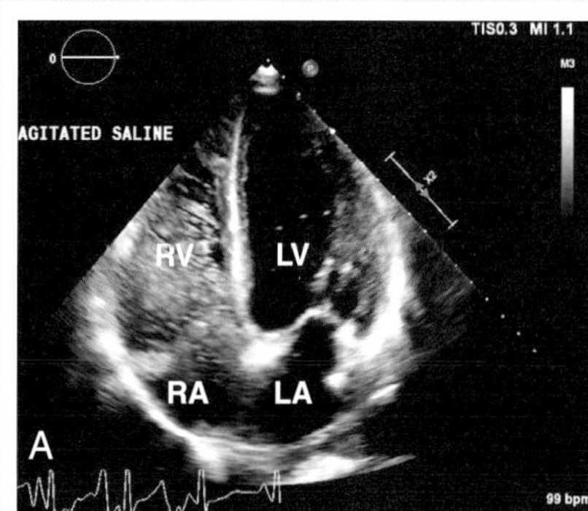


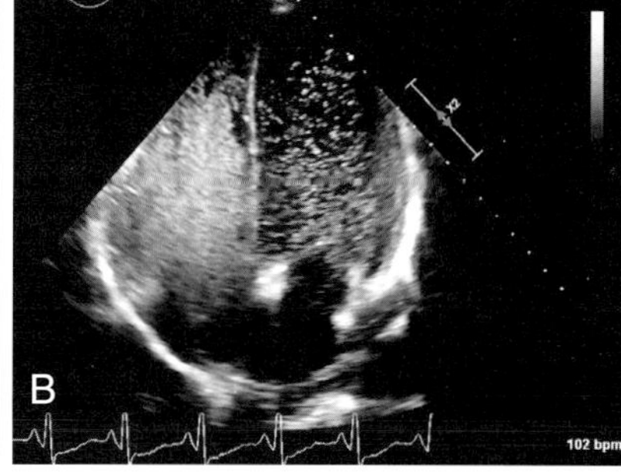


**Figure 46-2.** (Courtesy of Steven E. Mansoor, MD, PhD.)

***What is the most likely cause of hypoxemia in this patient?***

What is hypoxemia?

Hypoxemia refers to a physiologic state in which the partial pressure of oxygen in arterial blood ($Pao_2$) is low. Normal $Pao_2$ at room air is 80 to 100 mm Hg.[1,2]

Which noninvasive bedside instrument can be used to estimate the partial pressure of oxygen in arterial blood by spectrophotometrically measuring the fraction of oxygenated hemoglobin in peripheral arterial blood?

Pulse oximetry measures the fraction of oxygenated hemoglobin in peripheral arterial blood (expressed as % saturation, $Spo_2$), which can be used to provide an estimate of $Pao_2$.

**How accurate is pulse oximetry?**

Pulse oximetry is accurate to within ±3% when true oxygen saturation of hemoglobin in arterial blood ($Sao_2$) is above 70%.[3]

**Under what conditions is pulse oximetry unreliable?**

Pulse oximetry is unreliable in patients with carbon monoxide poisoning and methemoglobinemia. In the setting of methemoglobinemia, the reading rarely falls below 85%, which can be a clue to the diagnosis. Measurement of pulse oximetry requires a steady and fairly regular pulse, and therefore may be unreliable in the setting of poor circulation (eg, Raynaud's phenomenon) and cardiac dysrhythmias (eg, atrial fibrillation). Other conditions may compromise measurements by obstructing the pulse oximeter (eg, the presence of fingernail polish). The use of an oximetry probe on the earlobe may be helpful in some circumstances.[3]

**Which invasive test can directly measure the partial pressure of oxygen in arterial blood?**

$Pao_2$ can be directly measured with an arterial blood gas test. $Sao_2$ can be calculated based on the $Pao_2$ value and other factors (eg, blood pH).

**How does the partial pressure of oxygen in arterial blood relate to the true oxygen saturation of hemoglobin in arterial blood?**

Under normal circumstances, $Sao_2$ is dependent on $Pao_2$, and a predictable relationship has been established (oxygen-hemoglobin [or oxyhemoglobin] dissociation curve). Important numbers to recognize are $Pao_2$ of 27 mm Hg and $Pao_2$ of 60 mm Hg, which correspond to hemoglobin saturations of 50% and 90%, respectively (Figure 46-3).

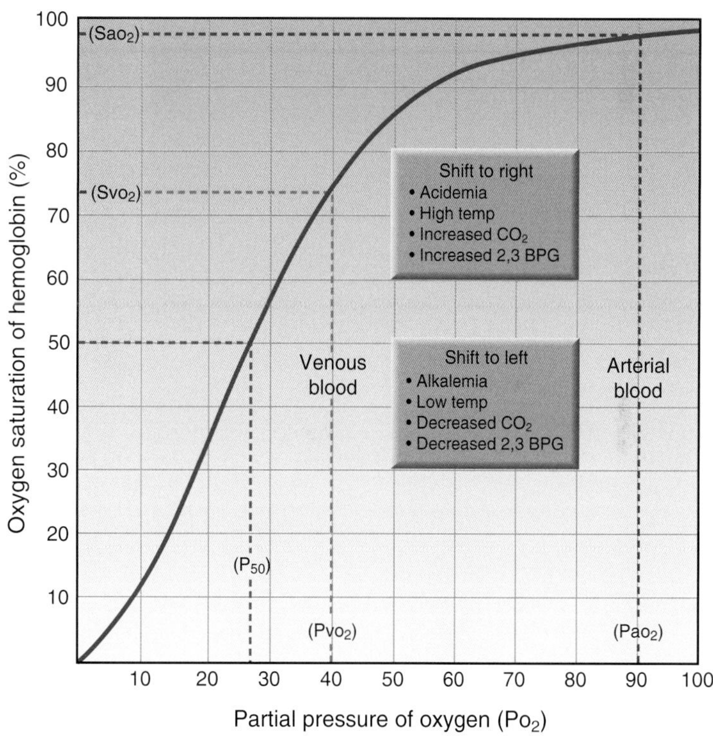


**Figure 46-3.** Oxyhemoglobin dissociation curve showing the normal relationship between the $Po_2$ in blood and the $O_2$ saturation of hemoglobin. The $P_{50}$ is the $Po_2$ that corresponds to 50% saturation of hemoglobin with $O_2$. (From Marino PL. *Marino's The ICU Book*. 4th ed. Philadelphia, PA: Wolters Kluwer Health/Lippincott Williams & Wilkins; 2014.)

**What physiologic conditions shift the oxyhemoglobin dissociation curve to the right, and what conditions shift the curve to the left?**

Conditions that shift the oxyhemoglobin dissociation curve to the right include increased temperature, acidemia, increased $Paco_2$, and increased 2,3-bisphosphoglycerate (2,3-BPG). Conditions that shift the curve to the left include decreased temperature, alkalemia, decreased $Paco_2$, and decreased 2,3-BPG (see Figure 46-3).[4]

**What formula describes the oxygen content of arterial blood ($CaO_2$)?**

$CaO_2 = SaO_2 \times [Hb] \times 1.34 + (0.003 \times PaO_2)$

*In the above formula, $CaO_2$ is expressed in mL $O_2$/dL blood, $SaO_2$ is expressed as a fraction, [Hb] is the hemoglobin concentration in blood (g/dL), 1.34 is the oxygen-binding capacity of hemoglobin (mL $O_2$/g Hb), 0.003 is the solubility coefficient of $O_2$ in blood (mL $O_2$/dL blood/ mm Hg $PaO_2$), and $PaO_2$ is expressed in mm Hg.*[3]

**Using the formula for the oxygen content of arterial blood as reference, what are the 2 main determinants of the oxygen content of arterial blood?**

The main determinants of oxygen content of arterial blood are hemoglobin concentration and hemoglobin saturation (which is largely determined by $PaO_2$).

**Which formula describes oxygen delivery ($DO_2$) to the tissues?**

$DO_2$ (mL/min) is dependent on $CaO_2$ (mL/L) and cardiac output (CO, L/min).[3]

$DO_2 = CaO_2 \times CO$

**Using the formula for oxygen delivery as reference, what are the 3 main determinants of oxygen delivery to the tissues?**

The main determinants of oxygen delivery to the tissues are hemoglobin concentration, hemoglobin saturation (which is largely determined by $PaO_2$), and cardiac output.

**What is hypoxia?**

Hypoxia refers to the deficiency or ineffective use of oxygen within tissues of the body. Causes include stroke, myocardial infarction, claudication, and intestinal ischemia. Hypoxia cannot be measured directly in the same way that hypoxemia can. However, blood lactate concentration is often elevated in the setting of tissue hypoxia, producing lactic acidosis. Hypoxemia is the most common cause of hypoxia, but these conditions can occur independently.[1,2]

**When can hypoxia occur in the absence of hypoxemia?**

Hypoxia can occur in the absence of hypoxemia when any of the following actions are impaired: oxygen delivery (eg, low cardiac output, anemia, thrombus), oxygen binding to hemoglobin (eg, methemoglobinemia), and oxygen uptake or use by the tissues (eg, carbon monoxide poisoning, sepsis, cyanide poisoning).

**What is the effect of increased tissue oxygen extraction on the partial pressure of oxygen in arterial blood?**

Conditions that reduce $DO_2$ (eg, anemia, heart failure) trigger a compensatory increase in oxygen extraction by the tissues, resulting in abnormally low oxygen content of mixed venous blood entering the pulmonary capillary bed. In the setting of abnormal gas exchange (eg, pulmonary edema), the presence of low oxygen content of blood entering the pulmonary capillary bed will have a significant impact on the oxygen content of blood leaving the pulmonary capillary bed, worsening the degree of hypoxemia.[3]

**What is the alveolar gas equation?**

$PAO_2 = (FIO_2 \times [P_B - P_{H_2O}]) - (PaCO_2/RQ)$

*In the above formula, $PAO_2$ is the partial pressure of alveolar oxygen (mm Hg), $FIO_2$ is the fraction of inspired oxygen, $P_B$ is the barometric pressure (atmospheric pressure) (mm Hg), $P_{H_2O}$ is water vapor pressure in the airways (mm Hg), $PaCO_2$ is the partial pressure of carbon dioxide in arterial blood (mm Hg), and RQ is the respiratory quotient.*

*Several underlying causes of hypoxemia can be readily identified using this equation, as demonstrated in subsequent sections.*

What is the fraction of inspired oxygen of room air?

$FIO_2$ of room air is 21%.[3]

What is the barometric pressure at sea level?

$P_B$ at sea level is 760 mm Hg.[3]

What is the water vapor pressure in the airways at 37°C?

$P_{H_2O}$ at 37°C is 47 mm Hg.[3]

What is normal partial pressure of carbon dioxide in arterial blood?

Normal $PaCO_2$ is 40 mm Hg.[3]

What is the respiratory quotient?

The RQ is the ratio of carbon dioxide produced by the tissues to oxygen consumed by the tissues. It is dependent on the patient's dietary fat, protein, and carbohydrate content. The average value for a balanced diet at resting state is 0.8 (range is 0.7-1.0).[3]

Based on the alveolar gas equation, what is the partial pressure of alveolar oxygen in a patient breathing room air with normal partial pressure of carbon dioxide in arterial blood?

$PAO_2 = (0.21 \times [760 - 47]) - (40/0.8) = \sim 100$ mm Hg.

The causes of hypoxemia can be separated into which 2 general categories?

Hypoxemia can occur in the setting of normal A-a gradient or elevated A-a gradient.

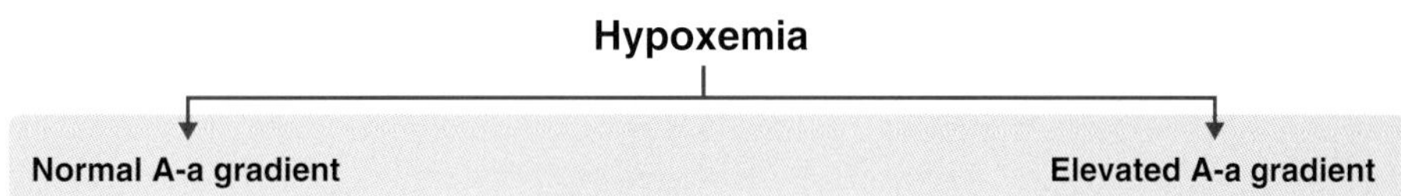


What is the A-a gradient?

The A-a gradient is the difference in partial pressure of oxygen between the alveolus (A) and arterial blood (a). $PAO_2$ is calculated using the alveolar gas equation, whereas $PaO_2$ is measured with a sample of arterial blood (arterial blood gas test) (Figure 46-4).

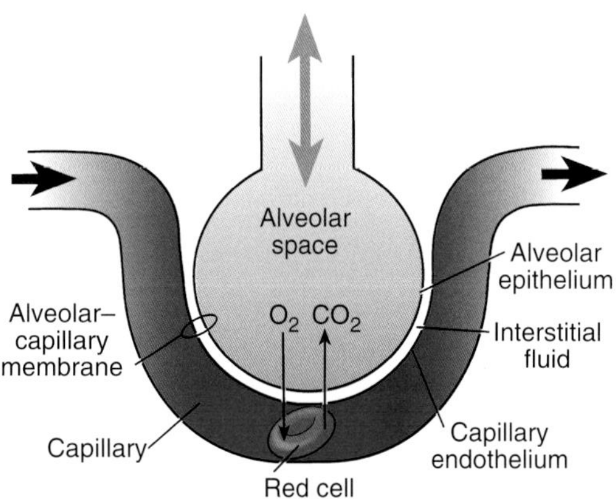


**Figure 46-4.** Gas exchange in the lung. The A-a gradient is the difference in partial pressure of oxygen between the alveolar space and arterial blood. (From Rhoades RA, Bell DR. *Medical Physiology: Principles for Clinical Medicine.* 5th ed. Philadelphia, PA: Wolters Kluwer; 2018.)

**What is a normal A-a gradient?**

Normal A-a gradient increases with age and $FIO_2$. The following table indicates the upper limits of normal A-a gradient at room air according to age:

**Table 46-1**

| Age (years) | A-a gradient (mm Hg) |
|---|---|
| 20 | 17 |
| 30 | 21 |
| 40 | 24 |
| 50 | 27 |
| 60 | 31 |
| 70 | 34 |
| 80 | 38 |

Normal A-a gradient increases 5 to 7 mm Hg for every 10% increase in $FIO_2$.[3,5]

## HYPOXEMIA ASSOCIATED WITH NORMAL A-a GRADIENT

**What are the 2 general causes of hypoxemia with normal A-a gradient?**

Hypoxemia associated with normal A-a gradient can be caused by reduced partial pressure of inspired oxygen ($PIO_2$) or hypoventilation.

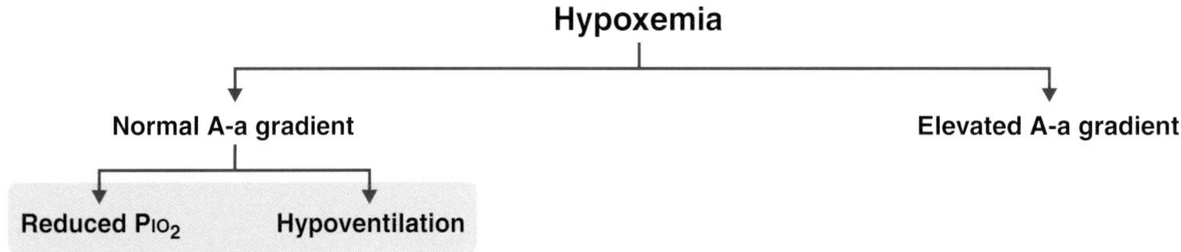


*These categories of hypoxemia are easily identified within the alveolar gas equation.*

## HYPOXEMIA RELATED TO REDUCED $PIO_2$

**What are the 2 main causes of reduced partial pressure of inspired oxygen?**

A reduction in either $FIO_2$ or $P_B$ can result in reduced $PIO_2$.

**What is the A-a gradient in a patient breathing air with a fraction of inspired oxygen of 16% at normal barometric pressure, with a normal partial pressure of carbon dioxide in arterial blood, and a partial pressure of oxygen in arterial blood of 58 mm Hg?**

$PAO_2 = (0.16 \times [760 - 47]) - (40/0.8) = \sim 64$ mm Hg. A-a gradient = 64 − 58 = 6 mm Hg. This value is normal, as expected in a patient with hypoxemia driven purely by reduced $PIO_2$.

**How does the hypoxemia related to reduced partial pressure of inspired oxygen respond to inhaled oxygen?**

Decreased $PaO_2$ related to reduced $PIO_2$ improves with inhaled oxygen.[6]

### What are the causes of hypoxemia related to reduced $PIO_2$?

**Firefighters are at increased risk.**

Inhalation of polluted air from smoke.

**A toddler passes out after playing with a large plastic bag.**

Suffocation.

**Aircraft cabins are pressurized for this reason.**

High altitude.

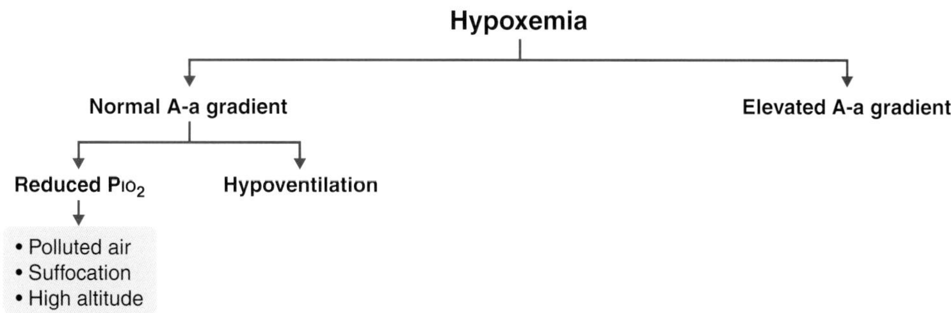


**What is the fraction of inspired oxygen in a patient with true oxygen saturation of hemoglobin in arterial blood of 50%, assuming an A-a gradient of 5 mm Hg and normal partial pressure of carbon dioxide in arterial blood?**

The $Pa_{O_2}$ at which hemoglobin is 50% saturated is 27 mm Hg (see Figure 46-3). If the A-a gradient is 5 mm Hg, then the $P_{AO_2}$ must be 32 mm Hg. Using the alveolar gas equation, $F_{IO_2}$ = ([40/0.8] + 32)/(760 – 47) = 0.115 (or 11.5% oxygen).

**What are some causes of suffocation that can lead to hypoxemia?**

Causes of suffocation include enclosed and poorly ventilated spaces (eg, a child left in a car with the windows rolled up), drowning, and accidental suffocation (eg, a toddler with a plastic bag).

**How is the partial pressure of alveolar oxygen affected by altitude?**

At increasing altitudes, $F_{IO_2}$ remains constant at 0.21 (21%) but $P_B$ decreases, resulting in reduced $P_{IO_2}$. For example, at 8400 m above sea level, $P_B$ is approximately 272 mm Hg. In a person with compensatory hyperventilation and a $P_{CO_2}$ of 20 mm Hg, $P_{AO_2}$ = (0.21 × [272 – 47]) – (20/0.8) = ~22 mm Hg. One of the lowest recorded $Pa_{O_2}$ values logged in a healthy individual was 19 mm Hg, which was recorded on Mount Everest at 8400 m (Figure 46-5).[7]

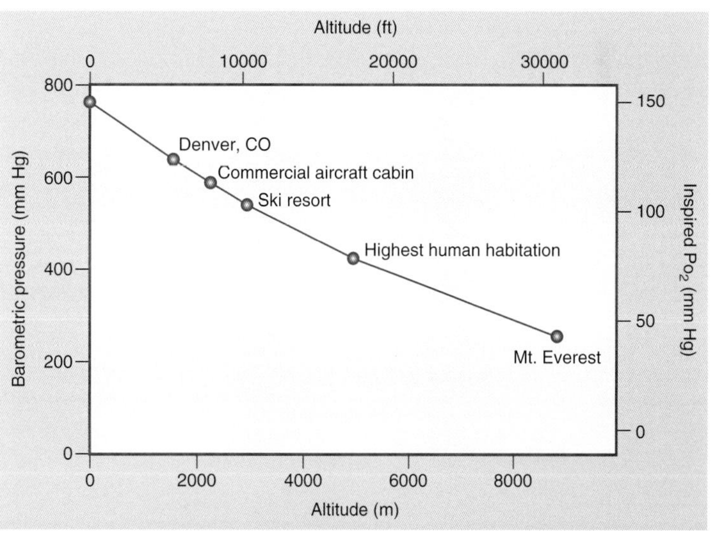


**Figure 46-5.** Relationship between altitude, barometric pressure (atmospheric pressure), and inspired oxygen. Note that at an altitude of 5000 m (~16,000 ft), the highest at which humans reside, the inspired $P_{IO_2}$ is approximately half of the value at sea level. On the summit of Mount Everest, at 8850 m (~29,030 ft), the inspired $P_{IO_2}$ is less than 30% of the value at sea level. (From West JB. The physiologic basis of high-altitude diseases. *Ann Intern Med*. 2004;141:789-800.)

## HYPOXEMIA RELATED TO HYPOVENTILATION

**How does hypoventilation affect the partial pressure of carbon dioxide in arterial blood?**

$Pa_{CO_2}$ increases as a result of hypoventilation.

**What is the A-a gradient in a patient breathing room air at sea level, with an elevated partial pressure of carbon dioxide in arterial blood of 80 mm Hg, and a measured partial pressure of oygen in arterial blood of 45 mm Hg?**

$P_{AO_2} = (0.21 \times [760 - 47]) - (80/0.8) = \sim 50$ mm Hg. A-a gradient = 50 – 45 = 5 mm Hg. This value is normal, as expected in a patient with hypoxemia driven purely by hypoventilation.

**How does the hypoxemia related to hypoventilation respond to inhaled oxygen?**

Decreased $Pa_{O_2}$ related to hypoventilation generally improves with inhaled oxygen, but it is more effective to increase ventilation.[6]

### What are the causes of hypoxemia related to hypoventilation?

**A 24-year-old man is brought to the emergency department with hypoventilation and hypoxemia and is noted to have track marks near the antecubital regions of his arms.**

Drugs and toxins.

**Large neck circumference is a significant risk factor for this condition.**

Obstructive sleep apnea (OSA).

**This patient was described in the Charles Dickens novel "*The Posthumous Papers of the Pickwick Club.*"**

Obesity hypoventilation syndrome (OHS, or Pickwickian syndrome).

**A 26-year-old woman with asthma presents with obtundation and $Pa_{CO_2}$ of 90 mm Hg after being exposed to cat dander.**

Severe airway obstruction related to asthma exacerbation.

**A 34-year-old woman presents with ascending paralysis complicated by shortness of breath and hypoxemia 2 weeks after a diarrheal illness.**

Neuromuscular weakness related to Guillain-Barré syndrome.

**Abnormal curvature of the spine in the coronal and sagittal planes.**

Mechanical obstruction related to kyphoscoliosis.

**Hypoventilation as a compensatory mechanism.**

Metabolic alkalosis.

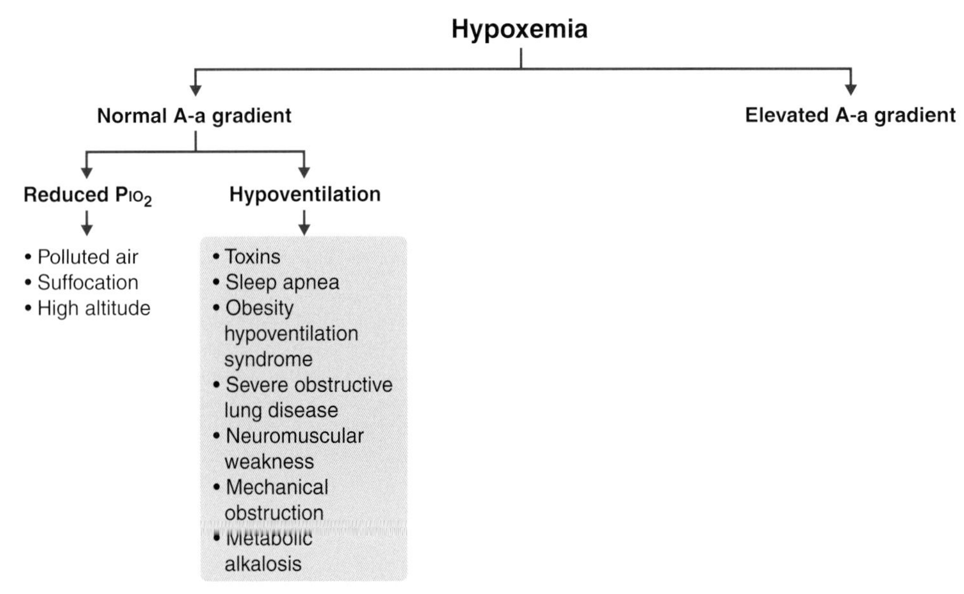

**Which 2 main classes of substances, used both as prescription medications and drugs of abuse, cause hypoventilation by depressing the respiratory drive?**

Narcotics and benzodiazepines are common causes of depressed respiratory drive. Naloxone may be given as an antidote for narcotic toxicity, whereas flumazenil is the antidote of choice for benzodiazepine toxicity.

**What are the common symptoms of obstructive sleep apnea?**

Symptoms of OSA include excessive daytime sleepiness, snoring, and morning headache. Weight loss and nocturnal continuous positive airway pressure (CPAP) are the initial treatments of choice.[8]

**How is obesity hypoventilation syndrome defined?**

OHS is defined by the constellation of obesity (body mass index > 30 kg/$m^2$), daytime hypoventilation (awake $Pa_{CO_2}$ > 45 mm Hg), and sleep-disordered breathing in the absence of other causes of hypoventilation. Weight loss and treatment of coexistent OSA with CPAP are the initial strategies of choice.[8]

**What are the main contributors to hypoventilation in patients with acute exacerbation of chronic obstructive pulmonary disease (COPD)?**

Hypoventilation in patients with acute exacerbation of COPD is related to worsening airflow obstruction from mucus or bronchoconstriction, combined with respiratory muscle fatigue. Noninvasive treatment strategies include inhaled short-acting bronchodilators (eg, albuterol), glucocorticoids (eg, prednisone), antibiotics (eg, azithromycin), and noninvasive positive pressure ventilation (NPPV) via CPAP or bilevel positive airway pressure (BiPAP).[8]

**What are some causes of neuromuscular weakness that can lead to hypoventilation?**

Neuromuscular weakness can occur as a result of the following conditions: upper motor neuron disease (eg, spinal cord injury), anterior horn cell disease (eg, amyotrophic lateral sclerosis), peripheral neuropathy (eg, Guillain-Barré syndrome), disorders of the neuromuscular junction (eg, myasthenia gravis), muscular dystrophy (eg, Duchenne), myopathy (eg, polymyositis), and electrolyte disturbance (eg, hypophosphatemia).

**What are the causes of mechanical obstruction that can lead to hypoventilation?**

Causes of mechanical obstruction include obesity, ascites, and restrictive chest wall disorders (eg, kyphoscoliosis, ankylosing spondylitis, fibrothorax, multiple rib fractures).[8]

**What is the expected partial pressure of carbon dioxide in arterial blood in a patient with primary metabolic alkalosis and serum bicarbonate of 48 mEq/L?**

The following formula, which is predominantly based on serum bicarbonate ($HCO_3^-$) concentration, can be used to predict the $Pa_{CO_2}$ in the setting of a metabolic alkalosis: Expected $Pa_{CO_2} = 0.7 \times ([HCO_3^-] - 24) + 40 \pm 2$. In this example, expected $Pa_{CO_2} = 0.7 \times (48 - 24) + 40 \pm 2 = 57 \pm 2$ mm Hg.[9]

## HYPOXEMIA ASSOCIATED WITH ELEVATED A-a GRADIENT

**What are the 4 general mechanisms of hypoxemia related to elevated A-a gradient?**

Hypoxemia associated with elevated A-a gradient can occur as a result of dead space (a form of ventilation-perfusion [V/Q] mismatch), physiologic shunt (a form of V/Q mismatch), impaired diffusion, or anatomic shunt.

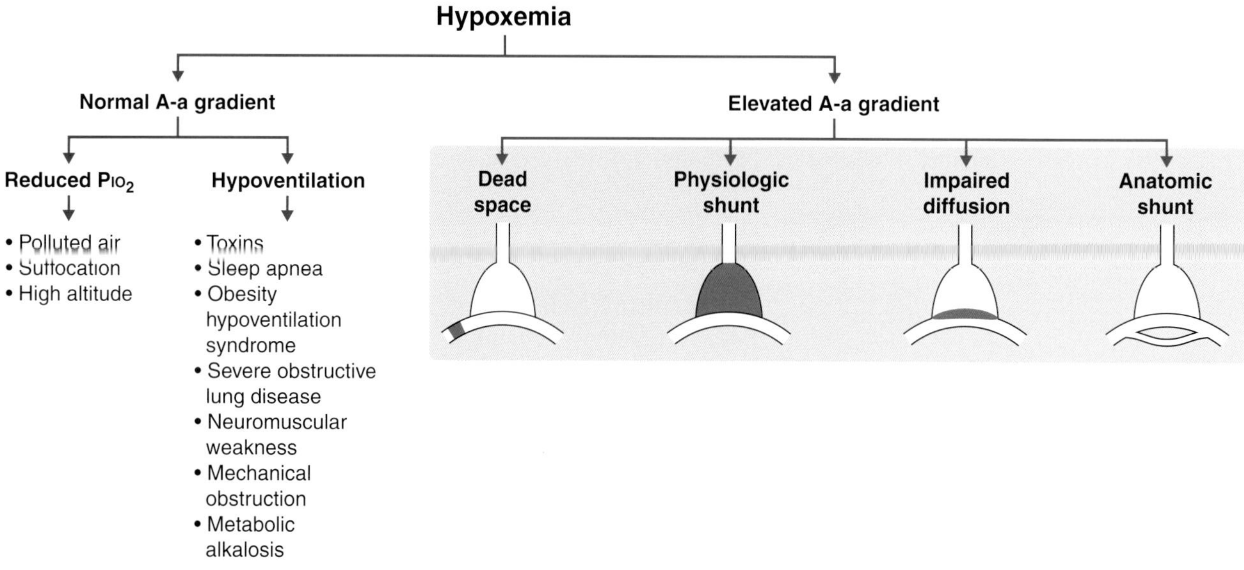


*Lung diseases often cause hypoxemia with elevated A-a gradient through a combination of these mechanisms (eg, emphysema is associated with increased dead space, shunt, and impaired diffusion). However, most etiologies predominantly act through 1 mechanism in particular, and that principle will be used in this chapter to organize the framework.*

**What is the ventilation-perfusion ratio?**

The V/Q ratio describes the relationship between ventilation of the alveoli and perfusion of the pulmonary capillaries. A perfect match between ventilation and perfusion (ie, V/Q of 1) is the reference point for defining normal and abnormal gas exchange in the lungs (Figure 46-6).[3]

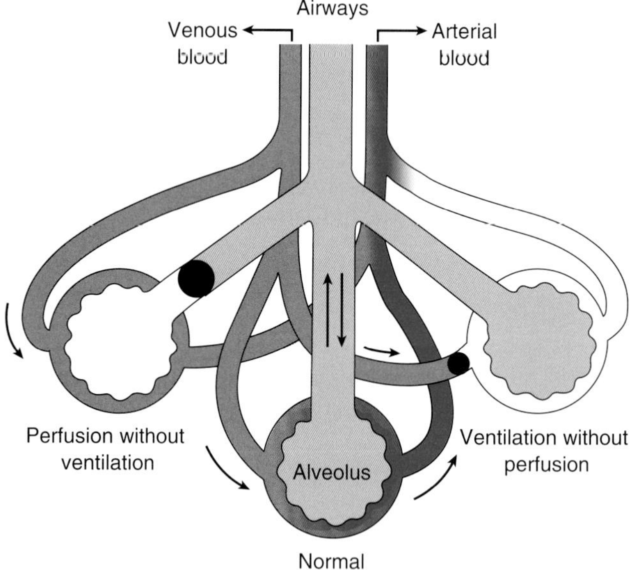


**Figure 46-6.** Matching of ventilation and perfusion. Center: normal matching of ventilation and perfusion; left: perfusion without ventilation (ie, shunt); right: ventilation without perfusion (ie, dead space). (From Porth CM. *Essentials of Pathophysiology: Concepts of Altered Health States*. 4th ed. Philadelphia, PA: Wolters Kluwer; 2015.)

## HYPOXEMIA RELATED TO INCREASED DEAD SPACE

**What is dead space?**

Dead space occurs when there is excess alveolar ventilation relative to pulmonary capillary perfusion (ie, V/Q > 1). Anatomic dead space is normal and refers to parts of the airway that are not normally involved in gas exchange (eg, the trachea); it accounts for 20% to 30% of total ventilation (roughly 1 mL per pound of body weight). Alveolar dead space is abnormal and refers to areas of the lung that are normally involved in gas exchange. The combination of anatomic and alveolar dead space is referred to as physiologic dead space (Figure 46-7). Increased physiologic dead space can result in both hypoxemia and hypercapnia. Because of compensatory hyperventilation, hypercapnia does not occur until dead space is >50% of total lung volume.[3]

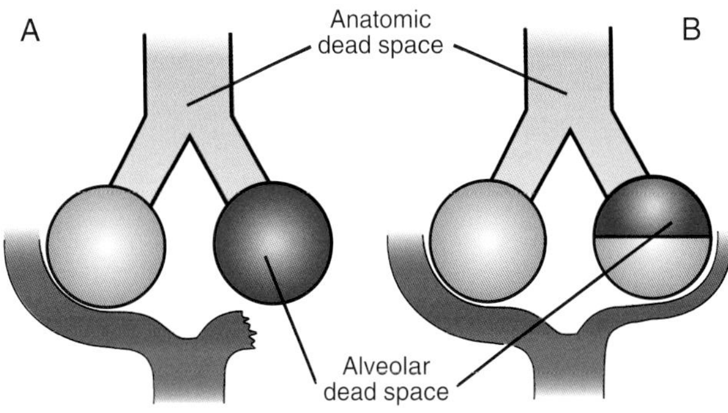


**Figure 46-7.** A, Absence of blood flow to an alveolar region. B, Reduced blood flow to an alveolar region. In both cases, a portion of alveolar air does not participate in gas exchange and constitutes alveolar dead space volume. Physiologic dead space is the sum of alveolar dead space plus anatomic dead space. (From Rhoades RA, Bell DR. *Medical Physiology: Principles for Clinical Medicine*. 5th ed. Philadelphia, PA: Wolters Kluwer; 2018.)

**What local compensatory mechanism occurs to offset the effects of pathologic dead space?**

In the setting of increased dead space, compensatory bronchoconstriction acts to normalize the V/Q ratio.[6,10]

**How does the hypoxemia related to dead space respond to inhaled oxygen?**

Decreased $Pa{O_2}$ related to dead space generally improves with inhaled oxygen.[6]

### What are the causes of increased physiologic dead space?

**Acute right-sided heart strain in a patient with an erythematous and edematous lower extremity.**

Pulmonary embolism (PE).

**Hyperinflation, bleb formation, and increased lung compliance.**

Emphysema.

**A global decrease in pulmonary capillary perfusion.**

Hypotension.

**Listen for a loud (and sometimes palpable) pulmonic component of the second heart sound (P2).**

Pulmonary hypertension.

**Often associated with small vessel vasculitis and glomerulonephritis.**

Pulmonary capillaritis (eg, granulomatosis with polyangiitis [GPA, or Wegener's granulomatosis]).

**Iatrogenic.**

Positive pressure ventilation (PPV).

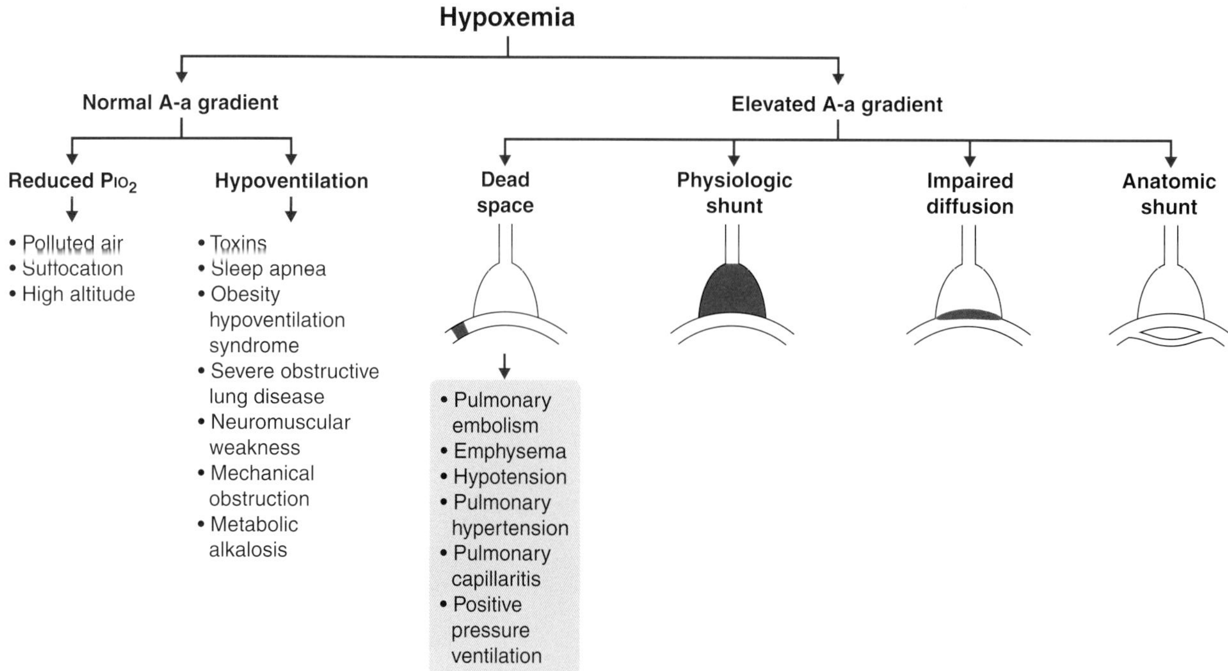


**What are the principal mechanisms of hypoxemia related to pulmonary embolism?**

In the setting of PE, there is a shift in blood flow to the unaffected parts of the lungs, causing a relative V/Q mismatch in the form of physiologic shunt, resulting in hypoxemia. In some patients, increased right-sided intracardiac pressures related to the PE lead to a right-to-left intracardiac shunt through the foramen ovale or a different atrial septal defect.[11,12]

**What additional mechanism of hypoxemia is often identified on pulmonary function testing in patients with emphysema?**

Emphysema is associated with impaired gas transfer.

**What cause of hypotension should be suspected in a patient with fever, normal central venous pressure, and decreased systemic vascular resistance?**

Septic shock is characterized by normal or low central venous pressure and decreased systemic vascular resistance, and should be suspected in patients who present with fever along with these hemodynamic changes.

**What are the additional mechanisms of hypoxemia related to pulmonary hypertension?**

In addition to increasing dead space, pulmonary hypertension causes hypoxemia through a variety of mechanisms, including impaired diffusion and anatomic shunt (increased right-sided heart pressures can force blood through the foramen ovale). Additionally, decreased cardiac output related to cor pulmonale can result in low mixed venous $Po_2$, contributing to hypoxemia.[13]

**What condition can occur in patients with pulmonary capillaritis that results in hemoptysis and physiologic shunt?**

Diffuse alveolar hemorrhage (DAH) is a severe complication of pulmonary capillaritis that can result in massive hemoptysis and physiologic shunt.

**Why does positive pressure ventilation cause increased physiologic dead space?**

Physiologic dead space is increased by PPV for the following 2 reasons: (1) increase in alveolar pressure with resultant overdistention and (2) reduced venous return to the right side of the heart, which causes a decrease in pulmonary blood flow.[3]

## HYPOXEMIA RELATED TO PHYSIOLOGIC SHUNT

**What is a physiologic shunt?**

Physiologic shunting occurs when there is excess pulmonary capillary perfusion relative to alveolar ventilation (ie, $V/Q < 1$) (see Figure 46-6). When there is partial gas exchange, it is referred to as "venous admixture." When there is total absence of any gas exchange, it is referred to as a "true shunt," which is equivalent to an anatomic shunt.[3]

**How does the hypoxemia related to physiologic shunt respond to inhaled oxygen?**

The response to inhaled oxygen in the setting of physiologic shunt depends on the degree of shunt present. As the shunt fraction increases from normal (<10%) to 50%, there is an incremental decrease in response to inhaled oxygen. At shunt fractions >50%, $Pao_2$ is independent of the fraction of inspired oxygen, behaving like a true or anatomic shunt. *Understanding this concept can prevent iatrogenic oxygen toxicity in these patients.*[3]

### What are the causes of physiologic shunt?

**Pus in the alveolar space.**

Pneumonia.

**Fluid in the alveolar space.**

Pulmonary edema.

**Alveolar collapse.**

Atelectasis.

**Wheezing is usually appreciated on auscultation of the chest.**

Airway constriction.

**Blood in the alveolar space.**

Diffuse alveolar hemorrhage.

**A patient with cirrhosis experiences dyspnea that worsens in the upright position and improves when lying supine.**

Hepatopulmonary syndrome.

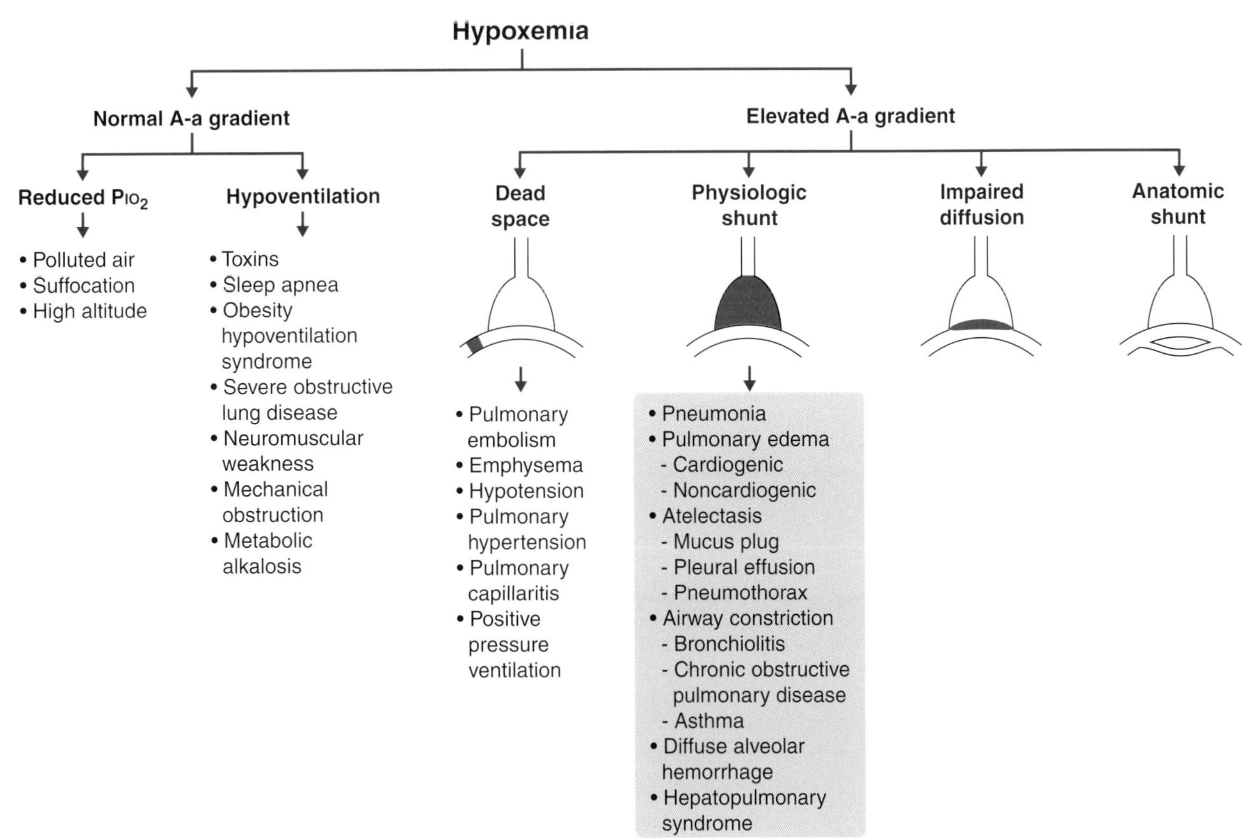

**In patients with acquired immunodeficiency syndrome who develop pneumonia from *Pneumocystis jirovecii* (PJP), why is it important to evaluate for hypoxemia?**

In patients with moderate-to-severe PJP pneumonia (defined as $PaO_2$ < 70 mm Hg or A-a gradient of >35), early treatment with glucocorticoids (within 72 hours after initiation of antipneumocystis therapy) is associated with a significant reduction in mortality.[14]

**What are the cardiogenic causes of pulmonary edema?**

Left-sided heart failure is by far the most common cardiogenic cause of pulmonary edema; others include mitral stenosis and mitral regurgitation with flail posterior leaflet (which results in focal right upper lobe pulmonary edema).

**What are the causes of noncardiogenic pulmonary edema?**

Causes of noncardiogenic pulmonary edema include acute respiratory distress syndrome (ARDS, which can be caused by a variety of underlying conditions), drug toxicity (eg, narcotic overdose), inhalation injury, high altitude pulmonary edema, neurogenic pulmonary edema, reexpansion pulmonary edema (ie, pulmonary edema following large-volume thoracentesis), and reperfusion pulmonary edema.[15]

**What are the key features of acute respiratory distress syndrome?**

ARDS is characterized by the acute development (within 1 week) of a respiratory illness associated with severe hypoxemia ($PaO_2/FIO_2$ ratio of ≤300) and bilateral opacities on chest imaging consistent with pulmonary edema that cannot be explained by cardiac disease.[15]

**What are the causes of acute respiratory distress syndrome?**

Bacterial and viral pneumonias are the most common causes of ARDS; others include sepsis, aspiration of gastric contents, acute pancreatitis, drug reactions (eg, methotrexate), inhalation of toxic fumes or particles (eg, massive smoke inhalation), and nonthoracic trauma.[16]

**How does the distribution of fluid on chest imaging differ between cardiogenic and noncardiogenic pulmonary edema?**

Cardiogenic pulmonary edema tends to occur in a dependent distribution.

**What lung conditions can predispose to mucous plugging of the small airways?**

Mucous plugging of the small airways commonly occurs in the setting of COPD, asthma, cystic fibrosis, and bronchiectasis.

**Which clue on the chest radiograph can be used to determine if complete hemithorax opacification is related to a mucous plug of a large airway or a pleural effusion?**

Tracheal deviation toward an opacified hemithorax suggests volume loss in that area (eg, atelectasis from a mucous plug); tracheal deviation away from an opacified hemithorax suggests a volume-occupying process (eg, pleural effusion).

**What condition associated with hypoxemia can develop in patients who undergo thoracentesis with large-volume drainage?**

Reexpansion pulmonary edema is an uncommon complication of thoracentesis that occurs within 24 hours of the procedure (usually within 1-2 hours). Risk factors include younger age, duration of lung collapse >72 hours, removal of large volumes of pleural fluid (>1500 mL), and rapid reexpansion. The vast majority of patients recover within 5 to 7 days.[17]

**Obliterative bronchiolitis is associated with which types of transplant procedures?**

Patients who have undergone either lung or hematopoietic stem cell transplantation are at risk for developing obliterative bronchiolitis. It is more common in lung transplant recipients, where it develops in most long-term survivors. Other associated conditions include autoimmune diseases (eg, rheumatoid arthritis) and exposure to inhalational toxins (eg, diacetyl).[18]

**What is the key difference between asthma and chronic obstructive pulmonary disease on pulmonary function testing?**

Unlike with COPD, airway obstruction related to asthma demonstrates reversibility. Hypoxemia can be a feature of severe asthma and COPD exacerbations, caused by shunt from airway constriction as well as hypoventilation. Pharmacologic management includes inhaled short-acting bronchodilators, glucocorticoids, and antibiotics in some cases. Noninvasive and invasive ventilation techniques may be necessary in some patients.[8]

**What is the treatment for diffuse alveolar hemorrhage?**

Most cases of DAH are related to pulmonary capillaritis (eg, GPA). Such cases may be responsive to immunosuppressive therapy (eg, glucocorticoids, cyclophosphamide, rituximab). Other etiologies of or contributors to DAH, such as infection and medications, should be specifically addressed.[19]

**What are the main clinical manifestations of hepatopulmonary syndrome?**

Dyspnea is the main symptom of hepatopulmonary syndrome and can be triggered by moving from a supine to an upright position (ie, platypnea). In addition to physical findings of cirrhosis (eg, spider angiomas), there may be digital clubbing, cyanosis, and orthodeoxia (defined by a decrease in $Pa{O_2}$ by ≥5% or by ≥4 mm Hg when moving from a supine to an upright position).[20]

## HYPOXEMIA RELATED TO IMPAIRED DIFFUSION CAPACITY

**What is diffusion capacity?**

Diffusion capacity describes the efficiency of gas transfer from the alveolar space to the pulmonary capillaries, which is principally dependent on the integrity of the alveolar-capillary membrane (Figure 46-8). In the laboratory, it is evaluated by measuring the diffusing capacity for carbon monoxide (DLCO).

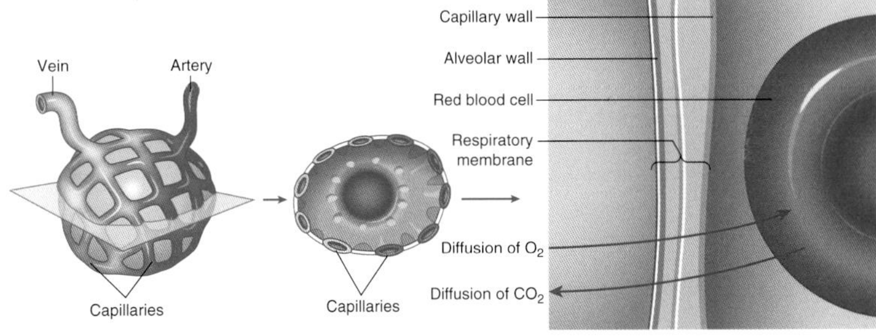


**Figure 46-8.** Gas exchange in the lung. Oxygen and carbon dioxide move across the alveolar capillary membrane via Fick's laws of diffusion. (From Kraemer WJ, Fleck SJ, Deschenes MR. *Exercise Physiology Integrating Theory and Application*. 2nd ed. Philadelphia, PA: Wolters Kluwer; 2016.)

**Why does impaired diffusion result in hypoxemia but not hypercapnia?**

$CO_2$ is approximately 20 times more soluble in water than $O_2$, making it significantly less likely to be affected by impaired diffusion. Furthermore, hyperventilation is often induced by hypoxemia, leading to a reduction in $Pa{CO_2}$.[6]

**What is the response to exercise in patients with impaired diffusion?**

Hypoxemia is significantly worsened during exercise in patients with impaired diffusion. This is principally related to an increase in cardiac output during exercise, which reduces pulmonary capillary transit time, further impairing oxygen diffusion. Moreover, tissue oxygen extraction increases during exercise, which results in decreased mixed venous oxygen content entering the pulmonary capillaries. *The 6-minute walk test and cardiopulmonary exercise testing are useful in the evaluation of patients with impaired diffusion.*[6]

**How does the hypoxemia related to impaired diffusion respond to inhaled oxygen?**

Decreased $Pa{O_2}$ related to impaired diffusion generally improves with inhaled oxygen.[6]

## What are the causes of impaired diffusion?

**A 54-year-old woman with dermatomyositis develops dyspnea and hypoxemia, and is found to have fine, end-inspiratory rales on auscultation of the lungs.**

Interstitial lung disease (ILD).

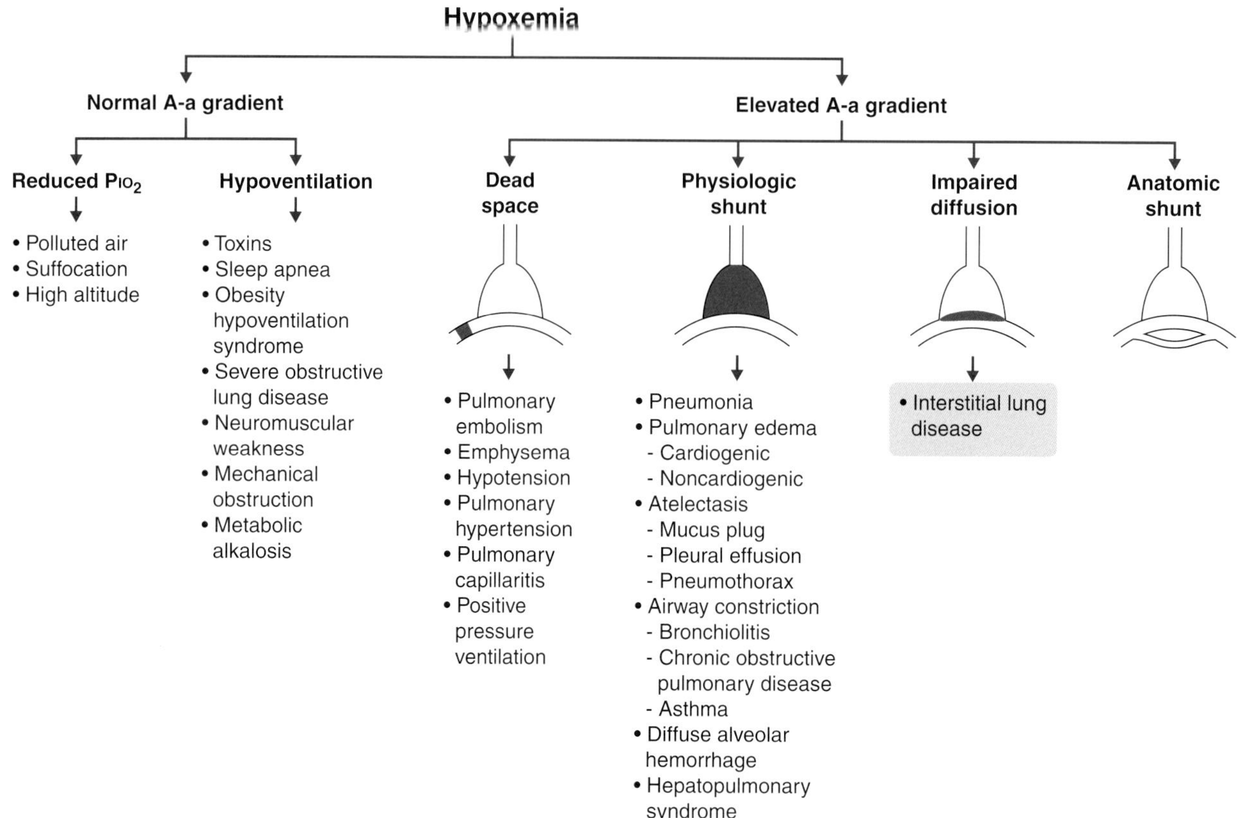


**What are the characteristic findings of interstitial lung disease on pulmonary function testing?**

Pulmonary function testing in a patient with ILD typically reveals a restrictive pattern (low forced vital capacity [FVC] and forced expiratory volume in 1 second [$FEV_1$] with normal $FEV_1$/FVC) in combination with impaired DLCO. Impaired diffusion may be the only abnormality in early ILD. The 6-minute walk test (which measures distance walked and oxygen desaturation) correlates with severity and can be prognostic in some forms of ILD. *Interstitial lung disease is discussed in depth in chapter 47, Interstitial Lung Disease.*[21]

*Other conditions can be associated with impaired diffusion, such as pulmonary hypertension and emphysema.*

## HYPOXEMIA RELATED TO ANATOMIC SHUNT

**What is an anatomic shunt?**

An anatomic shunt occurs when venous blood completely bypasses the pulmonary capillaries and enters the systemic circulation (Figure 46-9). A normal anatomic shunt occurs when the bronchial veins drain directly into the pulmonary veins (which amounts to 2%-3% of cardiac output).[6]

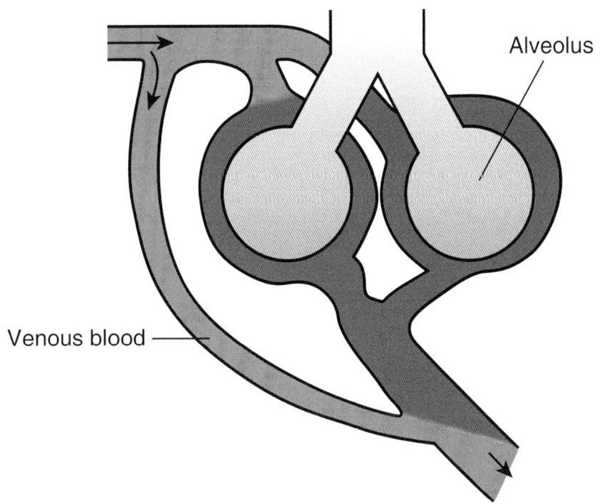


**Figure 46-9.** Illustration of an anatomic shunt, showing venous blood bypassing the alveoli and entering systemic circulation (arrows). (Adapted from Rhoades RA, Bell DR. *Medical Physiology: Principles for Clinical Medicine*. 5th ed. Philadelphia, PA: Wolters Kluwer; 2018.)

**How does the hypoxemia related to anatomic shunt respond to inhaled oxygen?**

The $Pa_{O_2}$ response to inhaled oxygen in the setting of an anatomic shunt is independent of the fraction of inspired oxygen. *This information can be useful in identifying the presence of an anatomic shunt.*[3]

### What are the causes of anatomic shunt?

**Echocardiography with agitated saline contrast results in the immediate appearance of bubbles in the left side of the heart.**

Intracardiac shunt.

**Echocardiography with agitated saline contrast results in the delayed appearance of bubbles in the left side of the heart.**

Pulmonary arteriovenous malformation.

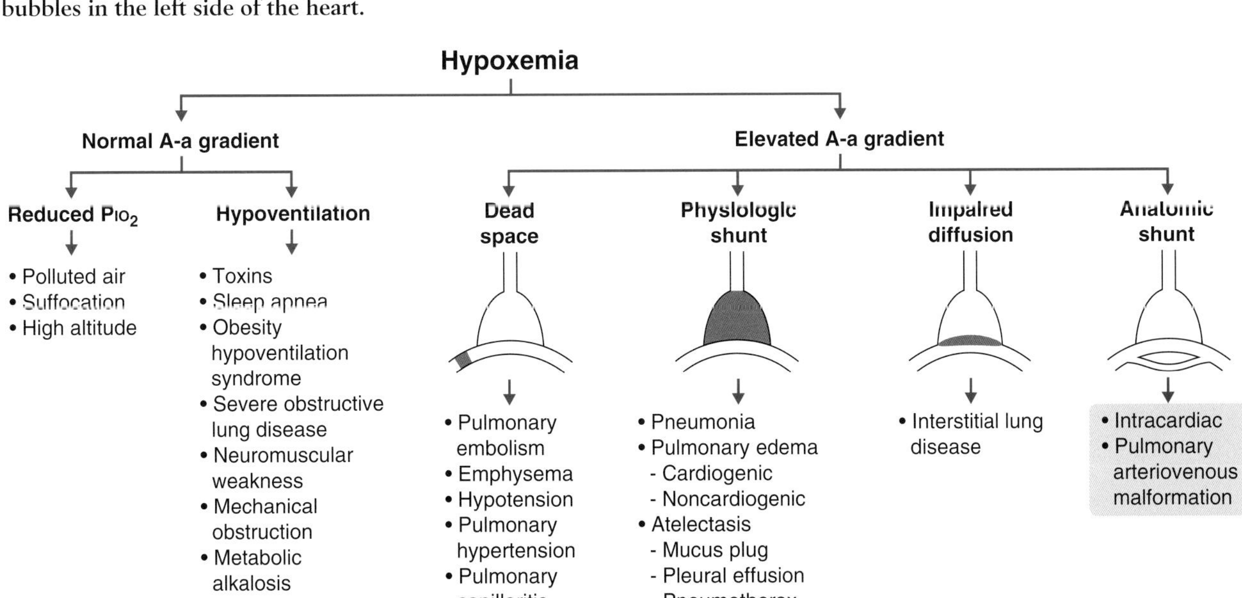

**What condition can occur with sudden-onset in patients with right-to-left intracardiac shunt, sometimes with devastating outcomes?**

Patients with right-to-left shunt are at risk for experiencing paradoxical embolism to critical organs such as the brain and kidneys.

**What is the relationship between pulmonary arteriovenous malformation and hereditary hemorrhagic telangiectasia (HHT, or Osler-Weber-Rendu syndrome)?**

The majority of cases of pulmonary AVM are congenital and associated with HHT; however, only a minority of patients with HHT develop pulmonary AVMs. Symptoms usually present between 30 and 60 years of age. An example of acquired pulmonary AVMs occurs in some patients with hepatopulmonary syndrome.[22]

## Case Summary

A 51-year-old man with cirrhosis presents with dyspnea and is found to have positional hypoxemia.

***What is the most likely cause of hypoxemia in this patient?***

Hepatopulmonary syndrome.

### BONUS QUESTIONS

***What is the A-a gradient in this case? (Recall ABG showed $Pao_2$ of 56 mm Hg and $Paco_2$ of 32 mm Hg.)***

$PAO_2$ = (0.21 × [760 − 47]) − (32/0.8) = 110 mm Hg. A-a gradient = 110 − 56 = 54 mm Hg. The upper limit of normal A-a gradient in a 50-year-old patient is approximately 27 mm Hg (see Table 46-1). The A-a gradient is therefore elevated, indicating that the mechanism of hypoxemia in this case involves 1 or more of the following: increased dead space, physiologic shunt, impaired diffusion capacity, and anatomic shunt.

***What finding is present in the photograph of the patient's hand in this case?***

The photograph of the patient's hand in this case (see Figure 46-1) demonstrates cyanosis and digital clubbing (one of the oldest signs in medicine originally described by Hippocrates in a patient with empyema).[23]

***What causes digital clubbing?***

Digital clubbing occurs when circulating megakaryocytes, normally trapped in the lung, bypass the filter through a right-to-left shunt and become lodged in the peripheral vasculature of the digits. There, the megakaryocytes release platelet-derived growth factor and vascular endothelial growth factor, which lead to the connective tissue changes found in clubbed digits.[23]

***What would be the expected findings if a chest radiograph were performed in this case?***

The chest radiograph in patients with pure hepatopulmonary syndrome is typically normal. *Patients with cirrhosis could have abnormalities related to other pathophysiologic processes (eg, pleural effusion [hepatic hydrothorax]).*

***What are the mechanisms of hypoxemia related to hepatopulmonary syndrome?***

Hypoxemia related to hepatopulmonary syndrome is caused by physiologic and/or anatomic shunt. The main mechanism is the dilation of pulmonary capillaries to 15 to 100 µm (normal is <8-15 µm), which increases perfusion relative to ventilation (ie, physiologic shunt). In addition, pulmonary arteriovenous communications can develop (ie, anatomic shunt).[20]

***How is hepatopulmonary syndrome diagnosed?***

Transthoracic echocardiography with agitated saline contrast is the most practical method for diagnosing hepatopulmonary syndrome. Normally, the microbubbles are unable to pass through the pulmonary capillary bed; however, when there is abnormal dilation of the capillary bed, with or without pulmonary AVMs, the bubbles are able to pass through, resulting in a positive study (see Figure 46-2). The administration of 100% oxygen in the pulmonary function laboratory can be used to calculate the shunt fraction.[20]

***What is the prognosis of hepatopulmonary syndrome?***

Liver transplantation is the only effective treatment for hepatopulmonary syndrome. Without it, median survival is around 24 months and 5-year survival rates are approximately 25%. Survival is significantly shorter in patients with a $Pao_2$ <50 mm Hg at the time of diagnosis. Identifying hepatopulmonary syndrome is important, as it may improve a patient's wait list status and candidacy for liver transplantation.[20]

***What additional pulmonary vascular condition that sometimes develops in patients with portal hypertension could be contributing to the hypoxemia in this case?***

Portopulmonary hypertension, which is defined as pulmonary arterial hypertension in association with portal hypertension of any etiology, should be suspected in patients with cirrhosis who develop hypoxemia. The diagnosis can be established with hemodynamic measurements from right heart catheterization.[24]

## KEY POINTS

- Hypoxemia is defined as low $Pao_2$ (<80 mm Hg).
- Hypoxia refers to the deficiency or ineffective use of oxygen within tissues of the body.
- Hypoxemia is the most common cause of hypoxia, but the two can occur independently.
- Hypoxia can occur in the absence of hypoxemia when any of the following actions are impaired: oxygen delivery (eg, low cardiac output), oxygen binding to hemoglobin (eg, methemoglobinemia), and oxygen uptake or use by the tissues (eg, sepsis).
- Pulse oximetry is a valuable noninvasive tool for the evaluation of hypoxemia.
- Arterial blood gas analysis allows for definitive evaluation of hypoxemia.
- Hemoglobin saturations of 50% and 90% correspond to $Pao_2$ values of 27 and 60 mm Hg, respectively.
- The alveolar gas equation, $PAO_2 = (FIO_2 \times [P_B - P_{H_2O}]) - (PaCO_2/RQ)$, allows for calculation of the A-a gradient, which is the first step in evaluating the cause of hypoxemia.
- Normal A-a gradient increases with age (eg, 17 mm Hg at age 20 years, 38 mm Hg at age 80 years).
- Hypoxemia associated with normal A-a gradient can be caused by reduced $PIO_2$ or hypoventilation.
- Hypoxemia associated with elevated A-a gradient can be caused by dead space, physiologic shunt, impaired diffusion, or anatomic shunt.
- Lung diseases often cause hypoxemia through a combination of mechanisms.
- Dead space occurs when there is excess ventilation relative to perfusion (eg, PE); physiologic shunt occurs when there is excess perfusion relative to ventilation (eg, pneumonia).
- Impaired diffusion is the abnormal transfer of gas across the alveolar-capillary membrane (eg, ILD).
- Anatomic shunt occurs when venous blood completely bypasses the pulmonary capillaries and enters the systemic circulation (eg, intracardiac shunt).

PULMONOLOGY

## REFERENCES


1. Hypoxemia vs. hypoxia. *N Engl J Med*. 1966;274(16):908-909.
2. Myers JA, Millikan KW, Saclarides TJ, eds. *Common Surgical Diseases: An Algorithmic Approach to Problem Solving*. 2nd ed. New York, NY: Springer New York; 2008.
3. Marino PL. *The ICU Book*. 3rd ed. Philadelphia, PA: Lippincott Williams & Wilkins – A Wolters Kluwer business; 2007.
4. Berne RML, Levy MN. *Physiology*. 4th ed. St. Louis, Missouri: Mosby, Inc.; 1998.
5. Morris AH, ed. *Clinical Pulmonary Function: A Manual of Uniform Laboratory Procedures*. 2nd ed. Salt Lake City: InterMountain Thoracic Society; 1984.
6. Sarkar M, Niranjan N, Banyal PK. Mechanisms of hypoxemia. *Lung India*. 2017;34(1):47-60.
7. Brown JPG, Michael PW. Humans at altitude: physiology and pathophysiology. *Contin Educ Anaesth Crit Care Pain*. 2013;13(1):17-22.
8. Chebbo A, Tfaili A, Jones SF. Hypoventilation syndromes. *Med Clin North Am*. 2011;95(6):1189-1202.
9. Berend K, de Vries AP, Gans RO. Physiological approach to assessment of acid-base disturbances. *N Engl J Med*. 2014;371(15):1434-1445.
10. Gurewich V, Thomas D, Stein M, Wessler S. Bronchoconstriction in the presence of pulmonary embolism. *Circulation*. 1963;27:339-345.
11. Jardin F, Gurdjian F, Desfonds P, Fouilladieu JL, Margairaz A. Hemodynamic factors influencing arterial hypoxemia in massive pulmonary embolism with circulatory failure. *Circulation*. 1979;59(5):909-912.

12. Kasper W, Geibel A, Tiede N, Just H. Patent foramen ovale in patients with haemodynamically significant pulmonary embolism. *Lancet*. 1992;340(8819):561-564.
13. Vodoz JF, Cottin V, Glerant JC, et al. Right-to-left shunt with hypoxemia in pulmonary hypertension. *BMC Cardiovasc Disord*. 2009;9:15.
14. Consensus statement on the use of corticosteroids as adjunctive therapy for pneumocystis pneumonia in the acquired immunodeficiency syndrome. The National Institutes of Health-University of California Expert Panel for Corticosteroids as Adjunctive Therapy for Pneumocystis Pneumonia. *N Engl J Med*. 1990;323(21):1500-1504.
15. Ferguson ND, Fan E, Camporota L, et al. The Berlin definition of ARDS: an expanded rationale, justification, and supplementary material. *Intensive Care Med*. 2012;38(10):1573-1582.
16. Matthay MA, Ware LB, Zimmerman GA. The acute respiratory distress syndrome. *J Clin Invest*. 2012;122(8):2731-2740.
17. Kasmani R, Irani F, Okoli K, Mahajan V. Reexpansion pulmonary edema following thoracentesis. *CMAJ*. 2010;182(18):2000-2002.
18. Barker AF, Bergeron A, Rom WN, Hertz MI. Obliterative bronchiolitis. *N Engl J Med*. 2014;370(19):1820-1828.
19. Park MS. Diffuse alveolar hemorrhage. *Tuberc Respir Dis (Seoul)*. 2013;74(4):151-162.
20. Rodriguez-Roisin R, Krowka MJ. Hepatopulmonary syndrome–a liver-induced lung vascular disorder. *N Engl J Med*. 2008;358(22):2378-2387.
21. Wallis A, Spinks K. The diagnosis and management of interstitial lung diseases. *BMJ*. 2015;350:h2072.
22. Gossage JR, Kanj G. Pulmonary arteriovenous malformations. A state of the art review. *Am J Respir Crit Care Med*. 1998;158(2):643-661.
23. Sarkar M, Mahesh DM, Madabhavi I. Digital clubbing. *Lung India*. 2012;29(4):354-362.
24. Porres-Aguilar M, Altamirano JT, Torre-Delgadillo A, Charlton MR, Duarte-Rojo A. Portopulmonary hypertension and hepatopulmonary syndrome: a clinician-oriented overview. *Eur Respir Rev*. 2012;21(125):223-233.

Chapter 47

# INTERSTITIAL LUNG DISEASE

## Case: A 58-year-old man with a tight skin

A 58-year-old man presents to the emergency department with difficulty breathing. He reports that he was healthy up until 10 years ago when he noticed that his fingers would turn white when exposed to cold environments. A few years later, he developed progressive skin tightening and decreased mobility of his hands, becoming dependent on his wife for help with most tasks. He lives in a rural town and has not previously sought medical care. Over the past year, he developed a dry cough and difficulty catching his breath; he is now short of breath at rest. Review of systems is notable for gastroesophageal reflux for which the patient takes over-the-counter medication.

Heart rate is 104 beats per minute, and respiratory rate is 26 breaths per minute. Hemoglobin oxygen saturation by pulse oximetry ($Spo_2$) is 86% on room air (using an earlobe probe). Jugular venous pressure is 12 cm $H_2O$. Cardiac auscultation reveals a loud P2 and an early decrescendo diastolic murmur over the second intercostal space along the left sternal border that is augmented with inspiration. There are fine end-inspiratory rales most pronounced at the bases of the lungs. The patient's hands are shown in Figure 47-1. High-resolution computed tomography (HRCT) imaging of the chest is shown in Figure 47-2A (coronal view) and Figure 47-2B (cross-sectional view of the lower lobes).

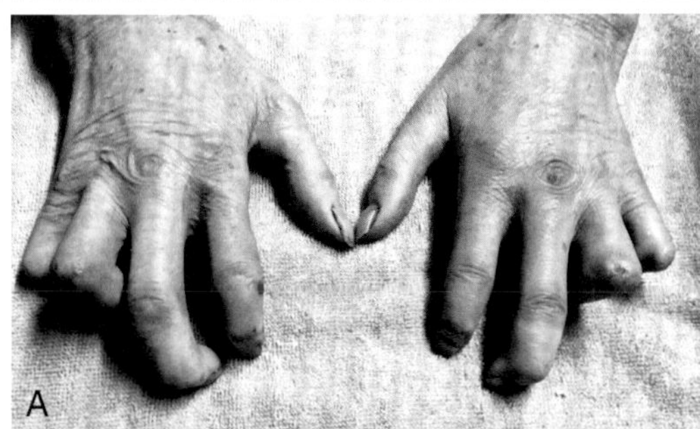

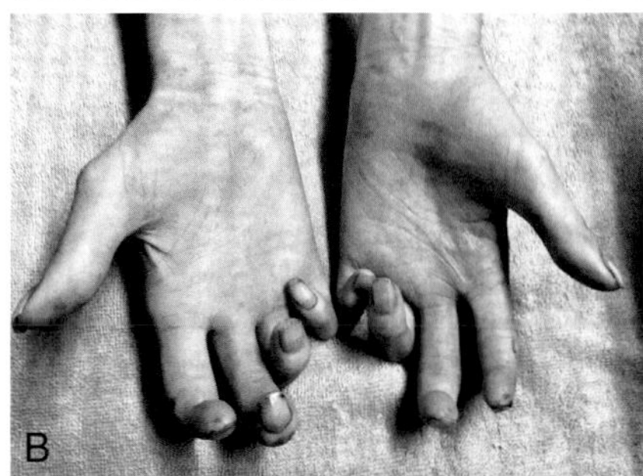


**Figure 47-1.**

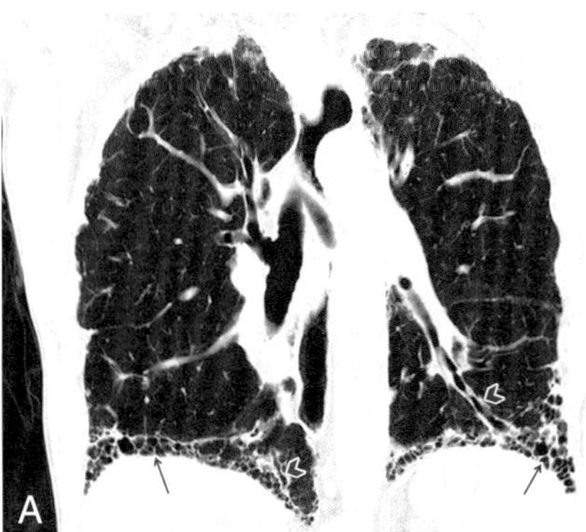

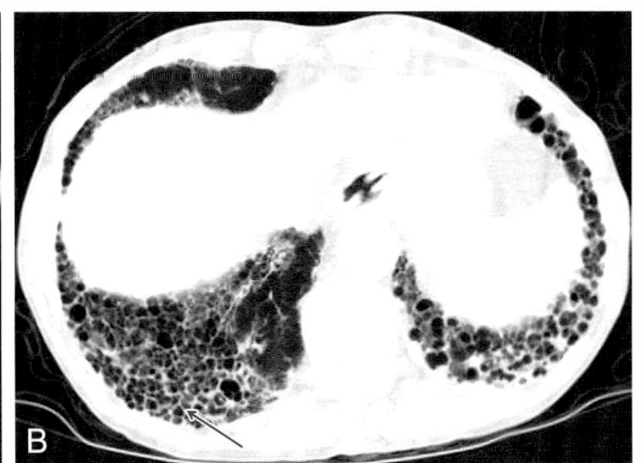


**Figure 47-2.**

***What is the most likely diagnosis in this patient?***

**What is interstitial lung disease (ILD)?**

ILD describes a heterogeneous group of diseases that affect the lung parenchyma, including the alveoli, pulmonary capillaries, and interstitial spaces, producing characteristic clinical, physiologic, imaging, and histologic manifestations (Figure 47-3).[1,2]

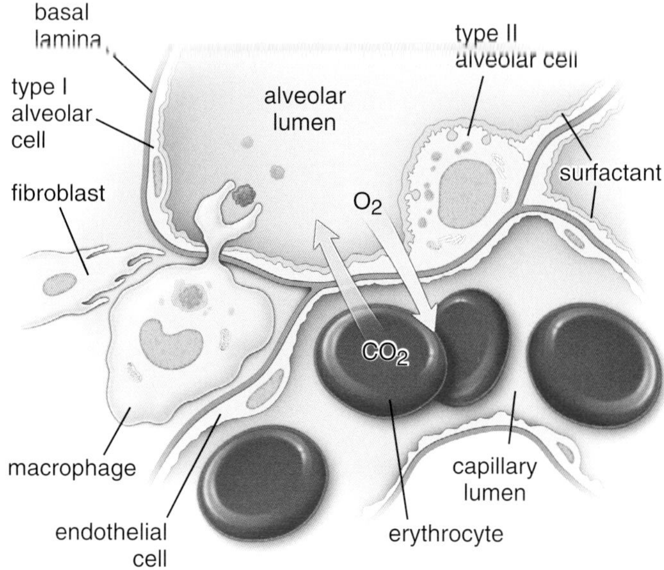


**Figure 47-3.** Microscopic elements of the pulmonary parenchyma. (From Ross MH, Pawlina W. *Histology: A Text and Atlas with Correlated Cell and Molecular Biology*. 7th ed. Philadelphia, PA: Wolters Kluwer Health; 2016.)

**What are the symptoms of interstitial lung disease?**

The most common symptoms of ILD include dyspnea, dry cough, fatigue, and weight loss. Additional symptoms may accompany specific etiologies of ILD (eg, dry eyes in Sjögren's syndrome). Symptom onset and disease course can be acute and rapidly progressive or insidious depending on the underlying etiology, and variability often exists between patients with the same etiology.[2]

**What are the physical findings of interstitial lung disease?**

Bilateral fine end-inspiratory rales are the hallmark of ILD. Other pulmonary findings may include pleural rubs and inspiratory squeaks or squawks. Extrapulmonary findings may include digital clubbing and signs of pulmonary hypertension (eg, loud P2). Additional findings may be associated with specific etiologies of ILD (eg, Gottron's papules in dermatomyositis).[2]

**What is the role of conventional radiography in the evaluation of interstitial lung disease?**

Conventional chest radiography is neither sensitive nor specific for the diagnosis of ILD. However, findings may include decreased lung volumes and increased reticulonodular markings. Particular etiologies of ILD may be suggested by the pattern of changes (eg, upper lobe predominance in sarcoidosis) or associated findings (eg, pleural plaques in asbestosis). The chest radiograph can also be helpful in evaluating for alternative or additional sources of symptoms such as pulmonary edema or pleural effusions.[2]

**What is the role of CT imaging in the evaluation of interstitial lung disease?**

HRCT imaging without contrast should be performed when ILD is suspected. The 2 main patterns of ILD on HRCT imaging are usual interstitial pneumonia (UIP) and nonspecific interstitial pneumonia (NSIP).[2]

**What are the characteristics of usual interstitial pneumonia on high-resolution CT imaging?**

The UIP pattern of ILD on HRCT imaging includes lower lung–predominant subpleural reticulations, traction bronchiectasis, honeycombing (ie, cystic dilation of distal bronchioles), and minimal ground glass opacities.[2]

**What are the characteristics of nonspecific interstitial pneumonia on high-resolution CT imaging?**

The NSIP pattern of ILD on HRCT imaging includes lower lung–predominant subpleural ground glass opacification and reticulations and traction bronchiectasis in the absence of honeycombing.[2]

**What are the findings of interstitial lung disease on pulmonary function testing?**

On pulmonary function testing, ILD typically manifests a restrictive pattern (ie, low forced vital capacity [FVC] and forced expiratory volume in 1 second [$FEV_1$] with normal $FEV_1$/FVC) in combination with impaired gas transfer testing (ie, impaired diffusing capacity for carbon monoxide [DLCO]). Impaired diffusion may be the only abnormality in early ILD. The 6-minute walk test (which measures distance walked and oxygen desaturation) correlates with severity and can be prognostic in some forms of ILD.[2]

**What is the role of bronchoscopy in the evaluation of interstitial lung disease?**

Bronchoscopy can be helpful in excluding infection in patients suspected of having ILD. In addition, bronchoalveolar lavage (BAL) can generate cell differentials that may be supportive of specific etiologies of ILD (eg, marked lymphocytic predominance in hypersensitivity pneumonitis). Endobronchial or transbronchial biopsies can occasionally establish the diagnosis and even the type of ILD (eg, sarcoidosis) but are generally too small to diagnose most cases.[2]

**What are the histologic findings of interstitial lung disease?**

Surgical lung biopsy can be helpful in identifying ILD and specific subtypes. As with HRCT imaging, there are 2 important histologic patterns of ILD: UIP and NSIP. Lung biopsy can be risky, particularly in older patients: open lung biopsy is associated with a mortality of approximately 4% at 30 days, whereas video-assisted thoracoscopic surgery (VATS) biopsy is associated with a mortality of about 2% at 30 days.[2]

**What are the 2 general categories of interstitial lung disease?**

ILD can be idiopathic or secondary to other conditions.

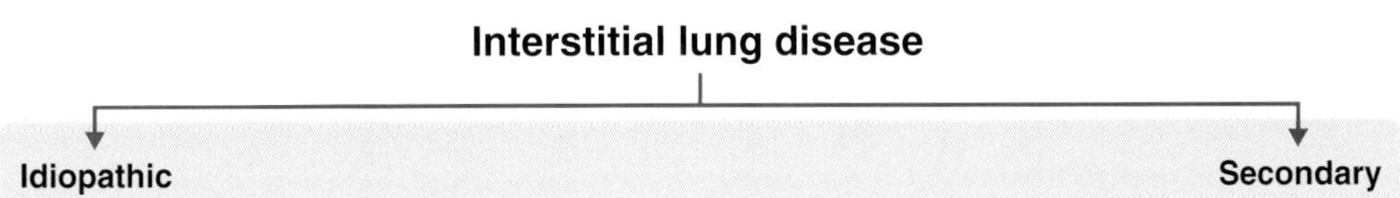


*Some secondary forms of ILD present with the imaging and histologic patterns of particular types of idiopathic ILD. In general, secondary ILD is more common than idiopathic ILD.*

## IDIOPATHIC INTERSTITIAL LUNG DISEASE

**What is idiopathic interstitial lung disease?**

The idiopathic forms of ILD present with characteristic clinical, imaging, and histologic patterns but are not related to known or identifiable systemic diseases or exposures.

### What are the idiopathic forms of interstitial lung disease?

**A previously healthy 68-year-old man develops slowly progressive dyspnea and dry cough over the course of a year and has fine end-inspiratory rales and digital clubbing on examination and a UIP pattern on HRCT imaging.**

Idiopathic pulmonary fibrosis (IPF). *Because IPF is the clinical correlate of the morphologic pattern of UIP, the terms are often paired (ie, IPF/UIP).*

**The second main morphologic pattern of ILD.**

NSIP.

PULMONOLOGY

**A 55-year-old woman presents to the emergency department with dyspnea, nonproductive cough, and fever for the third time in the past month despite several rounds of antibiotics and is found to again have a lung consolidation, but in a different location compared with prior episodes.**

Cryptogenic organizing pneumonia (COP, or bronchiolitis obliterans with organizing pneumonia).

**Diffuse interstitial infiltration with lymphocytes, plasma cells, and macrophages, often associated with peribronchiolar reactive lymphoid follicles.**

Lymphoid interstitial pneumonia (LIP).

**The only idiopathic form of ILD with acute-onset symptoms.**

Acute interstitial pneumonia (AIP, or Hamman-Rich syndrome).

**A 45-year-old woman with slowly progressive dyspnea and cough over a period of several months is found to have peripheral eosinophilia.**

Chronic eosinophilic pneumonia (CEP).

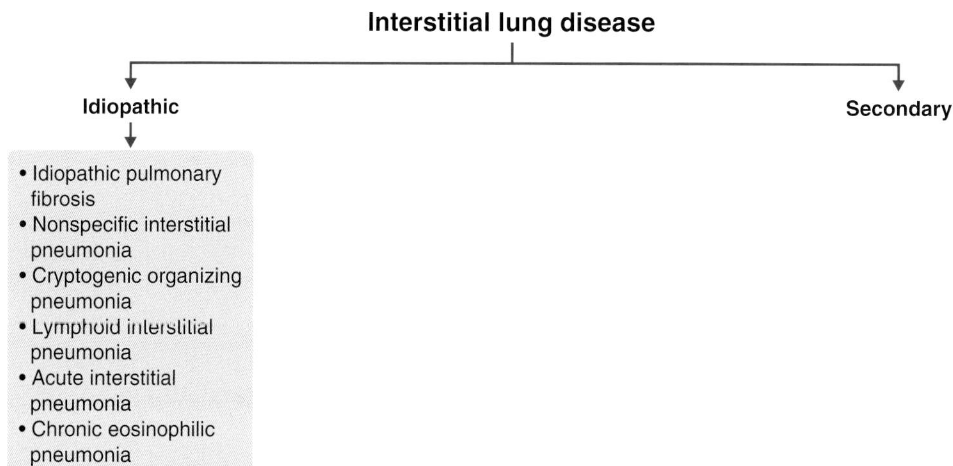


**What are the clinical characteristics of idiopathic pulmonary fibrosis?**

IPF is the most common type of ILD, with a prevalence in the industrialized world of around 65 cases per 100,000 persons. It typically occurs in patients older than 50 years with insidious onset and gradual progression over years. It is eventually fatal in most cases, but certain therapies may slow progression, including tyrosine kinase inhibitors (eg, nintedanib), antifibrotics (eg, pirfenidone), and supplemental oxygen. Other therapies such as pulmonary rehabilitation and treatment for asymptomatic gastroesophageal reflux disease may also be beneficial. Lung transplantation should be considered for appropriate patients. Acute exacerbations of IPF occur in some patients and may be responsive to glucocorticoids.[3,4]

**What are the clinical characteristics of nonspecific interstitial pneumonia?**

The onset of NSIP usually occurs between ages 40 and 50 years—about 10 years before the onset in the typical patient with IPF. Symptoms are similar to but milder than IPF. Treatment includes glucocorticoids and other immunosuppressive agents, and most patients stabilize or improve. Compared with IPF, prognosis of NSIP is better.[5]

**What are the imaging features of cryptogenic organizing pneumonia?**

The characteristic findings of COP on HRCT imaging are lung opacities, varying from ground glass to consolidation, located in a peripheral or peribronchial distribution, and most frequently involving the lower lobes. The opacities range in size from a few centimeters to an entire lobe and tend to be migratory on repeat imaging.[5]

**What are the clinical characteristics of lymphoid interstitial pneumonia?**

LIP is more common in women and typically presents in the fifth decade of life. There is insidious progression of symptoms, including dyspnea and cough, over a period of 3 years or more. *Idiopathic LIP is rare; it presents more commonly as a result of a secondary condition (eg, Sjögren's syndrome, acquired immunodeficiency syndrome).*[5]

**What are the clinical characteristics of acute interstitial pneumonia?**

Patients with AIP present at a mean age of 50 years, and symptoms typically develop within a 3-week time period, usually with an antecedent viral-like illness. Treatment is largely supportive, but glucocorticoids may be effective early in the course of the disease. Mortality rate is high, and most survivors develop lung fibrosis.[5]

**Which distinctive radiographic feature is associated with chronic eosinophilic pneumonia?**

On chest imaging, peripheral airspace consolidation often referred to as the "photographic negative shadow of pulmonary edema" may be seen in cases of CEP.[5]

*Some secondary forms of ILD present with the morphologic patterns of the idiopathic forms of ILD (eg, ILD associated with Sjögren's syndrome often presents in an LIP pattern). These secondary conditions must be ruled out before a diagnosis of idiopathic ILD is made.*

## SECONDARY CAUSES OF INTERSTITIAL LUNG DISEASE

**What are the 2 general causes of secondary interstitial lung disease?**

ILD can occur as a result of exposure or systemic disease.

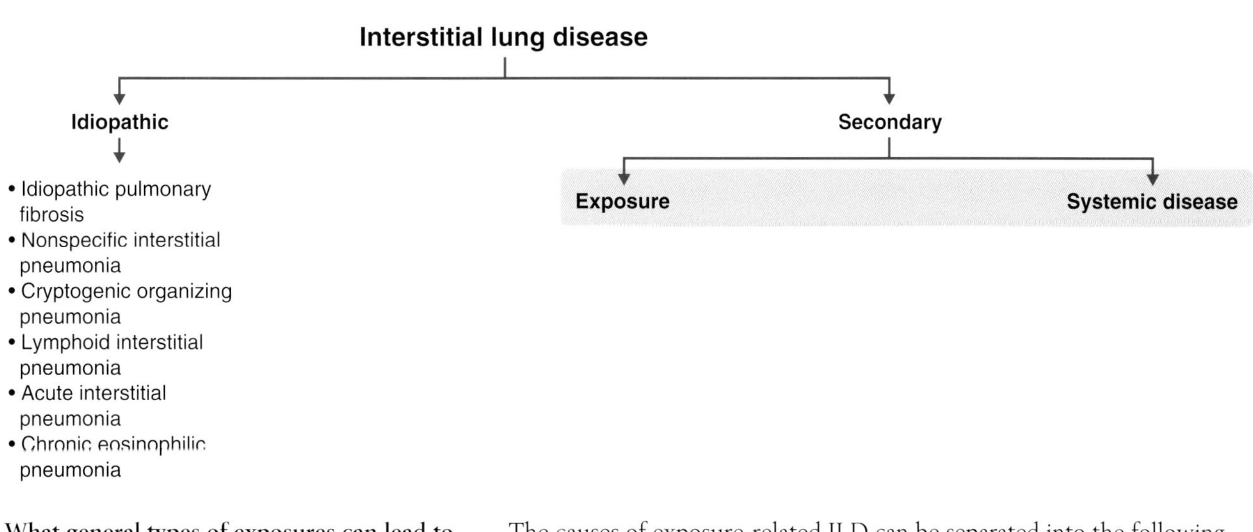


**What general types of exposures can lead to interstitial lung disease?**

The causes of exposure-related ILD can be separated into the following subcategories: iatrogenic, hypersensitivity, pneumoconiosis, and other.

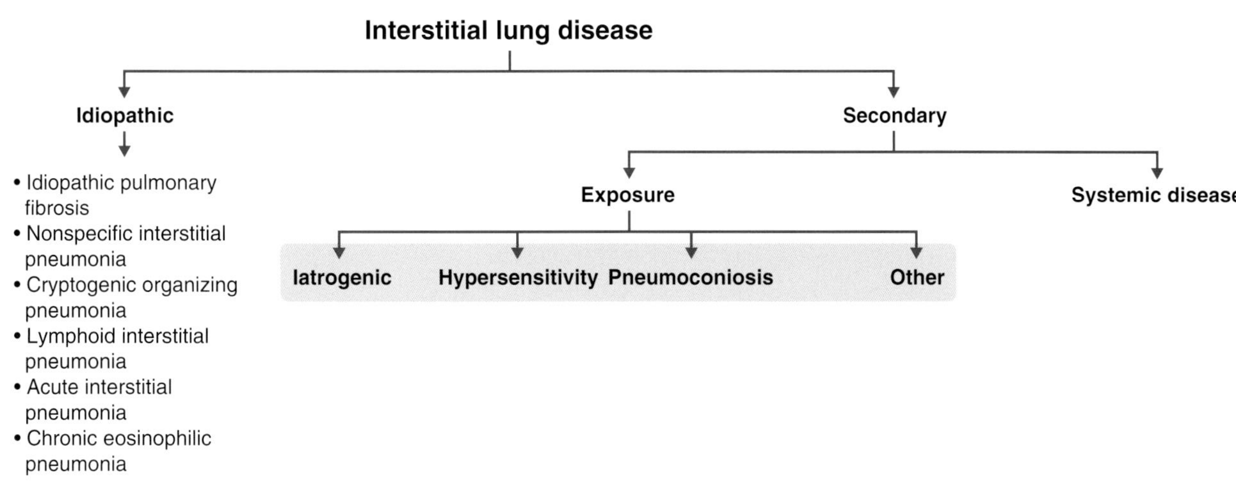


PULMONOLOGY

## INTERSTITIAL LUNG DISEASE RELATED TO IATROGENIC EXPOSURE

### What iatrogenic exposures are associated with interstitial lung disease?

**Sometimes it is not the underlying systemic disease that leads to interstitial lung disease but rather the treatment used.**

Medication.

**Look for tattoo marks on the chest.**

History of thoracic external beam radiation therapy.

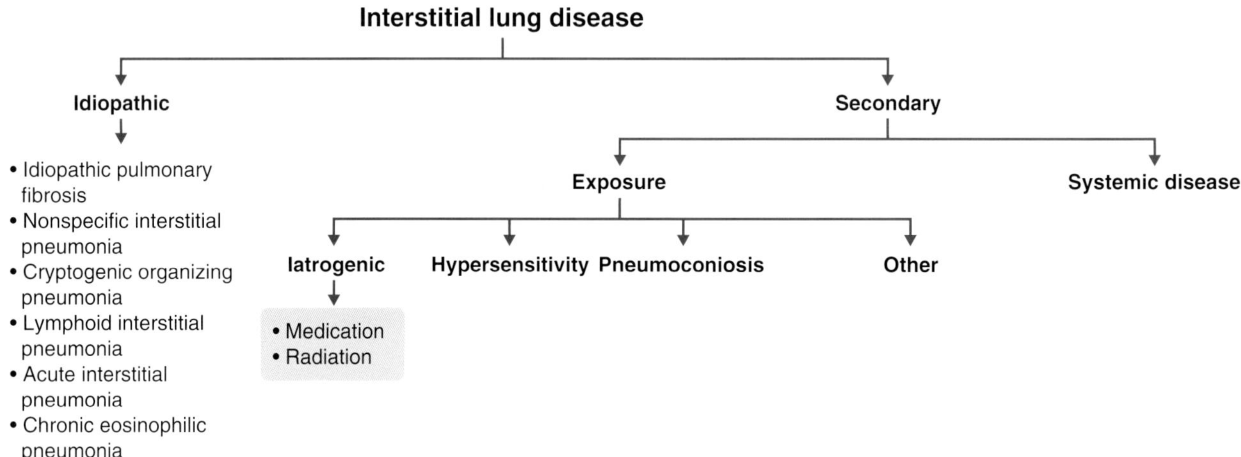


**What medications are associated with interstitial lung disease?**

Numerous drugs are associated with ILD, including drugs for rheumatic disorders (eg, methotrexate), chemotherapeutic agents (eg, bleomycin), biological modifiers (eg, etanercept), selective serotonin reuptake inhibitors (eg, fluoxetine), antibiotics (eg, nitrofurantoin), and cardiac agents (eg, amiodarone). In some cases, drug withdrawal is followed by complete resolution of ILD.[2]

**How often does thoracic external beam radiation therapy result in pulmonary toxicity?**

The occurrence and severity of lung disease after external beam radiation therapy is dependent on several factors, including dose delivered and volume of lung irradiated. Symptomatic radiation-induced pneumonitis typically develops 1 to 3 months after therapy. Some patients experience resolution of pneumonitis while others go on to develop pulmonary fibrosis. In some cases, pulmonary fibrosis develops in the absence of an acute phase. Fibrosis typically develops between 6 and 24 months post-treatment, achieving stability after 2 years. The radiographic pattern of disease tends to conform to the irradiation field, manifesting a variety of shapes (eg, rectangular).[6]

## INTERSTITIAL LUNG DISEASE RELATED TO HYPERSENSITIVITY PNEUMONITIS

**What is hypersensitivity pneumonitis (HP)?**

HP (ie, extrinsic allergic alveolitis) describes a syndrome related to repeated inhalation of and sensitization to aerosolized antigens in susceptible hosts, resulting in inflammatory changes in the lung parenchyma and airways. There is usually a history of exposure with compatible clinical, imaging, and histologic findings.[7]

**How common is hypersensitivity pneumonitis?**

HP accounts for up to 15% of all cases of ILD in the industrialized world. However, many cases are unrecognized or mischaracterized, so the true prevalence may be higher.[7]

**What are the main classes of antigens that cause hypersensitivity pneumonitis?**

The main classes of antigens associated with HP include bacterial antigens, fungal antigens, animal or bird proteins, insect proteins, and chemicals. Patients may be exposed to these antigens in a variety of environments, including at home and in the workplace.[7,8]

**What is the clinical course of hypersensitivity pneumonitis?**

The course of HP is highly variable, with some cases manifesting as an acute illness that resolves with no long-term sequelae and other cases manifesting with chronic pulmonary fibrosis. There is considerable overlap between the acute, subacute, and chronic forms of the disease (eg, a patient with chronic HP may have acute exacerbations with antigen exposure), and clinical criteria to distinguish the subtypes are lacking.[7,8]

**What are the clinical characteristics of acute hypersensitivity pneumonitis?**

The symptoms of acute HP typically occur within a few hours of antigen exposure and resemble an influenza-like illness. Wheezing is often present on examination. Acute HP is typical with thermophilic actinomycete species or fungal antigen exposure. Patients generally begin to improve over hours to days. Recurrences on antigen reexposure are common. Acute HP is usually nonprogressive.[8]

**What are the clinical characteristics of subacute hypersensitivity pneumonitis?**

The symptoms of subacute HP typically develop over weeks to months and include dyspnea, fatigue, and cough. Subacute HP is usually progressive.[8]

**What are the clinical characteristics of chronic hypersensitivity pneumonitis?**

The symptoms of chronic HP are typically insidious and slowly progressive in nature, often culminating in pulmonary fibrosis. This type of presentation is typical with bird antigen exposure. Patients with chronic HP, particularly male smokers, may experience acute exacerbations.[8]

**What is the role of serologic testing in the evaluation of hypersensitivity pneumonitis?**

Serum assays for precipitating antibodies (ie, precipitins) are available and support the diagnosis of HP when positive. However, results are positive in many patients who have been exposed to these antigens but do not have a compatible clinical syndrome of HP. Conversely, a negative result does not rule out HP because the particular antigen causing disease may not have been included in the assay.[7]

**What are the radiographic findings of hypersensitivity pneumonitis?**

Chest radiography in patients with HP can demonstrate variable findings. In acute and subacute HP, the chest radiograph can be normal but may also show nonspecific findings such as ground glass opacities and fine nodular opacities. The findings of chronic HP are more specific and consist of upper lobe–predominant fibrotic changes such as reticular opacities and honeycombing.[7]

**What are the findings of chronic hypersensitivity pneumonitis on high-resolution CT imaging?**

The typical findings of HP on HRCT imaging include a combination of reticular, ground glass, and centrilobular nodular opacities with fibrotic changes such as interlobular septal thickening, volume loss, traction bronchiectasis, and honeycombing. The fibrotic changes tend to spare the lower lobes, a distinguishing feature between chronic HP and UIP or NSIP.[8]

**What is the role of bronchoscopy in the evaluation of hypersensitivity pneumonitis?**

The characteristic finding of HP on bronchoscopy with BAL is an increase in total cell count with a dramatic elevation in the percentage of T lymphocytes (>20%, often >50%; normal <5%).[7,8]

**What is the treatment for hypersensitivity pneumonitis?**

Avoiding exposure to offending antigens is the cornerstone of therapy for HP. Glucocorticoids may alleviate acute symptoms in cases that do not resolve after eliminating antigen exposure, but do not appear to affect long-term outcomes.[7]

## What are the common types of hypersensitivity pneumonitis?

**Exposure to moldy hay and grain.**

Farmer's lung.

**Pet parakeets, parrots, or canaries.**

Bird fancier's lung.

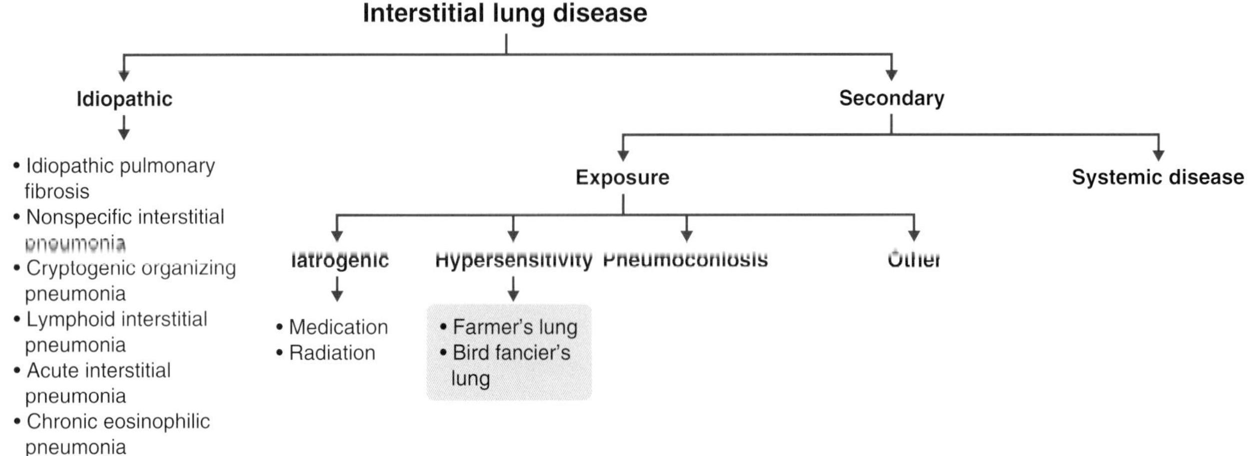


**What antigens are principally responsible for famer's lung?**

Farmer's lung is most commonly associated with antigens from the thermophilic actinomycete species and fungi (eg, *Aspergillus* species). *Farmer's lung is the prototype of acute HP.*[8]

**What antigens are principally responsible for bird fancier's lung?**

The antigens associated with bird fancier's lung come from a mixture of high- and low-molecular weight proteins in avian droppings and dried serum and on feathers. *Bird fancier's lung is the prototype of chronic HP (but can also cause acute HP).*[8]

**What are the other types of hypersensitivity pneumonitis?**

Many other types of HP have been described, some of which include woodworker's lung (from *Alternaria* species), hot tub lung (from *Mycobacterium avium-intracellulare*), and chemical worker's lung (eg, from diisocyanates).

## INTERSTITIAL LUNG DISEASE RELATED TO PNEUMOCONIOSIS

**What is pneumoconiosis?**

Pneumoconiosis describes a disease that occurs as a result of the lung reaction to various inhaled inorganic particles and dust, usually occurring in an occupational setting.[9]

### What are the most common pneumoconioses?

**Mining, quarrying, drilling, tunneling, and sandblasting.**

Silicosis.

**"Black lung."**

Coal worker's pneumoconiosis.

**Builders, plumbers, electricians, and shipyard workers.**

Asbestosis.

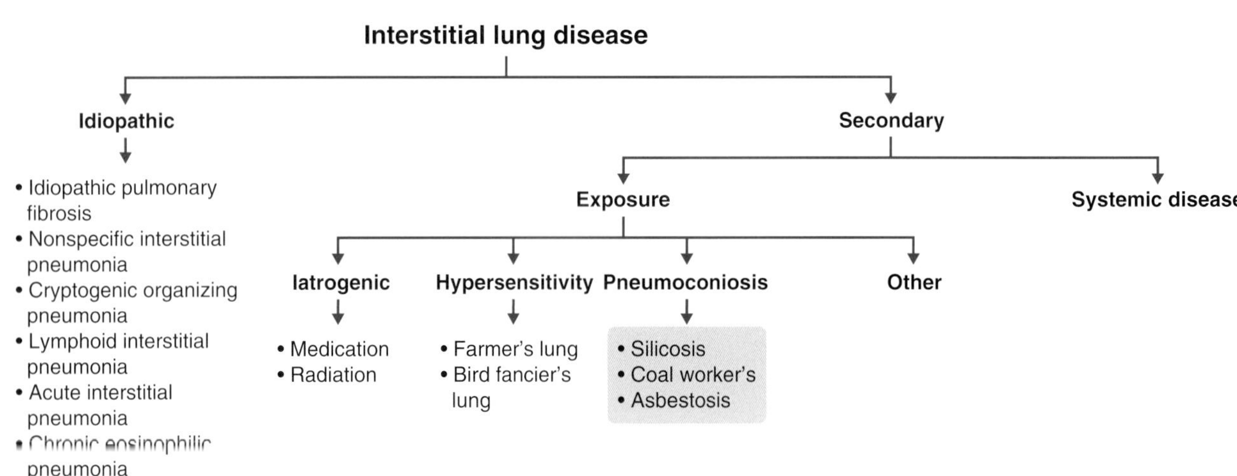

**When does silicosis typically develop after exposure?**

There are 3 main forms of silicosis: acute, chronic, and accelerated. Acute silicosis (ie, acute silicoproteinosis) is rare but can occur within weeks to a few years after initial high-level exposure. It is typically progressive with a poor prognosis. Chronic silicosis (ie, classic silicosis), the most common form, develops insidiously after 10 or more years of low-level exposure. The 2 subtypes of chronic silicosis are simple silicosis and progressive massive fibrosis (PMF); the clinical and imaging features of PMF are more severe. Accelerated silicosis develops 5 to 10 years after initial high-level exposure; clinical and imaging features are similar to chronic silicosis (usually PMF subtype).[10]

**When does coal worker's pneumoconiosis typically develop after exposure?**

Coal worker's pneumoconiosis usually presents >10 years after initial exposure and, like chronic silicosis, is characterized by simple and PMF subtypes.[11]

**What are the findings of silicosis and coal worker's pneumoconiosis on high-resolution CT imaging?**

The HRCT imaging features of silicosis and coal worker's pneumoconiosis are similar. The most common findings are nodular opacities that are well defined, uniform in shape, and located predominantly in the upper lung zones. The nodules are smaller (<1 cm) in milder forms (ie, simple) and larger (≥1 cm) in more severe forms (ie, PMF).[11]

**Which granulomatous infectious disease is associated with both silicosis and coal worker's pneumoconiosis?**

Pulmonary and extrapulmonary tuberculosis occur more frequently in patients with silicosis and coal worker's pneumoconiosis, and the risk increases with severity of lung disease. Cavitation on chest imaging is the strongest indicator of coexistent tuberculosis.[9]

**What is the spectrum of manifestations of asbestos-related lung disease?**

Asbestos inhalation can cause benign respiratory conditions (eg, pleural plaques and thickening and pleural effusions), interstitial lung disease (ie, asbestosis), and malignant disease (eg, mesothelioma and bronchogenic carcinoma). Asbestosis typically develops 20 to 30 years after exposure with a severity that is proportional to the magnitude and duration of exposure.[12]

**What are the other pneumoconioses?**

Less common pneumoconioses include berylliosis, hard-metal pneumoconiosis (eg, cobalt), talcosis, and siderosis.[9]

## INTERSTITIAL LUNG DISEASE RELATED TO OTHER EXPOSURES

### What are the other types of exposure-related interstitial lung disease?

**Smokers are at risk for these 3 types of ILD.**

Respiratory bronchiolitis–associated interstitial lung disease (RB-ILD), desquamative interstitial pneumonia (DIP), and pulmonary Langerhans cell histiocytosis (PLCH).

**High risk for right-sided infective endocarditis.**

Intravenous drug use.

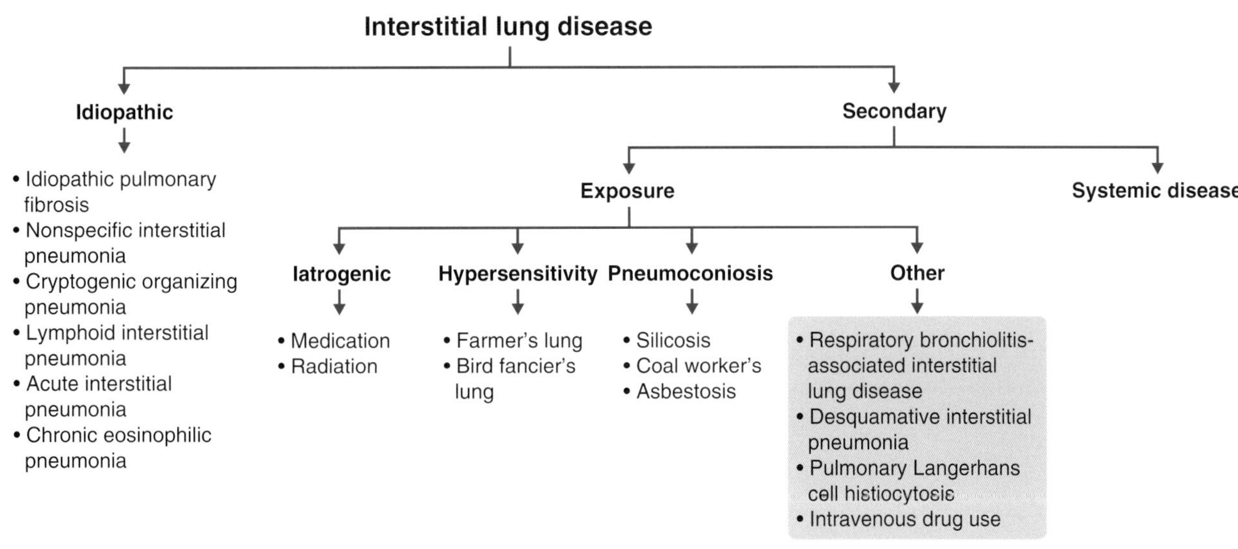


PULMONOLOGY

**What are the clinical characteristics of respiratory bronchiolitis–associated interstitial lung disease?**

RB-ILD typically affects active smokers between 30 and 40 years of age with ≥30-pack-year history, with a slight predominance in men. Dyspnea and mild cough are the most common symptoms. Inspiratory rales are present in about one-half of cases, whereas digital clubbing is rare. Smoking cessation is the cornerstone of management. The disease usually remains stable or improves, and long-term prognosis is good.[13]

**What are the clinical characteristics of desquamative interstitial pneumonia?**

DIP most commonly affects smokers (90% of cases) in the fourth and fifth decades of life, with a 2:1 predilection for men. Dyspnea and cough are the most common symptoms. Inspiratory rales are present in most, and digital clubbing occurs in about one-half of cases. Smoking cessation is the cornerstone of management, but glucocorticoids may be beneficial in some cases. Prognosis is mixed, with some patients experiencing complete recovery and others progressing despite treatment.[13]

**What are the clinical characteristics of pulmonary Langerhans cell histiocytosis?**

PLCH affects middle-aged smokers with a slight female predominance. Dyspnea and cough are the most common symptoms. In some cases, there may be involvement of other organ systems (eg, bone, skin, lymph nodes). Smoking cessation is the cornerstone of management and, when instituted early in the course of disease, is usually associated with good prognosis.[14]

**What is the mechanism of interstitial lung disease related to intravenous drug use?**

Talc, an agent used to maintain the integrity of medications in tablet form, can become lodged within the lung and cause a foreign-body granulomatous reaction when patients crush and intravenously inject prescription medications.[15]

## INTERSTITIAL LUNG DISEASE ASSOCIATED WITH SYSTEMIC DISEASE

### What systemic diseases are associated with interstitial lung disease?

**A noninfectious multisystem granulomatous disease that often affects the lungs, producing hilar and mediastinal lymphadenopathy with or without upper lobe–predominant parenchymal changes such as bronchial wall thickening, nodules along the bronchovascular bundles, ground glass opacities, cysts, and fibrosis.**

Sarcoidosis.

**Thickened and hardened skin.**

Scleroderma (ie, systemic sclerosis [SSc]).

**Associated with antibodies against cyclic-citrullinated peptide.**

Rheumatoid arthritis (RA).

**A 48-year-old woman with proximal muscle pain and weakness, elevated serum creatine kinase (CK), heliotrope rash, and "mechanic's hands" (Figure 47-4).**

Dermatomyositis (DM).

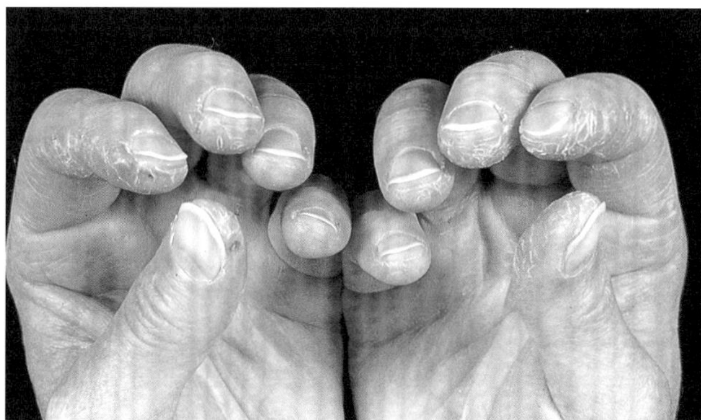

**Figure 47-4.** Drying and cracking of the skin over the lateral and palmar surfaces of the fingers, known as "mechanic's hands," is seen frequently in the antisynthetase syndrome that occurs in some patients with dermatomyositis or polymyositis. (From Koopman WJ, Moreland LW. *Arthritis and Allied Conditions A Textbook of Rheumatology*. 15th ed. Philadelphia, PA: Lippincott Williams & Wilkins; 2005.)

**A 45-year-old woman with proximal muscle weakness, elevated serum CK, and no skin findings or muscle pain.**

Polymyositis (PM).

**Among the connective tissue diseases, this is associated with the lowest relative frequency of ILD.**

Systemic lupus erythematosus (SLE).[16]

**A middle-aged woman with dry mouth, dry eyes, and parotitis is found to have serum anti-SSA (ie, anti-Ro) antibodies.**

Sjögren's syndrome.

**A 52-year-old woman with Raynaud's phenomenon, sclerodactyly, polyarticular inflammatory arthritis, and myositis.**

Mixed connective tissue disease (MCTD).

**Hemoptysis, glomerulonephritis, palpable purpura, and a foot drop.**

Vasculitis.

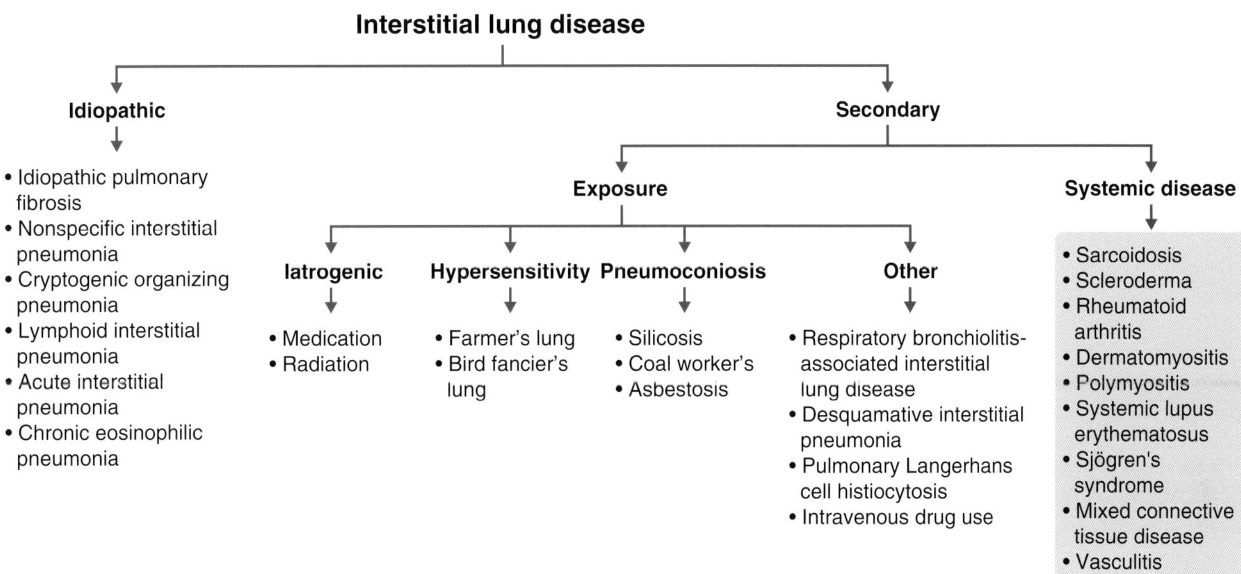


**What are the stages of pulmonary involvement of sarcoidosis?**

There are 4 stages of pulmonary involvement of sarcoidosis, according to radiographic evaluation: stage 1, bilateral hilar and mediastinal lymphadenopathy without parenchymal disease; stage 2, bilateral hilar lymphadenopathy with upper lobe–predominant parenchymal disease with distinctive features (eg, nodules along bronchovascular bundles); stage 3, parenchymal disease alone (shrinking or absent hilar lymphadenopathy); and stage 4, fibrosis, often upper lobe predominant, usually accompanied by volume loss, traction bronchiectasis, cysts, and diaphragmatic tenting (around 10% of patients progress to this stage). *The ILD of sarcoidosis is associated with a distinctive pattern on HRCT imaging.*[2,17]

**How common is interstitial lung disease in patients with systemic sclerosis?**

A significant proportion of patients with SSc develop ILD. It is more common in patients with diffuse SSc (approximately 55%) compared with those with limited SSc (approximately 35%). *The ILD of SSc most commonly manifests as NSIP or UIP.*[16]

**What are the characteristics of interstitial lung disease associated with rheumatoid arthritis?**

ILD is the most common pulmonary manifestation of RA, occurring more frequently in men (2:1), with onset most often in the fifth to sixth decades of life. The occurrence of ILD decreases survival in patients with RA from around 10 years to 2.5 years from the time of diagnosis. *The ILD of RA most commonly manifests as UIP or NSIP.*[18]

**How common is interstitial lung disease in patients with dermatomyositis or polymyositis?**

ILD occurs in up to half of patients with DM or PM and is predicted by the presence of autoantibodies to aminoacyl-tRNA synthetase enzymes (eg, anti-histidyl tRNA synthetase [anti-Jo-1]), which is associated with the antisynthetase syndrome. *The ILD of DM and PM most commonly manifests as NSIP, UIP, or COP.*[16]

**What populations with systemic lupus erythematosus are at higher risk for interstitial lung disease?**

Among patients with SLE, ILD is more common in those who are older, male, and have late-onset disease. *The ILD of SLE most commonly manifests as AIP. Given the higher prevalence of SLE in women, more women will be affected by ILD despite the relative higher frequency in men with SLE.*[19]

**What are the main risk factors for pulmonary involvement related to Sjögren's syndrome?**

Risk factors for pulmonary involvement in Sjögren's syndrome include male sex, smoking, late onset, and long evolution of disease. *The ILD of Sjögren's syndrome most commonly manifests as LIP, NSIP, UIP, or COP.*[20]

**How common is interstitial lung disease in patients with mixed connective tissue disease?**

ILD complicates MCTD in about one-half of patients (around 20% of these cases result in severe fibrosis). The occurrence of ILD in patients with MCTD results in increased mortality. *The ILD of MCTD most commonly manifests as NSIP.*[16,21]

**Which vasculitides are associated with interstitial lung disease?**

ILD is associated with antineutrophil cytoplasmic antibody–associated vasculitis, particularly microscopic polyangiitis—it is frequently present at the time of diagnosis. *The ILD of vasculitis most commonly manifests as UIP.*[22]

## Case Summary

A 58-year-old man presents with chronic and progressive dyspnea and weight loss and is found to have hypoxemia, abnormalities of the hands, a loud P2, a diastolic murmur, fine end-inspiratory rales, and abnormal cross-sectional imaging of the chest.

***What is the most likely diagnosis in this patient?***

Interstitial lung disease associated with scleroderma.

### BONUS QUESTIONS

***What is scleroderma?***

Scleroderma refers to a group of related conditions that result in cutaneous thickening and sclerosis (ie, hardening of the skin) and digital cutaneous ulcers. Depending on the subtype of scleroderma, there may be a variety of other manifestations, including internal organ involvement (eg, esophageal dysmotility).

***What are the 2 main types of scleroderma?***

Scleroderma can be localized (eg, morphea) or systemic (SSc), the latter of which is frequently associated with internal organ involvement. There are 2 main subtypes of SSc: limited cutaneous SSc (around 60% of cases) and diffuse cutaneous SSc (around 35% of cases). There can be considerable overlap between these subtypes.[23]

***What are the main features of limited cutaneous systemic sclerosis?***

Limited cutaneous SSc involves the skin but is typically limited to the hands, forearms, and face. Serum antinuclear antibodies and anticentromere antibodies are present in most cases.[23]

***What are the main features of diffuse cutaneous systemic sclerosis?***

Diffuse cutaneous SSc is more rapidly progressive than the limited form. Cutaneous involvement may extend to the proximal arms, trunk, and face. Other than antinuclear antibody, anti-Scl-70 is the most frequent antibody in diffuse cutaneous SSc. Early and severe internal organ involvement (eg, gastrointestinal tract, kidneys, lungs, heart) is typical.[23]

***What is the nature of lung involvement in limited and diffuse cutaneous systemic sclerosis?***

Limited cutaneous SSc is more closely associated with pulmonary hypertension, whereas diffuse cutaneous SSc is more closely associated with ILD. However, there is considerable overlap, and both manifestations may be present in some cases.[23,24]

***What findings are demonstrated in the image of the patient's hands in this case?***

The photograph of the patient's hands in this case (see Figure 47-1) shows sclerodactyly, which is characterized by skin thickening and hardening, giving the skin a shiny appearance and leading to curling of the fingers with loss of mobility. There is also evidence of digital skin pitting and poorly healing ulcerations.

***What are the major findings on high-resolution CT imaging of the chest in this case?***

HRCT imaging in this case (see Figure 47-2A and B) shows lower lobe–predominant subpleural reticular opacities and honeycombing (arrows), traction bronchiectasis (arrowheads), and the absence of ground glass opacities.

***The imaging pattern in this case is characteristic of which idiopathic form of interstitial lung disease?***

The pattern on HRCT imaging in this case is that of UIP, which is a common presentation of ILD associated with scleroderma.

***Based on the physical findings, which additional pulmonary condition is likely to be present in this case?***

The loud pulmonic component of the second heart sound (P2) is suggestive of pulmonary hypertension, which can be associated with SSc.

***What is the significance of the diastolic murmur in this case?***

Pulmonic valve insufficiency can occur as a result of pulmonary hypertension. In this setting, it is referred to as a Graham Steell murmur.

***How common is interstitial lung disease in patients with systemic sclerosis?***

Interstitial changes are found in the vast majority of patients with SSc, but clinically significant pulmonary fibrosis is seen in about one-quarter of cases.[24]

***What is the prognosis of interstitial lung disease associated with systemic sclerosis?[24]***

Treatment for scleroderma-associated ILD, typically with cyclophosphamide, is only of modest benefit. There is variability in prognosis, but overall, it is poor. Patients with an NSIP pattern tend to have better outcomes (median survival of 15 years) compared with those with a UIP pattern (median survival of 3 years).

## KEY POINTS

- ILD describes a group of heterogeneous diseases of the lung parenchyma that produce characteristic clinical, physiologic, imaging, and histologic manifestations.
- The most common clinical manifestations of ILD include dyspnea, dry cough, bibasilar fine end-inspiratory rales, and digital clubbing.
- ILD can be acute and rapidly progressive or insidious in onset, depending on the subtype.
- HRCT imaging is useful in the evaluation of ILD and can identify patterns of findings associated with particular subtypes of ILD.
- ILD usually manifests as a restrictive lung disease with impaired diffusion capacity on pulmonary function testing.
- Bronchoscopy or surgical biopsy (including VATS) can provide a histologic diagnosis and can also evaluate for alternative etiologies (eg, infection).
- ILD can be idiopathic or secondary to other conditions.
- Idiopathic ILD is not associated with any identifiable secondary condition.
- The various idiopathic forms of ILD are associated with distinctive imaging and histologic patterns.
- The 2 most common morphologic patterns of ILD are UIP and NSIP.
- Secondary ILD can occur as a result of exposure or systemic disease.
- The causes of exposure-related ILD can be separated into the following subcategories: iatrogenic, HP, pneumoconiosis, and other.
- The secondary forms of ILD, particularly systemic diseases, often present with the morphologic patterns of the idiopathic forms of ILD.
- Clinical manifestations and prognosis of ILD are highly variable and depend on the specific subtype, ranging from self-limited and reversible to rapidly progressive and fatal.

## REFERENCES


1. Longo DL, Fauci AS, Kasper DL, Hauser SL, Jameson JL, Loscalzo J, eds. *Harrison's Principles of Internal Medicine*. 18th ed. New York, NY: McGraw-Hill; 2012.
2. Wallis A, Spinks K. The diagnosis and management of interstitial lung diseases. *BMJ*. 2015;350:h2072.
3. Raghu G, Collard HR, Egan JJ, et al. An official ATS/ERS/JRS/ALAT statement: idiopathic pulmonary fibrosis: evidence-based guidelines for diagnosis and management. *Am J Respir Crit Care Med*. 2011;183(6):788-824.
4. Raghu G, Rochwerg B, Zhang Y, et al. An official ATS/ERS/JRS/ALAT clinical practice guideline: treatment of idiopathic pulmonary fibrosis. An update of the 2011 clinical practice guideline. *Am J Respir Crit Care Med*. 2015;192(2):e3-e19.
5. Mueller-Mang C, Grosse C, Schmid K, Stiebellehner L, Bankier AA. What every radiologist should know about idiopathic interstitial pneumonias. *Radiographics*. 2007;27(3):595-615.
6. Williams JP, Johnston CJ, Finkelstein JN. Treatment for radiation-induced pulmonary late effects: spoiled for choice or looking in the wrong direction? *Curr Drug Targets*. 2010;11(11):1386-1394.
7. Spagnolo P, Rossi G, Cavazza A, et al. Hypersensitivity pneumonitis: a comprehensive review. *J Investig Allergol Clin Immunol*. 2015;25(4):237-250; quiz follow 50.
8. Selman M, Pardo A, King TE Jr. Hypersensitivity pneumonitis: insights in diagnosis and pathobiology. *Am J Respir Crit Care Med*. 2012;186(4):314-324.
9. Chong S, Lee KS, Chung MJ, Han J, Kwon OJ, Kim TS. Pneumoconiosis: comparison of imaging and pathologic findings. *Radiographics*. 2006;26(1):59-77.
10. Leung CC, Yu IT, Chen W. Silicosis. *Lancet*. 2012;379(9830):2008-2018.
11. Laney AS, Weissman DN. Respiratory diseases caused by coal mine dust. *J Occup Environ Med*. 2014;56(suppl 10):S18-S22.
12. Currie GP, Watt SJ, Maskell NA. An overview of how asbestos exposure affects the lung. *BMJ*. 2009;339:b3209.
13. Attili AK, Kazerooni EA, Gross BH, Flaherty KR, Myers JL, Martinez FJ. Smoking-related interstitial lung disease: radiologic-clinical-pathologic correlation. *Radiographics*. 2008;28(5):1383-1396; discussion 96-98.
14. Elia D, Torre O, Cassandro R, Caminati A, Harari S. Pulmonary Langerhans cell histiocytosis: a comprehensive analysis of 40 patients and literature review. *Eur J Intern Med*. 2015;26(5):351-356.
15. Roberts WC. Pulmonary talc granulomas, pulmonary fibrosis, and pulmonary hypertension resulting from intravenous injection of talc-containing drugs intended for oral use. *Proc (Bayl Univ Med Cent)*. 2002;15(3):260-261.
16. Castelino FV, Varga J. Interstitial lung disease in connective tissue diseases: evolving concepts of pathogenesis and management. *Arthritis Res Ther*. 2010;12(4):213.
17. Iannuzzi MC, Rybicki BA, Teirstein AS. Sarcoidosis. *N Engl J Med*. 2007;357(21):2153-2165.
18. Shaw M, Collins BF, Ho LA, Raghu G. Rheumatoid arthritis-associated lung disease. *Eur Respir Rev*. 2015;24(135):1-16.
19. Cheema GS, Quismorio FP Jr. Interstitial lung disease in systemic lupus erythematosus. *Curr Opin Pulm Med*. 2000;6(5):424-429.
20. Flament T, Bigot A, Chaigne B, Henique H, Diot E, Marchand-Adam S. Pulmonary manifestations of Sjogren's syndrome. *Eur Respir Rev*. 2016;25(140):110-123.
21. Gunnarsson R, Aalokken TM, Molberg O, et al. Prevalence and severity of interstitial lung disease in mixed connective tissue disease: a nationwide, cross-sectional study. *Ann Rheum Dis*. 2012;71(12):1966-1972.
22. Katsumata Y, Kawaguchi Y, Yamanaka H. Interstitial lung disease with ANCA-associated vasculitis. *Clin Med Insights Circ Respir Pulm Med*. 2015;9(suppl 1):51-56.
23. Hinchcliff M, Varga J. Systemic sclerosis/scleroderma: a treatable multisystem disease. *Am Fam Physician*. 2008;78(8):961-968.
24. Schoenfeld SR, Castelino FV. Interstitial lung disease in scleroderma. *Rheum Dis Clin North Am*. 2015;41(2):237-248.

Chapter 48

# PLEURAL EFFUSION

## Case: A 62-year-old man with pleuritic chest pain

A 62-year-old Filipino man who underwent coronary artery bypass grafting (CABG) surgery 5 months ago presents to the emergency department with increasing shortness of breath. The patient had done well in the months after surgery until 1 week before presentation when he developed fever, chills, and dry cough. This was followed by progressive dyspnea on exertion. He also describes sharp left-sided chest discomfort that worsens with deep breathing and coughing. Other than coronary artery disease, the patient has no known medical problems. He takes aspirin and metoprolol but no other medications. The patient was born in the Philippines and lived there before emigrating to the United States 2 years ago. He has never smoked cigarettes.

Temperature is 38.3°C, and respiratory rate is 26 breaths per minute. The patient appears acutely ill and is diaphoretic. There is decreased inspiratory excursion of the left posterior chest wall along with dullness to percussion and absent tactile fremitus. There are tubular breath sounds just above the region of dullness but no inspiratory rales. Chest radiographs are shown in Figure 48-1A (current) and Figure 48-1B (before surgery).

A thoracentesis is performed, and pleural fluid analysis shows a leukocyte count of 2600 cells/μL with a lymphocyte fraction of 95%. Pleural fluid protein concentration is 5.8 g/dL (serum total protein concentration is 8.1 g/dL). Pleural fluid Gram stain and Ziehl-Neelsen stain for acid-fast bacilli do not show any organisms. Culture is pending. Cytologic examination of the fluid is negative for malignant cells. Pleural fluid adenosine deaminase level is 6.3 U/L (reference range 0 to 9.4 U/L).

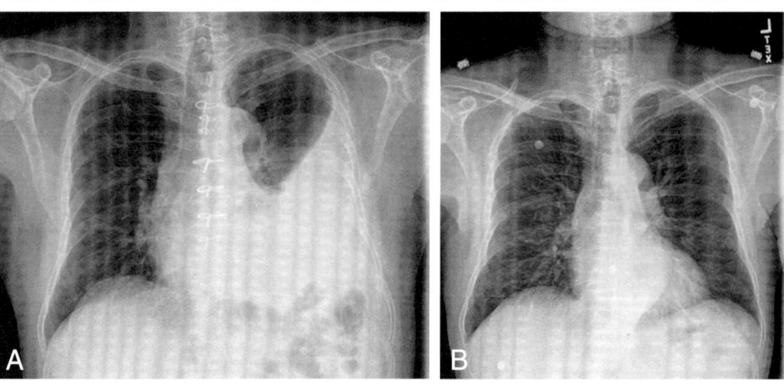

**Figure 48-1.**

***What is the most likely cause of the pleural effusion in this patient?***

**What is a pleural effusion?**

A pleural effusion is the abnormal accumulation of fluid in the pleural cavity, usually as a result of increased pleural fluid production, decreased pleural fluid absorption, or both (Figure 48-2).[1]

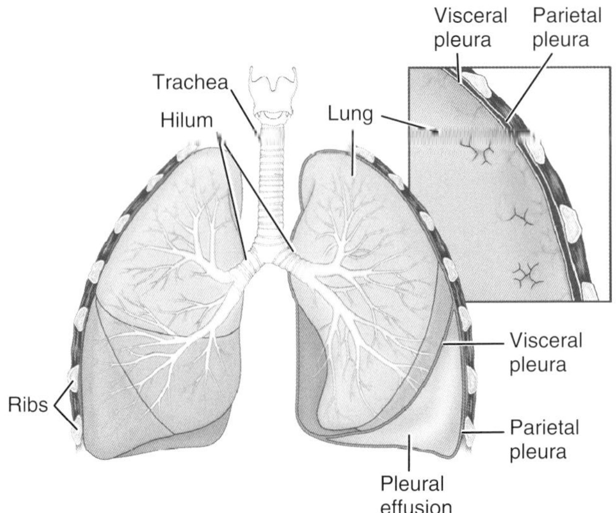


**Figure 48-2.** Pleural effusion describes the abnormal accumulation of fluid in the pleural space. (From Pellico LH. *Focus on Adult Health: Medical-Surgical Nursing*. Philadelphia, PA: Wolters Kluwer Health; 2013.)

**What are the mechanisms of pleural fluid accumulation?**

The main mechanisms of pleural effusion accumulation are increased pulmonary capillary and interstitial hydrostatic pressure, decreased capillary oncotic pressure, increased pleural membrane permeability, decreased intrapleural pressure, and obstruction to lymphatic flow.[2]

**How common are pleural effusions?**

Pleural effusions are common, with an incidence of approximately 400 cases per 100,000 persons per year in the industrialized world.[1]

**What are the symptoms of pleural effusions?**

Symptoms of pleural effusions depend on the size and rate of accumulation but may include dyspnea, nonproductive cough, and chest pain (usually pleuritic).[1,2]

**What physical findings are associated with pleural effusions?**

Physical findings of pleural effusions may include decreased inspiratory expansion of the chest wall on the affected side, dullness to percussion, decreased tactile fremitus, and reduced breath sounds over the effusion.

**What is the role of chest radiography in the evaluation of pleural effusions?**

Chest radiography is sensitive for the presence of a pleural effusion, which appears as a meniscus on the lateral view when the volume is >50 mL. A meniscus becomes visible on the posteroanterior view when the volume is >200 mL; obscuration of the hemidiaphragm occurs when the volume is >500 mL.[3]

**What is the definition of a large pleural effusion?**

A pleural effusion is considered large when it occupies more than one-quarter of the hemithorax.[4]

**What radiographic clue can be used to determine if complete hemithorax opacification is related to atelectasis or a space-occupying process?**

On a chest radiograph, tracheal deviation toward the opacified hemithorax suggests volume loss over that area (ie, collapsed lung); tracheal deviation away from the opacified hemithorax suggests a volume-occupying process (eg, pleural effusion).

**What is the role of computed tomography (CT) imaging in the evaluation of pleural effusions?**

Contrast enhanced CT imaging provides more information than conventional radiography. In addition to the pleural effusion(s), it may identify findings such as pleural thickening and nodularity, and parenchymal lesions not visible with chest radiography.[1]

**What is a loculated pleural effusion?**

A loculated pleural effusion does not flow freely within the pleural cavity and can be associated with certain types of effusions. A chest radiograph taken in the lateral decubitus position can identify whether the fluid is flowing freely or not (Figure 48-3). Ultrasonography and CT imaging have largely supplanted this technique and are now increasingly used to identify loculation.

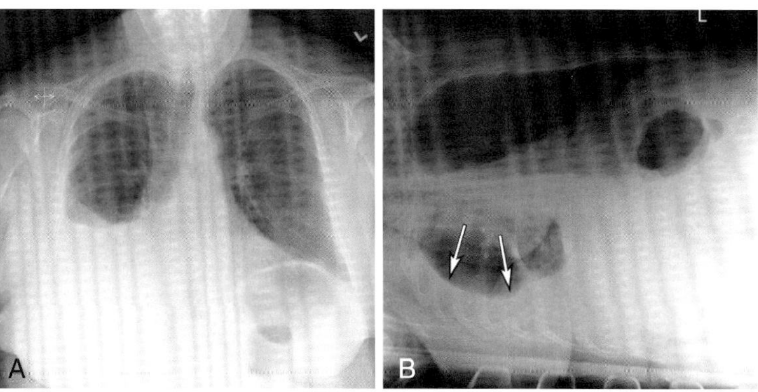


**Figure 48-3.** A, Chest radiograph showing a moderate right-sided pleural effusion. B, Right lateral decubitus radiograph confirming that the right pleural effusion (arrows) is free flowing and not loculated. (From Smith WL, Farrell TA. *Radiology 101: The Basics and Fundamentals of Imaging*. 4th ed. Philadelphia, PA: Lippincott Williams & Wilkins; 2014.)

**What is an empyema?**

An empyema is defined by the presence of pus in the pleural space. The fluid is thick, viscous, and purulent in appearance.[5]

**What are the 2 general types of pleural effusions?**

Pleural effusions can be transudative or exudative.

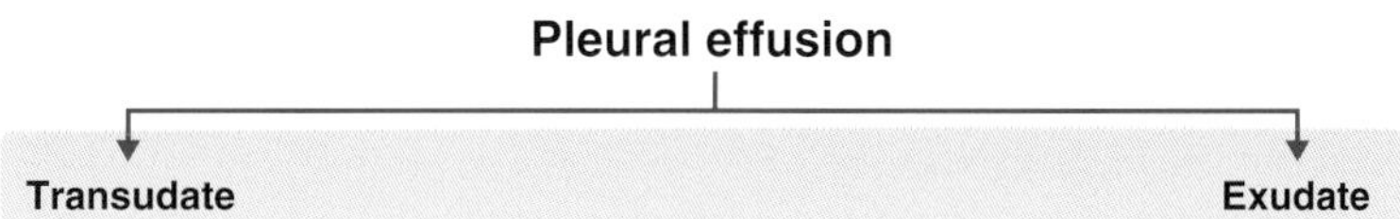


**What procedure must be performed to determine whether pleural fluid is transudative or exudative?**

Thoracentesis allows for the evaluation of pleural fluid, including the determination of its transudative or exudative nature. *Therapeutic thoracentesis can also be used to relieve symptoms in patients with refractory or recurrent pleural effusions.*

**What validated criteria can help determine whether pleural fluid is transudative or exudative?**

Pleural fluid is considered exudative when at least 1 of the following 3 conditions are met: (1) ratio of pleural fluid protein level to serum protein level >0.5, (2) ratio of pleural fluid lactate dehydrogenase (LDH) level to serum LDH level >0.6, or (3) pleural fluid LDH level >two-thirds the upper limit of normal for serum LDH level. These conditions are collectively known as Light's criteria.[6,7]

**What are the operating characteristics of Light's criteria?**

The use of Light's criteria is 98% sensitive for identifying exudates, but specificity is lower at 83%. This means that 17% of true transudates will be misclassified as exudates. In cases where an effusion is unexpectedly classified as an exudate by Light's criteria (ie, the clinical picture suggests a transudate), then the difference between albumin levels in serum and pleural fluid should be calculated by subtracting pleural fluid albumin from serum albumin. If the difference is >1.2 g/dL, the effusion is transudative in virtually all cases.[6]

**What basic fluid characteristics can be helpful in the evaluation of pleural effusions?**

Routine pleural fluid evaluation includes the gross appearance of the fluid (color, turbidity, viscosity); total and differential cell counts; protein, LDH, and glucose levels; and smear and culture. Other tests are available and should be used in the appropriate settings (eg, pH if empyema is suspected, cytology if malignancy is suspected, adenosine deaminase concentration if tuberculosis [TB] is suspected).

**What is the significance of the gross appearance of pleural fluid?**

The appearance of pleural fluid can help narrow the differential diagnosis. For example, bloody effusions are most commonly associated with hemothorax, malignancy, pulmonary embolism (PE), trauma, and pneumonia. Tenacious and cloudy fluid suggests infection. Fluid that is milky in appearance suggests chylothorax.[6]

**What is the significance of the differential cell count of pleural fluid?**

The predominant cell type in pleural fluid can help narrow the differential diagnosis. A predominance of neutrophils (>50%) suggests an acute process, such as pneumonia, PE, pancreatitis, or intra-abdominal abscess, whereas a predominance of mononuclear cells suggests a chronic process. A predominance of lymphocytes is suggestive of malignancy, tuberculous pleuritis, postcardiac injury syndrome (PCIS), or post-CABG (some of these conditions may be associated with an initial predominance of neutrophils). A predominance of eosinophils can be suggestive of drug-induced effusions, hemothorax, asbestos exposure, and eosinophilic granulomatosis with polyangiitis (EGPA, or Churg-Strauss syndrome).[6]

**What is the significance of the glucose concentration of pleural fluid?**

Low pleural fluid glucose concentration (<60 mg/dL) is suggestive of parapneumonic effusion or malignancy. Other less common causes include hemothorax, tuberculous pleuritis, and rheumatoid pleuritis.[6]

**What is the significance of Gram stain and culture of pleural fluid?**

Gram stain and culture of pleural fluid should be included in any infectious workup. Culture bottles should be inoculated at the bedside. Special smears and cultures may be indicated based on other clinical data (eg, acid-fast smear if TB is suspected).[6]

**What is the significance of cytologic examination of pleural fluid?**

Cytologic examination of pleural fluid can establish a diagnosis of malignancy. Yield is variable and dependent on the type of cancer. For example, the sensitivity of cytologic examination is as high as 70% for metastatic adenocarcinoma but as low as 10% for mesothelioma.[6]

## TRANSUDATIVE PLEURAL EFFUSIONS

**What are the 3 main mechanisms of transudative pleural effusions?**

Transudative pleural effusions can occur as a result of changes in hydrostatic pressure, changes in oncotic pressure, or diaphragmatic defects.

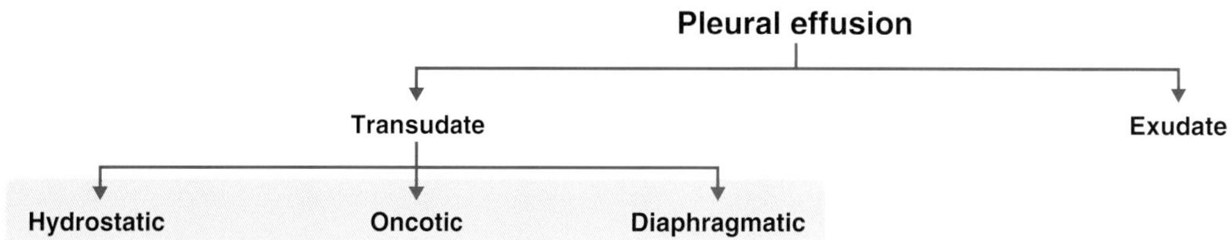


**What is the role of hydrostatic pressure in the development of a pleural effusion?**

An increase in capillary hydrostatic pressure, which opposes capillary oncotic pressure and intrapleural pressure, will lead to efflux of fluid from the capillaries to the pleural space.

**What is the role of intrapleural pressure in the development of a pleural effusion?**

Intrapleural pressure opposes both capillary and interstitial hydrostatic pressure, acting to prevent influx of fluid into the pleural space. A decrease in intrapleural pressure will lead to a relative increase in capillary and interstitial hydrostatic pressure and an efflux of fluid from the capillaries and interstitium to the pleural space.

**What is the role of capillary oncotic pressure in the development of a pleural effusion?**

Capillary oncotic pressure opposes capillary hydrostatic pressure, acting to maintain fluid within the capillaries. A decrease in capillary oncotic pressure will lead to efflux of fluid from the capillaries to the interstitial and pleural spaces.

**What is the role of the diaphragm in the development of a pleural effusion?**

Small defects in the diaphragm can allow peritoneal fluid to move into the pleural space.

## TRANSUDATIVE PLEURAL EFFUSIONS RELATED TO HYDROSTATIC PRESSURE

### What are the causes of transudative pleural effusions related to hydrostatic pressure?

More than 80% of effusions related to this condition are bilateral.

Congestive heart failure (CHF). *All causes of volume overload, including renal failure and intravenous fluid administration, are described by this term.*[6]

External cardiac restraint.

Constrictive pericarditis.

Elevated jugular venous pressure, dilated chest wall veins, and Horner's syndrome.

Superior vena cava (SVC) syndrome.

These entities result in decreased intrapleural pressure, creating a relative increase in capillary and interstitial hydrostatic pressure, resulting in the movement of fluid into the pleural space.

Atelectasis and pneumonectomy.

Drainage of pleural fluid related to this entity will invariably result in pneumothorax.

Trapped lung.

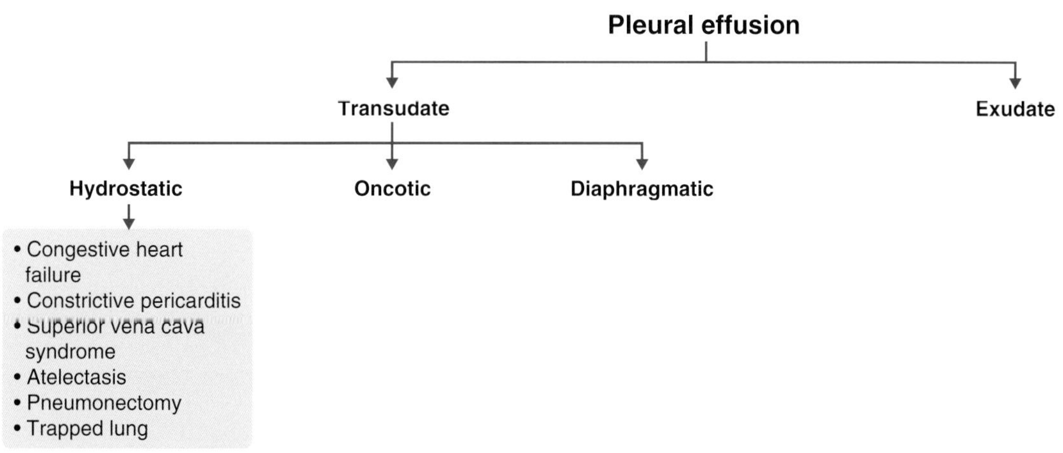


What is the management of pleural effusions related to congestive heart failure?

Diuretic therapy is the cornerstone of treating pleural effusions related to CHF. Within 48 hours of initiating diuresis, most effusions decrease or resolve. *Pleural effusions related to CHF may be exudative in patients with a history of CABG or may become exudative after aggressive diuretic therapy.*[6,8]

What are the characteristics of pleural effusions related to constrictive pericarditis?

Pleural effusions occur in about one-half of patients with constrictive pericarditis. Most are bilateral, but unilateral effusions affecting either the right or the left side occur.[9]

What types of pleural effusions can develop in patients with superior vena cava syndrome?

In addition to transudative effusions, exudative effusions (including chylous effusions) have been described in adult patients with SVC syndrome. The mechanisms are likely multifactorial, including lymphatic obstruction.[10]

Why are pleural effusions associated with atelectasis?

A pleural effusion of any cause can result in passive atelectasis, which can often be appreciated on physical examination as signs of consolidation (eg, egophony) just above the level of the effusion.

**When does pleural fluid usually accumulate after pneumonectomy?**

The rate of pleural fluid accumulation after pneumonectomy is variable. Typically, half of the pleural space is filled with fluid within the first 4 to 5 days after pneumonectomy; fluid gradually increases until the space is filled over a period of weeks to months. If more rapid filling is detected, a surgical complication resulting in hemothorax or chylothorax should be investigated. If filling is tardy or stops, a bronchial anastomotic leak should be suspected.[11]

**What is trapped lung?**

Trapped lung describes the inability of lung to re-expand as a result of fibrous visceral pleural thickening that can develop from a chronic inflammatory pleural process. As pleural fluid surrounding trapped lung is removed via thoracentesis, intrapleural pressures become increasingly negative because lung cannot re-expand to fill the space. This creates a vacuum within the pleural space that pulls in air from around the catheter (known as pneumothorax ex vacuo).[12]

## TRANSUDATIVE PLEURAL EFFUSIONS RELATED TO ONCOTIC PRESSURE

### What are the causes of transudative pleural effusions related to oncotic pressure?

**A reduction in albumin synthesis.**

Cirrhosis.

**A 38-year-old man with human immunodeficiency virus (HIV) infection presents with anasarca and foamy urine.**

Nephrotic syndrome.

**Albumin loss from the gastrointestinal tract.**

Protein-losing enteropathy (PLE).

**An endocrinopathy.**

Myxedema.

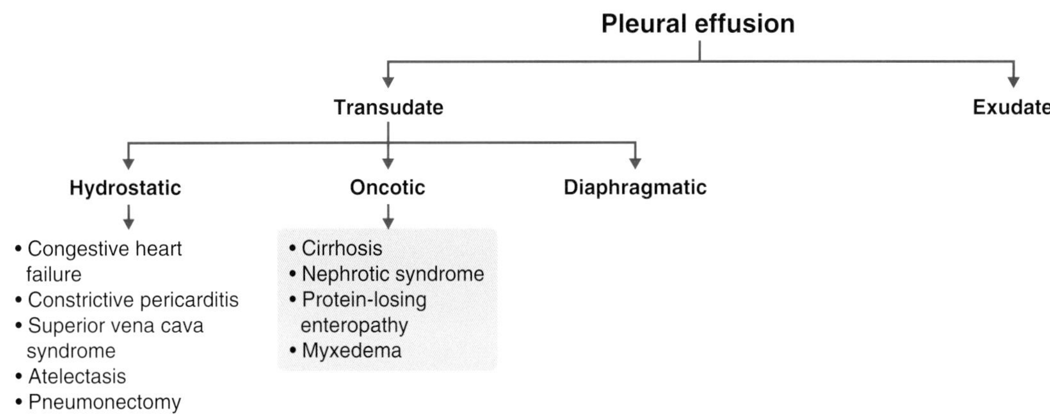


**Is hypoalbuminemia the only mechanism of pleural effusion formation related to cirrhosis?**

In addition to hypoalbuminemia, cirrhosis can also cause a pleural effusion via movement of ascitic fluid into the pleural space through diaphragmatic defects (ie, hepatic hydrothorax).

**What pulmonary condition should be suspected in patients with nephrotic syndrome who present with sudden-onset dyspnea and chest pain?**

Pulmonary embolism is a known complication of nephrotic syndrome (particularly membranous glomerulonephropathy) and should be suspected when these patients present with sudden-onset pulmonary symptoms. Pleural effusions associated with nephrotic syndrome tend to develop over time and are often associated with peripheral edema and ascites. The effusions are bilateral and usually responsive to diuretic agents in addition to management of the underlying kidney disease.[13]

**What stool study can be helpful in the diagnosis of protein-losing enteropathy?**

Increased fecal α-1 antitrypsin clearance is suggestive of PLE. The clinical characteristics of pleural effusions associated with PLE are similar to those of nephrotic syndrome.

**What is the treatment for pleural effusions related to myxedema?**

Most pleural effusions related to myxedema are not clinically relevant or symptomatic, and respond to thyroid replacement therapy. *Pleural effusions related to myxedema can be either transudative or exudative.*[14]

## TRANSUDATIVE PLEURAL EFFUSIONS RELATED TO DIAPHRAGMATIC DEFECTS

### What are the causes of transudative pleural effusions related to diaphragmatic defects?

**There is usually obvious ascites associated with this condition, but sometimes it is inconspicuous.**

Hepatic hydrothorax.

**An iatrogenic cause.**

Peritoneal dialysis.

**A middle-aged man presents with a new pleural effusion 1 month after percutaneous nephrolithotomy.**

Urinothorax.

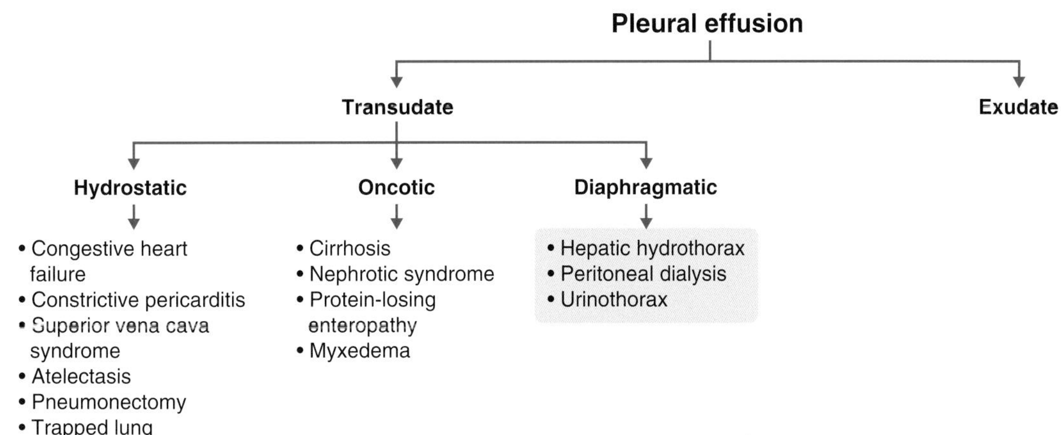


**What are the characteristics of hepatic hydrothorax?**

Hepatic hydrothorax occurs in up to 10% of patients with cirrhosis. Most cases occur on the right (approximately 85%) and are usually >500 mL in volume. As with ascitic fluid, spontaneous infection of the pleural fluid, called spontaneous bacterial empyema, can occur. It is defined as a nonparapneumonic pleural effusion with a polymorphonuclear (PMN) cell count >500 cells/μL, or a PMN cell count >250 cells/μL with positive culture.[15]

**What are the characteristics of pleural effusions related to peritoneal dialysis?**

Pleural effusions occur in around 2% of peritoneal dialysis patients. It typically occurs on the right but can occur on the left or on both sides in some cases. Sometimes referred to as "sweet hydrothorax," the fluid has characteristically high glucose content, which is a clue to the diagnosis.[16]

**What pleural fluid characteristic is pathognomonic for urinothorax?**

A fluid-to-serum creatinine ratio >1.0 is diagnostic of urinothorax.[17]

## EXUDATIVE PLEURAL EFFUSIONS

**What are the 2 main mechanisms of exudative pleural effusions?**

Exudative pleural effusions can occur as a result of increased capillary permeability or lymphatic obstruction.

**What are the 2 general types of exudative pleural effusions?**

Exudative pleural effusions can be infectious or noninfectious.

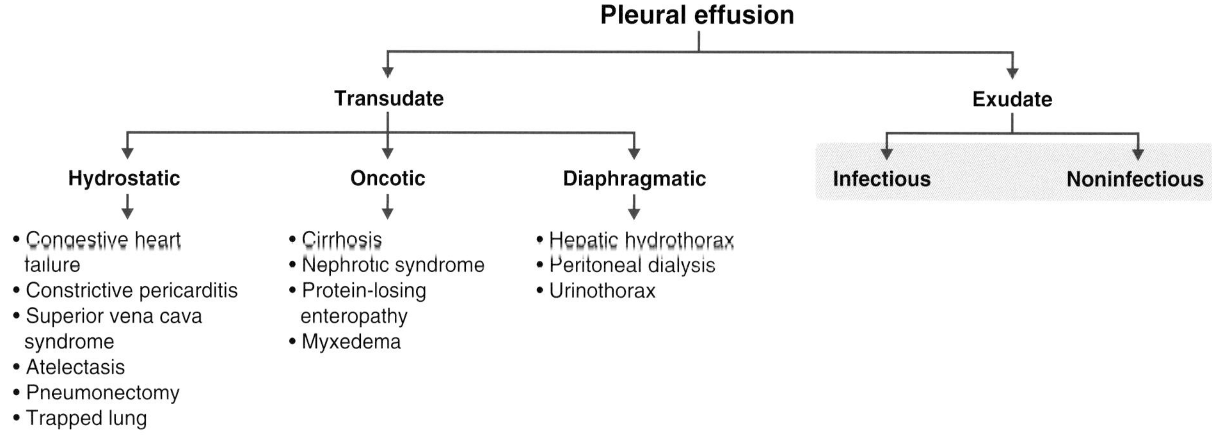


**Why is it important to distinguish infection from other causes of exudative pleural effusions?**

It is important to recognize infectious pleural effusions because urgent drainage may be necessary in some cases.

## INFECTIOUS PLEURAL EFFUSIONS

### What are the infectious causes of exudative pleural effusions?

**Fever, dyspnea, purulent cough, and consolidation with an associated pleural effusion on chest imaging.**

Pneumonia.

**One of the most common extrapulmonary manifestations of this granulomatous disease.**

Tuberculous pleuritis.

**A 60-year-old woman with immune thrombocytopenic purpura who recently underwent splenectomy is admitted with fever and abdominal pain and is found to have an exudative pleural effusion with a neutrophil cell fraction of 90% without evidence of an associated parenchymal consolidation.**

Subphrenic abscess.

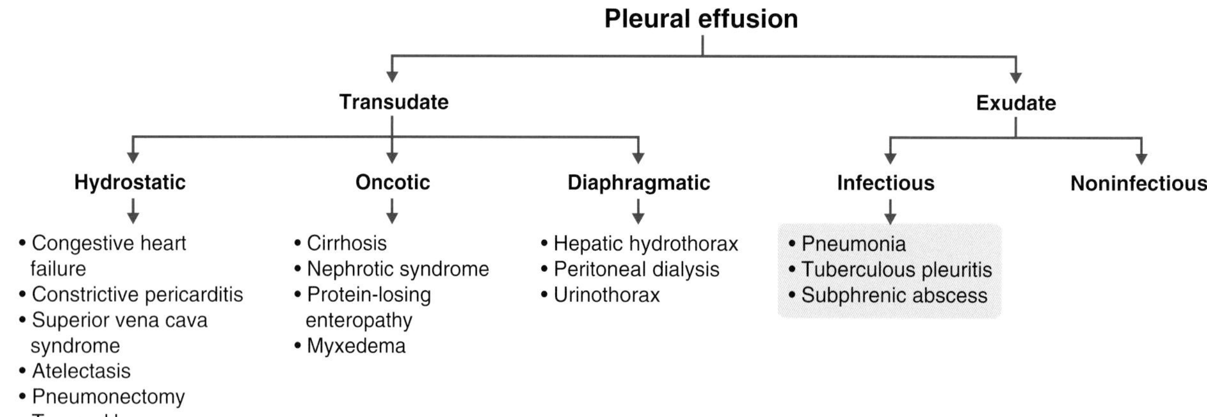


**What features of pleural effusions associated with pneumonia (ie, parapneumonic effusion) are important for deciding whether the fluid should be sampled?**

*It is said that "the sun should never set on a parapneumonic effusion."* Thoracentesis is indicated for all parapneumonic effusions except those that are free flowing and less than 10 mm thick on a lateral decubitus chest radiograph. These effusions are associated with low risk of poor outcomes and do not require drainage.[5,18]

**When a parapneumonic effusion is diagnosed and drained with thoracentesis, what urgent clinical determination must be made next?**

It must be determined if a parapneumonic effusion is complicated, as such effusions are likely to require an additional, more invasive procedure (eg, tube thoracostomy) for resolution and prevention of trapped lung. A pleural effusion is considered to be complicated if any of the following are present: (1) frank pus in the pleural space, (2) positive Gram stain or culture of the fluid, (3) fluid pH <7.2, (4) fluid glucose <60 mg/dL, or (5) the fluid occupies more than one-half the hemithorax, is loculated, or is associated with thickened parietal pleura on imaging.[5]

**Is mycobacterial culture from sputum samples helpful in the diagnosis of tuberculous pleuritis when there is no discernable parenchymal involvement?**

Sputum mycobacterial cultures can be helpful even in patients without obvious parenchymal involvement on chest imaging, with a yield of up to 55%. Pleural fluid studies are associated with variable sensitivity. Pleural biopsy may ultimately be necessary to make the diagnosis.[19]

**What are the characteristics of the pleural effusion related to a subphrenic abscess?**

A pleural effusion occurs in most cases of subphrenic abscess. It is typically small to moderate in size, and there is a predominance of neutrophils. The presentation is often dominated by thoracic symptoms, such as pleuritic chest pain; in fact, around one-third of patients with subphrenic abscess do not report any abdominal pain.[14]

## NONINFECTIOUS EXUDATIVE PLEURAL EFFUSIONS

### What are the noninfectious causes of exudative pleural effusions?

**A 65-year-old man who is an active smoker presents with hemoptysis, weight loss, and a new pleural effusion.**

Malignancy.

**Unilateral leg swelling, hemoptysis, and a pleural effusion.**

Pulmonary embolism.

**A young woman with malar rash, pleuritic chest pain, and a new pleural effusion.**

Systemic lupus erythematosus (SLE).

**A 44-year-old man with heavy alcohol use presents with epigastric abdominal pain radiating to the back and a new pleural effusion.**

Acute pancreatitis.

**A 24-year-old man presents to the emergency department with dyspnea and chest pain following a motor vehicle accident, during which he hit his chest against the dashboard, and is found to have dullness to percussion of the left hemithorax and decreased tactile fremitus.**

Hemothorax.

**Milky appearing pleural fluid.**

Chylothorax.

**A 56-year-old man who sustained a myocardial infarction 3 weeks ago presents with fever and pleuritic chest pain and is found to have pericarditis and a pleural effusion.**

Postcardiac injury syndrome (PCIS).

**A history of coronary artery disease is a prerequisite.**

Post-CABG.

**Medication review is part of taking a good history.**

Medication.

**Pleural effusions related to this treatment could be mistaken for disease recurrence.**

External beam radiation therapy for intrathoracic malignancy.

**An environmental exposure commonly associated with the development of pleural plaques.**

Asbestos.

**Associated with delirium and asterixis on examination.**

Uremia.

**Ascites, a pleural effusion, and a benign ovarian tumor.**

Meigs' syndrome.

**Yellow fingernails, lymphedema, and a pleural effusion.**

Yellow nail syndrome.

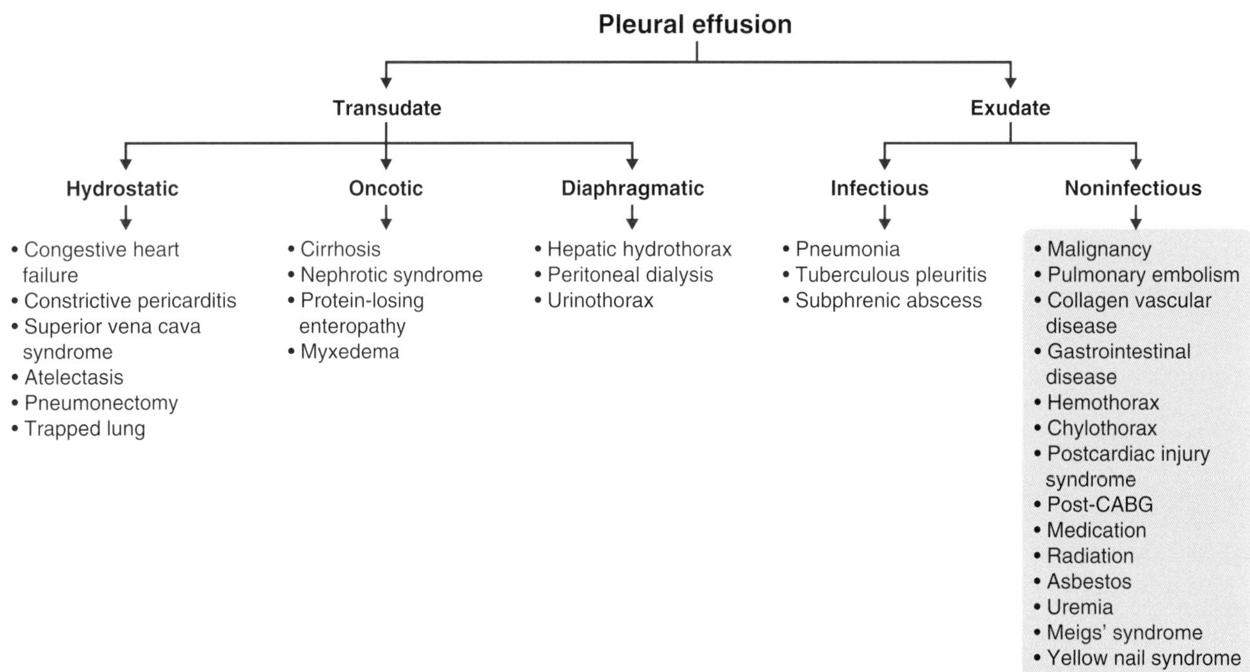


**What types of malignancies are most often associated with pleural effusions?**

In the industrialized world, lung cancer, breast cancer, and lymphoma cause the majority of malignant pleural effusions. Other causative malignancies include metastatic ovarian cancer, sarcoma, and melanoma. Fluid cytology examination may be diagnostic. The presence of a pleural effusion in a patient with lung cancer almost always indicates noncurable disease even in the absence of positive cytology.[14]

**What radiographic findings are associated with pulmonary embolism?**

The chest radiograph is typically clear in the setting of PE but may show a wedge-shaped opacity in the periphery of the lung abutting the pleura indicative of infarction (Hampton's hump) or oligemia distal to the embolus (Westermark sign). Pleural effusions associated with pulmonary embolism are typically small. *It is often asserted that pulmonary embolism can cause both transudative and exudative pleural effusions, but the vast majority are exudative.*[14]

**What additional tests should be considered in patients with Sjögren's syndrome who present with a pleural effusion?**

Because of the risk of lymphoma in patients with Sjögren's syndrome and the fact that lymphoma is a leading cause of malignant pleural effusion, additional tests such as cytology, flow cytometry, and pleural biopsy should be considered in these patients.

**What pleural fluid study can be useful in cases of acute pancreatitis or esophageal rupture?**

Pleural fluid amylase level can be elevated when the effusion is related to either acute pancreatitis or esophageal rupture (ie, Boerhaave's syndrome).[6]

**When hemothorax is suspected based on the appearance of the fluid, what laboratory test can confirm the diagnosis?**

When the pleural fluid hematocrit level is <1%, the presence of blood is insignificant. A pleural fluid hematocrit level above 1% is most often caused by malignancy with pleural involvement, pulmonary embolism, or trauma. Hemothorax can be confirmed when the pleural fluid hematocrit level is greater than one-half that of blood. Tube thoracostomy should be considered in cases of hemothorax. Although not always accurate, an estimate of the hematocrit of the fluid can be obtained by dividing the red blood cell (RBC) count by 100,000 (eg, RBC count of 1,000,000 = hematocrit of 10).[2,14]

**What pleural fluid study can be useful in the evaluation of chylothorax?**

The pleural fluid triglyceride level is helpful in diagnosing chylothorax. If the level is >110 mg/dL, there is a high likelihood of chylothorax; if the level is <50 mg/dL, chylothorax is ruled out. For values in between, lipoprotein electrophoresis can be performed.[14]

**What are some causes of postcardiac injury syndrome?**

PCIS can be caused by postmyocardial infarction syndrome (ie, Dressler's syndrome), cardiac surgery, blunt chest trauma, pacemaker implantation, and angioplasty.[4]

**Which hemithorax is most often involved in post-CABG pleural effusions?**

The left hemithorax is most often involved in post-CABG pleural effusions.[4]

**What medications can cause pleural effusions?**

Medications most commonly associated with pleural effusions include amiodarone, methotrexate, phenytoin, sirolimus, and nitrofurantoin.[2]

**What are the characteristics of radiation-induced pleural effusions?**

Radiation-induced pleural effusions most commonly occur in association with radiation pneumonitis, affecting the ipsilateral lung. Unlike malignant effusions, radiation-related effusions typically do not increase in size over time, which can help inform the diagnosis when considering cancer recurrence in patients who develop a pleural effusion after radiation therapy.[20]

**What is the prognosis of asbestos-related pleural effusions?**

The vast majority of asbestos-related pleural effusions are benign, but since asbestos is associated with lung cancer (including mesothelioma), the effusion should be thoroughly evaluated. Most benign asbestos effusions are small and unilateral, and resolve spontaneously after a few months. Recurrences are rare.[21]

**What are the characteristics of pleural effusions related to uremia?**

Pleural effusions occur in around 3% of uremic patients and are most frequently unilateral (approximately 20% are bilateral). Most patients are symptomatic with fever, chest pain, cough, and dyspnea. The size of the effusion can be variable but is frequently large.[14]

**What is the definitive treatment for the pleural effusion associated with Meigs' syndrome?**

Surgical removal of the ovarian tumor usually results in resolution of the pleural effusion associated with Meigs' syndrome.[22]

**What are the characteristics of pleural effusions related to yellow nail syndrome?**

The pleural effusions of yellow nail syndrome are bilateral in about one-half of cases and vary in size from small to massive. There is typically a predominance of lymphocytes. Persistence and rapid recurrence of the effusion after thoracentesis is typical. There is no specific treatment for the disease, but pleurodesis can be considered for symptomatic cases.[14]

## Case Summary

A 62-year-old Filipino man who recently underwent CABG surgery presents with fever, dyspnea, and chest pain and is found to have a large left pleural effusion.

***What is the most likely cause of the pleural effusion in this patient?***

Postcardiac injury syndrome.

### BONUS QUESTIONS

***How does the history shape the differential diagnosis in this case?***

The 2 most relevant pieces of history in this case include the patient's country of origin, which has a high burden of tuberculosis, and recent cardiac surgery, which can lead to PCIS.

***Based on the information provided in this case, is the pleural effusion transudative or exudative?***

The pleural fluid protein to serum protein ratio is >0.5, meeting Light's criteria for an exudative effusion.

***What is the significance of the lymphocytic predominance of the fluid in this case?***

A lymphocyte-predominant exudative pleural effusion narrows the differential diagnosis primarily to malignancy, tuberculous pleuritis, and PCIS. Based on the history in this case, tuberculosis and PCIS should already have been under consideration.

***What is the significance of the fluid adenosine deaminase test in this case?***

Pleural fluid adenosine deaminase level, which increases in the setting of TB, has excellent operating characteristics. A cutoff value of 40 U/L is associated with sensitivity and specificity that exceed 90% for the diagnosis of tuberculous pleuritis. The yield of pleural fluid smear for acid-fast bacilli is poor except in patients infected with HIV and those with tuberculous empyema. Pleural fluid culture has a low sensitivity and is limited by lengthy delays in obtaining results. Pleural fluid nucleic acid amplification tests are also associated with poor sensitivity. Sputum cultures are positive in up to one-half of cases, even in the absence of obvious parenchymal disease. Pleural biopsy may ultimately be necessary to definitively rule out tuberculous pleuritis in cases where suspicion remains high despite negative pleural fluid studies.[6,23]

***How common is postcardiac injury syndrome after cardiac surgery?***

Following cardiac surgery, PCIS occurs in up to one-third of cases.[4]

***What is the timing of postcardiac injury syndrome after cardiac surgery?***

On average, onset of PCIS occurs 3 weeks after surgery but can vary from 3 days to 1 year.[4]

***What are the main clinical manifestations of postcardiac injury syndrome?***

The clinical manifestations of PCIS may include fever, chest pain, pericarditis, pleuritis, and pneumonitis.[4]

***How common are pleural effusions in patients with postcardiac injury syndrome?***

A pleural effusion is present in about 80% of cases of PCIS.[4]

***What are the characteristics of pleural effusions associated with postcardiac injury syndrome?***

Pleural effusions are bilateral in one-half of patients with PCIS, and there is a predilection for the left side in cases of unilateral effusion. The fluid is bloody in around one-third of patients. PMNs are the dominant cell type in early PCIS, but this evolves to a lymphocytic predominance over time.[4]

***What are the key clinical differences between postcardiac injury syndrome and post-CABG pleural effusion?***

Although CABG can cause PCIS, it can also lead to a separate entity called post-CABG pleural effusion. The time course and fluid parameters are similar for both. The main distinguishing features are the absence of fever and chest pain in patients with post-CABG pleural effusion. Both of these features are present in this case, consistent with PCIS.[4]

***What is the treatment for postcardiac injury syndrome?***

There are no known methods of preventing PCIS from developing. Once the diagnosis is made, the cornerstone of treatment includes nonsteroidal anti-inflammatory drugs (eg, indomethacin 25-50 mg every 8 hours) or glucocorticoids (eg, prednisone).[4]

## KEY POINTS

- A pleural effusion is defined as excess fluid in the pleural cavity.
- Symptoms of pleural effusions include dyspnea, dry cough, and chest pain (usually pleuritic).
- The physical findings of pleural effusions include decreased inspiratory expansion of the chest wall on the affected side, dullness to percussion, decreased tactile fremitus, and reduced breath sounds over the effusion.
- A large pleural effusion occupies >25% of the hemithorax.
- A loculated pleural effusion does not flow freely within the pleural cavity and is best evaluated with ultrasonography or CT imaging.
- An empyema is defined by the presence of pus in the pleural space.
- Thoracentesis is helpful in characterizing the nature of pleural effusions.
- Pleural effusions can be transudative or exudative, determined by Light's criteria.
- Basic fluid features such as gross appearance; total and differential cell counts; protein, LDH, and glucose levels; and smears and cultures are helpful in narrowing the differential diagnosis.
- Supplementary fluid studies (eg, cytologic examination) can be helpful in certain cases.
- Transudative effusions can occur as a result of changes in hydrostatic pressure, changes in oncotic pressure, or diaphragmatic defects.
- The most common causes of transudative effusions are congestive heart failure, hepatic hydrothorax, and nephrotic syndrome.
- Exudative effusions can be infectious or noninfectious.
- The most common causes of exudative effusions are pneumonia, pulmonary embolism, and malignancy.
- Treatment for pleural effusions depends on the underlying etiology. Some infectious effusions require urgent drainage.

## REFERENCES


1. Bhatnagar R, Maskell N. The modern diagnosis and management of pleural effusions. *BMJ*. 2015;351:h4520.
2. McGrath EE, Anderson PB. Diagnosis of pleural effusion: a systematic approach. *Am J Crit Care*. 2011;20(2):119-127; quiz 28.
3. Blackmore CC, Black WC, Dallas RV, Crow HC. Pleural fluid volume estimation: a chest radiograph prediction rule. *Acad Radiol*. 1996;3(2):103-109.
4. Light RW. Pleural effusions following cardiac injury and coronary artery bypass graft surgery. *Semin Respir Crit Care Med*. 2001;22(6):657-664.
5. Light RW. Parapneumonic effusions and empyema. *Proc Am Thorac Soc*. 2006;3(1):75-80.
6. Light RW. Clinical practice. Pleural effusion. *N Engl J Med*. 2002;346(25):1971-1977.
7. Light RW, Macgregor MI, Luchsinger PC, Ball WC Jr. Pleural effusions: the diagnostic separation of transudates and exudates. *Ann Intern Med*. 1972;77(4):507-513.
8. Eid AA, Keddissi JI, Samaha M, Tawk MM, Kimmell K, Kinasewitz GT. Exudative effusions in congestive heart failure. *Chest*. 2002;122(5):1518-1523.
9. Doustkami H, Hooshyar A, Maleki N, Tavosi Z, Feizi I. Chronic constrictive pericarditis. *Case Rep Cardiol*. 2013;2013:957497.
10. Rice TW. Pleural effusions in superior vena cava syndrome: prevalence, characteristics, and proposed pathophysiology. *Curr Opin Pulm Med*. 2007;13(4):324-327.
11. Chae EJ, Seo JB, Kim SY, et al. Radiographic and CT findings of thoracic complications after pneumonectomy. *Radiographics*. 2006;26(5):1449-1468.
12. Albores J, Wang T. Images in clinical medicine. Trapped lung. *N Engl J Med*. 2015;372(19):e25.
13. Jenkins PG, Shelp WD. Recurrent pleural transudate in the nephrotic syndrome. A new approach to treatment. *JAMA*. 1974;230(4):587-588.
14. Light RW. *Pleural Diseases*. 5th ed. Philadelphia, PA: Lippincott Williams & Wilkins, A Wolters Kluwer Business; 2007.
15. Cardenas A, Kelleher T, Chopra S. Review article: hepatic hydrothorax. *Aliment Pharmacol Ther*. 2004;20(3):271-279.
16. Szeto CC, Chow KM. Pathogenesis and management of hydrothorax complicating peritoneal dialysis. *Curr Opin Pulm Med*. 2004;10(4):315-319.
17. Ferreira PG, Furriel F, Ferreira AJ. Urinothorax as an unusual type of pleural effusion – clinical report and review. *Rev Port Pneumol*. 2013;19(2):80-83.
18. Sahn SA, Light RW. The sun should never set on a parapneumonic effusion. *Chest*. 1989;95(5):945-947.
19. Vorster MJ, Allwood BW, Diacon AH, Koegelenberg CF. Tuberculous pleural effusions: advances and controversies. *J Thorac Dis*. 2015;7(6):981-991.
20. Choi YW, Munden RF, Erasmus JJ, et al. Effects of radiation therapy on the lung: radiologic appearances and differential diagnosis. *Radiographics*. 2004;24(4):985-997; discussion 98.
21. Chapman SJ, Cookson WO, Musk AW, Lee YC. Benign asbestos pleural diseases. *Curr Opin Pulm Med*. 2003;9(4):266-271.
22. Light RW. *Textbook of Pleural Diseases*. 3rd ed. Boca Raton, FL: Taylor & Francis Group; 2016.
23. Jeon D. Tuberculous pleurisy: an update. *Tuberc Respir Dis (Seoul)*. 2014;76(4):153-159.

# SECTION 12

# Rheumatology

## Chapter 49

# ARTHRITIS

### Case: A 62-year-old man with subcutaneous nodules

A 62-year-old man with a history of alcohol abuse and venous insufficiency presents to the clinic for evaluation of a painful left elbow. Medical history is notable for recurrent episodes of swelling and pain in various joints over a period of 15 years, mostly involving the bases of the great toes, ankles, and knees. The episodes involve one joint at any given time, usually last 7 to 10 days, and completely resolve between attacks. He stopped drinking alcohol 4 years ago, and the episodes abated. He had done well until the night before presentation when he was awoken from sleep with pain and swelling of the left elbow. Approximately 1 month ago, the patient was prescribed furosemide for lower extremity edema related to venous stasis, but he takes no other medication.

Temperature is 37.4°C. The left elbow is erythematous, warm, and swollen (Figure 49-1A), and there is exquisite tenderness with passive range of motion. There are multiple firm 1 to 2 cm nontender subcutaneous nodules overlying the interphalangeal (IP) joints of both hands (Figure 49-1B).

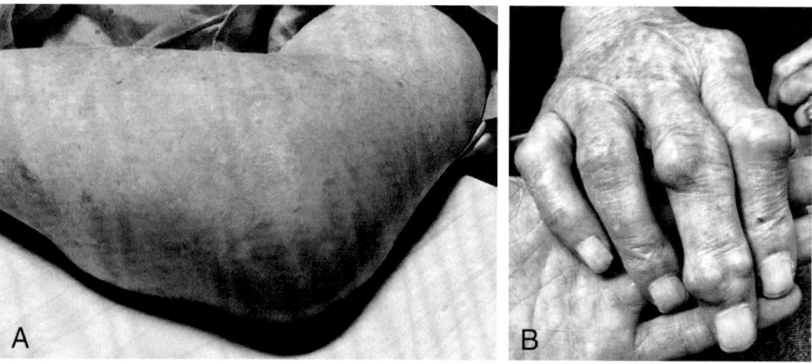


**Figure 49-1.**

***What is the most likely cause of arthritis in this patient?***

**What is the difference between arthralgia and arthritis?**

Arthralgia is the symptom of joint pain; arthritis is inflammation of any part of the joint. Arthralgia can be associated with arthritis and nonarthritic conditions.

**What are the articular structures?**

Articular structures include the synovium, synovial fluid, articular cartilage, intra-articular ligaments, joint capsule, and juxta-articular bone.[1]

**What are the periarticular structures?**

Periarticular structures include supportive extra-articular ligaments, tendons, bursae, muscle, fascia, bones, nerves, and overlying skin.[1]

**What are the mimics of arthritis?**

Conditions that can be confused for arthritis include bursitis, tendinitis, enthesitis, epicondylitis, ligament damage, cellulitis, deep vein thrombosis, polymyalgia rheumatica, myositis, and bone lesions (eg, metastasis).

**How can physical examination help localize the source of pain to the joint (arthritis) rather than neighboring tissue (periarthritis)?**

Articular involvement is more likely when there is pain and limited range of motion on both active and passive movement. Additional findings may include joint line tenderness on palpation, effusion, crepitation, instability, and locking. *These additional findings may be absent in deep-seated joints.* In contrast, nonarticular processes tend to be painful with active movement only; focal tenderness in regions adjacent to the joint may also be present.[1]

**What are the 2 general types of arthritis?**

Arthritis can be noninflammatory or inflammatory.

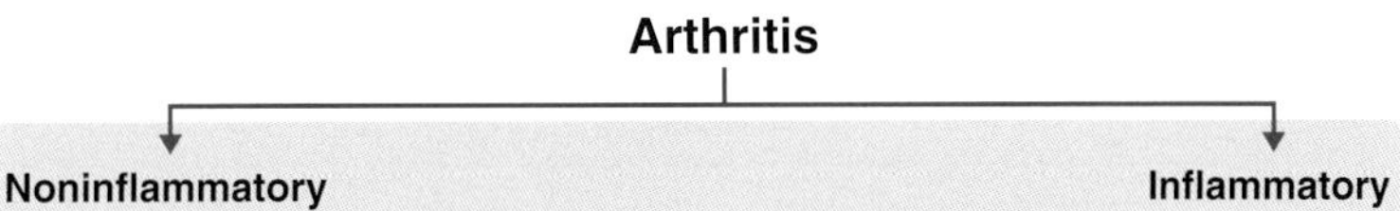


*It may seem contradictory to separate the term arthritis, which by definition implies the presence of inflammation, into inflammatory and noninflammatory categories. Although all forms of arthritis are associated with some degree of inflammation, the term "inflammatory arthritis" implies immune-mediated inflammation with special features that are discussed in more detail in this chapter.*

**What historical features are suggestive of inflammatory arthritis?**

The presence of systemic symptoms (eg, fever, weight loss, night sweats), morning stiffness lasting >30 minutes, worsened symptoms with rest, and improved symptoms with activity are suggestive of an inflammatory condition.[1]

**What physical findings are suggestive of inflammatory arthritis?**

Inflammatory arthritis is suggested by the presence of the cardinal physical findings of inflammation, which are erythema (rubor), warmth (calor), pain (dolor), and swelling (tumor).[1]

**What is crepitus?**

Crepitus is a palpable, sometimes audible, crackling or vibratory sensation that occurs with motion of the joint. It can be associated with noninflammatory arthritis, particularly osteoarthritis (OA). *The presence of crepitus, clicking, or snapping with joint movement commonly occurs as a result of ligamentous stretch in patients without arthritis.*[1]

**What is subluxation?**

Subluxation refers to joint misalignment such that articular surfaces are not in contact. It can be associated with certain types of noninflammatory arthritis (eg, OA) and inflammatory arthritis (eg, rheumatoid arthritis [RA]).

**What is synovitis?**

Synovitis is inflammation of the synovium. It is associated with inflammatory arthritis.

**What is tenosynovitis?**

Tenosynovitis is inflammation of a tendon and its sheath. It can be associated with certain types of inflammatory arthritis (eg, RA, disseminated gonorrhea).

**What is enthesitis?**

Enthesitis is inflammation of the site of attachment of tendons, ligaments, fascia, and joint capsule fibers to bone. It can be associated with certain types of inflammatory arthritis (eg, spondyloarthritis).[2]

**What is dactylitis?**

Dactylitis is inflammation of an entire finger or toe (often called a "sausage" digit) resulting from the combination of synovitis, tenosynovitis, and enthesitis (Figure 49-2). It can be associated with certain types of inflammatory arthritis (eg, spondyloarthritis, gout, septic arthritis).[2]

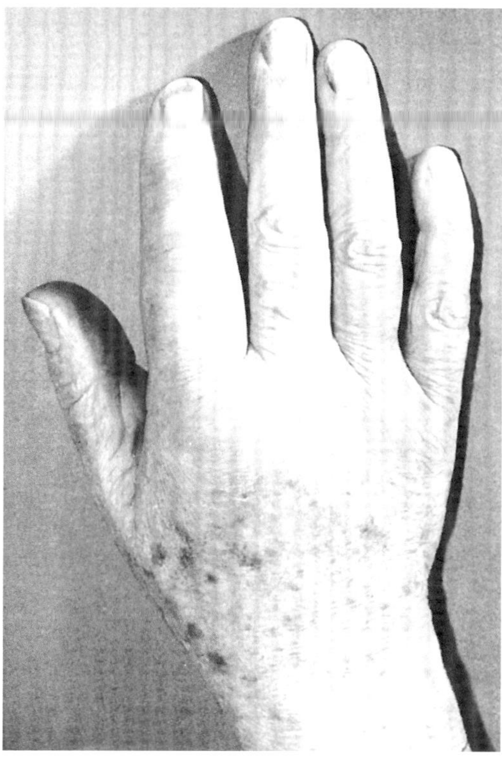

**Figure 49-2.** Psoriatic arthritis involving the metacarpophalangeal and proximal interphalangeal joints of the index finger with associated flexor tenosynovitis and enthesitis. This combination of involvement gives rise to dactylitis ("sausage" digit). (From Koopman WJ, Moreland LW. *Arthritis and Allied Conditions A Textbook of Rheumatology.* 15th ed. Philadelphia, PA: Lippincott Williams & Wilkins; 2005.)

**What is spondyloarthritis?**

Spondyloarthritis refers to a family of immune-mediated inflammatory diseases characterized by spondylitis (ie, inflammation of the axial skeleton including the vertebrae, entheseal attachments to the vertebral column, and axial synovial joints), along with inflammation of the peripheral joints. It is associated with extra-articular manifestations such as inflammation of the eye (eg, iris, conjuctiva), inflammatory bowel disease, and psoriasis.

**What is migratory arthritis?**

Migratory arthritis describes an arthritic process that begins in 1 or 2 joints, with subsequent improvement or resolution over a period of a few days, followed by involvement in a new joint. It can be associated with certain types of inflammatory arthritis (eg, acute rheumatic fever).

**What is symmetric arthritis?**

Symmetric arthritis describes an arthritic process that affects pairs of joints on either side of the body. It can be associated with certain types of noninflammatory arthritis (eg, OA) and inflammatory arthritis (eg, RA).

**What general blood tests are helpful in the evaluation of inflammatory arthritis?**

Inflammatory conditions can be suggested by peripheral leukocytosis and elevation of the acute phase reactants such as erythrocyte sedimentation rate (ESR) and C-reactive protein (CRP). Other blood tests can be useful in the evaluation of specific causes of arthritis (eg, serum ferritin is markedly elevated in patients with adult-onset Still's disease).[1]

**What imaging studies can be helpful in the evaluation of arthritis?**

Conventional radiography, ultrasonography, computed tomography, and magnetic resonance imaging can each be helpful in the evaluation of arthritis.

**What procedure is most helpful in the evaluation of arthritis?**

Arthrocentesis allows for the analysis of synovial fluid, which is essential in the evaluation of arthritis.

**What synovial fluid findings are suggestive of inflammatory arthritis?**

Common patterns of synovial fluid findings are provided in the table below.[1,3,4]

| | Normal | Noninflammatory | Inflammatory | Septic |
|---|---|---|---|---|
| Appearance | Clear/straw | Clear/amber | Opaque | Turbid |
| WBCs/µL | ≤200 | ≤2000 | >2000 | >25,000 |
| PMNs (%) | <50% | ≤75% | >75% | >90% |

*Total WBC count is the single most important synovial fluid test for identifying inflammatory arthritis. It is important to note that the numbers provided in the table represent a general rule of thumb, and there is considerable overlap, particularly between the inflammatory and septic categories (eg, it is not uncommon for septic arthritis to present with a synovial WBC count between 2000 and 25,000, particularly infections involving prosthetic joints). A diagnosis of septic arthritis cannot be made based on WBC count alone because nonseptic inflammatory arthritis is sometimes associated with a WBC count >25,000 (synovial fluid Gram stain and culture can be helpful in these situations).*

## NONINFLAMMATORY ARTHRITIS

### What are the causes of noninflammatory arthritis?

**A 64-year-old woman with obesity presents with chronic pain of the hips and knees when she shops and is found to have crepitus of both knees without overlying erythema or warmth.**

Osteoarthritis (ie, degenerative arthritis).

**A 32-year-old woman presents with a painful and swollen ankle after stepping in a hole while exercising.**

Trauma.

**A previously healthy 81-year-old woman presents with skin bruising and a swollen right knee without antecedent trauma and is found to have a positive mixing study (ie, there is no correction after mixing).**

Hemarthrosis related to an acquired factor inhibitor.

**Most commonly found in diabetic patients with peripheral neuropathy; the acute form of this joint condition can mimic cellulitis, septic arthritis, and deep vein thrombosis.**

Charcot joint.

**This condition, which is commonly associated with glucocorticoid use, predominates in middle-aged and older patients, and may be identified on conventional radiography by the presence of the crescent sign, a line of subchondral lucency.**

Osteonecrosis (ie, avascular necrosis).

**A combination of arthritis and digital clubbing, usually in the setting of lung cancer.**

Hypertrophic osteoarthropathy.

**A 26-year-old woman with cystic fibrosis experiences episodes of acute polyarthritis that typically resolve within a few days, but does not have evidence of clubbing.**

Episodic arthritis of cystic fibrosis. *Patients with cystic fibrosis can also develop hypertrophic osteoarthropathy.*

**Large doughy hands, protruding jaw (see Figure 41-4), and arthralgias.**

Acromegaly.

**Skin hyperpigmentation and elevated serum ferritin.**

Hemochromatosis.

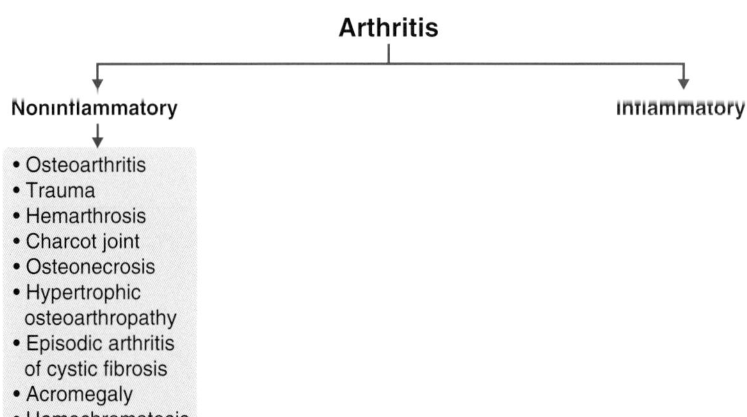


**Which joints are most commonly affected by osteoarthritis?**

OA is the most common cause of arthritis. The hallmark lesion in this condition is the loss of hyaline articular cartilage. Age and obesity are the most significant risk factors. The most commonly involved joints include those of the cervical and lumbosacral spine, hips, knees, hands, and feet. In the hands, the carpometacarpal joint at the base of the thumb, and the proximal interphalangeal (PIP) and distal interphalangeal (DIP) joints are more likely to be involved. In the feet, the first metatarsophalangeal (MTP) joint is usually symptomatic. The elbow, wrist, metacarpophalangeal (MCP), and ankle joints are typically spared. Pain is often episodic at first, mirroring activity levels, but later becomes persistent.[1]

**What clinical features are suggestive of traumatic arthritis?**

Traumatic arthritis is monoarticular in nature, usually associated with a history of antecedent trauma, and is often associated with additional pathology such as fractures or torn cartilage and ligaments.

**What are the causes of hemarthrosis?**

Common causes of hemarthrosis include trauma and bleeding diatheses (eg, anticoagulation use, hemophilia, factor inhibitors); other causes include osteoarthritis, tumors (especially villonodular synovitis), and septic arthritis.

**What is the typical presentation of Charcot joint?**

Charcot joint most commonly affects the joints of the foot and ankle. There is an acute phase characterized by rapid-onset erythema, warmth, and swelling; pain is variable because of neuropathy. A chronic phase follows, in which the acute inflammation subsides but permanent deformities of the foot develop (eg, arch collapse, dislocations, subluxations).[5]

**What is the most common and debilitating location of steroid-induced osteonecrosis?**

Hip involvement occurs most commonly in patients with steroid-induced osteonecrosis and is often bilateral. Typically, it is progressive and medical treatments are unsuccessful; resection of the femoral head and hip replacement may ultimately be necessary.[6]

**What are the 2 main forms of hypertrophic osteoarthropathy?**

The primary form of hypertrophic osteoarthropathy is hereditary and presents in childhood; the secondary (and more common) form occurs as a result of an underlying condition, most frequently intrathoracic malignancy. The associated arthritis usually involves the ankles, wrists, and knees. Digital clubbing is present in most patients.[1]

**What extra-articular manifestations often accompany the episodic arthritis of cystic fibrosis?**

Fever and erythema nodosum are commonly associated with the episodic arthritis of cystic fibrosis. As the name implies, attacks occur intermittently. Cystic fibrosis patients who develop persistent arthritis and digital clubbing may have hypertrophic osteoarthropathy, which is more common than episodic arthritis in adults.[7]

**What are the clinical characteristics of the arthritis related to acromegaly?**

Arthritis is a frequent manifestation of acromegaly and may be the first indication of the disease. The cervical and lumbar spines are the most common sites of involvement. The typical radiographic findings include widened joint spaces and severe osteophytosis.[8]

**What are the clinical characteristics of the arthritis related to hemochromatosis?**

Arthritis is a frequent manifestation of hemochromatosis, affecting up to 40% of patients, and may be the first indication of the disease. The second and third MCP joints are often the first and most severely affected joints (an important clue to the diagnosis). The other joints of the hands and the larger joints (eg, hips, knees, shoulders, ankles) are less likely to be affected, and their involvement is usually less severe. *Patients with hemochromatosis are also more likely to experience attacks of acute pseudogout.*[1]

## INFLAMMATORY ARTHRITIS

**What are the 3 subcategories of inflammatory arthritis based on the number of joints involved?**

Inflammatory arthritis can occur in a monoarticular, oligoarticular, or polyarticular pattern.

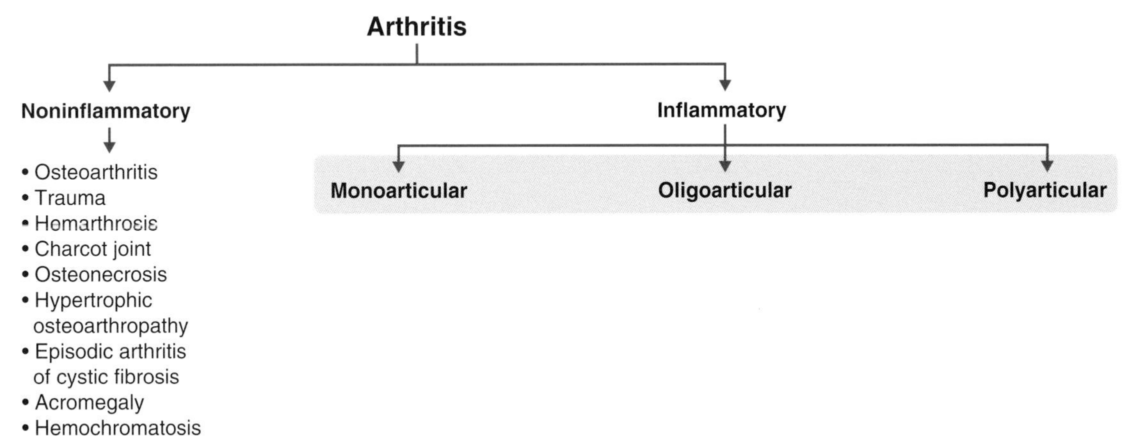


## MONOARTICULAR INFLAMMATORY ARTHRITIS

**How many joints are involved in monoarticular arthritis?**

Monoarticular arthritis involves 1 joint.

### What are the causes of monoarticular inflammatory arthritis?

**The diagnosis can be made using polarized light microscopy.**

Crystal arthropathy.

**A 24-year-old man with a history of intravenous drug use presents with a new heart murmur, Osler's nodes, and an exquisitely painful, erythematous, warm, and swollen right knee.**

Acute septic arthritis.

**A 36-year-old woman living in Connecticut complains of recurrent episodes of right knee swelling and pain following a tick bite.**

Chronic infectious arthritis from Lyme disease.

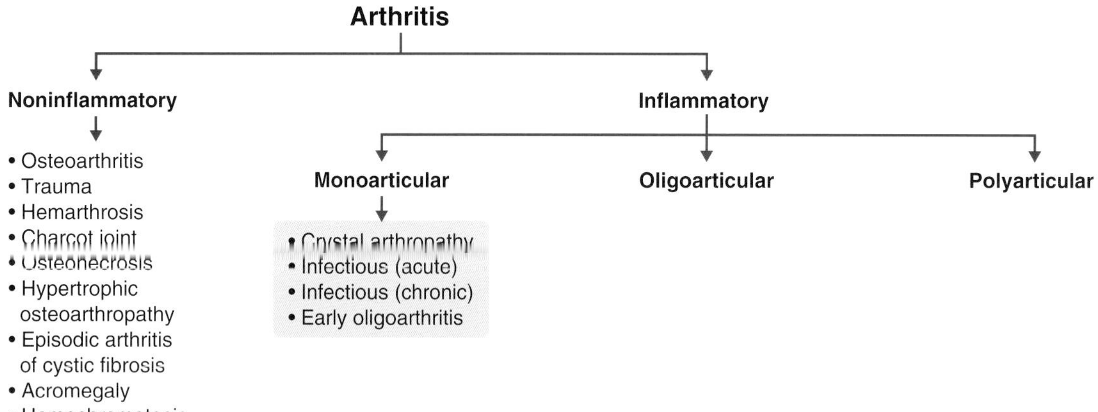


**What are the main types of crystals that deposit within joints and cause arthritis?**

Crystals that most commonly cause arthritis include monosodium urate (which causes gout) and calcium pyrophosphate dihydrate (which causes calcium pyrophosphate dihydrate disease [CPPD, or "pseudogout"]). *Crystal arthropathy can be oligoarticular or polyarticular, particularly in older patients (especially women) and in those with longstanding disease.*[1,9]

**What is the appearance of monosodium urate (gout) crystals under polarized light?**

Under polarized light, monosodium urate crystals are needle shaped with strongly negative birefringence.

**What is the appearance of calcium pyrophosphate dihydrate (pseudogout) crystals under polarized light?**

Under polarized light, calcium pyrophosphate dihydrate crystals are rhomboid shaped with weakly positive birefringence.

**What are the most common organisms involved in acute infectious monoarticular arthritis in adults?**

*Staphylococcus aureus* and *Neisseria gonorrhoeae* are the most common causes of acute infectious monoarticular arthritis in the industrialized world. Other organisms include *Streptococcus pneumoniae*, β-hemolytic streptococci (particularly groups A and B), and gram-negative bacilli (eg, *Haemophilus influenza*). *Septic arthritis related to infective endocarditis often involves more than 1 joint at the time of presentation.*[1]

**What are the most common organisms involved in chronic infectious monoarticular arthritis in adults?**

Organisms involved in chronic infectious monoarticular arthritis in adults include *Borrelia burgdorferi* (Lyme disease), *Mycobacterium tuberculosis* (tuberculosis), *Nocardia* species, *Brucella* species, and fungi (eg, *Candida* species, *Coccidioides immitis*, *Blastomyces dermatitidis, Sporothrix schenckii*, *Cryptococcus neoformans*).[1]

*Monoarticular arthritis can be an early manifestation of oligoarticular arthritis, particularly the peripheral spondyloarthritides (eg, psoriatic arthritis, reactive arthritis, enteropathic arthritis).*

## OLIGOARTICULAR INFLAMMATORY ARTHRITIS

**How many joints are involved in oligoarticular arthritis?**

Oligoarticular arthritis involves 2 to 4 joints.

### What are the causes of oligoarticular inflammatory arthritis?

**Sexually transmitted.**

Disseminated gonorrhea.

**A 29-year-old man with erythema nodosum (see Figure 15-3), bloody diarrhea, and inflammatory arthritis of the right knee and left ankle.**

Enteropathic arthritis.

**Corkscrew-shaped organisms (Figure 49-3).**

Spirochetal arthritis (eg, Lyme disease, syphilis).

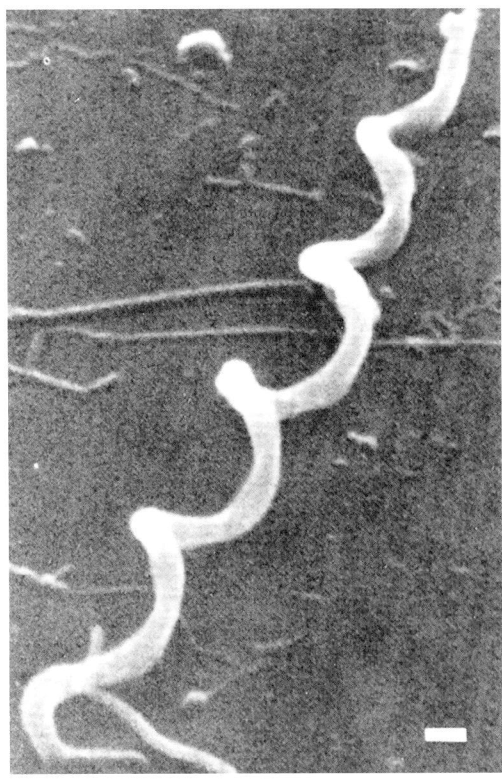

**Figure 49-3.** Electron micrograph demonstrating the "corkscrew" appearance of *Borrelia burgdorferi*. (From Johnson RC, Hyde FW, Rumpel CM. Taxonomy of the Lyme disease spirochetes. *Yale J Biol Med*. 1984;57:527-529, with permission.)

**A 38-year-old woman with erythema nodosum, bilateral ankle arthritis and periarthritis, and bilateral hilar lymphadenopathy (see Figure 21-4).**

Löfgren's syndrome (an acute form of sarcoidosis).

**More common in children than adults; this disease often presents with palpable purpura, acute kidney injury, and oligoarticular arthritis.**

Henoch-Schönlein purpura (HSP, or immunoglobulin A vasculitis).

**A 56-year-old man with chronic hepatitis C virus (HCV) infection develops palpable purpura and oligoarticular inflammatory arthritis.**

Cryoglobulinemia.

**Fever, erythema nodosum, recurrent aphthous ulcers of the mouth and genitalia, and oligoarticular inflammatory arthritis.**

Behçet's disease.

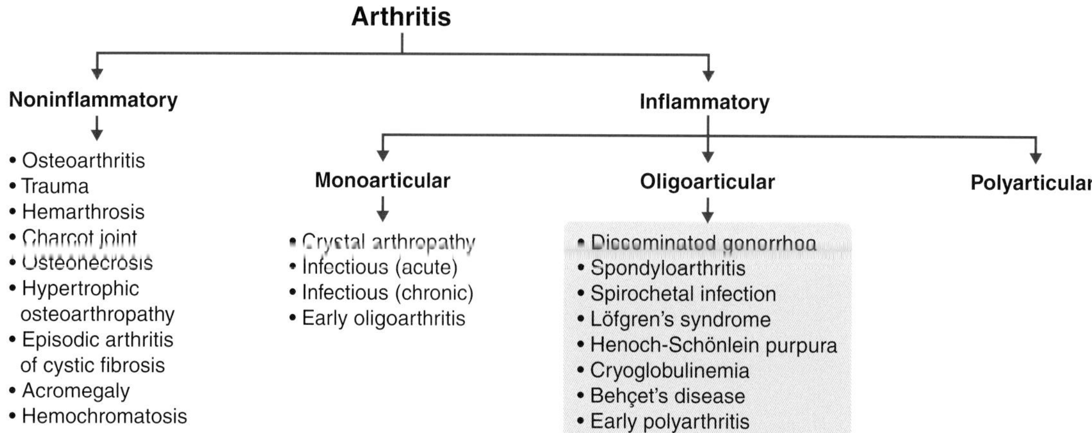


**What are the clinical features of disseminated gonorrhea?**

Disseminated gonorrhea is a common cause of inflammatory arthritis in young patients. It develops in the setting of bacteremia associated with acute infection or asymptomatic gonococcal colonization of the genitourinary tract or pharynx. Disseminated gonorrhea is characterized by a syndrome of fever, chills, pustular rash on the trunk and extensor surfaces of the distal extremities, and nonpurulent migratory oligoarticular inflammatory arthritis associated with tenosynovitis. True septic gonococcal arthritis may follow this syndrome, typically presenting as purulent monoarticular inflammatory arthritis involving the hip, knee, ankle, or wrist. In either syndrome, it is difficult to identify gonococci from synovial fluid Gram stain and culture. Nucleic acid amplification assays are more sensitive. Testing other sites such as skin lesions and oropharyngeal and genitourinary mucosa should also be performed to increase yield.[1]

**What are the spondyloarthritides?**

The spondyloarthritides (also referred to as spondyloarthropathies) are a group of inflammatory disorders that share certain clinical and genetic characteristics (eg, the presence of human leukocyte antigen [HLA]-B27). The main types include psoriatic arthritis, enteropathic arthritis, ankylosing spondylitis, and reactive arthritis.

**In addition to peripheral arthritis, what musculoskeletal inflammatory conditions can be associated with the spondyloarthritides?**

Musculoskeletal inflammatory conditions associated with the spondyloarthritides include spondylitis (particularly sacroiliitis), enthesitis, and dactylitis.[2]

**What nonmusculoskeletal inflammatory conditions can be associated with the spondyloarthritides?**

Nonmusculoskeletal inflammatory conditions associated with some of the spondyloarthritides include conjunctivitis, uveitis, pyoderma gangrenosum, erythema nodosum, aphthous stomatitis, urethritis, psoriasis, and inflammation of bowel mucosa.[1]

**Why should both the hands and feet be carefully examined when psoriatic arthritis is suspected?**

Involvement of the hands and feet are common in psoriatic arthritis, marked by synovitis (including the DIP joints, which are spared by most other inflammatory arthritides), dactylitis (more common in feet than hands), shortening of digits as a result of osteolysis, and certain fingernail and toenail changes (eg, pitting, horizontal ridging, onycholysis, yellow discoloration of the margins, dystrophic hyperkeratosis).[1,2]

**What are the 2 main subtypes of enteropathic arthritis?**

Enteropathic arthritis is subdivided based on the predominance of either axial or peripheral joint involvement. The axial subtype precedes enteritis in onset, and its course is largely independent of the bowel disease. The peripheral subtype may occur before, during, or after the enteritis, and its course usually parallels that of the bowel disease, becoming active with flares and improving with treatment.[10]

**What is the typical presentation of ankylosing spondylitis?**

Ankylosing spondylitis is more common in men than women (around 2.5:1) and typically presents in late adolescence or early adulthood with dull low-back pain that improves with activity, worsens with rest, peaks during the second half of the night, and is associated with significant morning stiffness (>30 minutes). Other associated symptoms may include enthesitis, osteitis, and peripheral inflammatory arthritis.[1]

**Which joints are most commonly involved in reactive arthritis?**

Reactive arthritis usually involves the joints of the lower extremities, including the knee, ankle, subtalar, MTP, and IP joints.[1]

**What are the characteristics of arthritis related to Lyme disease?**

Arthritis occurs in most patients with untreated disseminated Lyme disease. It typically begins as a migratory inflammatory arthritis early in the course of infection, evolving to monoarticular or oligoarticular inflammatory arthritis primarily affecting the knees and other large joints later in the disease course. Without treatment, symptoms typically wax and wane for months to years before eventually resolving. A small proportion of patients will develop joint erosions and damage. Polyarticular arthralgias without arthritis may also occur in patients with disseminated Lyme disease.[11]

**What are the characteristics of arthritis related to syphilis acquired in adulthood?**

The arthritis of syphilis is usually oligoarticular, inflammatory, symmetric and nonmigratory in nature. It occurs during secondary syphilis and is commonly associated with the typical nonpruritic papulosquamous rash of secondary syphilis, mucocutaneous lesions, and generalized lymphadenopathy. *Tertiary syphilis can be associated with* Charcot *joint related to tabes dorsalis.*[1,12]

**What is the prognosis of Löfgren's syndrome?**

Löfgren's syndrome is an acute form of sarcoidosis characterized by the triad of arthritis (most often involving both ankle joints), erythema nodosum, and bilateral hilar lymphadenopathy. It is more common in young white women of the Nordic countries and Spain; it is uncommon in blacks. Löfgren's syndrome is self-limited in most cases and has an excellent prognosis with >90% of patients experiencing resolution within 2 years.[1,13]

**What are the characteristics of arthritis related to Henoch-Schönlein purpura in adults?**

The arthritis of HSP usually presents as asymmetric oligoarticular inflammatory arthritis affecting the knees and ankles. It occurs in more than one-half of adult patients with HSP, and incidence decreases with age.[14]

**What are the characteristics of arthritis related to HCV-associated cryoglobulinemia?**

There are 2 distinct arthritic syndromes associated with chronic HCV infection: rheumatoid-like arthritis (two-thirds of patients) and cryoglobulin-related arthritis (one-third of patients). Rheumatoid-like arthritis is characterized by a symmetric polyarticular inflammatory arthritis. Cryoglobulin-related arthritis usually occurs in older patients with long-standing HCV infection. It is an oligoarticular inflammatory arthritis of the medium and large joints that typically follows an intermittent and benign course.[15]

**What are the characteristics of arthritis related to Behçet's disease?**

Oligoarticular inflammatory arthritis is found in most patients with Behçet's disease, including at the time of diagnosis. It occurs most frequently in women, and the knees are the most common sites, followed by the ankles and wrists. It is generally nonerosive.[16]

**In addition to Henoch-Schönlein purpura, cryoglobulinemia, and Behçet's disease, what other systemic vasculitides are associated with arthritis?**

Arthralgias are more common in systemic vasculitis, but arthritis does occur, particularly with antineutrophil cytoplasmic antibody (ANCA)-associated small vessel systemic vasculitis (eg, granulomatosis with polyangiitis [GPA, or Wegener's granulomatosis]) and polyarteritis nodosa. The typical presentation is migratory oligoarticular inflammatory arthritis of the large joints, but polyarticular inflammatory arthritis also occurs.[17]

*Oligoarticular arthritis can be an early manifestation of polyarticular arthritis.*

## POLYARTICULAR INFLAMMATORY ARTHRITIS

How many joints are involved in polyarticular arthritis?

Polyarticular arthritis involves >4 joints.

### What are the causes of polyarticular inflammatory arthritis?

Symmetric polyarticular inflammatory arthritis more common in women and associated with anti–cyclic citrullinated peptide antibodies and joint erosions on radiography.

Rheumatoid arthritis.

This etiology is associated with positive antinuclear and double-stranded deoxyribonucleic acid (dsDNA) antibody titers.

Systemic lupus erythematosus (SLE).

A 32-year-old woman develops symmetric polyarticular inflammatory arthritis of the hands and knees several weeks after one of her children was diagnosed with "slapped-cheek syndrome."

Parvovirus B19.

Proximal muscle weakness and elevated serum creatine kinase with or without skin manifestations.

Dermatomyositis (DM) or polymyositis (PM).

Associated with markedly elevated serum ferritin.

Adult-onset Still's disease.

A disease of developing countries caused by group A streptococcal infections of the upper respiratory tract, associated with migratory inflammatory arthritis.

Acute rheumatic fever.

A 25-year-old man with a history of lung transplantation for cystic fibrosis complicated by acute rejection is treated with horse antithymocyte globulin and a week later develops polyarticular inflammatory arthritis.

Serum sickness.

A granulomatous disease that most commonly affects the lung but can be associated with extrapulmonary manifestations, including polyarticular inflammatory arthritis.

Sarcoidosis.

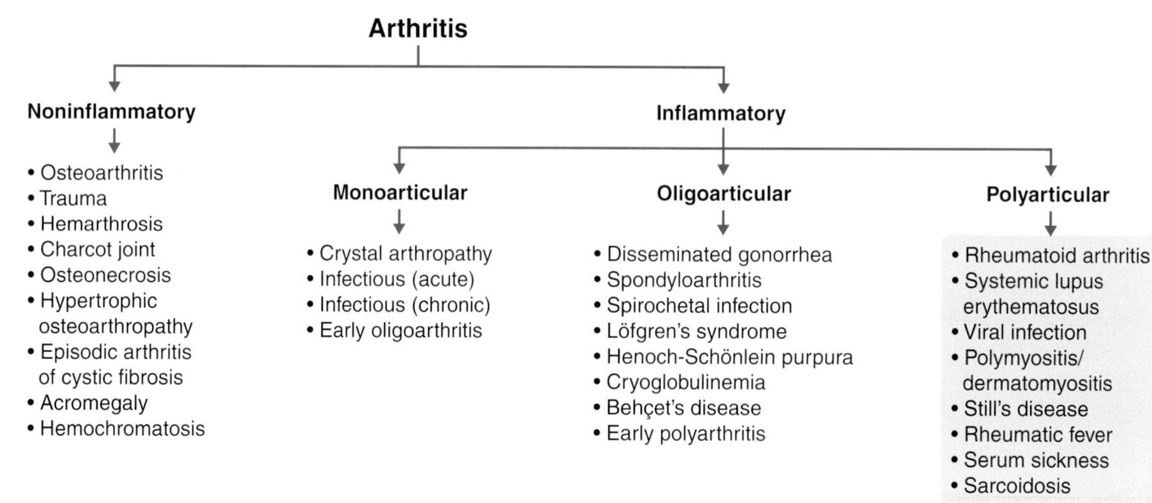

**Which joints are most often involved in rheumatoid arthritis?**

RA is a chronic systemic inflammatory condition characterized by symmetric destructive polyarticular inflammatory arthritis, as well as a host of periarticular and extra-articular manifestations. RA is more common in women (2 to 3:1). It affects up to 1% of adults worldwide, with some populations at higher risk (eg, Native American Yakima, Pima, and Chippewa tribes). The pathogenesis is not known. The wrist, MCP, PIP, and MTP joints are the most commonly involved in RA. Chronic joint destruction leads to several classic physical findings of the hands, including ulnar deviation and subluxation of the MCP joints, hyperextension of the PIP joint with flexion of the DIP joint (swan-neck deformity), and flexion of the PIP joint with hyperextension of the DIP joint (Boutonnière deformity) (Figure 49-4).[1]

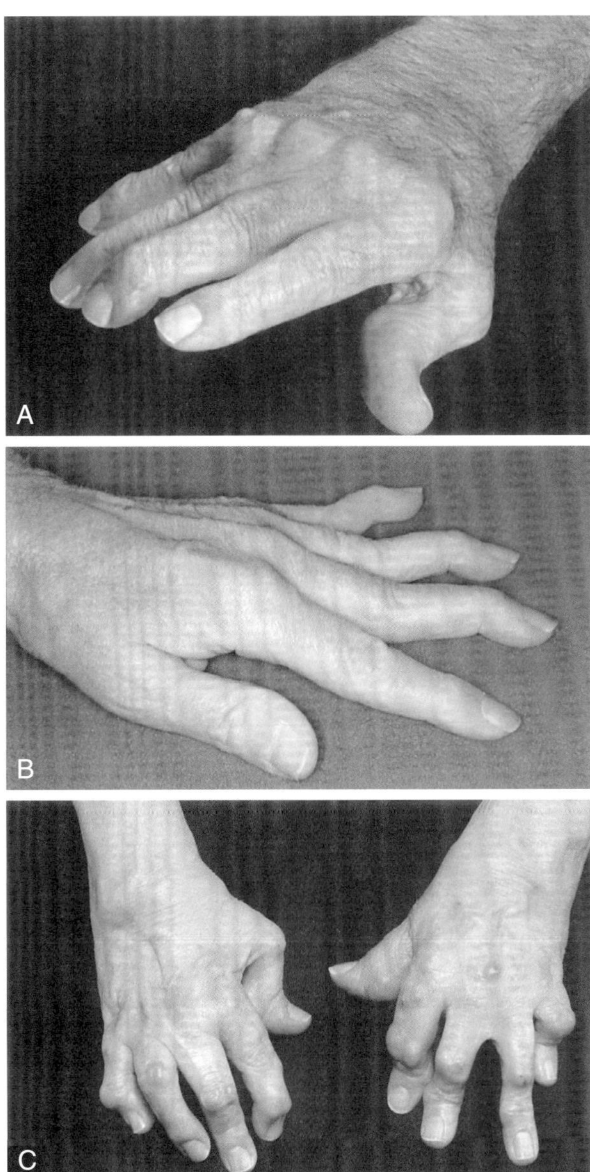


**Figure 49-4.** Rheumatoid arthritis. A, Ulnar deviation at the metacarpophalangeal joints. B, Swan-neck deformity. C, Boutonnière deformity. (From Hunder GG. *Atlas of Rheumatology*. 3rd ed. Philadelphia, PA: Lippincott Williams & Wilkins; 2000:11.)

**What are the characteristics of the arthritis associated with systemic lupus erythematosus?**

Arthritis is a common manifestation of SLE, affecting most patients. It is typically a nonerosive polyarticular inflammatory arthritis that most commonly affects the MCP, PIP, and knee joints.[18]

**Which viruses are associated with polyarticular inflammatory arthritis?**

Viruses most commonly associated with polyarticular inflammatory arthritis include human immunodeficiency virus (HIV), parvovirus B19, hepatitis B virus, HCV, rubella, and several vector-borne viruses such as chikungunya and dengue fever.[19]

**What is the antisynthetase syndrome?**

The antisynthetase syndrome occurs in some patients with DM or PM and significantly increases the likelihood of arthritis. It is associated with a constellation of clinical manifestations, including fever, interstitial lung disease, inflammatory myopathy, polyarticular inflammatory arthritis, Raynaud's phenomenon, and mechanic's hands (see Figure 47-4). Affected patients have serum autoantibodies to aminoacyl-tRNA synthetase enzymes, the most recognized of which is the anti-histidyl-tRNA synthetase (anti-Jo-1) antibody.[20]

**Which joints are most commonly involved in adult-onset Still's disease?**

Adult-onset Still's disease is a systemic inflammatory condition that is characterized by the triad of fever, arthralgias or arthritis, and salmon-colored evanescent skin rash. The arthritis most often affects the knees, wrists, ankles, and elbows. The DIP joints are also frequently involved (which are spared by most other inflammatory arthritides except for psoriatic arthritis).[21]

**How common is polyarticular inflammatory arthritis in patients with acute rheumatic fever?**

Arthritis occurs in most patients with acute rheumatic fever. It is classically asymmetric, migratory, and inflammatory and affects the large joints most frequently (eg, knees, ankles, hips, elbows). It is highly responsive to salicylates and other nonsteroidal anti-inflammatory drugs (NSAIDs). Polyarticular arthralgias without arthritis also occur in patients with acute rheumatic fever. *Note, because of the migratory nature of acute rheumatic fever, at any given time <4 joints may be involved, which would present as oligoarticular arthritis or monoarticular arthritis.*[1]

**What are the other clinical manifestations of serum sickness?**

Serum sickness is a flu-like illness that occurs as a result of tissue deposition of immune complexes, which form in response to the presence of foreign protein or serum (eg, horse antithymocyte globulin). It typically develops 1 to 2 weeks after exposure. In addition to polyarticular inflammatory arthritis, serum sickness presents with fever, cutaneous manifestations (eg, urticaria), and lymphadenopathy. Withdrawal of the offending agent usually results in resolution; however, severe cases may benefit from systemic glucocorticoids.[1]

**Which joints are most commonly involved in the chronic arthritis of sarcoidosis?**

Arthritis related to sarcoidosis most commonly occurs acutely in the setting of Löfgren's syndrome. However, chronic arthritis related to systemic sarcoidosis does occur in a small proportion of cases, usually involving the knees, ankles, wrists, hands, and feet.[22]

## Case Summary

A 62-year-old man with a history of alcohol abuse and recurrent episodes of monoarticular arthritis presents with acute monoarticular inflammatory arthritis of the left elbow after recently starting a diuretic medication, and is found to have non-tender subcutaneous nodules overlying the IP joints of the hands.

***What is the most likely cause of arthritis in this patient?***

Gout.

BONUS QUESTIONS

***What is gout?***

Gout is the manifestation of intra-articular deposition of urate crystals related to hyperuricemia. Under normal temperature and pH, the limit of urate solubility is around 6.8 mg/dL. Less than one-half of all patients with hyperuricemia experience gout.[9]

***What is the nature of the subcutaneous nodules in this case?***

The subcutaneous nodules in this case (see Figure 49-1B) are tophi, which are deposits of urate crystals in the joints and soft tissues.

***What is the significance of tophi?***

Tophi are a manifestation of longstanding and poorly controlled gout. Patients with tophaceous gout can experience polyarticular attacks and symptoms between attacks. Tophi are typically painless but may become acutely inflamed. Patients with tophaceous gout have erosive and destructive arthritis.[9]

***What other arthritic conditions are associated with subcutaneous nodules?***

OA is associated with osteophytes around the DIP joints (ie, Heberden's nodes) and the PIP joints (ie, Bouchard's nodes); RA is associated with subcutaneous nodules that appear in areas subject to repeated trauma such as the forearm, sacral prominences, and the Achilles tendon.[1]

***What was the most likely trigger for the episode of acute gout in this case?***

Triggers for acute flares of gout include alcohol use, hospitalization, surgery, and diuretic use. In this case, it is likely that alcohol served as the trigger for past flares, whereas the diuretic medication that was recently started triggered the current flare.[9]

***Is gout more common in men or women?***

Gout affects middle-aged men more frequently than women (3 to 4:1), related in part to the uricosuric effects of estrogen. The incidence of gout in women rises after menopause.[9]

***Should serum uric acid levels be measured in this case?***

At the time of an acute attack of gout, serum uric acid levels may not be elevated. If the underlying diagnosis of gout is proven, then serum uric acid levels should be evaluated between attacks with a goal of maintaining it within the normal range, often through a combination of lifestyle modification and pharmacologic agents.[9]

***How is the diagnosis of gout definitively made?***

Gout can be definitively diagnosed with arthrocentesis and evaluation of synovial fluid. The presence of needle-shaped crystals with strongly negative birefringence under polarized light is pathognomonic. Synovial WBC count >2000 cells/μL with a predominance of PMNs would also be expected.

***Should arthrocentesis be performed in this case?***

Arthrocentesis should be performed to prove the diagnosis and to rule out other crystal arthritides (eg, calcium pyrophosphate dihydrate) and septic arthritis (patients with joint damage from a history of aseptic inflammatory arthritis are predisposed to developing septic arthritis).

***What is the short-term pharmacologic management of acute gout?***

First-line pharmacologic agents used to control acute gout flairs include NSAIDs and colchicine. Systemic glucocorticoids can also be used when NSAIDs and colchicine are contraindicated or poorly tolerated. Monoarticular attacks can be managed with intra-articular glucocorticoids. Therapy with an interleukin-1 receptor antagonist (eg, anakinra) can be used in some circumstances (eg, recalcitrant disease).[9]

***What is the long-term management of gout?***

The prevention of recurrent attacks of gout by maintaining serum uric acid levels <6 mg/dL is the cornerstone of the long-term management of gout. Lifestyle modification, including reduction in alcohol consumption, is paramount. Pharmacologic urate-lowering therapy (eg, xanthine oxidase inhibitors, uricosuric agents, uricase agents) to prevent acute attacks and the development of tophi should be considered based on the frequency of attacks and other patient-specific factors (eg, patient preference).[9]

## KEY POINTS

- Arthritis describes inflammation involving any structure within a joint.
- Articular structures include the synovium, synovial fluid, articular cartilage, intra-articular ligaments, joint capsule, and juxta-articular bone.
- Mimics of arthritis include bursitis, tendinitis, enthesitis, epicondylitis, ligament damage, cellulitis, deep vein thrombosis, polymyalgia rheumatica, myositis, and periarticular bone lesions.
- An articular process is suggested by the presence of pain with both active and passive range of motion and joint line tenderness on palpation.
- Arthritis can be noninflammatory or inflammatory.
- The cardinal signs of inflammation include erythema, warmth, pain, and swelling.
- Other inflammatory musculoskeletal conditions such as tenosynovitis, enthesitis, and dactylitis can occur with certain types of inflammatory arthritis.
- Synovial fluid WBC count is the single most important laboratory test in the evaluation of inflammatory arthritis (WBC count >2000 cells/µL is consistent with inflammatory arthritis).
- The most common causes of noninflammatory arthritis include osteoarthritis and trauma.
- Inflammatory arthritis can occur in a monoarticular (1 joint), oligoarticular (2-4 joints), or polyarticular (>4 joints) pattern.
- Inflammatory arthritides can generally be classified by the number of joints involved, but exceptions occur (eg, monoarticular peripheral spondyloarthritis, polyarticular gout).

## REFERENCES


1. Longo DL, Fauci AS, Kasper DL, Hauser SL, Jameson JL, Loscalzo J, eds. *Harrison's Principles of Internal Medicine*. 18th ed. New York, NY: McGraw-Hill; 2012.
2. Mease PJ. Distinguishing inflammatory from noninflammatory arthritis, enthesitis, and dactylitis in psoriatic arthritis: a report from the GRAPPA 2010 annual meeting. *J Rheumatol*. 2012;39(2):415-417.
3. McGillicuddy DC, Shah KH, Friedberg RP, Nathanson LA, Edlow JA. How sensitive is the synovial fluid white blood cell count in diagnosing septic arthritis? *Am J Emerg Med*. 2007;25(7):749-752.
4. Shmerling RH, Delbanco TL, Tosteson AN, Trentham DE. Synovial fluid tests. What should be ordered? *JAMA*. 1990;264(8):1009-1014.
5. Gouveri E, Papanas N. Charcot osteoarthropathy in diabetes: a brief review with an emphasis on clinical practice. *World J Diabetes*. 2011;2(5):59-65.
6. Mankin HJ. Nontraumatic necrosis of bone (osteonecrosis). *N Engl J Med*. 1992;326(22):1473-1479.
7. Dixey J, Redington AN, Butler RC, et al. The arthropathy of cystic fibrosis. *Ann Rheum Dis*. 1988;47(3):218-223.
8. Killinger Z, Kuzma M, Sterancakova L, Payer J. Osteoarticular changes in acromegaly. *Int J Endocrinol*. 2012;2012:839282.
9. Neogi T. Clinical practice. Gout. *N Engl J Med*. 2011;364(5):443-452.
10. Peluso R, Di Minno MN, Iervolino S, et al. Enteropathic spondyloarthritis: from diagnosis to treatment. *Clin Dev Immunol*. 2013;2013:631408.
11. Puius YA, Kalish RA. Lyme arthritis: pathogenesis, clinical presentation, and management. *Infect Dis Clin North Am*. 2008;22(2):289-300, vi-vii.
12. Reginato AJ, Schumacher HR, Jimenez S, Maurer K. Synovitis in secondary syphilis. Clinical, light, and electron microscopic studies. *Arthritis Rheum*. 1979;22(2):170-176.
13. Mañá J, Gómez Vaquero C, Montero A, et al. Lofgren's syndrome revisited: a study of 186 patients. *Am J Med*. 1999;107(3):240-245.
14. Pillebout E, Thervet E, Hill G, Alberti C, Vanhille P, Nochy D. Henoch-Schonlein Purpura in adults: outcome and prognostic factors. *J Am Soc Nephrol*. 2002;13(5):1271-1278.
15. Kemmer NM, Sherman KE. Hepatitis C-related arthropathy: diagnostic and treatment considerations. *J Musculoskelet Med*. 2010;27(9):351-354.
16. Kim HA, Choi KW, Song YW. Arthropathy in Behcet's disease. *Scand J Rheumatol*. 1997;26(2):125-129.
17. Agard C, Mouthon L, Mahr A, Guillevin L. Microscopic polyangiitis and polyarteritis nodosa: how and when do they start? *Arthritis Rheum*. 2003;49(5):709-715.
18. Grossman JM. Lupus arthritis. *Best Pract Res Clin Rheumatol*. 2009;23(4):495-506.
19. Calabrese LH, Naides SJ. Viral arthritis. *Infect Dis Clin North Am*. 2005;19(4):963-980, x.
20. Katzap E, Barilla-LaBarca ML, Marder G. Antisynthetase syndrome. *Curr Rheumatol Rep*. 2011;13(3):175-181.
21. Gopalarathinam R, Orlowsky E, Kesavalu R, Yelaminchili S. Adult onset Still's disease: a review on diagnostic workup and treatment options. *Case Rep Rheumatol*. 2016;2016:6502373.
22. Sweiss NJ, Patterson K, Sawaqed R, et al. Rheumatologic manifestations of sarcoidosis. *Semin Respir Crit Care Med*. 2010;31(4):463-473.

# Chapter 50

# SYSTEMIC VASCULITIS

## Case: A 67-year-old man with hemoptysis

A previously healthy 67-year-old man presents to the emergency department after coughing up blood. He describes progressive shortness of breath over the past few weeks with dry cough and intermittent fever. He has been seen in the clinic several times over the past few months for persistent nasal congestion and sinusitis. The nasal and sinus symptoms have not responded to antibiotics. He has experienced weight loss of 12 pounds over this time. On the morning of presentation, the cough became productive of bloody sputum. The patient estimates that he has produced 2 tablespoons of blood over the past 6 hours.

Temperature is 37.5°C; heart rate, 103 beats per minute; blood pressure, 110/30 mm Hg; and respiratory rate, 28 breaths per minute. Breathing appears labored. There is marked depression of the midportion of the nasal bridge. There are multiple red-purple papules ranging from 5 mm to 2 cm in diameter with some areas of confluence over the shins and ankles. There is diffuse expiratory wheezing.

Serum creatinine is 1.9 mg/dL. Evaluation of urine sediment reveals the presence of dysmorphic red blood cells and red blood cell casts. Serum antibodies to PR3 (c-ANCA) are present. Computed tomography (CT) imaging of the chest is shown in Figure 50-1.

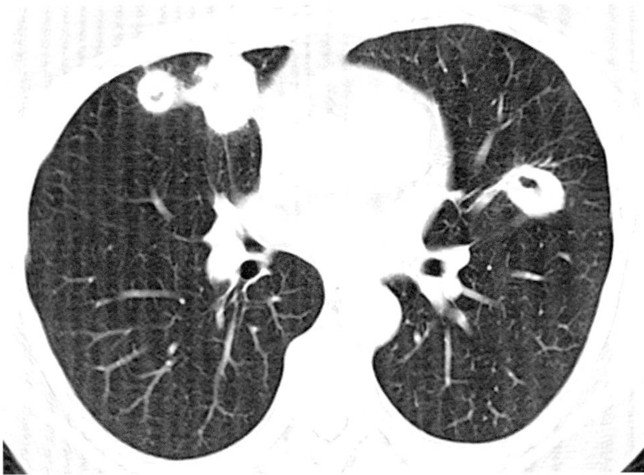

**Figure 50-1.** (From Elicker BM, Webb WR. *Fundamentals of High-Resolution Lung CT: Common Findings, Common Patterns, Common Diseases, and Differential Diagnosis*. Philadelphia, PA: Wolters Kluwer Health; 2013.)

***What is the most likely diagnosis in this patient?***

What is vasculitis?

Vasculitis describes a heterogeneous group of diseases that share the defining feature of blood vessel wall inflammation. The inflammatory process can involve blood vessels of virtually any type, size, and location in the body and can lead to partial or complete luminal compromise, with ensuing ischemia of the related tissues. Vasculitis can be a primary disorder or occur secondary to an underlying systemic disease.[1]

What is the difference between vasculitis and vasculopathy?

Vasculitis is a specific term that is defined by blood vessel wall inflammation. Vasculopathy is a broader term that includes conditions such as atherosclerosis and Buerger's disease (ie, thromboangiitis obliterans), where there is no histologic evidence of vessel wall inflammation.

**What are the clinical manifestations of vasculitis?**

The manifestations of vasculitis are protean owing to variability in the size and location of blood vessel involvement; it may be confined to a single organ (eg, skin), or it may affect a range of organ systems (eg, pulmonary-renal syndrome). Vasculitis should be considered when multiple systems are involved or characteristic physical findings are present.

**What is systemic vasculitis?**

Systemic vasculitis refers to a group of named primary vasculitides that are immune mediated and individually distinguished by the presence of unique clinicopathologic features (eg, giant cell arteritis [GCA], polyarteritis nodosa [PAN], microscopic polyangiitis [MPA]).

**What is limited systemic vasculitis?**

Limited systemic vasculitis refers to systemic vasculitis involving only 1 organ system, (eg, upper respiratory tract–limited granulomatosis with polyangiitis [GPA, or Wegener's granulomatosis]).[1]

**What is vasculitis associated with systemic disease?**

Vasculitis associated with systemic disease describes the occurrence of vasculitis in the setting of an underlying systemic disease known to cause vasculitis (eg, rheumatoid vasculitis).[1]

**What is vasculitis associated with probable etiology?**

Vasculitis associated with probable etiology describes the occurrence of systemic vasculitis in the setting of a known and likely provoking factor (eg, malignancy-associated vasculitis).[1]

**What is single-organ vasculitis?**

Single-organ vasculitis refers to vasculitis involving a single organ without any features suggestive of systemic vasculitis; it is distinct from limited systemic vasculitis. Distribution within the involved organ may be unifocal or multifocal (diffuse). Some patients initially diagnosed with single-organ vasculitis may go on to develop features of systemic vasculitis and should be reclassified accordingly (eg, cutaneous small vessel vasculitis [CSVV] over time may meet the diagnostic criteria of PAN).[1]

**What are the single-organ vasculitides?**

Examples of single-organ vasculitis include CSVV, primary angiitis of the central nervous system, and isolated aortitis (eg, related to thoracic radiation treatment). Importantly, these organs may be involved in systemic vasculitis.

**What is leukocytoclastic vasculitis (LCV)?**

LCV is a histologic term that describes neutrophilic infiltration within the walls of small-sized blood vessels. This term is often used synonymously with CSVV.[2]

**What are the physical findings of vasculitis?**

Physical findings of vasculitis are variable, depending on the type of vasculitis and extent of organ involvement. Particular findings can indicate involvement of certain types of blood vessels and, in some cases, specific vasculitides.

**What are the laboratory features of systemic vasculitis?**

Systemic vasculitis can be suggested by peripheral leukocytosis and elevation of acute phase reactants such as erythrocyte sedimentation rate (ESR) and C-reactive protein (CRP). Other laboratory studies can be useful in the evaluation of specific causes of systemic vasculitis (eg, serum antineutrophil cytoplasmic antibodies [ANCA]).

**What conditions can mimic the presentation of systemic vasculitis?**

Other systemic conditions with protean manifestations can be confused for systemic vasculitis, including infection (eg, bacterial endocarditis), malignancy (eg, lymphoma), drug toxicity (eg, amphetamines), connective tissue disease (eg, systemic lupus erythematosus), sarcoidosis, thrombotic microangiopathy (eg, thrombotic thrombocytopenic purpura), and atheroembolic disease.[3]

**What are the 3 categories of systemic vasculitis based on the size of involved blood vessels?**

Systemic vasculitis can involve the large vessels, medium vessels, or small vessels.

**Systemic vasculitis**

**Large vessel** | **Medium vessel** | **Small vessel**

**Which vessels are included within the large-, medium-, and small-sized categories?**

Large-sized vessels include the aorta and its branches and the analogous veins; medium-sized vessels are distal to large-sized vessels and include the main visceral arteries (eg, renal, hepatic, coronary, and mesenteric arteries) and their initial branches and the analogous veins; small-sized vessels are distal to medium-sized vessels, are microscopic in size, and refer to arterioles, capillaries, and venules.[1]

*Individual vasculitides are capable of affecting blood vessels of more than 1 size (eg, large and medium vessels or medium and small vessels). However, most conditions predominantly affect vessels of 1 particular size, and that principle will be used in this chapter.*

## LARGE VESSEL SYSTEMIC VASCULITIS

**What physical findings are associated with large vessel vasculitis?**

Physical findings of large vessel vasculitis may include asymmetric pulses, discrepancies in blood pressure between extremities, bruits, and thrills. In addition, specific findings can be associated with certain vasculitides (eg, tender and thickened superficial temporal artery in GCA). In some cases, large vessel vasculitis occurs in association with medium vessel vasculitis, which may lead to other findings.

### What are the causes of large vessel systemic vasculitis?

**A 67-year-old man complains of prandial headache and jaw pain and is found to have a palpable and tender subcutaneous cord-like mass in the lateral forehead (Figure 50-2).**

Giant cell arteritis (ie, temporal arteritis).

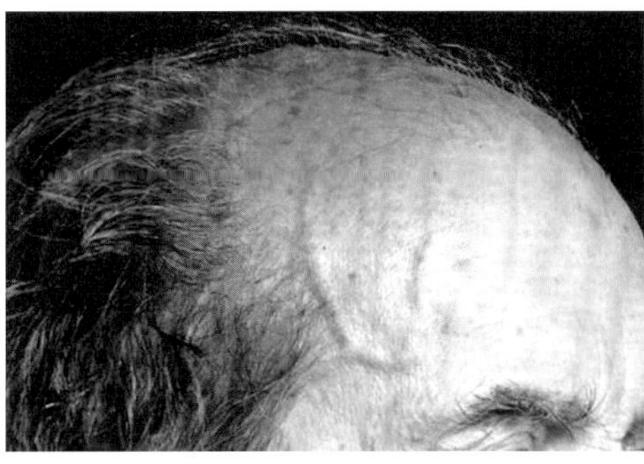

**Figure 50-2.** Temporal artery inflammation in a patient with giant cell arteritis. The temporal artery may be tender, red, enlarged, tortuous, or nodular, and can have decreased pulsation. (From Mackie SL, Pease CT. Diagnosis and management of giant cell arteritis and polymyalgia rheumatic: challenges, controversies, and practical tips. *Postgrad Med J.* 2013;89(1051):284-292, Copyright © 2013, British Medical Journal.)

**This entity can present in nonsmoking younger patients (<50 years of age) with pulseless extremities and discrepant blood pressure measurements between extremities.**

Takayasu arteritis.

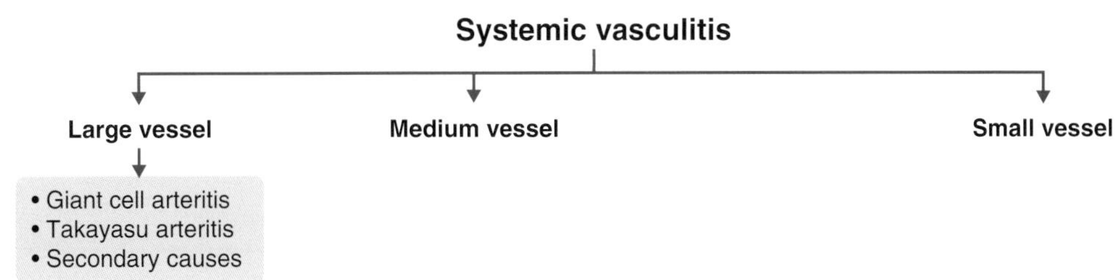

**What other rheumatologic disease often coexists with giant cell arteritis?**

GCA is a disease found almost exclusively in patients above 50 years of age, with a predilection for women. Patients develop inflammation of the extracranial branches of the aorta, typically sparing the intracranial vessels. Diagnosis is confirmed with biopsy of the temporal artery. GCA is associated with polymyalgia rheumatica (PMR), which is characterized by pain and stiffness of the muscles of the neck, shoulders, hips, and thighs. PMR most often occurs in isolation but develops in close to one-half of patients with GCA. Of those who present with isolated PMR, around 15% will ultimately develop GCA.[3,4]

**What populations are at highest risk of Takayasu arteritis?**

Individuals at highest risk for developing Takayasu arteritis include adolescent girls and women in their second and third decades of life from Japan, Southeast Asia, India, and Mexico. Involvement of the large elastic arteries can lead to dilatation, aneurysm formation, and thrombosis. Renal artery involvement can result in severe hypertension. Cardiac involvement occurs in some patients and can lead to manifestations such as aortic regurgitation and dilated cardiomyopathy. Carotid artery involvement can result in cerebral ischemia (eg, stroke).[4]

**What are the secondary causes of large vessel vasculitis?**

Secondary causes of large vessel vasculitis include aortitis associated with probable etiology, such as infection-associated vasculitis (eg, syphilis, tuberculosis, *Salmonella* species), and aortitis associated with systemic disease (eg, ankylosing spondylitis).[3]

**What is Cogan's syndrome?**

Cogan's syndrome is a chronic inflammatory condition that typically affects young white patients, characterized by interstitial keratitis, vestibulo-auditory symptoms, and, in some cases, vasculitis. Although the vasculitis can affect vessels of any size, there is a predilection for the aorta.[3,5]

## MEDIUM VESSEL SYSTEMIC VASCULITIS

**What physical findings are associated with medium vessel vasculitis?**

Physical findings of medium vessel vasculitis are related to nerve involvement (eg, mononeuritis multiplex, polyneuropathy, radiculopathy, plexopathy), vascular changes (eg, diminished peripheral pulses), and cardiac involvement (eg, pericardial friction rub). In some cases, medium vessel vasculitis occurs in association with large vessel or small vessel vasculitis, which may lead to other findings.

### What are the causes of medium vessel systemic vasculitis?

**A 49-year-old man with chronic hepatitis B infection presents with recurrent fever, weight loss, testicular pain, hypertension, livedo reticularis, and a foot drop.**

Polyarteritis nodosa.

**This entity usually occurs in children and presents with a constellation of findings such as fever, conjunctival injection, oral mucosal findings (eg, erythema and cracking of the lips, "strawberry" tongue), cervical lymphadenopathy, peripheral extremity changes (eg, swelling of the hands or feet), and skin rash.**

Kawasaki disease.[3]

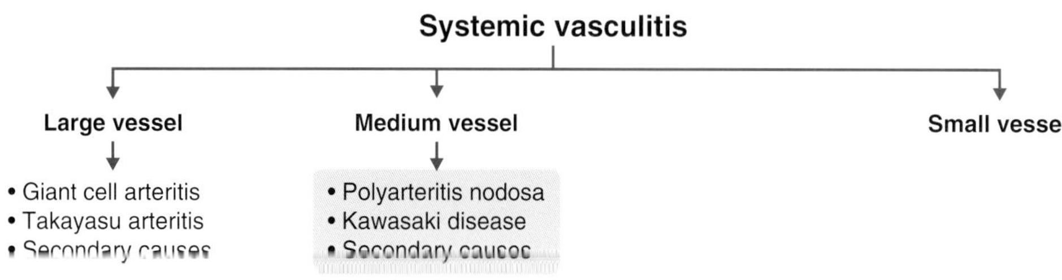

**What are the arteriographic findings of polyarteritis nodosa?**

PAN affects medium and small vessels, most frequently the renal and visceral arteries. The presence of microaneurysms (1-5 mm in diameter) is a hallmark of PAN but is not universal (Figure 50-3). Other findings include stenotic segments and obliteration of vessels. These changes mainly occur in the mesenteric, renal, and hepatic arteries.[3,6]

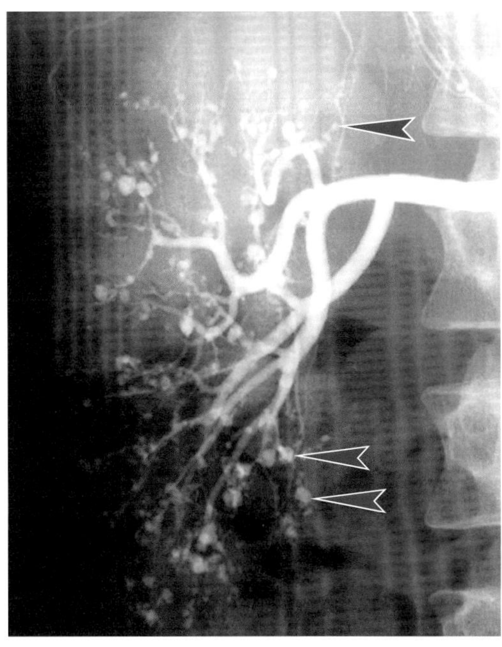

**Figure 50-3.** Right renal angiogram demonstrating multiple renal arterial microaneurysms (arrowheads) in a patient with polyarteritis nodosa. (From Brant WE, Helms CA. *Fundamentals of Diagnostic Radiology*, 4th ed. Philadelphia, PA: Wolters Kluwer Health; 2012.)

**What is the treatment for Kawasaki disease?**

Kawasaki disease typically occurs in children. It is generally self-limited but can be associated with long-term complications (eg, coronary artery aneurysms) and has an overall mortality rate of up to 3%. Early treatment with the combination of intravenous immunoglobulin (IVIG) and aspirin improves outcomes.[3,7]

**What are the secondary causes of medium vessel vasculitis?**

Secondary causes of medium vessel vasculitis include vasculitis associated with systemic disease (eg, rheumatoid vasculitis) and vasculitis associated with probable etiology (eg, hepatitis B–associated PAN).

## SMALL VESSEL SYSTEMIC VASCULITIS

**What physical findings are associated with small vessel vasculitis?**

Physical findings of small vessel vasculitis are usually related to cutaneous involvement (eg, palpable purpura), pulmonary involvement (eg, wheezing), and ocular involvement (eg, conjunctivitis). In addition, specific findings can be associated with certain vasculitides (eg, saddle nose deformity in GPA). In some cases, small vessel vasculitis occurs in association with medium vessel vasculitis, which may lead to other findings.[3]

**What is the typical distribution of palpable purpura?**

Palpable purpura usually occurs in dependent areas of the body (eg, lower extremities).[3]

**What are the cutaneous manifestations of small vessel vasculitis?**

While palpable purpura is the most common cutaneous finding of small vessel vasculitis, other potential manifestations include papules, petechiae, vesicles, ulcers, and subcutaneous nodules.[3]

**What are the 2 subcategories of small vessel systemic vasculitis based on serological testing?**

Small vessel systemic vasculitis can be ANCA-associated or non–ANCA-associated.

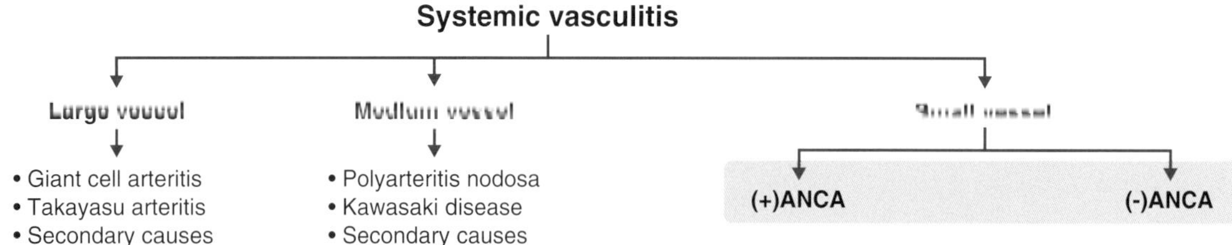


**What does ANCA refer to?**

Antineutrophilic cytoplasmic antibodies are a group of autoantibodies directed against proteins found in the cytoplasm of neutrophils, including proteinase 3 (PR3) and myeloperoxidase (MPO).

**In ANCA-positive patients, which 2 patterns may be seen on immunofluorescence microscopy?**

Under immunofluorescence microscopy, the presence of antibodies to PR3 results in a cytoplasmic pattern (c-ANCA), whereas antibodies to MPO are associated with a perinuclear pattern (p-ANCA). Enzyme-linked immunosorbent assays (ELISA) can specifically detect the presence of PR3 and MPO antibodies in the serum of affected patients.[2]

## ANCA-ASSOCIATED SMALL VESSEL SYSTEMIC VASCULITIS

### What are the causes of ANCA-associated small vessel systemic vasculitis?

**A 63-year-old man presents with hemoptysis, hematuria, and acute kidney injury and is found to have positive c-ANCA titers.**

Granulomatosis with polyangiitis.

**This condition, most commonly associated with p-ANCA, is distinguished from the other causes of ANCA-associated small vessel vasculitis by the absence of granulomatous inflammation.**

Microscopic polyangiitis.

**A 43-year-old woman with a recent diagnosis of asthma presents with palpable purpura and a wrist drop.**

Eosinophilic granulomatosis with polyangiitis (EGPA, or Churg-Strauss syndrome).

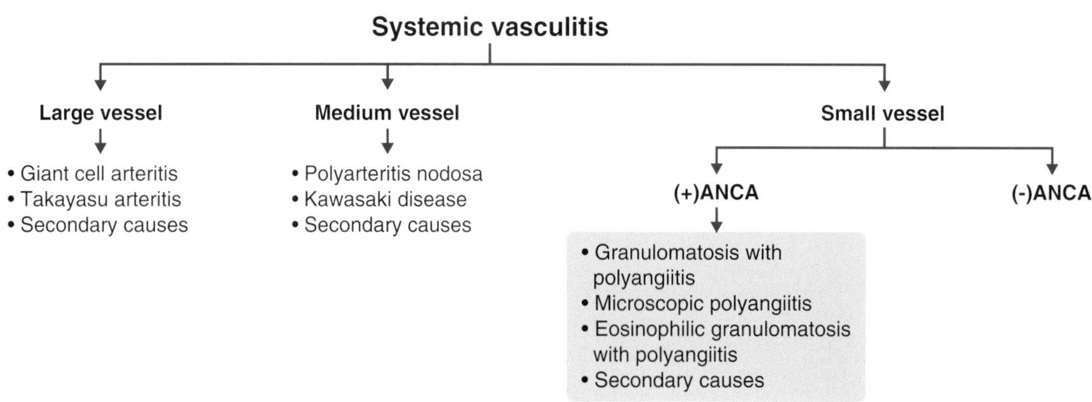

**What systems are most commonly involved in granulomatosis with polyangiitis?**

Upper airway involvement (eg, sinus disease) occurs in virtually all cases of GPA (around 95%) (Figure 50-4). Lower airway (eg, pulmonary capillaritis), renal (eg, glomerulonephritis), cutaneous (eg, palpable purpura), musculoskeletal (eg, arthralgias or arthritis), and eye involvement (eg, episcleritis) are also common. Nervous system involvement (eg, mononeuritis multiplex) and cardiac involvement (eg, pericarditis) occur less frequently. Notably, GPA commonly presents with limited disease (eg, sinus disease only).[3]

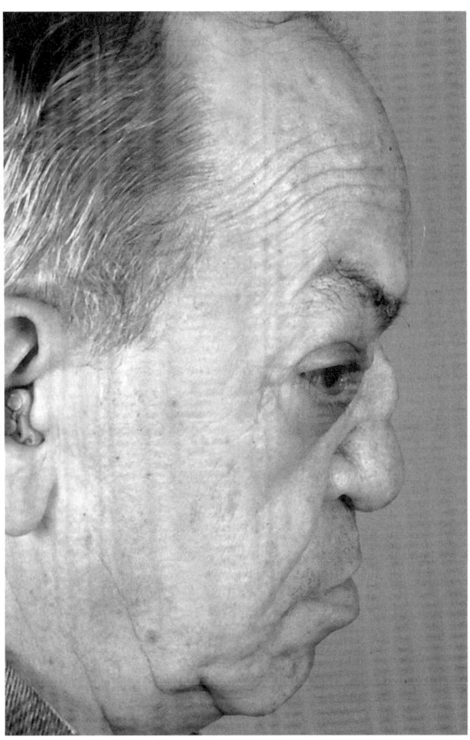

**Figure 50-4.** Saddle nose deformity in a patient with granulomatosis with polyangiitis (Wegener's granulomatosis). (From Rubin R, Strayer DS. *Rubin's Pathology: Clinicopathologic Foundations of Medicine*. 5th ed. Philadelphia, PA: Lippincott Williams & Wilkins; 2008.)

**What systems are most commonly involved in microscopic polyangiitis?**

MPA affects small and medium vessels. Renal involvement is by far the most common manifestation of MPA (>80%), ranging from asymptomatic proteinuria to rapidly progressive glomerulonephritis. Like GPA, other systems can be involved, including the nervous, cutaneous, gastrointestinal, and pulmonary systems.[8]

**Why is a complete blood count (with differential) helpful in the workup of eosinophilic granulomatosis with polyangiitis?**

Peripheral eosinophilia (typically >1500 cells/μL or >10%) often occurs in patients with active EGPA and can be supportive of the diagnosis. The presence and degree of peripheral eosinophilia correlates with disease activity; in patients with known EGPA, relapses can be predicted by the occurrence of or rise in peripheral eosinophilia. *Patients with asthma who do not have EGPA can develop peripheral eosinophilia, but it is typically mild (<10%).*[9]

**What are the secondary causes of ANCA-associated small vessel vasculitis?**

Secondary causes of ANCA-associated small vessel vasculitis include vasculitis associated with probable etiology, such as drug-associated p-ANCA vasculitis (eg, hydralazine, propylthiouracil) and levamisole-associated p-ANCA vasculitis (this entity should be considered in cocaine users who present with necrosis of the ears and nose). Some small vessel vasculitides associated with systemic disease can present with positive ANCA in a minority of cases (eg, rheumatoid vasculitis).[3]

*ANCA-associated small vessel systemic vasculitides can occur in the absence of ANCA positivity and should remain on the differential diagnosis of any small vessel systemic vasculitis until a clear diagnosis has been made.*

## NON–ANCA-ASSOCIATED SMALL VESSEL SYSTEMIC VASCULITIS

### What are the causes of non–ANCA-associated small vessel systemic vasculitis?

**Abdominal pain, palpable purpura, acute kidney injury, and arthritis in a patient with a normal platelet count.**

Henoch-Schönlein purpura (HSP, or immunoglobulin A vasculitis).

**A 54-year-old man with chronic hepatitis C virus (HCV) infection presents with palpable purpura and glomerulonephritis.**

Cryoglobulinemia.

**"Silk road disease."**

Behçet's disease.

**A 26-year-old man presents with hemoptysis, hematuria, and acute kidney injury, and immunofluorescence microscopy of renal tissue shows linear deposition of immunoglobulins along the glomerular basement membrane.**

Anti–glomerular basement membrane (anti-GBM) disease.

**Itchy and tender urticarial lesions that remain fixed for more than 24 hours.**

Urticarial vasculitis (UV).

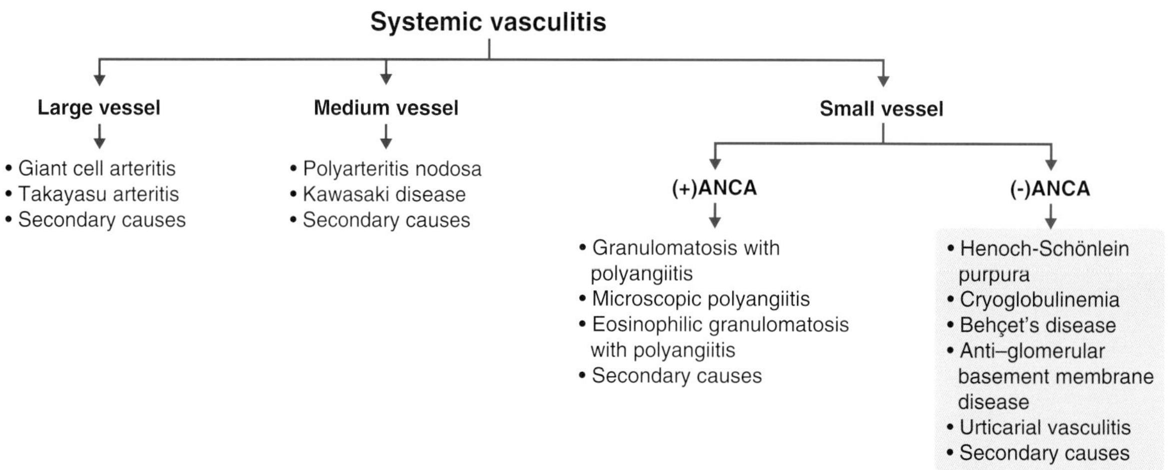


**What is the hallmark immunofluorescence finding from a skin biopsy in patients with Henoch-Schönlein purpura?**

HSP is more common in children, but does occur in adults. Palpable purpura is present in most patients, and is typically distributed over the buttocks and lower extremities. Other clinical manifestations include arthralgias or arthritis, abdominal pain, and glomerulonephritis. Immunofluorescence demonstrating IgA deposits within the walls of cutaneous blood vessels is pathognomonic of HSP.[3]

**What are the laboratory features of cryoglobulinemic vasculitis?**

Cryoglobulins refer to monoclonal or polyclonal immunoglobulins that precipitate on exposure to cold (ie, cryoprecipitates). Clinical manifestations include systemic vasculitis, arthritis, peripheral neuropathy, and glomerulonephritis. Hypocomplementemia is present in most patients with cryoglobulinemic vasculitis (around 90%); C4 is often more profoundly affected than C3. Rheumatoid factor is often positive, and circulating cryoprecipitates can be detected. Anemia and elevated ESR are also common. All patients with cryoglobulinemia should be tested for HCV.[3]

**What are the most common clinical manifestations of Behçet's disease?**

Recurrent painful oral ulcers are often the earliest manifestation of Behçet's disease (ultimately occuring in up to 90% of patients). Genital ulcers also affect most patients and are more specific than oral ulcers. Ocular disease involving the retina and uvea occurs commonly and can lead to blindness. Cutaneous manifestations are also common and include papulopustular rash, acne-like lesions, and erythema nodosum (especially in women). Neurologic, cardiovascular, pulmonary, gastrointestinal, and articular manifestations occur less commonly. Pulmonary artery aneurysm is one of the most dreaded complications of Behçet's disease (occurring in approximatley 1% of cases) and carries a high mortality rate.[10]

**How common is pulmonary involvement in patients with anti–glomerular basement membrane disease?**

In approximately one-half of patients with anti-GBM disease, pulmonary hemorrhage occurs along with glomerulonephritis (ie, Goodpasture's syndrome). In rare cases, there is pulmonary hemorrhage in the absence of glomerulonephritis. Goodpasture's syndrome has a predilection for 2 populations in particular: young men in the third decade of life and women in the seventh and eighth decades of life. Clinical manifestations tend to be more dramatic in the younger population (eg, fever, hemoptysis [particularly among smokers], dyspnea, hematuria). Prognosis is more favorable in patients with pulmonary hemorrhage when compared with older patients who tend to present with renal manifestations only, particularly when there is oliguria.[3,11]

**What is the role of serum complement levels in the diagnosis of patients with urticarial vasculitis?**

UV is ultimately diagnosed in around 10% of patients who present with chronic or recurrent urticarial lesions. An underlying systemic disease is present in the majority of cases. Serum complement levels have prognostic implications in patients with UV. Normal complement levels are more commonly associated with idiopathic UV and portend a more benign course; low complement levels often indicate a potentially serious underlying condition such as SLE, hypocomplementemic urticarial vasculitis syndrome (HUVS), or Sjögren's syndrome.[12]

**What are the secondary causes of non–ANCA-associated small vessel vasculitis?**

Secondary causes of non–ANCA-associated small vessel vasculitis include vasculitis associated with systemic disease and vasculitis associated with probable etiology. Vasculitis associated with systemic disease includes lupus vasculitis, rheumatoid vasculitis, sarcoid vasculitis, relapsing polychondritis vasculitis, and Sjögren's vasculitis. Vasculitis associated with probable etiology includes drug-associated vasculitis, infection-associated vasculitis (eg, subacute bacterial endocarditis, HCV, Epstein-Barr virus, human immunodeficiency virus, histoplasmosis), malignancy-associated vasculitis (eg, lymphoma), and serum sickness–associated vasculitis.[1]

## Case Summary

A previously healthy 67-year-old man with a recent history of subacute sinusitis, nasal congestion, dyspnea, and weight loss presents with acute-onset hemoptysis and is found to have a saddle nose deformity, palpable purpura, and abnormal findings on chest imaging.

***What is the most likely diagnosis in this patient?***

Granulomatosis with polyangiitis.

### BONUS QUESTIONS

***What general features in this case are suggestive of systemic vasculitis?***

The combination of multisystem involvement, including the upper and lower airways, skin, and kidneys, and the presence of constitutional features such as fever and weight loss raises the possibility of systemic vasculitis.

***Which clinical features in this case are consistent with the diagnosis of granulomatosis with polyangiitis?***

Upper airway involvement is present in virtually all patients with GPA, including sinusitis, purulent or bloody nasal discharge, and nasal septal perforation with associated saddle nose deformity (collapse of the nasal bridge, see Figure 50-4). In addition, active GPA is associated with c-ANCA in most patients (approximately 90%).[3]

***What findings are present on imaging of the chest in this case?***

CT imaging of the chest in this case (see Figure 50-1) demonstrates cavitary lesions. These lesions can be found in up to one-half of patients with pulmonary involvement of GPA. Pulmonary nodules, particularly subpleural in location, are even more common.[13]

***What is the typical age of onset of granulomatosis with polyangiitis?***

GPA can occur at any age, but the peak age of onset is between 65 and 75 years.[14]

***What are the 3 distinctive histopathologic features of granulomatosis with polyangiitis?***

The 3 distinctive histopathologic features of GPA are (1) vasculitis of small vessels or small and medium vessels, (2) granulomatous inflammation, and (3) tissue necrosis.[13]

***What is the treatment for active granulomatosis with polyangiitis?***

Active GPA is treated with immunosuppressive medications, with an induction phase followed by maintenance therapy. The choice of agents for either phase depends on severity and extent of disease (limited or generalized). Induction regimens for severe disease usually consist of glucocorticoids in combination with either cyclophosphamide or rituximab. Methotrexate or azathioprine is usually used for maintenance. Limited GPA can be treated with prednisone, methotrexate, or even trimethoprim-sulfamethoxazole.[13]

***What is the prognosis of granulomatosis with polyangiitis?***

Without treatment, generalized GPA is invariably fatal within months of diagnosis. In the era of immunosuppressive therapy, 5-year survival is approximately 75%. Relapse occurs in around one-half of cases.[3,13]

## KEY POINTS

- Vasculitis describes a heterogeneous group of diseases that share the defining feature of blood vessel wall inflammation.
- Vasculitis can involve blood vessels of virtually any type, size, and location in the body and can lead to partial or complete luminal compromise, with ensuing ischemia of the related tissues.
- Systemic vasculitis refers to a group of named primary vasculitides that are immune mediated and individually distinguished by the presence of unique clinicopathologic features.
- The clinical manifestations of systemic vasculitis are protean; it may be confined to a single organ or affect a range of organ systems.
- Systemic vasculitis should be considered when particular physical findings are present or multiple systems are involved.
- Systemic vasculitis can involve the large vessels, medium vessels, or small vessels.
- Individual vasculitides predominantly affect either small, medium, or large vessels, but are capable of affecting vessels of more than 1 size.
- The primary large vessel systemic vasculitides are giant cell arteritis and Takayasu arteritis.
- The primary medium vessel systemic vasculitides are polyarteritis nodosa and Kawasaki disease.
- Small vessel systemic vasculitis can be ANCA-associated or non–ANCA-associated.
- The primary ANCA-associated small vessel systemic vasculitides include granulomatosis with polyangiitis (Wegener's granulomatosis), microscopic polyangiitis, and eosinophilic granulomatosis with polyangiitis (Churg-Strauss syndrome).
- The primary non–ANCA-associated small vessel systemic vasculitides include Henoch-Schönlein purpura, cryoglobulinemia, Behçet's disease, anti-glomerular basement membrane disease, and urticarial vasculitis.
- Systemic vasculitis can be associated with a variety of secondary conditions (eg, systemic disease, infection, drugs).

## REFERENCES


1. Jennette JC, Falk RJ, Bacon PA, et al. 2012 revised International Chapel Hill Consensus Conference Nomenclature of Vasculitides. *Arthritis Rheum*. 2013;65(1):1-11.
2. Jennette JC, Falk RJ, Andrassy K, et al. Nomenclature of systemic vasculitides. Proposal of an international consensus conference. *Arthritis Rheum*. 1994;37(2):187-192.
3. Longo DL, Fauci AS, Kasper DL, Hauser SL, Jameson JL, Loscalzo J, eds. *Harrison's Principles of Internal Medicine*. 18th ed. New York, NY: McGraw-Hill; 2012.
4. Weyand CM, Goronzy JJ. Medium- and large-vessel vasculitis. *N Engl J Med*. 2003;349(2):160-169.
5. Migliori G, Battisti E, Pari M, Vitelli N, Cingolani C. A shifty diagnosis: Cogan's syndrome. A case report and review of the literature. *Acta Otorhinolaryngol Ital*. 2009;29(2):108-113.
6. De Virgilio A, Greco A, Magliulo G, et al. Polyarteritis nodosa: a contemporary overview. *Autoimmun Rev*. 2016;15(6):564-570.
7. Fraison JB, Seve P, Dauphin C, et al. Kawasaki disease in adults: observations in France and literature review. *Autoimmun Rev*. 2016;15(3):242-249.
8. Chung SA, Seo P. Microscopic polyangiitis. *Rheum Dis Clin North Am*. 2010;36(3):545-558.
9. Vaglio A, Buzio C, Zwerina J. Eosinophilic granulomatosis with polyangiitis (Churg-Strauss): state of the art. *Allergy*. 2013;68(3):261-273.
10. Zeidan MJ, Saadoun D, Garrido M, Klatzmann D, Six A, Cacoub P. Behcet's disease physiopathology: a contemporary review. *Auto Immun Highlights*. 2016;7(1):4.
11. Troxell ML, Houghton DC. Atypical anti-glomerular basement membrane disease. *Clin Kidney J*. 2016;9(2):211-221.
12. Wisnieski JJ. Urticarial vasculitis. *Curr Opin Rheumatol*. 2000;12(1):24-31.
13. Almouhawis HA, Leao JC, Fedele S, Porter SR. Wegener's granulomatosis: a review of clinical features and an update in diagnosis and treatment. *J Oral Pathol Med*. 2013;42(7):507-516.
14. Kubaisi B, Abu Samra K, Foster CS. Granulomatosis with polyangiitis (Wegener's disease): an updated review of ocular disease manifestations. *Intractable Rare Dis Res*. 2016;5(2):61-69.

# Educator's Appendix

## A BRIEF HISTORY OF MEDICAL EDUCATION AND INTRODUCTION TO THE CHALK TALK

The practice of medicine has evolved over thousands of years. It began in ancient Egypt with Imhotep, the world's first recognized physician. In the 5th century BC, medicine made epochal strides in the Hippocratic School. The fall of Rome gave way to the Golden Age of Islam, where groundbreaking innovations were felt across the Arab Empire, from Baghdad to Damascus to Córdoba, and beyond. Medicine blossomed in the Renaissance, making Europe the center of medical advance until the 20th century AD when it migrated to America, where, among other places, it has flourished. Evolution of this kind requires "high-fidelity" transference of current knowledge from one generation to the next. Physicians have viewed teaching as a duty since the 5th century BC. Hence the term "doctor," which derives from the Latin "docere," meaning "to teach."[1-5]

The methods of medical education have undergone complex and important changes over centuries. At the present time, 2 pillars support the curricular structure of most American medical schools: basic science and clinical medicine. The Age of Enlightenment led to the experimental method and the birth of the basic sciences. The impact of scientific discovery on the practice of clinical medicine began to burgeon. For example, in the mid-to-late 18th century, important respiratory gases were discovered in the laboratory: carbon dioxide was identified by Joseph Black, nitrogen by Daniel Rutherford, and oxygen by Carl Wilhelm Scheele and Joseph Priestley. These scientific breakthroughs were integrated by Antoine-Laurent Lavoisier, leading to the discovery of the nature of respiration. To this day, clinical decision-making is influenced by the measurement of these gases in arterial blood.[3-5]

The synergetic relationship between basic science and clinical medicine can be illustrated in a more recent example. In 1960, Nowell and Hungerford discovered the chromosomal abnormality underlying the terminal illness chronic myelogenous leukemia (CML). An aberrant reciprocal translocation between the long arms of chromosomes 9 and 22 (Philadelphia chromosome) produces a persistently activated protein tyrosine kinase that functions in the control of cellular replication. This leads to uninhibited replication of white blood cells, manifesting in the disease known as CML. In the 1990s, scientists envisioned a molecule capable of specifically targeting the abnormal protein tyrosine kinase responsible for uninhibited cellular replication, thereby shutting this process down. Following years of research in the laboratory, this vision was realized in 2001 when imatinib, a tyrosine kinase inhibitor, was approved for clinical use. This new approach to cancer therapy diverges from conventional chemotherapeutic agents that produce numerous side effects related to indiscriminant toxic effects on healthy cells in the body. The mechanism by which imatinib targets cancer cells is a paradigm for future therapies. The application of basic sciences to the practice of clinical medicine will continue to grow.[6-8]

Despite the powerful connection between basic science and clinical medicine, the integration of these 2 pillars into medical school curricula has been a contentious process. A chasm existed even in ancient Mesopotamian civilization, where the medical traditions of Sumer were divided into "scientific" and "practical" schools. In ancient Greece, there was disagreement about the most worthy candidates to learn the discipline of medicine. Plato and others advocated that those with interests in philosophy and science rather than those with practical experience were more suitable to become physicians. This debate continued centuries later during the latter part of the Middle Ages when medical education became more formalized with the establishment and rise of the universities, including the Schola Medica Salernitana, regarded as the world's first modern medical school. These institutions paved the way for the medical programs established in Europe during the 18th century. However, depending on location, the methods of these programs differed in important ways. Early medical education in Germany, for example, focused mostly on the basic sciences. The French and British, on the other hand, pioneered the concept of hospital schools, which focused education around clinical teaching. French medical students were advised to "read little, see much, do much."[1,3,5]

It was not until the 19th century in Germany that the relationship between basic science and clinical medicine was formally developed. This occurred after Wilhelm von Humboldt redesigned the medical education system in Germany. One important step in the process was the integration of scientific laboratories into both the preclinical and clinical years of medical training. This established correspondence between the two. Under Humboldt's leadership, medical schools remained part of the university. This system rose to preeminence and served as the model for many early American medical institutions, most notably Johns Hopkins University. Although Thomas Bond had planted the seeds of clinical instruction in America during the 18th century at Pennsylvania Hospital, it was Johns Hopkins that formally integrated clinical teaching into American medical education. Under the direction of William Osler, students were brought into the hospital to learn directly from the care of patients. The formal education of medical students became in large part the responsibility of clinicians.[3,9]

Since first modeled in the United States by Johns Hopkins, an equal emphasis on basic science and clinical acumen has been central to American medical education. Since the early 20th century, the curriculum of most American medical schools has been divided into 2 halves. The first 2 years consist of lecture-based courses and laboratory experience designed to instruct students in the basic sciences. The instructors of these courses typically hold a Doctor of Philosophy (PhD) and are trained and involved in basic science research. This is followed by 2 years of clinical-based training, mostly occurring in the hospital and the outpatient clinics. Most clinical instructors hold a Doctor of Medicine (MD). Despite sharing responsibility for nearly all of medical education, these groups of instructors usually do not receive any formal training in the art of teaching.[3,10]

Carl Ludwig, a German physician, professor of anatomy and physiology, and renowned teacher, once wrote in a letter to a former pupil, "Destiny has conferred on us professors the favor of helping the responsive heart of youth to find the right path. In the seemingly insignificant vocation of the schoolmaster there is enclosed a high, blessed calling; I know no higher."[11]

In the early years of formal clinical medical education, students learned by directly observing and working alongside attending physicians. Ludwig was lauded as a gifted clinical teacher who interacted directly with students. Osler spent hours with students at the bedside. This focus on learners was a hallmark of American medical education in the early 20th century. The substantial growth of academic medical centers across the United States, beginning in the latter half of the 20th century, generated a shift in focus from teaching to productivity, which has had a significant erosive effect on the education of medical students. The growing chasm between attending physicians and medical students has shifted the responsibility of clinical teaching to resident physicians.[3,10,12-14]

Coincident with the growing preoccupation of clinicians with nonteaching responsibilities, academic medical centers began to rely on team-based systems to educate medical students in the clinical environment. The internal medicine clerkship is the quintessential model of this relationship. Inpatient ward teams are comprised of learners with various levels of training, including residents, interns, third-year medical students, and physician assistant students. Medical students are introduced into this new environment with little prior experience. Having been removed from the classroom where the basic sciences were studied during the first 2 years, these students are now expected to learn clinical medicine in new ways. Observation and experience become the primary vehicles of education. As leaders of the team, resident physicians must guide these learners through the clerkship. Residents must be able to discuss and illustrate the clinical problems that learners observe in patients. Residents must teach.[12-14]

Within the discipline of internal medicine, there are myriad approaches to clinical teaching. The communication of ideas through illustration is deeply rooted in human history. One of the first recorded uses of this technique related to medicine dates back to the Paleolithic period, where a cave painting in Spain depicted the outline of a mammoth with a dark spot in the center, thought to represent the beast's heart (Figure A-1). There was almost certainly an audience intended to benefit from this anatomic drawing. In 1801, a teacher in Scotland used a large piece of slate to illustrate concepts to a group of students. On the medical ward, this technique is known as a "chalk talk."[3,15-17]

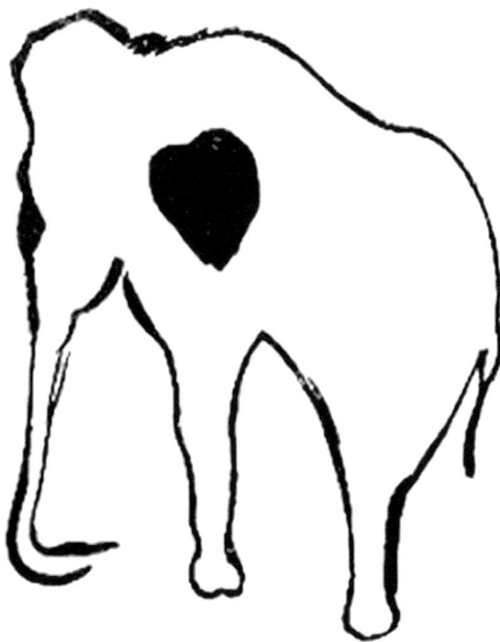

**Figure A-1.** A cave painting from the Paleolithic period (circa 15000 BC) depicting the heart of a mammoth, thought to be the first anatomic drawing.

Modern approaches to teaching include the use of computer programs to project prearranged lecture material. This technique is most suitable for the classroom-based lectures of the preclinical years of medical training. The dynamic nature of the medical ward demands a more flexible teaching modality. For internal medicine residents who must teach at a moment's notice, often during a rare period of downtime, the ability to pick up a writing instrument and begin teaching within a matter of seconds is essential.[16]

A chalk talk can be described as the use of a writing instrument on a canvas in real time to facilitate discussion between a leader and an audience. In medicine, chalk talks have particular qualities. Most commonly, the writing instrument is a dry-erase marker and the canvas is a whiteboard. The leaders are attending physicians or residents, and the audience usually consists of medical students, physician assistant students, and interns, in various combinations. Typical venues include physician workrooms, conference rooms, and anywhere else on the medical ward where a whiteboard may be found. The ability to deliver an informative and effective chalk talk is an acquired skill that requires understanding, preparation, and repetition.[16]

## REFERENCES


1. Magner LN. *A History of Medicine*. 2nd ed. Boca Raton, FL: Taylor & Francis Group; 2005.
2. Osler W. *The Evolution of Modern Medicine: A Series of Lectures Delivered at Yale University on the Stillman Foundation in April 1913*. New Haven, CT: Yale University Press; 1921.
3. Smith JJ, Shaker LS. *Looking Back Looking Ahead: A History of American Medical Education*. Chicago, IL: Adams Press; 2003.
4. Major RH. *A History of Medicine*. Springfield, IL: Charles C. Thomas; 1954.
5. Porter R. *The Greatest Benefit to Mankind: A Medical History of Humanity from Antiquity to the Present*. New York, NY: W. W. Norton & Company; 1999.
6. Druker BJ, Tamura S, Buchdunger E, et al. Effects of a selective inhibitor of the Abl tyrosine kinase on the growth of Bcr-Abl positive cells. *Nat Med*. 1996;2(5):561-566.
7. Iqbal N, Iqbal N. Imatinib: a breakthrough of targeted therapy in cancer. *Chemother Res Pract*. 2014;2014:357027.
8. Nowell PC, Hungerford DA. A minute chromosome in human chronic granulocytic leukemia. *Science*. 1960;132:1497.
9. Flexner A. Medical education in the United States and Canada. From the Carnegie Foundation for the Advancement of Teaching, Bulletin Number Four, 1910. *Bull World Health Organ*. 2002;80(7):594-602.
10. Ludmerer KM. Time and medical education. *Ann Intern Med*. 2000;132(1):25-28.
11. Lombard WP. The life and work of Carl Ludwig. *Science*. 1916;44(1133):363-375.
12. Chokshi BD, et al. A "Resident-as-Teacher" curriculum using a flipped classroom approach: can a model designed for efficiency also be effective? *Acad Med*. 2017;92(4):511-514.
13. Hill AG, et al. A systematic review of resident-as-teacher programmes. *Med Educ*. 2009;43(12):1129-1140.
14. Jafri W, et al. Improving the teaching skills of residents as tutors/facilitators and addressing the shortage of faculty facilitators for PBL modules. *BMC Med Educ*. 2007;7:34.
15. Hajar R. Medical illustration: art in medical education. *Heart Views*. 2011;12(2):83-91.
16. Muttappallymyalil J. et al. Evolution of technology in teaching: blackboard and beyond in medical education. *Nepal J Epidemiol*. 2016;6(3):588-592.
17. Orlander JD. Twelve tips for use of a white board in clinical teaching: reviving the chalk talk. *Med Teach*. 2007;29(2-3):89-92.

# THE SEVEN TENETS OF THE CHALK TALK

## TIMELINESS

Time is volatile on the inpatient medical ward; it must be maximized when possible. However, a talk must be of reasonable length. For the average audience, attention reaches a nadir after around 20 minutes (Figure A-2). Therefore, the maximum length of a talk should not stretch far beyond this limit. If we give medical learners more credit than the average audience, 30 minutes is a reasonable constraint. If time and energy for teaching remain after 30 minutes, it may be helpful to move on to a new topic that can recapture the full attention of the audience. Certain factors can prolong a talk beyond the optimal timeframe. It will be necessary to redirect the discussion at times, as questions from the audience, while encouraged, can occasionally derail the process. Strong leadership is necessary to ensure a timely talk.[1,2]

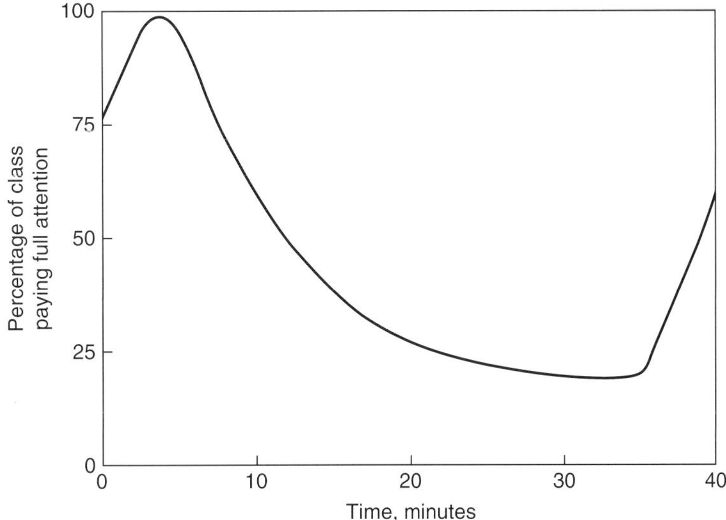


**Figure A-2.** Average audience attention as a function of time. (From Mills HR. *Techniques of Technical Training.* 3rd ed. London: Macmillan; 1977.)

## RELEVANCE

Unlike the predictable lecture-based curriculum of the preclinical years of medical school, the dynamic nature of the clerkship creates variable experiences. Some of the factors that define a learner's experience on the medical ward are not governable. For example, learning principally derives from the observation and study of diseases affecting the patients on the ward. However, over the period of a given clerkship, the breadth and severity of illness can be highly variable. This gives rise to heterogeneity as students are dispersed into different milieus. However, certain medical problems are pervasive. Examples include acute kidney injury, anemia, hypoxemia, pneumonia, heart failure, and delirium. It is most helpful to learners when talks are focused on these and other common problems.

It may be tempting to discuss with the team matters of personal interest. For example, a resident involved in research comparing plastic and metal biliary stents in patients with cholangiocarcinoma may wish to give a talk on this subject. Although important, it focuses on a small subset of patients suffering from an uncommon disease and is unlikely to strike a chord with learners on the medicine clerkship. On the other hand, a discussion of anemia, for example, which affects up to one-third of the world's population, is immediately applicable to the clerkship. It is particularly effective when a chalk talk is focused on active problems in patients cared for by the team. Students will be energized by the proximity of patients with the condition.[3]

## PARTICIPATION

*Tell me, and I will forget. Show me, and I may remember. Involve me, and I will understand.*

—Confucius, circa 450 BC[4]

It is important for the audience of a chalk talk to be involved in the discussion. The Socratic method should be used to engage learners and increase participation. Retention improves when audience members are actively engaged. For example, in a talk on arthritis, when the framework divides into inflammatory and noninflammatory categories, the audience should have the opportunity to identify the characteristics of inflammatory arthritis.

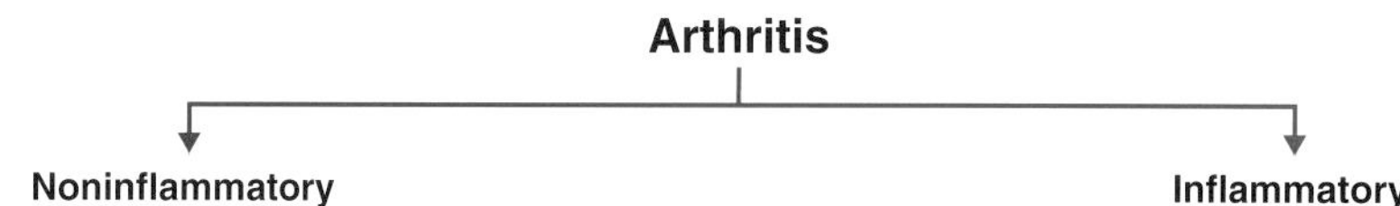


Rather than announce what the features of inflammation are, the leader should ask the audience, "How do you establish whether there is an inflammatory process?" If the audience is stuck, the skilled leader will supply hints until the correct answers are identified. For example, the original question might be followed with another, "Are there physical findings indicative of inflammation?" At this point, someone in the audience might use this hint and offer answers such as "erythema" or "edema," which are, of course, both correct. Using this strategy, the leader can go on to extract the bulk of the discussion from the audience.[2]

## VERBALIZATION

The majority of information discussed during a chalk talk should be spoken, not written. The canvas is simply an aid to highlight key points. If the leader transcribes all that is discussed during a talk, 2 things will occur. First, the volume of information must be unfavorably condensed to compensate for the time consumed by the slow process of writing. Second, the leader will spend too much time facing the whiteboard, leading to a loss of audience engagement.

The leader must verbally expand on components of the framework as it unfolds. As an example, recall the framework for arthritis, which divides into inflammatory and noninflammatory categories. During the talk, the skilled leader does more than simply write these categories on the board; the verbal discussion about the features of inflammatory arthritis must be richer than what is illustrated.

## RELIABILITY

There are many questions in the field of medicine that have yet to be answered. At academic medical centers all over the world, there is ongoing research exploring the frontier, making discoveries that pave the way for new and sometimes confusing questions. The edge of discovery gives rise to debate, of which there is no shortage in medicine. When the evidence is not clear, physicians rely on the opinions of experts. For example, what is the role of prostate specific antigen (PSA) screening in the primary care clinic? When considering the diagnosis of endocarditis, is it more cost-effective to obtain a transesophageal echocardiogram (TEE) before obtaining a transthoracic echocardiogram (TTE) in some patients? Discussing these questions is healthy and challenges learners to explore the information that supports different theories. However, for the purposes of a chalk talk, it is best to focus on "hard" findings in medicine that are widely accepted. For example, it has long been established that iron-deficiency anemia is associated with decreased mean corpuscular volume (MCV) of red blood cells; this is not debatable or controversial. Based on MCV, a construct can be designed to approach anemia. Foundations of medical knowledge should be built using these reliable principles.[5]

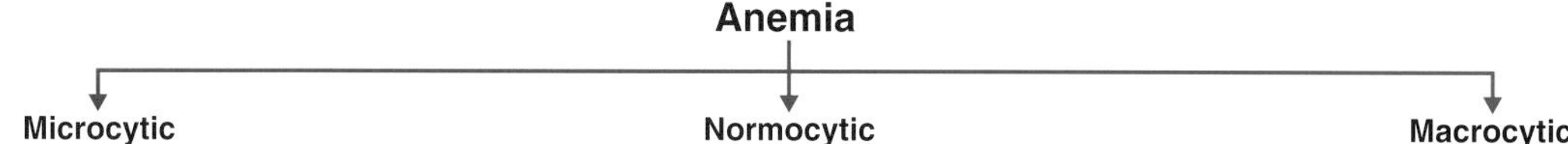


## ADAPTABILITY

Internal medicine chalk talks are usually given to diverse audiences that may include students, interns, residents, nurses, and faculty. The talk should be pitched at the appropriate level. Certain aspects of clinical problems are best discussed with learners at a particular level of training. For example, in a discussion of heart failure with third-year medical students, time spent identifying the physical findings of heart failure will be worthwhile. Advanced internal medicine residents may instead want to focus on more complex concepts, such as inotropic support or ventricular assist devices. The same framework for heart failure can be used to facilitate entirely different discussions, depending on the audience. When the group is mixed, as it often is, the leader should try to reach all learners by directing questions appropriately. This adaptability ensures that all audience members benefit from the talk.

## COMPLETENESS

A chalk talk must be timely, but it must also be complete. The talk should have a beginning and an end. With the large space of a clean whiteboard available, it is easy to become distracted by various ideas that arise during a talk, taking the discussion into directions that may only be narrowly related to the topic at hand. The disciplined leader will allow some flexibility but will quickly recover direction, to ensure that completeness is not sacrificed. To remain organized, a leader must be primed with an outline before the talk begins. This will ensure that, despite how extensive or tangential the discussion may be, the core components of the talk are addressed and a complete picture is provided.

The frameworks found in this text have been assembled to provide complete overviews of each topic. Certain elements of the talk may be expanded on if desired. Whether these liberties are taken or not, respecting the framework for the talk should ensure that the audience is left with a complete outline of the topic.

## REFERENCES

1. Mills HR. *Techniques of Technical Training.* 3rd ed. London: Macmillan; 1977.
2. Prince M. Does active learning work? A review of the research. *J Eng Educ.* 2004;93(3):223-231.
3. Sankaran VG, Weiss MJ. Anemia: progress in molecular mechanisms and therapies. *Nat Med.* 2015;21(3):221-230.
4. Ende J, ed. *Theory and practice of teaching medicine*. Philadelphia, PA: American College of Physicians; 2010.
5. Guyatt GH, Oxman AD, Ali M, Willan A, McIlroy W, Patterson C. Laboratory diagnosis of iron-deficiency anemia: an overview. *J Gen Intern Med*. 1992;7(2):145-153.

# CHALK TALKS AND THE FRAMEWORK SYSTEM

Modern technology-based lectures are guided by prearranged material, usually in the form of slides on a computer screen. For the presenter, it is not difficult to discuss a topic for any length of time because there are prompts to reinforce order and cue certain discussion points. Without that aid, lecturing becomes more challenging, even if only for 5 to 10 minutes. Indeed, some readers may have questioned whether discussing a topic for 30 minutes on a whiteboard without significant preparation is a realistic proposition. The framework system makes it possible. The presenter need only recollect the framework itself. The majority of the discussion, although guided by the framework, originates from the presenter's own fund of knowledge. As entities appear within the framework during a talk, the presenter will draw on this knowledge base to illuminate various teaching points. Importantly, these discussion items are not scripted and are subject to the discretion of the presenter. The discourse resulting from any given talk is dynamic, bound only by the outline of the framework. The latitude afforded by the framework system is uniquely suited to whiteboard teaching.

At the end of a successful chalk talk, the whiteboard will contain various remnants of the discussion. At the very least, the associated framework should be intact and clearly displayed. If nothing else, this provides the audience with an approach to a clinical problem. This alone is valuable for students. However, it is important to understand that a chalk talk is more than a simple illustration on a whiteboard. The teaching points found between the lines of the framework should generate most of the discussion. It is the responsibility of the leader to illuminate these teaching points. Using hints and questions, the leader should allow the audience members to identify as much of the content within a framework as possible. Going further, whenever a new concept is introduced on the board, the presenter should discuss it at the desired level of expertise. For example, during a talk on dyspnea, when the audience identifies cardiomyopathy as an etiology, the leader can then review that condition more closely.

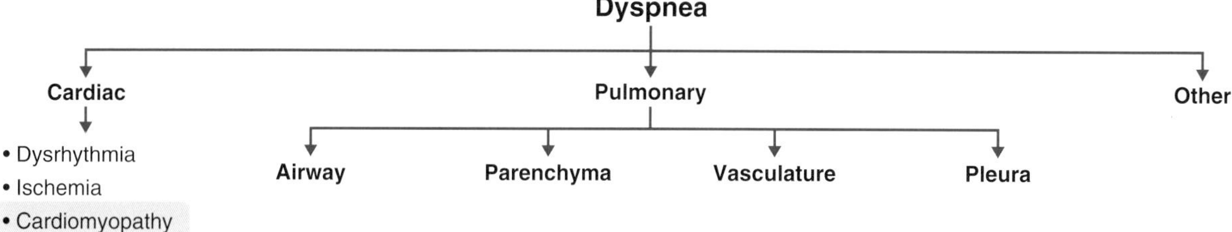


"What are the most common causes of cardiomyopathy in America?" "What physical findings are associated with heart failure?" When these questions are asked, the leader is facing and engaging the audience rather than simply writing on the whiteboard. Parts of the framework are used to launch segments of the talk that are entirely verbal. These questions are not etched in the framework; rather they are generated from the presenter's knowledge base. In this way, the tenet of *verbalization* is realized.

The number of teaching points that can be found within a single framework is astonishing. The leader is limited only by time and erudition and must select high-yield points to emphasize. The leader should direct questions to appropriate audience members. For example, consider the framework for hypotonic hyponatremia, which is largely based on volume status.

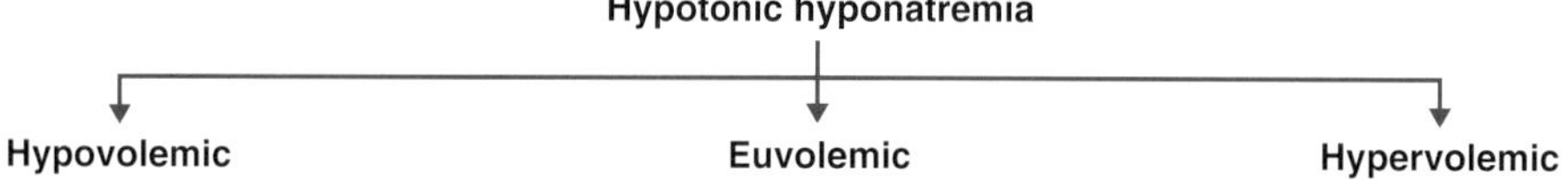


At this point in the talk, the medical students in the audience might be asked to identify the physical findings associated with hypovolemia and hypervolemia. While later in the talk, the residents might be asked to identify the laboratory studies that help differentiate primary polydipsia from the syndrome of inappropriate antidiuretic hormone, a more challenging inquiry. Here, the tenet of *adaptability* is exercised. When the audience initially struggles to identify the correct answer, the leader must provide guidance. Hints can be offered until the audience has enough information to achieve success. Not only does this interplay provide positive reinforcement for the audience, but it also ensures that there is active *participation*, which benefits learning and retention.[1]

When an entity arises within a framework and the presenter decides to discuss it in more detail, there are many options on which to focus. For most entities, it works well to generate questions from several fixed domains, including epidemiology, history of presentation, physical examination, laboratory tests, imaging, and other studies (eg, electrocardiography, echocardiography). Consider the diagnosis of gout, for example. When this entity arises within the arthritis framework, there are many potential high-yield teaching points to discuss with the audience.

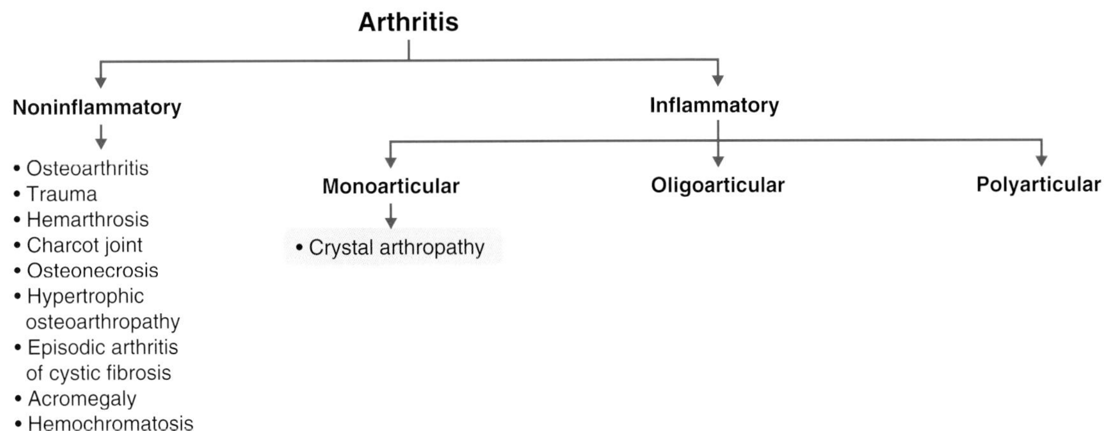


The leader can test the audience on the typical presentation of gout, pulling from each of the aforementioned domains. Specifically, the audience can be asked to describe the prototypical patient in terms of epidemiologic risk factors; the common historical narrative expressed by patients with an acute gout flare; the physical findings of acute and chronic gout; the relevant laboratory or radiographic findings of gout; and, finally, the unique tests associated with gout, such as the characteristics of synovial fluid during an acute flare. Whenever a new entity is introduced, following this simple order to generate questions for discussion is an effective way to raise key teaching points naturally while maintaining the fluidity of the talk. The quantity and quality of questions should be adapted to the time available, the goals of the presenter, the types of patients being cared for, and the degree of training of the audience members.

A framework is a critical component of a successful chalk talk. Without the outline of a talk in mind, discussing a topic on an empty whiteboard is a futile endeavor. Even if a presentation were memorized, its *adaptability* to an individual audience is lost. This is particularly true when facing a mixed audience, a common occurrence in medicine. Moreover, the amount of preparation required to deliver a scripted 30-minute talk puts a limit on the spontaneity with which it can occur and essentially requires the availability of preplanned didactic time. In reality, on the medical ward, residents and attending physicians are virtually never provided such luxury. Instead, teaching didactics must be cut, shaped, and carved to fit the available time. On the other hand, it is relatively easy to memorize or simply become familiar with a framework moments before delivering a talk, which serves as the catalyst for a discussion that develops mostly from the presenter's own knowledge base.

## USING THE CHAPTERS

A framework is effective when used as an outline for a chalk talk. Yet, alone, it is not enough for a successful presentation. The leader must improvise and create content between the lines of the framework. The final presentation depends on factors related to the presenter, the audience, the patients being cared for, and the amount of time available. For example, if the audience consists of new learners, then the questions and content explored by the facilitator should be basic. If the amount of time available for the talk is limited, then the facilitator must tailor the extent of discussion. In this way, chalk talks are customizable.

Each chapter in this book is a prototype of a talk on a particular clinical problem. Included in each are suggested high-yield, evidence-based concepts to discuss with an audience assumed to be students and interns. Ultimately, the leader can choose to use or disregard these suggestions. The leader may ask original questions to emphasize teaching points thought to be more suitable. The leader may choose to focus on entities within a framework that are *relevant* to the patients under the team's care. For example, if a patient on the team presents with dyspnea and is ultimately diagnosed with pulmonary hypertension, the leader may choose to spend more time discussing that particular entity when it arises within the dyspnea framework. The breadth and depth of these peripheral discussions are ultimately influenced by a number of factors, including the time available for teaching. There is a delicate balance to be achieved. On the one hand, when time is short, the leader must be mindful of the limitations the clock has set on the discussion. On the other, when time is plentiful, there must be consideration of the tenet of *timeliness*, or there is a risk of losing the attention of the audience.

The formula for the chapters is simple. Each begins with the top of the framework, which is then built over the course of the chapter using hints and questions. This is the general way in which a chalk talk should flow. From the moment the topic is introduced on the whiteboard, there must be dialogue between the presenter and audience. Opportunities to identify the next part of the framework, whether a diagnostic study, a differential diagnosis, or otherwise, should be given to the audience. To this end, the chapters offer suggested hints and questions to ask of the audience along the way. When a concept is introduced, there is opportunity for deeper discussion. This interaction between presenter and audience drives the discussion forward.

Nascent educators may find it helpful to follow the chapters more explicitly. With repetition, educators will begin to discover and use the questions and hints that bring out the best in audiences. After experience is gained, most will become so familiar with the formula that they will begin to generate original discussion points to supplement those that are tried and true. With enough experience, original frameworks may be built for other clinical problems within internal medicine or other disciplines.

For the first 20 scholastic years, physicians are primarily students. For all physicians this role continues throughout life. Upon the academic clinician, the additional responsibility of teaching is bestowed. This transition begins during residency training. It is there that the skills of teaching are learned, practiced, and sharpened. Many tools are available to the educator, but few are as important for the internal medicine resident as the chalk talk. As burgeoning teachers, residents must begin to "provide the favor of helping the responsive heart of youth to find the right path."[2]

In academic medicine, there is no higher calling.

## REFERENCES


1. Prince M. Does active learning work? A review of the research. *J Eng Educ*. 2004;93(3):223-231.
2. Lombard WP. The life and work of Carl Ludwig. *Science*. 1916;44(1133):363-375.

# INDEX

Note: Page numbers followed by "f" indicate figures and "t" indicate tables.


**A**

A-a gradient, 615, 615f
  elevated
    mechanisms of, 619
    ventilation-perfusion (V/Q) ratio, 620, 620f
  normal, reduced $PIO_2$
    causes of, 616
    high altitude, 617, 617f
    polluted air inhalation, 616
    suffocation, 616–617
Aanatomic shunt, hypoxemia, 627–628, 627f
Acetylcholinesterase inhibitor, 192
Acid-base disorders
  acidemia, 416
  alkalemia, 416
  arterial pH, 415
  carbonic anhydrase, 414
  diagnosis, 415
  extracellular buffer, 414
  Henderson-Hasselbalch equation, 414
  homeostasis, 417
  metabolic acidosis
    anion gap, 417, 420–422
    development of, 418, 418f
    lung function, 418
    non-anion gap, 418–420, 420f
  metabolic alkalosis, 426–428
  minute ventilation, 417
  persistent respiratory disorder, 417
  with polyuria, 414
  primary acid-base disorder, 416, 416f
  respiratory acidosis, 422–424, 422f
  respiratory alkalosis, 424–426
  serum concentration, 416
  types, 414
  volatile and nonvolatile acid elimination, 415, 415f
Acidemia, 101, 416
"Acid-loving" cells infiltration, 48
Acquired hemolytic anemia, 327
  immunologic, 333–335, 334f
  infectious, 337–339, 339f
  mechanisms, 332
  toxic, 335–336
  traumatic, 336–337
Acromegaly, 43, 107, 662
  cause of, 108
  clinical characteristics, 663
  high-output physiologic state, 44
Acute biliary obstruction, 219–220
Acute bronchitis, 607
  dyspnea, 253–254
Acute chest syndrome, 22
  chest imaging, 22
Acute coronary syndrome (ACS)
  acute myocardial infarction *vs.* myocardial ischemia, 16
  causes of
    coronary artery dissection, 18–19
    coronary artery embolism, 18–19
    coronary artery vasospasm, 18–19
    premature coronary artery disease, 19
    risk factors, 18
    stent thrombosis, 18–19
    unrelated to, 19–21, 20f
    unstable atherosclerotic plaque rupture, 18, 18f
  characteristic symptoms, 16
  clinical syndromes, 16
  contiguous ECG leads, 17
  diagnosis, 16
  ischemia, electrocardiographic features, 17
  non–ST-elevation myocardial infarction (NSTEMI), 16
    electrocardiographic findings, 17, 17f
    myocardial injury, 17
  ST-elevation myocardial infarction (STEMI), 16
    electrocardiographic manifestation of, 16–17, 17f
  unstable angina (UA), 16
    electrocardiographic findings, 17, 17f
    myocardial injury, 17
Acute hypersensitivity pneumonitis, 637
Acute interstitial nephritis (AIN), 439–441, 440f
Acute interstitial pneumonia (AIP), 634–635
Acute kidney injury (AKI)
  biochemical laboratory definition, 431
  blood urea nitrogen levels, 430
  with blue toes, 430, 430f
  causes of, 431
  classification, 432
  definition, 430
  history of, 431
  intrarenal
    acute interstitial nephritis (AIN), 439–441, 440f
    acute tubular necrosis (ATN), 437–439, 438f
    classification, 435
    cross-section of, 435, 435f
    vascular, 436–437
  physical findings, 431
  postrenal, 441–442
  prerenal, 432–434, 433f
  renal replacement therapy, 431
  risk factors, 431
  sequelae of, 431
  serum creatinine concentration, 431
  structures, 432
  symptoms of, 431
Acute (fulminant) liver failure, 151, 153
Acute mesenteric ischemia
  biochemical laboratory abnormalities, 225
  causes of, 225
  computed tomography (CT) imaging, 225
  diagnosis, 225
  mechanisms, 225
  nonocclusive, 227
  occlusive
    arterial embolism, 226
    arterial thrombosis, 226
    venous thrombosis, 226–227
  physical findings, 224
  prognosis of, 225
  symptoms of, 224
Acute myocardial infarction, definition, 16
Acute pancreatitis, 23, 120, 167, 653, 655
  characteristics of, 121
  diagnosis of, 24
Acute pericarditis, 19
  electrocardiographic findings, 20
Acute pulmonary arterial hypertension, 605
Acute respiratory distress syndrome (ARDS), 624
Acute rheumatic fever, 668, 670
Acute septic arthritis, 663
Acute tubular necrosis (ATN), 437–439, 438f
Adenoviruses, 57
  gastroenteritis, 179
Adrenal cortical tissue, 81
Adrenal hyperplasia, 97
  types of, 98
Adrenal insufficiency, 107
  with acute abdominal pain, 78, 78f
  adrenocorticotropic hormone (ACTH) stimulation, 80
    causes of, 81
    cortisol deficiency, 80

Adrenal insufficiency *(continued)*
false-negative result, 80
primary *vs.* central, 80
results of, 80
androgens, 79
catecholamines, 79
central
central process, 87
glucocorticoids, 88
hypothalamic dysfunction, 87
hypothalamus recovery, 88
mechanism of, 87
mineralocorticoid deficiency, 87
pituitary gland dysfunction, 87
characteristics of, 108
clinical condition, 80
clinical manifestations
acute, 80
chronic, 79
corticotropin-releasing hormone (CRH) stimulants, 79
definition, 79
glucocorticoids, 79
hypothalamic-pituitary-adrenal axis, 79, 79f
incidence of, 79
mineralocorticoids, 79
primary
adrenal cortical tissue, 81
adrenoleukodystrophy (ALD), 86–87
autoimmune causes, 81–82
bilateral adrenalectomy, 86–87
causes of, 81
external beam radiation, 87
hemorrhagic causes, 83–85
infectious causes, 82–83
infiltrative causes, 85–86
mechanism of, 81
medication, 86–87
mineralocorticoid deficiency, 81
radiotherapy, 86
serum cortisol levels, 79
Adrenal tumor, 97
characteristics of, 98
Adrenocortical hormones, 79
Adrenocorticotropic hormone (ACTH)
-dependent Cushing's syndrome, 94–97
diagnosis, 94
ectopic production, 95–97
eutopic production, 94–95
hypercortisolism, 94
prevalence of, 94
-independent Cushing's syndrome, 97–98
stimulation, 80
causes of, 81
cortisol deficiency, 80
false-negative result, 80
primary *vs.* central, 80
results of, 80
Adrenoleukodystrophy (ALD), 86–87
Adrenomyeloneuropathy (AMN), 87
Adult-onset Still's disease (AOSD), 668, 670
fever of unknown origin (FUO), 267
Afterload, 46
Aging, sinus bradycardia, 8
Agoraphobia, 25
Airways
constriction, 623–624
dyspnea
acute bronchitis, 253–254
anaphylaxis, 254
asthma, 253–254
bronchiectasis, 253–254, 253f
chronic obstructive pulmonary disease, 253–254
foreign body aspiration, 254–255
tracheomalacia, 254–255
hemoptysis
acute bronchitis, 607
bronchiectasis, 607
bronchovascular fistula, 607–608
causes of, 606
foreign body aspiration, 607–608
iatrogenic, 607–608
malignancy, 607
Alcohol consumption, 41
cardiomyopathy development, 42
chronic, 95, 122
Alcoholic hepatitis, 271–272
Alkalemia, 101, 121, 416
mechanism of, 122
Alloimmune hemolytic anemia, 333–334
Altered mental status, 236
Alveolar gas equation, 614
carbon dioxide, partial pressure of, 615
Aminotransferases, 212
abnormal level, 213
elevation, 213
severity of, 213
Amphetamines, 41
Amyloidosis, 48, 85, 115, 132–133, 193–194
characteristics of, 116
with renal involvement, 86
Anal fissure, 206
Anaphylaxis, dyspnea, 254
Androgens, 79
Anemia
conditions, 313
definition, 311
dyspnea, 258–259
macrocytic anemia
megaloblastic. *See* Megaloblastic anemia
nonmegaloblastic, 321–323, 322f
mean corpuscular volume (MCV), 313–314, 314f
microcytic anemia
iron deficiency, 314–315
lead poisoning, 314, 316
sideroblastic anemia, 314, 316
thalassemia, 314–315, 315f
normal hemoglobin concentration, 311
normocytic anemia
bone marrow, 316
hyperproliferative, 318–319
hypoproliferative, 316–318
reticulocytes, 316
physical findings, 313
physiologic adaptations, 313
with pleuritic chest pain, 310, 310f
prevalence, 313
red blood cell indices, 313
red blood cell production, 312, 312f
red blood cell, role of, 311
severity of, 311
symptoms of, 313
tissue oxygenation, 311
Angiodysplasia, 205, 206–207
Angiotensin-converting enzyme (ACE) inhibitors
coarctation, 46
hypertension, 46
reduced left ventricular systolic function, 39–40
Angiotensin II receptor blockers (ARBs)
coarctation, 46
hypertension, 46
reduced left ventricular systolic function, 39–40
Angiotensin receptor-neprilysin inhibitor (ARNi), 39–40
Ankylosing spondylitis, 667
Anorexia nervosa, 7
symptoms and signs, 142
Anthracycline chemotherapeutic agents, 41
treatment with, 42
Antiarrhythmic agents, 8
Anti–glomerular basement membrane (anti-GBM) disease, 680–681
Antineutrophil cytoplasmic antibodies (ANCA)
glomerulonephritis
ANCA-positive patients, 451
c-ANCA, 452–453
characteristic findings, 452
p-ANCA, 453–454
small vessel systemic vasculitis
eosinophilic granulomatosis with polyangiitis (EGPA), 678–679
granulomatosis with polyangiitis, 678–679, 679f
microscopic polyangiitis, 678–679
secondary causes of, 679
Antiretroviral therapy (ART), 43
Antisynthetase syndrome, 670
α-1 Antitrypsin deficiency, 218–219
Anxiety (panic disorder), 25
treatment for, 25
Aorta coarctation, 46
Aortic dissection, 19, 62, 62f
mechanism of, 63
risk factors, 20
Aortic regurgitation, 40–41
Aortic stenosis, 19
dyspnea, 250–251
echocardiographic criteria, 47
patient survival, without treatment, 20
Aortic valve endocarditis, 11
Arachnodactyly, 62, 62f
Arboviruses, 385–386
Arterial embolism, 226
Arterial thrombosis, 226
Arteriovenous malformation (AVM), 606
Arthralgia, 658
Arthritis
*vs.* arthralgia, 658
articular structures, 658
inflammatory arthritis
blood tests, 660

classification, 663
crepitus, 659
dactylitis, 660
enthesitis, 659
historical features, 659
imaging studies, 660
migratory arthritis, 660
monoarticular, 663–664
oligoarticular, 664–667, 665f
physical findings, 659
polyarticular, 668–670, 669f
procedure, 660
spondyloarthritis, 660
subluxation, 659
symmetric arthritis, 660
synovial fluid findings, 661
synovitis, 659
tenosynovitis, 659
mimics of, 659
noninflammatory arthritis
acromegaly, 662, 663
causes of, 661–662
charcot joint, 661–662
episodic arthritis, cystic fibrosis, 661, 663
hemarthrosis, 661–662
hemochromatosis, 662, 663
hypertrophic osteoarthropathy, 661–662
osteoarthritis (OA), 661–662
osteonecrosis, 661–662
trauma, 661–662
periarticular structures, 659
physical examination, 659
with subcutaneous nodules, 658, 658f
types, 659
Arthrocentesis, 660
Asbestos, 654–655
Asbestosis, 638–639
Ascariasis, 165–166
Ascites, 43
classification, 148
cytologic examination, 149
definition, 148
differential cell count, 149
fluid characteristics, 149
Gram stain and culture, 149
gross appearance, 149
lactate dehydrogenase (LDH) concentration, 149
peritoneal fluid volume, 148
physical findings, 148
portal hypertension, 148
classification, 150
clinical sequelae, 150
diagnosis, 150
hepatic, 151–153, 152f
mechanism of, 149
posthepatic, 154–155
prehepatic, 150–151
unrelated to, 155–159, 156f
severity of, 148
with shortness of breath, 147, 147f
spontaneous bacterial peritonitis, 149
symptoms of, 148
total protein concentration, 149
ultrasonography, 148, 148f
Aseptic meningitis, 393–394
*Aspergillus*, 59–60
Aspiration pneumonia
cause of, 410–411
clinical characteristics, 409, 409f
definition, 409
mechanism of, 408
methods, 410
risk factors, 409
treatment, 410
Asterixis, 63
Asthenia, 579
Asthma
dyspnea, 253–254
exacerbation, 618–619
Astrovirus gastroenteritis, 179
Atelectasis, 623–624, 649
Atherosclerotic plaque, 228
stable angina, 20, 20f
unstable rupture, 18, 18f
Atonic activity, 541
Atrial fibrillation
characteristics of, 71
coronary artery embolism, 19
irregular supraventricular tachycardia (SVT), 74
mitral stenosis, 47
with slow ventricular rate, 9
causes of, 10
tachyarrhythmia-induced cardiomyopathy, 41
Atrial flutter, 69
atrioventricular (AV) conduction ratio, 8
bradycardia, 7, 7f
characteristics of, 69
irregular supraventricular tachycardia (SVT), 74
with variable AV block, 9
atrioventricular (AV) conduction ratio, 10, 72
irregular bradycardia, 12
Atrial septal defect (ASD), 50
Atrial tachycardia, 69
with atrioventricular (AV) block, 8
characteristics of, 71
definition, 8
prognosis of, 10
with variable atrioventricular (AV) block, 9
Atrioventricular (AV) block
with atrial flutter, 7, 7f
atrioventricular (AV) conduction ratio, 8
with atrial tachycardia, 8
Atrioventricular nodal reentrant tachycardia (AVNRT), 69
characteristics of, 70
dual AV nodal pathways physiology, 70, 70f
Atrioventricular reentrant tachycardia (AVRT), 69
characteristics of, 70
short PR interval and delta wave, 70, 70f
Aura, 541
Autoimmune adrenalitis, 81–82
Autoimmune causes, primary adrenal insufficiency, 81–82
Autoimmune encephalitis, 238–239
Autoimmune hemolytic anemia (AIHA), 333–334, 334f
Autoimmune hepatitis, 219
Autoimmune-related hypoparathyroidism, 114–115
Automatisms, 541


## B


*Bacillus cereus*, 180–181
Bacterial meningitis
atypical, 389–391
typical, 386–389, 388f
Bacterial pericarditis
characteristics of, 58
management of, 58
mechanisms of, 58
*Mycobacterium tuberculosis* (TB), 58–59
*Staphylococcus aureus*, 58–59
*Streptococcus pneumoniae*, 58–59
zoonoses, 58–59
Bare metal stents, 19
Becker muscular dystrophy, 44
Behçet's disease, 62, 665, 680–681
characteristics of, 667
Bernard-Soulier syndrome (BSS), 355–356, 356f
Berylliosis, 106–107
Bilateral adrenalectomy, 86, 98
hormone replacement, 87
Bilateral macronodular adrenal hyperplasia, 98
Biliary colic, 23–24
Biliary system, extrahepatic cholestasis
anatomy of, 164, 164f
ascariasis, 165–166
biliary stricture, 165–166
choledochal cyst, 165–166
choledocholithiasis, 165, 165f
liver flukes, 165–166
malignancy, 165–166
Bird fancier's lung, 637–638
β-Blockers, 8
coarctation, 46
hypertension, 46
reduced left ventricular systolic function, 39–40
Boerhaave syndrome, 23–24
Bone marrow hypoplasia, pancytopenia
antithyroid medication, 345
arsenic poisoning, 345
characteristics of, 346
definition, 344
idiopathic aplastic anemia, 345, 347
infections, 346
inherited aplastic anemia, 345–346, 346f
medications, 345
paroxysmal nocturnal hemoglobinuria (PNH), 345–346
parvovirus B19 infection, 345
pregnancy, 345
Bone marrow infiltration, 348–349, 348f
Brachial-femoral pulse delay, 46
Bradycardia
coronary artery supplies
atrioventricular (AV) node, 6
sinoatrial (SA) node, 6

Bradycardia *(continued)*
 definition, 6
 electrical conduction, normal heart, 6, 6f
 heart rate
  and cardiac output (CO), 6
  regulation, 6
 hypothyroidism, 125, 125f
 narrow-complex bradycardia. *See* Narrow-complex bradycardia
 pacemakers, 12
 physical findings, 7
 QRS complex
  classification, 7
  definition, 7
 resting heart rate, in adults, 6
 rhythm disturbance, 5, 5f
 during sleep
  in elderly patients, 6
  in young healthy patients, 6
 symptoms, 7
 wide-complex bradycardia. *See* Wide-complex bradycardia
Bradykinesia, 579
Brain abscess, 243–244
Brain tumor, 237–238
"Broken-heart" syndrome, 43
Bronchiectasis, 607
 dyspnea, 253–254, 253f
Bronchoscopy, 607
 hemoptysis, 605
Bronchovascular fistula, 607–608
Bronze diabetes, 49
Brugada criteria, 73, 73f
Budd-Chiari syndrome, 154, 217
Bundle branch block, 11, 12, 74

## C

Calcimimetics, 114
Calcium channel blockers, 8
Calcium chelators, 101
Calcium pyrophosphate dihydrate (pseudogout) crystals, 664
Calcium-sensing receptor (CaSR), 116
 clinical manifestations, 117
 negative feedback loop, 115
Cameron lesion, 203–204
*Campylobacter* species, 183, 185
*Candida*, 59–60
Capillary hydrostatic pressure, peripheral edema
 characteristics of, 290
 chronic venous insufficiency, 291–292, 292f
 cirrhosis, 290–291
 constrictive pericarditis, 291–292
 deep vein thrombosis (DVT), 290–291
 mechanisms, 290, 290f
 medication, 291
 pregnancy, 291–292
 renal failure, 290–291
 right-sided heart failure, 290–291
 superior vena cava (SVC) syndrome, 291–292
 systemic arterial hypertension, 290
Capillary oncotic pressure, peripheral edema
 albumin synthesis, 293, 293f
 characteristics of, 293
 liver disease and malnutrition, 293
 nephrotic syndrome, 293–294
 plasma proteins, 292
 protein-calorie malnutrition, 293
 protein-losing enteropathy, 293–294
Capillary permeability, peripheral edema, 295–297
Carbonic anhydrase, 414
Carcinoid tumor, 96, 191–192
Cardiac chest pain
 acute coronary syndrome (ACS). *See* Acute coronary syndrome (ACS)
 causes, 15
Cardiac conduction system, 6, 6f
Cardiac dysrhythmia
 dyspnea, 250–251
 hyperkalemia, 461
 hypokalemia, 480
Cardiac output (CO), 6
 and heart rate, 29
 hypotension, 276
Cardiac tamponade
 dyspnea, 250, 252
 malignant pericarditis, 60
Cardiogenic hypotension
 acute aortic regurgitation, 281
 acute inferior ST-elevation myocardial infarction, 281
 acute pulmonary embolism (PE), 281–282
 cardiogenic shock, 280–281
 cardiomyopathy, 281
 dysrhythmia, 281
 left ventricular outflow tract obstruction, 281
 mechanism, 280
 patterns of, 280
 primary pulmonary hypertension, 281
Cardiogenic shock, 227
Cardiology
 bradycardia. *See* Bradycardia
 chest pain. *See* Chest pain
 heart block. *See* Heart block
 heart failure. *See* Heart failure
 pericarditis. *See* Pericarditis
 tachycardia. *See* Tachycardia
Cardiomyopathy, dyspnea, 250–251
Cardiothoracic ratio, 39
Cardiovascular causes, heart failure, 40–41
Carpal tunnel syndrome, 43
Carvallo's sign, 47
Case study
 acid-base disorders. *See* Acid-base disorders
 acute kidney injury (AKI). *See* Acute kidney injury (AKI)
 adrenal insufficiency. *See* Adrenal insufficiency
 anemia. *See* Anemia
 arthritis. *See* Arthritis
 bradycardia. *See* Bradycardia
 chest pain. *See* Chest pain
 cholestatic liver injury. *See* Cholestatic liver injury
 Cushing's syndrome. *See* Cushing's syndrome
 delirium. *See* Delirium
 diarrhea. *See* Diarrhea
 dyspnea. *See* Dyspnea
 endocarditis. *See* Endocarditis
 fever of unknown origin (FUO). *See* Fever of unknown origin (FUO)
 gastrointestinal (GI) bleeding. *See* Gastrointestinal (GI) bleeding
 glomerular disease. *See* Glomerular disease
 headache. *See* Headache
 heart block. *See* Heart block
 heart failure. *See* Heart failure
 hemolytic anemia. *See* Hemolytic anemia
 hepatocellular liver injury. *See* Hepatocellular liver injury
 hypercalcemia. *See* Hypercalcemia
 hyperkalemia. *See* Hyperkalemia
 hypernatremia. *See* Hypernatremia
 hypocalcemia. *See* Hypocalcemia
 hypokalemia. *See* Hypokalemia
 hyponatremia. *See* Hyponatremia
 hypotension. *See* Hypotension
 hypothyroidism. *See* Hypothyroidism
 hypoxemia. *See* Hypoxemia
 interstitial lung disease (ILD). *See* Interstitial lung disease (ILD)
 intestinal ischemia. *See* Intestinal ischemia
 meningitis. *See* Meningitis
 pancytopenia. *See* Pancytopenia
 pericarditis. *See* Pericarditis
 peripheral edema. *See* Peripheral edema
 platelet disorders. *See* Platelet disorders
 pleural effusion. *See* Pleural effusion
 pneumonia. *See* Pneumonia
 polyneuropathy. *See* Polyneuropathy
 secondary hypertension. *See* Secondary hypertension
 seizure. *See* Seizure
 stroke. *See* Stroke
 syncope. *See* Syncope
 systemic vasculitis. *See* Systemic vasculitis
 tachycardia. *See* Tachycardia
 thyrotoxicosis. *See* Thyrotoxicosis
 weakness. *See* Weakness
Catamenial hemoptysis, 609
Catecholamines, 79, 465
Cavotricuspid isthmus, 69
Celiac disease, 189–190, 219–220
Central adrenal insufficiency
 central process, 87
 glucocorticoids, 88
 hypothalamic dysfunction, 87
 hypothalamus recovery, 88
 mechanism of, 87
 mineralocorticoid deficiency, 87
 pituitary gland dysfunction, 87
Central hypothyroidism, 133
Central nervous system (CNS) vasculitis, 238–239
Cerebral hypoxia, 238
Cervical angina, 24–25
Chagas disease, 42
 acute and chronic, 43
Charcot joint, 661–662
Chest pain
 cardiac

acute coronary syndrome (ACS). *See* Acute coronary syndrome (ACS)
causes, 15
electrocardiogram (ECG), 15, 15f
noncardiac, 15
anxiety (panic disorder), 25
causes, 21
gastrointestinal, 23–24
herpes zoster, 25
musculoskeletal, 24–25
pulmonary, 21–22
pericarditis. *See* Pericarditis
sources of, 15
Chest wall trauma, 24–25
Chest wall tumor, 24–25
Choledochal cyst, 165–166
Choledocholithiasis, 165, 165f
Cholelithiasis, 24
Cholerheic diarrhea, 189–190
Cholestatic liver injury
aminotransferases, 163
bilirubin, 163
classification, 163
clinical manifestations, 163
computed tomography (CT), 164
elevated serum levels, 163
evaluation of, 164
extrahepatic cholestasis, 163
biliary tree, 164–166, 164f–165f
classification, 164
imaging modality, 163
life-threatening condition, 164
mechanism of, 163
pancreas, 164, 164f, 167–168, 168f
intrahepatic cholestasis, 163
clinical features of, 168
diagnosis, 168
imaging modality, 163
infection, 172–173, 173f
mechanisms of, 168
obstruction, 169–170
toxicity, 171–172
laboratory pattern, 162
serum alkaline phosphatase levels, 162
hepatic metabolism, 163
laboratory result, 163
sources of, 162
woman with pruritis, 162, 162f
Chronic anemia and shunt, 40–41
Chronic dilated cardiomyopathy, 43
Chronic eosinophilic pneumonia (CEP), 634–635
Chronic hypersensitivity pneumonitis, 637
Chronic kidney disease (CKD), 118, 431
Chronic mesenteric ischemia
atherosclerotic disease, 228
epidemiology of, 228
fibromuscular dysplasia, 228–229
imaging modalities, 228
indications, 228
physical finding, 228
symptoms of, 228
vasculitis, 228–229
Chronic obstructive pulmonary disease (COPD), 607
dyspnea, 253–254
Chronic pancreatitis, 167
Chronic systolic heart failure, 19
Chvostek's sign, 113
Chylothorax, 653, 654
Chylous ascites, 157–158
Cirrhosis, 43, 650
hepatic portal hypertension, 151–152, 152f
high-output physiologic state, 44
Citrate, 121
mechanism of, 122
Clonic activity, 541
Clonidine, 8
Clonus, 579
*Clostridium difficile,* 180–181
*Clostridium perfringens,* 180–181
Cluster headache, 511–512
Coagulopathy, 84
Coal worker's pneumoconiosis, 638–639
Cocaine, 41
myocardial ischemia/infarction, 42
*Coccidioides immitis,* 59
Cogan's syndrome, 676
Cognitive dysfunction, 102
Colchicine, 191
Collagen vascular diseases, 8
Colon cancer, 269, 271
Colorectal polyps, 206–207
Community-acquired pneumonia (CAP)
atypical pathogens, 401–403
causes, 399
endemic pathogens, 403–405, 404f
typical pathogens, 400–401, 401f
Concentric hypertrophy, 39, 39f
preserved left ventricular systolic function, 45
valvular disease, heart failure, 47
Concussion, 237
Conduction abnormalities, 461
Confusion, hypercalcemia, 100, 100f
Congestive hepatopathy, 217
Connective tissue disease (CTD)
mixed connective tissue disease (MCTD), 61
prevalence, 60
rheumatoid arthritis, 60–61
scleroderma, 61
seronegative spondyloarthritides, 61–62
systemic lupus erythematosus (SLE), 60–61
vasculitis, 61–62
Constrictive pericarditis, 51, 56, 154, 649
dyspnea, 250, 252
Kussmaul's sign, 56
Corkscrew-shaped organisms, 665, 665f
Coronary artery dissection, 18
in peripartum period, 19
Coronary artery embolism, 18
risk factor, 19
Coronary artery vasospasm, 18, 19
cause of, 21
risk factor, 19
substances with, 21
Cor pulmonale, 46
Corticotropin-releasing hormone (CRH), 79, 92
stimulants, 79, 92
Costochondritis, 24–25
Coxsackieviruses, 57
Crepitus, 659
Crescendo-decrescendo systolic murmur, 47
Crohn's disease, 106–107
Cryoglobulinemia, 665, 680
Cryptogenic organizing pneumonia (COP), 634
Cryptosporidiosis, 183
Crystal arthropathy, 663
types, 664
Culture-negative endocarditis, 264
Cushing's syndrome
ACTH-dependent process, 94
diagnosis, 94
ectopic production, 95–97
eutopic production, 94–95
hypercortisolism, 94
prevalence of, 94
ACTH-independent process, 97–98
clinical evaluation, 92
clinical manifestations, 92, 92f
corticotropin-releasing hormone (CRH), 92
stimulants, 92
definition, 92
delirium, 241, 243
with delusions, 91, 91f
exogenous glucocorticoids, 93
hypothalamic-pituitary-adrenal axis, 92
metabolic syndrome, obesity, 92
negative confirmatory test, 93
positive confirmatory test, 93
probability of, 92
serum cortisol levels, 92
urine free cortisol (UFC) test, 92
false-negative result, 93
Cyanosis, 49
*Cyclospora cayetanensis,* 182–183
Cystic fibrosis, 169–170, 668
*Cystoisospora belli,* 182–183
Cytomegalovirus (CMV), 57–58, 184, 186, 214–215


## D


Dactylitis, 660
Dead space, hypoxemia
anatomic and alveolar dead space, 621, 621f
causes of, 621–622
definition, 621
inhaled oxygen, 621
mechanism, 621
Deconditioning, 259–260
Delirium
altered mental status, 236
causes of, 237
clinical examination, 236
clinical features, 236
definition, 236
electroencephalography (EEG), 237
encephalitis, 236
with flushed skin, 235, 235f
hypertensive encephalopathy, 244–245
incidence of, 236
infectious, 243–244
insomnia, 244–245
limbic encephalitis, 236
lumbar puncture, 237

Delirium *(continued)*
- management, 237
- metabolic
  - Cushing's syndrome, 241, 243
  - hepatic encephalopathy, 241–242
  - hypercarbia, 241–242
  - hyperosmolar hyperglycemic state, 241–242
  - hyperthermia, 241, 243
  - hypoglycemia, 241
  - hypothermia, 241, 241f, 243
  - refeeding syndrome, 241–242
  - uremia, 241–242
  - Wernicke's encephalopathy, 241–242
- neuroimaging, 236
- neurologic
  - brain tumor, 237–238
  - central nervous system (CNS) vasculitis, 238–239
  - cerebral hypoxia, 238
  - concussion, 237
  - hydrocephalus, 237, 239, 239f
  - immune-mediated encephalitis, 238–239
  - intracranial hemorrhage, 237–238
  - seizure, 237–238
  - stroke, 237–238
- pharmacologic agents, 237
- posterior reversible encephalopathy syndrome (PRES), 244–245, 245f
- predisposing factors, 236
- psychosis, causes of, 236
- toxic, 240–241

Delusions, 91, 91f

Dermatomyositis (DM), 668, 670
- secondary interstitial lung disease, 640, 640f, 642

Desquamative interstitial pneumonia (DIP), 639–640

Diabetes mellitus, 192–193

Dialysis-related pericarditis, 63–64

Diarrhea
- definition, 177
- with dyspnea, 176, 176f
- inflammatory diarrhea. *See* Inflammatory diarrhea
- intestinal dysmotility, 192–194
- mechanisms of, 177
- osmotic diarrhea
  - celiac disease, 189–190
  - cholerheic diarrhea, 189–190
  - lactose intolerance, 188–189
  - laxatives, 188
  - medications, 189
  - pancreatic exocrine insufficiency, 189–190
  - short bowel syndrome, 189–190
  - small intestinal bacterial overgrowth, 189–190
  - sugar alcohol, 188, 190
  - tropical sprue, 189–190
- secretory diarrhea, 191–192
- water absorption, 177

Diastolic murmur, 603, 603f

Dietary fortification, 130

Dieulafoy's lesion, 203–204

Diffuse alveolar hemorrhage, 623, 625

Diffuse lymphadenopathy, 85

Digital clubbing, 662

Digoxin, 8

Dilated cardiomyopathy, 19, 39

Disseminated fungal infection, 82–83

Disseminated gonorrhea, 664
- clinical features of, 665

Distributive hypotension, 282–283

Diuretics, 39

Diverticulosis, 206–207

Dressler's syndrome, 63

Drug-eluting stents, 19

Drug-induced immune hemolytic anemia, 333–334

Drug-induced thyroiditis, 129

Duchenne muscular dystrophy, 44

Duodenitis, 204–205

Dysfunctional hypothalamic-pituitary axis, 81

Dysmorphic red blood cell, 451, 451f

Dyspnea
- anemia, 258–259
- breathing regulation, 249, 249f
- cardiac
  - aortic stenosis, 250–251
  - cardiac dysrhythmia, 250–251
  - cardiac output (CO) determinants, 250
  - cardiac tamponade, 250, 252
  - cardiomyopathy, 250–251
  - constrictive pericarditis, 250, 252
  - intracardiac shunt, 251–252
  - mechanisms, 250
  - myocardial ischemia, 250
  - myocarditis, 250, 252
  - oxygen delivery, 250
  - superior vena cava (SVC) syndrome, 251–252
- deconditioning, 259–260
- definition, 249
- with facial edema, 248, 248f
- heart and lungs, roles, 249
- hyperventilation, 249
- metabolic acidosis, 259–260
- myasthenia gravis, 259
- panic attack, 258–259
- pregnancy, 259–260
- pulmonary
  - airway, 253–255, 253f
  - causes of, 252
  - gas exchange, 252
  - mechanisms, 252
  - parenchyma, 255–256, 255f
  - pleura, 258
  - vasculature, 257–258
- reduced partial pressure of inspired oxygen, 258, 260
- tachypnea, 249
- thyrotoxicosis, 259–260

Dystonic activity, 541


## E


Eccentric hypertrophy, 39, 39f
- on chest radiography, 39

Echoviruses, 57

Ectopic ACTH production
- carcinoid tumor, 96
- diagnosis, 97
- electrolyte disturbance, 95
- hypokalemia, 95
- medullary thyroid carcinoma, 96
  - multiple endocrine neoplasia types 2a and 2b, 97
- pancreatic islet cell tumor, 96
  - characteristics of, 97
- pheochromocytoma, 96
  - multiple endocrine neoplasia types 2a and 2b, 96
- small cell lung cancer, 96
- source of, 97

Ectopic 1,25(OH)$_2$D secretion, 105

Electrolyte disturbances, 8

Embolism
- infarction pattern, 572
- mechanisms, 566, 572–573

Emery-Dreifuss muscular dystrophy, 44

Emphysema, 621–622

Empyema, 647

Encephalitis, 236
- delirium, 243–244

Endobronchial biopsy, 607

Endocardial fibrosis, 49

Endocarditis, 266
- classification, 365
- definition, 365
- infective endocarditis
  - classification, 370
  - clinical manifestations, 369
  - complications, 370
  - definition, 367
  - diagnosis, 369
  - heart valves, 367
  - intravenous drug use (IVDU), 377–379, 377f
  - Janeway lesions, 368, 368f
  - modified Duke criteria, 369, 369t
  - native valve, 370–373
  - physical findings, 368
  - prognosis of, 370
  - prosthetic valve, 373–377
  - Roth spots, 368, 368f
  - splinter hemorrhage, 368, 368f
  - symptoms of, 368
  - therapy, 369
- noninfective endocarditis
  - definition, 366
  - nonbacterial thrombotic endocarditis (NBTE). *See* Nonbacterial thrombotic endocarditis (NBTE)
- prevalence of, 366
- with pulsating nail beds, 365, 365f

Endocrine disorders, 132

Endocrinology
- adrenal insufficiency. *See* Adrenal insufficiency
- Cushing's syndrome. *See* Cushing's syndrome
- hypercalcemia. *See* Hypercalcemia
- hypocalcemia. *See* Hypocalcemia
- hypothyroidism. *See* Hypothyroidism
- PTH-independent hypercalcemia, 107–108
- thyrotoxicosis. *See* Thyrotoxicosis

End-stage renal disease, 102
*Entamoeba histolytica*, 184–185
Enterohemorrhagic *Escherichia coli* (EHEC), 183, 185
Enteroinvasive *Escherichia coli* (EIEC), 183, 185
Enteropathic arthritis, 664
 types, 666
Enterotoxigenic *Escherichia coli* (ETEC), 180–181
Enteroviruses, 384–385
Enthesitis, 659
Eosinophilia, 48–49
Eosinophilic granulomatosis with polyangiitis (EGPA), 62
 ANCA-associated small vessel systemic vasculitis, 678–679
Eosinophilic myocarditis. *See* Löffler endocarditis
Epilepsy
 antiepileptic drugs, 543
 causes of, 542
 definition, 542
 nonpharmacologic long-term treatment, 543
 prevalence, 542
 triggers for, 542
 types, 543
Episodic arthritis, cystic fibrosis, 661, 663
Epstein-Barr virus (EBV), 57–58, 214–215
Erythema nodosum, 664
Erythematous base, 25
Esophageal cancer, 201–202
Esophageal rupture, 23
 cause of, 24
Esophageal spasm, 23
 diagnosis of, 24
Esophagitis, 201–202
Essential hypertension, 502
Ethylenediaminetetraacetic acid (EDTA), 121
 mechanism of, 122
Eutopic ACTH production, 94–95
Euvolemic hypernatremia, 475
Euvolemic hyponatremia, 493–495
Exogenous glucocorticoids, 93
Exogenous thyroid hormone, 142
External beam radiation therapy, 131–132
Extracranial secondary headache disorders, 520–522
Extraglandular production, 142–143
Extrahepatic cholestasis, 163
 biliary system
  anatomy of, 164, 164f
  ascariasis, 165–166
  biliary stricture, 165–166
  choledochal cyst, 165–166
  choledocholithiasis, 165, 165f
  liver flukes, 165–166
  malignancy, 165–166
 classification, 164
 imaging modality, 163
 life-threatening condition, 164
 mechanism of, 163
 pancreas
  acute pancreatitis, 167
  anatomy of, 164, 164f
  chronic pancreatitis, 167
  pancreatic cancer, 167–168
  pancreatic pseudocyst, 167–168, 168f
Extrarenal hyperkalemia
 catecholamines, 465
 concentration gradient, 465
 factors, 465
 insulin effect, 465
 mechanism, 464, 465f
 medications, 466
 transcellular shift, 464–465, 465f
Extravascular consumption, 120–121
Extrinsic vessel compression, 227
Exudative pleural effusion
 causes of, 652
 infectious, 652–653
 mechanisms of, 651
 noninfectious, 653–655
 types, 651

## F

Fabry disease, 49–50
Facial weakness, 583
Factitious disorder, 271–272
Familial dilated cardiomyopathy, 43
 diagnosis, 44
Familial hypocalciuric hypercalcemia (FHH), 102
 mechanism of, 103
Familial Mediterranean fever (FMF), 267, 269
Fanconi anemia, 345–346, 346f
Farmer's lung, 637–638
Fever of unknown origin (FUO)
 alcoholic hepatitis, 271–272
 causes of, 264
 definition, 263
 drug fever, 271–272
 factitious disorder, 271–272
 incidence of, 263
 infectious
  causes of, 264
  culture-negative endocarditis, 264
  endocarditis, 266
  intra-abdominal abscess, 264–265
  leptospirosis, 265, 265f
  miliary tuberculosis (TB), 264, 266
  osteomyelitis, 265–266
  viral infection, 265–266
  zoonotic infection, 266
 intra-abdominal hematoma, 271–272
 malignant
  atrial myxoma, 269, 271
  causes of, 269
  colon cancer, 269, 271
  hepatocellular carcinoma (HCC), 269, 271
  leukemia, 269–270
  lymphoma, 269–270
  metastatic breast cancer, 269
  myelodysplastic syndrome (MDS), 269–270, 270f
  renal cell carcinoma, 269, 271
 noninfectious inflammatory
  adult-onset Still's disease (AOSD), 267
  causes of, 266
  familial Mediterranean fever (FMF), 267, 269
  inflammatory bowel disease (IBD), 267, 269
  polyarteritis nodosa, 267
  polymyalgia rheumatica (PMR), 267, 269
  reactive arthritis, 267–268
  rheumatoid arthritis (RA), 267–268, 268f
  sarcoidosis, 267–268, 268f
  systemic lupus erythematosus (SLE), 267–268
 with oral ulcers, 263, 263f
 postpartum thyroiditis, 271
 prevalence of, 264
 prognosis of, 264
 venous thromboembolism, 271–272
Fibromuscular dysplasia, 228–229
First-degree atrioventricular (AV) block
 atria and ventricles conduction, 30
 causes of, 30
 coronary artery supplies, 30
 electrocardiographic findings, 30, 30f
 nonconducted beats, 30
 prevalence of, 30
 PR interval measures, 30
 prognosis of, 31
 symptoms of, 30
 treatment for, 31
Focal seizures, 543–544, 543f
 subtypes, 544–545
Foreign body aspiration, 607–608
 dyspnea, 254–255
Foscarnet, 121
 mechanism of, 122
Fungal meningitis, 391–393, 392f
Fungal pericarditis, 59–60

## G

Gain-of-function genetic mutations, 117
α-Galactosidase A, 49
Gallavardin phenomenon, 47
Gastric antral vascular ectasia (GAVE), 203–204
Gastric cancer, 203–204
Gastric varices, 203–204
Gastrinoma, 191–192
Gastritis, 202–203
Gastroenterology and hepatology
 ascites. *See* Ascites
 cholestatic liver injury. *See* Cholestatic liver injury
 diarrhea. *See* Diarrhea
 gastrointestinal (GI) bleeding. *See* Gastrointestinal (GI) bleeding
 hepatocellular liver injury. *See* Hepatocellular liver injury
 intestinal ischemia. *See* Intestinal ischemia
Gastroesophageal reflux disease (GERD), 23
 lifestyle modifications, 23
Gastrointestinal (GI) bleeding
 capsule endoscopy, 200
 catheter angiography, 200

Gastrointestinal (GI) bleeding *(continued)*
  characteristics, 199
  classification, 199
  coffee-ground emesis, 199
  CT angiography, 200
  deep enteroscopy, 201
  definition, 198
  hematemesis, 198
  hematochezia, 199
    upper gastrointestinal bleeding, 200
  with hypotension, 198, 198f
  incidence of, 199
  lower gastrointestinal tracts, 199. *See also* Lower gastrointestinal bleeding
  management, 199
  melena, 199, 199f
    lower gastrointestinal bleeding, 200
  push enteroscopy, 201
  radionuclide imaging, 200
  source of, 200
  upper gastrointestinal tracts, 199. *See also* Upper gastrointestinal bleeding
Gastrointestinal calcium absorption, 117
Gastrointestinal malabsorption, 118, 120
Gastrointestinal noncardiac chest pain, 21
  acute pancreatitis, 23–24
  biliary colic, 23–24
  esophageal rupture, 23–24
  esophageal spasm, 23–24
  gastroesophageal reflux disease (GERD), 23
  peptic ulcer disease (PUD), 23–24
Gastropathy, 202, 204
Generalized lymphadenopathy, 48
Generalized seizures, 543–544, 543f
  subtypes, 545–546
Genetic disorders, heart failure
  congenital heart disease, 49
  Fabry disease, 49–50
  glycogen storage disease, 49
  hemochromatosis, 49
  hypertrophic cardiomyopathy, 49
Giant cell arteritis, 62
  large vessel systemic vasculitis, 675–676, 675f
Giant cell myocarditis, 44
*Giardia lamblia*, 182
Giardiasis, 183
Glomerular disease
  clinical syndromes, 446
  definition, 446
  effects of, 446
  glomerulus, anatomy, 446, 446f
  with hematuria, 445, 445f
  nephritic syndrome
    characteristic urinary findings, 447
    glomerulonephritis. *See* Glomerulonephritis
  nephrotic syndrome
    characteristic urinary findings, 446
    classification, 448
    infection, 447
    laboratory features, 447
    pathophysiology, 447
    pharmacologic agents, 448
    physical findings, 447
    primary, 448–449
    secondary, 449–450
    symptoms, 447
    thromboembolism, 447
  renal biopsy, 447
Glomerulonephritis
  ANCA, 451–454
  anti-GBM antibodies, 454
  classification, 451
  dysmorphic red blood cell, 451, 451f
  Henoch-Schönlein purpura (HSP), 456–457
  immunoglobulin A nephropathy, 456–457
  laboratory findings, 451
  low serum complement levels, 454–456
  physical findings, 450
  secondary hypertension, 506–507
  symptoms, 450
Glucagonoma, 191–192
Glucocorticoids, 79, 87
Glucose-6-phosphate dehydrogenase (G6PD) deficiency, 330, 330f
Glycogen storage disease, 49
  hypoglycemia, 50
Graft-*versus*-host disease (GVHD), 169–170
Graham Steell murmur, 48
Granulomatosis with polyangiitis, 678–679, 679f
Granulomatosis with polyangiitis (GPA), 62, 106
  prognosis of, 107
Granulomatous disease, 48, 85, 115
  hypoparathyroidism, 116
  polyarticular inflammatory arthritis, 668
  PTH-independent hypercalcemia
    berylliosis, 106–107
    Crohn's disease, 106–107
    granulomatosis with polyangiitis (GPA), 106–107
    histoplasmosis, 106–107
    sarcoidosis, 106
    tuberculosis (TB), 106–107
Graves' disease, 131
  diffusely increased radioactive iodine uptake, 140–141
Guillain-Barré syndrome, 618–619

## H

Hamman-Rich syndrome, 634
Hashimoto's thyroiditis, 128
  diagnosis of, 129
HCV-associated cryoglobulinemia, 667
Headache
  classification, 511
  prevalence, 510
  primary disorders, 511. *See also* Primary headache disorders
  secondary disorders, 511. *See also* Secondary headache disorders
  with tinnitus, 510, 510f
Heart block
  abnormal jugular venous waveform, 29, 29f
  definition, 29
  electrical conduction path, normal heart, 29
  first-degree atrioventricular (AV) block, 30–31, 30f
  heart rate
    and cardiac output (CO), 29
    regulation, 29
  physical findings, 30
  second-degree atrioventricular (AV) block, 31–33, 31f–33f
  symptoms of, 29
  third-degree atrioventricular (AV) block, 34, 34f
  types, 30
  with ventricular escape rhythm, [illegible]
Heart failure
  definition, 38
  hemoptysis, 605–606
  left-sided heart failure
    physical findings, 38
    pulmonary lymphatic vessel dilation, 38
  left ventricular function, 38
  with orthostatic hypotension, 37, 37f
  preserved systolic function, 38. *See also* Preserved left ventricular systolic function
  prognosis of, 38
  reduced systolic function, 38. *See also* Reduced left ventricular systolic function
  right-sided heart failure, physical findings, 38
  risk factors, 38
  symptoms of, 38
Heart rate
  and cardiac output (CO), 29
  regulation, 29
HELLP syndrome, 219–220
Hemangioma, 206–207
Hemarthrosis, 661
  causes of, 662
Hematemesis, 198, 604
Hematochezia, 199–200
Hematology
  anemia. *See* Anemia
  hemolytic anemia. *See* Hemolytic anemia
  pancytopenia. *See* Pancytopenia
  platelet disorders. *See* Platelet disorders
Hematopoiesis, 343, 343f
  ineffective, 347
Hemiparesis, 583
Hemochromatosis, 49, 85, 662
  characteristics of, 86
  clinical characteristics, 663
  primary hypothyroidism, 132
  treatment, 50
Hemoglobin C disease, 328–329
Hemolytic anemia
  acquired hemolytic anemia, 327
    immunologic, 333–335, 334f
    infectious, 337–339, 339f
    mechanisms, 332
    toxic, 335–336
    traumatic, 336–337
  average life span, 326
  causes of, 327
  clinical sequelae, 327
  with dark urine, 326, 326f
  definition, 326
  inherited hemolytic anemia, 327

cell membrane defects, 331–332, 332f
classification, 328
hemoglobin defects, 328–329, 329f
intracellular enzyme defects, 330–331, 330f
intravascular hemolysis, 326
laboratory features, 327
mechanisms, 327
physical findings, 327
symptoms of, 327
Hemoperitoneum ascites, 157–158
Hemoptysis
arterial system, 604
bronchoscopy, 605
cardiovascular causes
arteriovenous malformation (AVM), 606
heart failure, 605–606
infarction, 605, 605f
pulmonary embolism (PE), 605–606, 605f
valvular disease, 606
vasculitis, 606
catamenial hemoptysis, 609
chest radiography, 605
computed tomography (CT) imaging, 605
definition, 604
with diastolic murmur, 603, 603f
historical features, 604
idiopathic pulmonary hemosiderosis, 609
mimic conditions, 604
pulmonary arteries, blood supply, 604, 604f
pulmonary causes
acute bronchitis, 607
bronchiectasis, 607
bronchovascular fistula, 607–608
causes of, 606
foreign body aspiration, 607–608
iatrogenic, 607–608
lung abscess, 608–609
malignancy, 607
pneumonia, 608
pulmonary aspergillosis, 608–609
pulmonary paragonimiasis, 608–609
pulmonary tuberculosis (TB), 608–609
quantity of, 605
severity of, 604
Hemorrhagic causes, primary adrenal insufficiency
bilateral adrenal hemorrhage, 83
adrenal vein thrombosis, 84
causes of, 84
critical illness, 84
diagnosis of, 83
immune thrombocytopenic purpura, 84
prognosis of, 84
traumatic injuries, 84–85, 85f
Waterhouse-Friderichsen syndrome, 84–85
vascular anatomy, 83
Hemorrhagic stroke
causes and treatment, 559
intracerebral hemorrhage, 560–562, 560f
occurence, 559, 559f
relative rates, 560
subarachnoid hemorrhage, 562–564, 563f
Hemorrhoids, 206
Hemothorax, 653, 655
Henderson-Hasselbalch equation, 414
Henoch-Schönlein purpura (HSP), 456–457, 665
characteristics of, 667
non–ANCA-associated small vessel systemic vasculitis, 680
Hepatic encephalopathy, 241–242
Hepatic hydrothorax, 651
Hepatic portal hypertension
acute (fulminant) liver failure, 151, 153
cirrhosis, 151–152, 152f
hepatocellular carcinoma, 151, 153
idiopathic noncirrhotic portal hypertension, 151, 153
primary biliary cholangitis (PBC), 151, 153
primary sclerosing cholangitis (PSC), 151, 153
schistosomiasis, 151, 153
sinusoidal obstruction syndrome (SOS), 152, 153
Hepatic tuberculosis (TB), 172–173, 173f
Hepatitis A and B viruses, 57
Hepatitis A virus (HAV), 213–214
Hepatitis B virus (HBV), 213–214
Hepatitis C virus (HCV), 213, 215
Hepatitis D virus (HDV), 214–215
Hepatitis E virus (HEV), 213–214
Hepatocellular carcinoma (HCC), 169–170, 269, 271
hepatic portal hypertension, 151, 153
Hepatocellular liver injury
abnormal aminotransferase level, 213
acute biliary obstruction, 219–220
aminotransferases, 212
elevation, 213
severity of, 213
autoimmune hepatitis, 219
biochemical laboratory pattern, 212
causes of, 213
Celiac disease, 219–220
HELLP syndrome, 219–220
hereditary, 218–219, 218f
infectious, 213–215
laboratory tests, 213
life-threatening condition, 213
nonalcoholic fatty liver disease (NAFLD), 219
with skin rash, 212, 212f
toxic, 216–217
vascular, 217
Hepatopulmonary syndrome, 623, 625
Hereditary elliptocytosis, 331–332, 332f
Hereditary hemochromatosis, 218
Hereditary hemorrhagic telangiectasia (HHT), 606, 628
Hereditary polyneuropathy, 535–536, 536f
Hereditary spherocytosis, 331
Hereditary stomatocytosis, 331–332
Hereditary xerocytosis, 331–332
Herpes simplex virus (HSV), 57, 214–215
Herpes simplex virus types 1 (HSV-1) and 2 (HSV-2), 384–385, 385f
Herpes zoster, 25
High-altitude pulmonary edema (HAPE), 259
His-Purkinje system, 32
*Histoplasma capsulatum*, 59, 107
Histoplasmosis, 106–107
Holosystolic murmur, 40–41
Hormonal cycle, 79
Hospital-acquired pneumonia (HAP), 405–407
Human chorionic gonadotropin (hCG), 140–141
Human immunodeficiency virus (HIV), 42
antiretroviral therapy (ART), 43
primary adrenal insufficiency, 82–83
viral meningitis, 384, 386
viral pericarditis, 57–58
Hungry bone syndrome, 120–121
Hydrocephalus, delirium, 237, 239, 239f
11β-Hydroxysteroid dehydrogenase type 2, 95
Hyperalbuminemia, 101
Hypercalcemia
calcium distribution, 100
clinical manifestations, 102
cognitive dysfunction, 102
with confusion, 100, 100f
electrocardiographic manifestations, 102
etiology of, 102
gastrointestinal symptoms, 102
ionized calcium, 101
neuropsychiatric symptoms, 102
PTH actions, 101, 101f
PTH-dependent
familial hypocalciuric hypercalcemia (FHH), 102–103
mechanism of, 102
primary hyperparathyroidism, 102–103
secondary hyperparathyroidism, 103
tertiary hyperparathyroidism, 102–103
PTH-independent
causes of, 103
endocrinopathy, 107–108
granulomatous disease, 106–107
immobility, 108
malignancy, 105
mechanism of, 103
medication, 104
rhabdomyolysis, 108–109
renal symptoms, 102
total serum calcium concentration, 100
measurement of, 101
vitamin D, 101
Hypercarbia, delirium, 241–242
Hypercortisolism, 94
ACTH-dependent Cushing's syndrome, 94
Hypereosinophilic syndrome (HES), 49
Hyperkalemia
cardiac dysrhythmias, 461
classification, 461
conduction abnormalities, 461
with dark urine, 460, 460f

Hyperkalemia *(continued)*
  electrocardiographic manifestations, 461, 461f
  extrarenal
    catecholamines, 465
    concentration gradient, 465
    factors, 465
    insulin effect, 465
    mechanism, 464, 465f
    medications, 466
    transcellular shift, 464–465, 465f
  glomerular filtration rate, 462
  normal serum $K^+$ concentration, 460
    regulation, 461
  pseudohyperkalemia, 460
  renal function, 462
    decreased renal clearance, 462–463
    normal renal clearance, 463–464, 464f
  serum creatinine concentration, 462
  symptoms, 461
Hypermagnesemia, 116
Hypernatremia
  acute and chronic, 472, 472f
  adaptive mechanisms, 471
  clinical manifestations, 472
  definition, 469
  euvolemic, 475
  hypervolemic, 475–476
  hypovolemic, 473–475, 474f
  physical findings, 472
  with polyuria, 469
  serum $Na^+$ concentration, 469
    effects of, 471
  water homeostasis, 470, 470f
Hyperosmolar hyperglycemic state, 241–242
Hyperphosphatemia, 120
  mechanism of, 121
Hyperproliferative normocytic anemia, 318–319
Hypersensitivity pneumonitis (HP)
  antigens classes, 636
  bird fancier's lung, 637–638
  bronchoscopy, 637
  characteristics, 637
  clinical course, 637
  definition, 636
  farmer's lung, 637–638
  high-resolution CT imaging, 637
  prevalence, 636
  serologic testing, 637
  treatment for, 637
Hypersplenism, 333–334, 349–350
Hypertension
  encephalopathy, 244–245
  preserved systolic function, 46
Hyperthermia, delirium, 241, 243
Hypertonic/isotonic hyponatremia, 490
Hypertrophic cardiomyopathy, 49
  without outflow obstruction, 50
Hypertrophic obstructive cardiomyopathy (HOCM), 19
  preserved systolic function, 46
  squatting position, murmur quality change, 21
Hypertrophic osteoarthropathy, 661–662
Hyperventilation, dyspnea, 249
Hypervolemic hypernatremia, 475–476
Hypervolemic hyponatremia, 495–497
Hypoalbuminemia, 101
Hypocalcemia
  calcium distribution, 112
    in blood, 112
  with chest pain, 112
  Chvostek's sign, 113
  clinical manifestations, 113
  etiology of, 113
  PTH-dependent
    autoimmune causes, 114–115
    calcium-sensing receptor, 116–117
    causes of, 113
    iatrogenic causes, 114
    infiltrative causes, 115–116
    laboratory pattern, 113
    magnesium derangement, 116
    mechanism of, 113
  PTH-independent
    causes of, 117
    extravascular consumption, 120–121
    hypomagnesemia, 122
    intravascular consumption, 121–122
    laboratory pattern, 117
    mechanism of, 117
    medication, 122
    pseudohypoparathyroidism, 122
    vitamin D deficiency, 117–120, 118f–119f
  serum ionized calcium concentration, 113
  serum PTH value, 113
  total serum calcium concentration, 112
    hypoalbuminemia, 112
    ionized calcium, 112
  Trousseau's sign, 113
Hypoglycemia, 50
  delirium, 241
Hypokalemia, 95
  cardiac dysrhythmias, 480
  with dry mouth, 479, 479f
  electrocardiographic manifestations, 480, 480f
  extracellular $K^+$ concentration, 479
  mechanisms, 480
  normal serum $K^+$ concentration, 479
  potassium
    excess loss, 481, 481f
    extrarenal loss, 482–483
    low oral intake, 480–481
    renal loss, 481–482
    transcellular shift, 483–484
  symptoms, 480
Hypomagnesemia, 116, 122
Hyponatremia
  acute and chronic, 489
  adaptive mechanisms, 488, 488f
  clinical manifestations, 489
  definition, 487
  with hemoptysis, 487, 487f
  hypertonic/isotonic, 490
  hypotonic, 489
    cause of, 490
    euvolemic, 493–495
    hypervolemic, 495–497
    hypovolemic, 491–493
    laboratory test, 491
    physical findings, 491
  laboratory definitions, 489
  serum $Na^+$ concentration, 487
    effects of, 488
  serum osmolality *vs.* tonicity, 489
  severity of, 487
  water homeostasis regulation, 488
Hypoparathyroidism
  autoimmune causes, 114–115
  calcium-sensing receptor, 116–117
  causes of, 113
  iatrogenic causes, 114
  infiltrative causes, 115–116
  laboratory pattern, 113
  magnesium derangement, 116
  mechanism of, 113
Hypoproliferative normocytic anemia, 316–318
Hypotension, 621–622
  blood pressure
    measurement, 277
    regulation, 277, 277f
  cardiac output (CO), 276
  cardiac tamponade, 56, 56f
  cardiogenic, 280–282
  with cool extremities, 276, 276f
  distributive, 282–284
  hypotensive shock, 278
  hypovolemic, 278–280, 279f
  Korotkoff sounds, 277
  mean arterial pressure (MAP), 276
  mechanisms, 278
  obstructive, 284–285, 285f
  physical findings, 278
  prevalence of, 278
  symptoms of, 278
Hypotensive shock, 278
Hypothalamic-pituitary-adrenal axis, 79, 79f
  Cushing's syndrome, 92
Hypothalamic-pituitary-thyroid axis, 126, 126f
Hypothermia, 8
  delirium, 241, 241f, 243
Hypothyroidism, 8
  with bradycardia, 125, 125f
  causes of, 127
  central, 133
  clinical condition, 127
  clinical entity, 127
  definition, 126
  function, 127
  hypothalamic-pituitary-thyroid axis, 126, 126f
  life-threatening complication, 127
  overt hypothyroidism, 127
  pericarditis, 63–64
  physical findings of, 127
  prevalence of, 126, 128
  primary
    causes of, 128
    iatrogenesis, 131–132
    infiltrative disorders, 132–133
    iodine, 130–131
    mechanism of, 128
    thyroiditis, 128–130

subclinical, 127
symptoms of, 126
$T_3$ and $T_4$, 126
thyroid-releasing hormone (TRH), 126
thyroid-stimulating hormone (TSH), 126
treatment, 127
Hypotonic hyponatremia
cause of, 490
euvolemic, 493–495
hypervolemic, 495–497
hypovolemic, 491–493
laboratory test, 491
physical findings, 491
Hypovolemic hypernatremia, 473–475, 474f
Hypovolemic hyponatremia, 491–493
Hypovolemic hypotension
gastrointestinal losses, 279
hemorrhagic shock, 279
hypovolemic shock, 278
isotonic fluid, 279, 279f
mechanisms, 278
patterns of, 278
poor oral intake, 279
renal salt wasting, 279–280
severe burn injury, 279–280
Hypoxemia
A-a gradient, 615, 615f
elevated, 619–620, 620f
normal, 616, 616t. *See also* A-a gradient
alveolar gas equation, 614
partial pressure of, 615
anatomic shunt, 627–628, 627f
barometric pressure, 615
causes of, 615
dead space
anatomic and alveolar dead space, 621, 621f
causes of, 621–622
definition, 621
inhaled oxygen, 621
mechanism, 621
definition, 612
hypoventilation
A-a gradient, 618
asthma exacerbation, 618–619
drugs and toxins, 618–619
Guillain-Barré syndrome, 618–619
inhaled oxygen, 618
kyphoscoliosis, 618–619
obesity hypoventilation syndrome (OHS), 618–619
obstructive sleep apnea (OSA), 618–619
partial pressure of carbon dioxide, 618
primary metabolic alkalosis, 619
hypoxia, 614
impaired diffusion capacity, 625–626, 625f
inspired oxygen fraction, 615
invasive test, 613
oxygen content, arterial blood, 614
determinants, 614
oxygen delivery, 614
oxyhemoglobin dissociation curve, 613, 613f
partial pressure of carbon dioxide, 615
partial pressure of oxygen, 613
physiologic conditions, 613
physiologic shunt
acute respiratory distress syndrome (ARDS), 624
airway constriction, 623–624
atelectasis, 623–624
definition, 623
diffuse alveolar hemorrhage, 623, 625
hepatopulmonary syndrome, 623, 625
inhaled oxygen, 623
pneumonia, 623–624
pulmonary edema, 623–624
with positional dyspnea, 612, 612f
pulse oximetry, 612
conditions, 613
respiratory quotient (RQ), 615
tissue oxygen extraction, 614
water vapor pressure, 615

## I

Iatrogenesis, 86
hypoparathyroidism, 114
primary hypothyroidism
external beam radiation therapy, 131–132
Graves' disease, 131
lithium, 131–132
thyroidectomy/radioactive iodine ablation, 131
Idiopathic dilated cardiomyopathy, 44
Idiopathic interstitial lung disease
acute interstitial pneumonia (AIP), 634–635
chronic eosinophilic pneumonia (CEP), 634–635
cryptogenic organizing pneumonia (COP), 634
definition, 633
idiopathic pulmonary fibrosis (IPF), 633–634
lymphoid interstitial pneumonia (LIP), 634–635
non-specific interstitial pneumonia (NSIP), 633–634
pattern of, 633
Idiopathic noncirrhotic portal hypertension, 151, 153
Idiopathic pulmonary fibrosis (IPF), 633–634
Idiopathic pulmonary hemosiderosis, 609
Idiopathic restrictive cardiomyopathy, 50
prognosis of, 51
Immune-mediated encephalitis, 238–239
Immune-mediated inflammatory diseases, 660
Immune-mediated parathyroid destruction, 115
Immunoglobulin A nephropathy, 456–457
Immunoglobulin light chain (AL) amyloidosis, 48
Impaired diffusion capacity, 625–626, 625f
Impaired sensitivity, 143–144
Infarction, hemoptysis, 605, 605f
Infarct pericarditis, 63
Infectious colitis, 208–209
Infectious diseases, 8
endocarditis. *See* Endocarditis
heart failure, 42–43
meningitis. *See* Meningitis
pneumonia. *See* Pneumonia
primary adrenal insufficiency, 82–83
Infectious exudative pleural effusion, 652–653
Infectious pericarditis
bacterial pericarditis, 58–59
causes of, 57
clinical presentation, 57
fungal pericarditis, 59–60
viral pericarditis, 57–58
Infectious thyroiditis, 129
risk factors for, 130
Infective endocarditis
classification, 370
clinical manifestations, 369
complications, 370
definition, 367
diagnosis, 369
heart valves, 367
intravenous drug use (IVDU), 377–379, 377f
Janeway lesions, 368, 368f
modified Duke criteria, 369, 369t
native valve, 370–373
physical findings, 368
prognosis of, 370
prosthetic valve, 373–377
Roth spots, 368, 368f
splinter hemorrhage, 368, 368f
symptoms of, 368
therapy, 369
Inferior vena cava (IVC) obstruction, 154–155
Infiltrative causes, primary adrenal insufficiency, 85–86
Infiltrative disorders, 169–170
amyloidosis, 48
eosinophilia, 48–49
iron overload, 48–49
lymphoma, 48–49
primary hypothyroidism
amyloidosis, 132–133
hemochromatosis, 132
Riedel's thyroiditis, 132–133
sarcoidosis, 132–133
thyroid gland, 133
sarcoidosis, 48–49
sinus bradycardia, 8
Inflammatory bowel disease (IBD), 267, 269
Inflammatory diarrhea
diagnosis, 178f, 187
historical features, 177
invasive infectious diarrhea, 183–186
life-threatening complication, 178
mechanism of, 177
noninfectious inflammatory diarrhea, 186–188, 186f
noninvasive bacterial diarrhea, 180–182
noninvasive infectious diarrhea, 178
noninvasive protozoal diarrhea, 182–183
noninvasive viral diarrhea, 178–179
stool study, 177

Inflammatory polyneuropathy
causes of, 532
classification, 532
infectious causes, 532–533
noninfectious causes, 533–535
pathophysiologic/electrophysiologic pattern, 532
Influenza A and B viruses, 57
Inherited hemolytic anemia, 327
cell membrane defects, 331–332, 332f
classification, 328
hemoglobin defects, 328–329, 329f
intracellular enzyme defects, 330–331, 330f
In situ occlusion ischemic stroke
of large vessel, 567–569
mechanisms, 566
of small vessel, 570–571, 570f
Insomnia, delirium, 244–245
Internal medicine
delirium. *See* Delirium
dyspnea. *See* Dyspnea
fever of unknown origin (FUO). *See* Fever of unknown origin (FUO)
hypotension. *See* Hypotension
peripheral edema. *See* Peripheral edema
syncope. *See* Syncope
Interstitial lung disease (ILD)
bronchoscopy, 633
classification, 633
CT imaging, 632
characteristics, 633
definition, 632
histologic findings, 633
idiopathic, 633–635
microscopic elements, pulmonary parenchyma, 632, 632f
physical findings of, 632
pulmonary function testing, 633
radiography, 632
secondary
causes of, 635
desquamative interstitial pneumonia (DIP), 639–640
exposures, types, 635
hypersensitivity pneumonitis (HP), 636–638
iatrogenic exposure, 636
pneumoconiosis, 638–639
pulmonary Langerhans cell histiocytosis (PLCH), 639–640
respiratory bronchiolitis–associated interstitial lung disease (RB-ILD), 639–640
systemic disease, 640–642, 640f
symptoms of, 632
with tight skin, 631, 631f
Interstitial oncotic pressure, peripheral edema, 294–295, 295f
Intestinal ischemia
definition, 223
ischemic colitis, 224. *See also* Ischemic colitis
mesenteric ischemia, 224
acute. *See* Acute mesenteric ischemia
blood vessels supply, 224, 224f
chronic, 228–229
subtypes of, 224
with testicular pain, 223, 223f
types, 223
Intra-abdominal abscess, 264–265
Intracardiac shunt, 627
dyspnea, 251–252
Intracerebral hemorrhage stroke, 560–562, 560f
Intracranial hemorrhage, 237–238
Intracranial secondary headache disorders
cerebrospinal fluid, 518–519, 518f
infectious, 515–517
post-traumatic headache, 519–520
trigeminal neuralgia, 519–520
tumor, 517–518
vascular, 513–515
Intrahepatic cholestasis, 163
clinical features of, 168
diagnosis, 168
imaging modality, 163
infection, 172–173, 173f
mechanisms of, 168
obstruction, 169–170
toxicity, 171–172
Intrarenal acute kidney injury
acute interstitial nephritis (AIN), 439–441, 440f
acute tubular necrosis (ATN), 437–439, 438f
classification, 435
cross-section of, 435, 435f
vascular, 436–437
Intrathoracic malignancy, 654
Intravascular consumption, 121–122
Intravenous drug use (IVDU), 377–379, 377f
Invasive infectious diarrhea, 183–186
Iodine-induced hypothyroidism
cause of, 131
characteristics of, 131
dietary fortification, 130
Wolff-Chaikoff effect, 130
Ionized calcium, 101
Ionizing radiation therapy, 114
Iron deficiency, 314–315
Iron infiltration, 115–116
Iron overload, 48
causes of, 49
Irritable bowel syndrome (IBS), 192–193
Ischemia
cardiomyopathy, 40
electrocardiographic features, 17
sinus bradycardia, 8
Ischemic colitis, 208–209, 209f, 224
biochemical laboratory abnormalities, 230
blood vessels supply, 229, 229f
collateral circulation, 229
diagnosis, 230
endoscopy, 230
epidemiology of, 230
mechanism, 229–230
nonocclusive, 231
occlusive, 231–232
physical findings, 230
prognosis of, 230
symptoms of, 230
Ischemic hepatitis, 217
Ischemic stroke
anterior and posterior circulations, 565
classification, 566
embolism
infarction pattern, 572
mechanisms, 566, 572–573
internal carotid arteries (ICAs), 565, 565f
in situ occlusion
of large vessel, 567–569
mechanisms, 566
of small vessel, 570–571, 570f
treatment, 567
Watershed
causes of, 574
clinical manifestations, 573–574
mechanisms, 566
prevalence, 573


## J


Janeway lesions, 368, 368f
Jaundice, 43
Jod-Basedow phenomenon, 142–143
Jugular venous waveform
constrictive pericarditis, 51
tricuspid regurgitation, 48
tricuspid stenosis, 48
Junctional escape rhythm, 8
rate of, 9
Junctional tachycardia, 69
digitalis toxicity, 71


## K


Kaposi sarcoma, 206–207
Kawasaki disease, 676
treatment for, 677
Kussmaul's sign, 56
Kyphoscoliosis, 618–619


## L


Lactate, 121
mechanism of, 122
Lactose intolerance, 188–189
Lancisi's sign, 48
Large vessel systemic vasculitis
Cogan's syndrome, 676
giant cell arteritis, 675–676, 675f
physical findings, 675
secondary causes of, 676
Takayasu arteritis, 675–676
Laxatives, 188
Lead poisoning, microcytic anemia, 314, 316
Leptospirosis, 265, 265f
Leukemia, 269–270
Limb-girdle muscular dystrophy, 44
Limbic encephalitis, 236
*Listeria monocytogenes*, 180–181
Lithium-induced hypercalcemia, 104, 131–132
Liver disease, 118
Liver flukes, 165–166
Loculated pleural effusion, 647, 647f

Löffler endocarditis, 49
Löfgren's syndrome, 665
  prognosis of, 667
Long-chain fatty acids, 86
Lower gastrointestinal bleeding
  classification, 205
  diagnostic modality, 205
  inflammatory, 208–209, 209f
  structural, 206–207
  vascular, 207–208
Lower motor neuron lesions
  anatomic structures, 588
  anterior horn cell, 589–591
  definition, 588
  motor nerve fibers, 589, 589f
  peripheral nerve, 593–594
  root/plexus, 591–593
Lung abscess, 608–609
Lyme disease, 663, 667
Lymphocytic choriomeningitis virus (LCMV), 385–386
Lymphoid interstitial pneumonia (LIP), 634–635
Lymphoma, 48, 85, 105
  clinical syndrome, 49
  fever of unknown origin (FUO), 269–270

## M

Macrocytic anemia
  megaloblastic. *See* Megaloblastic anemia
  nonmegaloblastic, 321–323, 322f
Macroglossia, 48
Major depression, 25
Malignancy, 653–654
  extrahepatic cholestasis, 165–166
  fever of unknown origin (FUO)
    atrial myxoma, 269, 271
    causes of, 269
    colon cancer, 269, 271
    hepatocellular carcinoma (HCC), 269, 271
    leukemia, 269–270
    lymphoma, 269–270
    metastatic breast cancer, 269
    myelodysplastic syndrome (MDS), 269–270, 270f
    renal cell carcinoma, 269, 271
  lower gastrointestinal bleeding, 206
  PTH-independent hypercalcemia, 105
Malignant pericarditis, 60
Mallory-Weiss tear, 201–202
Marfan syndrome, 62, 62f
Mean arterial pressure (MAP), 276
Mean corpuscular volume (MCV), 313–314, 314f
Mediastinal radiation therapy, 50–51
Medium vessel systemic vasculitis
  Kawasaki disease, 676
    treatment for, 677
  physical findings, 676
  polyarteritis nodosa (PAN), 676
    arteriographic findings of, 677, 677f
  secondary causes, 677
Medullary thyroid carcinoma, 96
  multiple endocrine neoplasia types 2a and 2b, 97
Megaloblastic anemia
  on bone marrow evaluation, 320
  copper deficiency, 320–321
  definition, 319
  features, 320, 320f
  folate deficiency, 320–321
  nitrous oxide inhalation, 320–321
  vitamin B12 deficiency, 320–321
Meigs' syndrome, 654–655
Melena, 199–200, 199f
Meningitis
  with agitated delirium, 382, 382f
  antimicrobial therapy, 383
  aseptic meningitis, 393–394
  bacterial meningitis
    atypical, 389–391
    typical, 386–389, 388f
  characteristics, 383, 384t
  classification, 383
  definition, 382
  delirium, 243–244
  diagnostic procedure, 383
  *vs.* encephalitis, 383
  fungal meningitis, 391–393, 392f
  meningoencephalitis, 383
  neuroimaging, 383
  physical findings of, 383
  pleocytosis, 384
  symptoms of, 382
  viral meningitis
    arboviruses, 385–386
    characteristic cerebrospinal fluid, 384
    diagnosis, 384
    enteroviruses, 384–385
    herpes simplex virus types 1 (HSV-1) and 2 (HSV-2), 384–385, 385f
    human immunodeficiency virus (HIV), 384, 386
    lymphocytic choriomeningitis virus (LCMV), 385–386
    with lymphocytic pleocytosis, 384
    mumps, 385–386
    pressure of, 384
    treatment, 384
Meningococcemia, 84
Meningoencephalitis, 383
Mesenteric ischemia, 224
  acute. *See* Acute mesenteric ischemia
  blood vessels supply, 224, 224f
  chronic, 228–229
  subtypes of, 224
Mesenteric vasospasm, 227
Mesotheliomas, 60
Metabolic acidosis, 416
  anion gap, 417, 420–422
  development of, 418, 418f
  dyspnea, 259–260
  lung function, 418
  non-anion gap, 418–420, 420f
Metabolic alkalosis, 416, 426–428
Metabolic pericarditis, 63–64
Metabolic polyneuropathy, 528–530, 529f
Metabolic provoked seizure, 552–553, 552f
Metastatic breast cancer, 269
Metastatic infiltration, 86
Methamphetamine-associated cardiomyopathy, 42
Microcytic anemia
  iron deficiency, 314–315
  lead poisoning, 314, 316
  sideroblastic anemia, 314, 316
  thalassemia, 314–315, 315f
Micronodular adrenal hyperplasia, 98
Microscopic polyangiitis, 678–679
Migraine headache, 511–512
Migratory arthritis, 660
Miliary tuberculosis (TB), 264, 266
Milk-alkali syndrome, 104
Mineralocorticoid, 79, 87, 81
  receptor, 95
Minute ventilation, 417
Mitral regurgitation, 40–41
Mitral stenosis, 47
  atrial fibrillation, 47
Mitral valve prolapse (MVP), 19
  symptoms, 21
Mixed connective tissue disease (MCTD), 61
  secondary interstitial lung disease, 641–642
Mobitz type II second-degree atrioventricular (AV) block, 9
  AV conduction ratio, 33
  block location, 32
  bundle branch blocks, 12
  causes of, 32
  electrocardiographic findings, 32, 32f
  prognosis of, 32
  symptomatic AV block, 12
  symptoms of, 32
  treatment for, 32
  wide QRS complex, 10
  with myocardial infarction, 32
Mobitz type I second-degree atrioventricular (AV) block, 9
  AV conduction ratio, 33
  block location, 31
  causes of, 32
  electrocardiographic findings, 31, 31f
  with myocardial infarction, 31
  nonconducted P wave, 10
  prognosis of, 32
  symptoms of, 32
  treatment for, 32
Modified Duke criteria, 369, 369t
Monoarticular inflammatory arthritis
  acute infectious, 664
  acute septic arthritis, 663
  chronic infectious, 664
  crystal arthropathy, 663
    types, 664
  Lyme disease, 663
  *Neisseria gonorrhoeae*, 664
  under polarized light
    calcium pyrophosphate dihydrate (pseudogout) crystals, 664
    monosodium urate (gout) crystals, 664
  *Staphylococcus aureus*, 664
Monomorphic wide-complex tachycardia
  irregular rhythm, 72
  regular rhythm, 72
    causes of, 72–74
  types, 72
Mononeuritis multiplex, 527

Mononeuropathy, 526
Monosodium urate (gout) crystals, 664
Multifocal atrial tachycardia (MAT)
  characteristics of, 71
Multiple myeloma, 85, 101
Mumps, 385–386
Muscular dystrophy, 44
  types, 44
Musculoskeletal noncardiac chest pain, 21, 24–25
Myasthenia gravis, dyspnea, 259
*Mycobacterium tuberculosis*, 58, 83
  characteristics of, 59
Myelodysplastic syndrome (MDS), 269–270, 270f
Myocardial infarction
  coronary artery vasospasm, 19
  Mobitz type I second-degree atrioventricular (AV) block, 31
  Mobitz type II second-degree atrioventricular (AV) block, 32
Myocardial ischemia, 16–17, 250
  *vs.* acute myocardial infarction, 16
Myocardial oxygen demand, 20
Myocardial scar, 72
Myocarditis, 19, 42
  acute, 43
  dyspnea, 21, 250, 252
Myoclonus, 540
Myopathy, weakness, 597–599
Myotonic dystrophy, 8, 44
Myxedema, 650–651
  ascites, 157–158
  coma, 127
  interstitial oncotic pressure, 294–295, 295f

**N**

Narrow-complex bradycardia
  with irregular rhythm, 7
    causes, 9–10, 10f
  with regular rhythm
    causes, 7–9, 7f
    electrocardiographic characteristics, 7
Narrow-complex tachycardia
  irregular rhythm, 68, 71–72
  regular rhythm
    causes of, 69–71, 70f
    electrocardiographic characteristics, 68
Native valve infective endocarditis
  acute, 371–372
  clinical differences, 371
  diagnosis, 370
  subacute, 372–373
  types, 370
Negative cardiac stress test, 19
*Neisseria gonorrhoeae*, 664
Nephritic syndrome
  characteristic urinary findings, 447
  glomerulonephritis. *See* Glomerulonephritis
Nephrology
  acid-base disorders. *See* Acid-base disorders
  acute kidney injury (AKI). *See* Acute kidney injury (AKI)
  glomerular disease. *See* Glomerular disease
  hyperkalemia. *See* Hyperkalemia
  hypernatremia. *See* Hypernatremia
  hypokalemia. *See* Hypokalemia
  hyponatremia. *See* Hyponatremia
  secondary hypertension. *See* Secondary hypertension
Nephrotic syndrome, 155–156, 650
  characteristic urinary findings, 446
  classification, 448
  infection, 447
  laboratory features, 447
  pathophysiology, 447
  pharmacologic agents, 448
  physical findings, 447
  primary, 448–449
  secondary, 449–450
  symptoms, 447
  thromboembolism, 447
Neurally-mediated reflexes, 8
Neuroendocrine tumor, 96
Neurology
  headache. *See* Headache
  polyneuropathy. *See* Polyneuropathy
  seizure. *See* Seizure
  stroke. *See* Stroke
  weakness. *See* Weakness
Neuromuscular junction (NMJ), 595–597, 595f
Neuropathy, definition, 526, 526f
Nonalcoholic fatty liver disease (NAFLD), 219
Non–ANCA-associated small vessel systemic vasculitis
  anti–glomerular basement membrane (anti-GBM) disease, 680–681
  Behçet's disease, 680–681
  cryoglobulinemia, 680
  Henoch-Schönlein purpura (HSP), 680
  secondary causes of, 681
  urticarial vasculitis (UV), 680–681
Nonbacterial thrombotic endocarditis (NBTE)
  autoimmune conditions, 367
  clinical manifestations, 366
  heart valves, 366
  infection, 366–367
  lung cancer, 366
  malignancies, 367
  systemic lupus erythematosus (SLE), 366
  treatment options, 366
Noncardiac chest pain, 15
  anxiety (panic disorder), 25
  causes, 21
  gastrointestinal, 21
    acute pancreatitis, 23–24
    biliary colic, 23–24
    esophageal rupture, 23–24
    esophageal spasm, 23–24
    gastroesophageal reflux disease (GERD), 23
    peptic ulcer disease (PUD), 23–24
  herpes zoster, 25
  musculoskeletal, 21, 24–25
  pulmonary
    acute chest syndrome, 22
    pleurisy, 21–22
    pneumonia, 21–22
    pneumothorax, 21–22
    pulmonary embolism (PE), 21–22
    pulmonary hypertension, 22
Noncaseating granulomas, 132
Noninfectious exudative pleural effusion, 653–655
Noninfectious inflammatory diarrhea, 186–188, 186f
  arsenic poisoning, 187–188
  colorectal cancer (CRC), 186–187
  external beam radiation therapy, 187
  inflammatory bowel disease, 186–187, 186f
  ischemic colitis, 186–187
Noninvasive bacterial diarrhea, 180–182
Noninvasive infectious diarrhea, 178
Noninvasive protozoal diarrhea, 182–183
Noninvasive viral diarrhea, 178–179
Nonmegaloblastic macrocytic anemia, 321–323, 322f
Non-specific interstitial pneumonia (NSIP), 633–634
Non–ST-elevation myocardial infarction (NSTEMI), 16
  electrocardiographic findings, 17, 17f
  myocardial injury, 17
Normal pressure hydrocephalus (NPH), 237, 239, 239f
Normocytic anemia
  bone marrow, 316
  hyperproliferative, 318–319
  hypoproliferative, 316–318
  reticulocytes, 316
Norovirus gastroenteritis, 178–179

**O**

Obesity hypoventilation syndrome (OHS), 618–619
Obliterative bronchiolitis, 624
Obstructive hypotension, 284–285, 285f
Obstructive sleep apnea (OSA), 618–619
  secondary hypertension, 506–507
Oligoarticular inflammatory arthritis, 61
  ankylosing spondylitis, 667
  Behçet's disease, 665
    characteristics of, 667
  causes of, 664
  cryoglobulinemia, 665
  disseminated gonorrhea, 664
    clinical features of, 665
  enteropathic arthritis, 664
    types, 666
  HCV-associated cryoglobulinemia, 667
  Henoch-Schönlein purpura (HSP), 665
    characteristics of, 667
  Löfgren's syndrome, 665
    prognosis of, 667
  Lyme disease, 667
  nonmusculoskeletal inflammatory conditions, 666
  psoriatic arthritis, 666
  reactive arthritis, 667
  spirochetal arthritis, 665, 665f

spondyloarthritides, 666
syphilis, 667
systemic vasculitides, 667
Orthostatic hypotension, heart failure, 37, 37f
Osmotic diarrhea
celiac disease, 189–190
cholerheic diarrhea, 189–190
lactose intolerance, 188–189
laxatives, 188
medications, 189
pancreatic exocrine insufficiency, 189–190
short bowel syndrome, 189–190
small intestinal bacterial overgrowth, 189–190
sugar alcohol, 188, 190
tropical sprue, 189–190
Osteoarthritis (OA), 659, 661–662
Osteoblastic bone metastases, 120
characteristics of, 121
Osteolytic metastases, 105, 105f
Osteomalacia, 118
Osteomyelitis, 265–266
Osteonecrosis, 661
location of, 662
Overlap syndrome, 61
Overt hypothyroidism, 127

**P**

Pacemaker-facilitated tachycardia, 72
mechanisms of, 74
Pacemakers, 12
Paget disease, 43
high-output physiologic state, 44
Painless thyroiditis, 129
characteristics of, 130
Palpable purpura, 61
Pancreas, extrahepatic cholestasis
acute pancreatitis, 167
anatomy of, 164, 164f
chronic pancreatitis, 167
pancreatic cancer, 167–168
pancreatic pseudocyst, 167–168, 168f
Pancreatic islet cell tumor, 96
characteristics of, 97
Pancreatic pseudocyst, 167–168, 168f
Pancreatitis ascites, 157–158
Pancytopenia
bone marrow evaluation, 344, 344f
bone marrow hypoplasia
antithyroid medication, 345
arsenic poisoning, 345
characteristics of, 346
definition, 344
idiopathic aplastic anemia, 345, 347
infections, 346
inherited aplastic anemia, 345–346, 346f
medications, 345
paroxysmal nocturnal hemoglobinuria (PNH), 345–346
parvovirus B19 infection, 345
pregnancy, 345
bone marrow infiltration, 348–349, 348f
bruising, 342, 342f
definition, 343
hematopoiesis, 343, 343f
ineffective, 347
hypersplenism, 349–350
investigation of, 344
mechanisms, 344
physical findings, 343
symptoms of, 343
Panic attack, dyspnea, 258–259
*Paragonimus westermani*, 609
Paralysis, 580
Paraneoplastic encephalitis, 239
Paraparesis, 583
Parasympathetic nervous system, 6, 29, 67
Parathyroid hormone (PTH)
-dependent hypercalcemia
familial hypocalciuric hypercalcemia (FHH), 102–103
mechanism of, 102
primary hyperparathyroidism, 102–103
secondary hyperparathyroidism, 103
tertiary hyperparathyroidism, 102–103
-dependent hypocalcemia
autoimmune causes, 114–115
calcium-sensing receptor, 116–117
causes of, 113
iatrogenic causes, 114
infiltrative causes, 115–116
laboratory pattern, 113
magnesium derangement, 116
mechanism of, 113
-independent hypercalcemia
causes of, 103
endocrinopathy, 107–108
granulomatous disease, 106–107
immobility, 108
malignancy, 105
mechanism of, 103
medication, 104
rhabdomyolysis, 108–109
-independent hypocalcemia
causes of, 117
extravascular consumption, 120–121
hypomagnesemia, 122
intravascular consumption, 121–122
laboratory pattern, 117
mechanism of, 117
medication, 122
pseudohypoparathyroidism, 122
vitamin D deficiency, 117–120, 118f–119f
Parathyroid hormone–related peptide (PTHrP), 96, 105
Paresis, 580
Paroxysmal nocturnal hemoglobinuria (PNH), 333, 335, 345–346
Parvovirus B19 infection, 345, 668, 670
Peptic ulcer disease (PUD), 23, 202–204
with pain, 24
Perforated viscus, 157, 159
Pericardial coccidioidomycosis, 59
Pericardial disease, 50–51
Pericardiocentesis, 56
Pericarditis
acute
characteristic features, 55
diagnosis, 64
electrocardiographic manifestations, 55
occurence ratio, 56
with pericardial effusion, 56
physical findings, 55
symptoms of, 55
cardiac causes, 62–63
cardiac tamponade, 56, 56f
chest radiography, 56
connective tissue disease (CTD), 60–62
constrictive pericarditis, 56
Kussmaul's sign, 56
definition, 55
infectious causes, 57–60
malignant causes, 60
medications, 64
metabolic causes, 63–64
pericardiocentesis, 56
pleuritic chest pain, 55
with positional chest pain, 55, 55f
radiation therapy, 64
Peripartum cardiomyopathy, 43–44
during pregnancy, 44
Peripheral edema
capillary hydrostatic pressure
characteristics of, 290
chronic venous insufficiency, 291–292, 292f
cirrhosis, 290–291
constrictive pericarditis, 291–292
deep vein thrombosis (DVT), 290–291
mechanisms, 290, 290f
medication, 291
pregnancy, 291–292
renal failure, 290–291
right-sided heart failure, 290–291
superior vena cava (SVC) syndrome, 291–292
systemic arterial hypertension, 290
capillary oncotic pressure
albumin synthesis, 293, 293f
characteristics of, 293
liver disease and malnutrition, 293
nephrotic syndrome, 293–294
plasma proteins, 292
protein-calorie malnutrition, 293
protein-losing enteropathy, 293–294
capillary permeability, 295–297
definition, 288
dependent edema, 289
fluid balance, regulation factors, 289, 289f
generalized edema, 289
interstitial oncotic pressure, 294–295, 295f
mechanisms, 289
with palmar erythema, 288, 288f
pitting edema, 288
total body water distribution, 289
Peripheral neuropathy, 526
Peritoneal dialysis, 651
Persistent respiratory disorder, 417
Pes cavus with hammertoes, 536, 536f

Pheochromocytoma, 96, 107
  mechanisms of, 108
  multiple endocrine neoplasia types 2a and 2b, 96
Phlebotomy, 50
Physiologic shunt, hypoxemia
  acute respiratory distress syndrome (ARDS), 624
  airway constriction, 623–624
  atelectasis, 623–624
  definition, 623
  diffuse alveolar hemorrhage, 623, 625
  hepatopulmonary syndrome, 623, 625
  inhaled oxygen, 623
  pneumonia, 623–624
  pulmonary edema, 623–624
Pickwickian syndrome, 618
Pituitary adenoma, 94, 143–144
  characteristics of, 95, 95f
Pituitary gland dysfunction, 87, 133
Pituitary macroadenomas, 133
Platelet disorders
  classification, 355
  clinical manifestations, 354
  with fever and skin rash, 353, 353f
  function of, 354, 354f
  laboratory tests, 355
  petechiae and purpura, 354
  production, 354
  qualitative platelet disorders
    mechanisms, 355
    platelet adhesion, 355–356, 356f
    platelet aggregation, 358
    platelet secretion, 356–357
  quantitative platelet disorders
    decreased platelet production, 359–360
    increased platelet destruction, 360–361
    normal peripheral platelet count, 358
    pseudothrombocytopenia, 359
Plegia, 580
Pleocytosis, 384
Pleural effusion
  abnormal fluid accumulation, 646, 646f
  chest radiography, 646
  computed tomography (CT) imaging, 646
  criteria for, 647
  cytologic examination, 648
  definition, 646
  differential cell count, 648
  dyspnea, 258
  empyema, 647
  exudative
    causes of, 652
    infectious, 652–653
    mechanisms of, 651
    noninfectious, 653–655
    types, 651
  fluid characteristics, 647
  glucose concentration, 648
  Gram stain and culture, 648
  gross appearance of, 648
  hemithorax opacification, 646
  incidence of, 646
  large pleural effusion, 646
  loculated pleural effusion, 647, 647f
  mechanisms of, 646
  operating characteristics, Light's criteria, 647
  physical findings, 646
  with pleuritic chest pain, 645, 645f
  symptoms of, 646
  thoracentesis, 647
  transudative
    capillary oncotic pressure, 648
    diaphragm, 648
    diaphragmatic defects, 651
    hydrostatic pressure, 648, 649–650
    intrapleural pressure, 648
    mechanisms of, 648
    oncotic pressure, 650–651
  types, 647
pleurisy, 21–22
Plexopathy, 526
Pneumoconiosis, 638–639
*Pneumocystis jirovecii* (PJP), 624
Pneumonectomy, 649–650
Pneumonia, 21, 608
  aspiration pneumonia
    cause of, 410–411
    clinical characteristics, 409, 409f
    definition, 409
    mechanism of, 408
    methods, 410
    risk factors, 409
    treatment, 410
  cardiac events, 399
  clinical presentation, 398
  community-acquired pneumonia (CAP)
    atypical pathogens, 401–403
    causes, 399
    endemic pathogens, 403–405, 404f
    typical pathogens, 400–401, 401f
  definition, 398
  delirium, 243–244
  hospital-acquired pneumonia (HAP), 405–407
  infectious exudative pleural effusion, 652
  microbial pathogens, 399
  noninfectious conditions, 399
  pericardial coccidioidomycosis, 59
  physical findings of, 398
  physiologic shunt, hypoxemia, 623–624
  with shaking chills, 398, 398f
  *Streptococcus pneumoniae*, 58
  symptoms of, 398
  tactile fremitus, 22
  ventilator-associated pneumonia (VAP), 407–408
Pneumothorax, 21
  dyspnea, 258
  treatment for, 22
Polyarteritis nodosa (PAN), 62, 676
  arteriographic findings of, 677, 677f
  fever of unknown origin (FUO), 267
Polyarticular inflammatory arthritis
  acute rheumatic fever, 668, 670
  adult-onset Still's disease, 668, 670
  dermatomyositis (DM), 668, 670
  parvovirus B19, 668, 670
  polymyositis (PM), 668, 670
  rheumatoid arthritis, 668–669, 669f
  sarcoidosis, 668, 670
  serum sickness, 668
    clinical manifestations, 670
  systemic lupus erythematosus (SLE), 668
    characteristics of, 670
Polyglandular autoimmune syndrome type 1 (PAS-1), 82
Polyglandular autoimmune syndrome type 2 (PAS-2), 82
Polymorphic wide-complex tachycardia
  polymorphic ventricular tachycardia (VT), 74
    characteristics of, 75
    Torsades de pointes, 75, 75f
  ventricular fibrillation (VF), 75
Polymyalgia rheumatica (PMR), 267, 269
Polymyositis (PM), 668, 670
  secondary interstitial lung disease, 641–642
Polyneuropathy
  autonomic dysfunction, 528
  axonal degeneration and demyelinating disease, 527, 527f
  causes of, 528
  classification, 528
  definition, 527
  diagnosis, 528
  electrodiagnostic testing, 528
  genetic studies, 528
  hereditary causes, 535–536, 536f
  inflammatory
    causes of, 532
    classification, 532
    infectious causes, 532–533
    noninfectious causes, 533–535
    pathophysiologic/electrophysiologic pattern, 532
  metabolic, 528–530, 529f
  motor disturbance, 528
  neurologic examination, 527
  painful tongue, 525, 525f
  pathophysiologic and electrophysiologic patterns, 527
  physical findings of, 528
  symptoms of, 527
  toxic, 530–531, 530f
Portal hypertension ascites, 148
  classification, 150
  clinical sequelae, 150
  diagnosis, 150
  hepatic, 151–153, 152f
  mechanism of, 149
  posthepatic, 154–155
  prehepatic, 150–151
  unrelated to, 155–159, 156f
Portal vein thrombosis (PVT), 150–151
Positive pressure ventilation (PPV), 621–622
Postcardiac injury syndrome (PCIS), 62, 653, 655
  causes of, 63
Posterior reversible encephalopathy syndrome (PRES), 244–245, 245f
Posthepatic portal hypertension ascites, 154–155

Postpartum thyroiditis, 128
  fever of unknown origin (FUO), 271
Postrenal acute kidney injury, 441–442
Posttransplant complications, 169–170
Post-traumatic headache, 519–520
Potassium
  excess loss, 481, 481f
  extrarenal loss, 482–483
  low oral intake, 480–481
  renal loss, 481–482
  transcellular shift, 483–484
Pregnancy
  dyspnea, 259–260
  secondary hypertension, 506–507
Prehepatic portal hypertension ascites, 150–151
Prerenal acute kidney injury, 432–434, 433f
Preserved left ventricular systolic function
  afterload, 46
  causes of, 45
  concentric hypertrophy, 45
  enlarged cardiac silhouette, chest radiograph, 45
  genetic causes, 49–50
  idiopathic restrictive cardiomyopathy, 50–51
  infiltrative causes, 48–49
  mediastinal radiation therapy, 50–51
  pericardial disease, 50–51
  restrictive cardiomyopathy, 45
  scleroderma, 50–51
  S4 gallop, 45, 45f
  treatment for, 45
  valvular causes, 47–48
Primary adrenal insufficiency
  adrenal cortical tissue, 81
  adrenoleukodystrophy (ALD), 86–87
  autoimmune causes, 81–82
  bilateral adrenalectomy, 86–87
  causes of, 81
  external beam radiation, 87
  hemorrhagic causes, 83–85
  infectious causes, 82–83
  infiltrative causes, 85–86
  mechanism of, 81
  medication, 86–87
  mineralocorticoid deficiency, 81
  radiotherapy, 86
Primary biliary cholangitis (PBC), 169–170
  hepatic portal hypertension, 151, 153
Primary headache disorders
  cluster headache, 511–512
  migraine headache, 511–512
  tension headache, 511
  trigeminal autonomic cephalalgias (TACs), 512
Primary hyperparathyroidism, 102
  characteristics of, 103
  clinical features, 103
  parathyroid carcinoma, 103
Primary hypothyroidism
  causes of, 128
  iatrogenesis
    external beam radiation therapy, 131–132
    Graves' disease, 131
    lithium, 131–132
    thyroidectomy/radioactive iodine ablation, 131
  infiltrative disorders
    amyloidosis, 132–133
    hemochromatosis, 132
    Riedel's thyroiditis, 132–133
    sarcoidosis, 132–133
    thyroid gland, 133
  iodine
    cause of, 131
    characteristics of, 131
    dietary fortification, 130
    Wolff-Chaikoff effect, 130
  mechanism of, 128
  thyroiditis
    definition, 128
    drug-induced thyroiditis, 129
    Hashimoto's thyroiditis, 128–129
    infectious thyroiditis, 129
    medications, 130
    painless thyroiditis, 129
    phase of, 128
    postpartum thyroiditis, 128
    radiation-induced thyroiditis, 129
    subacute thyroiditis, 129
Primary metabolic alkalosis, 619
Primary sclerosing cholangitis (PSC), 169–170
  hepatic portal hypertension, 151, 153
Prinzmetal's angina, 19
Prosthetic valve infective endocarditis
  diagnosis, 374
  early, 374–375
  late, 376–377
  mechanical valves, 373
  microbiological differences, 374
  mortality rate, 373
  time course, 374
  types, 374
Protein-calorie malnutrition, 155–156, 156f
Protein-losing enteropathy (PLE), 155–156, 650–651
Protein-poor ascites
  capillary oncotic pressure, 155
  mechanism, 155
  nephrotic syndrome, 155–156
  protein-calorie malnutrition, 155–156, 156f
  protein-losing enteropathy, 155–156
Protein-rich ascites
  chylous ascites, 157–158
  hemoperitoneum, 157–158
  intraperitoneal malignancy, 157
  mechanisms, 157
  myxedema, 157–158
  pancreatitis, 157–158
  perforated viscus, 157, 159
  tuberculosis, 157–158
Provoked seizure, 542
  causes of, 546
  infectious, 551–552
  metabolic, 552–553, 552f
  nonstructural conditions, 546
  structural, 550
  toxic, 549–550
  vascular, 546–549, 547f
Pseudohyperkalemia, 460
Pseudohypoparathyroidism, 122
Psoriatic arthritis, 660, 660f, 666
Psychogenic pseudosyncope
  syncope, 306–307
Psychosis, causes of, 236
Pulmonary arteriovenous malformation, 627
Pulmonary aspergillosis, 608–609
Pulmonary capillaritis, 621–622
Pulmonary causes, hemoptysis
  airways
    acute bronchitis, 607
    bronchiectasis, 607
    bronchovascular fistula, 607–608
    causes of, 606
    foreign body aspiration, 607–608
    iatrogenic, 607–608
    malignancy, 607
  pulmonary parenchyma
    lung abscess, 608–609
    pneumonia, 608
    pulmonary aspergillosis, 608–609
    pulmonary paragonimiasis, 608–609
    pulmonary tuberculosis (TB), 608–609
Pulmonary edema, 623–624
Pulmonary embolism (PE), 21, 621–622, 653–654
  acute, electrocardiographic findings, 22
  hemoptysis, 605–606, 605f
Pulmonary hypertension, 22, 46, 621–622
  diagnosis, 22
Pulmonary Langerhans cell histiocytosis (PLCH), 639–640
Pulmonary noncardiac chest pain
  acute chest syndrome, 22
  pleurisy, 21–22
  pneumonia, 21–22
  pneumothorax, 21–22
  pulmonary embolism (PE), 21–22
  pulmonary hypertension, 22
Pulmonary paragonimiasis, 608–609
Pulmonary parenchyma
  lung abscess, 608–609
  pneumonia, 608
  pulmonary aspergillosis, 608–609
  pulmonary paragonimiasis, 608–609
  pulmonary tuberculosis (TB), 608–609
Pulmonary tuberculosis (TB), 608–609
Pulmonic stenosis, 47
  causes, 48
Pulmonology
  hemoptysis. *See* Hemoptysis
  hypoxemia. *See* Hypoxemia
  interstitial lung disease (ILD). *See* Interstitial lung disease (ILD)
  pleural effusion. *See* Pleural effusion
Pulse oximetry, 612
  conditions, 613
Pulsus parvus et tardus, 19
Pyruvate kinase deficiency, 330–331

**Q**

Quadriparesis, 583
Qualitative platelet disorders
  mechanisms, 355
  platelet adhesion, 355–356, 356f
  platelet aggregation, 358
  platelet secretion, 356–357
Quantitative platelet disorders
  decreased platelet production, 359–360
  increased platelet destruction, [illegible]
  normal peripheral platelet count, 358
  pseudothrombocytopenia, 359

**R**

Radiation coloproctitis, 208–209
Radiation-induced thyroiditis, 129
  types of, 130
Radiculopathy, 24–25, 526
Radioactive iodine ablation, 131
Radioactive iodine uptake, 140–143, 140f
Rash, 25
Reactive arthritis, 667
  fever of unknown origin (FUO), 267–268
Reduced left ventricular systolic function
  acromegaly, 43–44
  cardiovascular causes, 40–41
  causes of, 40
  cirrhosis, 43–44
  dilated cardiomyopathy, 39
  eccentric hypertrophy, 39f
    on chest radiography, 39
  familial dilated cardiomyopathy, 43–44
  giant cell myocarditis, 44
  idiopathic dilated cardiomyopathy, 44
  infectious causes, 42–43
  muscular dystrophy, 44
  myocardial hypertrophy, types, 39, 39f
  Paget disease, 43–44
  peripartum cardiomyopathy, 43–44
  pharmacologic agents
    improved patients survival, 40
    improved symptoms, 39
  S3 gallop, 39, 39f
  Takotsubo cardiomyopathy, 43–44
  thiamine deficiency, 43–44
  toxic causes, 41–42
Refeeding syndrome, 241–242
Regular rhythm, definition, 7
Relative bradycardia, 8
  pacemaker-dependent patient, 12
Renal cell carcinoma, 269, 271
Renal replacement therapy, 431
Respiratory acidosis, 416, 422–424, 422f
Respiratory alkalosis, 416, 424–426
Respiratory bronchiolitis–associated interstitial lung disease (RB-ILD), 639–640
Respiratory quotient (RQ), 615
Respiratory syncytial virus, 57
Restrictive cardiomyopathy, 45
Rhabdomyolysis, 108–109
Rheumatoid arthritis (RA), 60, 668–669, 669f
  clinical features, 60
  fever of unknown origin (FUO), 267–268, 268f
  secondary interstitial lung disease, 640, 642
Rheumatology
  arthritis. *See* Arthritis
  systemic vasculitis. *See* Systemic vasculitis
Rib fracture, 24–25
Rickets, 118, 118f
Riedel's thyroiditis, 132–133
"Ripping" chest pain, 19
Rotavirus gastroenteritis, 178–179
Roth spots, 368, 368f

**S**

Saddle nose deformity, 106
*Salmonella* species, 183–184
Sarcoidosis, 48–49, 106, 668, 670
  characteristics of, 86
  fever of unknown origin (FUO), 267–268, 268f
  primary hypothyroidism, 132–133
  secondary interstitial lung disease, 640
Sarcomas, 60
Schistosomiasis, 151, 153
Scleroderma, 50–51, 61, 193–194
  secondary interstitial lung disease, 640–641
Secondary headache disorders
  causes of, 512
  classification, 512
  extracranial, 520–522
  intracranial
    cerebrospinal fluid, 518–519, 518f
    infectious, 515–517
    post-traumatic headache, 519–520
    trigeminal neuralgia, 519–520
    tumor, 517–518
    vascular, 513–515
Secondary hypertension
  blood pressure regulation, 502
  causes of, 502
  clinical characteristics, 502
  with discordant peripheral pulses, 501, 501f
  endocrinologic causes, 503–505
  essential hypertension, 502
  glomerulonephritis, 506–507
  obstructive sleep apnea (OSA), 506–507
  pregnancy-associated hypertension, 506–507
  prevalence, 502
  toxic causes, 505–506
  vascular causes, 502–503, 503f
  white-coat hypertension, 506–507
Secondary interstitial lung disease
  causes of, 635
  desquamative interstitial pneumonia (DIP), 639–640
  exposures, types, 635
  hypersensitivity pneumonitis (HP)
    antigen classes, 636
    bird fancier's lung, 637–638
    bronchoscopy, 637
    characteristics, 637
    clinical course, 637
    definition, 636
    farmer's lung, 637–638
    high-resolution CT imaging, 637
    prevalence, 636
    serologic testing, 637
    treatment for, 637
  iatrogenic exposure, 636
  pneumoconiosis, 638–639
  pulmonary Langerhans cell histiocytosis (PLCH), 639–640
  respiratory bronchiolitis–associated interstitial lung disease (RB-ILD), 639–640
  sarcoidosis, 640–641
  systemic disease
    dermatomyositis (DM), 640, 640f, 642
    mixed connective tissue disease (MCTD), 641–642
    polymyositis (PM), 641–642
    rheumatoid arthritis (RA), 640, 642
    sarcoidosis, 640–641
    scleroderma, 640–641
    Sjögren's syndrome, 641–642
    systemic lupus erythematosus (SLE), 641–642
    vasculitis, 641–642
Second-degree atrioventricular (AV) block
  Mobitz type I (Wenckebach), 31–32, 31f
  Mobitz type II, 32–33, 32f
  second-degree 2:1 AV block, 33, 33f
  types, 31
Seizure
  atonic activity, 541
  aura, 541
  automatisms, 541
  classification, 542
  clonic activity, 541
  conditions, 540
  definition, 540
  delirium, 237–238
  dystonic activity, 541
  electroencephalography (EEG), 541
  emergency neuroimaging, 541
  focal seizures, 543–544, 543f
    subtypes, 544–545
  generalized seizures, 543–544, 543f
    subtypes, 545–546
  myoclonus, 540
  pharmacologic treatment, 541
  physical examination, 541
  postictal state, 541
  with pronator drift, 540, 540f
  provoked seizure, 542
    causes of, 546
    infectious, 551–552
    metabolic, 552–553, 552f
    nonstructural conditions, 546
    structural, 550
    toxic, 549–550
    vascular, 546–549, 547f
  status epilepticus, 541
  symptoms and signs, 540
  tonic activity, 541
  unprovoked seizure, 542
    epilepsy, 542
Sepsis, 42
  delirium, 243–244

intrahepatic cholestasis, 172
prognosis of, 43
Seronegative spondyloarthritides, 61
reactive arthritis, 62
Serum sickness, 668
clinical manifestations, 670
S3 gallop, 39, 39f, 154
S4 gallop, 45, 45f
Sheehan's syndrome, 87
*Shigella* species, 183, 185
Short bowel syndrome, 189–190
Sickle cell anemia, 22, 169–170
inherited hemolytic anemia, 328–329, 329f
Sideroblastic anemia, 314, 316
Silicosis, 638–639
Sinoatrial exit block, 9
definition, 10
type I, 10
type II, 10, 10f
Sinus arrest, 9
definition, 10
Sinus arrhythmia, 9
Sinus bradycardia, 7
bundle branch block, 11
causes of, 8
mechanism of, 8
medications of, 8
pulse-temperature pattern, 8
ventricular escape rhythms, 11
Sinusoidal obstruction syndrome (SOS), 152, 153
Sinus tachycardia, 69
Sjögren's syndrome, 653
secondary interstitial lung disease, 641–642
Skin hyperpigmentation, 662
Slapped-cheek syndrome, 668
Small cell lung cancer, 96
Small vessel systemic vasculitis
ANCA-associated
eosinophilic granulomatosis with polyangiitis (EGPA), 678–679
granulomatosis with polyangiitis, 678–679, 679f
microscopic polyangiitis, 678–679
secondary causes of, 679
manifestations of, 677
non–ANCA-associated
anti–glomerular basement membrane (anti-GBM) disease, 680–681
Behçet's disease, 680–681
cryoglobulinemia, 680
Henoch-Schönlein purpura (HSP), 680
secondary causes of, 681
urticarial vasculitis (UV), 680–681
palpable purpura distribution, 677
physical findings, 677
serological testing, 678
Smoking, 96
Soft tissue sarcoma, 25
Spider angiomas, 43
Spirochetal arthritis, 665, 665f
Splanchnic arteriovenous fistula, 150–151
Splenic vein thrombosis, 150–151
Splinter hemorrhage, 368, 368f
Spondylitis, 660
Spondyloarthritides, 666
Spondyloarthritis, 660
Spur cell anemia, 333, 335
Stable angina pectoris, 19
mechanism of, 20, 20f
*Staphylococcus aureus*, 58–59, 180–181, 664
Status epilepticus, 541
ST-elevation myocardial infarction (STEMI), 16
electrocardiographic manifestation of, 16–17, 17f
Stent thrombosis, 18
timing of, 19
*Streptococcus pneumoniae*, 58–59
Stroke
CT imaging, 559
definition, 557
delirium, 237–238
with flank pain, 557, 557f
hemorrhagic, 559. *See also* Hemorrhagic stroke
ischemic, 559. *See also* Ischemic stroke
mechanisms of, 558, 558f
prevalence, 558
prognosis of, 558
relative rates, 558
risk factors, 558
transient ischemic attack (TIA), 557
conditions, 558
risk of, 558
types, 558
Structural provoked seizure, 550
Subacute hypersensitivity pneumonitis, 637
Subacute thyroiditis, 129
Subarachnoid hemorrhagic stroke, 562–564, 563f
Subclavian steal syndrome, 303, 303f
Subcutaneous emphysema, 23
Subluxation, 659
Subphrenic abscess, 652–653
Substance abuse, 25
Sugar alcohol, 188, 190
Superior vena cava (SVC) syndrome, 649
dyspnea, 251–252
Supraventricular rhythm
irregular, 12
regular, 11
Supraventricular tachycardia (SVT)
irregular, 74
wide QRS complex, 74
regular, 72
*vs.* baseline wide QRS complex, 73
Surgical trauma, 8
Surreptitious thyroid hormone ingestion, 142
Symmetric arthritis, 660
Symmetric hypertrophy, 39, 39f
Symmetric inflammatory polyarticular arthritis, 60
Sympathetic nervous system, 6, 29, 67
Syncope
α-blocker medication, 306
cardiovascular, 301–303, 303f
causes of, 300
definition, 300
enlarged cardiac silhouette, 300, 300f
hyperventilation, 306
hypoxemia and anemia, 306
incidence of, 300
mechanism of, 300
neurocardiogenic, 303–305
neurologic, 305
prognosis of, 300
psychogenic pseudosyncope, 306–307
tension pneumothorax, 306–307, 307f
Syndrome of inappropriate antidiuretic hormone (SIADH), 96
Synovial fluid, 661
Synovitis, 659
Syphilis, 667
Systemic disease
dermatomyositis (DM), 640, 640f, 642
mixed connective tissue disease (MCTD), 641–642
polymyositis (PM), 641–642
rheumatoid arthritis (RA), 640, 642
sarcoidosis, 640–641
scleroderma, 640–641
Sjögren's syndrome, 641–642
systemic lupus erythematosus (SLE), 641–642
vasculitis, 641–642
Systemic lupus erythematosus (SLE), 60, 653, 668
characteristics of, 670
clinical features, 61
fever of unknown origin (FUO), 267–268
nonbacterial thrombotic endocarditis (NBTE), 366
secondary interstitial lung disease, 641–642
Systemic mastocytosis, 191–192
Systemic vasculitides, 667
Systemic vasculitis
classification, 674
conditions, 674
definition, 674
with hemoptysis, 673, 673f
laboratory features of, 674
large vessel, 675–676
limited systemic vasculitis, 674
medium vessel, 676–677, 677f
occurrence of, 674
small vessel
ANCA-associated, 678–679, 679f
manifestations of, 677
non–ANCA-associated, 680–681
palpable purpura distribution, 677
physical findings, 677
serological testing, 678
Systolic ejection murmur, 19

**T**

Tachyarrhythmia-induced cardiomyopathy, 40–41
Tachycardia
definition, 68
electrical conduction, normal heart, 67
heart rate
and cardiac output (CO), 68
regulation, 67

Tachycardia *(continued)*
mechanisms of, 68
narrow QRS complex, 68. *See also* Narrow-complex tachycardia
physical findings of, 68
resting heart rate, adults, 68
symptoms of, 68
wide QRS complex, 68. *See also* Wide-complex tachycardia
definition, 68
woman with palpitations, 67, 67f
Tachypnea, 249
Tactile fremitus, 22
Takayasu arteritis, 675–676
Takotsubo cardiomyopathy, 43
echocardiographic finding, 44
sepsis, 43
Telangiectasias, 206–207
Tenosynovitis, 659
Tension headache, 511
Tension pneumothorax, 22
syncope, 306–307, 307f
Tertiary hyperparathyroidism, 102–103
Thalassemia, 115
inherited hemolytic anemia, 328–329
microcytic anemia, 314–315, 315f
Thiamine deficiency, 43–44
Thiazide diuretics, 104
Third-degree atrioventricular (AV) block, 34, 34f
Thoracentesis, 647
Thrombocytopenia
clinical manifestations, 359
decreased platelet production, 359–360
immature platelets, 359
increased platelet destruction, 360–361
laboratory test, 359
mechanisms, 359
normal peripheral platelet count, 358
pseudothrombocytopenia, 359
Thromboembolism, nephrotic syndrome, 447
Thymic carcinoid tumors, 96
Thyroid adenomas, 142
Thyroidectomy, 131
Thyroiditis, 142–143
Thyroid-releasing hormone (TRH), 126, 137
Thyroid-stimulating hormone (TSH), 126, 137
-dependent thyrotoxicosis
impaired sensitivity, 143–144
mechanism of, 143
pituitary adenoma, 143–144
-independent thyrotoxicosis
with decreased radioactive iodine uptake, 142–143
diagnosis, 139
diffusely increased radioactive iodine uptake, 140–141
with focally increased radioactive iodine uptake, 141–142
increased radioactive iodine uptake, 140, 140f
mechanism of, 139
Thyrotoxicosis, 41, 107, 127, 192, 194
cardiovascular conditions, 42
characteristics, 139
characteristics of, 108
clinical evaluation, 138
definition, 137
dyspnea, 259–260
hypothalamic-pituitary-thyroid axis, 137
life-threatening complication, 138
with palpitations, 137, 137f
physical findings of, 138, 138f
prevalence, 138
serum thyroid hormone levels, 139
symptoms of, 138
$T_3$ and $T_4$, 137, 139
thyroid function, 139
thyroid-releasing hormone (TRH), 137
thyroid-stimulating hormone (TSH), 137
-dependent thyrotoxicosis, 143–144
-independent thyrotoxicosis, 139–143, 140f
Thyrotoxicosis factitia, 142
Tissue ischemia, 121
Tissue oxygen extraction, 614
Tonic activity, 541
Torsades de pointes, 75, 75f
characteristics of, 75
Total parenteral nutrition (TPN), 171–172
Toxic adenoma, 141
Toxic causes, heart failure, 41–42
Toxic multinodular goiter (TMNG), 141
Toxic polyneuropathy, 530–531, 530f
Toxic provoked seizure, 549–550
Tracheomalacia, 254–255
Transient ischemic attack (TIA), 557
conditions, 558
risk of, 558
Transsphenoidal adenectomy, 95
Transthyretin amyloidosis, 48
Transudative pleural effusion
capillary oncotic pressure, 648
diaphragm, 648
diaphragmatic defects, 651
hydrostatic pressure, 648, 649–650
intrapleural pressure, 648
mechanisms of, 648
oncotic pressure, 650–651
Transverse incision scar, 114
Trapped lung, 649–650
Traumatic arthritis, 661
clinical features, 662
Tricuspid regurgitation, 47
Lancisi's sign, 48
Tricuspid stenosis, 47
jugular venous waveform, 48
Trigeminal autonomic cephalalgias (TACs), 512
Trigeminal neuralgia, 519–520
*Tropheryma whipplei*, 180, 182
Trousseau's sign, 113
Tuberculosis (TB), 82, 85, 106
antimicrobial treatment, 106
percentage of, 83
pleuritis, 652–653
protein-rich ascites, 157–158

**U**

Ultraviolet B radiation, 119
Unprovoked seizure, 542
epilepsy, 542
Unstable angina (UA), 16
electrocardiographic findings, 17, 17f
myocardial injury, 17
Unstable hemoglobins, 328–329
Upper gastrointestinal bleeding
blood urea nitrogen (BUN) level, 201
classification, 201
diagnostic modality, 201
duodenal, 204–205
esophageal, 201–202
gastric, 202–204
procedure, 201
Upper motor neuron lesions, 580
anatomic structures, 581
of brain, 583–584
characteristics, 582
definition, 581
effects of, 581
facial weakness, 583
hemiparesis, 583
ipsilateral cranial nerve signs, 583
neurologic manifestations, 583
paraparesis, 583
pathways, 582, 582f
quadriparesis, 583
restricted weakness, 583
of spinal cord, 584–588
Uremia, 654–655
delirium, 241–242
pericarditis, 63
Urinary tract infection, 243–244
Urine calcium concentration, 102
Urine free cortisol (UFC) test, 92
false-negative result, 93
Urinothorax, 651
Urticarial vasculitis (UV), 680–681

**V**

Valvular disease
heart failure
aortic stenosis, 47
concentric hypertrophy, 47
mitral stenosis, 47
pulmonic regurgitation, 47–48
pulmonic stenosis, 47–48
tricuspid regurgitation, 47–48
tricuspid stenosis, 47–48
hemoptysis, 606
Variceal hemorrhage, 201–202
Varicella-zoster virus (VZV), 214–215
Vascular provoked seizure, 546–549, 547f
Vasculitis, 61–62
chronic mesenteric ischemia, 228–229
clinical manifestations of, 674
definition, 673
etiology, 674
hemoptysis, 606
leukocytoclastic vasculitis (LCV), 674
physical findings of, 674
secondary interstitial lung disease, 641–642
single-organ vasculitides, 674
*vs.* vasculopathy, 673
Venous thromboembolism, 271–272
Venous thrombosis, 226–227
Ventilation-perfusion (V/Q) ratio, 620, 620f

Ventilator-associated pneumonia (VAP), 407–408
Ventricular escape rhythm
  heart block with, 11
  rate of, 11
  sinus bradycardia, 11
Ventricular fibrillation (VF), 75
Ventricular tachycardia (VT), 72
  Brugada criteria, electrocardiographic (ECG) algorithm, 73, 73f
  monomorphic, characteristics of, 73
Vesicular skin lesions, 25
*Vibrio cholerae*, 180–181
*Vibrio parahaemolyticus*, 184, 186
VIPoma, 191–192
Viral hepatitis, 172–173
Viral infection, 265–266
Viral meningitis
  arboviruses, 385–386
  characteristic cerebrospinal fluid, 384
  diagnosis, 384
  enteroviruses, 384–385
  herpes simplex virus types 1 (HSV-1) and 2 (HSV-2), 384–385, 385f
  human immunodeficiency virus (HIV), 384, 386
  lymphocytic choriomeningitis virus (LCMV), 385–386
  with lymphocytic pleocytosis, 384
  mumps, 385–386
  pressure of, 384
  treatment, 384
Viral pericarditis
  causes of, 57
  characteristics, 58
  incidence of, 58
  occurence, 57
Vitamin A, 101
Vitamin D, 101, 104
  deficiency
    antiepileptic medication, 118
    calcium resorption, 117
    chronic kidney disease, 118
    $D_2$ and $D_3$, 117, 120
    gastrointestinal calcium absorption, 117
    gastrointestinal malabsorption, 118, 120
    liver disease, 118
    measurement of, 117
    mechanism of, 120
    osteomalacia, 118
    rickets, 118, 118f
    sunlight deprivation, 118–119, 119f
Von Willebrand disease (VWD), 355–356

**W**

Water homeostasis, 470, 470f
Watershed stroke
  causes of, 574
  clinical manifestations, 573–574
  mechanisms, 566
  prevalence, 573
Weakness
  asthenia, 579
  bradykinesia, 579
  characteristics, 581
  classification, 580, 580f
  clonus, 579
  fatigability, 579
  grade muscle strength, 580
  lower motor neuron lesions
    anatomic structures, 588
    anterior horn cell, 589–591
    definition, 588
    motor nerve fibers, 589, 589f
    peripheral nerve, 593–594
    root/plexus, 591–593
  motor unit, 579, 579f
  muscle bulk, 579
  muscle fasciculation, 579
  muscle fibrillation, 579
  muscle tone, 579
  muscle weakness, 578
  myopathy, 597–599
  neuromuscular junction (NMJ), 595–597, 595f
  paralysis, 580
  paresis, 580
  physical examination, 581
  plegia, 580
  resistance testing, 580
  upper motor neuron lesions, 580
    anatomic structures, 581
    of brain, 583–584
    characteristics, 582
    definition, 581
    effects of, 581
    facial weakness, 583
    hemiparesis, 583
    ipsilateral cranial nerve signs, 583
    neurologic manifestations, 583
    paraparesis, 583
    pathways, 582, 582f
    quadriparesis, 583
    restricted weakness, 583
    of spinal cord, 584–588
  "waddling" gait, 578, 578f
Wernicke's encephalopathy, 241–242
Wet beriberi, 43
Whipple disease, 180, 182
White-coat hypertension, 506–507
Wide-complex bradycardia
  classification, 10
  with irregular rhythm, 10
    causes, 12
  with regular rhythm, 10
    causes, 11
Wide-complex tachycardia
  uniform QRS morphology, 72. *See also* Monomorphic wide-complex tachycardia
  variable QRS morphology, 72. *See also* Polymorphic wide-complex tachycardia
Wide QRS complex, definition, 7
Wilson's disease, 218, 218f
Wolff-Chaikoff effect, 130
Wolff-Parkinson-White syndrome, 69

**X**

X-linked disease, 86
X-linked lysosomal storage disorder, 49

**Y**

Yellow nail syndrome, 654–655
*Yersinia* species, 184–185

**Z**

Zoonoses, 58–59
Zoonotic infection, 266